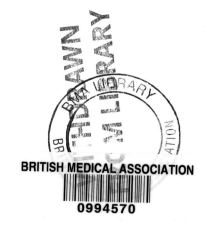

Urinary Tract Stone Disease

P. Nagaraja Rao • Glenn M. Preminger
John P. Kavanagh
Editors

Urinary Tract Stone Disease

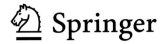 Springer

Editors

P. Nagaraja Rao, Ch.M., F.R.C.S (Ed)
Formerly Director
Total Stone Management Centre
University Hospital of South Manchester
Manchester, UK
Currently Visiting Professor of Urology
NTR University of Health Sciences
Vijayawada, India

John P. Kavanagh
Department of Urology
University Hospital of South Manchester
Manchester, UK

Glenn M. Preminger
Division of Urologic Surgery
Duke University Medical Center
Durham, NC, USA

ISBN 978-1-84800-361-3   e-ISBN 978-1-84800-362-0
DOI 10.1007/978-1-84800-362-0
Springer London Dordrecht Heidelberg New York

British Library Cataloguing in Publication Data
A catalogue record for this book is available from the British Library

Library of Congress Control Number: 2010937973

Printed on acid-free paper

Springer is part of Springer Science+Business Media (www.springer.com)

Preface

The surgical management of urinary stone disease has advanced quite dramatically since the introduction of shock wave lithotripsy (SWL), percutaneous nephrolithotomy (PCNL), ureteroscopy (URS), and more recently retrograde intrarenal surgery (RIRS) with small, flexible fiber-optic ureteroscopes. As a result, "cutting for stones" has become a rare procedure. These minimally invasive techniques are now used in the pediatric population as well with great safety and success.

In the practice of medicine, it is far more important to prevent a disease than try to treat it once the symptoms have manifested. In this respect, our understanding on how stones form has also advanced significantly, particularly in the last decade. It is also being recognized that while it is possible to remove the stones with minimal morbidity, it is far better and more economical if stones can be prevented.

Given such advances, there is the need for a "text book" that brings together all aspects of urinary stone disease, and we have been fortunate to be able to recruit experts and opinion leaders from 15 countries across the globe to contribute. The book consists of 60 chapters divided into nine sections. The first three sections are devoted to basic sciences on subjects ranging from epidemiology of urinary calculi to shock wave physics. The fourth section deals with diagnostic, laboratory, and research methods in the diagnosis and investigation of stones. Stone disease in children is dealt with in Chap. 5 followed by three sections on surgical management of stones. Finally there is an entire section on medical management of stones. Most of the chapters are highly illustrated with diagrams, photographs, and X-rays.

We believe that this is the most comprehensive reference book on urinary stones currently available. In a work of this nature, there is bound to be some overlap between some of the chapters. However, this only enhances the information provided rather than being repetitive. We hope that this book would be of value and interest to urological surgeons, physicians with an interest in urolithiasis, scientists with a research interest as well as other health care professionals dealing with stones.

P. Nagaraja Rao
Glenn M. Preminger
John P. Kavanagh

Contents

Part II   Basic Sciences

Part III   Basic Sciences

Part X   Medical Management

Contributors

Reem Al-Bareeq, M.D., F.R.C.S.I., C.A.B.U.
Department of Urology, The University of Western Ontario, London, ON, Canada

Peter Alken, M.D.
Department of Urology, University Clinic Mannheim, Heidelberg Medical School,
Mannheim, Germany

Dean G. Assimos, M.D.
Department of Urology, Wake Forest University School of Medicine,
Winston-Salem, NC, USA

Brian K. Auge, M.D., F.A.C.S.
Department of Urology, Naval Medical Center San Diego, San Diego, CA, USA

Thorsten Bach, M.D.
Department of Urology, Asklepios Hospital Barmbek, Hamburg, Germany

Dominique C. Bazin, Ph.D.
Laboratoire de Physique des Solides, Bat 510, Université Paris XI, Orsay, France

Mustafa Berber, M.D.
Department of Pediatrics, Yeditepe University Hospital, Istanbul, Turkey

Vincent C. Biourge, D.V.M., Ph.D., Diplomate A.C.V.N. & E.C.V.C.N.
Health and Nutrition Scientific Director, Royal Canin, Centre de Recherche,
BP4, 650 Avenue de la Petite Camargue, Aimargues, 30470, France

Chandra Shekhar Biyani, M.B.B.S., M.S. (Gen Surg), D.Urol., F.R.C.S. (Urol), F.E.B.U.
Department of Urology, Pinderfields General Hospital, Wakefield, West Yorkshire, UK

Loris Borghi, M.D.
Department of Clinical Sciences, University of Parma, Parma, Italy

Alison J. Bradley, M.B., Ch.B., M.R.C.P., F.R.C.R.
Department of Radiology, University Hospital of South Manchester,
Manchester, Lancashire, UK

Noor N.P. Buchholz, M.B.B.S., M.D., F.S.S.U., F.K.N.M.G.
Department of Urology, Barts and The London NHS Trust, London, UK

Kin Foong Chan, Ph.D.
Reliant Technologies, Inc., Mountain View, CA, USA

F. Hadley Cocks, B.S., M.S., Ph.D.
Department of Mechanical Engineering and Materials Science,
Duke University, Durham, NC, USA

Gary C. Curham, M.D., Sc.D.
Department of Medicine and Epidemiology, Brigham and Women's Hospital,
Harvard Medical School/Harvard School of Public Health, Boston, MA, USA

Christopher J. Danpure, B.Sc., Ph.D.
Department of Cell and Developmental Biology, University College London, London, UK

Michel Daudon, Ph.D.
Department of Biochemistry, Stone Laboratory, Necker Hospital, Paris, France

Kim Davenport, M.D., F.R.C.S. (Urol)
North Bristol NHS Trust, Bristol Urological Institute, Bristol, Avon, UK

John D. Denstedt, M.D.
Division of Urology, The University of Western Ontario, London, ON, Canada

Mahesh Desai, M.S., F.R.C.S. (Eng.), F.R.C.S. (Edinburgh)
Department of Urology, Muljibhai Patel Urological Hospital, Nadiad, Gujarat, India

Tamer El-Husseiny, M.B.B.Ch., M.Sc. (Urol), M.R.C.S. (Ed)
Department of Urology, Barts and the London NHS Trust, London, UK

Denise A. Elliott, B.V.S.C. (Hons), Ph.D., Dipl. A.C.V.I.M., Dipl. A.C.V.N.
Department of Research and Development, Royal Canin, Aimarges, France

Tarık Esen, M.D.
Department of Urology, Istanbul Faculty of Medicine,
Istanbul University, Istanbul, Turkey

Michael Ferrandino, M.D.
Division of Urology and Department of Surgery, Duke University Medical Center,
Zootrent Drive, DUMC 2803, Durham, North Carolina, 27713, USA

Gerhard J. Fuchs, M.D., F.A.C.S.
Department of Surgery, Cedars-Sinai Medical Center, Los Angeles, CA, USA

Giovanni Gambaro, M.D., Ph.D.
Dipartimento di Medicina Interna e di Scienze Mediche Specialistiche,
Università Cattolica del Sacro Cuore, Rome, Italy

Aldrin Joseph R. Gamboa, M.D.
Department of Urology, University of California, Irvine, UCI Medical Center,
Paranaque City, Philippines

Mary Garthwaite, M.B.B.S., Ph.D., F.R.C.S. (Urol)
Department of Urology, St James' University Hospital, Leeds, West Yorkshire, UK

Yehoshua Gdor, M.D.
Department of Urology, University of Michigan Health System, Ann Arbor, MI, USA

David S. Goldfarb, M.D.
Nephrology Section, New York Harbor VA Medical Center, New York, NY, USA

Andreas J. Gross, M.D.
Department of Urology, Asklepios Hospital Barmbek, Hamburg, Germany

Narmada P. Gupta, M.S., M.Ch., D.Sc.
Department of Urology, All India Institute of Medical Sciences, New Delhi, India

Jorge Gutierrez-Aceves, M.D.
Department of Urology, Hospital Civil Nuevo, Universidad de Guadalajara,
Guadalajara, México

George E. Haleblian, M.D.
Division of Urology, The Warren School of Brown University,
Rhode Island Hospital, Providence, RI, USA

Bernhard Hess, M.D.
Department of Internal Medicine & Nephrology/Hypertension,
Klinik Im Park, Zurich, Switzerland

Albrecht Hesse, M.D.
Klinik und Poliklinik für Urologie, Universitätsklinikum Bonn, Bonn, Germany

Doreen M. Houston, D.V.M., D.V.Sc., Diplomate A.C.V.I.M. (Internal Medicine)
Division of Scientific Communication and Clinical Trials,
Medi-Cal Royal Canin Veterinary Diets, Guelph, ON, Canada

Katharine A. Jamieson, M.A., B.M.B.Ch.
Department of Paediatrics, North London Deanery, London, UK

Katharine V. Jamieson, M.A., M.D., F.R.C.S.
Department of Transplantation Surgery, Addenbrooke's Hospital, Cambridge,
Cambridgeshire, UK

Adrian D. Joyce, M.S., F.R.C.S., (Urol)
Pyrah Department of Urology, St. James' University Hospital, Leeds,
West Yorkshire, UK

Paul Jungers, M.D.
Department of Nephrology, Necker Hospital, Paris, France

John P. Kavanagh, Ph.D.
Department of Urology, University Hospital of South Manchester, Manchester, UK

Francis X. Keeley, M.D., F.R.C.S. (Urol)
Department of Urology, Southmead Hospital, Bristol, UK

Saeed R. Khan, M.Sc., Ph.D.
Departments of Pathology and Urology, University of Florida, College of Medicine,
Gainesville, FL, USA

Lisa Kleinen, Dipl. Phys.
Kaiserslautern University of Technology, Institute of Thin Film Technology,
Rheinbreitbach, Germany

Jack G. Kleinman, M.D.
Department of Nephrology, Veterans Affairs Medical Center
and the Medical College of Wisconsin, Milwaukee, WI, USA

Thomas Knoll, M.D., Ph.D., M.Sc.
Department of Urology, Sindelfingen-Böblingen Medical Center, Sindelfingen, Germany

Kai Uwe Köhrmann, M.D.
Department of Urology, Theresienkrankenhaus, Mannheim, Germany

Dirk J. Kok, Ph.D.
Department of Pediatric Urology, Erasmus Medical Center, Rotterdam, The Netherlands

Amy E. Krambeck, M.D.
Department of Urology, Mayo Clinic Rochester, Rochester, MN, USA

Patrick Krombach, M.D.
Urologische Klinik, Universitätsmedizin Mannheim, Mannheim, Germany

Anup Kumar, M.Ch. (Urol)
Department of Urology, All India Institute of Medical Sciences, New Delhi, India

Norbert Laube, Ph.D.
Medizinisches Zentrum Bonn Friedensplatz, Academic Teaching Center
of the University of Bonn, Bonn, Germany

James E. Lingeman, M.D.
Department of Research, Methodist Hospital Institute for Kidney Stone Disease,
Indianapolis, IN, USA

Achim M. Loske, Ph.D.
Centro de Física Aplicada y Tecnología Avanzada,
Universidad Nacional Autónoma de México, Querétaro, México

Umberto Maggiore, M.D.
Department UO Nefrologia, Azienda Ospedaliero – Universitaria di Parma, Parma, Italy

Andrew J. Marks
Division of Urology, Department of Urologic Sciences, St. Paul's Hospital,
Providence Healthcare, University of British Columbia, Vancouver, BC, Canada

Junaid Masood, M.B.B.S., F.R.C.S. (Eng), M.Sc. (Urol), F.R.S.C. (Urol)
Department of Urology, Barts and the London NHS Trust, London, UK

Brian R. Matlaga, M.D., M.P.H.
James Buchanan Brady Urological Institute, The Johns Hopkins Hospital,
Baltimore, MD, USA

Elspeth M. McDougall, M.D., F.R.C.S.C., M.H.P.E.
Department of Urology, UCI Medical Center, Orange, CA, USA

Tiziana Meschi, M.D.
Department of Clinical Sciences, University of Parma, Parma, Italy

Thomas E. Milner, Ph.D.
Department of Biomedical Engineering, The University of Texas at Austin,
Austin, TX, USA

Marnes Molina-Torres, M.D.
Instituto de Endourología, Centro Medico Puerta de Hierro
and Nuevo Hospital Civil, Zapopan, Jalisco, México

Manoj Monga, M.D., F.A.C.S.
Department of Urologic Surgery, University of Minnesota, Minneapolis, MN, USA

Andrew Moore, B.Sc., M.Sc.
Canadian Veterinary Urolith Centre, University of Guelph,
Laboratory Services, Guelph, ON, Canada

Stephen Y. Nakada, M.D.
Department of Urology, University of Wisconsin School of Medicine
and Public Health, Madison, WI, USA

Oscar Negrete-Pulido, M.D.
Instituto de Endourología, Centro Medico Puerta de Hierro
and Nuevo Hospital Civil, Zapopan, Jalisco, México

Antonio Nouvenne, M.D.
Department of Clinical Sciences, University of Parma, Parma, Italy

Tayfun Oktar
Istanbul Faculty of Medicine Department of Urology,
Division of Pediatric Urology, Istanbul University, Istanbul, Turkey

Athanasios Papatsoris, M.D., M.Sc., Ph.D., F.E.B.U.
Department of Urology, Barts and The London NHS Trust, London, UK

Margaret S. Pearle, M.D., Ph.D.
Department of Urology, University of Texas Southwestern Medical Center,
Dallas, TX, USA

Aaron Potretzke, M.D.
Department of Urology, University of Minnesota Medical Center,
Minneapolis, MN, USA

Glenn M. Preminger, M.D.
Division of Urologic Surgery, Duke University Medical Center, Durham, NC, USA

Eric C. Pua
Department of Mechanical Engineering and Materials Science,
Duke University, Durham, NC, USA

Jinze Qiu, M.A.
Department of Biomedical Engineering, The University of Texas
at Austin, Austin, TX, USA

Jay D. Raman, M.D.
Department of Surgery, Penn State Milton S. Hershey Medical Center,
Hershey, PA, USA

P. Nagaraja Rao, Ch.M., F.R.C.S. (Ed)
Formerly Director, Total Stone Management Centre, University Hospital of South
Manchester, Manchester, UK;
Currently Visiting Professor of Urology, NTR University of Health Sciences,
Vijayawada, India

Jens Rassweiler
Department of Urology, SLK Kliniken Heilbronn GMBH, Heilbronn, Germany

José Manuel Reis-Santos, M.D.
Faculdade De Engenharia, Universidade Católica Portuguesa, Rio de Mouro, Portugal

William G. Robertson, Ph.D., D.Sc.
Department of Physiology (Centre for Nephrology), Royal Free and University College
Medical School, Rowland Hill Street, London NW3 2PF, UK

Allen Rodgers, M.Sc., Ph.D.
Department of Chemistry, University of Cape Town, Cape Town Western Cape,
South Africa

Gregory S. Rosenblatt, M.D.
Department of Surgery, Cedars-Sinai Medical Center, Los Angeles, CA, USA

Rosemary Lyons Ryall, B.Sc. (Hons), Ph.D., D.Sc.
Department of Surgery, Flinders Medical Centre and Flinders University,
5042, Adelaide, SA, Australia

Khashayar Sakhaee, M.D.
Department of Internal Medicine, University of Texas Southwestern Medical Center,
Dallas, TX, USA

Kemal Sarica, M.D.
Department of Urology, University of Yeditepe, Medical School, Istanbul, Turkey

Gernot Schubert Dipl. Kristallograph
Institute of Laboratory Diagnostics, Vivantes Klinikum im Friedrichshain,
Berlin, Germany

Michelle Jo Semins, M.D.
The Brady Urological Institute, The Johns Hopkins Medical Institution,
Baltimore, MD, USA

Roswitha Siener, Ph.D.
Department of Urology, University of Bonn, Bonn, Germany

W. Neal Simmons
Department of Mechanical Engineering and Materials Science,
Duke University, Durham, NC, USA

Laura Soldati, Ph.D.
Department of Medicine, Surgery, and Dentistry,
Università degli Studi di Milano, Milano, Italy

Samuel P. Sterrett, DO
Department of Urology, University of Wisconsin, Madison, WI, USA

Walter Ludwig Strohmaier, M.D., Ph.D., F.E.B.U.
Department of Urology and Paediatric, RegioMed, Klinikum Coburg,
Coburg, Bayern, Germany

Sean P. Stroup, M.D.
Department of Urology, Naval Medical Center San Diego, San Diego, CA, USA

Stephanie J. Symons, F.R.C.S. (Urol)
Department of Urology, Pinderfields General Hospital, Wakefield, West Yorkshire, UK

Joel M.H. Teichman, M.D., F.R.C.S.
Department of Urologic Sciences, St. Paul's Hospital, University of British Columbia,
Vancouver, BC, Canada

Ben Thomas, M.D., F.R.C.S. (Urol)
Department of Urology, Western General Hospital, Scottish Lithotripter Centre,
Edinburgh, UK

Hans-Göran Tiselius, M.D., Ph.D.
Department of Urology, Karolinska University Hospital Huddinge,
Stockholm, Sweden

David Tolley, M.B., F.R.C.S., F.R.C.S. (Ed)
Department of Urology, Western General Hospital, Scottish Lithotripter Centre,
Edinburgh, UK

Olivier Traxer, M.D.
Department of Urology, Hôpital Tenon, Paris, France

Alberto Trinchieri, M.D.
Department of Urology, Lecco, Italy

Giuseppe Vezzoli
Istituto Scientifico San Raffaele, Università Vita Salute, Milan, Italy

Gunnar Wendt-Nordahl, M.D.
Department of Urology, Sindelfingen-Böblingen Medical Center,
Sindelfingen, Germany

James C. Williams, Jr. Ph.D.
Department of Anatomy and Cell Biology, Indiana University,
Indianapolis, IN, USA

J. Stuart Wolf, Jr. M.D.
Department of Urology, The University of Michigan, Ann Arbor, MI, USA

Yifei Xing
Department of Mechanical Engineering and Materials Science,
Duke University, Durham, NC, USA

J. Graham Young, M.A., B.M., B.Ch., Ph.D., F.R.C.S., (Urol)
Department of Minimally, Invasive Surgery, and Stone Disease,
University Hospital of South Manchester, Manchester, UK

Joseph E. Zerwekh, Ph.D.
University of Texas Southwestern Medical Center,
Charles and Jane Pak Center for Mineral Metabolism and Clinical Research,
Dallas, TX, USA

Pei Zhong, Ph.D.
Department of Mechanical Engineering and Materials Science,
Duke University, Durham NC, USA

Jack M. Zuckerman, B.S.
Department of General Surgery, Wake Forest University School of Medicine,
Winston-Salem NC, USA

Epidemiology

Gary C. Curham

1

Abstract Substantial progress has been made in our understanding of the epidemiology of nephrolithiasis. Epidemiologic studies have quantified the burden of this common and painful condition, and they have expanded our understanding of risk factors for stone disease. A variety of dietary, non-dietary, and urinary risk factors contribute to the risk of stone formation, and the importance of these varies by age, sex, and body mass index (BMI). Scientifically, results from these studies have forced a reappraisal of our view of risk factors for stone disease. Importantly, the results from epidemiologic studies can be considered in the clinical setting when devising treatment plans for reducing the likelihood of stone formation.

1.1 Introduction

Nephrolithiasis is a common and complex disorder. Epidemiologic studies have quantified the burden of disease and have identified a variety of risk factors, which may help improve our understanding of the pathophysiology as well as lead to new approaches to reduce the risk of stone formation.

1.2 Prevalence

The prevalence of nephrolithiasis – defined as a history of stone disease – varies by age, sex, race, and geography. The prevalence increases with age, and the lifetime risk of stone formation in the USA exceeds 12% in men and 6% in women.[1,2] The prevalence appeared to be increasing in the last quarter of the twentieth century for men and women, whether black or white[2] (see Figs. 1.1 and 1.2). A history of stone disease in the USA is most common among older white males (~12%) and lowest in younger black females (~1%); frequencies for Asians and Hispanics fall in between.[2,3] Increased detection of asymptomatic stones resulting from

the increasing use and sensitivity of radiologic studies may explain, in part, the rise in prevalence.

Few population-based studies of the prevalence of nephrolithiasis have been conducted outside of the USA. Prevalence of stone disease has increased in Japan[4] and Germany.[5]

A study of more than one million individuals found geographic variability with a north–south and west–east gradient; the highest prevalence of self-reported nephrolithiasis was in the Southeastern USA.[6]

A decrease in the male-to-female ratio was suggested by a recent study of hospital discharges.[7] Data from the Nationwide Inpatient Survey between 1997 and 2002 found

G.C. Curham (✉)
Department of Medicine and Epidemiology, Brigham and Women's Hospital, Harvard Medical School/Harvard School of Public Health, Boston, MA, USA
e-mail: gcurham@partners.org

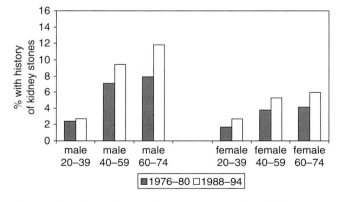

Fig. 1.1 Prevalence of stone disease by sex and age (Adapted and reprinted from Ref.[2] Copyright 2003, with permission from Nature Publishing Group)

P.N. Rao et al. (eds.), *Urinary Tract Stone Disease*,
DOI 10.1007/978-1-84800-362-0_1, © Springer-Verlag London Limited 2011

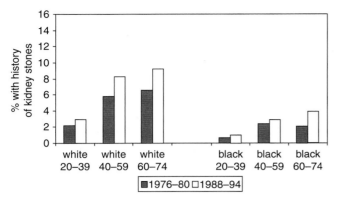

Fig. 1.2 Prevalence of stone disease by race and age (Adapted and reprinted from Ref.[2] Copyright 2003, with permission from Nature Publishing Group)

a male to female ratio 1.3:1; substantially lower than the commonly reported ratio of 2–3:1. Population-based studies of this interesting observation are needed.

1.3 Incidence

The incidence of nephrolithiasis – defined as the first stone event – varies by age, sex, and race. As with prevalence, white males have the highest incidence rates. In men, the incidence begins to rise after age 20, peaks between 40 and 60 years at ~3/1,000/year and then declines.[1,8,9] In women, the incidence is higher in their late twenties at 2.5/1,000/year and then decreases to 1/1,000/year by age 50, remaining at this rate for the next several decades.[1,9–11]

A recent study from Rochester, Minnesota, raised the possibility that incidence rates may be decreasing. Using the same methodology as a study performed 30 years earlier, the recent study reported incidence rates since 1990 may be falling in men and have leveled off in women.[12] Because there were only 157 cases in men and 91 in women, additional larger studies are needed to explore this important issue.

1.4 Recurrence Rates

Few studies provide reliable information on recurrence rates. Case series suggested 30–40% percent of untreated individuals will form another stone within 5 years after the initial episode.[1] Obviously, the risk of recurrence is influenced by a variety of factors including stone type and urinary composition. Fortunately, randomized trials demonstrated that interventions can reduce the likelihood of recurrence by 50% or more.[13–16] These interventions emphasize that prevention of stone recurrence is possible.

1.5 Risk Factors

Information on the importance of a variety of risk factors for stone formation has increased substantially over the past several decades. Risk factors are generally divided into non-dietary, dietary, and urinary.

1.5.1 Non-dietary

1.5.1.1 Family History

Studies of twins and populations have demonstrated that the common forms of stone disease are heritable.[17] The risk of stone formation is twofold higher in individuals with a family history of stone disease.[18] The increased risk is likely due to both genetic predisposition and similar environmental exposures (e.g., diet). Genetic causes of rare forms of nephrolithiasis (e.g., cystinuria, Dent disease) have been identified, but information is still limited on genes that contribute to risk of the common forms of stone disease.

1.5.1.2 Race/Ethnicity

In a cross-sectional Canadian study, individuals of Arabic, west Indian, west Asian, and Latin American descent were more likely to be stone formers than those of European descent.[19] Overall, in the general population, African-Americans have a lower frequency of stones; however, among individuals with end-stage renal disease, African-Americans had a higher than expected prevalence of stone disease.[20]

1.5.1.3 Systemic Disorders

There is substantial evidence that nephrolithiasis is a systemic disorder. Well-known conditions associated with calcium-containing stones include primary hyperparathyroidism, renal tubular acidosis, and Crohn's disease.

Several other common conditions, including obesity, gout, and diabetes mellitus (DM), have recently been convincingly linked to nephrolithiasis. Increasing body size, assessed by weight, body mass index (BMI), or waistline, increases the risk of stone formation independent of other risk factors including diet[21]; for unexplained reasons, the impact is greater in women than in men. For example, the risk of stone formation for individuals with a BMI $\geq$ 30 kg/m^2 compared to those with a BMI 21–23 was 30% higher among men but nearly twofold higher among women. Urinary composition by body size; for example, higher BMI, is associated with higher urine oxalate and lower urine pH, changes that would increase risk for calcium oxalate or uric acid stones.[22]

In a cross-sectional study, individuals with gout were 50% more likely to have a history of stones.[23] When examined prospectively, individuals with a history of gout had a twofold higher risk of incident nephrolithiasis, independent of diet, weight, and medications.[24] Possible mechanisms for this relation include insulin resistance and acidification defects.

Diabetes mellitus (DM) has also been associated with an increased risk of stone formation, independent of diet and body size.[25] Cross-sectionally, individuals with a history of diabetes were more than 30% more likely also to have a history of nephrolithiasis. Prospectively, a history of DM increased the risk of stone formation by 30–50% in women but not in men.[26,27] In support of these findings, a recent study based on National Health and Nutrition Examination Survey (NHANES) III data found that the risk of being a stone former increased with an increasing number of metabolic syndrome traits.[28]

1.5.1.4 Environmental Factors

Occupations or settings with higher insensible fluid losses, such as a hot environment, increase the risk of stone formation.[29] The risk will also be higher when individuals have restricted access to water or bathroom facilities, leading to lower fluid intake and lower urine volume.

1.5.2 Dietary Factors

Dietary intake influences urine composition, thereby modifying the risk of nephrolithiasis. Implicated nutrients include calcium, animal protein,[30] oxalate,[31] sodium,[32] sucrose,[33] fructose,[34] magnesium,[35] and potassium.[36] Care must be taken when interpreting studies of diet and stone risk. Retrospective studies may be biased because individuals who develop stones may subsequently change their diet. Results from studies that use change in urine composition as a surrogate for actual stone formation should be viewed with caution because the composition of the urine does not completely predict risk and not all the components that modify risk are included in the calculation of supersaturation (e.g., urine phytate). Thus, prospective studies that assess a variety of nutrients are best suited for examining the associations between dietary factors and risk of actual stone formation.

1.5.2.1 Calcium

The associations between dietary factors and the risk of incident stone disease have been examined prospectively in three large cohorts: Health Professionals Follow-up Study (HPFS) involving more than 45,000 male health professionals aged 40–75 years at baseline; Nurses' Health Study I (NHS I) involving more than 80,000 female nurses aged 34–59 at baseline; and NHS II involving more than 80,000 female nurses aged 27–44 at baseline.[8,10,11] Prior to these studies, higher calcium intake had been strongly suspected of raising the risk of stone disease. However, these studies demonstrated that individuals with a higher intake of dietary calcium actually had a *lower* risk of incident nephrolithiasis independent of other risk factors.[8,10,11] Although this may seem counter-intuitive, lower calcium intake increases dietary oxalate absorption and urinary oxalate excretion.[37] Another possible explanation is that there is some other protective factor present in milk (dairy products are the major source of dietary calcium in the USA). Even among individuals with a family history of nephrolithiasis, lower dietary calcium intake was associated with an increased risk of stone formation.[18]

Borghi and colleagues performed a randomized controlled study diet that confirmed these observational findings. Men with elevated urine calcium and a history of calcium oxalate stones were randomized to one of two diets: a low calcium diet (400 mg/day) or a diet containing 1,200 mg of calcium along with low sodium and low animal protein intake.[13] Men in the higher calcium intake group had a 50% lower risk of recurrence. The evidence is now overwhelming that calcium restriction is not beneficial and may in fact be harmful, both for stone formation and bone loss.

In contrast to dietary calcium, supplemental calcium does not appear to reduce risk in men or younger women[8,11] and may in fact increase the risk of stone formation in older women. In an observational study[10] and randomized trial,[38] calcium supplement users were ~20% more likely to form a stone than women who did not take supplements, after adjusting for dietary factors. However, the results from the randomized trial should be interpreted cautiously as the participants were instructed to take their supplements with meals, and the supplements contained both calcium and vitamin D. The timing of the supplemental calcium intake may account for the differences in risk. In the cohort studies, calcium supplements were typically not taken with meals, which would diminish binding of dietary oxalate in the intestine.

1.5.2.2 Oxalate

Urine oxalate is clearly an important risk factor for calcium oxalate stone formation; however, the role of dietary oxalate in the pathogenesis of calcium oxalate nephrolithiasis is less clear.[39] The proportion of dietary oxalate that is absorbed is estimated to range from 10% to 50%.[39] The factors influencing the absorption are incompletely characterized but likely include other dietary factors (e.g., calcium), genetic factors, and possibly intestinal flora. In addition, the bioavailability of oxalate in food is unknown. Urinary oxalate is also derived from the endogenous metabolism of glycine, glycolate, hydroxyproline, and vitamin C. A recent study found individuals with a history of calcium oxalate nephrolithiasis were less likely to be colonized with *Oxalobacter formigenes*, an intestinal bacterium that degrades oxalate.[40] Prospective studies of dietary oxalate and stone risk were performed after modern approaches to measure the oxalate content of food provided information on the oxalate content of many foods.[41,42] Surprisingly the impact of dietary oxalate was minimal in men and older women and not associated with stone formation in younger women.[43]

1.5.2.3 Other Nutrients

A variety of other nutrients have been implicated in stone formation. Of note, the magnitudes of the associations often vary by age, sex, or body mass index. For example, higher animal protein intake may increase urinary calcium and decrease urinary citrate,[44] thereby increasing the risk of stone formation. However, when studied prospectively, animal protein was associated with an increased risk in men but not in women.[8,10,11] Further, the increased risk in men was only found among men with BMI < 25 kg/m[2].[45] Higher dietary potassium intake decreased risk in men and older women[8,10,45] possibly by reducing urine calcium excretion[36] or increasing urine citrate. Higher intake of sodium[32] or sucrose[33] increases urinary calcium excretion independent of calcium intake. In prospective studies, sucrose was associated with an increased risk in women and fructose increased risk in men and women.[10,11,34] Phytate, found in whole grains and beans, was observed to reduce risk of stone formation in younger women,[11] possibly by directly inhibiting calcium oxalate crystal formation.

Although magnesium may reduce dietary oxalate absorption, randomized trials of magnesium supplements did not find a protective effect on stone recurrence, though the dropout rates were high. In prospective observational studies, higher dietary magnesium was associated with a lower risk of stone formation in men[45] but not women.[10,11]

Vitamin C (ascorbic acid) can be metabolized to oxalate. Consumption of 1,000 mg of supplemental vitamin C twice daily increased urinary oxalate excretion by 22%.[46] In a prospective observational study, men who consumed 1,000 mg or more per day of vitamin C had a 40% higher risk of stone formation compared to men who consumed less than 90 mg/day (the recommended dietary allowance).[45] While restricting *dietary* vitamin C is not recommended (because foods high in vitamin C contain inhibitory factors such as potassium), calcium oxalate stone formers should avoid vitamin C supplements.

Although high-dose vitamin B6 (pyridoxine) may reduce oxalate production in selected patients with type 1 primary hyperoxaluria, it is unclear if there would be benefit from the use of vitamin B6 supplements to prevent common stone disease. In observational studies, higher intake of vitamin B6 was associated with a reduced risk of kidney stone formation in women[47] but not in men.[48]

1.5.2.4 Fluid Intake and Beverages

The main determinant of urine volume is fluid intake. Urine volume, and therefore fluid intake, is an important determinant of stone risk. When the urine output is less than 1 L/day, risk of stone formation is markedly higher. Higher fluid intake has been demonstrated to reduce the likelihood of stone formation in observational studies[8,10,11] and a randomized controlled trial.[49]

Patients with stone disease often ask which beverages they should drink and which they should avoid. Coffee, tea, beer, and wine were associated with a *reduced* risk of stone formation in prospective studies.[50,51] Although citrus juices theoretically could reduce the risk of stone formation by increasing urine citrate,[52] the prospective studies did not find an independent association with orange juice and grapefruit juice was associated with a significantly higher risk.[50,51] Grapefruit juice is known to affect several intestinal enzymes, but the mechanism for the observed increased risk of stone formation is unknown. Consumption of sugared soda was not associated with a higher risk of stone formation.[50,51] Milk intake reduces the risk of calcium kidney stone formation.

1.6 Urinary Factors

The 24-h urine collection is the cornerstone of the metabolic evaluation and the urine chemistries provide important prognostic information and guide preventive recommendations. Like many laboratory tests, urine results have traditionally been categorized into "normal" and "abnormal." However, recent data has revealed this grouping is unsatisfactory. Urine values are continuous so the dichotomization into "normal" and "abnormal" is arbitrary and potentially misleading. In addition, stone formation is a disorder of *concentration*, not just the absolute amount excreted. Although terms of abnormal excretion, such as "hypercalciuria" or "hypocitraturia" are often used clinically and in the scientific literature, the limitations of these terms should be acknowledged.

Hypercalciuria is commonly defined as urine calcium excretion ≥ 300 mg/day (7.5 mmol/day) in men and ≥ 250 mg/day (6.25 mmol/day) in women[53] on a 1,000-mg/day calcium diet (but a variety of definitions are in use). Using these traditional definitions, approximately 20–40% of patients with calcium stone disease will have hypercalciuria. Although possibly reasonable from a calcium balance perspective, there is insufficient justification for different thresholds for males and females. In fact, the sex-based definitions are particularly concerning because nephrolithiasis is a disorder of concentration and 24-h urine volumes are slightly higher in women than in men.[54]

Hyperoxaluria is typically defined as urinary oxalate excretion >45 mg/day (0.5 mmol/day), though here too a variety of thresholds are in use. Elevated urinary oxalate excretion is three to four times more common among men (~40%) than in women (~10%).[54] Mean urinary oxalate levels are only slightly higher in cases than in controls, but in multivariate models oxalate is clearly an important independent risk factor for stone formation.[54] Of note, the risk begins to rise well below the 45 mg/day level.

The relation between uric acid excretion and calcium stone disease is unsettled. Some early cross-sectional studies reported that *hyperuricosuria* (typically defined as greater than 800 mg/day (4.76 mmol/day) in men or 750 mg/day (4.46 mmol/day) in women) is more frequent in patients who form calcium stones than controls.[55] However, a recent study of more than 2,200 stone formers and 1,100 non-stone formers reported that a higher urine uric acid was associated with a lower likelihood of being a stone former in men, and there was no increase in risk for women.[54] A double-blind trial of allopurinol successfully decreased recurrence rates of calcium stones in patients with hyperuricosuria suggesting that uric acid is important,[16] but it is possible that the beneficial effect of allopurinol was through a mechanism unrelated to lowering of urine uric acid.

Hypocitraturia, often defined as 24-h excretion≤ 320 mg/day (1.67 mmol/day), increases risk of stone formation[56] and is found in 5–11% of first-time stone formers.[54] There is suggestive evidence that increasing urinary citrate into the high-normal range provides additional protection.[54]

Low urine volume, for which a variety of definitions have been used, is a common and modifiable risk factor. When defined as 24-h urine volume less than 1 L/day, 12–25% of first-time stone formers will have this abnormality.[54] Observational studies and a randomized trial have demonstrated the risk of stone formation decreases with increasing total urine volume.[49,54]

1.7 Conclusions

Epidemiologic studies have expanded our understanding of the magnitude and risk factors for stone disease. A variety of dietary, non-dietary, and urinary risk factors contribute to the risk of stone formation and the importance of these varies by age, sex, and BMI. Scientifically, results from these studies have forced a reappraisal of our view of risk factors for stone disease. Importantly, the results from epidemiologic studies can be considered in the clinical setting when devising treatment plans for reducing the likelihood of stone formation.

Acknowledgment This work was supported by grant DK070756 from the National Institutes of Health.

References

1. Johnson CM, Wilson DM, O'Fallon WM, Malek RS, Kurland LT. Renal stone epidemiology: a 25-year study in Rochester, Minnesota. *Kidney Int.* 1979;16(5):624-631.
2. Stamatelou KK, Francis ME, Jones CA, Nyberg LM, Curhan GC. Time trends in reported prevalence of kidney stones in the United States: 1976-1994. *Kidney Int.* 2003;63(5):1817-1823.
3. Soucie JM, Thun MJ, Coates RJ, McClellan W, Austin H. Demographic and geographic variability of kidney stones in the United States. *Kidney Int.* 1994;46(3):893-899.
4. Yoshida O, Okada Y. Epidemiology of urolithiasis in Japan: a chronological and geographical study. *Urologia Internationalis.* 1990;45:104-111.
5. Hesse A, Brändle E, Wilbert D, Köhrmann KU, Alken P. Study on the prevalence and incidence of urolithiasis in Germany comparing the years 1979 vs. 2000. *Eur Urol.* 2003;44(6):709-713.
6. Soucie J, Coates RJ, McClellan W, Austin H, Thun M. Relation between geographic variability in kidney stones prevalence and risk factors for stones. *Am J Epidemiol.* 1996;143:487-495.
7. Scales CD Jr, Curtis LH, Norris RD, et al. Changing gender prevalence of stone disease. *J Urol.* 2007;177(3):979-982.
8. Curhan GC, Willett WC, Rimm EB, Stampfer MJ. A prospective study of dietary calcium and other nutrients and the risk of symptomatic kidney stones. *N Engl J Med.* 1993;328:833-838.
9. Hiatt RA, Dales LG, Friedman GD, Hunkeler EM. Frequency of urolithiasis in a prepaid medical care program. *Am J Epidemiol.* 1982;115:255-265.
10. Curhan G, Willett WC, Speizer FE, Spiegelman D, Stampfer MJ. Comparison of dietary calcium with supplemental calcium and other nutrients as factors affecting the risk for kidney stones in women. *Ann Intern Med.* 1997;126:497-504.
11. Curhan GC, Willett WC, Knight EL, Stampfer MJ. Dietary factors and the risk of incident kidney stones in younger women: Nurses' Health Study II. *Arch Intern Med.* 2004;164(8):885-891.
12. Lieske JC, de la Vega LS Peña, Slezak JM. Renal stone epidemiology in Rochester, Minnesota: an update. *Kidney Int.* 2006;69(4):760-764.
13. Borghi L, Schianchi T, Meschi T, et al. Comparison of two diets for the prevention of recurrent stones in idiopathic hypercalciuria. *N Engl J Med.* 2002;346(2):77-84.
14. Ettinger B, Citron JT, Livermore B, Dolman LI. Chlorthalidone reduces calcium oxalate calculous recurrence but magnesium hydroxide does not. *J Urol.* 1988;139(4):679-684.
15. Ettinger B, Pak CY, Citron JT, Thomas C, Adams-Huet B, Vangessel A. Potassium-magnesium citrate is an effective prophylaxis against recurrent calcium oxalate nephrolithiasis. *J Urol.* 1997;158(6):2069-2073.
16. Ettinger B, Tang A, Citron JT, Livermore B, Williams T. Randomized trial of allopurinol in the prevention of calcium oxalate calculi. *N Engl J Med.* 1986;315(22):1386-1389.

17. Goldfarb DS, Fischer ME, Keich Y, Goldberg J. A twin study of genetic and dietary influences on nephrolithiasis: a report from the Vietnam Era Twin (VET) Registry. *Kidney Int.* 2005;67(3): 1053-1061.

18. Curhan G, Willett WC, Rimm EB, Stampfer MJ. Family history and risk of kidney stones. *J Am Soc Nephrol.* 1997;8:1568-1573.

19. Mente A, Honey RJ, McLaughlin JR, Bull SB, Logan AG. Ethnic differences in relative risk of idiopathic calcium nephrolithiasis in North America. *J Urol.* 2007;178(5):1992-1997. discussion 1997.

20. Stankus N, Hammes M, Gillen D, Worcester E. African American ESRD patients have a high pre-dialysis prevalence of kidney stones compared to NHANES III. *Urol Res.* 2007;35(2):83-87.

21. Taylor EN, Stampfer MJ, Curhan GC. Obesity, weight gain, and the risk of kidney stones. *Jama.* 2005;293(4):455-462.

22. Taylor EN, Curhan GC. Body size and 24-hour urine composition. *Am J Kidney Dis.* 2006;48(6):905-915.

23. Kramer HM, Curhan G. The association between gout and nephrolithiasis: the National Health and Nutrition Examination Survey III, 1988-1994. *Am J Kidney Dis.* 2002;40(1):37-42.

24. Kramer HJ, Choi HK, Atkinson K, Stampfer M, Curhan GC. The association between gout and nephrolithiasis in men: The Health Professionals' Follow-Up Study. *Kidney Int.* 2003;64(3): 1022-1026.

25. Taylor EN, Stampfer MJ, Curhan GC. Diabetes mellitus and the risk of nephrolithiasis. *Kidney Int.* 2005;68(3):1230-1235.

26. Daudon M, Traxer O, Conort P, Lacour B, Jungers P. Type 2 diabetes increases the risk for uric acid stones. *J Am Soc Nephrol.* 2006;17(7):2026-2033.

27. Lieske JC, de la Vega LS, Gettman MT, et al. Diabetes mellitus and the risk of urinary tract stones: a population-based case-control study. *Am J Kidney Dis.* 2006;48(6):897-904.

28. West B, Luke A, Durazo-Arvizu RA, Cao G, Shoham D, Kramer H. Metabolic syndrome and self-reported history of kidney stones: the National Health and Nutrition Examination Survey (NHANES III) 1988-1994. *Am J Kidney Dis.* 2008;51(5):741-747.

29. Atan L, Andreoni C, Ortiz V, et al. High kidney stone risk in men working in steel industry at hot temperatures. *Urology.* 2005;65(5): 858-861.

30. Robertson WG, Peacock M, Hodgkinson A. Dietary changes and the incidence of urinary calculi in the U.K. between 1958 and 1976. *J Chron Dis.* 1979;32:469-476.

31. Larsson L, Tiselius HG. Hyperoxaluria. *Miner Electrolyte Metab.* 1987;13(4):242-250.

32. Muldowney FP, Freaney R, Moloney MF. Importance of dietary sodium in the hypercalciuria syndrome. *Kidney Int.* 1982;22(3): 292-296.

33. Lemann J Jr, Piering WF, Lennon EJ. Possible role of carbohydrate-induced calciuria in calcium oxalate kidney-stone formation. *N Engl J Med.* 1969;280(5):232-237.

34. Taylor EN, Curhan GC. Fructose consumption and the risk of kidney stones. *Kidney Int.* 2008;73(2):207-212.

35. Johansson G, Backman U, Danielson BG, Fellström B, Ljunghall S, Wikström B. Biochemical and clinical effects of the prophylactic treatment of renal calcium stones with magnesium hydroxide. *J Urol.* 1980;124:770-774.

36. Lemann J Jr, Pleuss JA, Gray RW, Hoffmann RG. Potassium administration reduces and potassium deprivation increases urinary calcium excretion in healthy adults [corrected]. *Kidney Int.* 1991;39(5): 973-983.

37. Bataille P, Charransol G, Gregoire I, et al. Effect of calcium restriction on renal excretion of oxalate and the probability of stones in the various pathophysiological groups with calcium stones. *J Urol.* 1983;130(2):218-223.

38. Jackson RD, LaCroix AZ, Gass M, et al. Women's Health Initiative Investigators. Calcium plus vitamin D supplementation and the risk of fractures. *N Engl J Med.* 2006;354(7):669-683.

39. Holmes RP, Assimos DG. The impact of dietary oxalate on kidney stone formation. *Urol Res.* 2004;32(5):311-316.

40. Kaufman DW, Kelly JP, Curhan GC, et al. Oxalobacter formigenes May Reduce the Risk of Calcium Oxalate Kidney Stones. *J Am Soc Nephrol.* 2008;19(6):1197-1203.

41. Holmes R, Kennedy M. Estimation of the oxalate content of foods and daily oxalate intake. *Kidney Int.* 2000;57:1662-1667.

42. Siener R, Hönow R, Voss S, Seidler A, Hesse A. Oxalate content of cereals and cereal products. *J Agric Food Chem.* 2006;54(8): 3008-3011.

43. Taylor EN, Curhan GC. Oxalate intake and the risk for nephrolithiasis. *J Am Soc Nephrol.* 2007;18(7):2198-2204.

44. Breslau N, Brinkley L, Hill KD, Pak CY. Relationship of animal protein-rich diet to kidney stone formation and calcium metabolism. *J Clin Endocrinol Metab.* 1988;66:140-146.

45. Taylor EN, Stampfer MJ, Curhan GC. Dietary factors and the risk of incident kidney stones in men: new insights after 14 years of follow-up. *J Am Soc Nephrol.* 2004;15(12):3225-3232.

46. Traxer O, Huet B, Poindexter J, Pak CY, Pearle MS. Effect of ascorbic acid consumption on urinary stone risk factors. *J Urol.* 2003;170(2 Pt 1):397-401.

47. Curhan GC, Willett WC, Speizer FE, Stampfer MJ. Intake of vitamins B6 and C and the risk of kidney stones in women. *J Am Soc Nephrol.* 1999;10(4):840-845.

48. Curhan GC, Willett WC, Rimm EB, Stampfer MJ. A prospective study of the intake of vitamins C and B6, and the risk of kidney stones in men. *J Urol.* 1996;155(6):1847-1851.

49. Borghi L, Meschi T, Amato F, Briganti A, Novarini A, Giannini A. Urinary volume, water and recurrences in idiopathic calcium nephrolithiasis: a 5-year randomized prospective study. *J Urol.* 1996;155: 839-843.

50. Curhan GC, Willett WC, Rimm EB, Spiegelman D, Stampfer MJ. Prospective study of beverage use and the risk of kidney stones. *Am J Epidemiol.* 1996;143(3):240-247.

51. Curhan GC, Willett WC, Speizer FE, Stampfer MJ. Beverage use and risk for kidney stones in women. *Ann Intern Med.* 1998;128(7): 534-540.

52. Wabner C, Pak C. Effect of orange juice consumption on urinary stone risk factors. *J Urol.* 1993;149:1405-1409.

53. Hodgkinson A, Pyrah LN. The urinary excretion of calcium and inorganic phosphate in 344 patients with calcium stone of renal origin. *Br J Surg.* 1958;46(195):10-18.

54. Curhan GC, Taylor EN. 24-h uric acid excretion and the risk of kidney stones. *Kidney Int.* 2008;73(4):489-496.

55. Coe FL. Hyperuricosuric calcium oxalate nephrolithiasis. *Kidney Int.* 1978;13(5):418-426.

56. Pak CY. Citrate and renal calculi: an update. *Miner Electrolyte Metab.* 1994;20(6):371-377.

Genetics and Molecular Biology of Renal Stones

Giovanni Gambaro, Laura Soldati, and Giuseppe Vezzoli

Abstract Genetic studies of calcium kidney stones have hitherto assessed single candidate genes by testing for linkage disequilibria or associations between a locus and stone disease. They have identified the potential involvement of the calcium-sensing receptor (CaSR), vitamin D receptor, (VDR), and bicarbonate-sensitive adenylyl cyclase genes. In addition to research in humans, studies on different strains of knock-out mice have enabled us to include the phosphate reabsorption carrier NPT2 gene, the caveolin-1 gene, the protein NHERF-1 gene modulating calcium and urate reabsorption, osteopontin, and Tamm–Horsfall protein among the possible determinants. Interactions between genes, and between environmental factors and genes, are generally considered fundamental to calcium stone formation, however. To date, therefore, genetic studies have failed to significantly advance our understanding of the causes of calcium kidney stones, though they have enabled us to assess the dimension of the problem and establish criteria for facing it. Further progress in our knowledge of what causes calcium stones may derive from using the tools afforded to researchers by modern biotechnology and bioinformatics.

2.1 Introduction

Metabolic studies on patients have established that calcium kidney stones can be associated with various defects of mono- and bivalent electrolyte excretion. The most well known of these conditions is primary hypercalciuria, detected in 50% of patients with stones.[1] Others, such as hypo-citraturia, renal hypophosphatemia, hyperuricuria, and an elevated sodium and chloride excretion accompany stone-forming disease less frequently. It is consequently impossible to predict the onset of a calcium stone on the strength of these conditions alone, which leads us to assume that a number of factors interact and/or combine together to predispose an individual to calcium kidney stones.

In the last decade, nephrological research has focused on establishing the genetic causes of calcium nephrolithiasis. Our understanding of this topic has not improved substantially, however, and it has consequently not been possible to develop effective prevention and treatment criteria. Among the predisposing factors, we tend to consider those of genetic and environmental origin, though the distinction between the two is hazy because kidney stones are probably the outcome of an interaction between genes and environment.[1–4] Nephrolithiasis is consequently among the complex diseases with a multifactorial pathogenesis, like hypertension, diabetes, ischemic cardiopathy, and osteoporosis. Studying its causes is bound to be difficult, although advances in our biological/molecular knowledge and new biotechnologies have provided us with powerful analytical tools. These methods have certainly enabled progress to be made in genetic research, but our awareness of the complexity of the pathogenic picture, and of the commitment that will be needed to fully understand it, has likewise grown.

2.2 Genetic Linkage Studies

The genetic study of calcium kidney stones developed starting from the latter half of the 1990s. Early studies were conducted using linkage methods that assess the cosegregation of the nephrolithiasis with a chromosomal locus in members of stone-forming families. These methods are strong and

G. Gambaro (✉)
Dipartimento di Medicina Interna e di Scienze Mediche Specialistiche, Università Cattolica del Sacro Cuore, Rome, Italy
e-mail: giovanni.gambaro@rm.unicatt.it

P.N. Rao et al. (eds.), *Urinary Tract Stone Disease*,
DOI 10.1007/978-1-84800-362-0_2, © Springer-Verlag London Limited 2011

accurate in pointing to the genes involved in a given disease, especially in monogenic diseases, which is why they were applied to nephrolithiasis.[5] Some studies also evaluated the phenotypes implicated in the disease, such as hypercalciuria.

Some linkage studies considered the loci of candidate genes believed to have a pathogenic role in the light of the prevailing pathophysiological hypotheses. This strategy was applied to a sample of more than 300 pairs of French–Canadian brothers suffering from kidney stones, whose chromosomal loci coding for renal 1α (alpha)-hydroxylase of 25(OH) vitamin D, the vitamin D receptor (VDR), or the calcium-sensing receptor (CaSR) were tested. Each region was assayed using specific polymorphic markers. The locus of the 1α (alpha)-hydroxylase of 25-dihydroxy-vitamin D (chromosomal locus 12q13.1-q13.3) was the first to be studied in this sample, but the results could confirm no role for it.[6] The locus of the VDR on chromosome 12q12–14 was analyzed using six different markers, four of which emerged in linkage disequilibrium with nephrolithiasis and only one with hypercalciuria, but with only a low significance.[7] Finally, no linkage was found between the locus of the CaSR (3q13.3–21) and the onset of nephrolithiasis in the series of French–Canadian brothers.[8]

Linkage studies have produced more significant results when members of stone formers' families were studied, by generation. One study reconsidered the locus of the VDR in Indian families and substantially confirmed the results obtained in the French–Canadian brothers.[9] Another confirmed the absence of CaSR gene mutations in seven European families.[10] Only one family-based study used chromosomal markers covering the whole genome (a genome-wide scan): this method enabled them to proceed without any preliminary pathogenic hypothesis or definition of a candidate gene. After exploring the whole genome with polymorphic markers, the results of the study suggested the loci where the genes implicated in nephrolithiasis could be found. In other words, a genome-wide scan enables a pathogenic hypothesis to be developed on the strength of the results obtained. Taking this approach, a linkage was identified between chromosome 1q23.3-q24 and hypercalciuria in three families suffering from absorptive hypercalciuria and kidney stones.[11] The interpretation of this finding was entrusted to a subsequent case-control study, which found an association between hypercalciuria and six polymorphisms of the soluble (bicarbonate-sensitive) adenylate cyclase (sAC) gene. The same polymorphisms were also associated with a low bone mineral mass.[12] The functional role of the sAC gene has yet to be clarified, though we know that it is expressed in the kidney, intestine, and bone cells, and that its function is activated by bicarbonate and modulated by bivalent cations.[13] The linkage between the sAC gene and hypercalciuria was not confirmed, however, in a European study of nine families.[14]

Despite the greater reliability of linkage studies, studies conducted using other strategies, such as analyzing the association between genotype and calcium nephrolithiasis, have been far more numerous. The reasons for this tendency lie in the numerous practical and theoretical problems involved. First, there is the difficulty of finding family groups covering at least three generations and numerically large enough to enable linkage studies. Another problem lies in the inability of linkage studies to identify genes with a scarce phenotypic effect.[3,5] This problem applies particularly to nephrolithiasis because stones may be caused not by a mutation in one or a few genes with a strongly predominant effect, but by compound changes induced by numerous genes, each incapable alone of giving rise to the disease.[15] This being the case, the causal substrate might be so variable and heterogeneous as to make it extremely difficult to conduct genetic studies and identify individual genes.

In addition to these specific problems, there is also the more general difficulty of classifying an individual as a stone-former; in fact, a kidney stone can develop at any age, and may even go unrecognized. It may also be that an individual possessing the predisposing genetic heritage forms no stones because other genes or nutrients with an antilithogenic effect prevail over the lithogenic factors.[16] A clear example of this phenomenon in the kidney stone setting is the low-sodium diet prescribed for hypercalciuric individuals. The lithogenic risk in these people is increased by their higher calcium excretion levels, but restricting their dietary intake of sodium and chloride reduces their stone-forming potential related to their hypercalciuria, which is known to have a genetic component.[17] It may also be that several genetic causes come into play in patients with recurrent kidney stones, but not in those who produce only one stone in a lifetime.[18]

2.3 Genetic Association Studies

The studies associating a genotype with calcium kidney stones are the most common alternative to genetic linkage studies. They assess whether an allele or a genotype is more or less common in patients with kidney stones than in those without them. The search for this association can involve analyzing of the whole genome or only a candidate gene. In the nephrolithiasis setting, only candidate genes have been tested to date,[2] but analyses with genome-wide markers represent the way forward.[19] In association studies, patients and controls are genotyped for single-base polymorphisms arranged along the sequence of candidate genes. These polymorphisms have a mean frequency of one for every 1,200 bases and contribute to the variability of the phenotype. They can be placed in coding regions and cause an amino acid change, or in untranscribed regions and leave the amino acid sequence in the protein unchanged. Their potential influence on the phenotype often remains unknown and this is a crucial drawback of such analyses.[20]

The first gene to be analyzed using this method was the VDR gene, considering the polymorphisms of the untranscribed 3′ region or of the transcription start codon. These polymorphisms emerged as being associated with calcium kidney stones in various studies, and some also observed that patients carrying allele variants to 3′-terminal region polymorphisms developed stones earlier in life and had a more aggressive form of the disease and lower urinary citrate excretion levels.[21–23] Although some works have not confirmed these associations,[24] overall the results obtained give the impression that VDR gene polymorphisms can play a part in the onset of calcium nephrolithiasis. It remains to be seen whether the VDR gene polymorphisms identified have an important functional effect on the disease or whether the association is simply due to their cosegregation (i.e., they are in linkage disequilibrium) with other functionally relevant polymorphisms. Their functional link to nephrolithiasis is generally justified by the fact that the VDR-vitamin D complex activates intestinal calcium absorption (Fig. 2.1). It seems, however, that the VDR-vitamin D complex

is also capable of reducing urinary citrate excretion. In fact, it can derepress the expression of phosphoenolpyruvate carboxyl kinase that can limit its renal excretion by stimulating the citrate reabsorption carrier on the luminal membrane of the proximal tubule cells.[25]

Particular results were obtained by analyzing the CaSR gene, studying its polymorphisms of exon 7 (3′-terminal) and the polymorphisms of the first intron and of the untranscribed 5′ region near the promoter. The Arg990Gly polymorphism of exon 7 is associated with hypercalciuria in patients with and without kidney stones. Results in vitro on HEK293 embryonal renal cells transfected with the CaSR gene indicate that the Arg990Gly polymorphism can give rise to a functional gain for the CaSR gene.[26,27] This hypothesis is confirmed by the fact that patients with primary and secondary hyperparathyroidism carrying the allele variant have lower mean circulating levels of PTH than carriers of the arginine allele.[28] It is consequently feasible that the glycine allele at codon 990 is less effective in inhibiting calcium reabsorption in the cells of the thick ascending limb of the Henle's loop, predisposing carriers to higher calcium excretion levels (Fig. 2.2). This poses the question of why these same individuals are not hypocalcemic too, like the carriers of CaSR gene activating mutations: maybe the Arg990Gly polymorphism has a different influence on the signaling systems used by parathyroid and renal cells, so it could inhibit tubular calcium reabsorption and PTH production in

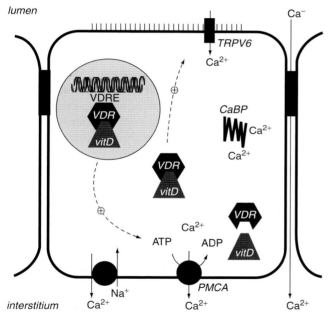

Fig. 2.1 Intestinal absorption of calcium is considered particularly important in stone formation. Transcellular absorption is mediated by a transport system involving the transfer of calcium from the lumen into the enterocyte through the calcium channel TRPV6, while on the basolateral membrane the calcium pump (PMCA) and sodium–calcium exchange carry the calcium ion into the interstitium. PMCA is only involved in absorption in the jejunum and duodenum, where absorption is active. In the cytoplasm, calbindin 9k (*CBP*) binds the calcium ions absorbed and guides them toward the carriers of the basolateral membrane. The vitamin D receptor (*VDR*) complex controls the gene expression of all these carriers and CBP, and it regulates TRPV6 activity via a non-genomic effect. The VDR complex binds to a specific gene sequence called *VDRE* (vitamin D response element), which derepresses the genes of the vitamin-D-dependent proteins. Alongside these mechanisms, there is also a paracellular calcium absorption

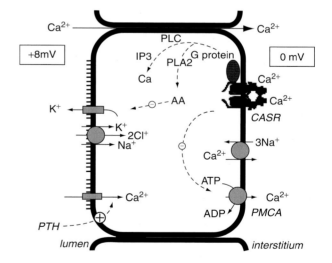

Fig. 2.2 The figure schematically shows a cell of the thick ascending limb, illustrating the effects of the calcium-sensing receptor (*CaSR*) gene, which inhibits Na–K–Cl cotransport and sodium reabsorption via phospholipase A2 (*PLA2*) activation and the production of arachidonic acid (*AA*) and eicosatetraenoic acid. This inhibitory effect reduces the electric potential between the interstitium and the lumen, which in itself obstructs the passive paracellular reabsorption of calcium and other cations. In addition, the activation of calcium reabsorption has a direct effect on the calcium pump (*PMCA*), which inhibits the active reabsorption of calcium

parathyroid cells to a different degree. The importance of this polymorphism in calciuria has also been confirmed in patients with primary hyperparathyroidism, because patients who carry the 990Gly allele variant have higher urinary calcium excretion levels and form stones more frequently.[28]

Polymorphisms of the CaSR gene promoter region located in the first intron or the untranscribed 5′ region were recently associated with nephrolithiasis in the Italian population.[29] They do not entail an amino acid change and they can presumably take effect by modifying the gene's transcription and the expression of the CaSR in the tubule cells of the renal papilla, given the nearness of the gene promoter. With high calcium concentrations in the renal papilla, a different cell expression of the CaSR is likely to be crucial to the precipitation of calcium salts and the formation of oxalate stones.[30]

Polymorphisms of the genes coding for osteopontin, urokinase, interleukin receptor-1, intestinal transient receptor potential cation channel (TRPV6), E-cadherin and epidermal growth factor have also been associated with kidney stones.[14,31–36] The physiopathological role of these genes in nephrolithiasis is still not clear and there are still no works to confirm the preliminary results. On the other hand, a functional result has been obtained for the gene *TRPV6*, coding for the calcium channel expressed in the intestinal mucosa, according to which the activating mutations would be associated with nephrolithiasis[32] via an increase in intestinal calcium absorption (Fig. 2.2).

Association studies are certainly easier to perform than linkage analyses, but they are not without their problems. The previously mentioned difficulties in classifying an individual as affected apply in this case too; and they suffer from a poor repeatability of the results in different populations due to differences in genetic substrate or environmental factors that can lead to unrecognized stratifications, which make the various populations unsuitable for comparison.[37] This can also apply in the opposite sense; that is, creating the conditions for false-positive results due to unwitting favorable stratifications. These studies can nonetheless also reveal genes with a limited effect on the phenotype, as is probably the case of the relationship between hypercalciuria and the CaSR gene Arg990Gly polymorphism. The allele variant 990Gly was found associated with hypercalciuria and explained 4% of the phenotypic variability of calciuria in one study population[24]; vice versa, the locus of the CaSR gene was not in linkage with hypercalciuria or nephrolithiasis in the pairs of French–Canadian brothers.[8] This scarce influence of the Arg990Gly polymorphism on the variability of calciuria is probably responsible for the negative outcome of the linkage studies.

The association and linkage studies conducted to date chose the genes and polymorphisms to investigate in advance. While the choice of genes was generally based on physiopathological knowledge, the choice of polymorphisms was only rarely guided by functional knowledge.[20] This important

weakness can now be avoided thanks to the introduction of genome-wide scanning methods, which can now be undertaken at a still considerable but sustainable cost, but this demands technologies and bioinformatic software products capable of testing and processing massive numbers of samples and amounts of data. Finally, irrespective of the study strategy adopted, it is fundamental for genetic findings to be confirmed by functional studies on cell and animal models. These potential developments and the previously mentioned experiences have led to association studies being progressively reconsidered in recent years.

2.4 Animal Models of Genetic Disease

Knockout mice are animals genetically programmed not to express a given gene. The development of kidney stones in the phenotype of a knockout strain indicates that the silenced gene is important in preventing the onset of nephrolithiasis. Five strains of knockout mice are known to develop kidney stones. The mice without the *slc26a13* gene lack the carrier that secretes oxalate in the intestinal lumen. As a consequence, these animals accumulate oxalate in the organism and its renal excretion is increased, leading to urinary precipitation and stone formation.[38] *Caveolin-1* knockout mice are incapable of producing caveol in the renal cells; that is, the plasma membrane invaginations where proteins important to cell functions (such as the calcium pump, CaSR, and VDR) collect. These mice fail to absorb calcium from the tubular lumen and consequently become hypercalciuric, developing calcium–phosphate deposits in the tubule.[39] The third knockout mouse strain lacks a protein, Na⁺/H⁺ exchanger regulatory factor (NHERF-1), that modulates sodium, calcium, and uric acid reabsorption. Calcium and urate excretion increases with the consequent formation of papillary calcium deposits.[40] In the double knockout mouse strain, for osteopontin and the Tamm–Horsfall protein, papillary interstitial deposits are found in 39% of the animals, presumably because of their urine's inability to inhibit calcium salt precipitation. The two proteins seem to have a synergetic antilithogenic effect, since knocking out only one or the other induces papillary deposits in only 10–15% of the animals.[41]

Finally, knockout mice for the renal sodium/phosphate cotransporter (NPTa) are an interesting model with a phenotype characterized by hypophosphatemia secondary to renal phosphate loss, high renal vitamin D synthesis, hypercalciuria, and renal stone formation.[42] This picture is similar to the one that develops in patients with autosomal dominant hereditary hypophosphotemic rickets with hypercalciuria (HHRH). Knockout mice for *NPT2a* have consequently been considered as a model of the renal impairment in patients with HHRH. No *NPT2a* gene mutation has been found, however, in patients with HHRH, while mutations have been identified in the proximal phosphate NPT2c carrier.[43] This means that there is a different organization of proximal phosphate reabsorption in humans and mice: while the former probably uses NPT2c as the main carrier for phosphate reabsorption in the proximal tubule cell (Fig. 2.3), the latter uses NPT2a. The two carriers differ functionally because NPT2a sustains the electrogenic cotransport of three sodium ions and one phosphate, while NPT2c produces an electroneutral cotransport that reabsorbs two sodium ions and one phosphate. NPT2a or NPT2c deficiency seems to differently affect bone, since the phenotype in mice does not include the rickets observed in humans. It may be that the two phosphate carriers are differently expressed in the bone cells: in particular, NPT2a occurs in the osteoclasts and the NPT2a knockout mice seem to have fewer, less active osteoclasts.[44]

Experience gained with the previously mentioned animal strains shows that knockout mice are a source of useful information and relatively easy to obtain. They may pave the way to new research hypotheses, but they do not represent a cornerstone for research because in any case transferring findings from mice to humans demands knowledge of the role played by the proteins under study in human physiology. Osteopontin and Tamm–Horsfall protein are known for their antilithogenic activity in humans, while the role of the slc26a13 oxalate carrier and NHERF-1 have yet to be ascertained. The studies on NPT2 go to show that transferring data obtained in the mouse to human beings is not always possible.

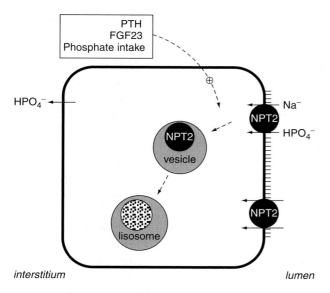

Fig. 2.3 The NPT2 transporter/carrier in humans serves the purpose of reabsorbing phosphate in the proximal tubule. To be specific, the NPT2c isoform is responsible for 85% of phosphate reabsorption, while 15% is mediated by NPT1. Phosphate, FGF23, and PTH intake inhibits NPT2 expression on the luminal membrane because their presence causes NPT2 to be internalized and lysed in the lysosomes. This is the mechanism by which they reduce phosphate reabsorption

2.5 Future Areas of Study

It is easy to see from the previous considerations that the genes involved in nephrolithiasis and how the disease is transmitted have yet to be explained. In choosing candidate genes to investigate, researchers have focused on genes specifically related to calcium metabolism, among which the *VDR, CaSR,* and *sAC* genes seem to contribute to the formation of calcium stones, though the extent of the contribution is not yet clear. These genes may be involved in the onset of primary hypercalciuria and osteoporosis, so the association of these disorders with nephrolithiasis emphasizes the importance of hypercalciuria as a pathogenic factor and explains the high frequency of osteoporosis among stone formers, irrespective of calciuria levels.

It is nonetheless highly likely that, in addition to calcium metabolism, other aspects of renal electrolyte metabolism remaining to be explored are also important in the pathogenesis behind stone formation. An example comes from studies indicating the potentially stone-forming role of the sAC gene. Genome-wide scans are consequently awaited with much interest; specifically for the opportunity they will give us to formulate new hypotheses and research perspectives that overcome the limits of our current understanding.

In the main, the studies listed here considered a single gene, while the interactions between different genes, and between genes and the environment are generally considered fundamental to the development of kidney stones. Stone-forming genes can interact with the environment in a more or less complex manner, giving rise to multiple forms of interaction. As at the current state of research, the most interesting interactions are of epigenetic type, in which environmental influences can modify the phenotype in a stable manner, transmissible to subsequent generations, without changing the genotype.[45] They do so by modifying gene expression through various mechanisms. In humans, the most common of these consists in the methylation of the gene promoter regions, which can mean that gene transcription is repressed or rearranged, respectively, in the event of hyper- or hypo-methylation.[46] In fetal and perinatal life, different environmental conditions are thought to be able to produce epigenetic changes, thereby influencing the newborn's susceptibility to chronic diseases. Studies on interactions between genes and the environment are destined to expand progressively in the nephrolithiasis setting, also thanks to epigenetic analyses, but such research is yet to be conducted at either epidemiological level or in animal models.

2.6 Conclusions

In conclusion, we might say that 10 years of genetic studies on nephrolithiasis have been unable to substantially improve our understanding of what causes calcium kidney stones.

But this conclusion would be ungenerous to all those who have committed themselves to this difficult, insidious area of research, and anyway the same could be said, more in general, of all complex diseases. In fact, the genetic investigation tools available up until not long ago produced exciting results for the monogenic, Mendelian-transmission diseases, but disappointing results for more complex diseases. New human genome scanning methods, less expensive high throughput gene investigation tools, and bio-informatic software capable of managing the body of data collected from large population samples (in terms of numerosity) have all become available in recent years, however. The studies conducted so far have served as preliminary investigations and, despite their limits, they can be used to provide the basis on which to found future research efforts. The results obtained relate mainly to changes in calcium metabolism in nephrolithiasis, but they have also produced criteria and tested the dimension of the problem. In the light of these studies, modern biotechnological and bioinformatic tools, provided they are put to good use, should be able to help us make further advances in our knowledge of the genetic causes behind calcium kidney stones. In this effort, however, it is important to acknowledge that a fundamental step concerns sample collection, to make it as phenotypically homogeneous as possible. To obtain significant results with our modern tools, we still need to rely on the ancient art of clinical patient assessment and our ability to obtain precise and standardized information on their characteristics.

References

1. Hodkinson A, Pyrah LN. The urinary excretion of calcium and inorganic phosphate in 344 patients with calcium stones of renal origin. *Brit J Surg*. 1958;46:10-18.
2. Manolio TA, Bailey-Wilson JE, Collins FS. Genes, environment and the value of prospective cohort studies. *Nature Rev Genet*. 2006;7:812-820.
3. Colhourn HM, McKeigue PM, Smith JD. Problems of reporting genetics associations with complex outcomes. *Lancet*. 2003;361:865-872.
4. Loredo-Osti JC, Roslin NM, Tessier J, et al. Segregation of urine calcium excretion in families ascertained for nephrolithiasis: evidence for a major gene. *Kidney Int*. 2005;68:966-971.
5. Lander ES, Schork NJ. Gentic dissection of complex traits. *Science*. 1994;265:2037-2048.
6. Scott P, Ouimet D, Proulx Y, et al. The 1 alpha hydroxylase locus is not linked to calcium stone formation or calciuric phenotype in French-Canadian families. *J Am Soc Nephrol*. 1998;9:425-432.
7. Scott P, Ouimet D, Valiquette L, et al. Suggestive evidence for a susceptibility gene near the vitamin D receptor locus in idiopathic calcium stone formation. *J Am Soc Nephrol*. 1999;10:1007-1013.
8. Petrucci M, Scott P, Ouimet D, et al. Evaluation of the calcium-sensing receptor gene in idiopathic hypercalciuria and calcium nephrolithiasis. *Kidney Int*. 2000;58:38-42.
9. Khullar M, Relan V, Singh SK. VDR gene and urinary calcium excretion in nephrolithiasis. *Kidney Int*. 2006;69:943.
10. Lerolle N, Coulet F, Lantz B, et al. No evidence for point mutations of the calcium-sensing receptor in familial idiopathic hypercalciuria. *Nephrol Dial Transplant*. 2001;16:2317-2322.
11. Reed BY, Heller HJ, Gitomer WL, et al. Mapping a gene defect in absorptive hypercalciuria to chromososme 1q23.3-q24. *J Clin Endocrinol Metab*. 1999;84:3907-3913.
12. Reed BY, Gitomer WL, Heller HJ, et al. Identification and characterization of a gene with base substitutions associated with the absorptive hypercalciuria phenotype and low spine bone density. *J Clin Endocrinol Metab*. 2002;87:1476-1485.
13. Geng W, Wang Z, Zhang J, et al. Cloning and characterization of the human soluble adenylyl cyclase. *Am J Physiol Cell Physiol*. 2005;288:C1305-C1316.
14. Muller D, Hoenderop JGJ, Vennekens R, et al. Epithelial Ca channel (ECAC1) in autosomal dominant idiopathic hypercalciuria. *Nephrol Dial Transplant*. 2002;17:1614-1620.
15. Goodman HO, Holmes RP, Assimov DG. Genetic factors in calcium oxalate stone disease. *J Urol*. 1995;153:301-307.
16. Wright A, Charlesworth B, Rudan I, et al. A polygenic basis for late-onset disease. *Trends Genet*. 2003;19:97-106.
17. Borghi L, Schianchi T, Meschi T, et al. Comparison of two diets for the prevention of recurrent stones in idiopathic hypercalciuria. *N Engl J Med*. 2002;346:77-84.
18. Gambaro G, Vezzoli G, Casari G, et al. Genetics of hypercalciuria and calcium nephrolithiasis: from the rare monogenic to the common polygenic forms. *Am J Kidney Dis*. 2004;44:963-986.
19. Wang WYS, Barratt BJ, Clayton DG, et al. Todd JA. Genome-wide associtation studies: theoretical and practical concerns. *Nature Rev Genet*. 2005;6:109-118.
20. Tabor HK, Risch NJ, Myers RM. Candidate-gene approaches for studying complelx genetic traits: practical considerations. *Nature Rev Genet*. 2002;3:1-7.
21. Soylemezoglu O, Ozkaya O, Gonen S, et al. Vitamin D receptor gene polymorphism in hypercalciuric children. *Pediatr Nephrol*. 2004;19:724-727.
22. Rendina D, Mossetti G, Viceconti R, et al. Association between vitamin D receptor gene polymorphisms and fasting idiopathic hypercalciuria in recurrent stone-forming patients. *Urology*. 2004;64:833-838.
23. Relan V, Khullar M, Singh SK, et al. Association of vitamin D receptor genotypes with calcium excretion in nephrolithiatic subjects in northern India. *Urol Res*. 2004;32:236-240.
24. Vezzoli G, Soldati L, Proverbio MC, et al. Polymorphism of vitamin D receptor gene start codon in patients with calcium kidney stones. *J Nephrol*. 2002;15:158-164.
25. Sugiyama T, Wang JC, Scott DK, Granner DK. Transcription activation by the orphan nuclear receptor, chicken ovalbumin upstream promoter-trascription factor I (COUP-TFI). *J Biol Chem*. 2000;275:3446-3454.
26. Vezzoli G, Tanini A, Ferrucci L, et al. Influence of calcium-sensing receptor gene on urinary calcium excretion in stone-forming patients. *J Am Soc Nephrol*. 2002;13:2517-2523.
27. Vezzoli G, Terranegra A, Arcidiacono T, et al. R990G polymorphism of calcium-sensing receptor does produce a gain-of-function and predispose to primary hypercalciuria. *Kidney Int*. 2007;71:1155-1162.
28. Corbetta S, Eller-Vainicher C, Filopanti M, et al. The A990G polymorphism of calcium sensing receptor gene (CaSR) is associated with nephrolithiasis in patients with primary hyperparathyroidism (PHPT). *Eur J Endocr*. 2006;155:687-692.
29. Terranegra A, Arcidiacono T, Biasion R, et al. Calcium-sensing receptor (CaSR), a candidate gene for calcium kidney stone disease. *Nephrol Dial Transplant*. 2006;21(suppl 4):292.
30. Bushinsky DA. Nephrolithiasis: site of the initial solid phase. *J Clin Invest*. 2003;111:602-605.

31. Gao B, Yasui T, Itoh Y. Association of osteopontin gene haplotypes with nephrolithiasis. *Kidney Int.* 2007;72:592-598.

32. Suzuki Y, Pasch A, Bonny O, et al. Gain of function haplotype in the epithelial calcium channel TRPV6 is a risk factor for renal calcium stone formation. *Hum Mol Genet.* 2008;17(11):1613-8.

33. Chen WC, Wu HC, Chen HY, et al. Interleukin-1beta gene and receptor antagonist gene polymorphisms in patients with calcium oxalate stones. *Urol Res.* 2001;29:321-324.

34. Tsai FJ, Lin CC, Lu HF, et al. Urokinase gene 3'-UTR T/C polymorphism is associated with urolithiasis. *Urology.* 2002;59:458-461.

35. Tsai FJ, Wu HC, Chen HY, et al. Association of E-cadherin gene 3-UTR C/T polymorphism with calcium oxalate stone disease. *Urol Int.* 2003;70:278-281.

36. Chen WC, Chen HY, Wu HC, et al. Vascular endothelial growth factor gene polymorphism is associated with calcium oxalate stone disease. *Urol Res.* 2003;31:218-222.

37. Freedman ML, Reich D, Penney KL, et al. Assessing the impact of population stratification on genetic association studies. *Nat Genet.* 2004;36:388-993.

38. Jiang Z, Asplin JR, Evan AP, et al. Calcium oxalate urolithiasis in mice lacking anion transporter Slc26a6. *Nat Genet.* 2006; 38:474-478.

39. Cao G, Yang G, Timme TL, et al. Disruption of the caveolin-1 gene impairs renal calcium reabsorption and leads to hypercalciuria and urolithiasis. *Am J Pathol.* 2003;162:1241-1248.

40. Weinman EJ, Mohanlal V, Stoycheff N, et al. Longitudinal study of urinary excretion of phosphate, calcium, and uric acid in mutant NHERF-1 null mice. *Am JPhysiol Renal Physiol.* 2006;290:F838-843.

41. Mo L, Liaw L, Evan AP, et al. Renal calcinosis and stone formation in mice lacking osteopontin, Tamm-Horsf all protein, or both. *Am J Physiol Renal Physiol.* 2007;293:F1935-1943.

42. Chau H, El-Maadawy S, McKee M, et al. Renal calcification in mice homozygous for the disrupted type Iia Na/Pi cotransporter gene Npt2. *J Bone Miner Res.* 2003;18:64-657.

43. Lorenz-Depiereux B, Benet-Pages A, Eckstein G, et al. Hereditary hypophosphatemic rickets with hypercalciuria is caused by mutations in the sodium-phosphate cotransporter gene SLC34A3. *Am J Hum Genet.* 2006;78:193-201.

44. Gupta A, Tenenhouse HS, Hoag HM, et al. Identification of the type II Na+–Pi cotransporter (Npt2) in the osteoclast and the skeletal phenotype of *Npt2–/–* mice. *Bone.* 2001;29:467-476.

45. Jirtle RL, Skinner MK. Environmental epigenomics and disease susceptibility. *Nature Rev Genet.* 2007;8:253-262.

46. Robertson KD. DNA metilation and human disease. *Nature Rev Genet.* 2005;6:597-610.

Physicochemical Aspects of Uro-crystallization and Stone Formation

3

John P. Kavanagh

Abstract Urinary stones are predominantly crystalline and the precipitation of uro-crystals must obey the physical-chemical principles applicable to crystallization in a broader sense. Key amongst these is the requirement for supersaturation to be generated, providing the necessary thermodynamic driving force for crystallization. The three main processes of nucleation, growth, and aggregation are all dependent on the degree of supersaturation. Nucleation of uro-crystals will be heterogeneous (occurring at a surface) and can only be sustained at a supersaturation above the equilibrium condition. Once nucleation has occurred, growth and aggregation can proceed until a saturated equilibrium is achieved, although in the continuous flow of the urinary system the supersaturation may be maintained by replenishment with fresh solute. A new crystallization process has recently been recognized involving the ordered clustering of nanocrystals, which brings together elements of nucleation, growth, and aggregation. The relevance of this to uro-crystallization is not yet clear. Of established significance is the presence of crystallization inhibitors and promoters in urine. These might act through changes in supersaturation or directly at the interface between crystals and solution or crystals and their nucleating substrate.

Symbols and Abbreviations

a	activity
Δa	activity driving force (supersaturation)
A	pre-exponential factor (in Arrhenius reaction rate equation)
c	concentration
Δc	concentration driving force (supersaturation)
CaOx	calcium oxalate (crystalline)
ΔG	Gibbs energy change
ΔG_{het}	Gibbs energy change for heterogeneous nucleation
ΔG_{hom}	Gibbs energy change for homogeneous nucleation
ΔG_s	Gibbs energy change for production of new crystal surface
ΔG_v	Gibbs energy change for production of new crystal volume
ΔG_{crit}	Gibbs energy change for production of a critical nucleus
g	growth rate
I	ionic strength
J	nucleation rate
k	growth rate constant
k_{sp}	solubility product
$\boldsymbol{k}$	Boltzmann constant
FP	formation product
L	particle size
L_{crit}	size of critical nucleus
M	strength factor of aggregation bridge
ML	metastable limit
N	Avogadro's number
n	growth rate reaction order
pK_a	−log (acid dissociation constant)
r	radius
r_{crit}	radius of critical nucleus
$\mathbf{R}$	gas constant
R_{agg}	aggregation rate
R_{coll}	aggregate collision rate
R_{con}	aggregate consolidation rate
R_{disp}	aggregate dispersion rate
S	supersaturation ratio
T	absolute temperature
v_m	molecular volume
(x)	concentration of species x

J.P. Kavanagh
Department of Urology, University Hospital of South Manchester, Manchester, UK
e-mail: john.p.kavanagh@btinternet.com

P.N. Rao et al. (eds.), *Urinary Tract Stone Disease*,
DOI 10.1007/978-1-84800-362-0_3, © Springer-Verlag London Limited 2011

$[x]$	activity of species x
z	valency
α	volume shape factor
β	surface shape factor
γ	activity coefficient
γ_{Ss}	interfacial energy (between substratum and solution phase)
γ_{cs}	interfacial energy (between crystal and solution phase)
γ_{Sc}	interfacial energy (between substratum and crystal phase)
θ	contact angle
μ^0	chemical potential at the standard state
μ	chemical potential
$\Delta\mu$	thermodynamic driving force
σ	relative supersaturation
τ	induction time
Φ	reaction affinity (positive form of $\Delta\mu$)
$\Phi_{/N}$	reaction affinity per molecule
φ	heteronucleation factor
Ψ	aggregation efficiency factor

Subscripts

c	crystals
eq	equilibrium
s	solution
S	substratum

3.1 Introduction

Stones in the urinary tract are usually predominantly crystalline and the exceptions (rare matrix stones) will not be considered in this chapter. Crystallization is a physicochemical process involving a change of phase and this has been extensively written about elsewhere, either as a subject in its own right[1,2] or with particular attention to urinary/biomineral crystallization.[3–7] The intention of this chapter is to introduce the important concepts and their theoretical background, concentrating on relevance to stones but without attempting to encompass the whole of the crystallization field. In particular, crystal morphology and how modifiers (often urinary macromolecules) of crystallization act will barely be touched upon.

Whatever the chemical nature and wherever in the urinary system that uro-crystallization takes place, it is an absolute requirement that there is sufficient free energy to drive the reaction. This only occurs when the solution is supersaturated; that is, the concentration of the crystallizing species in the solution is higher than its solubility in that solution. For all those rare components that make up only 1% or 2% of stones (e.g., the metabolically derived cystine, xanthine, dihydroxyadenosine,

or drug-induced stones such as indinavir), supersaturation with the relevant species is absent from the urine of the general population and is only found in those who form these stones. In these cases the presence of supersaturation is sufficient to explain the consequent stone disease.[7] Similarly, urine is normally undersaturated with struvite, and this only forms stones when supersaturation is developed by the action of urea-splitting bacteria. By contrast, the more common stone components, calcium oxalate (CaOx), calcium phosphate (in the form of carboxy- or hydroxyapatite), and, to a lesser extent, uric acid are often found at supersaturated levels in the urine of healthy people.[7] It follows that, while supersaturation is an essential requirement for stone formation, it is possible for persistently supersaturated urine to be produced without any ill effects. In part, this is achieved by crystallization inhibitors, but it also reflects the fundamental physical chemistry of crystallization, where the energy barrier to be overcome for initiation of crystallization is greater than that required to sustain it.

The most important crystallization processes are crystal nucleation, crystal growth, and crystal aggregation. Nucleation is the first stage and involves the formation of small crystal nuclei. These will be made up of only a small number of atoms (some tens or hundreds) and therefore contribute a negligible amount toward the total crystal mass or volume. Crystal growth is the incorporation of molecules or ions from solution into the crystal lattice and is the most important contributor to the total mass and volume. Aggregation is the bringing together and consolidation of individual crystals into a polycrystalline body. Although this may involve a small amount of incorporation of material from solution, it can be thought of as essentially a redistribution of the volume with little change in mass. All three of these processes are dependent on the degree of supersaturation.

3.2 Supersaturation

3.2.1 Different States of Saturation

Different degrees of saturation are recognized (Fig. 3.1). A solute is *undersaturated* if it is in solution below its solubility, and in this case further solute, when added in

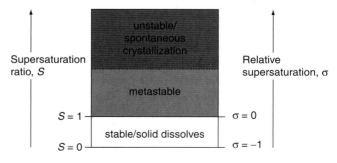

Fig. 3.1 Different regions of saturation can be distinguished (Reprinted with kind permission from Springer Science+Business Media[7])

crystalline form, will dissolve. At the point when no more solid will dissolve, the solution is in equilibrium with the crystals and is *saturated*. In this state, the chemical potential of the substance in solution (μ_s) is equal to the chemical potential of the crystals (μ_c). If a saturated solution, in equilibrium with crystals, is cooled (lowering the solubility or decreasing μ_c) or evaporated (with the aim of increasing the solute concentration and thereby increasing μ_s) then the crystals will grow (taking solute from the solution) and maintain an equilibrium position with μ_s and μ_c matched. Conversely, if the saturated solution in equilibrium with crystals is heated or diluted, then some of the crystals will dissolve, again preserving the balance between the chemical potentials.

At first sight, it might be thought that a supersaturated solution should not be attainable because any means used to generate a chemical potential difference between the solution and solid phase will be resisted by crystallization to the equilibrium condition. It is, however, possible to produce a *supersaturated* solution by cooling or evaporating an undersaturated solution (which, of course, will not contain any crystals). This is because the chemical energy required for crystallization to begin (nucleation) is greater than that needed to maintain crystallization, once crystals are already present. As long as the solution remains free of crystals then a supersaturated state can persist. As soon as crystals are introduced, or a nucleation event takes place, then these crystals will grow until the equilibrium condition is reached. This relatively stable supersaturated condition is described as being *metastable*. Another way to produce a supersaturated solution is to mix two solutions of soluble salts, each of which contains one part of an insoluble salt (for example, sodium oxalate and calcium chloride); if both of these are sufficiently concentrated then CaOx will immediately begin to crystallize when they are mixed. This is because the high supersaturation formed is sufficient to induce spontaneous nucleation. It is also possible to mix less concentrated solutions of two soluble salts to produce a metastable (supersaturated) solution of calcium oxalate. Forming supersaturated and crystallizing solutions of calcium oxalate in this way is a common experimental method,[8,9] but it is not how urine becomes supersaturated. In the urinary tract, supersaturation is achieved largely by water removal, which gradually increases the solution concentration.

3.2.2 Supersaturation Equations

The extent of supersaturation can be expressed in a number of ways, all involving the concentration of the crystallizing species in the solution and the solubility of the species (i.e., the concentration in a solution, which is in equilibrium with crystals).

The concentration driving force (Δc) is simply the difference between the solution and equilibrium concentrations (c_s and c_{eq} respectively):

$$\Delta c = c_s - c_{eq} \qquad (3.1)$$

The supersaturation ratio (S) is defined by

$$S = \frac{c_s}{c_{eq}} \qquad (3.2)$$

and the relative supersaturation (σ) is

$$\sigma = \frac{\Delta c_s}{c_{eq}} = S - 1 \qquad (3.3)$$

In the urolithiasis community and literature, the term *supersaturation* is often not clearly explained. It is rarely expressed as the concentration driving force and when explicitly defined Eq. 3.2 is most commonly used. The phrases *supersaturation ratio* and *relative supersaturation* have sometimes been used as though they are synonymous. Within a particular piece of work and when used for internal comparisons this need not be a particular problem, but it can cause some confusion when comparing across different publications, especially when the supersaturation ratio or relative supersaturation have been quantified with the same tool (e.g., Equil2). Of course, one major distinction is the equilibrium condition, at which $S = 1$ and $\sigma = 0$ (Fig. 3.1).

When the crystallizing species is a salt, such as calcium oxalate, then the concentrations in the previous equations are replaced by the concentration products of the components; for example,

$$S = \frac{\left(Ca^{2+}\right)_s \times \left(Ox^{2-}\right)_s}{\left(Ca^{2+}\right)_{eq} \times \left(Ox^{2-}\right)_{eq}} \qquad (3.4)$$

Strictly speaking, it is the *effective* concentrations (i.e., the activities) of the relevant species that are the decisive factors. While this distinction is not very important in dilute solutions (close to the solubility limit for poorly soluble salts) and in the absence of other solutes, it becomes very significant when other salts are present, as in urine. This is clearly demonstrated if one considers the denominator in Eq. 3.4 (i.e., the solubility product, k_{sp}), which for CaOx (monohydrate) in water at 37°C is 2.24×10^{-9} M (calculated).[10] In a solution of 0.2 M NaCl this increases to 3.84×10^{-8} M (measured), and in a urine-like solution further increases to 1.00×10^{-7} M (measured) or 1.10×10^{-7} M (calculated).[10] Based on concentrations, CaOx is therefore about 50 times more soluble in urine than in pure water. The reason for these changes will be considered later. The previous equations can be expressed in terms of activities (a or [x]):

$$\Delta a = a_s - a_{eq} \qquad (3.5)$$

$$S = \frac{a_s}{a_{eq}} \qquad (3.6)$$

$$\sigma = \frac{\Delta a_s}{a_{eq}} = S - 1 \qquad (3.7)$$

$$S = \frac{\left[Ca^{2+}\right]_s \times \left[Ox^{2-}\right]_s}{\left[Ca^{2+}\right]_{eq} \times \left[Ox^{2-}\right]_{eq}} \qquad (3.8)$$

Of these equations for supersaturation, the supersaturation ratio (S) is most clearly evident in the expression of the thermodynamic driving force for crystallization. This derives from consideration of the chemical potentials of the substance in the crystal state and solution state, with the difference between them being the force available:

$$\Delta\mu = \mu_c - \mu_s \qquad (3.9)$$

Because the reactions we are concerned with take place at constant temperature and pressure, this is equivalent to the familiar Gibbs energy (ΔG) and it is only when $\Delta\mu$ (and ΔG) are negative that crystallization can take place. It is more convenient to express this driving force for crystallization as a positive quantity by defining the reaction affinity as

$$\Phi = -\Delta\mu \qquad (3.10)$$

The chemical potentials are indirectly related to the concentrations and are defined by their relationship to their activities. The chemical activity of a component is its *effective* concentration and takes into account the effect of interactions between itself and between the surrounding solvent and other solutes. The chemical potential of this particular component (μ) in a mixture is

$$\mu = \mu^0 + \mathbf{R}T \ln(a) \qquad (3.11)$$

where μ^0 is its chemical potential in the standard state (at a defined temperature and concentration), $\mathbf{R}$ is the gas constant, and T is the absolute temperature.

Combining Eqs. 3.9–3.11 leads to

$$\Phi = \mathbf{R}T \ln\left(\frac{a_s}{a_{eq}}\right) \qquad (3.12)$$

Substituting from Eq. 3.6, the reaction driving force is seen to be directly proportional to the logarithm of the supersaturation ratio

$$\Phi = \mathbf{R}T \ln(S) \qquad (3.13)$$

3.2.3 Estimating Urinary Supersaturation

There is no great value in estimating S for those stone components that are only found at supersaturated levels in the urine of the corresponding stone formers. In these cases, either stone analysis or urine analysis showing a urease positive infection or cystine levels consistent with a homozygous cystinuria gene defect will be sufficient to determine a primary diagnosis and treatment regime. For the more common stone types, especially where stone analysis is not available, estimating S can provide some clinically useful information, over and above that given by simply measuring the concentrations of the individual components such as uric acid, calcium, oxalate, etc.

It is possible to apply the appropriate version of Eq. 3.4 or 3.8. Finlayson[3] referred to these two approaches as semiempirical and ab initio methods respectively. If applying Eq. 3.4, it is necessary to recognize that the concentration - k_{sp} will vary from urine to urine. This can be determined for the particular sample by equilibrating the urine with the appropriate crystals and measuring the concentrations remaining in solution. This approach has been described fully for CaOx and brushite,[11] but has rarely been applied in recent years, largely from practical considerations. A simplified method for brushite has recently been described.[12] The other approach is to calculate the activities of the various species from their measured concentrations and take into account the ionic strength and the known interactions between the various species. These calculations are not trivial and are accomplished with speciation computer programs. Equil2[13] is the best known of these for use in urolithiasis investigations while a more generalized program, JESS, has also been applied in this field.[10,14–17] A comparison of Equil2, JESS, and the semiempirical method for brushite suggests that Equil2 overestimates the supersaturation because it does not allow for some calcium complexes, particularly $Ca_2H_2(PO_4)_2$.[18]

Use of these speciation programs requires measurement of all the urinary components that will affect the activity of the species in question. This may include all the major electrolytes, specific species (such as citrate), and pH. A potential flaw is that interactions between species not included in the program may be significant, particularly calcium-binding macromolecules. Tiselius has provided simplified equations[19–21] for calcium oxalate and calcium phosphates that produce approximate activity products. These are based on comparing the urine analysis of many samples with the outcome from Equil2 and include only the most relevant species. For calcium oxalate, these are limited to calcium, oxalate, citrate, and magnesium and the volume. By the same approach a similar equation for the activity product of calcium and oxalate, without including the volume, has been proposed.[22]

3.2.4 Solubility

One of the obvious factors in determining solubility is the temperature, but for the urinary system we can consider this to be fixed at 37°C. For many simple systems such as a single, poorly soluble salt in water, it may be appropriate to consider the solubility expressed in terms of concentration (c_{eq}) despite the awareness that the more fundamental description should be in activities (a_{eq}). In mixtures such as urine, the influence of the other components in solution must be considered as they will affect the activity through ionic strength effects and the formation of complexes, amongst which are the many equilibrium reactions involving H^+.

The solubility of stone components is very dependent on pH. Uric acid becomes more likely to crystallize as the pH decreases while calcium oxalate can be solubilized by strong acid. Calcium phosphate, in the form of brushite, is least soluble around pH 7, but as hydroxy- or carboxy-apatite its solubility decreases as the pH rises further and becomes more alkaline. Struvite also becomes more insoluble in alkaline conditions while cystine becomes more soluble. All these effects can be understood by considering the relevant protonation/deprotonation reactions and the pH at which they occur (Fig. 3.2). The pH of urine will also have less direct effects on the solubility of stone components as, for example, the changes in the protonation state of citrate/citric acid changes will have consequent changes in its ability to form soluble complexes with calcium.

The formation of soluble complexes effectively removes free ions from solution and therefore increases the solubility expressed as a concentration. This will be particularly important for CaOx and calcium phosphates. Not only must one consider the direct complexes with the precipitating species but also the interactions between the counter ions. Thus for CaOx in the presence of citrate and magnesium it would be necessary to account for soluble calcium oxalate, calcium citrate species, soluble magnesium oxalate, *and* magnesium citrate species. This is why speciation programs, such as Equil2 or JESS, require the concentration of all the major electrolytes as part of their input. By the same token, if an important equilibrium reaction is not included in the program then it will necessarily result in some error.

At the concentration of electrolytes in urine, the ionic strength effects on activity are very significant. Ionic strength (I) is calculated from the sum of the concentrations of the various ions and their valencies

$$I = \frac{1}{2}\sum_i c_i z_i^2 \qquad (3.14)$$

where z_i is the valency of the ith ion. The activity coefficient (γ) is then usually calculated by some variation of the Debye–Hückel equation such as the Davies modification

$$\text{Log}\,\gamma = -0.523 z^2 \left\{ \left(\frac{I^{1/2}}{1+I^{1/2}} \right) - 0.3I \right\} \qquad (3.15)$$

where the factor 0.523 is a temperature dependent constant (for 37°C) and 0.3 is the usual empirical constant, although Equil2 uses 0.286.[13] This equation is approximately valid for I up to about 0.1 or 0.2 mol/L; that is, it will become increasingly unreliable at the higher concentrations sometimes encountered in urine. Equation 3.15 gives a value of γ for divalent ions of 0.303 in 0.2M NaCl. So for CaOx monohydrate, assuming complete dissociation and no complex formation, the solubility product (at 37°C and zero ionic strength) of 2.24×10^{-9} would increase to 2.44×10^{-8}. The difference between this and the measured value[10] of 3.83×10^{-8} is mainly due to complexes (soluble calcium oxalate, sodium oxalate [anion], and $CaCl_2$).

Changing the solubility through addition of electrolytes is often referred to as "salting in" (increasing solubility) or "salting out" (decreasing solubility). For calcium salts in urine, the effects of ionic strength and complex formation discussed previously will generally lead to salting in. A relevant example of salting out was provided by Grover et al.,[23] who showed that adding dissolved sodium urate to urine could bring about crystallization of CaOx or lower its metastable limit (ML). Although they did not directly measure CaOx solubilities in urate solutions, they showed that the effect was not dependent on decreasing the barrier for nucleation. As they pointed out,[23] Equil2 does not accommodate this effect and they discuss more fully possible mechanisms to account for it.[24]

3.3 Classical Crystallization Processes

3.3.1 Nucleation

Nucleation is the initial process in crystallization in which a small number (some tens or hundreds) of molecules come together to form a crystal nucleus, which can then grow by further deposition from the solution. It can be described as primary when crystals of the precipitating phase are not involved

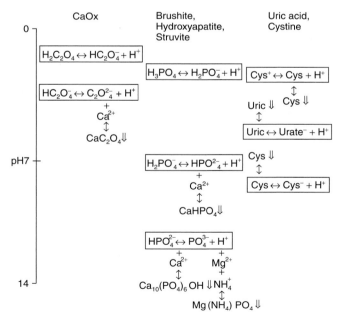

Fig. 3.2 pH and solubility of urinary stone species. Protonation reactions are shown in boxes, located on the pH axis at their pK_a; that is, where the equilibrium is at 50%. The precipitating species are shown by ⇓ (ignoring any water of crystallization)

or secondary when the nuclei form at preexisting crystal surfaces. Primary nucleation can be further divided into homogeneous and heterogeneous nucleation. Homogeneous nucleation occurs spontaneously when the supersaturation is sufficient. This is difficult to achieve in practice because of the need to exclude all foreign particles and surface imperfections. Nucleation that occurs at a surface (of a foreign body or the container) is known as heterogeneous. In the absence of preformed crystals, all nucleation in the urinary system will almost certainly be heterogeneous.

3.3.1.1 Homogeneous Nucleation

Although homogeneous nucleation is not expected to be relevant to urinary crystallization, it is helpful to consider classical nucleation theory because heterogeneous nucleation can then be described as an accelerated or catalyzed version of the homogeneous nucleation rate (J). As mentioned in the introduction, there is an additional energy barrier to be overcome before crystal initiation can be achieved at any significant rate. This is because when very small nuclei increase in size, the energy difference between the surface and the particle bulk (ΔG_s, which is positive) increases faster than the decrease in energy difference between the solute occupying the volume of the particle and the solute in solution (ΔG_v, which is negative). ΔG_s is proportional to the surface area while ΔG_v is proportional to the particle volume. When the nuclei reach a critical size, the overall energy change ($\Delta G_v + \Delta G_s$) begins to decrease (Fig. 3.3a). Thus particles below this critical size will tend to dissolve, while those above will continue to grow. For spherical nuclei of radii r, the energy change for homogeneous nucleation is

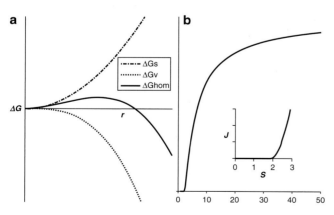

Fig. 3.3 Classical homogeneous nucleation. (**a**) The change in energy associated with formation of new surface and fresh volume as the size of the nucleus increases. The net energy change reaches a maximum at a critical nucleus size and thereafter decreases. Particles above this size will tend to grow and below this size will tend to dissolve. (**b**) The nucleation rate is dependent on the supersaturation. It is initially very low and at some point (the metastable limit) will start to increase very rapidly with higher supersaturations

$$\Delta G_{hom} = \Delta G_v + \Delta G_s = \frac{4}{3}\pi r^3 \frac{\Phi_{/N}}{v_m} + 4\pi r^2 \gamma_{cs} \quad (3.16)$$

where v_m is the molecular volume and γ_{cs} is the interfacial energy between the crystal surface and the solution. $\Phi_{/N}$ is the affinity expressed per molecule (i.e., Φ/N, where N is Avogadro's number).

ΔG_{hom} passes through a maximum value (ΔG_{crit}) when the derivative of Eq. 3.16 with respect to r is zero and the size of the critical nucleus is r_{crit}

$$\frac{d\Delta G_{hom}}{dr} = 4\pi r^2 \frac{\Phi_{/N}}{v_m} + 8\pi r \gamma_{cs} = 0 \quad (3.17)$$

$$\therefore r_{crit} = -\frac{2\gamma_{cs} v_m}{\Phi_{/N}} \quad (3.18)$$

Substituting the value for r_{crit} into Eq. 3.16 simplifies to

$$\Delta G_{crit} = \frac{16\pi \gamma_{cs}^3 v_m^2}{3\Phi_{/N}^2} \quad (3.19)$$

This can be expressed more generally than for a spherical nucleus by using shape factors (α for the volume, β for the surface) and L for the particle size, leading to

$$L_{crit} = \frac{2\beta \gamma_{cs} v_m}{3\alpha \Phi_{/N}} \quad (3.20)$$

and

$$\Delta G_{crit} = \frac{4\beta^3 \gamma_{cs}^3 v_m^2}{27\alpha^2 \Phi_{/N}^2} \quad (3.21)$$

The energy requirement for formation of the critical nucleus can be seen as equivalent to the activation energy for a chemical reaction and the Arrhenius reaction equation can therefore be applied to express the nucleation rate:

$$J = A \exp\left(-\Delta G_{crit} / kT\right) \quad (3.22)$$

where A is the pre-exponential factor, k is the Boltzmann constant. The homogeneous nucleation rate can therefore be expressed as

$$J = A \exp\left(-\frac{16\pi \gamma_{cs}^3 v_m^2}{3k^3 T^3 (\ln S)^2}\right) \quad (3.23)$$

and

$$J = A \exp\left(-\frac{4\beta^3 \gamma_{cs}^3 v_m^2}{27\alpha^2 k^3 T^3 (\ln S)^2}\right) \quad (3.24)$$

for spherical and general particles respectively. J is dependent on the particle surface tension and the supersaturation and the characteristics of the rate equation mean that the rate will initially be undetectable and will start to increase very rapidly at some supersaturation ratio greater than 1 (Fig. 3.3b).

3.3.1.2 Heterogeneous Nucleation

Heterogeneous nucleation can be viewed as a catalyzed form of homogeneous nucleation in which the nuclei form on some foreign surface or particle and the Gibbs energy change is reduced:

$$\Delta G_{het} = \varphi \Delta G_{hom} \qquad (3.25)$$

where φ is a factor that is less than 1. It is usual[1,2,25] to describe heterogeneous nucleation of a crystal from solution by analogy with the heterogeneous nucleation of a liquid from a vapor in which the contact angle (θ) is critical (Fig. 3.4). This angle can be expressed in terms of the interfacial tensions between the crystal and solution phase (γ_{cs}), the crystal and the nucleating substratum (γ_{cS}), and the substratum and solution (γ_{Ss}) (Fig. 3.4):

$$\cos\theta = \frac{\gamma_{Ss} - \gamma_{cS}}{\gamma_{cs}} \qquad (3.26)$$

The factor φ in Eq. 3.25, which expresses the catalytic nucleating efficiency of the substratum, depends on the contact angle, with

$$\varphi = \left(2 - 3\cos\theta + \cos^3\theta\right)/4$$

or, equivalently,

$$\varphi = \left(2 + \cos\theta\right)\left(1 - \cos\theta\right)^2/4 \qquad (3.27)$$

As the angle θ increases from 0° through to 180°, the factor φ increases from 0 to 1; that is, the surface moves from having no nucleating effect through to there being no energy barrier to nucleation. The physical meaning of the contact angle for a nucleating crystal on a solid is not clear but the analogy with a liquid on a surface leads to the idea that as θ decreases, so too does the volume of material required to form a critical nucleus; for example, compare the volumes of the two nuclei in Fig. 3.4. The better the match between the lattice dimensions of the crystal nucleus and the nucleating surface, the better will be the nucleating efficiency. The limit of $\theta = 180°$ can be thought of as equivalent to the presence of seed crystals of the crystallizing compound.

Of particular interest in uro-crystallization is the potential for crystals of one component to have similar lattice parameters to another and thereby act as a promoter of nucleation. This can be thought of as a special form of heteronucleation and is known as epitaxy. Many different possible matches have been described between the dimensions of different uro-crystal types[26] that offer support to the idea that this might be relevant. Experimentally, enhanced nucleation of stone forming crystals by different uro-crystals has been demonstrated (e.g., Refs. 36–39 from Finlayson[3] and many others since). It is also clear that many (or most) stones contain more than one crystalline component and that the center or apparent initiation point of stones is often distinctly different from the majority of the material.[27]

Secondary nucleation occurs in the presence of crystals of the crystallizing component. If seed crystals are introduced into a metastable supersaturated solution they would be expected to grow without a change in particle number, but if the particle number increases this suggests that secondary

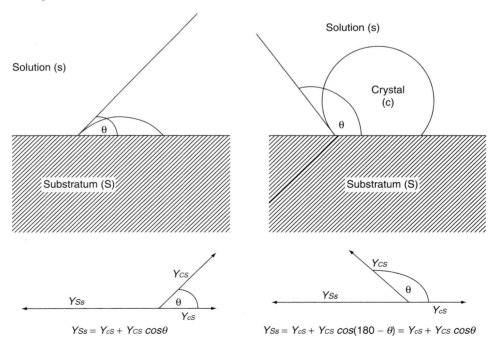

Fig. 3.4 Heterogeneous nucleation occurs with the nucleating crystal, c, forming on another surface, S, from solution, s. As the contact angle between them (θ) increases so too does the volume of crystal required to form a critical nucleus. Resolving the three interfacial forces in the horizontal direction allows this angle to be expressed as $\cos\theta = (\gamma_{Ss} - \gamma_{cS})/\gamma_{cs}$

nucleation has taken place. This can arise through direct solution – crystal interaction or through crystals colliding with each other or their surroundings. By definition this cannot be the process to initiate crystallization within the urinary system, but it could be important in the later stages of stone formation.[28,29]

There have been relatively few attempts to apply an understanding of nucleation theory, particularly interfacial energies and contact angles, to stone research, although Wu and Nancollas have discussed the theories and their application in some detail.[4,25,30] This lack of application is disappointing because, as the initial process required to kick-start crystallization, it is of fundamental significance, as was highlighted by Finlayson more than 30 years ago.[3]

3.3.1.3 The Metastable Limit and Induction Time

Two aspects of nucleation of uro-crystals that have received considerable practical attention are the metastable limit (ML) and the induction time (τ). The ML is the supersaturation at which spontaneous nucleation occurs (i.e., it reflects the magnitude of ΔG_{crit}) and the induction time is the delay between generating the nucleation and the measurable onset of crystallization. The ML is a much less well-defined boundary than the supersaturated/undersaturated point (Fig. 3.1). It is very difficult to ensure that truly homogeneous nucleation takes place and it is difficult to control reproducibly the nature and quantity of heterogeneous nucleators. Even if it were possible to achieve homogeneous nucleation, this will not generally be appropriate for the study of uro-crystals where urine is often the preferred medium. Measurement of the onset of nucleation will be technically demanding and, in practice, the observed onset point will usually have included crystal growth. This time taken for the nucleated crystals to grow sufficiently to produce a detectable change in the system will be part of τ. The timing of the observations will therefore be important, as it may or may not be sufficient to include the induction time (Fig. 3.5), with consequences for the interpretation of the results.

Despite these practical limitations, use of ML or τ can be useful to explore the differences between different urines in their nucleating potential or to examine particular crystals for epitaxy and the ability of additives to modify nucleating activity. Under these circumstances, it is comparisons of results that matter rather than the absolute values. τ can simply be expressed as a time but a number of ways of expressing the ML are employed, often dependent on the methods being used. Rather than calculating the supersaturation, it may be more convenient to state the results by the extent the supersaturation was raised; for example, by the amount of

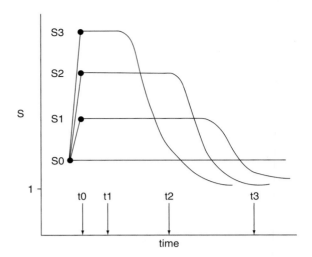

Fig. 3.5 Estimation of metastable limit (*ML*) and the influence of the induction time. If metastable solutions with a supersaturation of S0 are raised to supersaturations of S1, S2, and S3 at t0 and observed for onset of crystallization at t1, t2, and t3 different conclusions would be reached. At t1, ML > S3. At t2, ML > S2 and ≤ S3. At t3, ML > S0 and ≤ S1

added oxalate required to initiate crystallization of CaOx. If urines, which will vary in their ionic composition, are being tested and compared, it would be preferable to calculate the ML from the known composition and the added oxalate; but it is often seen as sufficient to calculate a formation product (*FP*),[11,12] for example,

$$FP = (Ca) \times (Ox) \qquad (3.28)$$

Because estimates of ML or τ are likely to include a period of crystal growth as well as nucleation, it is important to recognize that it may not be possible to conclude that any observed changes are restricted to changes in nucleating activity.

Measurements of τ (and to a lesser degree, ML) can be used to investigate not only comparative nucleation activity but also the nucleation kinetics more directly. If τ is considered to be inversely proportional to the nucleation rate, then

$$\ln \tau \propto -\ln A + \frac{4\beta^3 \gamma_{cs}^3 v_m^2}{27\alpha^2 k^3 T^3 (\ln S)^2} \qquad (3.29)$$

and plotting $\ln \tau$ against $1/(\ln S)^2$ should give a straight line from which γ_{cs} can be calculated. In practice, there may be different regions of the plot, corresponding to two straight lines, reflecting heterogeneous and homogeneous nucleation. An example of this approach to CaOx nucleation is given by El-Shall et al.[31]

Together, the ML and τ can allow supersaturated urine to be produced without resulting in cyrstalluria. τ may be especially important within the renal tubules where the developing urine passes from one region to the next, being modified as it moves along. In regions where conditions are right for nucleation to take place, τ could prolong the process until conditions have changed so as not to be so favorable.

3.3.2 Crystal Growth

Crystal growth is usually taken to mean the incorporation of solute into the crystal lattice; that is, it does not necessarily equate to an increase in average particle size, which can also happen by aggregation. While nucleation is a crucial first step in crystallization, it is crystal growth that accounts for the bulk of the material precipitated. Without growth, clinically significant stones would not form.

It is usual to consider two processes that must be performed in sequence to achieve crystal growth: transport of the crystallizing component or ions from the solution to the surface and their incorporation into the lattice. If the rates of these two processes are dissimilar, then the process with the slower rate will control the overall crystal growth rate; while if they are similar, then both will contribute to the growth kinetics.

As the crystallizing species are integrated into the solid crystal, the local solution concentration at the surface is decreased and a concentration gradient between the crystal and the bulk solution can develop. Transport across this region is dependent upon the concentration gradient, the diffusion coefficient, and the thickness of the layer. The thickness in vitro would depend on the agitation imposed, but in the renal system the fluid flow rate and any crystal immobilization (e.g., to a cell membrane) would be expected to be important factors.

Various models for the integration of new material into the lattice have been proposed. Units of the crystallizing substance at the surface of the crystal may form an adsorption layer in which, although they may have lost solvated water, they have not yet become firmly integrated into the lattice. Under these conditions they can undergo surface diffusion. They can then become incorporated when they find themselves coming up to an active center such as a step. The surface diffusing units may also come together at a point on the surface in sufficient numbers to act as a two-dimensional nucleus, which then acts as an active center for further units. Kinks and dislocations on the crystal surface can also act as active centers from which growth can propagate. The kinetics of growth are usually described by the empirical relationship to the relative supersaturation (σ):

$$g = k\sigma^n \tag{3.30}$$

where g is the crystal growth rate, k is a rate constant, and n is referred to as the reaction order. The value of n is indicative of the growth mechanism with, for example, $n = 1$ suggesting diffusion from solution as the controlling process and $n = 2$ suggesting surface diffusion and integration dominate.[4,5] A reaction order of 2 has commonly, but not always, been reported for CaOx crystal growth.[3,32–36] Since the advent of atomic force microscopy, it has been possible to visualize and measure crystal growth directly, and it is clear that measurement of growth rates and reaction orders from a crystallizing solution can only give information about the overall process. At the level of individual crystallographic faces, atomic force microscopy reveals that different mechanisms and rates can apply in specific crystallographic directions of CaOx monohydrate.[37,38]

3.3.2.1 Desaturation Profile

During the course of crystallization the incorporation of solute into the crystal lattice will deplete the solution supersaturation (unless it is replenished) and this can have a significant effect on the relative significance of different crystallization processes as they proceed toward the equilibrium position.[1] The way that supersaturation is developed and allowed to decay can be a helpful way of distinguishing between different laboratory crystallization methods.[8,9] As uro-crystals form, they may be swept along with the surrounding urine, which will therefore undergo desaturation; but if they have become fixed, their milieu will be continually replenished by fresh urine. Once beyond the ducts of Bellini, any suspended crystals and developing stones will be in urine that is being continually refreshed and they can be thought of as being in a mixed suspension mixed product removal system in which a characteristic supersaturation is dynamically maintained.[39]

3.3.2.2 Stoichiometry

When two or more ions combine to produce the crystal then their stoichiometry in solution and solid phases can be very important. For example, calcium and oxalate are present at 1:1 in the crystal, but in urine the ratio may typically be anything between about 5:1 and 50:1. It seems self-evident that the ion in the minority would have a rate controlling influence and Robertson found that the volume of CaOx crystallized from solutions with the same initial supersaturation but different stoichiometries followed a bell-shaped curve against the log of the ratio, reaching a peak when the ratio was 1:1.[40] It should be remembered that in a desaturating system, such as was used in this case, the ratio of ions remaining in solution will also change during the course of the crystallization. Zhang and Nancollas[41] analyzed and discussed the effect of the ionic ratio for a simple crystal and showed that symmetrical curves of rate against the log of the ratio are expected for crystal growth governed by transport processes or by surface integration. The effect for both mechanisms becomes more pronounced with increasing supersaturation (Fig. 3.6). Chernov et al.[42,43] measured growth of steps on CaOx monohydrate crystals by atomic force microscopy and found approximately symmetrical profiles for growth against log calcium:oxalate ratio at a constant supersaturation, which is consistent with the theoretical predictions with the assumption that the attachment of calcium and oxalate each have the same proportional relationship to their concentrations.

In the case of urine, a small increase in calcium will increase the calcium:oxalate ratio while a small increase in oxalate will decrease the calcium:oxalate ratio, and these opposing changes in ratio will push the growth rate in opposite directions. For a kink propagation model, one can calculate that for typical urine values an increase in calcium by 10% might increase the crystal growth rate by 10%, but a 10% increase in oxalate would have a corresponding increase in growth rate of 23% (Table 3.1).

The large calcium:oxalate ratios in urine have been widely held to be responsible for realistic changes in oxalate changes having a disproportionately large effect on the supersaturation compared to changes in calcium. It is suggested that as the calcium and oxalate in urine are in equilibrium with soluble calcium–oxalate complex, then an increase in calcium will, to some extent, be offset by a reduction in ionized oxalate; on the other hand, an increase in oxalate will have a negligible effect on the ionized calcium, which is present in comparative excess.[40] The magnitude of this effect has been disputed[45] and the difference in opinion ascribed to the dissociation constant used for the soluble calcium–oxalate complex. The higher the value used the greater will be the disproportionate effect of calcium and oxalate changes. The recent reanalysis[45] uses a lower (and widely accepted) value for this dissociation complex and concluded that, over physiological meaningful ranges, changes in the calcium and oxalate would have very similar effects on the supersaturation. While the similarity of response in S to changes in Ca and oxalate is true over most of their range, the discrepancy grows with increasing concentrations. Changes in calcium in a hypercalciuric sample will have a smaller effect on S than changes in oxalate in a hyperoxaluric sample of the same volume.

3.3.3 Aggregation

When crystals are observed in urine, naturally occurring or produced in vitro, they are commonly seen to be clumped together. This aggregation is a means of rapidly increasing the average particle volume and, as stones are clearly polycrystalline aggregates, the process is widely seen as crucial in enabling uro-crystals to become entrapped and to develop into macroscopic stones.[46,47] Because aggregation of crystals is likely to take place at the same time as growth and nucleation, changes in particle numbers or volumes will reflect all three processes. In a continuously crystallizing mixed suspension mixed product removal system a steady state crystal size distribution is achieved from which it is possible to isolate and quantify the different processes.[35,48] If a metastable solution is seeded with the appropriate crystals then nucleation events can largely be excluded, and the growth and aggregation contributions can be separately extracted from the change in crystal size distribution during the crystallization.[49]

The aggregation process can be described as the outcome of a series of collision events between two crystal masses, which either results in their dispersion or consolidation by local crystal growth to establish a cementing bridge or neck.[50,51] The consolidation rate (R_{con}) is thus an expression of the aggregation rate (R_{agg}), which is the difference between the collision rate (R_{coll}) and the dispersion rate (R_{disp})

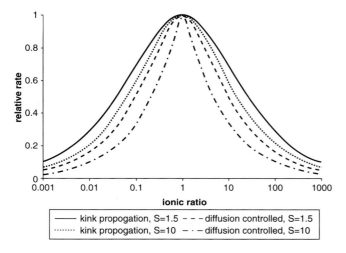

Fig. 3.6 The effect of changing the ionic ratio on the relative crystal growth rate for two different mechanisms and supersaturations. Curves calculated from equations B1 and B8 of Zhang and Nancollas[41]

Table 3.1 Example of effects of 10% changes in calcium and oxalate concentrations on crystal growth rate (g)

Ca (mM)	Oxalate (mM)	S	Ionic ratio	Correction factor	g	Change in g (%)
6.0	0.30	9.8	20.0	0.54	52	
6.6	0.30	10.5	22.0	0.51	57	10
6.0	0.33	10.8	18.2	0.55	64	23

S is calculated with Equil2[13] using an artificial urine composition[44] and g (in undefined units) is taken to be proportional to $(S - 1)^2$ (Eq. 3.30) times the correction factor for kink propagation given by equation B1 of Zhang and Nancollas[41]

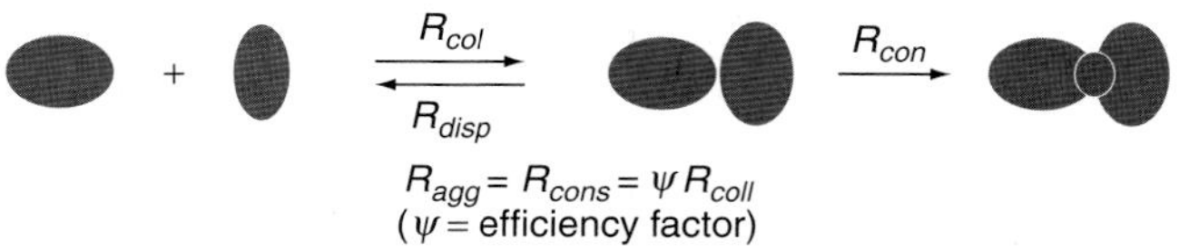

Fig. 3.7 The rate of aggregation (R_{agg}) reflects the rates of collision and dispersion (R_{coll} and R_{disp}), where the difference between R_{coll} and R_{disp} is the rate of consolidation (R_{cons}) (Reprinted with kind permission from Springer Science+Business Media[7])

(Fig. 3.7). R_{con} can also be expressed in terms of an R_{coll} aggregation efficiency factor Ψ and if consolidation is seen as dependent on growth one would expect the aggregation rate to be similarly dependent on growth:

$$R_{agg} = R_{con} = R_{coll} - R_{disp} = \Psi R_{coll} \quad (3.31)$$

The collision rate will depend on the particle sizes and the hydrodynamics. Small (e.g., <0.2 μm) particles dispersed in a static environment can be described by perikinetic coagulation, and larger crystals in a stirred vessel correspond to orthokinetic aggregation,[1] where the rate is proportional to the average diameter and square of the particle number (the Smoluchowski equation). The hydrodynamics in the renal system will be complex and variable throughout and have not been rigorously applied to aggregation models. On the other hand, aggregation in stirred crystallizers is the norm for experimental studies.

Following a series of papers on experimental CaOx monohydrate aggregation, with a developing theoretical basis, Hounslow and colleagues have reached a point where they can explain their data in terms of the Smoluchowski orthokinetic equation governing the collision rate and a dimensionless strength factor (M) that determines the efficiency factor Ψ.[50,52] According to this analysis,

$$\Psi = \frac{M / M_{50}}{1 + M / M_{50}} \quad (3.32)$$

where M_{50} is the value of M for which $\Psi = 0.5$ and M is directly proportional to the crystal growth rate and the length of the initial edge of contact. A recent reanalysis of Hounslow's data[53] uses a theory that considers that there will be a thin film of liquid between the two approaching crystals and consolidation as an aggregate requires the formation of nucleus-bridges across the gap. A satisfactory fit between the data and model was found with a suggested gap width of 1–1.5 nm. In this model, the efficiency factor is related to the supersaturation.

Whatever the physical details of the consolidation activity and despite the fact that large stirred chambers will behave differently from in vivo renal spaces, these approaches demonstrate the dependence of aggregation on crystal growth and supersaturation. They also offer experimental and theoretical tools to assess and compare aggregation inhibitors.

3.4 Nonclassical Crystallization

The previous description of uro-crystallization and stone formation as being essentially a sequential process of nucleation, growth, and aggregation follows the classical description of crystallization. Recently, new concepts and experimental evidence have emerged, particularly related to controlled biomineralization and bio-inspired crystallization, which may be applicable to the (relatively) uncontrolled biomineralization of urinary stones.[54] In contrast to the classical view of growth being an ion by ion incorporation at energetically favored sites on a face growing from a critically sized nucleus, an alternative model is clustering and assembly of nanoparticles.[5, 55] The ordered assembly of small units has been described as mesocrystallization[56–58] where the controlled alignment of the units can give x-ray scattering properties and a well-faceted appearance similar to a single crystal. Through fusion of the aligned units, a mesocrystal may transform into a single crystal, in which case the mesocrystal would be considered an intermediate stage. This view of subunit assembly is better able to accommodate inclusion of macromolecules within the crystalline structure because it can overcome the objection that such inclusions would be expected to absorb at kinks and edges of the crystal and thereby inhibit further growth.[56]

Copper and cobalt oxalates are among the quoted examples of mesocrystals that have been well studied where the presence of additives is important in directing the outcome.[56–58] The assembly of the nanoparticles into a mesocrystal structure can be seen as an ordered aggregation phenomenon. A number of processes have been suggested to direct aggregation such as removal of solvent or adsorbed modifiers from particular faces or the generation of electrical dipoles, which might also arise from absorbed molecules in surface-specific locations.[59] Working with calcite crystals ($CaCO_3$), a continuity of polymer mediated crystallization has been proposed with single crystals as one extreme, disordered aggregates as another, and ordered mesocrystals in between.[59] In this scheme the polymer concentration, the supersaturation, and ion stoichiometry are all important in determining which morphology from the continuum available is produced. A low supersaturation favored single crystals and higher supersaturation (with greater nucleating potential) progressively supported aggregation of nanocrystals with increasing disorder. From this example and extrapolating to the urinary environment, with its continuous replenishment of substrates, the potential for production of mesocrystal forms seems worthy of investigation. There are a number of reports on CaOx crystals in urine and in stones that suggest an ordered ultrastructure and face specific inclusions consistent with the picture of mesocrystallization.[60–64] On the other hand, the observation of a crystal substructure does not necessarily imply an ordered assembly of nanoscale subunits; for example, the appearance of a nanostructural morphology of CaOx monohydrate by inclusion of small amount of europium or terbium has been interpreted as changes in the orientation of ion-by-ion growth.[65]

3.5 Other Crystallization Processes

3.5.1 Promotion/Inhibition

Promotion and inhibition of uro-crystallization have for many years been at the forefront of urolithiasis research because of the potential for diminished inhibition or enhanced promotion to explain uro-crystallization in some individuals but not others. As has been made clear previously, any means of increasing or decreasing the urinary supersaturation would be expected to promote or inhibit crystallization. Although some authors include this in their definition of promoters and inhibitors, these terms are more commonly reserved for modification of crystallizing activity through more direct effects at the nucleus–substratum or crystal–solution interface. Crystallization inhibitors, particularly citrate and macromolecules will be dealt with elsewhere in this book. From what has been said previously about aggregation, one would expect inhibitors of crystal growth would also inhibit aggregation, and this seems to be generally the case. Promotion of uro-crystallization usually equates to enhancement of heterogeneous nucleation. Epitaxy as a particular form of this has been discussed previously, and there are reports of other nucleation promoters such as lipids and membrane fragments.[66,67] Adsorption of urinary macromolecules onto nucleating particles can also enhance their catalytic effects (e.g., albumin on hydroxyapatite as an inducer of CaOx nucleation).[30]

A fuller understanding of promotion/inhibition, the related phenomenon of crystal interactions with cells or with each other and how these are modified by urinary constituents is likely to emerge from further use of atomic force microscopy and molecular modeling. This may expose details of the site, orientation, and specificity of modifiers at the crystal surface.

3.5.2 Morphology/Aging

Much of what has been written previously in this chapter pays scant regard to crystal size, shape, form, or packing, or how these may change and evolve during a crystallization process. These are clearly a very important aspect of stone formation because calculi are the products of uro-crystallization over a prolonged (but not necessarily continuous) period. Although much of the activity in which we are interested is not amenable to realistic experimental interrogation, the processes must still operate according to physical-chemical principles that apply in simpler systems. Amongst these is Ostwald's rule of stages which predicts that, generally, the first form to crystallize will be the least stable, followed by transformation through to the most stable. For CaOx, the trihydrate is the least stable form (rarely seen as uro-crystals or in stones), followed by the dihydrate (often found in stones), then the monohydrate (most stable and most common form in stones). The stabilities of different forms of calcium phosphate are pH dependent, which can account for the dominant forms changing with pH[5] and why hydroxyapatite is much more common as a stone component than brushite. The transformation between polymorphs may involve dissolution and recrystallization, and another scenario where this occurs is in Ostwald ripening, when smaller crystals may dissolve and support the growth of larger neighbors.

An experimental example of many of these processes has recently appeared[68] in which brushite crystals were dissolving in slightly supersaturated calcium oxalate. The dissolution locally raised the calcium concentration enabling CaOx monohydrate to be nucleated on the brushite crystals. During these reactions a dehydrated form of brushite and CaOx trihydrate appeared as intermediates.

3.6 Conclusions

Uro-crystals and stones can only form when supersaturation has developed and even then there is a further energy barrier to overcome in order for nucleation to be initiated. For rare stones such as cystine, most people are safely behind the lines of supersaturation and the metastable limit, while those few at risk are well into enemy territory. For more common stones (uric or calcium phosphates) the general state is to be behind the front line with occasional forays over the top into no-man's-land, while for calcium oxalate most people are regularly in the danger zone of no-man's-land and it may only take a modest change in urine composition to bring them into contact with enemy lines. This can be seen as a necessary outcome of our need to regulate calcium and to excrete oxalate, a toxic product that we take in with our food and produce as an end result of some metabolic pathways.

Crystallization processes, similar in most respects to uro-crystallization, have been widely studied by chemists, crystallographers, and engineers and they have given us many of the theoretical and practical tools we need to describe, understand, and further investigate the events leading to stone formation.

References

1. Sohnel O, Garside J. Precipitation. In: *Basic Principles and Industrial Applications*. Oxford: Butterworth-Heinemann Ltd; 1992.
2. Mullin JW. *Crystallization*. 3rd ed. Oxford: Butterworth-Heinemann Ltd; 1993.
3. Finlayson B. Physicochemical aspects of urolithiasis. *Kidney Int*. 1978;13:344–360.
4. Wu WJ, Nancollas GH. Determination of interfacial tension from crystallization and dissolution data: a comparison with other methods. *Adv Coll Interface Sci*. 1999;79:229–279.
5. Wang LJ, Nancollas GH. Calcium orthophosphates: crystallization and dissolution. *Chem Rev*. 2008;108:4628–4669.
6. Kok D. Clinical implications of physicochemistry of stone formation. *Endocrinol Metab Clin N Am*. 2002;31:855.
7. Kavanagh JP. Supersaturation and renal precipitation: the key to stone formation? *Urol Res*. 2006;34:81–85.
8. Kavanagh JP. Methods for the study of calcium-oxalate crystallization and their application to urolithiasis research. *Scan Microsc*. 1992;6:685–705.
9. Kavanagh JP. In vitro calcium oxalate crystallization methods. *Urol Res*. 2006;34:139–145.
10. Streit J, Tran-Ho LC, Konigsberger E. Solubility of the three calcium oxalate hydrates in sodium chloride solutions and urine-like liquors. *Monatshefte Chem*. 1998;129:1225–1236.
11. Pak CYC, Holt K. Nucleation and growth of brushite and calcium-oxalate in urine of stone-formers. *Metab-Clin Exp*. 1976;25:665–673.
12. Pak CYC, Rodgers K, Poindexter JR, et al. New methods of assessing crystal growth and saturation of brushite in whole urine: effect of pH, calcium and citrate. *J Urol*. 2008;180:1532–1537.
13. Werness PG, Brown CM, Smith LH, et al. Equil2 – a basic computer-program for the calculation of urinary saturation. *J Urol*. 1985;134:1242–1244.
14. Laube N, Rodgers A, Allie-Hamdulay S, et al. Calcium oxalate stone formation risk – a case of disturbed relative concentrations of urinary components. *Clini Chem Lab Med*. 2008;46:1134–1139.
15. Rodgers A, Allie-Hamdulay S, Jackson G. Therapeutic action of citrate in urolithiasis explained by chemical speciation: increase in pH is the determinant factor. *Nephrol Dial Transplant*. 2006;21:361–369.
16. Grases F, Villacampa AI, Sohnel O, et al. Phosphate composition of precipitates from urine-like liquors. *Crystal Res Technol*. 1997;32:707–715.
17. Rodgers AL, Allie-Hamdulay S, Jackson GE. JESS: what can it teach us? *Renal Stone Dis*. 2007;900:183–191.
18. Pak CYC, Moe OW, Maalouf NM, et al. Comparison of semi-empirical and computer derived methods for estimating urinary saturation of brushite. *J Urol*. 2009;181:1423–1428.
19. Tiselius HG. Aspects on estimation of the risk of calcium-oxalate crystallization in urine. *Urol Int*. 1991;47:255–259.
20. Tiselius HG, Ferraz RRN, Heilberg IP. An approximate estimate of the ion-activity product of calcium oxalate in rat urine. *Urol Res*. 2003;31:410–413.
21. Tiselius HG. A simplified estimate of the ion-activity product of calcium-phosphate in urine. *Eur Urol*. 1984;10:191–195.
22. Ogawa Y, Hatano T. Comparison of the Equil2 program and other methods for estimating the ion-activity product of urinary calcium oxalate: a new simplified method is proposed. *Int J Urol*. 1996;3:383–385.
23. Grover PK, Marshall VR, Ryall RL. Dissolved urate salts out calcium oxalate in undiluted human urine in vitro: Implications for calcium oxalate stone genesis. *Chem Biol*. 2003;10:271–278.
24. Grover PK, Ryall RL. Critical appraisal of salting-out and its implications for chemical and biological sciences. *Chem Rev*. 2005;105:1–10.
25. Nancollas GH, Wu WJ. Biomineralization mechanisms: a kinetics and interfacial energy approach. *J Crystal Growth*. 2000;211:137–142.
26. Lonsdale K. Epitaxy as a growth factor in urinary calculi and gallstones. *Nature*. 1968;217:56–.
27. Grases F, Costa-Bauza A, Ramis M, et al. Simple classification of renal calculi closely related to their micromorphology and etiology. *Clin Chim Acta*. 2002;322:29–36.
28. Kavanagh JP. Enlargement of a lower pole calcium oxalate stone: a theoretical examination of the role of crystal nucleation, growth, and aggregation. *J Endourol*. 1999;13:605–610.
29. Sohnel O, Grases F, March JG. Experimental-technique simulating oxalocalcic renal stone generation. *Urol Res*. 1993;21:95–99.
30. Wu WJ, Gerard DE, Nancollas GH. Nucleation at surfaces: the importance of interfacial energy. *J Am Soc Nephrol*. 1999;10:S355–S358.
31. El-Shall H, Jeon JH, Abdel-Aal EA, et al. A study of primary nucleation of calcium oxalate monohydrate: II. Effect of urinary species. *Crystal Res Technol*. 2004;39:222–229.
32. Curreri PA, Onoda G, Finlayson B. A comparative appraisal of adsorption of citrate on whewellite seed crystals. *J Crystal Growth*. 1981;53:209–214.
33. Nancollas GH, Gardner GL. Kinetics of crystal growth of calcium oxalate monohydrate. *J Crystal Growth*. 1974;21:267–276.
34. Nancollas GH, Smesko SA, Campbell AA, et al. Physical-chemical studies of calcium-oxalate crystallization. *Am J Kidney Dis*. 1991;17:392–395.
35. Zauner R, Jones AG. Determination of nucleation, growth, agglomeration and disruption kinetics from experimental precipitation data: the calcium oxalate system. *Chem Eng Sci*. 2000;55:4219–4232.
36. Skrtic D, Markovic M, Komunjer L, et al. Precipitation of calcium oxalates from high ionic-strength solutions .1. Kinetics of spontaneous precipitation of calcium-oxalate trihydrate. *J Crystal Growth*. 1984;66:431–440.
37. Gvozdev NV, Petrova EV, Chernevich TG, et al. Atomic force microscopy of growth and dissolution of calcium oxalate monohydrate (COM) crystals. *J Crystal Growth*. 2004;261:539–548.
38. Guo SW, Ward MD, Wesson JA. Direct visualization of calcium oxalate monohydrate crystallization and dissolution with atomic force microscopy and the role of polymeric additives. *Langmuir*. 2002;18:4284–4291.
39. Finlayson B. Concept of a continuous crystallizer – its theory and application to in-vivo and in-vitro urinary-tract models. *Investig Urol*. 1972;9:258–263.
40. Robertson WG, Scurr DS, Bridge CM. Factors influencing the crystallization of calcium-oxalate in urine – critique. *J Crystal Growth*. 1981;53:182–194.
41. Zhang JW, Nancollas GH. Kink density and rate of step movement during growth and dissolution of an AB crystal in a nonstoichiometric solution. *J Colloid Interface Sci*. 1998;200:131–145.
42. Chernov AA, Rashkovich LN, Vekilov PG. Steps in solution growth: dynamics of kinks, bunching and turbulence. *J Crystal Growth*. 2005;275:1–18.
43. Chernov AA, Petrova E, Rashkovich LN. Dependence of the CaOx and MgOx growth rate on solution stoichiometry. Non-Kossel crystal growth. *J Crystal Growth*. 2006;289:245–254.
44. Kavanagh JP, Jones L, Rao PN. Calcium oxalate crystallization kinetics at different concentrations of human and artificial urine, with a constant calcium to oxalate ratio. *Urol Res*. 1999;27:231–237.
45. Pak CYC, Adams-Huet B, Poindexter JR, et al. Relative effect of urinary calcium and oxalate on saturation of calcium oxalate. *Kidney Int*. 2004;66:2032–2037.
46. Kok DJ, Khan SR. Calcium-oxalate nephrolithiasis, a free or fixed particle disease. *Kidney Int*. 1994;46:847–854.
47. Saw NK, Rao PN, Kavanagh JP. A nidus, crystalluria and aggregation: key ingredients for stone enlargement. *Urol Res*. 2008;36:11–15.
48. Falope GO, Jones AG, Zauner R. On modelling continuous agglomerative crystal precipitation via Monte Carlo simulation. *Chem Eng Sci*. 2001;56:2567–2574.

49. Bramley AS, Hounslow MJ, Ryall RL. Aggregation during precipitation from solution: A method for extracting rates from experimental data. *J Coll Interface Sci.* 1996;183:155–165.

50. Liew TL, Barrick JP, Hounslow MJ. A micro-mechanical model for the rate of aggregation during precipitation from solution. *Chem Eng Technol.* 2003;26:282–285.

51. David R, Espitalier F, Cameirao A, et al. Developments in the understanding and modeling of the agglomeration of suspended crystals in crystallization from solution. *KONA.* 2001;21:40–53.

52. Andreassen JP, Hounslow MJ. Growth and aggregation of vaterite in seeded-batch experiments. *AIChE J.* 2004;50:2772–2782.

53. Linnikov OD. Mechanism of aggregation and intergrowth of crystals during bulk crystallization from solutions. *Crystal Res Technol.* 2008;43:1268–1277.

54. Ryall RL. The future of stone research: rummagings in the attic, Randall's plaque, nanobacteria, and lessons from phylogeny. *Urol Res.* 2008;36:77–97.

55. Navrotsky A. Energetic clues to pathways to biomineralization: Precursors, clusters, and nanoparticles. *Proc Natl Acad Sci USA.* 2004;101:12096–12101.

56. Colfen H, Antonietti M. Mesocrystals: Inorganic superstructures made by highly parallel crystallization and controlled alignment. *Angew Chem Int Ed.* 2005;44:5576–5591.

57. Niederberger M, Colfen H. Oriented attachment and mesocrystals: Non-classical crystallization mechanisms based on nanoparticle assembly. *Phys Chem Chem Phys.* 2006;8:3271–3287.

58. Xu AW, Ma YR, Colfen H. Biomimetic mineralization. *J Mater Chem.* 2007;17:415–449.

59. Kulak AN, Iddon P, Li YT, et al. Continuous structural evolution of calcium carbonate particles: A unifying model of copolymer-mediated crystallization. *J Am Chem Soc.* 2007;129:3729–3736.

60. Webber D, Chauvet MC, Ryall RL. Proteolysis and partial dissolution of calcium oxalate: a comparative, morphological study of urinary crystals from black and white subjects. *Urol Res.* 2005;33:273–284.

61. Sandersius S, Rez P. Morphology of crystals in calcium oxalate monohydrate kidney stones. *Urol Res.* 2007;35:287–293.

62. Dorian HH, Rez P, Drach GW. Evidence for aggregation in oxalate stone formation: Atomic force and low voltage scanning electron microscopy. *J Urol.* 1996;156:1833–1837.

63. Ryall RL, Chauvet MC, Grover PK. Intracrystalline proteins and urolithiasis: a comparison of the protein content and ultrastructure of urinary calcium oxalate monohydrate and dihydrate crystals. *BJU Int.* 2005;96:654–663.

64. Ryall RL, Cook AF, Thurgood LA, et al. Macromolecules relevant to stone formation. *Renal Stone Disease.* 2007;900:129–140.

65. Touryan LA, Lochhead MJ, Marquardt BJ, et al. Sequential switch of biomineral crystal morphology using trivalent ions. *Nat Mater.* 2004;3:239–243.

66. Fasano JM, Khan SR. Intratubular crystallization of calcium oxalate in the presence of membrane vesicles: An in vitro study. *Kidney Int.* 2001;59:169–178.

67. Khan SR. Heterogeneous nucleation of calcium-oxalate crystals in mammalian urine. *Scan Microsc.* 1995;9:597–616.

68. Guan XY, Wang LJ, Dosen A, et al. An understanding of renal stone development in a mixed oxalate-phosphate system. *Langmuir.* 2008;24:7058–7060.

The Possible Roles of Inhibitors, Promoters, and Macromolecules in the Formation of Calcium Kidney Stones

4

Rosemary Lyons Ryall

Abstract The formation of kidney stones depends, absolutely, on the nucleation of sparingly soluble salts – principally calcium oxalate – in the urinary tract. Under everyday conditions, urine is supersaturated with calcium oxalate, and occasionally we all pass calcium oxalate crystals in our urine. Yet, we do not all suffer from kidney stones. Why? Because urine contains a range of low and high molecular weight components that are able to inhibit the nucleation of crystals or, if crystals do nucleate, which prevent their enlargement by growth or aggregation into particles large enough to block the renal collecting tubules. The same molecules may also affect the likelihood that crystals attach to, or nucleate directly upon, the renal epithelium. Some are also occluded within the mineral bulk of urinary crystals, and by disrupting their crystalline structure they may assist their intra-renal degradation, dissolution, and disposal. This chapter reviews what is known about the possible, and paradoxical, roles of urinary low molecular weight components and macromolecules in the formation of stone mineral crystals and their potential functions in the development of human kidney stones.

Abbreviations

BALB/c3T3	mouse cell line
BSC-1	African green monkey kidney cell line
CAK1-1	human kidney cancer cell line
CaOx	calcium oxalate
CaP	calcium phosphate
COD	calcium oxalate dihydrate
COM	calcium oxalate monohydrate
EDTA	ethylenediamine-tetra-acetic acid
FN	fibronectin
GAG	glycosaminoglycan
Gla	γ-carboxyglutamic acid
HA	hyaluronic acid
HPLC-MS	high pressure liquid chromatography/tandem mass spectrometry
HS	heparan sulfate
HSA	human serum albumin
IαI	inter-α-trypsin inhibitor inter-α-inhibitor

IMCD	inner medullary collecting duct
kDa	kiloDalton
MALDI-TOF	matrix-assisted laser desorption ionization-time of flight
MDCK	Madin-Darby canine kidney cells
mRNA	messenger RNA
NRK-52E	normal rat kidney cell line
OPN	osteopontin
PTF1	prothrombin fragment 1
SDS-PAGE	Sodium dodecyl sulfate polyacrylamide gel electrophoresis
SELDI-TOF	surface-enhanced laser desorption ionization-time of flight
THG	Tamm–Horsfall glycoprotein

4.1 Introduction

Although most information presented in this chapter is concerned principally with calcium oxalate (CaOx), because it is the most abundant and ubiquitous mineral component of human kidney stones, in many instances it applies equally to other calcium salts. I use the term *inhibitor* broadly to describe molecules or ions that retard any aspect of the crystallization

R.L. Ryall (✉)
Department of Surgery, Flinders Medical Centre and Flinders University, 5042, Adelaide, SA, Australia
e-mail: rose.ryall@flinders.edu.au

P.N. Rao et al. (eds.), *Urinary Tract Stone Disease*,
DOI 10.1007/978-1-84800-362-0_4, © Springer-Verlag London Limited 2011

process or the attachment of crystals to cells, despite the fact that, in the strictest sense, it should be used to describe only those substances that bind to crystal surfaces.[1] I have omitted reports of plant products other than phytate, and have left detailed discussion of the basic physicochemical mechanisms of inhibitory action to the experts, such as Chap. 3 by Kavanagh and published reviews.[2–4] The promotion of crystallization by increasing supersaturation is not included, since that is also dealt with in the previous chapter.

4.2 Calcium Oxalate Crystallization in the Urinary Tract

Stone formation involves a cascade of several crucial events beginning with supersaturation of urine with a sparingly soluble salt – most frequently CaOx. The degree of supersaturation of urine with CaOx fluctuates constantly, depending upon the state of hydration and the dietary intake of foods containing calcium and oxalate. Nonetheless, under everyday conditions, the urine of most individuals is supersaturated with the salt, which can lead to nucleation of crystals within the urinary collecting system. Although stones will not form without crystals, their nucleation is not synonymous with stone disease, since all of us occasionally experience crystalluria.[5] The fact that only about 10% of us get stones suggests that most crystals pass unimpeded through the kidney and are expelled innocuously in the urine. Progression from crystal nucleation to stones therefore requires retention of the crystals within the kidney, which is thought to occur by either a *free particle* or a *fixed particle* mechanism. The principal, and critical, difference between these two mechanisms is that free particle stone formation is hypothesized to be a physical process – mechanical, log-jamming blockage of renal tubules caused by large numbers of crystals. On the other hand, fixed particle stone formation is seen as the product of a battery of physiological processes involving epithelial cell surface injury and interactions between molecular motifs on their surfaces and atomic arrays, ions, and macromolecules on crystal surfaces.

4.2.1 Free-Particle Stone Formation

Figure 4.1 shows the events involved in the "Free Particle" theory of stone formation.4.1. Supersaturation of urine with CaOx leads to nucleation of crystals, which, provided the urine remains supersaturated, can enlarge both by deposition of additional solute upon their surfaces (growth) and by aggregating to form clusters. Each process is depicted separately in Fig. 4.1, but both can occur simultaneously. Growth

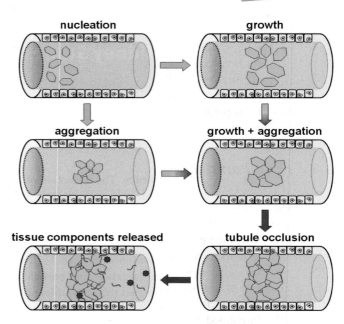

Fig. 4.1 Illustration depicting the events involved in "Free Particle" stone formation. Supersaturation of urine with calcium oxalate (CaOx) leads to nucleation of crystals, which can then grow and aggregate to form clusters of larger crystals. If the degree of supersaturation is sufficiently high, large numbers of crystals could nucleate and occlude a tubule by a process of log-jamming, which could abrade the epithelial membrane and cause the release of low (*red stars*) and high (*red "worms"*) molecular weight blood and tissue components

alone will not cause intrarenal crystal entrapment, because even high degrees of supersaturation are unable to permit sufficient deposition of new CaOx upon the surfaces of newly formed crystals to cause tubule blockage.[6] On the other hand, aggregation enables the formation of larger crystalline particles in a short period of time and is therefore regarded as the more important of the two mechanisms of particle enlargement.[7] Although this is supported by the observation that recurrent stone formers excrete greater quantities of large CaOx crystal clusters than do healthy subjects,[5] aggregation alone is also unlikely to block a tubule during short periods of time without high degrees of supersaturation and large crystal numbers. However, as shown in Fig. 4.1, the simultaneous occurrence of both processes could cause crystal retention, particularly under conditions producing large crystal showers, which will produce local inflammation, injury, and the release of tissue and blood components into the urine.

Thus, the free-particle theory proposes that tubular occlusion occurs by spontaneous nucleation of crystals, which subsequently grow and aggregate to a size that could block a collecting duct. The theory has been challenged, on the basis that newly formed crystals do not remain in the kidney for long enough to allow growth to produce sufficient particle enlargement to enable tubular occlusion.[6] However, it is certainly theoretically feasible,[7] has never been disproved, and is supported by work demonstrating that the enlargement of artificial stones to physiologically troublesome sizes correlates with high physiological concentrations of calcium and oxalate, as well as the number of crystals suspended in the surrounding medium.[8] Nevertheless, at the present time, there is general consensus that most stones are more likely to arise from a "fixed-particle" mechanism.

4.2.2 Fixed-Particle Stone Formation

The "Fixed Particle" theory of stone formation favors nucleation of crystals directly on to the renal epithelium, or attachment of previously precipitated crystals to the renal epithelial brush border membrane, as illustrated in Fig. 4.2.

The presence of crystals on the epithelial surface would effectively reduce the luminal diameter, impede the flow of urine and the passage of any crystals formed upstream, and increase the likelihood that they will adhere to crystals already attached to the tubular walls. With time, the tubule would become blocked with crystals, which as mentioned above, would cause local irritation and injury and the release of blood and structural molecules into the urine. Nucleation of CaOx dihydrate (COD) occurs on cultured renal cells,[9] and many studies have shown that the same cells bind CaOx monohydrate (COM)[10–15] and COD.[16] Intratubular binding has been confirmed to occur in vivo in lithogenic rats[17] and a patient suffering from primary hyperoxaluria.[18] Readers are referred to Chap. 5 by Khan for a detailed account of factors leading to cellular injury and adhesion of crystals to renal epithelial cells. Here, discussion will be confined principally to urine itself and selected molecules that inhibit or mediate crystal adhesion.

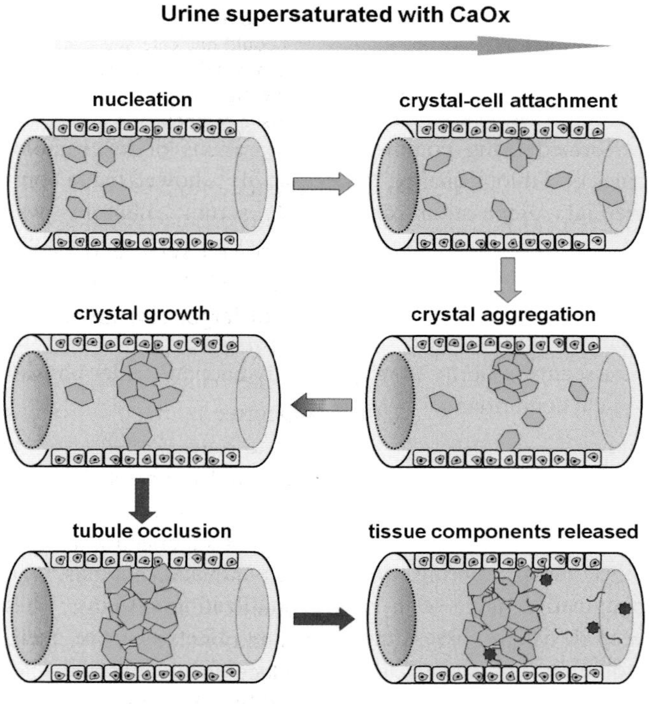

4.2.3 The Inhibitor Theory of Stone Formation

It is clear that the progression from supersaturated urine to crystal to stone proceeds through several intermediate steps involving a free- or fixed-particle mechanism. However, irrespective of which mechanism operates in vivo, relatively few of us form stones, despite the fact that our urine is ordinarily supersaturated with CaOx. The human body must therefore be able to prevent nucleation of crystals within the urinary tract, or if crystals do nucleate, their retention in the kidney. This notion is not novel.

Fifty years ago Howard and Thomas[19] showed that urine from healthy individuals could inhibit the calcification of rachitic rat cartilage while that from stone formers could not. They proposed that the urine of healthy individuals contained "preventers" that prevented calcification, which were absent from, or deficient in, the urine of stone formers. The quaint term "preventers" was later replaced by "inhibitors," which quickly became the principal protagonists in what has become known as the inhibitor theory of stone formation. The basis of the theory is illustrated in Fig. 4.3, which shows CaOx crystals newly precipitated from supersaturated urine. Low and high molecular weight inhibitors immediately attach to the crystal surfaces and retard or prevent enlargement of the crystalline particles by aggregation or deposition of additional calcium and oxalate ions.

Prompted by the exciting possibility that stones could be prevented by correcting a person's inhibitory deficit by dietary or pharmacological manipulation, researchers embarked upon a quest to discover natural and synthetic agents capable of preventing the formation of kidney stones. This has been achieved principally by testing the effects of those agents on (1) the formation of stone crystals induced in experimental animals; (2) the attachment of stone crystals to renal epithelial cells in culture; or (3) the crystallization of stone salts in a simple crystallization system in vitro.

Urine supersaturated with CaOx

Fig. 4.2 Diagrammatic representation of "Fixed Particle" stone formation. Supersaturation of urine with CaOx leads to nucleation of crystals, which can then attach directly to the epithelial cell membrane, where they can act as barriers for crystals nucleating later. During successive periods of urinary supersaturation, the bound crystals can then grow and also aggregate with other crystals that subsequently nucleate. The combination of attachment, growth, and aggregation then leads to tubule occlusion, epithelial damage, and the release of low (*red stars*) and high (*red "worms"*) molecular weight blood and tissue components

Fig. 4.3 Diagram depicting the putative role of inhibitors in stone prevention. Urine contains low molecular weight (*stars*) and high molecular weight (*"worms"*) components, which attach to the surfaces of newly formed crystals and inhibit or retard their growth and aggregation, allowing them to be passed harmlessly in the urinary stream

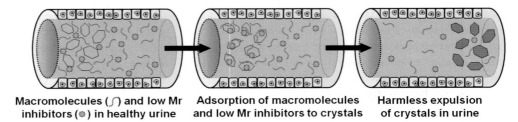

Macromolecules (∩) and low Mr inhibitors (◉) in healthy urine

Adsorption of macromolecules and low Mr inhibitors to crystals

Harmless expulsion of crystals in urine

These approaches have yielded a monumental amount of valuable information, but it is essential to remember that they are still just models, and it is hardly surprising that the vast amount of information collected to date has not always been consistent. There are various reasons for this:.

4.3 Measuring Inhibition and Promotion of Crystallization and Cell Adhesion

4.3.1 The Complexity of Crystallization

As is shown in Figs. 4.1 and 4.2, in stone pathogenesis the phenomenon of "crystallization" actually comprises several distinct, but interdependent, steps, namely, nucleation, growth, and aggregation, each of which could be influenced to different extents by a given molecule. For instance, nucleation could be promoted by a particular macromolecule that acts as a heterogeneous seed, or which sequesters calcium and oxalate ions to produce high local supersaturation levels of CaOx. It could also be prevented by molecules that bind either calcium or oxalate and thereby reduce supersaturation to levels at which precipitation is unlikely to occur. A single agent could inhibit the growth and aggregation of embryonic crystals by binding to their surfaces; or it may influence aggregation, but have no effect on growth. Or it may inhibit even without attaching irreversibly to the crystal surface, such as occurs with Tamm–Horsfall glycoprotein (THG), which prevents collisions between crystals simply by getting in the way.[20]

4.3.1.1 Uncertainty About Working Material: Identity, Purity, and Source

Except for those involving low molecular weight materials, which can be obtained in a state of high purity from reputable companies, many studies have used macromolecules whose identities have not been unambiguously demonstrated, either by Western blotting using specific antibodies, or by direct sequence analysis using other conclusive techniques. Even when a molecule's identity is known, and it has been purified from human urine, blood, or tissues, it may not be pure. Nor is it necessarily in its physiologically active form. For instance, fully intact urinary osteopontin (OPN) migrates on SDS-PAGE at 50–60 kDa,[21] but multiple bands are usually evident,[22] because the protein is digested by endogenous urinary serine proteases.[23,24] Full phosphorylation of OPN is required for inhibition of hydroxyapatite formation[25] and CaOx crystal growth,[26] but the degree of phosphorylation of OPN used in inhibition studies is rarely, if ever, mentioned.

The very process of purifying a protein, especially if it involves repeated freeze-thaw steps, can cause irreversible molecular fragmentation and removal of functional groups essential for its activity in vivo. Yet, the effects of proteins in various crystallization systems are often presented without any information about their state of purity. Work is also often performed using commercial preparations of macromolecules of dubious quality. Rodgers et al.[27] showed that a commercial preparation of human serum albumin was contaminated with other proteins and its inhibitory effects differed from those of the protein purified to homogeneity from human urine. Macromolecules may even be derived from foreign species.[28] Published findings may therefore bear scant similarity to what actually happens under physiological conditions.

4.3.1.2 A Multiplicity of Methodologies

Since the pioneering work of Howard and Thomas,[19] an imaginative range of in vitro crystallization systems[2,29] has been devised to assess the inhibitory effects of urine itself, inorganic ions and small molecules, fractionated and total urinary macromolecules, lipids, individual urinary proteins and glycosaminoglycans (GAGs), and artificial polymers. Those experimental models have been based on simple inorganic solutions, artificial inorganic urines, gels, and whole or processed urines, and have entailed the use of closed batch, continuous or constant composition crystallizers, and other less conventional techniques, including freezing[30] and a very novel "stone farm."[31] Using these techniques, investigators have measured rates and extents of nucleation, growth, aggregation, or combinations of these processes, based on particle size analysis, turbidity, radioactive tracers, and atomic absorption spectrophotometry, to name a few – mute testimony to the fertile inventiveness of urolithiasis researchers! As would be expected from the use of such a disparate assortment of methodologies, most of which have involved the use of aqueous inorganic media instead of urine, findings have often been inconclusive, physiologically irrelevant, confusing, and occasionally, downright contradictory. THG is again a useful example. Depending upon which particular method is used to induce crystallization, THG promotes *and* inhibits CaOx crystal formation.[32]

4.3.1.3 Necessary but Imperfect: Experimental Cell Models

It will never be possible to reproduce faithfully all the physical or biochemical conditions operating in the human nephron, so it will always be necessary to infer what *might* occur under physiological conditions from data generated in experiments conducted in vitro.

Obviously, immortalized cultured cells are not representative of epithelial cells actually lining the urinary tract, so we cannot be sure that crystal adhesion to cultured cells steeped in synthetic media truly reflects what happens in the human kidney. Furthermore, studies have used different cultured cell lines derived, for example, from murine inner medullary collecting duct (IMCD),[33] human renal cancer (CAKI-I),[34] normal rat kidney (NRK-52E),[35] African green monkey kidney (BSC-1), dog kidney (MDCK), and mouse fibroblasts BALB/c3T3.[36] Reaction conditions (pH, time, reagent concentrations, culture media) have varied, as well as the origin of the cells used – proximal, distal, or collecting duct.[37,38] Adhesion also depends upon whether the cells are damaged or intact,[39–41] proliferating, regenerating, or confluent.[10,38,40,42] Finally, most cell attachment systems have used aqueous solutions as the binding medium, which are no substitute for urine itself. And even when urine has been used, it has been passed from the bladder after several hours of static storage, only to be subjected to various clean-up procedures, some of which are well recognized to alter its macromolecular content. All these differences conspire against direct comparison of experimental findings.

4.3.1.4 What You See Is What You Get: Not Necessarily What Actually Happens in Real Life

Given the obvious and unavoidable inadequacies of experimental models, it must *never* be assumed that an inhibitor's

effects on crystallization, or attachment of crystals to cells under experimental conditions, accurately reproduce those it actually has on crystallization in vivo. Most important of all, crystallization or attachment of crystals to cells in vitro, or even in an animal model, is "not" synonymous with stone formation. This axiom of stone research, along with the advantages and deficiencies of models, have been emphasized for years;[29] so it is disappointing to see conclusions such as]*bovine* serum albumin plays an important role in suppressing urine stone formation in *humans* (my emphases) – based on data obtained from an inorganic model[28]!

Collectively, these factors must raise reasonable doubts about the relevance of experimental findings to physiological conditions. It is simply not valid to extrapolate from data generated in work performed in vitro, often using materials and conditions light years removed from real life, to make assumptions about the expected role of a promoter or inhibitor, not only in whole urine within the kidney, but also in stone formation. The fact will always remain that effects in vitro ≠ effects in vivo ≠ specific role in stone formation.

Nonetheless, putting aside any justifiable misgivings we may have about experimental methodology, there is overwhelming evidence that urine contains a variety of low and high molecular weight substances that have profound effects on the formation, growth, and aggregation of CaOx crystals, as well as on the attachment of those crystals to renal cells. Certainly, extravagant claims about the physiological significance of some urinary components should be viewed with caution, but to deny that all of them are probably inert under physiological conditions is to fly in the face of many years of carefully performed experimental work, chemical and physical principles, and homespun commonsense.

4.4 Inhibitors and Promoters of CaOx Crystallization

4.4.1 Promoters of CaOx Crystal Nucleation

As shown in Figs. 4.1 and 4.2, the first requisite for stone formation is crystal nucleation. It is widely acknowledged that precipitation of CaOx crystals in vivo must be heterogeneous, since levels of supersaturation in urine are only rarely sufficient to permit crystals to form homogeneously (spontaneously). Urine is not a clear solution. It contains numerous particles, including whole cells, membrane vesicles, and other cellular fragments – debris sloughed off the urothelium as a result of normal metabolic turnover, or as a consequence of cellular damage caused by high oxalate concentrations[43,44] or crystals themselves.[45]

Membrane fragments and lipids are common components of calculi and urinary crystals.[46] Lipids extracted from stone matrix can catalyze precipitation of CaOx from inorganic metastable solutions[47] and urinary particles and membrane vesicles can nucleate CaOx crystals in human urine.[48] However, at the present time there is limited evidence from in vitro studies that lipid assemblies act as initiating sites for COM crystal nucleation as a first step in stone formation. Nonetheless, there is some indication that glycoproteins and lipids conjugated to sialic acid moieties on cell surfaces may act as nucleation templates. For instance, COD crystals can nucleate directly on to the surfaces of cultured renal cells in culture,[9] almost exclusively via the (001) face, unless the cells are first treated with protease or neuraminidase, which causes a switch to the (100) crystal face.[49] It is possible, therefore, that under conditions of high supersaturation in vivo, molecular arrays on the surfaces of urothelial cells might control the nucleation of CaOx crystals of a specific habit and orientation.

To my knowledge, no study has demonstrated conclusively that any individual urinary macromolecule actively induces nucleation of CaOx specifically by molecular templating. Unfractionated urinary macromolecules[50] and chondroitin sulfate (CS)[51] can promote CaOx nucleation from inorganic media, and THG[32,52] enhances the deposition of CaOx from urine. There is also indirect evidence that urinary macromolecules are actively involved in CaOx crystal formation *at the point of nucleation*, since fractured urinary COM crystals clearly contain organic material concentrated at their centers.[53–55] Indeed, it is possible that they may actually initiate the process, though whether this occurs by molecular templating or heterogeneous nucleation remains moot. Nucleation in vivo is therefore likely to be induced by lipids or cellular debris[46,48] or perhaps by macromolecules that have bound and sequestered calcium ions. However, almost all urinary components whose effects have been examined have been shown to act as inhibitors.

4.4.2 Inhibitors of CaOx Crystallization

Innumerable natural and synthetic substances retard CaOx crystallization. The list includes metal ions – particularly magnesium; simple di- and tri-carboxylic acids like tartaric and citric acids; other low molecular weight compounds such as pyrophosphate and phytate; macromolecules, including proteins and GAGs; extracts of various plants and vegetables; synthetic peptides of varying lengths; and a galaxy of dyes.[56] Because our goal is to discover how stones form, it would seem obvious to suppose that only the naturally occurring inhibitors in urine deserve attention. However, nontoxic, low molecular weight compounds that are easily absorbed and excreted into the urine, and which inhibit CaOx crystallization, offer the possibility of preventing stones by being administered as therapeutic agents. Nonetheless, the information that follows is concerned mainly with inhibitory

substances found in renal cells and/or present in human urine, and I will begin with studies on urine itself.

4.4.2.1 The Effect of Urine on CaOx Crystallization

Urine is a potent inhibitor of CaOx crystallization – irrespective of how it is measured. The early 1970s began the publication of a number of papers that compared the inhibitory effect of urine from stone formers and healthy controls on at least one aspect of CaOx crystallization. Some of them[5,50,57–59] reported deficient inhibitory activity in the urine of stone patients, although not consistently. For instance, Springmann et al.[59] showed that 5% urine from control subjects inhibited crystal aggregation significantly more potently than did urine from stone patients, but no such difference was observed with nucleation rates, linear growth, or final crystal mass. Many others have also been unable to find differences,[60–66] which is probably not unexpected given that most reports involved the use of low concentrations of urine in inorganic reaction systems. Moreover, in most studies the urine samples were not screened to confirm the absence of blood, which, particularly in stone formers, would unavoidably alter the macromolecular content of the urine and, therefore, the inhibitory activity.

With increasing awareness that diluted samples are inadequate for assessing the inhibitory capacity of urine, and that results are highly dependent upon the methodology used, measurement of the overall inhibitory activity of individual urine samples was generally abandoned by the end of the 1980s. Although it was revisited briefly in 1999[67] and the early 2000s,[68,69] the shortcomings of methodology have never been overcome. Consequently, a difference between the inhibitory activities of urines from healthy subjects and stone formers has never been unequivocally demonstrated and the focus has shifted largely to measuring the effects on CaOx or calcium phosphate (CaP) crystallization of individual agents, as well as their excretion patterns in stone patients. Results of those studies will be discussed in a subsequent section.

4.5 Inhibitors and Promoters of CaOx Crystal–Cell Adhesion

4.5.1 Urine and Generic Urinary Macromolecules

Human urine inhibits crystal adhesion.[70] Furthermore, samples from children have been reported to inhibit more strongly than those from adults,[71] and those from healthy adults show greater potency than those from stone formers.[72] Activity is associated with the macromolecular fractions,[71,73,74] whose effects are proportional to the protein concentration[73] and related to the pH of the binding medium.[75] Crystals precipitated and grown in urine bind less avidly to cells than those generated from artificial urine,[73] in keeping with the observation that naturally formed stone crystals cause less injury to renal epithelial cells than inorganic crystals.[76] Nonetheless, approximately half of the observed inhibitory effect of urine can be attributed to small molecules,[73] at least two of which are likely to be citrate, which reduces attachment of COM[77] and hydroxyapatite[78] crystals to cultured renal epithelial cells and magnesium, which also reduces binding.[79,80]

The studies just described examined the effects of urine itself or macromolecular "soups" – undifferentiated preparations of total urinary macromolecules remaining after ultrafiltration – or urine fractions containing different amounts of macromolecules. Although they have shown that undifferentiated preparations of generic urinary macromolecules, as well as unidentified low molecular weight urinary components, inhibit the binding of CaOx crystals to renal cells in vitro, most work has involved the testing of specific, individual macromolecules.

4.5.2 Macromolecular Inhibitors of Cell Adhesion

Increasing numbers of naturally occurring and synthetic macromolecules have been reported to inhibit the attachment of COM, COD, or hydroxyapatite crystals to cultured renal cells. These include fibronectin,[36,81,82] OPN,[77] bikunin,[83] heparan sulfate/syndecan-1,[43] hepatocyte growth factor,[36] THG,[36] chondroitin sulfates A and B,[12,77] heparan sulfate,[12,77] transforming growth factor β-2,[36] and an assortment of molecules not present in the human kidney, such as heparin, pentosan polysulfate, polyaspartate, and polyglutamate.[12] Synthetic molecules have been tested because they could, at least in theory, form the basis of future preventive therapy. For instance, Atorvastin, the cholesterol antagonist, has been shown to inhibit retention of CaOx crystals in a rat model of urolithiasis.[84] Alterations in the levels of many proteins accompany the attachment of COM[85] and COD[86] crystals to MDCK cells. Although those findings may suggest that synthesis of natural macromolecules is a protective response to crystal attachment and could prevent stone formation, they may also simply represent a reaction to inflammation induced by the crystals. And some of them are promoters, not inhibitors.

4.5.3 Macromolecular Promoters of Crystal–Cell Adhesion

In contrast to other reports[12,77] *increased* attachment of CaOx crystals to cultured renal cells has been shown to occur in the presence of osteopontin,[35,87] and the effect is mitigated by agents that interfere with the protein's expression.[88] The transmembrane receptor protein CD44, together with two of its ligands, hyaluronic acid and again, OPN, have been strongly implicated as mediators of crystal retention in the kidney.[39,40,42] There is also evidence that Annexin II,[74] a 100 kDa protein related to nucleolin,[89] β-tubulin,[90] and collagen types I and IV[34] mediate the binding of COM to renal cells, a process that also appears to involve the presence of sialic acid residues.[91,92] Disrupting the expression of the chloride channel CLC-5, which is involved in the internalization of CaOx crystals, prevents internalization of crystals and causes them to remain upon the cell surface.[93,94] While this might at first seem to protect against stone formation by enabling their removal in excreted urine, their presence upon the epithelial surface could potentially provide centers for further crystal accumulation and agglomeration. Internalization is not, therefore, necessarily a bad thing. In fact, it has been proposed, paradoxically, to constitute a form of defense against urolithiasis.

4.5.4 A Fortunate Adversity: Phagocytosis, Intracrystalline Proteins, and Crystal Dissolution

Because stone formation can occur only if crystals remain within the kidney, it has been assumed that crystal adhesion encourages stone pathogenesis. However, once attached, crystals do not necessarily remain upon the cell surfaces. The same studies that reported adhesion of crystals to cells[10,11,13,14,95] also showed that binding is followed by phagocytosis of the crystals into the cytoplasm of epithelial cells. CaOx crystals are also engulfed by cultured macrophages,[96] as well as by renal macrophages and multinucleated cells recruited in response to acute and chronic oxalosis in rats and humans.[97]

After internalization, crystals dissolve within lysosomal inclusion bodies,[9,12,96,98,99] as depicted in Fig. 4.4. After attachment, the crystal is transferred into the cell by phagocytosis, a process succeeded by formation of a phagolysosome, whose internal environment is highly acidic and contains a potent cocktail of lysosomal proteases. Eventually, the crystal is degraded, the mineral dissolved, and the waste removed by exocytosis through either the apical or basolateral membranes. Inorganic crystals can take up to 7 weeks to dissolve in cultured epithelial cells[9,12,98,99] and only 4 days in macrophages.[96] But urinary crystals are degraded and dissolved more rapidly, because they are riddled with proteins.

4.5.4.1 Intracrystalline Proteins

All CaOx crystals precipitated from urine contain intracrystalline proteins[54,55,100,101] that bind irreversibly to the surfaces

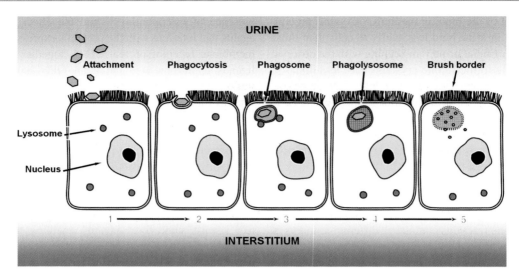

Fig. 4.4 Diagram illustrating possible events occurring in the kidney following adhesion of a crystal to the wall of a renal tubule. (*1*) attachment of a COM crystal to the apical brush border membrane of a renal tubular cell, followed by (*2*) phagocytosis of the crystal into the cytoplasm; (*3*) formation of phagosome containing the crystal, and migration of lysosomes to the phagosome; (*4*) fusion of phagosome and lysosomes to form a phagolysosome; and (*5*) destruction of intracrystalline proteins by lysosomal proteases and mineral dissolution by acid pH. Waste products would then be removed by exocytosis through either the apical or basolateral membranes. In the absence of phagocytosis, large numbers of crystals attached to the epithelium could cause tubular occlusion via a log-jamming mechanism

of crystals as they grow and become an integral component of the mineral bulk as they are engulfed by successive layers of solute. The incorporation of proteins into CaOx crystals is highly specific. For instance, urinary prothrombin fragment 1 (PTF1) is a major component of the organic matrix of COM,[22,102,103] but it barely binds to COD.[22] The opposite is true for OPN, which binds irreversibly to COD, but not COM.[22] Human serum albumin (HSA) is absent from demineralized COD crystal extracts, but is found inside COM, having arrived there by attaching to the side faces of inorganic crystals, but to the end faces of urinary ones.[104]

Once trapped, intracrystalline proteins form flaws in the mineral lattice by creating holes filled with organic material. Such crystals would be more vulnerable to attack by proteases in urine, and also by those contained within the phagolysosome following their internalization into the cell, as shown in Fig. 4.4. Lysosomal proteases would digest the protein phase and open channels throughout the mineral, thus enabling further excavation into the structure. This would increase the area of exposed crystal surface and thus facilitate crystal mineral dissolution in the acidic interior of the phagolysosome.[105] Intracrystalline proteins should therefore assist in the dismantling and dissolution of internalized crystals and thereby provide a natural defense against stone pathogenesis. This notion is supported by qualitative studies[53] and quantitative data confirming that urinary COM crystals are degraded and dissolved more rapidly than inorganic crystals, the rates of both processes being proportional to the quantity of intracrystalline proteins incarcerated within them.[106]

Thus, intrarenal fixation of crystals – a prerequisite for stone formation – appears also to protect against the disease by providing a means of removing obstructing crystals from the tubular lumen and then destroying them completely inside the cell. Therefore, macromolecules that promote attachment of cells to the urothelium could, paradoxically, also be regarded as inhibitors of stone formation.

4.5.4.2 Summary

From the foregoing discussion, it is evident that various small and large molecules occurring naturally in urine profoundly influence in vitro all the key processes occurring during kidney stone formation. While it is currently impossible to identify, unequivocally, any one of them as a key promoter or inhibitor of stone pathogenesis, several have been subjected to such intense scrutiny over many years that they warrant specific and detailed attention.

4.6 Low Molecular Weight Inhibitors

4.6.1 Pyrophosphate

4.6.1.1 Effect of Pyrophosphate on Crystallization

The first inhibitory component of urine to be identified and isolated was pyrophosphate.[107] Pyrophosphate is present in stones[108] and in inorganic solutions, inhibits CaOx crystal nucleation,[109] growth,[110,111] aggregation,[112] and a combination of growth and aggregation[113] by binding irreversibly to the CaOx crystal surface. In undiluted urine pyrophosphate does not affect the amount of oxalate required to induce detectable spontaneous CaOx crystal formation or the degree of crystal aggregation.[114] However, it does reduce the mass of CaOx deposited[114] from undiluted urine, except when crystallization is induced by evaporation of whole urine,[115] under which circumstances it has no influence on the precipitation of CaOx or CaP. Such inconsistencies emphasize the invalidity of extrapolating data obtained from inorganic solutions to expected outcomes in urine, and also illustrate that measured values depend greatly on the type of methodology used to obtain them.

It is difficult therefore to draw any definite conclusion about the effects of pyrophosphate under physiological conditions, although we might conclude that it perhaps might inhibit CaOx deposition in vivo – unless the urine is very concentrated. However, if pyrophosphate is an important urinary inhibitor of CaOx crystallization in vivo, it is reasonable to expect that its urinary concentration or output might be reduced in stone formers.

4.6.1.2 Urinary Excretion of Pyrophosphate

Pyrophosphate excretion has been reported by some authors to be significantly reduced in stone formers compared with healthy controls,[116–120] but not by others.[121–123] Thus, even if pyrophosphate does inhibit CaOx crystallization in urine under physiological conditions, stone formation cannot be unequivocally attributed to a reduction in its urinary output.

4.6.1.3 Summary

With increasing emphasis being placed on the role of inhibitors in the prevention of ectopic calcification[124] and on connections between bone metabolism and stone formation,[125] pyrophosphate has enjoyed a comeback in the medical literature. Nonetheless, despite its undoubted ability to inhibit CaOx crystallization in urine and aqueous solutions, as well as the regrowth of CaOx stone fragments in vitro,[126] it has not yet been demonstrated to be a major player in stone pathogenesis or a useful therapeutic agent.

4.6.2 Magnesium

4.6.2.1 Effect of Magnesium on Crystallization

Magnesium's association with urolithiasis began in 1932 when Cramer showed that dietary magnesium deficiency induced intrarenal calcification and tubular degeneration in rats.[127] Although magnesium forms strong ion complexes with oxalate, which undoubtedly explains its inhibitory effect on CaOx crystal nucleation,[128] growth,[109,116] and aggregation,[112,129] it might also act by binding to the surface of CaOx crystals and becoming incorporated into the crystal lattice, as occurs with hydroxyapatite.[130] Whatever the basis for magnesium's influence, experimental findings have not been consistent, even when all studies have used inorganic solutions as the reaction medium. Magnesium has been reported to have no effect on CaOx nucleation,[109] growth,[110,111,131] or combined growth and aggregation.[113] In urine, magnesium inhibits growth[132,133] and increases the amount of oxalate required to induce detectable spontaneous CaOx precipitation, but has no apparent effect on aggregation.[132]

4.6.2.2 Urinary Excretion of Magnesium

Magnesium's contradictory effects on CaOx crystallization, along with the logical conclusion that it plays no *significant* role in stone pathogenesis, probably explain failures to demonstrate unequivocal differences in the ion's output between stone formers and healthy controls. Several studies found that stone formers excrete less magnesium than healthy controls,[134–136] but many more were unable to detect any difference.[63,111,137–141] Repeated failure to demonstrate abnormally low urinary magnesium concentrations in stone patients prompted investigators to discover whether the important factor was not magnesium itself, but rather the ratio of magnesium to calcium output. However, the correlation between a reduced Mg/Ca ratio and stone frequency observed in at least 11 separate studies[138] is just as likely to have resulted from the fact that the stone formers tended to have raised Ca levels.

4.6.2.3 Effect of Magnesium in Experimental Models

Dietary administration of magnesium to experimental animals has provided little clarification. Su et al.[142] observed no effect on CaOx deposition of magnesium administration to hyperoxaluric rats at normal urinary magnesium concentrations, but the same group later concluded using the same model that magnesium given as MgO is beneficial.[143] The effect of magnesium on CaOx deposition in hyperoxaluric rats also appears to depend upon the form in which it is administered, namely, as the oxide, hydroxide, sulfate, trisilicate, or citrate, and, curiously, its beneficial effects appear to result from an increase in citrate concentration.[144]

4.6.2.4 Summary

Despite magnesium's long historical association with calcium urolithiasis, and the performance of numerous investigations, we are still none the wiser about its true involvement with the disease, especially since a number of trials in humans have failed to prove conclusively that magnesium administration reduces calcium stone recurrences.[145,146] Thus, on the basis of available evidence, the effect of magnesium on the formation of stones is likely to be relatively minor.

4.6.3 Citrate

4.6.3.1 Effect of Citrate on Crystallization

Studies have demonstrated that citrate inhibits CaOx crystal nucleation,[109] growth[112,131] and aggregation[112] in aqueous media, and CaOx deposition in undiluted[114] and concentrated urine.[147] Although such effects can be attributed at least partly to its ability to chelate calcium, citrate also binds to the CaOx crystal surface. Recent atomic force microscopy studies have demonstrated that it binds specifically to the large flat face of COM crystals,[148,149] which must also contribute to its inhibition of COM crystal growth and aggregation. Thus, citrate is both a chelator and a crystal poison. However, despite its well documented inhibition of CaOx crystallization in inorganic media, citrate has no apparent effect on crystal aggregation in urine,[114] despite the reported clinical association between large aggregate formation and low citrate excretion in vivo.[150] Nevertheless, it is clear that citrate is a potent inhibitor of CaOx deposition both in urine and under inorganic conditions and evidence accumulated over many years has now established hypocitraturia as a key contributor to the formation of CaOx stones.

4.6.3.2 Urinary Excretion of Citrate and Effects in Experimental Models

The suggestion that calcium stones are the product of a renal defect that prevents the kidney from adjusting citrate output to compensate for rises in urinary calcium excretion was proposed more than 60 years ago.[151] If true, stone formers would be expected to excrete abnormally low levels of urinary citrate, and correction of the deficit by citrate administration should prevent further episodes. A number of authors have reported that stone formers excrete normal levels of citrate,[122,140,152–154] but hypocitraturia in stone formers has been reported more frequently.[135,141,155–158] Goldberg et al.[159] cite 11 papers that report decreased citrate excretion by stone formers.

As long as polemic persists about the diagnostic accuracy of single or multiple 24-h urine analysis as well as the definition of normal ranges,[160] justifiable doubts will always remain as to the existence of unambiguous differences in the output or concentration of *any* urinary metabolite between stone patients and healthy controls. And citrate is no exception.

However, even though clear-cut differences have not always been demonstrable, epidemiological data obtained from large numbers of subjects have shown that stone risk rises inversely in relation to urinary citrate levels,[160] suggesting that citrate is an important natural inhibitor of stone formation. That conclusion is bolstered by results of clinical trials confirming its efficacy in preventing stone recurrences (see Chap. 14 by Hess) by scientific studies demonstrating that it reduces attachment of COM[77] and hydroxyapatite[78] crystals to cultured renal epithelial cells, and by work showing that it retards crystal deposition in experimentally induced nephrocalcinosis.[161–164]

4.6.3.3 Summary

It would be difficult to argue that citrate is not an effective inhibitor of CaOx crystallization, both in vitro and in vivo, and it is no surprise that this simple tricarboxylic acid is now an established agent for stone therapy. Still, there is at least one other natural, low molecular weight urinary component that also shows therapeutic promise for the treatment of urolithiasis.

4.6.4 Phytic Acid (Inositol 1,2,3,4,5,6-Hexakisphosphate)

Phytic acid is a natural sugar present in most seeds and cereal grains, where it functions as a major phosphorus sink.[165] The compound contains six phosphate groups, each with two hydroxyl moieties which, when ionized, enable the molecule to chelate divalent metal ions, including Zn^{2+}, Mg^{2+}, Fe^{2+}, and, most pertinent to this review, Ca^{2+}. Complexes formed between phytate and metal ions tend to be insoluble, and are consequently poorly absorbed from the gastrointestinal tract,[165] a property of great potential advantage to calcium stone formers, since it relieves the kidneys of having to dispose of excess calcium by transferring the responsibility to the bowel. Following the suggestion that dietary phytate might play a significant role in stone pathogenesis,[166] several attempts were made to establish a link between the two.[161,167,168] More recently, however, studies of the possible role of phytic acid in calcium stone formation have been performed principally by Grases and his colleagues.[169,170]

Urinary phytate excretion is directly related to dietary intake[171] and has been reported to be lower in stone formers than in healthy controls.[172] Consumption of the compound is well documented to reduce urinary calcium excretion in humans with hypercalciuria[168] and in lithogenic rats,[167,173,174] particularly when administered as the potassium salt.[173] Phytate also reduces CaOx nephrocalcinosis in lithogenic rats[161,169,175] to inhibit the regrowth in vitro of COM[126] and COD[176] stone particles resulting from extracorporeal shock wave lithotripsy and to decrease the growth rate of artificial stones.[8]

4.6.4.1 Summary

Prima facie, therefore, phytate appears to be an ideal means of preventing stone recurrences, especially in individuals who excrete excessive quantities of calcium in their urine. But it also has its drawbacks – which can be severe. Any recommendation for its use in stone prevention would rely on its ability to bind tightly to calcium ions. However, its affinity for other divalent ions, such as iron and zinc, is equally strong. They, too, are essential minerals, and their excretion in the form of insoluble phytate complexes can lead to mineral depletion and deficiency,[177] a factor that has led to the development of low-phytate cereal and legume strains for populations whose staple diets are based largely on grains and legumes. For the same reason vegetarian diets are recommended for CaOx stone formers only if they ingest sufficient quantities of calcium and avoid foods high in phytate, since too great a reduction in calcium excretion carries the risk of increasing the urinary output of oxalate.[178]

4.6.5 Summary: Low Molecular Weight Inhibitors

The low molecular weight inhibitors discussed above are easily purified and administered, and are excreted in the urine intact. However, at the present time it is not known with certainty whether they play a definitive role in preventing CaOx crystallization in vivo, and, with the exception of citrate, have not yet been used routinely for stone prevention.

4.7 Macromolecular Promoters and Inhibitors

The inclusion of a section on macromolecules in a chapter on urinary inhibitors is mandated by two simple facts: thousands of macromolecules are present in urine and *all* stones contain them. Collectively known as the organic matrix, macromolecules comprise only 2–3% of the weight of kidney stones. The organic matrix, which is distributed throughout the entire stone structure,[179] consists principally of GAGs and proteins, as well as three types of lipids: phospholipids, cholesterol, and glycolipids.[180] Here, we will consider only GAGs and proteins, most of which until recently had not been specifically identified and whose effects on CaOx crystallization had not been examined.

4.7.1 Glycosaminoglycans (GAGs)

4.7.1.1 GAGs in Kidney Stones

A major class of urinary macromolecules, GAGs migrate electrophoretically as three major bands[181] divisible into fast and slow-moving fractions.[182] The most abundant GAGs are chondroitin sulfates A and C[181–183] and heparan sulfate (HS),[181–183] which is excreted in the form of a proteoglycan.[184] Depending upon the urine sample, little or no keratan sulfate[183,185] or dermatan sulfate[181,183] is excreted in urine. Hyaluronic acid is excreted by healthy subjects and stone formers,[186] but some authors have detected it in only small quantities, if at all.[182,183,185] The GAGs heparan sulfate[187] and hyaluronic acid[187,188] have been shown to be present in CaOx kidney stone matrix, but chondroitin sulfate, the most abundant urinary GAG, has been detected only in apatite stones.[187]

4.7.1.2 Chondroitin Sulfate (CS)

By all accounts, CS would appear to be an active inhibitor of CaOx crystallization, since it reportedly inhibits crystal growth,[51,112,189] though to varying extents depending upon the crystal face to which it binds.[190] It also inhibits CaOx crystal aggregation,[112] a combination of growth and aggregation,[113] nucleation,[191] *promotes*[192] agglomeration,[51,193] mass deposition,[51] and attachment of COM to cultured renal cells.[12] But CS also *promotes* nucleation,[51] particularly that from healthy subjects,[192] as well as crystal growth rate and suspension density.[191] It would seem that CS is an effective inhibitor of CS crystallization – at least under inorganic conditions. However, other, more physiologically relevant data tell a different story. CS promotes large calculus formation in rats,[194] has no effect on CaOx deposition in rat kidneys,[195] and does not influence CaOx mass deposition, aggregation, or the amount of oxalate required to induce spontaneous CaOx precipitation in undiluted urine.[20]

4.7.1.3 Heparan Sulfate (HS)

HS, the second most abundant urinary GAG, is present in stones[187] and is the only natural one other than CS to have been studied in any detail. HS proteoglycans are major components of the glomerular basement membrane and play a key role in its molecular organization and function.[184] HS is incorporated into CaOx crystals at the expense of the more abundant CS[196] and enhances CaOx crystal nucleation and inhibits growth in frozen urine.[182,197] It does not affect the urinary CaOx metastable limit, or mass deposition of the salt in undiluted, ultrafiltered urine, but does inhibit crystal aggregation[196] and attachment of COM to cultured cells.[12] However, inhibition of crystal adhesion occurs only at concentrations far above those found in urine.[12] Crystal attachment is also reduced in cultured cells genetically engineered to synthesize high levels of HS proteoglycans[198] and renal HS proteoglycan mRNA increases in lithogenic rats.[199,200] The presence of HS in crystals and stones, combined with its inhibitory influence on crystal aggregation and cell adhesion, suggests that it may play a role in inhibiting CaOx crystallization in urine in vivo; but at the present time, a defined function for this GAG remains to be unambiguously demonstrated.

4.7.1.4 Hyaluronic Acid (HA)

Hyaluronic acid is present in CaOx stones,[187,188] and although it is present in urine in minor amounts it is a major component of the extracellular matrix in the renal medullary interstitium.[201] Like that of CS and HS,[202] the production of HA by cultured renal tubular cells is activated during cell proliferation and following physical injury, apparently as part of the cellular repair mechanism.[39] The structure and large size of the exposed HA molecule allow it to form hydrated gel-like matrices or "coats," which extend several microns from the surfaces of migrating and proliferating MDCK cells[40] and which, combined with its electronegativity, enable it to bind COM crystals.[42] It has been proposed that this HA-mediated binding of the crystals promotes their entrapment within the renal tubules, as well as the formation of Randall's plaques in the renal interstitium,[201] though both processes have yet to be unambiguously demonstrated to cause stone formation.

4.7.1.5 Heparin

Heparin is not present in human urine. Nonetheless, it was also tested in most of the studies that examined the properties of CS perhaps as a possible therapeutic agent, but probably because it is freely available and was just easy to include! Heparin inhibits CaOx crystal growth,[112] crystal aggregation,[112] both processes combined,[113] nucleation,[191,192] growth and agglomeration,[51] agglomeration,[193] and mass deposition.[191,193]

4.7.1.6 Synthetic GAGs

Several synthetic GAGs (sodium pentosan polysulfate [SPP], G871, G872) have been tested as potential treatments for stone prevention. Most attention has been focused on SPP, although one study reported that G871 and 872 inhibit CaOx crystal growth and agglomeration in inorganic media.[203] SPP inhibits growth[195,203–207] and agglomeration[203,206] under the same conditions, although it has also been reported to promote agglomeration.[204] Justification for studying synthetic GAGs can be found in reports that, unlike that of CS, the inhibitory potency of SPP is retained in urine and in vivo. It retards CaOx crystal growth in undiluted urine[207] and CaOx crystal deposition in lithogenic rats.[195,207,208] However, those findings must remain academic until the clinical usefulness of SPP is demonstrated beyond doubt by the performance of randomized, placebo-controlled studies.[209]

4.7.1.7 Urinary Excretion of GAGs

The literature is replete with many papers attempting to demonstrate that the urinary concentration or output of GAGs can be used as a marker for stone disease. Several papers have shown that undifferentiated stone formers,[122,210–212] recurrent stone formers,[213] and stone formers with type I hypercalciuria[214] excrete abnormally low levels of GAGs, but they are overwhelmed by reports that GAGs excretion by stone formers is indistinguishable from that of healthy controls,[213–219] including children.[220,221] Children have been reported to excrete larger quantities of GAGs than adults[211] and CS in particular,[185] although their output of HS is less than that of their parents.[185] Harangi et al.[220] showed that pediatric stone formers with renal hypercalciuria excreted significantly less keratan sulfate than did the controls or patients with absorptive hypercalciuria. They did, however, excrete much greater quantities of dermatan sulfate, making the total GAG excretion equal in all groups.

4.7.1.8 Summary: Are Urinary GAGs Important in Stone Formation?

Throughout the previous 40 years, a great deal of effort has been expended to discover whether or not urinary GAGs play a protective role in stone pathogenesis. Certainly, there is ample evidence that CS can inhibit CaOx crystallization, as do heparin and several synthetic GAGs, but only in inorganic solutions. Furthermore, it is clear that a low GAG excretion is not a consistent hallmark of urolithiasis, either in children or in adults. Why then does the impression persist that urinary GAGs are inhibitors not only of CaOx crystallization but of stone pathogenesis, when a *critical* appraisal of past literature leads to the conclusion that, as a group, they are not. And why, therefore, bother measuring the urinary excretion of GAGs when, as with proteins, their urinary concentration will alter in response to any cellular inflammation or damage leading to or resulting from stone formation? Perhaps available data might justify the measurement of HS excretion in the investigation of stone formers, but there is currently no scientific basis for routinely determining CS or *total* GAG excretion as a marker of stone disease, and the practice should be discontinued.

4.8 Proteins

Only proteins that have been unambiguously identified immunologically or by amino acid sequence analysis or other proteomic techniques are presented in detail in the following section. Thus, despite its prominence in past literature,[222] no information on nephrocalcin is included, because it has never been confirmed to be a substantive protein and because of the confusion regarding its relationship to THG and albumin,[223] and inter-α-trypsin inhibitor.[224]

4.8.1 Proteins in Kidney Stones

By 2004, approximately 30 proteins had been unambiguously detected in kidney stone matrix (Fig. 4.5) using techniques such as gel electrophoresis, Western blotting, or amino acid sequencing analysis.[105,180]

However, the last decade has seen increasing use of more sophisticated proteomic tools for analyzing urine. While this has been principally to discover protein markers of various diseases,[229] proteomic tools have been increasingly used to identify proteins present in kidney stones.[85] Such techniques include high pressure liquid chromatography and tandem mass spectrometry (HPLC-MS), surface-enhanced laser desorption ionization–time of flight (SELDI-TOF), and matrix-assisted laser desorption ionization–time of flight (MALDI-TOF). Because these techniques, in combination with rapid automated computer searches of published protein data bases, can quickly separate and analyze large numbers of peptides at exceedingly low concentrations, the number of proteins identified in stones has risen hyperbolically in the previous few years. In 2007, Mushtaq et al.[228] added myeloperoxidase and α-defensin to the list of known constituents of stone matrix, while Canales et al.[225] identified 68 different proteins, of which more than 50 had not previously been observed. Chen et al.[230] detected 11 low

α-1-acid glycoprotein • acidic (leucine - rich) nuclear phosphoprotein 32 family member A • α1 actinin • α2 actinin • β actinin • albumin • AMP-activated protein kinase β2 on-catalytic subunit • amphoterin • amyloid precursor protein homolog HSD -2 • amyloid βA4 protein precursor isoform b • ankyrin repeat and SOCS box-containing 17 ankyrin repeat domain 30A • α-1-antitrypsin • Ap-3 complex β-3A subunit • apolipo-protein A1 • apolipoprotein A - IV precursor • apolipoprotein B precursor • apolipoprotein C-1 precursor • apolipoprotein D • apolipoprotein E precursor • ARG99 protein • arginine / serine - rich splicing factor 6 • argininosuccinate lyase • argininosuccinate synthetase • ATP synthase H+ transporting mitochondrial F1 complex α subunit isoform a • azurocidin precursor • biglycan • calcium - activated potassium channel β2 subunit • calgranulin • calgranulin A • calgranulin B • calgranulin C • calprotectin • cAMP-dependent protein kinase regulatory subunit α 2 • carbonic an-hydrase • cathepsin G2 • cathepsin G preprotein • CD59 protein (protectin) • ceruloplasmin • chain α isoform α preprotein • chromosome 14 open reading frame 49 • chromosome 18 open reading frame 34 • clusterin isoform • clusterin α chain • collagen α1 (I) chain • collagen α1 (VI) chain • collagen α2 (I) chain • complement C3 • complement component 3 precursor • complement component 4 • binding protein α • comple-ment factor H • cyclophilin • cytokeratin 1 • cytokeratin 7 • cytokeratin 14 • cytokeratin 18 • cytoplasmic linker 2 isoform 2 • α - defensin • DEA (Asp-Glu-Ala-His) box polypeptide 15 • defensin α-1DEK gene • dimethylarginine-dimethylaminohydrolase • dishevelled-associated activator of morphogenesis 1 • DKFZP4341092 protein • dystrobrevin β isoform 1 • eosinophilic cationic protein • epidermal growth factor • erythrocyte membrane protein band 4.1 - like 3 • eukaryotic translation elongation factor 1 α 1 • eukaryotic translation initiation factor 3 subunit 8 • extra-cellular prosaposin • factor IX • factor X • F-box and leucine-rich repeat protein 18 • fibrinogen α chain • fibrinogen β chain • fibrinogen γ chain • glyceraldehyde - 3 - phosphate - dehydrogenase • fibrinogen β chain preprotein • fibrinogen γ chain isoform γ-B precursor • fibronectin • G patch domain and KOW motifs • α - globulin • γ - globulin • α1B glycoprotein • α-2HS-glycoprotein • β -1B glycoprotein (hemopexin) • GTF21 repeat domain containing 1 isoform 2 • H4 histone family member E • haemoglobin • haemoglobin α chain • haemoglobin β chain • haptoglobin • heat shock 27 kDa protein • heat shock 70kDa protein binding protein • heat shock 90 kDa protein 1 α • heat shock protein 75 • heparin - binding EGF - like growth factor • heterogeneous nuclear ribonucleoprotein C isoform a • hexokinase domain containing 1 AT-hook transcription factor • hypothetical protein DKFZP434G1411 • hypothetical protein FLJ11036 • hypothetical protein FLJ13089 • hypothetical protein FLJ35382 • hypo-thetical protein XP373506 similar to RIKEN cDNA 4732495G21 gene • hypothetical protein XP-499085 • I(3)mbt - like 2 isoform a • Ig heavy chain • Ig κ chain • Ig κ light chain • IgA light chain • IgG light chain • IgG2 heavy chain • insulin - like growth factor 1 • insulin - like growth factor binding protein 5 • inter - α - trypsin inhibitor H1 • inter - α -trypsin inhibitor H2 • inter-α-trypsin inhibitor bikunin • keratin 9 • kininogen • kinin-ogen 1 • lactoferrin • lectin • leukocyte elastase precursor • limbin • limitrin • longation factor 1 • lymphocyte antigen 64 homolog radioprot-ective 105 kDa • lysozyme • lysozyme C precursor • man9 - mannosidase • mannose - binding 2 • MASP – 2 • matrix Gla protein • MICAL - like 2 isoform 2 • α - 1 - microglobulin • β - 2-microglobulin • myeloblastin precursor • myeloperoxidase • myeloperoxidase chain A • MYL - 1 • myosin heavy chain IIa (non-muscle) • myosin heavy polypeptide 9 non-muscle • N - acylsphingosine amidohydrolase 1 preprotein isoform a • NAPSA gene product • nascent - polypeptide - associated complex α polypeptide • neutrophil defensin 3 precursor • neutrophil elastase • novel protein (transcription factor) • nucleophosmin 1 • origin recognition complex subunit 4 • orosomucoid • osteopontin • PABP1-dependent poly A-specific ribonuclease subunit PAN3 • periaxin • perioxiredoxin • peroxisome biogenesis factor 1 • phosphoprotein 75 • plasminogen • polymerase (DNA directed) κ • porin • PREDICTED similar to RIKEN cDNA 9330196J05, KIAA1529 • proline - rich tyrosine kinase 2 • proteasome 26S ATPase sub-unit 5 • protein C • protein C inhibitor • protein disulfide isomerise - related protein • protein 2 • prothrombin • prothrombin fragment 1 • proto-oncogene Wnt7 protein • PWP2 periodic tryptophan protein homolog • RAB13 member RAS oncogene family • RAB6 interacting protein 1 • RAD50 homolog isoform 1 • Ras association and pleckstrin homology domains 1 isoform 2 • renal lithostathine • retinol-binding protein • RNA polymerase • S100 calcium-binding protein • S100 calcium -binding protein P • S100 calcium - binding protein A8 • S100 calcium-binding protein A9 • scaffold attachment factor B • secreted phosphoprotein 2 24kDa • serum amyloid P • serum amyloid P component precursor • SET translocation, histidine - rich glycoprotein • splicing factor, arginine / serine rich 3 • superoxide dismutase • superoxide dismutase 3 • synapto-nemal complex protein 1 • syndecan 4 precursor • Tamm-Horsfall glycoprotein • ATA element modulatory factor 1 • tight junction protein 2 iso-form 2 • tight junction protein 4 (peripheral) • TIP120 protein • transferrin • Treacher Collins - Franceschetti syndrome protein 1 • trinucleotide repeat containing 15 • tumor necrosis factor α – induced protein • tumour rejection antigen (gp96) 1 • type 2 cytoskeletal 8, non-POU domain containing octamer binding, cytochrome P450 family 4 subfamily X polypeptide S-adenosylhomocysteine hydrolyase - like • ubiquitin B precurs-or • unactive progesterone receptor 23kDa • urogastrone • urokinase plasminogen activator • vacuolar protein sorting 16 isoform 1 • vitronectin (S-protein) • voltage-dependent calcium channel (α1c) • zinc finger transcription factor TRPS1

Fig. 4.5 Proteins known to be present in human kidney stones by 2008. Those highlighted in yellow were detected in CaOx stones up to and including 2007 (Compiled from[105,180,225–228])

molecular mass proteins in the matrix of 10 CaOx stones. However, all those studies have since been eclipsed by a recent report[227] demonstrating the presence in stone matrix of a mind-boggling 158 proteins, including 28 that were classified as common.

It is becoming difficult to state with any surety exactly how many and which individual proteins are now known to occur in stone matrix, since many detected peptides are precursor molecules or different chains or fragments of the same parent protein. Nonetheless, it is now clear that more than 200 proteins can occur in the organic matrix of calcium kidney stones (Fig. 4.5). But are they all active protagonists in stone development? Hardly. While commonsense allows us to accept that the properties of say, OPN, calgranulin, and prothrombin fragment 1 would seem to equip them for an active role in CaOx crystallization and stone formation, it is probably pushing the limits of credulity to suggest that *hypothetical proteins FLJ11036, FLJ13089, FLJ35382,* or *XP373506,* or *disheveled-associated activator of morphogenesis 1,* are likely to carry much responsibility for development of the disease! In fact, it is likely that *almost all* of the proteins listed in Fig. 4.5 have absolutely nothing whatsoever to do with dictating the direction of stone formation. It is possible, of course, that presence in stones of a select few of them could result from their inducing CaOx nucleation by acting as heterogeneous seeds or by sequestering calcium and oxalate ions to produce high local concentrations of CaOx. However, they could just as easily arrive in stones by incompletely inhibiting crystallization or as inflammatory molecules released by intratubular injury, as shown in Figs. 4.1 and 4.2 and suggested by the findings of Merchant et al.[227]

Confusion generated by our newfound ability to identify proteins with ease is complicated further by modern genomic technology. As will be seen in the following sections, one yardstick used to assess the likelihood that a protein is a significant participant in stone formation is to measure changes in its gene expression in animal models of renal calcification or in cultured cells. But again, we are overwhelmed with information. In one study alone[231] at least 173 genes were found to be at least twofold regulated at one or more time points during experimental nephrocalcinosis in rats!

Thus the simple fact that a macromolecule is in a stone, or that its mRNA or cDNA rises under lithogenic conditions, does not allow us to draw unambiguous conclusions about its anatomical origin, how it found its way into the stone, or whether it played a specific role in the stone's formation, because it is just as probable that it is a *product* of the stone, rather than a cause. Many stone macromolecules are components of blood and are not normally found in urine. This problem has been surmounted to a large extent by studying the organic matrix of CaOx crystals freshly precipitated from

urine.[232,233] Such crystals contain no macromolecules arising secondarily from cellular injury, and therefore allow the study of the macromolecules normally found in urine that participate in the crucial crystallization stage of stone formation. That approach, combined with better technology and the commercial availability of specific antibodies, has enabled the study of several macromolecules in sufficient detail to allow us at least to speculate whether they are maybe true functionaries in the process or just adventitious inclusions, and it is to these that we will now turn.

4.8.2 Tamm–Horsfall Glycoprotein (THG)

THG has been, undoubtedly, the most intensely studied protein associated with urolithiasis. Described in at least two comprehensive reviews,[234,235] early work will not be presented here in detail.

Despite its predominance in urine and in renal casts, the precise function of THG remains unknown. Its abundance in stone matrix[227] probably reflects its excretion in urine in higher quantities than any other protein, but seems inconsistent with its complete absence from CaOx crystals precipitated from whole human urine.[100,101,233] Reports that THG is incorporated into CaOx urinary crystals,[236–239] that it is more abundant in CaP crystals than COM,[236] and that it binds to COM crystals and prevents their attachment to cultured renal cells[72,74] undoubtedly stem from a failure in those studies to completely wash off superficial, loosely bound THG prior to EDTA demineralization and protein analysis.[101] The fact that THG is not incorporated into CaOx crystals indicates that it does not bind irreversibly to their surfaces. That observation is in keeping with the observation that it does not alter the habit or diffraction patterns of CaOx crystals or nucleate them in vitro[240] or in vivo,[241] and that calcium crystals form spontaneously in adult kidneys following inactivation of the THP gene in mouse embryonic stem cells.[242]

4.8.2.1 Effect of THG on Crystallization

Depending upon ambient conditions and methodology, THG exhibits a frustrating range of effects on CaOx crystallization, which probably reflect its ability to self-associate into polymeric behemoths with molecular masses of several millions. Although there are many reports that THG has no effect on CaOx deposition in synthetic inorganic media,[243] it has been reported to inhibit deposition of CaOx.[189,244] In urine, however, it promotes both CaOx[32,52] and CaP[245] precipitation. Nonetheless, it is a potent inhibitor of CaOx crystal aggregation in undiluted, ultrafiltered urine,[30,246] a property that probably results from steric hindrance,[20] since it does not bind to the crystal surface.

4.8.2.2 Effect of THG on Crystal–Cell Interaction

THG's inconsistent effects on CaOx crystallization also extend to the binding of CaOx crystals to renal cells. The sialic acid content of THG is crucial in defending the urinary tract against disease,[247] and sialic acid residues of cell surface proteins are thought to play a decisive role in the attachment of crystals to renal epithelial cells.[34,91] The protein has been reported to have no influence on[77] and to inhibit[36] crystal adhesion to cultured renal cells, and also to protect against oxalate-induced radical injury in MDCK cells, which has been attributed, at least in part, to its degree of glycosylation and its ability to adhere to the cell membrane.[248]

4.8.2.3 Structural Features of THG

Studies examining the molecular structure and excretion of THG have also generated confusing findings. It has been suggested that stone formers may synthesize and excrete THG with different physicochemical features (see[234,235]), one being an altered electrophoretic migration pattern.[249] One study reported that THG from stone patients was deficient in sialic acid,[250] a consequence of which is the promotion of crystal aggregation.[251] However, more recently[252] THG from stone formers was found to contain more sialic acid than did that from healthy subjects, and to inhibit crystallization less potently. Therefore, if differences do exist between THG from stone formers and controls, they are certainly not consistent, which might explain the failure of at least two groups of investigators to detect any disparities at all.[253,254]

4.8.2.4 Expression of THG in Animal and Cell Models

There has been one report that the expression of THG in cultured renal epithelial cells was unaffected by CaOx crystals and that it did not induce CaOx crystal formation in lithogenic rats,[241] while another paper showed that its gene expression, urinary excretion, biochemical properties, and function are unaffected in lithogenic rats.[255] Other studies, however, have demonstrated that renal THG mRNA and protein expression *decrease* in ethylene glycol treated rats,[256] and that the normal renal distribution of the protein is altered,[257] now appearing in the form of a fine, fibrillar meshwork surrounding individual crystals and their aggregates.[258] Strong expression of THG in lithogenic rats was induced not by crystals, but by renal tubular damage caused by tubular dilatation, leading to speculation that THG might promote stone

formation by acting as a crystal adhesive,[241] which again seems at odds with its inability to bind irreversibly to CaOx crystals.[100,101,233]

4.8.2.5 Urinary Excretion of THG

Excretion of THG by stone formers and healthy subjects has been generally shown not to differ,[219,259–261] in contrast to recent studies that have reported a significantly lower THG in calcium[262–264] and pure uric acid[265] stone formers than in healthy controls. Urinary THG levels increase in calcium stone formers after treatment with potassium citrate,[266] and also in healthy subjects in response to raised calcium and oxalate levels, a "self-protective" mechanism lacking in stone formers.[262]

4.8.2.6 Summary

The true role of THG in human stone formation remains somewhat of an enigma, principally because it exhibits contradictory effects in different milieu and different experimental models. However, even if it does fulfil some function in urolithiasis, it is undoubtedly not the only protein likely to be involved. With the advent of proteomic technology and the realization that other urinary proteins also have properties that equip them for a role in urolithiasis, interest in THG has tended to wane in recent years, and it is possible that the real basis of any association between THG and urolithiasis may never be fully elucidated.

4.8.3 Osteopontin

Osteopontin (OPN), a glycophosphoprotein rich in aspartic acid residues, is an abundant[227] component of kidney stone matrix[267–269] and is present in particles of Randall's plaque.[270] The protein is secreted in the luminal epithelia of the distal nephron[271] and the thick ascending loop of Henlé,[272] where urine is most concentrated and the likelihood of nucleation is highest.[267] Although OPN has traditionally been associated principally with bone mineralization,[273] it is now recognized to be a multifunctional molecule manufactured and secreted by various cell types, and to fulfil diverse roles ranging from cell adhesion, chemotaxis, cell signaling, prevention of apoptosis and invasion, to migration and anchorage-independent growth of tumor cells.[274] Given its ubiquity and wide-ranging physiological roles, it is not surprising that it has been the subject of a number of extensive reviews.[267,275–279] It is also the most extensively studied of any of the proteins implicated in stone formation.

4.8.3.1 Effect of OPN on Crystallization

OPN potently inhibits CaOx crystal growth[271,280] and nucleation and aggregation[281] under inorganic conditions: its effects in urine have not been reported. The protein's ability to induce preferential nucleation of COD[33] and to retard CaOx deposition results from step-pinning,[148] which it achieves by specific interactions with the growing crystal surface. Although OPN has been reported to attach preferentially to the edges between the top and apical faces of the inorganic COM crystal,[282] and also to the side faces,[148] it does not become incorporated to a significant extent into the mineral bulk of COM crystals precipitated from inorganic solutions [our own unpublished observations] or human urine.[22] Binding of OPN to the surface of crystals does however cause them to aggregate under certain conditions.[283] OPN's ability to increase the adhesiveness of crystals to which it is bound has also been observed in an atomic force microscopy study,[190] as well as in experiments in which its presence on the surface of collagen granules promoted the deposition and aggregation of COM from inorganic solutions.[284] Thus, OPN appears to possess an ability to increase the adhesiveness of surfaces, a property that also extends to those of cultured cells.

4.8.3.2 Effect of OPN on Crystal–Cell Interaction

In spite of reports that OPN has no effect on the attachment of uric acid crystals to cultured renal cells[285] and reduces the attachment of CaOx[77] and CaP[98] crystals, the evidence that it actually *increases* crystal adhesion is more convincing,[72,87,286] especially since the effect is mitigated by OPN antisense oligonucleotide in both MDCK[88] and NRK-52E cells.[35] Indeed, as mentioned previously, OPN has been strongly implicated as an important mediator of crystal retention in the kidney,[39,40,42] a property that depends upon its degree of phosphorylation[24] and its own molecular configuration, which, in turn, is affected by the features of the surface to which it binds.[287] On balance, the prevailing view is that OPN, whose expression in cultured monkey renal cells is stimulated by exposure to COM crystals,[12] is a major mediator of crystal attachment to cells in vivo. Therefore, despite the fact that it encourages retention of crystals, paradoxically, it could act as a defense mechanism by facilitating their removal by phagocytosis and intracellular destruction.

4.8.3.3 Expression of OPN in Animal and Cell Models

The increase in OPN observed in cell culture models in response to a CaOx crystal challenge is also observed in animals treated with various lithogenic agents. In rats, OPN is secreted at two sites in the kidney where the likelihood of stone mineral precipitation is greatest.[288] OPN mRNA and expression of the protein itself increase markedly following induction of renal CaOx crystal deposition.[289–296] This increase is, however, inhibited by estradiol, progesterone and/or testosterone,[295,298–300] vitamin K,[298] allopurinol,[301] and green tea[302]! Similar increases have been reported in mice,[303,304] including genetic hypercalciuric mice.[289] However, OPN knockout mice in which CaOx crystal formation was elicited by the injection of glyoxylate retained fewer crystals than did wild type mice, which is entirely in keeping with the protein's documented ability to promote crystal binding in cultured epithelial cells.[305]

4.8.3.4 Urinary Excretion of OPN

Urinary OPN levels are difficult to measure. Even normal ranges in healthy controls[21,23,281,306–309] have varied wildly, with average values from as low as 0.76 mg/L[21] to as high as 10 mg/L.[308] Despite such huge variability, most authors have reported that the urinary output of OPN is significantly decreased in the patient group.[309–312] However, Bautista et al.[23] did not observe a difference, nor did Hedgepeth et al.,[313] who used a semiquantitative approach. Where a reduced OPN output has been observed, it has been interpreted as a *cause* of the stone's formation, although in one instance, the authors speculated that it may have resulted from the protein's incorporation into the stone.[309] This is very likely to have been the case.

As discussed above, OPN binds to COM and COD crystals, and is incarcerated within the latter. Thus, any crystals in urine will effectively remove the protein from solution and cause its concentration to be significantly underestimated, as was recently demonstrated.[314] Measured values also vary with ambient calcium concentration, probably because of alterations in the Ca-dependent conformation of the molecule.[314] Of course, these problems are not confined to OPN: the measurement of *any* molecule that binds irreversibly to stone minerals, or whose molecular configuration is affected by Ca, will be unavoidably affected by the presence of any crystals in the urine, irrespective of whether they were formed spontaneously in vivo or later during storage in vitro. Obviously, calcium concentration and the formation of CaOx crystals in urine in vivo cannot be controlled: The potential for serious error will therefore be greatest in recurrent stone formers in whom hypercalciuria and crystalluria are especially prevalent. Reports comparing the urinary excretion in stone formers and healthy subjects of *any* macromolecule that binds CaOx or other stone crystals, or advocating the measurement of urinary proteins as markers of urolithiasis, must therefore be regarded with circumspection, particularly if the absence of hematuria has not been confirmed.

4.8.3.5 Summary

There is good evidence that OPN could fulfill an important role in stone formation. Nonetheless, at the present time it is true to say that unequivocal demonstration of a role for OPN in the pathogenesis of stones depends upon the generation of further information.

4.8.4 Prothrombin Fragment 1 (PTF1)

The first clue that a blood clotting protein might be associated with stone disease was unearthed more than 30 years ago, when a protein rich in γ-carboxyglutamic acid (Gla) was first detected in calcium stones.[315] However, it was not until 1991 that urinary PTF1, initially called crystal matrix protein, was discovered to be the principal band in gels of the soluble organic matrix of CaOx crystals freshly precipitated from whole human urine.[233] Crystal matrix protein was subsequently shown to be related to prothrombin,[103,316] and later confirmed to be its F1 activation fragment.[102,316]

Urinary PTF1 is a glycoprotein with a molecular mass of approximately 31 kDa, with different chromatographic properties from those of its cousin in serum.[102] The protein is present in calcium, but not struvite calculi, demonstrating that its occurrence there is not a consequence of intrarenal bleeding induced by the stone itself,[317] and is localized to the thick ascending limb of the loops of Henlé and the distal convoluted tubules, where its expression is greater in stone formers than in controls.[318] Contrary to the long-held belief that prothrombin is synthesized exclusively in the liver, it is clear that it is also manufactured in the kidney, since mRNA encoding the protein has been detected in both the human kidney[319,320] and rat[320–322] kidney.

4.8.4.1 Effect of PTF1 on Crystallization

PTF1 is a very strong inhibitor of both CaOx crystal growth and aggregation in inorganic solutions[280,323] and in undiluted, ultrafiltered human urine.[324] The protein's potency in both media can be attributed to its Gla (γ-carboxyglutamic acid) domain.[323,325] This domain, located at the N-terminus of PTF1 and its parent, prothrombin, contains 10 residues of Gla, full γ-carboxylation of which is indispensable for the efficient clotting of blood, and also for the binding of PTF1 to CaOx crystals. Warfarin reduces blood coagulation by inhibiting γ-carboxylation of prothrombin, and therefore that of the PTF1 fragment. It has been shown that Gla-deficient forms of the protein resulting from warfarin therapy are not incorporated into CaOx crystals,[326] while chemical reduction of the number of Gla residues also reduces the protein's

inhibitory effect on CaOx crystallization in inorganic media.[327] It has been reported that the Gla content of PTF1 from stone formers is less than that of healthy subjects, as is its inhibitory activity.[328]

PTF1's binding properties and inhibitory potency appear to depend, in addition to its Gla domain, upon the degree of sialylation of the molecule's o-glycan groups,[329] while its carbohydrate moieties affect its influence on crystal nucleation and aggregation, but not growth.[330] However, it is also apparent that the inhibitory potency of PTF1 in urine is related to the composition of the urine itself, since the activities of PTF1 isolated from the urines of black and white subjects differ when tested in urine obtained from each group,[331] despite the lack of any structural difference between them.[332] This observation is consistent with modeling studies suggesting that inhibitory activity is dictated by factors other than, or in addition to, the number of possible points of contact between various protein molecules and the COM crystal surface.[104,333]

PTF1 binds to CaOx in a highly selective manner. It attaches avidly to COM crystals, both in inorganic media[104] and urine,[22] but binds reluctantly to COD and only at low calcium concentrations.[22] The protein binds specifically to the end, apical faces of the COM crystal, a preference that cannot be explained simply in terms of interactions between the protein's Gla residues and Ca or oxalate arrays on the COM crystal surface.[104] In binding to the apical faces, PTF1 competes successfully with HSA (which also prefers to attach to those faces) forcing it to bind instead to the side faces of the crystal.[104]

4.8.4.2 Effect of PTF1 on Crystal–Cell Interaction

Although the concentration of PTF1 was not directly quantified in the study, COM crystal coating by the protein has been reported to correlate with decreased binding of the crystals to cultured renal epithelial cells.[72] Nonetheless, unpublished data from our laboratory have shown that PTF1 attached to the surfaces of COM crystals potently inhibits their binding to MDCK cells, and intracrystalline PTF1 facilitates their degradation and dissolution – both in a dose-dependent manner. PTF1 may therefore help to reduce the likelihood of crystal attachment, and thereby, the progression from crystalluria to stone formation. Moreover, if attachment and internalization do occur, it could also help to prevent the development of stones by encouraging intracellular crystal dissolution.

4.8.4.3 Expression of PTF1 in Animal and Cell Models

The expression of PTF1 has been shown to increase in MDCK cells challenged with oxalate[334] and two studies have examined the gene expression of prothrombin in animal models of urolithiasis. One reported a significant increase in the protein's mRNA in the kidneys of rats rendered hyperoxaluric by the administration of ethylene glycol,[320] but the other reported the exact opposite.[335] This discrepancy can probably be attributed to methodological differences in standardizing mRNA extraction.

4.8.4.4 Urinary Excretion of PTF1

Although at least two attempts have been made to quantify the excretion of PTF1 in urine, the results are almost certainly unreliable. As discussed above, the presence in urine of CaOx crystals formed either before or after voiding will unavoidably cause underestimation of any protein that binds irreversibly to them. A reduction in the measured concentration of PTF1 in the presence of crystals has been demonstrated,[336] an undoubted consequence of its extraordinary affinity for the COM crystal surface. Apart from a semiquantitative study that was unable to demonstrate any difference between the PTF1 content of urine from stone formers and controls,[313] there has been only one other report of the measurement of urinary PTF1 concentration.[308] Although that study observed a reduced concentration in the urine of stone formers, it did not take account of the possibility that CaOx crystals may have been present in the urine samples before or after voiding.

4.8.4.5 Summary

There is good evidence that PTF1 may play a significant regulatory role in stone formation. However, as with all other proteins to which have been putatively assigned similar functions, there is currently no unambiguous evidence that it is an obligate participant in stone pathogenesis.

4.8.5 Inter-α-Inhibitor (IαI)

It is now almost 20 years since Sørensen and his colleagues isolated from urine a glycoprotein related to inter-α-trypsin inhibitor, now more commonly known as inter-α-inhibitor (IαI), which inhibited the growth of CaOx in an inorganic medium.[337] IαI is a complex Kunitz-type proteinase inhibitor consisting of four heavy chains – H1, H2, H3, and H4. These are linked to a proteoglycan complex comprising bikunin and chondroitin sulfate, which is the predominant protease inhibitor in urine.[338] Heavy chain 3 is found in spherules comprising Randall's plaque and in the collecting ducts, thin loops of Henlé, and interstitial matrix of stone formers'

kidneys, while bikunin is present only in the collecting duct apical membranes and the loop cell cytoplasm.[339] The IαI family of peptide chains is encoded by at least five different genes.[338] Although the heavy chains are directly related to the physiological functions of intact IαI through transfer to hyaluronic acid,[338] it is the bikunin portion of the molecule that has so far attracted most attention. Bikunin appears to fulfil disparate physiological functions as a protease inhibitor, growth factor, regulator of intracellular calcium levels, a component of the extracellular matrix, and most relevant to this review, a potential modifier of calcium urolithiasis.[340]

Atmani and his coworkers extended the initial work of Sørensen et al.[337] Working on a closely related 35 kDa urinary protein that inhibited CaOx crystal growth, which they originally called uronic acid-rich protein,[341] they later showed that it shared homology with IαI.[342] Uronic acid-rich protein was eventually identified as bikunin.[343] Both H1 and H2[344] and bikunin[227] have been positively identified in the organic matrix of calcium stones, as well as in CaOx crystals precipitated from urine.[345,346]

4.8.5.1 Effect of IαI on Crystallization

Although inhibitory studies have shown that bikunin is a proficient inhibitor of CaOx crystallization in inorganic media,[342,347–352] it has little effect at expected physiological concentrations.[349] Its effects in undiluted human urine have never been reported. There is in agreement, however, that neither IαI itself nor its heavy chains significantly reduce CaOx crystallization, even in inorganic media[349,350]; activity appears to be confined to the bikunin fragment of IαI, where it is localized to the carboxy-terminal domain of the molecule.[350] The protein from the urine of stone formers has been reported to be a less efficient inhibitor of CaOx crystallization than that isolated from healthy subjects.[348]

4.8.5.2 Effect of IαI on Crystal–Cell Interaction

In the only study examining the effect of bikunin on crystal–cell attachment, the protein was reported to inhibit COM adhesion to MDCK cells.[83]

4.8.5.3 Expression of IαI in Animal and Cell Models

Bikunin is present in rat urine[353] and is expressed in the normal rat kidney, mainly in the proximal tubules and the thin descending segment near the loop of Henlé,[352] though the protein is redistributed to the corticomedullary junction under lithogenic conditions.[354] Levels of expression of bikunin mRNA rise in the kidneys and urine of rats during experimental CaOx nephrolithiasis[355–357] as well as in MDCK cells exposed to oxalate.[358] Gene expression does not, however, increase in MDCK cells challenged with CaOx crystals.[358]

4.8.5.4 Urinary Excretion of IαI

Although it has been reported that the intact IαI trimer molecule as well as dimers of two of its heavy chains with bikunin are detected more frequently in stone formers than healthy men,[313,359] this may simply represent a nonspecific inflammatory response to the presence of stones or crystals in the urinary tract, rather than synthesis of the protein as a specific form of defense against lithogenic conditions. In any event, findings have been inconsistent, since other studies have shown that bikunin levels in the urine of stone formers are decreased relative to controls.[351,360] Of course, as discussed above, reports of decreased bikunin levels in urine may simply reflect binding of the protein to urinary crystals, since in neither study[361,359] were allowances made for the possible presence of urinary crystals.

4.8.5.5 Summary

As with the other proteins discussed above, evidence continues to accumulate that suggests an association between IαI and calcium stone formation. However, the nature of that association is still uncertain, and it is not presently possible to state with any assurance whether the protein is a product of inflammation induced by oxalate, crystals, or stones, or whether it plays a directive role in the process.

4.8.6 Calgranulin (Calprotectin)

Calgranulin (24 kDa) is a heterodimer of two calcium-binding proteins comprising light and heavy chains, which is present in the cytoplasm of neutrophils and expressed on the membranes of monocytes.[361] Its involvement in inflammatory conditions has encouraged its measurement as a urinary marker of several diseases, including rheumatoid arthritis, pulmonary conditions, and bowel cancer.[361] The protein is present in the organic matrix of struvite[362] and CaOx stones[228,230,269,363] and is expressed by MDCK cells in the vicinity of CaP deposits formed when the cells are inoculated into nude mice.[364] The human urinary protein has been shown to inhibit CaOx crystal growth and aggregation at nanomolar concentrations[365] and suggested to be one of several marker proteins for urolithiasis,[366] although its usefulness is again tempered by the ever-present problem of crystalluria. Although calgranulin's properties and presence

in stone matrix strongly suggest an involvement in stone formation, it is a relative newcomer to the stone scene and little information has been collected thus far: more information will need to be collected before it will be possible to decide whether or not it fulfils a directive role in urolithiasis.

4.8.7 Human Serum Albumin (HSA)

After THG, HSA is the most abundant protein in urine. It has long been known to be present in stone matrix[367] and its detection in all the five kidney stones in which it was bound to other urinary proteins led to speculation that it fulfils a specific role in the formation of stone matrix.[368] HSA is incorporated into inorganic COM crystals, binding specifically to their end apical faces, but it attaches to the side faces of COM crystals precipitated from urine, because of competition from the more strongly binding PTF1.[104] Most HSA in stone matrix probably results, therefore, from nonspecific inclusion resulting from damage caused by the stone itself – together with its physiological ubiquity. HSA has only a weak affinity for the COM mineral, since it is included into COM crystals in much smaller quantities than would be expected from its high concentration in urine[232,233] and it is not detectable in COD crystal matrix [our own unpublished observations], despite the fact that its presence in solution tends to favor the formation of COD.[369]

HSA has very little effect on CaOx crystal growth in either inorganic solutions[223,243,370,371] or undiluted ultrafiltered human urine.[20] However, it retards crystal aggregation strongly in seeded metastable solutions,[223,243,372] but only relatively weakly in urine.[20,27] HSA derived from black subjects inhibits aggregation more potently than that from whites, which has been attributed to structural differences between the protein from each source.[27] There have been several papers showing that CaOx crystal nucleation from inorganic solutions is facilitated by HSA,[369,373] especially when it is adsorbed to solid supports,[369,374] and one report that HSA from normal controls is a stronger nucleator than is that from stone formers.[369] A raised HSA concentration in the urine of stone formers[261] may have been symptomatic of renal bleeding caused by the stone, rather than indicative of a crucial role for the protein in stone formation, particularly since it was accompanied by an increase in urinary excretion of transferrin – another blood protein.

4.8.7.1 Summary

Evidence that HSA plays a specific role in calcium stone formation is not convincing, and its invariable occurrence in stones is perhaps more likely to reflect its plenitude in urine, blood, and tissues, than to result from specific interactions with crystals or other proteins.

4.8.8 Fibronectin

Fibronectin (FN) is a relatively recent player in the stone saga. Present in high concentration in plasma, FN is a multifunctional protein that mediates various cellular interactions with the extracellular matrix and is an important protagonist in cell adhesion, migration, growth, and differentiation.[375] Although FN adsorbs to CaOx crystals,[376] its ability to inhibit COM crystal binding to cultured renal epithelial cells,[81] as well as subsequent internalization,[36,81] depends on interactions with the cells – not on coating of the crystals. These effects of FN appear to be related to the type of cells used, since it *promotes* binding of crystals to the human renal cancer cell line CAKI-1.[34]

FN also inhibits MDCK cell injury induced by exposure to oxalate and COM crystals,[377] and the FN content of the cells rises proportionately with the amount of crystals bound to them.[376] In a lithogenic rat model, the protein is found expressed on tubules to which crystals are attached.[375] Although it inhibits CaOx crystal aggregation in an inorganic seeded crystallization system,[376] it has only a slight effect on crystal growth.[284,376] Reports of a raised urinary FN concentration in recurrent stone formers with silent stones and a decreased concentration in those without silent stones[378] are more likely to reflect the presence of hematuria in the former group, rather than enhanced renal secretion of the protein.

4.9 Conclusions

This chapter reviews published literature on human stones up to the beginning of 2009. However, many reports have not been cited; not because they are irrelevant or unimportant, but because the relevant literature is simply too extensive. Nonetheless, the vast wealth of accumulated knowledge has told us a great deal about the low and high molecular weight components that have come to be regarded as promoters or inhibitors. But inhibitors or promoters of what? Calcium oxalate crystallization in an inorganic solution? In urine? Adhesion of crystals to renal epithelial cells? Stone formation itself? Of course, the aim of the studies reported here was to clarify the function of inhibitors and promoters in the formation of calculi, but currently, with the possible exception of citrate, there is no unequivocal evidence that any single molecule is directly instrumental in preventing or advancing stones. And we should not expect there to be.

I have previously described stone formation as an example of chaos – with good reason.[379] Literally countless factors affect the likelihood that sparingly soluble crystals will precipitate in the urinary tract and initiate stone pathogenesis – from genetics to diet, water quality to climate, and geography to urine and cellular composition. And even if we single out one group of factors – so-called inhibitors or promoters – we find that their influences are manifold and contradictory. Figure 4.6 shows the various ways in which urinary molecules could influence events leading to stone formation, both extracellularly in the urinary stew, and intracellularly within the kidney.

Fig. 4.6 The possible extra- and intracellular effects of urinary macromolecules in stone formation

Extracellular	Cellular
Promote nucleation in urine	Promote nucleation on epithelium
Inhibit nucleation in urine	Inhibit nucleation on epithelium
Inhibit growth in urine	⇧ Protein & gene expression
Promote growth in urine	⇩ Protein & gene expression
Inhibit aggregation in urine	Inhibit crystal attachment
Promote aggregation in urine	Promote crystal attachment
Facilitate crystal destruction	Facilitate crystal destruction

According to published literature, depending upon the experimental system used, it seems they can do just about *everything*. For instance, stones cannot form without the nucleation of crystals. But enhanced nucleation could actually be protective, because higher nucleation rates produce smaller crystals less likely to become trapped in the renal tubules. Attachment of crystals to the renal epithelium is required for stone formation, but their attachment does not inevitably lead to stones, because cells can swallow and demolish them. Thus, promoters can inhibit and inhibitors can promote.

Where does this leave the hapless stone former? It is likely that we have exhausted the range of natural low molecular weight molecules suitable for preventing stones, although the chemical agents responsible for the apparent success of some plant extracts have not yet been fully investigated. Proteins may well yield information about molecular motifs that could be synthesized and used to tailor stone treatment, but we are currently swamped with proteins which, though in stones, did not contribute actively to their formation. So which ones should we study? The most likely candidates are osteopontin, prothrombin fragment 1, calgranulin, hyaluronan, annexin, fibronectin, matrix Gla protein, fetuin, and osteocalcin. Why? Because Nature is economical. The macromolecules – especially proteins – involved in CaOx crystal formation and retention will almost certainly be the same ones already known in humans and other organisms to bind calcium, and its salts avidly regulate healthy calcium-dependent physiological functions, control the deposition and assembly of healthy bone, dentine, and cartilage, and prevent other ectopic calcification.[276]

Acknowledgments The support of Grant No. NDDK 1 R01 DK064050-01A1 from the National Institutes of Health, USA, in the preparation of this chapter is gratefully acknowledged.

References

1. Kok DJ. Inhibitors of calcium oxalate crystallization. In: Khan SR, ed. *Calcium Oxalate in Biological Systems*. Boca Raton, New York, London, Tokyo: CRC; 1995:23-36.
2. Kavanagh JP. Supersaturation and renal precipitation: the key to stone formation? *Urol Res.* 2006;34:81-85.
3. Kok DJ. Clinical implications of physicochemistry of stone formation. *Endocrinol Metabl Clin North Am.* 2003;31:855-867.
4. Kok DJ, Papapoulos SE. Physicochemical considerations in the development and prevention of calcium oxalate urolithiasis. *Bone Miner.* 1993;20:1-15.
5. Robertson WG, Peacock M. Calcium oxalate crystalluria and inhibitors of crystallisation in recurrent renal stone-formers. *Clin Sci.* 1972;43:499-506.
6. Finlayon B, Reid F. The expectation of free and fixed particles in urinary stone disease. *Invest Urol.* 1978;15:442-448.
7. Kok DJ, Khan SR. Calcium oxalate nephrolithiasis, a free or fixed particle disease. *Kidney Int.* 1994;46:847-854.
8. Saw NK, Chow K, Rao PN, Kavanagh JP. Effects of inositol hexaphosphate (phytate) on calcium binding, calcium oxalate crystallization and in vitro stone growth. *J Urol.* 2007;177:2366-2370.
9. Lieske JC, Toback FG, Deganello S. Direct nucleation of calcium oxalate dihydrate crystals onto the surface of living renal epithelial cells in culture. *Kidney Int.* 1998;54:796-803.
10. Bigelow MW, Wiessner JH, Kleinman JG, Mandel NS. Calcium oxalate crystal attachment to cultured kidney epithelial cell lines. *J Urol.* 1998;160:1528-1532.
11. Lieske JC, Swift H, Martin T, Patterson B, Toback GF. Renal epithelial cells rapidly bind and internalize calcium oxalate monohydrate crystals. *PNAS.* 1994;91:6987-6991.
12. Lieske JC, Norris R, Swift H, Toback FG. Adhesion, internalization and metabolism of calcium oxalate monohydrate crystals by renal epithelial cells. *Kidney Int.* 1997;52:1291-1301.
13. Lieske JC, Huang E, Toback GF. Regulation of renal epithelial cell affinity for calcium oxalate crystals. *Am J Physiol Renal Physiol.* 2000;278:F130-F137.
14. Riese RJ, Riese JW, Kleinman JG, Wiessner JH, Mandel GS, Mandel NS. Specificity in calcium oxalate adherence to papillary epithelial cells in cultures. *Am J Physiol.* 1988;255:F1025-1032.
15. Verkoelen CF, Van Der Boom BG, Kok DJ, Schröder FH, Romijn JC. Attachment sites for particles in the urinary tract. *J Am Soc Nephrol Suppl.* 1999;14:S430-S435.
16. Lieske JC, Toback FG, Deganello S. Face-selective adhesion of calcium oxalate dihydrate crystals to renal epithelial cells. *Calcif Tissue Int.* 1996;58:195-2000.
17. Khan SR. Calcium oxalate crystal interaction with renal tubular epithelium, mechanism of crystal adhesion and its impact on stone development. *Urol Res.* 1995;23:71-79.
18. Lieske JC, Spargo BH, Toback FG. Endocytosis of calcium oxalate crystals and proliferation of renal tubular epithelial cells in a patient with type 1 primary hyperoxaluria. *J Urol.* 1992;148:1517-1519.
19. Howard JE, Thomas WC. Some observations on rachitic rat cartilage of probable significance in the etiology of renal calculi. *Trans Am Clin Climatol Assoc.* 1958;70:94-102.
20. Ryall RL, Harnett RM, Hibberd CM, Edyvane KA, Marshall VR. Effects of chondroitin sulphate, human serum albumin and Tamm-Horsfall mucoprotein on calcium oxalate crystallization in undiluted human urine. *Urol Res.* 1991;19:181-188.
21. Hoyer JR, Pietrzyk RA, Liu H, Whitson PA. Effects of microgravity on urinary osteopontin. *J Am Soc Nephrol.* 1999;10:389-393.
22. Ryall RL, Chauvet MC, Grover PK. Intracrystalline proteins and urolithiasis: A comparison of the protein content and ultrastructure of urinary calcium oxalate monohydrate and dihydrate crystals. *BJU Int.* 2005;96:654-663.
23. Bautista DS, Densteldt J, Chambers AF, Harris JF. Low molecular weight variants of osteopontin generated by serine proteases in urine of patients with kidney stones. *J Cell Biochem.* 1996;61:402-409.
24. Christensen B, Petersen TE, Sørensen ES. Post-translational modification and proteolytic processing of urinary osteopontin. *Biochem J.* 2008;411:53-61.
25. Hunter GK, Kyle CL, Goldberg HA. Modulation of crystal formation by bone phosphoproteins: structural specificity of the osteopontin-mediated inhibition of hydroxyapatite formation. *Biochem J.* 1994;300:723-728.
26. Hoyer JR, Asplin JR, Otvos L. Phosphorylated osteopontin peptides suppress crystallization by inhibiting the growth of calcium oxalate crystals. *Kidney Int.* 2001;60:77-82.
27. Rodgers AL, Mensah PD, Schwager SL, Sturrock ED. Inhibition of calcium oxalate crystallization by commercial human serum albumin and human urinary albumin isolated from two different race groups: evidence for possible molecular differences. *Urol Res.* 2006;34:373-380.
28. Liu J, Jiang H, Liu XY. How does bovine serum albumin prevent the formation of kidney stone? A kinetics study. *J Phys Chem.* 2006;110:9085-9089.
29. Hess B, Ryall RL, Kavanagh JP, et al. Methods for measuring crystallization in urolithiasis research: why, how and when? *Eur Urol.* 2001;40:220-230.

30. Gohel MD, Shum DK, Li MK. The dual effect of urinary macromolecules on the crystallization of calcium oxalate endogenous in urine. *Urol Res.* 1992;20:13-17.

31. Chow K, Dixon J, Gilpin S, Kavanagh JP, Rao PN. A stone farm: development of a method for simultaneous production of multiple calcium oxalate stones in vitro. *Urol Res.* 2004;32:55-60.

32. Grover PK, Ryall RL, Marshall VR. Does Tamm-Horsfall mucoprotein inhibit or promote calcium oxalate crystallization in human urine? *Clin Chim Acta.* 1990;190:223-238.

33. Wesson JA, Worcester EM, Wiessner JH, Mandel NS, Kleinmann JG. Control of calcium oxalate crystal structure and cell adherence by urinary macromolecules. *Kidney Int.* 1998;53:952-957.

34. Kramer G, Steiner GE, Prinz-Kashani M, Bursa B, Marberger M. Cell-surface matrix proteins and sialic acids in cell-crystal adhesion; the effect of crystal binding on the viability of human CAKI-1 renal epithelial cells. *BJU Int.* 2003;91:554-559.

35. Yasui T, Fujita K, Asai K, Kohri K. Osteopontin regulates adhesion of calcium oxalate crystals to renal epithelial cells. *Int J Urol.* 2002;9:100-109.

36. Lieske JC, Toback GF. Regulation of renal epithelial cell endocytosis of calcium oxalate monohydrate crystals. *Am J Physiol.* 1993;264:F800-F807.

37. Schepers MSJ, Duim RAJ, Asselman M, Romijn JC, Schröder FH, Verkoelen CF. Internalization of calcium oxalate crystals by renal tubular cells: A nephron segment-specific process? *Kidney Int.* 2003;64:493-500.

38. Verkoelen CF, van der Boom BG, Kok DJ, et al. Cell type-specific acquired protection from crystal adherence by renal tubule cells in culture. *Kidney Int.* 1999;55:1426-1433.

39. Asselman M, Verhulst A, De Broe ME, Verkoelen CF. Calcium oxalate crystal adherence to hyaluronan-, osteopontin-, and CD44-expressing injured/regenerating tubular epithelial cells in rat kidneys. *J Am Soc Nephrol.* 2003;14:3155-3166.

40. Verhulst A, Asselman M, Persy VP, et al. Crystal retention capacity of cells in the human nephron: involvement of CD44 and its ligands hyaluronic acid and osteopontin in the transition of a crystal binding- into a nonadherent epithelium. *J Am Soc Nephrol.* 2003;14:107-114.

41. Wiessner JH, Hasegawa AT, Hung LY, Mandel GS, Mandel NS. Mechanisms of calcium oxalate crystal attachment to injured renal collecting duct cells. *Kidney Int.* 2001;59:637-644.

42. Verkoelen CF, Van Der Boom BG, Romijn JC. Identification of hyaluronan as a crystal-binding molecule at the surface of migrating and proliferating MDCK cells. *Kidney Int.* 2000;58:1045-1054.

43. Khan SR. Hyperoxaluria-induced oxidative stress and antioxidants for renal protection. *Urol Res.* 2005;33:349-357.

44. Scheid CR, Cao LC, Honeyman T, Jonassen JA. How elevated oxalate can promote kidney stone disease: changes at the surface and in the cytosol of renal cells that promote crystal adherence and growth. *Front Biosci.* 2004;9:797-808.

45. Guo C, McMartin KE. The cytotoxicity of oxalate, metabolite of ethylene glycol, is due to calcium oxalate monohydrate formation. *Toxicology.* 2005;208:347-355.

46. Khan SR, Atmani F, Glenton P, Hou Z, Talham DR, Khurshid M. Lipids and membranes in the organic matrix of urinary calcific crystals and stones. *Calcif Tissue Int.* 1996;59:357-365.

47. Khan SR, Shevock PN, Hackett RL. In vitro precipitation of calcium oxalate in the presence of whole matrix or lipid components of the urinary stones. *J Urol.* 1988;139:418-422.

48. Khan SR, Maslamani SA, Atmani F, et al. Membranes and their constituents as promoters of calcium oxalate crystal formation in human urine. *Calcif Tissue Int.* 2000;66:90-96.

49. Lieske JC, Toback FG, Deganello S. Sialic acid-containing glycoproteins on renal cells determine nucleation of calcium oxalate dihydrate crystals. *Kidney Int.* 2001;60:1784-1791.

50. Drach GW, Thorson S, Randolph AD. Effects of urinary organic macromolecules on crystallisation of calcium oxalate: enhancement of nucleation. *J Urol.* 1980;123:519-523.

51. Robertson WG, Scurr DS. Modifiers of calcium crystallization found in urine I. Studies with a continuous crystallizer using an artificial urine. *J Urol.* 1986;135:1322-1326.

52. Rose GA, Sulaiman S. Tamm-Horsfall mucoproteins promote calcium oxalate crystal formation in urine: quantitative studies. *J Urol.* 1982;127:177-179.

53. Chauvet MC, Ryall RL. Intracrystalline proteins and calcium oxalate crystal degradation in MDCK II cells. *J Struct Biol.* 2005;151:12-17.

54. Ryall RL, Fleming DE, Grover PK, Chauvet MC, Dean CJ, Marshall VR. The hole truth: intracrystalline proteins and calcium oxalate kidney stones. *Mol Urol.* 2000;4:391-402.

55. Ryall RL, Fleming DE, Doyle IR, Evans NA, Dean CJ, Marshall VR. Intracrystalline proteins and the hidden ultrastructure of calcium oxalate urinary crystals: Implications for kidney stone formation. *J Struct Biol.* 2001;134:5-14.

56. Sutor DJ, Wooley SE. Growth studies of calcium oxalate in the presence of various compounds and ions II. *Br J Urol.* 1970;42:296-301.

57. Dent CE, Sutor DJ. Presence or absence of inhibitor of calcium oxalate crystal growth in urine of normals or stone formers. *Lancet.* 1971;ii:772-778.

58. Sarig S, Garti N, Azoury R, Wax Y, Perlberg S. A method for discrimination between calcium oxalate kidney stone formers and normals. *J Urol.* 1982;128:645-649.

59. Springmann KE, Drach GW, Gottung B, Randolph AD. Effects of human urine on aggregation of calcium oxalate crystals. *J Urol.* 1986;135:69-71.

60. Baumann JM, Bisaz S, Felix R, Fleisch H, Ganz U, Russell RGG. The role of inhibitors and other factors in the pathogenesis of calcium-containing renal stones. *Clin Sci Mol Med.* 1977;53:141-148.

61. Crassweller PO, Oreopoulos DG, Toguri A, Husdan H, Wilson DR, Rapoport A. Studies in inhibitors of calcification and levels of urine saturation with calcium oxalate in recurrent stone patients. *J Urol.* 1978;120:6-10.

62. Oreopoulos DG, Walker D, Akriotis DJ, et al. Excretion of inhibitors of calcification in urine, part I. Findings in control subjects and patients with renal stones. *Can Med Assoc J.* 1975;112:827-832.

63. Pylypchuk G, Ehrig V, Wilson DR. Differences in urine crystalloids, urine saturation with brushite and urine inhibitors of calcification between persons with and persons without recurrent kidney stone formation. *Can Med Assoc J.* 1979;120:658-665.

64. Ryall RL, Darroch JN, Marshall VR. The evaluation of risk factors in male stone formers attending a general hospital out-patient clinic. *Br J Urol.* 1984;56:116-121.

65. Ryall RL, Hibberd CM, Mazzachi BC, Marshall VR. Inhibitory activity of whole urine: a comparison of urines from stone formers and normal subjects. *Clin Chim Acta.* 1986;154:59-68.

66. Ryall RL, Harnett RM, Hibberd CM, Mazzachi BC, Mazzachi RD, Marshall VR. Urinary risk factors in calcium oxalate stone disease: a comparison of men and women. *Br J Urol.* 1987;60:480-488.

67. Asplin JR, Parks JH, Chen MS, et al. Reduced crystallization inhibition by urine from men with nephrolithiasis. *Kidney Int.* 1999;56:1505-1516.

68. Asplin JR, Parks JH, Nakagawa Y, Coe FL. Reduced crystallization inhibition by urine from women with nephrolithiasis. *Kidney Int.* 2002;61:1821-1829.

69. Bergsland KJ, Kinder JM, Asplin JR, Coe BJ, Coe FL. Influence of gender and age on calcium oxalate crystal growth inhibition by urine from relatives of stone forming patients. *J Urol.* 2002;167:2372-2376.

70. Ebisuno S, Umehara M, Kohjimoto Y, Ohkawa T. The effects of human urine on the adhesion of calcium oxalate crystals to Madin-Darby canine kidney cells. *BJU Int.* 1999;84:118-122.

71. Miyake O, Kakimoto K, Tsujihata M, Yoshimura K, Takahara S, Okuyama A. Strong inhibition of crystal-cell attachment by pediatric urinary macromolecules: a close relationship with high urinary citrate secretion. *Urology.* 2001;58:493-497.

72. Kumar V, Peña de la Vega L, Farell G, Lieske JC. Urinary macromolecular inhibition of crystal adhesion to renal epithelial cells is impaired in male stone formers. *Kidney Int.* 2005;68:1784-1792.

73. Grover PK, Thurgood LA, Ryall RL. Effect of urine fractionation on the attachment of calcium oxalate crystals to renal epithelial cells: implications for studying renal calculogenesis. *Am J Physiol Renal Physiol.* 2007;292:F1396-F1403.

74. Kumar V, Farell G, Lieske JC. Whole urinary proteins coat calcium oxalate monohydrate crystals to greatly decrease their adhesion to renal cells. *J Urol.* 2003;170:221-225.

75. Wiessner JH, Hung LY, Mandel NS. Crystal attachment to injured renal collecting duct cells: influence of urine proteins and pH. *Kidney Int.* 2003;63:1313-1320.

76. Escobar C, Byer KJ, Khan SR. Naturally produced crystals obtained from kidney stones are less injurious to renal tubular epithelial cells than synthetic crystals. *BJU Int.* 2007;100:891-897.

77. Lieske JC, Leonard R, Toback FG. Adhesion of calcium oxalate monohydrate crystals to renal epithelial cells is inhibited by specific anions. *Am J Physiol.* 1995;268:F604-F612.

78. Lieske JC, Norris R, Toback FG. Adhesion of hydroxyapatite crystals to anionic sites on the surface of renal epithelial cells. *Am J Physiol.* 1997;273:F224-F233.

79. Lieske JC, Farell G, Deganello S. The effect of ions at the surface of calcium oxalate monohydrate crystals on cell-crystal interactions. *Urol Res.* 2004;32:117-123.

80. Rabinovich YI, Daosukho S, Byer KJ, El-Shall HE, Khan SR. Direct AFM measurements of adhesion forces between calcium oxalate monohydrate and kidney epithelial cells in the presence of Ca^{2+} and Mg^{2+} ions. *J Colloid Interface Sci.* 2008;325:594-601.

81. Tsujihata M, Yoshimura K, Tsujikawa K, Tei N, Okuyama A. Fibronectin inhibits endocytosis of calcium oxalate crystals by renal tubular cells. *Int J Urol.* 2006;13:743-746.

82. Tsujikawa K, Tsujihata M, Tei N, Yoshimura K, Nonomura N, Okuyama A. Elucidation of the mechanism of crystal-cell interaction using fibronectin-overexpressing Madin-Darby canine kidney cells. *Urol Int.* 2007;79:157-163.

83. Ebisuno S, Nishihata M, Inagaki T, Umehara M, Kohjimoto Y. Bikunin prevents adhesion of calcium oxalate crystals to renal tubular cells in human urine. *J Am Soc Nephrol Suppl.* 1999;14:S436-440.

84. Tsujihata M, Momohara C, Yoshioka I, Tsujimura A, Nonomura N, Okuyama A. Atorvastatin inhibits renal crystal retention in a rat stone forming model. *J Urol.* 2008;180:2212-2217.

85. Thongboonkerd V, Semangoen T, Sinchaikul S, Chen ST. Proteomic analysis of calcium oxalate monohydrate crystal-induced toxicity in distal renal tubular cells. *J Proteome Res.* 2008;7:4689-4700.

86. Semangoen T, Sinchaikul S, Chen ST, Thongboonkerd V. Altered proteins in MDCK renal tubular cells in response to calcium oxalate dihydrate crystal adhesion: a proteomics approach. *J Proteome Res.* 2008;7:2889-2896.

87. Yamate T, Kohri K, Umekawa T, et al. The effect of osteopontin on the adhesion of calcium oxalate crystals to Madin-Darby Canine Kidney cells. *Eur Urol.* 1996;30:388-393.

88. Yamate T, Kohri K, Umekawa T, Iguchi M, Kurita T. Osteopontin antisense oligonucleotide inhibits adhesion of calcium oxalate crystals in Madin-Darby canine kidney cells. *J Urol.* 1998;160:1506-1512.

89. Sorokina EA, Wesson JA, Kleinman JG. An acidic peptide sequence of nucleolin-related protein can mediate the attachment of calcium oxalate to renal tubule cells. *J Am Soc Nephrol.* 2004;15:2057-2065.

90. Koul HK, Koul S. β-tubulin is the major cell membrane COM-crystal binding protein in renal epithelial cells. In: Gohel MDI, Au DWT, eds. *Kidney Stones: Inside and Out.* Hong Kong: The Hong Kong Polytechnic University; 2004:123-126.

91. Farell G, Huang E, Kim SY, Horstkorte R, Lieske JC. Modulation of proliferating renal epithelial cell affinity for calcium oxalate monohydrate crystals. *J Am Soc Nephrol.* 2004;15:3052-3062.

92. Kramer G, Steiner GE, Neumayer C, et al. Over-expression of anti-CD75 reactive proteins on distal and collecting renal tubular epithelial cells in calcium oxalate stone-forming kidneys in Egypt. *BJU Int.* 2004;93:822-826.

93. Sayer JA, Carr G, Pearce SH, Goodship TH, Simmons NL. Disordered calcium crystal handling in antisense CLC-5-treated collecting duct cells. *Biochem Biophys Res Commun.* 2003;300:305-10.

94. Sayer JA, Carr G, Simmons NL. Calcium phosphate and calcium oxalate crystal handling is dependent upon CLC-5 expression in mouse collecting duct cells. *Biochim Biophys Acta.* 2004;1689:83-90.

95. Verkoelen CF, Romijn JC, de Bruijn WC, Boevé ER, Cao LC, Schröder FH. Association of calcium oxalate monohydrate crystals with MDCK cells. *Kidney Int.* 1995;48:129-138.

96. de Water R, Leenen PJM, Nordermeer C, et al. Cytokine production induced by binding and processing of calcium oxalate crystals in cultured macrophages. *Am J Kidney Dis.* 2001;38:331-338.

97. de Water R, Noordermeer C, van der Kwast TH, et al. Calcium oxalate nephrolithiasis: effect of renal crystal deposition on the cellular composition of the renal interstitium. *Am J Kidney Dis.* 1999;33:761-771.

98. Lieske JC, Deganello S. Nucleation, adhesion and internalization of calcium-containing urinary crystals by renal cells. *J Am Soc Nephrol.* 1999;10:S422-S429.

99. Lieske JC, Deganello S, Toback FG. Cell-crystal interactions and kidney stone formation. *Nephron.* 1999;81(Suppl 1):8-17.

100. Fleming DE, van Riessen A, Chauvet MC, et al. Intracrystalline proteins and urolithiasis: A synchrotron X-ray diffraction study of calcium oxalate monohydrate. *J Bone Miner Res.* 2003;18:1282-1291.

101. Ryall RL, Grover PK, Thurgood LA, Chauvet MC, Fleming DE, van Bronswijk W. The importance of a clean face: The effect of different washing procedures on the association of Tamm-Horsfall glycoprotein and other urinary proteins with calcium oxalate crystals. *Urol Res.* 2007;35:1-14.

102. Stapleton AMF, Ryall RL. Blood coagulation proteins and urolithiasis are linked: crystal matrix protein is the F1 activation peptide of human prothrombin. *Br J Urol.* 1995;75:712-719.

103. Stapleton AMF, Simpson RJ, Ryall RL. Crystal matrix protein is related to human prothrombin. *Biochem Biophys Res Commun.* 1993;195:1199-1203.

104. Cook AF, Grover PK, Ryall RL. Face-specific binding of prothrombin fragment 1 and human serum albumin to inorganic and urinary calcium oxalate monohydrate crystals. *BJU Int.* 2008;103(6):826-835.

105. Ryall RL. Macromolecules and urolithiasis: parallels and paradoxes. *Nephron Physiol.* 2004;98:37-42.

106. Grover PK, Thurgood LA, Fleming DE, van Bronswijk W, Wang T, Ryall RL. Intracrystalline urinary proteins facilitate degradation and dissolution of calcium oxalate crystals in cultured renal cells. *Am J Physiol Renal Physiol.* 2007;278:F130-F137.

107. Fleisch H, Bisaz S. Isolation from urine of pyrophosphate, a calcification inhibitor. *Am J Physiol.* 1962;203:671-675.

108. March JG, Simonet BM, Grases F. Determination of pyrophosphate in renal calculi and urine by means of an enzymatic method. *Clin Chim Acta*. 2001;314:187-194.

109. Doremus RH, Teich S, Silvis PX. Crystallization of calcium oxalate from synthetic urine. *Invest Urol*. 1978;15:469-472.

110. Sutor DJ. Growth studies of calcium oxalate in the presence of various ions and compounds. *Br J Urol*. 1969;41:171-178.

111. Welshman SG, McGeown MG. A quantitative investigation of the effects on the growth of calcium oxalate crystals of potential inhibitors. *Br J Urol*. 1972;44:677-680.

112. Ryall RL, Harnett RM, Marshall VR. The effect of urine, pyrophosphate, citrate, magnesium and glycosaminoglycans on the growth and aggregation of calcium oxalate crystals in vitro. *Clin Chim Acta*. 1981;112:349-356.

113. Robertson WG, Peacock M, Nordin BEC. Inhibitors of the growth and aggregation of calcium oxalate crystals in vitro. *Clin Chim Acta*. 1973;43:31-37.

114. Ryall RL, Hibberd CM, Marshall VR. A method for studying inhibitory activity in whole urine. *Urol Res*. 1985;13:285-289.

115. Hallson PC, Rose GA, Sulaiman S. Pyrophosphate does not influence calcium oxalate or calcium phosphate crystal formation in concentrated whole human urine. *Urol Res*. 1983;11:151-154.

116. Fleisch H, Bisaz S. Mechanism of calcification: inhibitory role of pyrophosphate. *Nature*. 1962;195:911.

117. Roberts NB, Dutton J, Helliwell T, Rothwell PJ, Kavanagh JP. Pyrophosphate in synovial fluid and urine and its relationship to urinary risk factors for stone disease. *Ann Clin Biochem*. 1992;29:529-534.

118. Schwille PO, Rümenapf G, Wölfel G, Köhler R. Urinary pyrophosphate in patients with recurrent calcium urolithiasis and in healthy controls: a re-evaluation. *J Urol*. 1988;140:239-245.

119. Sharma S, Vaidyanathan S, Thind SK, Nath R. Urinary excretion of inorganic pyrophosphate by normal subjects and patients with renal calculi in north-western India and the effect of diclofenac sodium upon urinary excretion of pyrophosphate in stone formers. *Urol Int*. 1992;48:404-408.

120. Wikström B, Danielson BG, Ljunghall S, McGuire M, Russell RGG. Urinary pyrophosphate excretion in renal stone formers with normal and impaired renal function. *World J Urol*. 1983;1:150-154.

121. O'Brien MM, Uhlemann I, McIntosh HW. Urinary pyrophosphate in normal subjects and in stone formers. *Can Med Assoc J*. 1967;96:100-103.

122. Robertson WG, Peacock M, Heyburn PJ, Marshall DH, Clark PB. Risk factors in calcium stone disease of the urinary tract. *Br J Urol*. 1978;50:449-454.

123. Russell RGG, Hodgkinson A. The urinary excretion of inorganic pyrophosphate by normal subjects and patients with renal calculus. *Clin Sci*. 1966;31:51-62.

124. Schlieper G, Westenfeld R, Brandenberg V, Ketteler M. Inhibitors of calcification in blood and urine. *Semin Dial*. 2007;20:113-121.

125. Moochhala SH, Sayer JA, Carr G, Simmons NL. Renal calcium stones: insights from the control of bone mineralization. *Exp Physiol*. 2007;93(1):43-49.

126. Costa-Bauzá A, Isern B, Perelló J, Sanchis P, Grases F. Factors affecting the regrowth of renal stones in vitro: a contribution to the understanding of renal stone development. *Scand J Urol Nephrol*. 2005;39:194-199.

127. Cramer W. Experimental production of kidney lesions by diet. *Lancet*. 1932;ii:174-175.

128. Li MK, Blacklock NJ, Garside J. Effects of magnesium on calcium oxalate crystallization. *J Urol*. 1985;133:123-125.

129. Azoury R, Garside J, Robertson WG. Calcium oxalate precipitation in a flow system: an attempt to simulate the early stages of stone formation in the renal tubules. *J Urol*. 1986;136:150-153.

130. Bertoni E, Bigi A, Cojazzi G, Gandolfi M, Panzavolta S, Roveri N. Nanocrystals of magnesium and fluoride substituted hydroxyapatite. *J Inorganic Biochem*. 1998;72:29-35.

131. Meyer JL, Smith LH. Growth of calcium oxalate crystals. II. Inhibition by natural crystal growth inhibitors. *Invest Urol*. 1975;13:36-39.

132. Ryall RL, Grover PK, Harnett RM, Hibberd CM, Marshall VR. Small molecular weight inhibitors. In: Walker VR, Sutton RAL, Cameron EC, Pak CYC, Robertson WG, eds. *Urolithiasis*. New York: Plenum; 1989:91-96.

133. Hallson PC, Rose GA, Sulaiman S. Magnesium reduces calcium oxalate crystal formation in human whole urine. *Clin Sci*. 1982;62:17-19.

134. Atakan IH, Kaplan M, Seren G, Aktoz T, Gül H, Inci O. Serum, urinary and stone zinc, iron, magnesium and copper levels in idiopathic calcium oxalate stone patients. *Int Urol Nephrol*. 2007;39:351-356.

135. Ogawa Y, Yonou H, Hokama S, Oda M, Morozumi M, Sugaya K. Urinary saturation and risk factors for calcium oxalate stone disease based on spot and 24-hour urine specimens. *Front Biosci*. 2003;8:a167-76.

136. Trinchieri A, Mandressi A, Luongo P, Rovera F, Longo G. Urinary excretion of citrate, glycosaminoglycans, magnesium and zinc in relation to age and sex in normal subjects and in patients who form calcium stones. *Scand J Urol Nephrol*. 1992;26:379-386.

137. Bach D, Hesse A, Strenge A, Vahlensieck W. Magnesium excretion in urine on condition of individual standard diet in healthy controls and calcium oxalate stone formers. In: Smith LH, Robertson WG, Finlayson B, eds. *Urolithiasis: Clinical and Basic Research*. New York: Plenum; 1981:45-49.

138. Johansson G, Backman U, Danielson BG, Fellström B, Ljunghall S. Biochemical and clinical effects of the prophylactic treatment of renal calcium stones with magnesium hydroxide. *J Urol*. 1980;124:770-774.

139. Resnick MI, Munday D, Boyce WH. Magnesium excretion and calcium oxalate urolithiasis. *Urology*. 1982;20:385-389.

140. Robertson WG, Peacock M, Nordin BEC. Activity products in stone-forming and non-stone-forming urines. *Clin Sci*. 1968;34:579-594.

141. Stejskal D, Karpisek M, Vrtal R, et al. Urine fetuin-A values in relation to the presence of urolithiasis. *BJU Int*. 2008;101:1151-1154.

142. Su CJ, Shevock PN, Khan SR, Hackett RL. Effect of magnesium on calcium oxalate urolithiasis. *J Urol*. 1991;145:1092-1095.

143. Khan SR, Shevock PN, Hackett RL. Magnesium oxide administration and prevention of calcium oxalate nephrolithiasis. *J Urol*. 1993;149:412-416.

144. Ogawa Y, Yamaguchi K, Morozumi M. Effects of magnesium salts in preventing experimental urolithiasis in rats. *J Urol*. 1990;144:385-389.

145. Ryall RL, Marshall VR. The value of the 24hr urine analysis in the assessment of stone formers attending a general hospital outpatient clinic. *Br J Urol*. 1983;55:1-5.

146. Massey L. Magnesium therapy for nephrolithiasis. *Magnes Res*. 2005;18:123-126.

147. Hallson PC, Rose GA, Sulaiman S. Raising urinary citrate lowers calcium oxalate and calcium phosphate crystal formation in whole urine. *Urol Int*. 1983;38:179-181.

148. Qiu SR, Wierzbicki A, Orme CA, et al. Molecular modulation of calcium oxalate crystallization by osteopontin and citrate. *PNAS*. 2004;101:1811-1815.

149. Qiu SR, Wierzbicki A, Salter A, et al. Modulation of calcium oxalate monohydrate crystallization by citrate through selective binding to atomic steps. *J Am Chem Soc*. 2005;127:9036-9044.

150. Kok DJ, Papapoulos SE, Bijvoet OLM. Excessive crystal agglomeration with low citrate excretion in recurrent stone formers. *Lancet*. 1986;i:1056-1058.

151. Shorr E, Almy TP, Sloan MH, Taussky H, Toscani V. The relation between the urinary excretion of citric acid and calcium: its implications for urinary calcium stone formation. *Science*. 1942;96:587-588.

152. Curhan GC, Willett WC, Speizer FE, Stampfer MJ. Twenty-four-hour urine chemistries and the risk of kidney stones among women and men. *Kidney Int*. 2001;59:2290-2298.

153. Mithani S, Zaidi Z. Comparison of 24 hours urinary citrate levels in urolithiasis patients and healthy controls. *J Pak Med Assoc*. 2005;55:371-373.

154. Shah O, Assimos DG, Holmes RP. Genetic and dietary factors in urinary citrate excretion. *J Endourol*. 2005;19:177-181.

155. Cupisti A, Morelli E, Lupetti S, Meola M, Barsotti G. Low urine citrate excretion as a main risk factor for recurrent calcium oxalate nephrolithiasis in males. *Nephron*. 1992;61:73-76.

156. Domrongkitchaiporn S, Stitchantrakul W, Kochakarn W. Causes of hypocitraturia in recurrent stone formers: focusing on urinary potassium excretion. *Am J Kidney Dis*. 2006;48:546-554.

157. Pak CYC. Citrate and renal calculi: an update. *Min Electrolyte Metab*. 1994;20:371-377.

158. Rudman D, Kutner MH, Redd SC, Waters WC, Gerron GG, Bleier J. Hypocitraturia in calcium nephrolithiasis. *J Clin Endocrinol Metab*. 1982;55:1050-1057.

159. Goldberg H, Grass L, Vogl R, Rapoport A, Oreopoulos DG. Urine citrate and renal stone disease. *CMAJ*. 1989;141:217-221.

160. Curhan GC, Taylor EN. 24-h uric acid excretion and the risk of kidney stones. *Kidney Int*. 2008;73:489-496.

161. Ebisuno S, Morimoto S, Yoshida T, Fukatani T, Yasukawa S, Ohkawa T. Effect of dietary calcium and magnesium on experimental tubular deposition of calcium oxalate crystals induced by ethylene glycol administration and its prevention with phytin and citrate. *Urol Int*. 1987;42:330-337.

162. Ogawa Y, Tanaka T, Yamaguchi K, Morozumi M, Kitagawa R. Effects of sodium citrate, potassium citrate, and citric acid in preventing experimental calc oxalate urolithiasis in rats. *Hinyokika Kiyo*. 1987;33:1772-1777.

163. Selvam R, Bijikurien T. Effect of citrate on free radical induced changes in experimental urolithiasis. *Indian J Exp Biol*. 1992;30:705-710.

164. Yasui T, Sato M, Fujita K, Tozawa K, Nomura S, Kohri K. Effects of citrate on renal stone formation and osteopontin expression in a rat urolithiasis model. *Urol Res*. 2001;29:50-56.

165. Zhou JR, Erdman JW. Phytic acid in health and disease. *Crit Rev Food Sci Nutr*. 1995;35:495-508.

166. Modlin M. Urinary phosphorylated inositols and renal stone. *Lancet*. 1980;2:1113-1114.

167. Ohkawa T, Ebisuno S, Kitagawa M, Morimoto S, Miyazaki Y, Yasukawa S. Rice bran treatment for patients with hypercalciuric stones: experimental and clinical studies. *J Urol*. 1984;132:1140-1145.

168. Shah PJ, Green NA, Williams G. Unprocessed bran and its effect on urinary calcium excretion in idiopathic hypercalciuria. *Br Med J*. 1980;281:426.

169. Grases F, Garcia-Gonzalez R, Torres JJ, Llobera A. Effects of phytic acid on renal stone formation in rats. *Scan J Urol Nephrol*. 1998;32:261-265.

170. Grases F, Costa-Bauzá A. Phytate (IP6) is a powerful agent for preventing calcifications in biological fluids: usefulness in renal lithiasis treatment. *Anticancer Res*. 1999;19:3717-3722.

171. Grases F, Simonet BM, March JG, Prieto RM. Inositol hexakisphosphate in urine: the relationship between oral intake and urinary excretion. *BJU Int*. 2000;85:138-142.

172. Grases F, March JG, Prieto RM, et al. Urinary phytate in calcium oxalate stone formers and healthy people – dietary effects on phytate excretion. *Scan J Urol Nephrol*. 2000;34:162-164.

173. Grases F, Perelló J, Simonet BM, Prieto RM, García-Raja A. Study of potassium phytate effects on decreasing urinary calcium in rats. *Urol Int*. 2004;72:237-243.

174. Wu N, Thon WF, Krah H, Schlick R, Jonas U. Effects of magnesium citrate and phytin on reducing urinary calcium excretion in rats. *World J Urol*. 1994;12:323-328.

175. Grases F, Isern B, Sanchis P, Perello J, Torres JJ, Costa-Bauza A. Phytate acts as an inhibitor in formation of renal calculi. *Front Biosci*. 2007;12:2580-2587.

176. Costa-Bauzá A, Perelló J, Isern B, Sanchis P, Grases F. Factors affecting calcium oxalate dihydrate fragmented regrowth. *BMC Urol*. 2006;5:6-16.

177. Raboy V. Progress in breeding low phytate crops. *J Nutr*. 2002;132:503S-505S.

178. Thomas E, von Unruh GE, Hesse A. Influence of a low- and a high-oxalate vegetarian diet on intestinal absorption and urinary excretion. *Eur J Clin Nutr*. 2008;62:1090-1097.

179. Boyce WH. Organic matrix of human urinary concretions. *Am J Med*. 1968;45:673-683.

180. Khan SR, Kok DJ. Modulators of urinary stone formation. *Front Biosci*. 2004;9:1450-1482.

181. Nagatsuka Y, Sato K, Ototani N, Yosizawa Z. A method of screening test for excretion pattern of urinary glycosaminoglycans and its application to normal human urine. *Tohoku J Exp Med*. 1980;132:159-171.

182. Gohel MD, Shum DK, Tam PC. Electrophoretic separation and characterization of urinary glycosaminoglycans and their roles in urolithiasis. *Carbohydr Res*. 2007;342:79-86.

183. Goldberg JM, Cotlier E. Specific isolation and analysis of mucopolysaccharides (glycosaminoglycans) from human urine. *Clin Chim Acta*. 1972;41:19-27.

184. Heintz B, Stöcker G, Mrowka C, et al. Decreased glomerular basement membrane heparan sulphate proteoglycan in essential hypertension. *Hypertension*. 1995;25:399-407.

185. Manley G, Severn M, Hawksworth J. Excretion patterns of glycosaminoglycans and glycoproteins in normal human urine. *J Clin Pathol*. 1968;21:339-345.

186. Shum DK, Gohel MD, Tam PC. Hyaluronans: crystallization-promoting activity and HPLC analysis of urinary excretion. *J Am Soc Nephrol Suppl*. 1999;14:S397-S403.

187. Nishio S, Abe Y, Wakatsuki A, et al. Matrix glycosaminoglycan in urinary stones. *J Urol*. 1985;143:503-505.

188. Roberts SD, Resnick MI. Glycosaminoglycans content of stone matrix. *J Urol*. 1986;135:1078-1083.

189. Fellström B, Danielson BG, Ljunghall S, Wikström B. Crystal inhibition: the effects of polyanions on calcium oxalate crystal growth. *Clin Chim Acta*. 1986;158:229-235.

190. Sheng X, Jung T, Wesson JA, Ward MD. Adhesion at calcium oxalate crystal surfaces and the effect of urinary constituents. *PNAS*. 2005;102:267-272.

191. Kohri K, Garside J, Blacklock NJ. The effect of glycosaminoglycans on the crystallization of calcium oxalate. *Br J Urol*. 1989;63:584-590.

192. Pak CYC, Holt K, Zerwekh JE. Attenuation by monosodium urate of the inhibitory effect of glycosaminoglycans on calcium oxalate nucleation. *Invest Urol*. 1979;17:138-140.

193. Scurr DS, Robertson WG. Modifiers of calcium oxalate crystallization found in urine. II. Studies on their mode of action in an artificial urine. *J Urol*. 1986;136:128-131.

194. Michelacci YM, Boim MA, Bergamaschi CT, Rovigatti RM, Schor N. Possible role for chondroitin sulfate in urolithiasis: in vivo studies in an experimental model. *Clin Chim Acta*. 1992;208:1-8.

195. Osswald H, Weinheimer G, Schütt I-D, Ernst W. Effective prevention of calcium-oxalate crystal formation in vitro and in vivo by pentosan polysulfate. In: Walker VR, Sutton RAL, Cameron ECB, Pak CYC, Robertson WG, eds. *Urolithiasis*. New York and London: Plenum; 1989:141-144.

196. Suzuki K, Ryall RL. The effect of heparan sulphate on the crystallization of calcium oxalate in undiluted, ultrafiltered human urine. *Br J Urol.* 1996;78:15-21.

197. Shum DK, Gohel MD. Separate effects of urinary chondroitin sulphate and heparan sulphate on the crystallization of urinary calcium oxalate: differences between stone formers and normal control subjects. *Clin Sci.* 1993;85:33-39.

198. Takazono I. Role of heparan sulphate proteoglycans (syndecan 1) on the renal epithelial cells during calcium oxalate monohydrate crystal attachment. *Kurume Med J.* 2002;49:201-210.

199. Iida S, Inoue M, Yoshii S, et al. Molecular detection of heparan sulphate proteoglycan mRNA in rat kidney during calcium oxalate nephrolithiasis. *J Am Soc Nephrol.* 1999;14:S412-S416.

200. Eguchi Y, Inoue M, Iida S, Matsuoka K, Noda S. Heparan sulfate (HS)/heparan sulfate proteoglycan (HSPG) and bikunin are up-regulated during calcium oxalate nephrolithiasis in rat kidney. *Kurume Med.* 2002;49:99-107.

201. Verkoelen CF. Crystal retention in renal stone disease: a crucial role for the glycosaminoglycan hyaluronan. *J Am Soc Nephrol.* 2006;17:1673-1687.

202. Borges FT, Michelacci YM, Aguiar JA, Dalboni MA, Garófalo AS, Schor N. Characterization of glycosaminoglycans in tubular epithelial cells: calcium oxalate and oxalate ions effects. *Kidney Int.* 2005;68:1630-1642.

203. Cao LC, Boevé ER, Schröder FH, Robertson WG, Ketelaars GAM, Bruijn D. The effect of two new semi-synthetic glycosaminoglycans (G871, G872) on the zeta potential of calcium oxalate crystals and on growth and agglomeration. *J Urol.* 1992;147:1643-1646.

204. Grases F, Gil JJ, Conte A. Glycosaminoglycans inhibition of calcium oxalate crystalline growth and promotion of crystal aggregation. *Coll Surf.* 1989;36:29-38.

205. Martin X, Werness PG, Bergert JH, Smith LH. Pentosan polysulfate as an inhibitor of calcium oxalate crystal growth. *J Urol.* 1984;132:786-788.

206. Norman RW, Scurr DS, Robertson WG, Peacock M. Inhibition of calcium oxalate crystallisation by pentosan polysulphate in control subjects and stone formers. *Br J Urol.* 1984;56:594-598.

207. Suzuki K, Miyazawa K, Tsugawa R. Inhibitory effect of sodium pentosan polysulfate on the formation, growth and aggregation of calcium oxalate in vitro. *Jpn J Urol.* 1989;80:526-531.

208. Miyazawa K, Suzuki K, Tsugawa R. The quantitative study of inhibitory effect of pentosan polysulfate and chlorophyllin on the experimental calcium oxalate stone. *Jpn J Urol.* 1989;80:861-869.

209. Jones M, Monga M. Is there a role for pentosan polysulfate in the prevention of calcium oxalate stones? *J Endourol.* 2003;17:855-858.

210. Baggio B, Gambaro G, Cicerello E, et al. Urinary excretion of glycosaminoglycans in urological disease. *Clin Biochem.* 1987;20:449-450.

211. Michelacci YM, Glashan RQ, Schor N. Urinary excretion of glycosaminoglycans in normal and stone forming subjects. *Urol Int.* 1989;44:218-221.

212. Nesse A, Garbossa G, Romero MC, Bogardo CE, Zanchetta JR. Glycosaminoglycans in urolithiasis. *Nephron.* 1992;62:36-39.

213. Nikkilä MT. Urinary glycosaminoglycan excretion in normal and stone-forming subjects: significant disturbance in recurrent stone formers. *Urol Int.* 1989;44:157-159.

214. Hwang TIS, Preminger GM, Poindexter J, Pak CYC. Urinary glycosaminoglycans in normal subjects and patients with stones. *J Urol.* 1988;139:995-997.

215. Akinci N, Esen T, Kocak T, Ozsoy C, Tellaloglu S. The role of inhibitor deficiency in urolithiasis. I. Rationale of urinary magnesium, citrate, pyrophosphate and glycosaminoglycan determinations. *Eur Urol.* 1992;19:240-243.

216. Caudarella R, Stefani F, Rizzoli E, Malavolta N, D'Antuono G. Preliminary results of glycosaminoglycans excretion in normal and stone forming subjects: Relationship with uric acid excretion. *J Urol.* 1983;129:665-667.

217. Hesse A, Wuzel H, Vahlensieck W. The excretion of glycosaminoglycans in the urine of calcium-oxalate-stone patients and healthy persons. *Urol Int.* 1986;41:81-87.

218. Ryall RL, Marshall VR. The relationship between urinary inhibitory activity and endogenous concentrations of glycosaminoglycans and uric acid: comparison of urines from stone formers and normal subjects. *Clin Chim Acta.* 1984;141:197-204.

219. Samuell CT. A study of glycosaminoglycan excretion in normal and stone-forming subjects using a modified cetylpyridinium chloride technique. *Clin Chim Acta.* 1981;117:63-73.

220. Harangi F, Györke Z, Melegh B. Urinary glycosaminoglycan excretion in healthy and stone forming children. *Pediatr Nephrol.* 1996;10:555-558.

221. Lama G, Carbone MG, Marrone N, Russo P, Spagnolo G. Promoters and inhibitors of calcium urolithiasis in children. *Child Nephrol Urol.* 1990;10:81-84.

222. Nakagawa Y, Margolis HC, Yokoyama S, Kézdy FJ, Kaiser ET, Coe FL. Purification and characterization of a calcium oxalate monohydrate crystal growth inhibitor from human kidney tissue culture medium. *J Biol Chem.* 1981;256:3936-3944.

223. Worcester EM, Nakagawa Y, Wabner CL, Kumar S, Fl C. Crystal adsorption and growth slowing by nephrocalcin, albumin, and Tamm-Horsfall protein. *Am J Physiol Renal Physiol.* 1988;255:F1197-F1205.

224. Tang Y, Grover PK, Moritz RL, Simpson RJ, Ryall RL. Is nephrocalcin related to the urinary derivative (bikunin) of inter-a-trypsin inhibitor? *Br J Urol.* 1995;76:425-30.

225. Canales BK, Anderson L, Higgins L, et al. Comprehensive proteomic analysis of human calcium oxalate monohydrate kidney stone matrix. *αJ Endourol.* 2008;22:1161-1167.

226. Kaneko K, Yamanobe T, Nakagomi K, Mawatari K, Onoda M, Fujimori S. Detection of protein Z in a renal calculus composed of calcium oxalate monohydrate with the use of liquid chromatography-mass spectrometry/mass spectrometry following two-dimensional polyacrylamide gel electrophoresis separation. *Anal Biochem.* 2004;324:191-196.

227. Merchant M, Cummins T, Wilkey D, et al. Proteomic analysis of renal calculi indicates an important role for inflammatory processes in calcium stone formation. *Am J Physiol Renal Physiol.* 2008;295:F1254-258.

228. Mushtaq S, Siddiqui AA, Naqvi ZA, et al. Identification of myeloperoxidase, alpha-defensin and calgranulin in calcium oxalate renal stones. *Clin Chim Acta.* 2007;284:41-47.

229. González-Buitrago JM, Ferreira L, Lorenzo I. Urinary proteomics. *Clin Chim Acta.* 2007;375:49-56.

230. Chen WC, Lai CC, Tsai Y, Lin WY, Tsai FJ. Mass spectroscopic characteristics of low molecular weight proteins extracted from calcium oxalate stones: preliminary study. *J Clin Lab Anal.* 2008;22:77-85.

231. Miyazawa K, Domiki C, Moriyama M, Suzuki K. cDNA macroarray analysis of genes in renal epithelial cells exposed to calcium oxalate crystals. In: Gohel MDI, Au DWT, eds. *Kidney Stones: Inside and Out.* Hong Kong: The Hong Kong Polytechnic University; 2004:130-131.

232. Morse RM, Resnick MI. A new approach to the study of urinary macromolecules as a participant in calcium oxalate crystallization. *J Urol.* 1988;139:869-873.

233. Doyle IR, Ryall RL, Marshall VR. Inclusion of proteins into calcium oxalate crystals precipitated from human urine: A highly selective phenomenon. *Clin Chem.* 1991;37:1589-1594.

234. Hess B. The role of Tamm-Horsfall glycoprotein and nephrocalcin in calcium oxalate monohydrate crystallization processes. *Scan Microsc.* 1991;5:689-696.

235. Hess B. Tamm-Horsfall glycoprotein – Inhibitor or promoter of calcium oxalate monohydrate crystallization processes? *Urol Res.* 1992;20:83-86.

236. Atmani F, Khan SR. Quantification of proteins extracted from calcium oxalate and calcium phosphate crystals induced in vitro in the urine of healthy controls and stone-forming patients. *Urol Int.* 2002;68:54-59.

237. Atmani F, Glenton PA, Khan SR. Identification of proteins extracted from calcium oxalate and calcium phosphate crystals in the urine of healthy and stone forming subjects. *Urol Res.* 1998;26:201-207.

238. Maslamani S, Glenton PA, Khan SR. Changes in urine macromolecular composition during processing. *J Urol.* 2000;164:230-236.

239. Walton RC, Kavanagh JP, Heywood BR, Rao PN. The association of different urinary proteins with calcium oxalate hydromorphs. Evidence for non-specific interactions. *Biochim Biophys Acta.* 2005;1723:175-183.

240. Deganello S. The interaction between nephrocalcin and Tamm-Horsfall proteins with calcium oxalate dihydrate. *Scan Microsc.* 1993;7:1111-1118.

241. Miyake O, Yoshioka T, Yoshimura K, et al. Expression of Tamm-Horsfall protein in stone-forming rat models. *Br J Urol.* 1998;81:14-19.

242. Mo L, Huang HY, Zhu XH, Shapiro E, Hasty DL, Wu XR. Tamm-Horsfall protein is a critical renal defense factor protecting against calcium oxalate crystal formation. *Kidney Int.* 2004;66:1159-1166.

243. Grover PK, Moritz RL, Simpson RJ, Ryall RL. Inhibition of calcium oxalate crystal growth and aggregation in vitro. A comparison of four human proteins. *Eur J Biochem.* 1998;253:637-644.

244. Kitamura T, Pak CYC. Tamm and Horsfall glycoprotein does not promote spontaneous precipitation and crystal growth of calcium oxalate in vitro. *J Urol.* 1982;127:1024-1026.*Eur J Biochem*

245. Rose GA, Sulaiman S. Tamm-Horsfall mucoprotein promotes calcium phosphate crystal formation in urine: quantitative studies. *Urol Res.* 1984;12:217-221.

246. Grover PK, Ryall RL, Marshall VR. Tamm-Horsfall mucoprotein reduces promotion of calcium oxalate crystal aggregation induced by urate in human urine in vitro. *Clin Sci.* 1994;87:137-144.

247. Serafini-Cessi F, Monti A, Cavallone D. N-Glycans carried by Tamm-Horsfall glycoprotein have a crucial role in the defense against urinary tract disease. *Glycoconj J.* 2005;22:383-394.

248. Hsieh N, Shih CH, Chen HY, Wu MC, Chen WC, Li CW. Effects of Tamm-Horsfall protein on the protection of MDCK cells from oxalate induced free radical injury. *Urol Res.* 2003;31:10-16.

249. Schnierle P. A simple diagnostic test for the differentiation of Tamm-Horsfall glycoproteins from healthy probands and those from recurrent calcium oxalate renal stone formers. *Experientia.* 1995;51:1068-1072.

250. Knörle R, Schnierle P, Koch A, et al. Tamm-Horsfall glycoprotein: role in inhibition and promotion of renal calcium oxalate stone formation studied with Fourier transform infrared spectroscopy. *Clin Chem.* 1994;40:1739-1743.

251. Hallson PC, Choong SK, Kasidas GP, Samuell CT. Effects of Tamm-Horsfall protein with normal and reduced sialic acid content upon the crystallization of calcium phosphate and calcium oxalate in human urine. *Br J Urol.* 1997;80:533-538.

252. Jaggi M, Nakagawa Y, Zipperle L, Hess B. Tamm-Horsfall protein in recurrent calcium kidney stone formers with positive family history: abnormalities in urinary excretion, molecular structure and function. *Urol Res.* 2007;35:55-62.

253. Grover PK, Resnick MI. Evidence for the presence of abnormal proteins in the urine of recurrent stone formers. *J Urol.* 1995;153:1716-1721.

254. Trewick AL, Rumsby G. Isoelectric focusing of native urinary uromodulin (Tamm-Horsfall protein) shows no physicochemical differences between stone formers and non-stone formers. *Urol Res.* 2000;27:250-254.

255. Gokhale JA, Glenton PA, Khan SR. Characterization of Tamm-Horsfall protein in a rat nephrolithiasis model. *J Urol.* 2001;166:L1492-1497.

256. Marengo SR, Chen DH, Kaung HL, Resnick MI, Yang L. Decreased renal expression of the putative calcium oxalate inhibitor Tamm-Horsfall protein in the ethylene glycol rat model of calcium oxalate urolithiasis. *J Urol.* 2002;167:2192-2197.

257. Gokhale JA, McKee MD, Khan SR. Localization of Tamm-Horsfall protein and osteopontin in a rat nephrolithiasis model. *Nephron.* 1996;73:456-461.

258. Gokhale JA, McKee MD, Khan SR. Immunocytochemical localization of Tamm-Horsfall protein in the kidneys of normal and nephrolithic rats. *Urol Res.* 1996;24:201-209.

259. Bichler KH, Kirchner C, Ideler V. Uromucoid excretion of normal individuals and stone formers. *Br J Urol.* 1976;47:733-738.

260. Grant AMS, Baker LRI, Neuberger A. Urinary Tamm-Horsfall glycoprotein in certain kidney disease and its content in renal and bladder calculi. *Clin Sci.* 1973;44:377-384.

261. Pourmand G, Nasseh H, Sarrafnejad A, et al. Comparison of urinary proteins in calcium stone formers and healthy individuals: a case-control study. *Urol Int.* 2006;76:163-168.

262. Glauser A, Hochreiter W, Jaeger P, Hess B. Determinants of urinary excretion of Tamm-Horsfall protein in non-selected kidney stone formers and healthy subjects. *Nephrol Dial Transplant.* 2000;15:1580-1587.

263. Lau WH, Leong WS, Ismail Z, Gam LH. Qualification and application of an ELISA for the determination of Tamm-Horsfall protein (THP) in human urine and its use for screening of kidney stone disease. *Int J Biol Sci.* 2008;4:215-222.

264. Romero MC, Nocera S, Nesse AB. Decreased Tamm-Horsfall protein in lithiasic patients. *Clin Biochem.* 1997;30:63-67.

265. Bichler K, Mittermüller B, Strohmaier WL, Feil G, Eipper E. Excretion of Tamm-Horsfall protein in patients with uric acid stones. *Urol Int.* 1999;62:87-92.

266. Fuselier HA, Ward DM, Lindberg JS, et al. Urinary Tamm-Horsfall protein increased after potassium citrate therapy in calcium stone formers. *Urology.* 1995;45:942-946.

267. Hoyer JR. Uropontin in urinary calcium stone formation. *Miner Electrolyte Metab.* 1995;20:385-392.

268. McKee MD, Nanci A, Khan SR. Ultrastructural immunodetection of osteopontin and osteocalin as major matrix components of renal calculi. *J Bone Miner Res.* 1995;10:1913-1929.

269. Tawada T, Fujita K, Sakakura T, et al. Distribution of osteopontin and calprotectin as matrix protein in calcium-containing stone. *Urol Res.* 1999;27:238-242.

270. Evan AP, Coe FL, Rittling SR, et al. Apatite plaque particles in inner medulla of kidneys of calcium oxalate stone formers: osteopontin localization. *Kidney Int.* 2005;68:145-154.

271. Shiraga H, Min W, VanDusen WJ, et al. Inhibition of calcium oxalate crystal growth in vitro by uropontin: another member of the aspartic acid-rich protein superfamily. *PNAS.* 1992;89:426-430.

272. Xie Y, Sakatsume M, Nishi S, Narita I, Arakawa M, Gejyo F. Expression, roles, receptors, and regulation of osteopontin in the kidney. *Kidney Int.* 2001;60:1645-1657.

273. Reinholt FP, Hultenby K, Oldberg A, Heingard D. Osteopontin – a possible anchor of osteoblasts to bone. *PNAS.* 1990;87:4473-4475.

274. Johnston NI, Gunasekharan VK, Ravindranath A, O'Connell C, Johnston PG, El-Tanani MK. Osteopontin as a target for cancer therapy. *Front Biosci.* 2008;13:4361-4372.

275. Asakura H. Osteopontin and stone formation. *Int J Urol.* 2002;9:108.

276. Jahnen-Dechent W, Schäfer C, Ketteler M, McKee MD. Mineral chaperones: a role for fetuin-A and osteopontin in the inhibition and regression of pathologic calcification. *J Mol Med.* 2008;86:389-389.

277. Kleinman JG, Wesson JA, Hughes J. Osteopontin and calcium stone formation. *Nephron Physiol.* 2004;98:43-47.

278. Mazzali M, Kipari T, Ophascharoensuk V, Wesson JA, Johnson R, Hughes J. Osteopontin – A molecule for all seasons. *QJM.* 2002;95:3-13.

279. Scatena M, Liaw L, Giachelli CM. Osteopontin: a multifunctional molecule regulating chronic inflammation and vascular disease. *Arterioscler Thromb Vasc Biol.* 2007;27:2302-2309.

280. Nishio S, Iseda T, Takeda H, Iwata H, Yokoyama M. Inhibitory effect of calcium phosphate-associated proteins on calcium oxalate crystallization: alpha2-HS-glycoprotein, prothrombin-F1 and osteopontin. *BJU Int.* 2000;86:543-548.

281. Asplin JR, Arsenault D, Parks JH, Coe FL, Hoyer JR. Contribution of uropontin to inhibition of calcium oxalate crystallization. *Kidney Int.* 1998;53:194-199.

282. Taller A, Grohe B, Rogers KA, Goldberg HA, Hunter GK. Specific adsorption of osteopontin and synthetic polypeptides to calcium oxalate monohydrate crystals. *Biophys J.* 2007;93:1768-1777.

283. Wesson JA, Ganne V, Beshensky AM, Kleinman JG. Regulation by macromolecules of calcium oxalate crystal aggregation in stone formers. *Urol Res.* 2005;33:206-212.

284. Konya E, Umekawa T, Iguchi M, Kurita T. The role of osteopontin on calcium oxalate crystal formation. *Eur Urol.* 2003;43:564-571.

285. Koka RM, Huang E, Lieske JC. Adhesion of uric acid crystals to the surface of renal epithelial cells. *Am J Physiol Renal Physiol.* 2000;278:F989-F998.

286. Yamate T, Kohri K, Umekawa T, et al. Interaction between osteopontin on madin darby canine kidney cell membrane and calcium oxalate crystal. *Utol Int.* 1999;62:81-86.

287. Liu L, Chen S, Giachelli CM, Ratner BD, Jiang S. Controlling osteopontin orientation on surfaces to modulate endothelial cell adhesion. *J Biomed Mater Res A.* 2005;74:23-31.

288. Kleinman JG, Beshensky A, Worcester EM, Brown D. Expression of osteopontin, a urinary inhibitor of stone mineral growth, in rat kidney. *Kidney Int.* 1995;47:1585-1896.

289. Evan AP, Bledsoe SB, Smith SB, Bushinsky DA. Calcium oxalate crystal localization and osteopontin immunostaining in genetic hypercalciuric stone-forming rats. *Kidney Int.* 2004;65:154-161.

290. Khan SR, Johnson JM, Peck AB, Cornelius JG, Glenton PA. Expression of osteopontin in rat kidneys: induction during ethylene glycol induced calcium oxalate nephrolithiasis. *J Urol.* 2002;168:1173-1181.

291. Jiang XJ, Feng T, Chang LS, et al. Expression of osteopontin mRNA in normal and stone-forming rat kidney. *Urol Res.* 1998;26:389-394.

292. Kohri K, Nomura S, Kitamura Y, et al. Structure and expression of the mRNA encoding urinary stone protein (osteopontin). *J Biol Chem.* 1993;268:15180-15184.

293. Marengo SR, Chen DH, MacLennan GT, Resnick MI, Jacobs GH. Minipump induced hyperoxaluria and crystal deposition in rats: a model for calcium oxalate urolithiasis. *J Urol.* 2004;171:1304-1308.

294. Okamoto N, Aruga S, Tomita K, Takeuchi T, Kitamura T. Chronic acid ingestion promotes renal stone formation in rats treated with vitamin D3. *Int J Urol.* 2007;14:60-66.

295. Umekawa T, Kohri K, Kurita T, Hirota S, Nomura S, Kitamura Y. Expression of osteopontin messenger RNA in the rat kidney on experimental model of renal stone. *Biochem Mol Biol Int.* 1995;35:223-230.

296. Yagisawa T, Chandhoke PS, Fan J, Lucia S. Renal osteopontin expression in experimental urolithiasis. *J Endourol.* 1998;12:171-176.

297. Yasui T, Fujita K, Sasaki S, et al. Expression of bone matrix proteins in urolithiasis model rats. *Urol Res.* 1999;27:255-261.

298. Chang L, Feng T, Li J, Dou C, Wei J, Guo Y. Regulation of osteopontin expression in a rat model of urolithiasis. *Chin Med J.* 2001;114:829-832.

299. Iguchi M, Takamura C, Umekawa T, Kurita T, Kohri K. Inhibitory effects of female sex hormones on urinary stone formation in rats. *Kidney Int.* 1999;56:479-485.

300. Yagisawa T, Ito F, Osaka Y, Amano H, Kobayashi C, Toma H. The influence of sex hormones on renal osteopontin expression and urinary constituents in experimental urolithiasis. *J Urol.* 2001;166:1078-1082.

301. Yasui T, Sato M, Fujita K, Ito Y, Nomura S, Kohri K. Effects of allopurinol on renal stone formation and osteopontin expression in a rat urolithiasis model. *Nephron.* 2001;87:170-176.

302. Itoh Y, Yasui T, Okada A, Tozawa K, Hayashi Y, Kohri K. Preventive effects of green tea in renal stone formation and the role of oxidative stress in nephrolithiasis. *J Urol.* 2005;173:271-275.

303. Wesson JA, Johnson RJ, Mazzali M, et al. Osteopontin is a critical inhibitor of calcium oxalate crystal formation and retention in renal tubules. *J Am Soc Nephrol.* 2003;14:139-147.

304. Okada A, Nomura S, Higashibata Y, et al. Successful formation of calcium oxalate crystal deposition in mouse kidney by intra-abdominal glyoxylate injection. α*Urol Res.* 2007;35:89-99.

305. Okada A, Nomura S, Saeki Y, et al. Morphological conversion of calcium oxalate crystals into stones is regulated by osteopontin in mouse kidney. *J Bone Miner Res.* 2008;23:1629-1637.

306. Kon S, Maeda M, Segawa T, et al. Antibodies to different peptides in osteopontin reveal complexities in the various secreted forms. *J Cell Biochem.* 2000;77:487-498.

307. Min W, Shiraga H, Chalko C, Goldfarb S, Krishna GG, Hoyer JR. Quantitative studies of human urinary excretion of uropontin. *Kidney Int.* 1998;53:189-193.

308. Nishio S, Hatanaka M, Takeda H, Iseda T, Iwata H, Yokoyama M. Analysis of urinary concentrations of calcium phosphate-associated proteins: a2-HS-glycoprotein, prothrombin F1 and osteopontin. *J Am Soc Nephrol.* 1999;10:S394-S396.

309. Yasui T, Fujita K, Hayashi Y, et al. Quantification of osteopontin in the urine of healthy and stone-forming men. α*Urol Res.* 1999;4:225-230.

310. Nishio S, Hatanaka M, Takeda H, et al. Calcium phosphate crystal-associated proteins: alpha-2-HS-glycoprotein, prothrombin fragment 1 and osteopontin. *Int J Urol.* 2001;8:S58-S62.

311. Huang HS, Ma MC, Chen CF, Chen J. Lipid peroxidation and its correlations with urinary levels of oxalate, citric acid, and osteopontin in patients with renal calcium oxalate stones. *Urology.* 2003;62:1123-1128.

312. Tsuji H, Tohru U, Hirotsugu U, Masanori I, Yuji H, Takashi K. Urinary concentration of osteopontin and association with urinary supersaturation and crystal formation. *Int J Urol.* 2007;14:630-634.

313. Hedgepeth RC, Yang L, Resnick MI, Marengo SR. Expression of proteins that inhibit calcium oxalate crystallization in vitro in the urine of normal and stone-forming individuals. *Am J Kidney Dis.* 2001;37:104-112.

314. Thurgood LA, Grover PK, Ryall RL. High calcium concentration and calcium oxalate crystals cause significant inaccuracies in the measurement of urinary osteopontin by enzyme linked immunosorbent assay. *Urol Res.* 2008;36:103-110.

315. Lian JB, Prien EL, Glimcher MJ, Gallop PM. The presence of protein-bound gamma-carboxylic acid in calcium-containing renal calculi. *J Clin Invest.* 1977;59:1151-1157.

316. Suzuki K, Moriyama M, Nakajima C, et al. Isolation and partial characterization of crystal matrix protein as a potent inhibitor of calcium oxalate crystal aggregation: evidence of activation peptide of human prothrombin. *Urol Res.* 1994;22:45-50.

317. Stapleton AMF, Dawson CJ, Grover PK, et al. Further evidence linking urolithiasis and blood coagulation: Urinary prothrombin fragment 1 is present in stone matrix. *Kidney Int.* 1996;49:880-888.

318. Stapleton AMF, Seymour AE, Brennan JS, Doyle IR, Marshall VR, Ryall RL. The immunohistochemical distribution and quantification of crystal matrix protein. *Kidney Int.* 1993;44:817-824.

319. Stapleton AMF, Timme TL, Ryall RL. Gene expression of prothrombin in the human kidney and its potential relevance to kidney stone disease. *Br J Urol.* 1998;81:666-672.

320. Suzuki K, Tanaka T, Miyazawa K, et al. Gene expression of prothrombin in human and rat kidneys: Basic and clinical approach. *J Am Soc Nephrol.* 1999;10:S408-S411.

321. Grover PK, Stapleton AMF, Ryall RL. Prothrombin gene expression in rat kidneys provides an opportunity to examine its role in urinary stone pathogenesis. *J Am Soc Nephrol.* 1999;10: S404-S407.

322. Grover PK, Dogra SC, Davidson BP, Stapleton AMF, Ryall RL. The prothrombin gene is expressed in the rat kidney. Implications for urolithiasis research. *Eur J Biochem.* 2000;267:61-67.

323. Grover PK, Ryall RL. Inhibition of calcium oxalate crystal growth and aggregation by prothrombin and its fragment in vitro. Relationship between protein structure and inhibitory activity. *Eur J Biochem.* 1999;263:50-56.

324. Ryall RL, Grover PK, Stapleton AMF, et al. The urinary F1 activation peptide of human prothrombin is a potent inhibitor of calcium oxalate crystallization in undiluted human urine in vitro. *Clin Sci.* 1995;89:533-541.

325. Grover PK, Ryall RL. Inhibition of calcium oxalate crystal growth and aggregation by prothrombin and its activation fragments in undiluted human urine in vitro: Relationship between protein structure and inhibitory activity. *Clin Sci.* 2002;102:425-434.

326. Buchholz NP, Kim DS, Grover PK, Dawson CJ, Ryall RL. The effect of warfarin therapy on the charge properties of urinary prothrombin fragment 1 and crystallization of calcium oxalate in undiluted human urine. *J Bone Miner Res.* 1999;14:1003-1012.

327. Liu J, Wang T, Chen J, Wang S, Ye Z. Decreased inhibitory activity of prothrombin to calcium oxalate crystallization by specific chemical modification of its gamma-carboxyglutamic acid residues. *Urology.* 2006;67:201-203.

328. Liu J, Chen J, Wang T, Wang S, Ye Z. Effects of urinary prothrombin fragment 1 in the formation of calcium oxalate calculus. *J Urol.* 2005;173:113-116.

329. Webber D, Radcliffe CM, Royle L, et al. Sialylation of urinary prothrombin fragment 1 is implicated as a contributory factor in the risk of calcium oxalate kidney stone formation. *FEBS J.* 2006;273:3024-3037.

330. Webber D, Rodgers AL, Sturrock ED. Glycosylation of prothrombin fragment 1 governs calcium oxalate crystal nucleation and aggregation, but not crystal growth. *Urol Res.* 2007;35:277-285.

331. Webber D, Rodgers AL, Sturrock ED. Synergism between urinary prothrombin fragment 1 and urine: a comparison of inhibitory activities in stone-prone and stone-free population groups. *Clin Chem Lab Med.* 2002;40:930-936.

332. Durrbaum D, Rodgers AL, Sturrock ED. A study of crystal matrix extract and urinary prothrombin fragment 1 from a stone-prone and stone-free population. *Urol Res.* 2001;29:83-88.

333. Gul A, Rez P. Models for protein binding to calcium oxalate surfaces. *Urol Res.* 2007;35:63-71.

334. Moriyama MT, Domiki C, Miyazawa K, Tanaka T, Suzuki K. Effects of oxalate exposure on Madin-Darby canine kidney cells in culture: renal prothrombin fragment-1 mRNA expression. *Urol Res.* 2005;33:470-475.

335. Grover PK, Miyazawa K, Coleman M, Stahl J, Ryall RL. Renal prothrombin mRNA is significantly decreased in a hyperoxaluric rat model of nephrolithiasis. *αJ Pathol.* 2006;210:273-281.

336. Dean CJ, Macardle PJ, Ryall RL. The effect of the presence of calcium oxalate crystals on the measurement of prothrombin fragment 1 in urine. In: Rodgers AL, Hibbert BE, Hess B, Khan SR, Preminger GM, eds. *Urolithiasis 2000.* Cape Town: University of Cape Town; 2000:150-152.

337. Sørensen S, Hansen K, Bak S, Justesen SJ. An unidentified macromolecular inhibitory constituent of calcium oxalate crystal growth in human urine. *Urol Res.* 1990;18:373-379.

338. Zhuo L, Hascall VC, Kimata K. Inter-a-trypsin inhibitor, a covalent protein-glycosaminoglycan-protein complex. *J Biol Chem.* 2004;279:38079-28082.

339. Evan AP, Bledsoe S, Worcester EM, Coe FL, Lingeman JE, Bergsland KJ. Renal inter-alpha-trypsin inhibitor heavy chain 3 increases in calcium oxalate stone-forming patients. *Kidney Int.* 2007;72:1503-1511.

340. Fries E, Blom AM. Bikunin – not just a plasma proteinase inhibitor. *αInt J Biochem Cell Biol.* 2000;32:125-137.

341. Atmani F, Lacour B, Drüeke T, Daudon M. Isolation and purification of a new glycoprotein from human urine inhibiting calcium oxalate crystallization. *αUrol Res.* 1993;21:6.

342. Atmani F, Lacour B, Strecker G, Parvy P, Drüeke T, Daudon M. Molecular characteristics of uronic-acid-rich protein, a strong inhibitor of calcium oxalate crystallization in vitro. *Biochem Biophys Res Commun.* 1993;91:1158-1165.

343. Atmani F, Mizon J, Khan SR. Identification of uronic-acid-rich protein as urinary bikunin, a light chain of inter-α-trypsin inhibitor. *Eur J Biochem.* 1996;236:984-990.

344. Dawson CJ, Grover PK, Ryall RL. Inter-a-inhibitor in urine and calcium oxalate urinary crystals. *Br J Urol.* 1998;81:20-26.

345. Atmani F, Opalko FJ, Khan SR. Association of urinary macromolecules with calcium oxalate crystals induced in vitro in normal human and rat urine. *Urol Res.* 1996;24:45-50.

346. Dawson CJ, Grover PK, Kanellos J, Pham H, Kupczyk OA, Ryall RL. Inter-α-inhibitor in calcium stones. *Clin Sci.* 1998;95:187-193.

347. Atmani F, Khan SR. Role of urinary bikunin in the inhibition of calcium oxalate crystallization. *αJ Am Soc Nephrol Suppl.* 1999;14:S385-8.

348. Atmani F, Lacour B, Jungers P, Drüeke T, Daudon M. Reduced inhibitory activity of uronic-acid-rich protein (UAP) in the urine of stone formers. *Urol Res.* 1994;22:257-260.

349. Dean CJ, Kanellos J, Pham H, et al. The effect of inter-a-inhibitor and several of its derivatives on calcium oxalate crystallization in vitro. *Clin Sci.* 2000;98:471-480.

350. Kobayashi H, Shibata K, Fujie M, Sugino D, Terao T. Identification of structural domains in inter-a-trypsin inhibitor involved in calcium oxalate crystallization. *Kidney Int.* 1998;53:1727-1735.

351. Médétognon-Benisson J, Tardivel S, Hennequin C, Daudon M, Drüeke T, Lacour B. Inhibitory effect of bikunin on calcium oxalate crystallization in vitro and urinary bikunin decrease in renal stone formers. *Urol Res.* 1999;27:69-75.

352. Okuyama M, Yamaguchi S, Yachiku S. Identification of bikunin isolated from human urine inhibits calcium oxalate crystal growth and its localization in the kidneys. *Int J Urol.* 2003;10:530-5.

353. Atmani F, Khan SR. Characterization of uronic-acid-rich inhibitor of calcium oxalate crystallization isolated from rat urine. *Urol Res.* 1995;23:95-101.

354. Atmani F, Glenton PA, Khan SR. Role of inter-alpha-inhibitor and its related proteins in experimentally induced calcium oxalate urolithiasis. Localization of proteins and expression of bikunin gene in the rat kidney. *Urol Res.* 1999;27:63-67.

355. Iida S, Peck AB, Johnson-Tardieu J, et al. Temporal changes in mRNA expression for bikunin in the kidneys of rats during calcium oxalate nephrolithiasis. *J Am Soc Nephrol.* 1999;10:986-996.

356. Moriyama MT, Glenton PA, Khan SR. Expression of inter-alpha inhibitor related proteins in kidneys and urine of hyperoxaluric rats. *J Urol.* 2001;165:1687-1692.

357. Eguchi Y, Inoue M, Iida S, Matsuoka K, Noda S. Heparan sulphate (HS)/heparan sulfate proteoglycan (HSPG) and bikunin are upgraded during calcium oxalate nephrolithiasis in rat Kidney. *Kurume Med.* 2002;49:99–107.

358. Iida S, Peck AB, Byer KJ, Khan SR. Expression of bikunin mRNA in renal epithelial cells after oxalate exposure. *J Urol.* 1999;162:1480-1486.

359. Marengo SR, Resnick MI, Yang L, Chung JY. Differential expression of urinary inter-a-trypsin inhibitor trimers and dimers

in normal compared to active calcium oxalate stone forming men. *J Urol.* 1998;159:1444-1450.

360. Suzuki M, Kobayashi H, Kageyama S, Shibata K, Fujie M, Terao T. Excretion of bikunin and its fragments in the urine of patients with renal stones. *J Urol.* 2001;166:268-274.

361. Stříž I, Trabichavský I. Calprotectin – a pleiotropic molecule in acute and chronic inflammation. *Physiol Res.* 2004;53:245-253.

362. Bennet J, Dretler SP, Selengut J, Orme-Johnson WH. Identification of the calcium-binding protein calgranulin in the matrix of struvite stones. *J Endourol.* 1994;8:95-98.

363. Umekawa T, Kurita T. Calprotecin-like protein is related to soluble organic matrix in calcium oxalate urinary stone. *Biochem Mol Biol Int.* 1994;34:309-313.

364. Sakakura T, Fujita K, Yasui T, et al. Calcium phosphate stones produced by Madin-Darby canine kidney (MDCK) cells inoculated in nude mice. *Urol Res.* 1999;27:200-205.

365. Pillay SN, Asplin JR, Coe FL. Evidence that calgranulin is produced by kidney cells and is an inhibitor of calcium oxalate crystallization. *Am J Physiol.* 1998;275:F255-F261.

366. Bergsland KJ, Kelly JK, Coe BJ, Coe FL. Urine protein markers distinguish stone-forming from non-stone-forming relatives of calcium stone formers. *Am J Physiol Renal Physiol.* 2006;291:F530-F536.

367. Boyce WH, King J, Fielden M. Total non-dialyzable solids (TNDS) in human urine XIII. Immunological detection of a component peculiar to renal calculous matrix and to urine of calculous patients. *J Clin Invest.* 1962;41:1180-1189.

368. Dussol B, Geider S, Lilova A, et al. Analysis of the soluble matrix of five morphologically different kidney stones. *Urol Res.* 1995;23:45-51.

369. Cerini C, Geider S, Dussol B, et al. Nucleation of calcium oxalate crystals by albumin: involvement in the prevention of stone formation. *Kidney Int.* 1999;55:1776-1786.

370. Edyvane KA, Ryall RL, Marshall VR. The influence of serum and serum proteins on calcium oxalate crystal growth and aggregation. *Clin Chim Acta.* 1986;157:81-88.

371. Honda M, Yoshioka T, Yamaguchi S, et al. Characterization of protein components of human urinary crystal surface binding substance. *Urol Res.* 1997;25:355-360.

372. Hess B, Meinhardt U, Zipperle L, Giovanoli R, Jaeger P. Simultaneous measurements of calcium oxalate crystal nucleation and aggregation: impact of various modifiers. *Urol Res.* 1995;23:231-238.

373. Chen WC, Lin HS, Chen HY, Shih CH, Li CW. Effects of Tamm-Horsfall protein and albumin on calcium oxalate crystallization and importance of sialic acids. *Mol Urol.* 2001;5:1-5.

374. Wu W, Gerard DE, Nancollas GH. Nucleation at surfaces: the importance of interfacial energy. *J Am Soc Nephrol Suppl.* 1999;14:S355-S358.

375. Pankov R, Yamada KM. Fibronectin at a glance. *J Cell Sci.* 2002;115:3861-3863.

376. Tsujihata M, Miyake O, Yoshimura K, Kakimoto KI, Takahara S, Okuyama A. Fibronectin as a potent inhibitor of calcium oxalate urolithiasis. *J Urol.* 2000;164:1718-1723.

377. Tsujihata M, Miyake O, Yoshimura K, Tsujikawa K, Tei N, Okuyama A. Renal tubular injury and fibronectin. *Urol Res.* 2003;31:368-373.

378. Tsujihata M, Miyake O, Yoshimura K, Kakimoto K, Takahara S, Okuyama A. Comparison of fibronectin content in urinary macromolecules between normal subjects and recurrent stone formers. *Eur Urol.* 2001;40:458-462.

379. Ryall RL. Chaos, crystals and calculi. In: Jungers P, Daudon M, eds. *Renal Stone Disease. Crystallization Process, Pathophysiology, Metabolic Disorders and Prevention.* Paris: Elsevier; 1997: 113-117.

Renal Cellular Dysfunction/Damage and the Formation of Kidney Stones

5

Saeed R. Khan

Abstract Supersaturation is the driving force behind crystal formation in the kidneys. It can, however, result only in the formation of crystals that can often be harmlessly excreted. For stone formation, crystals must form, grow, and be retained in the kidneys, which is indeed a rare occurrence. Crystalluria is universal while stone formation is not. Only pathological changes in the kidneys and renal cell dysfunction and injury can accomplish crystal retention and formation of stone nidus. Cellular dysfunction can be intrinsic or provoked. Lethal epithelial cellular injury promotes crystal nucleation, aggregation, and retention. Sublethal injury or dysfunctional cells may produce ineffective crystallization modulators and localized areas of supersaturation in the interstitium. The former will affect crystallization in the urine while the latter may cause precipitation in the interstitium and development of Randall's plaques. In addition, dysfunctional cells affect supersaturation, by influencing the excretion of participating ions such as calcium, oxalate, and citrate, and modulating urinary pH and production and excretion of macromolecular promoters and inhibitors of crystallization.

5.1 Introduction

Kidney stone formation is a common urological disorder in the USA with a lifetime risk of nearly 13% in men and 7% in women.[1] Recurrence of stone formation is common. Probability of recurrence in idiopathic stone formers is 40–50% within 5 years of the initial episode, and 50–60% by 10 years. Thus approximately 40% of the stone formers do not produce another stone. Stone formers with systemic diseases such as cystinuria, primary hyperoxaluria (PH), and primary hyperparathyroidism have a higher rate of recurrence. Calcium oxalate (CaOx) is the major constituent of most stones and is generally found mixed with calcium phosphate (CaP). Hypercalciuria, hyperoxaluria, and hypocitraturia, alone or in combination, are the main abnormalities in most idiopathic calcium oxalate stone formers. Obviously, stone formation is episodic and stone formers have specific abnormalities: some innate resulting in regular and frequent stone recurrences, and others that require triggering and activation leading to long intervals between stone events. It is our hypothesis that abnormalities are the result of cellular dysfunctions; some inherited and endogenous and others extrinsic and environmental.

That renal cellular and tubular dysfunction may be involved in stone formation was first suggested in 1884 by clinical and experimental observations of Ebstein, who examined the human stones as well as experimentally produced oxamide stones.[2] Ebstein showed that urinary stones contained a framework of albuminous substances (organic matrix). He believed that this substance, the matrix, was produced as a result of "inflammation or catarrh of the urinary tract, which lead to sloughing of the epithelium" and the formation of a "ground work for the impregnation of inorganic urinary components." In 1923, Keyser replicated Ebstein's experimental studies and found that oral administration of oxamide resulted in its hyperexcretion, and produced a "diffuse tubular nephritis" and bilateral stones, which were composed of oxamide and organic matrix. He suggested that urine contains "protective colloids," which keep the "crystalloids" in solution. Calculi develop as a result of the "abnormal colloidal mechanism."

Urinary stones can form anywhere in the urinary system, from kidneys to the bladder, but in the industrialized and affluent societies, they are generally restricted to the kidneys. Kidney stones generally form attached to the renal papillary

S.R. Khan (✉)
Departments of Pathology and Urology, University of Florida, College of Medicine, Gainesville, FL, USA
e-mail: khan@pathology.ufl.edu

P.N. Rao et al. (eds.), *Urinary Tract Stone Disease*,
DOI 10.1007/978-1-84800-362-0_5, © Springer-Verlag London Limited 2011

tips. Randall first emphasized the importance of renal papilla when he described minute tubular calculi and subepithelial calcium plaques within and on human renal papillae and suggested that these could serve as focal points for stone development.[3] He suggested that interstitial subepithelial deposits of calcium phosphate or calcium carbonate arising from pathological conditions of the renal papilla erode through to the papillary surface forming a lesion, which he called type 1. He further suggested that excessive urinary supersaturation in association with tubular cell death results in crystal deposition in the collecting ducts producing a type 2 lesion. Both types of lesions acted as foci for further stone growth in the pelvis or papillary ducts. Thus Randall proposed a theory in which both urinary supersaturation and renal tubular damage play a part in stone formation. This chapter will review clinical and experimental data and examine the role of renal dysfunction/damage and urinary supersaturation in the formation of CaOx kidney stones.

5.2 Supersaturation and Crystallization of Calcium Oxalate

The formation of kidney stones or nephrolithiasis is a result of crystal formation in the kidneys. Crystallization is modulated by a number of urinary inhibitors and promoters, which determine whether a crystal will nucleate and grow into a stone or excreted as a crystalluria particle. The driving force for crystallization is the development of supersaturation with respect to the precipitating salt.[4] However, supersaturation alone cannot explain stone formation because people who have never formed stones can also pass highly supersaturated urine.[5] Human urine is a complex solution containing not only calcium (Ca) and oxalate (Ox) but also other ions and macromolecules that can interact with Ca and/or Ox and modulate crystallization. Thus urinary CaOx supersaturation depends not only on the concentration of Ca and Ox but also the presence of ions such as citrate and magnesium; and hypercalciuria, hyperoxaluria, and hypocitraturia are major risk factors for calcific stone formation. Supersaturation and crystallization in the urine also depend upon the presence of macromolecules such as many proteins and lipids[6,] which can bind or form complexes with Ca and/or Ox. Any cellular defect or dysfunction that can affect participating urinary ions and macromolecules can also influence CaOx supersaturation and crystallization in the kidneys. Some defects are innate and the result of genetic modifications, while others are the result of exposure to various stimuli.

Crystal formation within the urinary tract, particularly of calcium phosphate (CaP) and CaOx, is widespread. Humans excrete millions of urinary crystals daily, indicating at least transient development of supersaturation. However, few develop kidney stones; probably because either the crystals do not form in the kidneys or the crystals that form do not stay there. It has been suggested that with a transit time across the kidney of 5–10 min, residence time for the crystals to nucleate and grow large enough to be trapped[7] is not enough. The inner diameter of various segments of renal tubules ranges from 15–60 μm (micrometers).[8] The crystals of CaOx, growing at the rate of 1–2 μm/min cannot grow bigger than a few micrometers and are therefore excreted with urine without causing any stone episode.

Even though crystals do not form without supersaturation, it is only one step in the process of stone formation. In order for stone to be formed, not only do the crystals need to be retained within the kidney but they should also be positioned at sites where crystals can ulcerate to renal papillary surface to form a stone nidus. It is hypothesized that renal injury promotes crystal retention and the development of stone nidus on renal papillary surface.[9] In addition, renal epithelial injury supports crystal nucleation at lower supersaturation.[10] Injury can be of any origin. Persistent mild hyperoxaluria by itself or through crystallization of CaOx is injurious to the renal epithelium.[11,12] Hypercalciuria may similarly be injurious.[13] Shock wave lithotripsy (SWL) is injurious to the renal tissue including tubular as well as vascular epithelium.[14]

5.3 Intrinsic Factors: Genetic Basis of Cellular Dysfunction

The fact that stone disease has a genetic basis has long been appreciated. There is however no agreement as to which genes are involved and to what extent.

5.3.1 Calciuria

Hypercalciuria is one of the major risk factors for the formation of idiopathic kidney stones. Genes encoding for soluble adenylate cyclase (sAC), vitamin D receptor (VDR), calcium sensing receptor (CaSR), sodium phosphate cotransporter-2 (NPT-2), chloride channel-5 (CLC-5), transient receptor potential cations channel V (TRPV5), and claudin-16 have been implicated in hypercalciuria and idiopathic nephrolithiasis (Table 5.1); many divergent results notwithstanding.[15] sAC is expressed in kidneys, intestine, and bone.[16] In the kidneys the expression is seen in epithelia lining distal tubules, thick ascending limbs (TALs), and collecting ducts.[17] sAC is suggested to be a bicarbonate exchanger.[16,17] Individuals with sAC mutations are hypercalciuric osteopenic stone formers.[18–20]

Table 5.1 Various genes involved in hypercalciuria and stone formation

Gene	Gene Product/Function	Renal Tubular Expression	Renal Phenotype
CLCN5	Cl/H antiporter	PT, TAL, αIC	Inactivating mutation causes hypercalciuria, hyperphosphaturia, low molecular weight proteinuria, nephrocalcinopsis, stones
CASR	Calcium sensing receptor	PT (apical), MCD (principal cell, apical), TAL (basal), DCT (basal)	Gain of function mutation produces hypercalciuria, nephrocalcinosis, stones
CLDN16	Tight junction protein	TAL, DCT	Hypercalciuria, magnesium wasting, nephrocalcinosis, stones
NPT2a/c	Sodium phosphate cotransporter	PT	Hypercalciuria, hypophosphatemia, phosphate wasting, nephrocalcinosis, stones
TRPV5	Calcium selective transient receptor potential channel	DCT, Connecting Tubule	Hypercalciuria, hyperphosphaturia
sAC	Soluble adenylate cyclase/bicarbonate exchanger	DCT, TAL, CD	Hypercalciuria, stones
KLOTHO	Aging Suppression protein/regulator of calcium homeostasis	DCT	Hypercalciuria

CD collecting duct; *DCT* distal convoluted tubule; *IC* intercalated cell; *PT* proximal tubule; *MCD* medullary collecting duct; *TAL* thick ascending limb

VDR is expressed in vitamin D sensitive tissues and VDR genes and their polymorphisms are suggested to play significant roles in hypercalciuria and stone formation.[15,20–25] The concept of VDR involvement in hypercalciuria and stone formation is strengthened by investigations of hypercalciuric rats produced by selective breeding of normal Sprague-Dawley rats over 60 generations. These rats have high intestinal expression of VDR, increased calcium absorption in the intestine, increased bone resorption, decreased calcium reabsorption in the kidney, and produce calcium phosphate stones in the urinary space.[21] The hypercalciuric rats produce CaOx stones when made hyperoxaluric through dietary manipulation.[26] Human investigations of VDR gene and polymorphism have, however, led to conflicting data. Increased numbers of vitamin D receptors were found on peripheral blood lymphocytes of some hypercalciuric patients but no abnormality of the VDR gene was detected.[27] In a study of French-Canadian sibling pairs a susceptibility locus associated with stones and hypercalciuria was identified on chromosome 12q12–14 near the VDR gene.[28] Somewhat similar results were obtained investigating Indian families with hypercalciuric stone forming members.[13] In another study, this time with European hypercalciuric stone forming families, no linkage was found between chromosome 12q12–14 and hypercalciuria.[29]

Several of the restriction fragment length polymorphisms (RFLPs) of the VDR gene have been implicated in hypercalciuria and stone formation. Links have been established in some cases and not confirmed in others. An association between *FokI* polymorphism and calcium oxalate stone disease[24,30,31] and *TaqI* polymorphism and severe recurrent stone disease[19] has been suggested. No association between stone formation and *FokI* or *TaqI* polymorphism has been reported.[20,32,33] In one study *ApaI* and *BsmI* polymorphisms coincided only with fasting hypercalciuria.[20]

CaSR is expressed in kidneys, intestine, parathyroid, and bone,[34,35] and among other functions is involved in renal handling of calcium and water. In the kidneys it is expressed in the apical membranes of proximal tubular epithelial cells and principal cells of the medullary collecting ducts and basolateral membranes of epithelial cells lining the thick ascending limb of the loop of Henle as well as the distal tubules. Polymorphism of CaSR gene has been shown to be associated with calcific stone formation. The relative risk of hypercalciuria is increased in individuals with gain of function mutation.[36,37] Activating CaSR mutation in a mice model leads to ectopic calcification.[38]

Renal phosphate wasting with nephrolithiasis is reported in hereditary hypophosphatemic rickets with hypercalciuria as well as Dent's disease. Since *NPt2a* encodes for proximal tubular sodium phosphate cotransporter, which is involved in reabsorption of filtered phosphate, this gene is considered a candidate gene for hereditary renal phosphaturia. Mutation in NPT-2 gene encoding sodium phosphate cotransporter in proximal tubule has been implicated in hypophosphatemia and kidney stone.[39] Variant Npt2a were found in two of 20 study subjects with osteoporosis or recurrent stone disease with renal phosphate leak. A later study of a cohort of 98 families of hypercalciuric stone formers found a number of genetic variations in the gene. But the variations were not associated with significant abnormalities of phosphate or calcium handling.[40] Recently, mutations in genes encoding NPT2c transporter have been identified in consanguineous kindreds and additional families with hereditary hypophosphatemic rickets and hypercalciuria indicating that NPT2c may play a significant role in the kidneys.[41] Mice with disrupted NPT-2a cotransporter gene created by targeted mutagenesis exhibit increased urinary excretion of phosphate, ~80% decrease in renal brush border membrane Na/phosphate cotransport, and hypophosphatemia, which leads to increased serum 1,25 (OH) 2D levels, overexpression of intestinal calcium channels, intestinal calcium hyperabsorption, and development of hypercalciuria.[42] NPT-2a -/- mice develop renal deposits of apatitic calcium phosphate in their kidneys,[43] present in newborn, weanling, as well as adult mice (Fig. 5.1).

Chloride/proton antiporter CLC-5 is encoded by the *CLCN5* gene and is expressed in the renal epithelial lining proximal tubule and thick ascending limb of the loop of Henle and alpha intercalated cells of the collecting ducts. Inactivating mutations of *CLCN5* cause Dent's disease, an X-linked recessive tubulopathy characterized by low molecular weight proteinuria, hypercalciuria, nephrocalcinosis, nephrolithiasis, and progressive renal failure.[44] CLC-5 is critical in endosome acidification and involved in membrane trafficking via receptor-mediated endocytic pathway. Loss of chloride channel ClC-5 impairs endocytosis by defective trafficking of megalin and cubilin in kidney proximal tubules.[45] Mice lacking CLC-5 gene show endocytic disruption[46,47] and develop renal tubular defects with low molecular weight proteinuria, hypercalciuria, and nephrocalcinosis.[47,48]

One cause of hypercalciuria is decreased calcium reabsorption by renal tubules, which occurs by passive entry of Ca^{2+} through apical Ca^{2+} channels (TRPV5 and TRPV6) followed by diffusion through the cytosol facilitated by calbindin-D28K with eventual extrusion across the basolateral membrane. Currently, it is thought that the primary rate-limiting step for transepithelial Ca^{2+} reabsorption is the apical entry step. TRPV5 is the main channel responsible for apical Ca^{2+} entry. TRPV5 is a calcium-selective channel expressed in distal convoluted tubule and connecting tubule and a member of the transient receptor potential (TRP) channel family, which includes 28 ion channels that act as cellular sensors and regulate a variety of cell functions.[49,50] TRPV5 channels mediate calcium reabsorption in the kidneys and their expression is regulated by parathyroid hormone; 1,25 di-hydroxyvitamin D3; estrogen; and dietary calcium. TRPV5 -/- mice have impaired Ca reabsorption and high plasma 1,25 di-hydroxyvitamin D3 with compensatory hyperabsorption of dietary calcium and severe calcium wasting.[51] Despite elevated urinary calcium excretion there is no renal calcification because of significant polyuria. Human mutations of *TRPV5* have so far not been reported. Thus the importance of this gene in idiopathic hypercalciuria is unknown. TRPV5-mediated calcium reabsorption could, however, be regulated by other molecules such as "with no kinase" 4 (WNK4).[52] Mutation of WNK4 causes autosomal dominant pseudohypoaldosteronism type II, which is characterized by hypercalciuria associated with hyperkalemic hypertension.

Claudins are present in membranes of tight junctions in a number of epithelia.[53] Claudin-16 also called paracellin-1 (PCLN-1) is exclusively expressed in thick ascending limb of the loop of Henle and plays a role in paracellular transport of calcium and magnesium.[54] Loss of function mutations in *CLDN16* gene encoding for claudin-16 have been identified in patients with familial hypomagnesemia with hypercalciuria and nephrocalcinosis.[55] Results of a study showed that many heterozygous relatives of patients with familial hypomagnesemia with hypercalciuria and nephrocalcinosis produced stones, but the prevalence of nephrolithiasis or

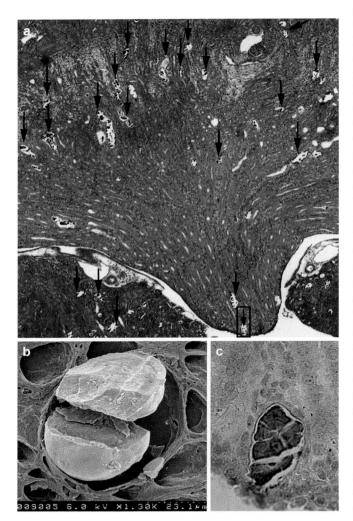

Fig. 5.1 Calcium phosphate deposition in kidneys of Npt2a -/- mice (**a**) H&E stained section showing intratubular calcium phosphate deposits (*arrows*) in both the medullary and papillary collecting ducts of 5-day-old male mice. (**b**) *SEM* of a calcium phosphate deposit showing both surface and interior. (**c**) Kidney section was stained with von Kossa to show that deposits are made of calcium phosphate. Deposit present in the papillary collecting duct seen in (**a**) (*inside the box*) is positively stained and concentrically laminated

hypercalciuria was not significantly different from that in the general population.[55] A missense mutation of *CLDN16* found in two families was associated with self-limiting childhood hypercalciuria, which decreased with age and was not associated with progressive renal decline.[56]

Klotho is an aging suppression protein predominantly expressed in renal distal convoluted tubules, parathyroid gland, and epithelial cells of the choroid plexus.[57–59] Overexpression of klotho increases the life span in mice.[58] In humans, a correlation between polymorphisms of klotho gene and life span, osteoporosis, and coronary artery disease has been shown.[59] Klotho-deficient mice are hypercalcemic and hypercalciuric, show reduced renal absorption of calcium and reduced TRPV5 expression, and have higher circulating levels of 1,25 dihydroxyvitamin D (1,25-D). Klotho inhibits the expression of 25-hydroxyvitamin D 1alpha hydroxylase, a key enzyme for synthesis of 1,25-D.[60] The treatment of cells in culture with klotho increases expression of TRPV5 channels.[61] Based on these and other observations, klotho is considered a critical regulator of calcium homeostasis. Klotho is also known to serve as a co-receptor for bone-derived fibroblast growth factor-23 (FGF23)[62], which promotes renal phosphate wasting and vitamin D activation. The Klotho-fibroblast growth factor receptor (FGFR) complex binds to FGF23 with a higher affinity than FGFR or Klotho alone.

5.3.2 Oxaluria

Urinary oxalate, the critical risk factor in CaOx nephrolithiasis, is derived from dietary as well as endogenous sources and its concentration is controlled by production in the liver, by the erythrocytes, conversion of ascorbate, and absorption and secretion in the gut and kidneys, involving many enzymes, transporters, and exchangers.[63] Glyoxylate is the immediate precursor of endogenous oxalate in the liver as well as erythrocytes. In the liver, glycolate is oxidized by peroxisomal glycolate oxidase to glyoxylate, which is further oxidized to oxalate by lactate dehydrogenase. Under normal conditions, glyoxylate is catalyzed by peroxysomal enzyme alanine glyoxylate aminotransferase (AGT) into glycine, which is metabolized to serine. Alternatively, glycoxylate is reduced to glycolate by the widely distributed cytosolic enzyme D-glyoxylate reductase/d-glycerate dehydrogenase/hydroxypyruvate reductase. Deficient AGT activity due to mutation or mistargeting results in failure to detoxify glyoxylate, which is either oxidized to oxalate or reduced to glycolate, leading to significantly increased urinary excretion of oxalate – a condition called primary hyperoxaluria type 1.[64] Deficiency of the enzyme d-glycerate dehydrogenase leads to increased oxidation of glyoxylate to oxalate and its significantly increased urinary excretion. This condition is called primary hyperoxaluria type 2.[65]

A null mutant mouse was generated by targeted mutagenesis of the homologous alanine-glyoxylate amino transferase gene, *Agxt*, in embryonic stem cells. Mutant mice, though developed normally, exhibited hyperoxaluria and CaOx crystalluria.[66] Urinary oxalate was normalized and CaOx crystalluria stopped by hepatic expression of human AGT1, the protein encoded by *Agxt*, by adenoviral vector-mediated gene transfer in *Agxt*(-/-) mice. The expression of wild-type human AGT1 was predominantly localized in peroxisomes of the mouse liver, while that of the most common mutant form of AGT1 (G170R) was primarily localized in the mitochondria.

Glyoxylate is also suggested to be the precursor of oxalate in the erythrocytes, where oxalate is transported via Band3 anion exchanger protein (AE1), whose gene is the solute linked carrier *Slc4a1*. In the kidneys, *Slc4a1* is expressed on the basolateral membrane of type A acid secretory intercalated cells of the collecting duct epithelium and is responsible for chloride/bicarbonate exchange.[67] Mice lacking *Slc4a1* develop nephrocalcinosis, hypercalciuria, hyperphosphaturia, and hypocitraturia.[68] Mutations in human gene *Slc4a1* that encodes for band 3 protein causes distal renal tubular acidosis, which is associated with hypercalciuria and considered one of the risk factors of recurrent nephrolithiasis.

A significant amount of urinary oxalate is derived from diet and some stone formers may be hyperabsorbers of oxalate.[69,70] Results of a study showed that idiopathic calcium oxalate stone formers with hyperoxaluria had significantly increased oxalate excretion after a 5 mmol oral oxalate load compared to those with normal urinary oxalate excretion.[70] Three members of the solute-linked carrier 26 (Slc26) family of anion exchangers with role in oxalate absorption are expressed along the intestinal tract.[71–73] Slc26a3 is localized to the apical membrane of the epithelial lining of the colon. Slc26a6 is localized in the apical membrane of the small intestine and stomach epithelial cells. Slc26a7 is localized to the basolateral membrane of the stomach's parietal cells.

Several members of the Slc26 family of anion exchangers are also expressed in the kidneys.[74] In the proximal tubules Slc26a1 (Sat-1) mediates the transport of sulfate and oxalate across the basolateral membrane.[75] Slc26a6 (CFEX, Pat-1) is located in the apical membrane of the proximal tubular epithelial cells and primarily mediates chloride–oxalate exchange.[76] Targeted deletion of oxalate/anion exchanger gene Slc26a6 in two separate lines of mice led to hyperoxaluria attributable to defective intestinal excretion.[77,78] In one model of *Slc26a6* -/- mice hyperoxaluria is attributed to loss of secretion in the distal ileum accompanied by increased oxalate absorption.[77] In the other model, loss of most duodenal oxalate secretion without change in the oxalate absorption[78] leads to hyperoxaluria, hyperoxalemia, and calcium oxalate nephrolithiasis. Results of the studies with *Slc26a6* -/- mice indicate that factors regulating these genes may affect oxalate homeostasis and possibly promote CaOx nephrolithiasis.

So far no polymorphism of the gene or its variants have, however, been identified among stone formers. But species-specific differences between mouse and human genes exist. Mouse *Slc26a6* and human *SLC26A6* share only 78% amino acid identity and exhibit significant differences in anion selectivity. The Slc26a6 in the mouse mediates bidirectional electrogenic chloride/oxalate transport while the same mediated by SLC26A6 in humans is electroneutral.

5.3.3 Citraturia

Urinary citrate is another significant determinant of CaOx supersaturation and an important risk factor for CaOx neph-rolithiasis. Citrate in the urine binds to calcium forming a soluble compound thereby lowering free ionic calcium, reducing urinary supersaturation with respect to CaOx and CaP, and inhibiting their precipitation.[4] In addition, urinary citrate is shown to inhibit crystal nucleation, as well as growth and aggregation.[79] Results of several studies indicate that stone formers excrete less citrate in their urine than the non-stone formers.[80–82] The incidence of hypocitratuiria in the stone-forming population is reported to range from 19% to 63%.[79] Any cellular abnormality that leads to altered urinary excretion of citrate impacts on CaOx supersaturation and nephrolithiasis. Low urinary citrate levels are found in many conditions such as potassium depletion and renal tubular acidosis.[83]

Citrate is derived from intestinal absorption as well as endogenous metabolism.[79,83–85] It is filtered freely by the glomerulus and its urinary excretion is regulated primarily by rate of its reabsorption in the proximal tubules. Sixty-five percent to 90% of the filtered citrate is reabsorbed in the proximal tubules with the assistance of sodium-citrate cotransporter present in the apical membrane.[86] The transporter is encoded by 3Na-citrate^{2-} cotransporter-1(*NaDc-1*), which has been isolated from human as well as rat and rabbit kidneys. Examination of an association between citrate excretion and single nucleotide polymorphism (SNP) in exon 12 of *hNaDC-1* in recurrent stone formers suggests that the B allele of 1550V polymorphism of *hNaDC-1* may be associated with reduction in urinary excretion of citrate and hypocitratuiria.[87] Similar polymorphism was also found in hypocitraturic non-stone formers indicating that factors other than hypocitraturia are also involved in the formation of kidney stones. Involvement of NaDC-1 in citrate excretion was also investigated in an animal model of CaOx ner-phrolithiasis.[88] Hyperoxaluria was induced in male Wistar rats by the administration of ethylene glycol, which is known

to lead to hypocitraturia and coax nephrolithiasis. NaDC-1 mRNA levels in the kidneys were determined by Northern blot analyses and its protein expression was examined by immunohistochemistry. Both mRNA and protein levels increased significantly in hyperoxaluric rats. Administration of potassium citrate significantly elevated urinary citrate and downregulated NaDC-1 expression in the kidneys.

5.3.4 Pyrophosphaturia

Pyrophosphate is present in urine at concentrations of 15–100 µM (micromolar). In a seeded crystal growth system, it inhibits calcium oxalate monohydrate (COM) crystal growth by 50% at 16–20 µM (micromolar).[89–92] It can also inhibit COM crystal growth inside a gel matrix[93] and effectively inhibits the growth of CaPs.[94,95] If it is equally efficient in urine it can contribute 50% crystal COM growth inhibition in the collecting ducts (five times dilution) and up to 80% in the urine.

Hypopyrophosphaturia is postulated to be a metabolic risk factor for recurrent kidney stone formers.[96] Mutations in the human homologue of the mouse progressive ankylosis (*ANKH*) gene, a pyrophosphate transporter, are associated with defects of calcification such as craniometaphyseal dysplasia and chodrocalcinosis and *ANKH* polymorphism has been associated with changes in bone mineral density and with ankylosing spondylitis (AS). A family-based association analyses of 201 multiplex AS families with nine *ANKH* intragenetic and two flanking microsatellite markers showed that two variants located in two different regions of the *ANKH* gene were associated with AS.[97] Association also revealed gender-genotype specificity. Renal stone prevalence is increased in AS patients. Likelihood of renal stone formation is also increased with extension of the disease duration.[98]

5.3.5 Macromoleculuria

In addition to small molecules such as citrate and pyrophosphate, crystallization in the kidneys is also modulated by a number of macromolecules.[6] Osteopontin (OPN), Tamm–Horsfall protein (THP), bikunin (BK), and urinary prothrombin fragment-1 are four of the more extensively examined crystallization modulators (Table 5.2). OPN is synthesized in the kidneys and excreted in the urine at levels sufficient to inhibit CaOx crystallization.[99] Stone formers have been reported to excrete less OPN in their urine than the normal healthy non-stone forming individuals.[100] OPN's role as an inhibitor of stone formation was further strengthened by

Table 5.2 Crystallization modulating macromolecules, their expression and production in renal epithelial cells under normal conditions as well as in response to an exposure to oxalate and CaOx crystals

Name	Role in CaOx crystallization and nephrolithiasis	Other features and functions	Expression on Ox and CaOx exposure
Tamm–Horsfall protein (THP)	Inhibitor of aggregation	Inflammation, renoprotective	+, −, ±
Osteopontin (OPN)	Free OPN inhibits crystal nucleation, growth, aggregation and attachment, immobilized OPN promotes crystal attachment	Calcium binding, renoprotective, tissue repair and inflammation, Chemoattractant for monocytes/macrophages (M/M)	+
Prothrombin fragment-1	Inhibitor of growth, and aggregation	Calcium binding, coagulation	+, −
Bikunin (BK) and Inter-α-Inhibitor	Inhibitor of nucleation, growth, aggregation and attachment	Metastasis, tissue repair and remodeling	+
α-1-microglobulin	Inhibitor of crystallization	Immunosuppressive, mitogenic	+
CD-44	Promoter of crystal attachment	Tissue repair and remodeling	+
Calgranulin	Inhibitor of crystal growth and aggregation	Calcium binding, tissue remodeling, and inflammation	+
Heparan sulfate (HS)	Inhibitor of crystal aggregation and attachment	Tissue remodeling	+
Osteonectin		Calcium binding, tissue remodeling	+
Fibronectin	Inhibitor of crystal aggregation, attachment and endocytosis	Morphogenesis, wound healing, and metastasis	+
Matrix Gla protein	Inhibitor of crystal deposition	Inhibitor of mineralization	+

Results of tissue culture and animal model. + upregulation, − downregulation, ± no change

observations that experimental induction of hyperoxaluria in OPN knockout mice leads to significant deposition of CaOx crystals in the kidneys, whereas OPN wild type mice showed upregulation of OPN production and were not affected.[101] Mutations in the genes regulating the synthesis of OPN could be a predisposing genetic factor for stone formation.

Recently an association between kidney stone risk and a single nucleotide polymorphism (SNP) of the human *OPN* gene has been reported. The entire human *OPN* gene of Japanese stone patients and matching controls was sequenced, haplotype-tagging SNPs searched, and association between haplotypes and nephrolithiasis determined.[102] Six novel polymorphisms were identified and a significant association was found between relative probability of stone formation and two haplotypes located in the *OPN* promoter. Interestingly OPN appeared to be dually associated with nephrolithiasis risk. One haplotype (T-G-T-G) was associated with reduced risk while another (G-T-T-G) one with the increased risk. Role of polymorphism in protein production, molecular structure, and crystallization inhibition and nephrolithiasis risk is not known. The post-translational modifications of OPN including phosphorylation, glycosylation, and sulfation[103,104] appear directly pertinent to stone formation. Inhibition of hydroxyapatite crystal growth by OPN was markedly reduced after dephosphorylation[105], and phosphorylation of OPN peptides markedly enhanced the inhibition of CaOx crystal growth.[106]

THP is a kidney-specific protein, synthesized in cells of the thick ascending limbs of the loop of Henle. It coats the luminal side of the epithelium and is the most abundant protein in the human urine (50–100 mg/day). It is consistently present in the stone matrix and has high affinity with calcium phosphate crystals. An analysis of proteins associated with CaOx and CaP crystals experimentally induced in vitro in the human urine showed THP as the most abundant protein in the matrix of the CaP crystals.[107] Normal THP is a potent inhibitor of CaOx crystal aggregation[108] and reduced urinary excretion of THP by stone formers has been reported.[109] In addition, stone formers are shown to produce THP with abnormal molecular structure which promotes crystal aggregation.[110] First direct evidence for THP's involvement in stone formation was provided by ablating the murine THP gene.[111,112] Kidneys of 16% of mice lacking THP gene and protein production contained intratubular as well as interstitial CaP deposits in the medullary and papillary collecting ducts. Induction of hypercalciuria and hyperoxaluria by the administration of vitamin D_3 and ethylene glycol, respectively, lead to copious crystal deposition in the kidneys of 76% of the THP knockout mice. There was no crystal deposition in kidneys of the wild-type mice, with or without the excessive intake of calcium and oxalate. Ablation of both the THP and OPN genes showed spontaneous deposition of CaP crystal deposition in 39% of the THP/OPN double knockout mice. Induction of hypercalciuria and hyperoxaluria resulted in

95% of the mice lacking both OPN and THP to suffer from deposition of CaOx crystals in their kidneys.[112] These results indicate that defects in both THP and OPN may contribute to crystallization in the kidneys and stone formation.

A number of naturally occurring THP mutations have been reported and linked to autosomal dominant medullary cystic disease and familial juvenile hyperurecemic nephropathy. Mutations lead to intracellular trafficking defects, retention within the endoplasmic reticulum, and reduction in THP secretion and excretion.[113,114] Renal stone disease has so far not been described in patients with any of these mutations.

Bikunin is the so-called light chain of Inter alpha inhibitor (IαI) and related molecules collectively referred to as the IαI family.[115] These molecules are normally synthesized in the liver and are common in plasma. They are composed of a combination of heavy chains, H1 (60 kDa), H2 (70 kDa), H3 (90 kDa) covalently linked via a chondroitin sulfate bridge to bikunin (35–45 kDa). Separate genes located on three different chromosomes encode these chains. Bikunin originates from a precursor that also codes for alpha (α)1-microglobulin (α1-m). The heavy and light chains also exist independently as single molecules. IαI (180–240 kDa (kilodalton)) is a heterotrimer consisting of bikunin linked to heavy chains H1 and H2. Pre-alpha(α)-inhibitor (PαI, 125 kDa) is composed of bikunin and heavy chain H3. Both heavy and light chains have been identified in the urine. Bikunin isolated from the stone patients, contained less sialic acid and exhibited less crystallization inhibitory activity than that purified from the urine of healthy subjects.[116] A significantly higher proportion of stone patients had a 25 kDa bikunin in their urine in addition to the normal 40 kDa species.[117] Twenty-five kilodalton bikunin was similar to the deglycosylated bikunin and was less inhibitory. Yet another study found decreased urinary excretion of bikunin by stone forming patients.[63]

IαI proteins have been shown to inhibit CaOx crystallization in vitro.[63,90,116,118,119] The inhibitory activity is confined to the carboxy terminal of the bikunin fragment of IαI. Both rat and human urinary bikunin inhibited nucleation and growth of CaOx crystals. Treatment with chondroitinase AC had no effect on this inhibitory activity, which was destroyed by pronase treatment indicating that the activity lies not with the chondroitin chain but with the peptide. Bikunin has also been implicated in modulating adhesion of CaOx crystals to the renal epithelial cells.[120] Madin–Darby canine kidney (MDCK) cells were exposed in culture to CaOx monohydrate crystals in the presence or absence of various protein fractions isolated from normal human urine. A single fraction with a molecular weight of 35 kDa was found to be most inhibitory of crystal adhesion. This protein inhibited crystal adhesion at the minimum concentration of 10 ng/mL and completely blocked it at 200 ng/mL. Amino acid sequence of the first 20 amino acids of the N-terminal was structurally homologous with bikunin.

Alpha (α)1-microglobulin (α1-m) is also an inhibitor of CaOx crystallization in vitro.[121] Alpha 1-m was isolated from human urine. Two species of 30 and 60 kDa, recognized by the antibody against α1-m, were isolated. Both inhibited CaOx crystallization in a dose-dependent manner. Using an ELISA assay, urinary concentration of α1-m was found to be significantly lower in 31 CaOx stone formers than in 18 healthy subjects (2.95 + 0.29 vs 5.34 + 1.08 mg/L, respectively, $P = 0.01$). As mentioned previously, genes at three different chromosomes are involved in encoding for various IαI-related proteins. The alpha-1-microglobulin/bikunin precursor gene that encodes for both bikunin and α1-m is regulated by a number of transcription factors. Mutations in any of the genes may produce structural and secretory variations seen in the kidney stone formers.

5.4 Extrinsic Factors: Renal Injury and Cellular Dysfunction

The kidneys, during performance of their normal duties, are challenged by substances and circumstances, which alter cellular functions, injure the cells, and may lead to cell death and degradation. Both clinical and animal model studies have provided evidence for the association between hyperoxaluria, crystal deposition in the kidneys, and renal dysfunction and injury. Abnormal renal cellular functions and cell death have an enormous impact upon crystal nucleation, growth, aggregation, and retention within the kidneys with obvious repercussions for kidney stone formation.

5.4.1 Clinical Studies

Calcium oxalate crystals have been observed in the kidneys of patients with a variety of hyperoxaluria-inducing disorders. Hyperoxaluria is caused either by overproduction or intestinal overabsorption of oxalate.[122–127] The three main types of hyperoxaluria are (1) primary hyperoxaluria, (2) enteric hyperoxaluria (EH), and (3) idiopathic or mild hyperoxaluria.

Primary hyperoxaluria (PH), in which oxalate is overproduced because of disturbances in the oxalate biosynthetic pathway, is rare. PH is an inherited disorder of glyoxylate metabolism characterized by the overproduction of oxalate (>200 mg/day [2.2 mmol/day]) and glycolate. Recent studies have estimated PH incidence of 1–2.7% in children with end-stage renal disease. In most patients, PH leads to chronic renal failure in mid to late childhood or early adulthood. However, in some the disease is more aggressive resulting in metabolic acidosis, nephrocalcinosis, end-stage renal disease, and death by the age of 1. Increased oxalate production after the onset of renal failure leads to systemic oxalosis. At this time, CaOx crystal deposits are seen in all parts of the kidneys including the interstitium and the cortex, and in all segments of the nephron including the proximal tubules.[123] Renal biopsies from patients with primary hyperoxaluria regularly demonstrate crystals within tubular epithelial cells as well as interstitium.[128] Crystal deposition is associated with cell proliferation, the formation of multinucleated giant cells, as well as vascular and interstitial inflammation.

Enteric hyperoxaluria (EH), characterized by severe hyperoxaluria ($\geq$ 80 mg/day [0.88 mmol/day]), is due to enhanced absorption of oxalate secondary to gastrointestinal problems such as diarrhea, cystic fibrosis, irritable bowel syndrome, colitis or ileal resection, jejuno-ileal bypass or Roux-n-Y gastric bypass surgery for obesity.[129–137] EH accounts for 5% of all cases of hyperoxaluria and their numbers appear to be increasing because of obesity-related complications and surgeries. Obesity is one of the major public health problems in the USA and nearly 20% of the US population can now be described as obese (body mass index (BMI) > 30 kg/m^2).[131] Above all, the population of morbidly obese (BMI > 40kg/m^2) is growing at an alarming rate and has grown 80% since 1988.[132] Comorbidities associated with morbid obesity include type II diabetes, hypertension, sleep apnea, hyperlipidemia, cardiovascular diseases, and osteoarthritis.[135] In the absence of effective therapy for sustainable weight loss, an increasing number of patients are choosing bariatric surgeries such as Roux-n-Y gastric bypass surgery. Such bariatric surgeries increased more than fivefold from 1998 to 2000.[136] Hyperoxaluria is a potential complicating factor for modern bariatric surgeries.[129] Results of a recent study showed mean urinary oxalate excretion of 83 mg/day (0.92 mmol/day) by the patients treated with modern bariatric surgeries compared to 39 mg/day (0.43 mmol/day) for idiopathic stone formers and 34 mg/day (0.38 mmol/day) for normal subjects.[133] Renal biopsies from patients with increased urinary excretion of oxalate secondary to enteric hyperoxaluria, such as Crohn's disease and after an intestinal bypass demonstrate crystals within the kidneys.[138–140]

Idiopathic or mild hyperoxaluria (40 mg/day (0.44 mmol/day)) is most common and is seen in the patients with idiopathic CaOx urolithiasis. Higher than normal levels of renal enzymes, gamma (γ)-glutamyl transpeptidase (GGTP), angiotensin 1 converting enzyme (ACE), beta (β)-galactosidase (GAL), and N-acetyl-beta (β)-glucosaminidase (NAG) were found in the urine of idiopathic CaOx stone formers.[141] Since elevation of these enzymes in the urine is considered an indication of renal proximal tubular injury, it was concluded that the stone patients had damaged renal tubules. Results of recent studies also describe CaOx kidney stone patients to be under oxidative stress[142,143] and renal injury. Urine from stone patients had increased NAG and significantly higher alpha (α)-glutathione S-transferase (α-GST),

malondialdehyde (MDA), and thiobarbituric acid-reactive substances (TBARS), indicating that CaOx kidney stone-associated renal injury is most likely caused by the production of reactive oxygen species (ROS).

5.4.2 Animal Model Studies

Experimental CaOx crystal deposition in the kidneys or nephrolithiasis can be induced by the administration of hyperoxaluria-causing agents such as sodium oxalate, ammonium oxalate (AOx), ethylene glycol (EG), or hydroxy-L-proline (HLP).[9,144–151] We have studied many aspects of urolithiasis in male and female Sprague-Dawley rats.[152–154] Kidneys of nephrolithic rats show the deposition of CaOx crystals in renal calyces and at papillary tips. Many deposits are located subepithelially and often anchored to the basement membrane.[9,145,146] These deposits formed in the terminal papillary collecting ducts appear as nodules on papillary surface (Fig. 5.2). Covering epithelium appears stretched. Disruption of the surface epithelium appears to expose the underlying crystals and lead to the development of stone nidus as a type 2 Randall's plaque.[146,147,155] Crystal deposition provoked inflammatory response. Ultrastructural examination of the kidneys revealed damage to the epithelial cells lining the renal tubules, which contained crystals. In addition there was intracellular edema, widened intercellular spaces, and many cells contained dividing nuclei. The clubbing of microvilli and focal loss of brush border distorted the luminal cell surfaces. Cells often appeared to have burst open and released their contents into the tubular lumen. Evidence has also been provided for apoptotic cell death of the tubular epithelial cells in the presence of high oxalate and CaOx crystals.[156]

The earliest noticeable changes were detected in cells of the proximal tubules, which appeared more sensitive to hyperoxaluria. This injury resulted in death and detachment of many epithelial cells, thus resulting in exposure of the basal lamina. Most crystals were intraluminal and invariably associated with cellular degradation products, indicating the possibility of membrane-induced nucleation of CaOx crystals. Crystal deposition was associated with the migration of inflammatory cells such as monocytes, macrophages, and polymorphonuclear leukocytes to the adjacent interstitium. In addition, interstitial crystals were often seen surrounded by macrophages and giant cells.[151,157]

Our study, in which kidneys were examined at different times after sodium oxalate injection induced acute hyperoxaluria, showed that crystals appeared first in the tubular lumen, then moved to inter- and intracellular locations and eventually into the interstitium. After a few weeks time interstitial crystals disappeared indicating the existence of a removal mechanism.[150] Other studies also showed that, in experimental CaOx

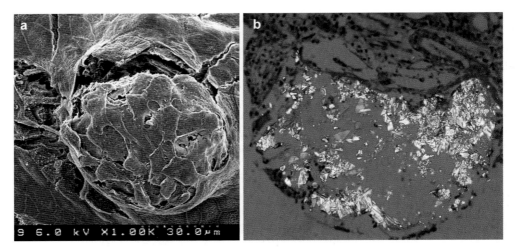

Fig. 5.2 Calcium oxalate deposition in kidneys of male rats made hyperoxaluric by the feeding hydroxyl-L-proline with rat chow. (**a**) Birefringent calcium oxalate crystals present in papillary collecting ducts. Subepithelial deposits are formed by crystal retention within the tubules. A layer of crystals appears attached to the basal lamina. Crystal deposition results in inflammatory response. Crystals become exposed by disruption of the surface epithelium leading to the formation of the Type 2 Randall's plaque. (**b**) *SEM* of an area similar to that illustrated in (**a**). Surface epithelium is stretched. Cells are separating along the intercellular junctions exposing the underlying crystals (Modified from[147], p. 914)

nephrolithiasis, crystals form in the tubular lumen and eventually move into the interstitium causing inflammation and attracting many inflammatory cells including leukocytes, monocytes, and macrophages.[158–160] Multinucleated giant cells were also identified in the interstitium (Fig. 5.2). The interstitial infiltrate around crystals may play an important role in renal tissue damage through the production of proteolytic enzymes, cytokines, and chemokines.[161,162] The mechanism by which the inflammatory cells enter the renal interstitium of the hyperoxaluric rats is not known, but it is likely that chemotactic factors and adhesion molecules are involved. Products of interaction between renal tubular cells and Ox or CaOx crystals under hyperoxaluric conditions might play an important role in the attraction and accumulation of infiltrating inflammatory cells.

5.4.3 Renal Cell Injury and Crystal Nucleation

CaP and CaOx crystalluria is widespread, an indication that human urine is often sufficiently supersaturated with respect to these salts for their nucleation and adequate growth.[122] But such crystalluria is temporary and crystals are mostly small and single. Stone formers on the other hand produce large and aggregated crystals. Studies performed in vivo in animal models have shown that renal epithelial injury promotes crystallization of calcific crystals, which are continuously excreted in the urine and excreted crystals are large aggregates.[9] Both urinary as well as renal CaOx crystals are seen associated with cellular degradation products.[9,12,150] Factors that cause renal epithelial injury and shedding of membranes into the urine promote crystallization in conditions that normally would not support it. When rats were made hyperoxaluric in the presence or absence of membrane shedding, those rats who had membrane vesicles in their urine quickly produced crystal deposits in their kidneys and crystal aggregates in their urine.[124] Cell degradation following renal epithelial injury produces numerous membrane vesicles, which act as substrates for heterogeneous nucleation. Interestingly, membranes of injured but intact cells also have the capacity to nucleate CaOx crystals.[163] Such direct nucleation on cell surfaces can also promote crystal retention within the tubules.[163]

Membrane vesicles isolated from renal epithelial cells have been shown in vitro to be good nucleators (Fig. 5.3) of both CaP and CaOx crystals[164,165] and eventually become incorporated in the matrix of the calcified products. Membranes and their lipids have also been implicated in other crystal deposition diseases.[166] The organic matrix of kidney stones contains both membrane vesicles and lipids. Lipids isolated from the kidney stone matrix promote the nucleation of CaOx crystals.[11,167]

5.4.4 Renal Cell Injury and Crystal Retention

Humans normally relieve urinary supersaturation by producing and excreting small crystals, perhaps the reason for rarity of stone disease in the presence of continuous urinary supersaturation with respect to many sparingly soluble salts. Crystals even when they form in the renal tubules are generally small (Fig. 5.4a) and move with the urine to be eventually excreted. The formation of kidney stones

Fig. 5.3 Nucleation of *CaOx* crystals. Brush border membrane was isolated from the tubules of normal rat kidneys and incubated in vitro in a metastable solution of CaOx. Crystals were isolated and examined. (**a**) *SEM* showing plate-like crystals of CaOx monohydrate associated with the substrate. (**b**) *TEM* of crystal aggregate showing an association between the membrane vesicles and CaOx crystal ghosts. Crystals are arranged as a rosette around a central nucleation site (N)

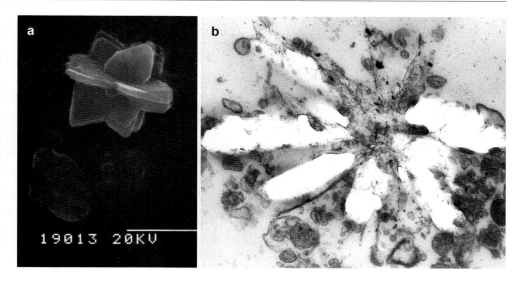

requires crystals to not only form within the kidneys but to stay there and grow. Crystal retention within kidneys can be accomplished by:

1. Formation in the renal interstitium or relocating there (Fig. 5.4b)
2. Attachment to the renal epithelial cells after crystal formation in the renal tubules (Fig. 5.4c)
3. Not moving with the urinary flow and growing large enough to be trapped
4. Aggregating with other crystals and thus accreting mass (Fig. 5.4d)

5.4.4.1 Crystal Formation in the Interstitium

Based on the concentration profile of calcium and oxalate in the urine, tubular fluid, and renal tissue, it was suggested that interstitium of the inner medulla had the highest Ox concentration and the best chance of being the primary nucleation site for CaOx.[51] In the absence of any convective flow in the interstitium, the crystals had unlimited time to grow and develop into a kidney stone. However, CaOx crystals have not been reported in the renal interstitium of idiopathic stone patients.[168,169] Even when hyperoxaluria is experimentally induced in an animal, deposition of CaOx crystals begins in the renal tubular lumen.[9,43,144–147,170] CaOx crystals can, however, migrate from tubular location to the interstitium[9,147] as illustrated in Fig. 5.4b.

Calcium phosphate crystals are frequently seen in the human renal interstitium.[155,168] They are most probably formed as a result of renal cellular dysfunction or pathology and when ulcerated to the papillary surface support stone formation.

5.4.4.2 Crystal Attachment to Renal Epithelium

Animal model and tissue culture studies have provided the evidence for crystal retention within the kidneys by attachment to renal epithelial cells (Fig. 5.4c). Experimental induction of CaOx nephrolithiasis starts with hyperoxaluria followed by crystalluria and crystal deposition in the kidney.[144–150] Hyperoxaluria alone triggers increased urinary excretion of enzymes such as N-acetyl-β(beta)-glucosaminidase, γ(gamma)-glutamyl transpeptidase, and alkaline phosphatase, indicating epithelial injury.[149] Crystal deposition is associated with overt injury as indicated by cellular death and degradation. Morphological injury appears to be mostly confined to the epithelium of crystal-containing renal tubules.[9,144] The degree of renal injury and the amount of crystal buildup are dependent upon the intensity and length of hyperoxaluria. Interestingly, human stone formers with mild hyperoxaluric display enzymuria of proximal tubular origin.[141]

Further support for crystal adherence to injured epithelia comes from studies with epithelial lining of the rat bladder.[171] Exposure of the bladder epithelium, after removal of surface glycosaminoglycans by triton X100 or hydrochloric acid, to CaOx crystals promoted their adherence to the exposed surfaces. Since heparin treatment reduced crystal attachment to the injured epithelium it was concluded that sulfated moieties were involved in crystal adherence.

Tissue culture studies provided evidence not only for the crystal adherence to the renal epithelium but also the possible mechanisms involved. When primary cultures of inner medullary collecting duct cells were exposed to crystals of CaOx, uric acid, or hydroxyapatite, crystals preferentially adhered to cells with impaired tight junctions.[172] It was concluded that crystals adhered to basolateral components, which moved to the cell surface after damage to the tight junctions. Recently, similar conclusions were made when MDCK-1 cell monolayers were first

Fig. 5.4 Crystal retention within the kidneys. Hyperoxaluria was induced in male Sprague-Dawley rats by intraperitoneal administration of oxalate. (**a**) A *CaOx* dihydrate crystal appears to be moving freely in the renal tubule. (**b**) CaOx monohydrate crystals are present in the papillary renal interstitium and are associated with fibrous and cellular material. (**c**) Plate-like crystals of calcium oxalate monohydrate appear attached to renal epithelium (*arrow*). They may have actually nucleated on the cell surface. (**d**) CaOx crystals have blocked the tubular lumen by aggregation and becoming entangled in slender projections (*arrow*) of the microvillous brush border (Modified from Khan SR, Finlayson B, Hackett RL. Scanning electron microscopy of calcium oxalate crystal formation in experimental nephrolithiasis. *Lab Invest* 1979, 41: 504)

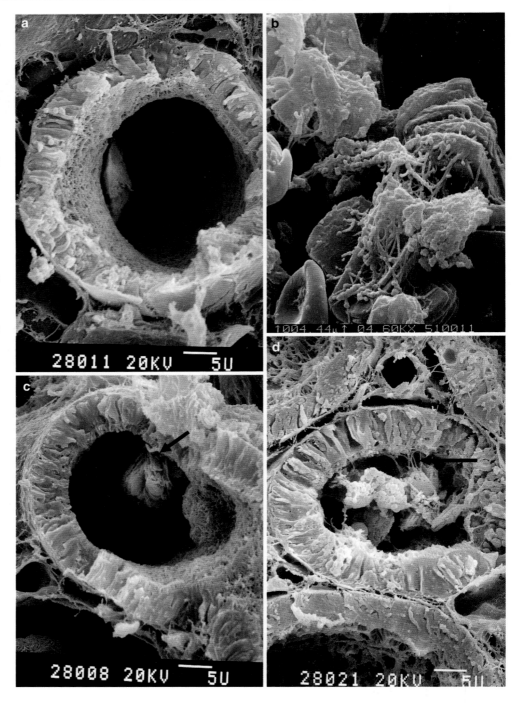

physically injured by removal of a strip of cells and then exposed to CaOx crystals. Crystals specifically adhered to residues on the growth substrate and surfaces of injured and regenerating cells. It was concluded that both mature and immature cell surfaces express crystal binding molecules, but while they are available on surfaces of immature cells, in mature cells these molecules become available only after injury.[173] These results strongly support the suggestions that epithelial damage promotes crystal adherence to the renal epithelium.

It is hypothesized that a regenerating/dedifferentiated tubular epithelium – characterized by luminal expression of crystal binding molecules (annexin-2 [ANX2], nucleolin-related-protein [NRP], hyaluronan [HA], and OPN) – plays an important role in the development of intratubular nephrocalcinosis.[174–176] Molecules, which become available on cell surfaces on exposure to high Ox and CaOx crystals include phosphatidylserine, CD44, OPN, and HA.[148,177–179] All have been shown to promote crystal adherence to renal epithelial cell surfaces.

5.4.4.3 Crystals Not Travelling with the Urinary Flow

It is assumed that urinary flow through the renal tubules is laminar, in which case the flow velocity should be very small near the epithelium and may even be zero at the epithelium. Thus crystals near the epithelial surface would be travelling, if at all, at a much slower speed.[180] Crystal movement can also be influenced by their morphology because of the Stokes drag. Calcium oxalate crystallizes both as CaOx monohydrate and dihydrate, which have different morphologies, and thus have different magnitudes of drag. Even the spherulitic form of calcium oxalate monohydrate is not a compact unit. Urine trapped between the crystallites would put a drag on crystal movement. Gravity will also have an effect upon particles travelling upward. There is also the possibility that urinary flow through the renal tubules is not laminar because urine in the papillary collecting ducts is suggested to move as discreet boluses and is propelled by peristaltic waves that occur at regular time intervals.

In animal models of nephrolithiasis, crystals preferentially deposit at cortico-medullary junctions where loops meet proximal tubules, in collecting ducts near renal fornices, and at papillary tips, where there is a change in luminal diameter of the renal tubules.[8,170] In the cortico-medullary junction area proximal tubules with wider luminal diameter meet slightly narrower thin loops of Henle. Distal tubules and collecting ducts have acute $70°$ angles and z-bends in renal fornices at the papillary base. Openings of the 60–100 µm diameter ducts of Bellini at the renal papillary tip are slit like and only 7–23 µm wide. At these sites, changing luminal diameter would disturb the urinary flow and impede the movement of crystals. Perhaps these architectural characteristics of the mammalian kidneys play a role in the development of human stones on renal papillary tips and in the lower calices and fornices of the kidneys.

Thus it is theoretically possible for crystals to be retained by their size alone, but to date single crystals larger than 10–12 µm have not been reported from either kidneys or urine of humans or rats. Five- to ten-micrometer crystals have been seen attached to the renal epithelium of hyperoxaluric rats. It is possible that as a result of fluid or particle drag close to the tubule wall, crystal/cell contact is increased, facilitating both physiological and pathological responses of cells to the presence of crystals. This prolonged contact may actually promote crystal adherence to the renal epithelium.

5.4.4.4 Crystal Aggregation

All models of CaOx nephrolithiasis concede that crystal aggregation is probably involved in crystal retention within the kidneys since aggregation of crystals can have a considerable effect on the particle size (Fig. 5.4d) and aggregated crystals are commonly found in urine and stones. Although CaOx crystalluria is common in both stone formers and healthy people, stone formers excrete more crystal aggregates.[5,181] When precipitation is induced, urine from stone formers produces larger crystal aggregates. Stone formers' urine is less inhibitory of crystal aggregation, and reduction in aggregation inhibition is proportional to severity of stone disease.

Animal model studies have shown that production of certain crystallization modulators, such as osteopontin and bikunin, is increased in kidneys with CaOx crystal deposits and become incorporated in the growing deposits. Ultrastructural examination of crystal aggregates in the kidneys, as well as urine, displays membranous cellular material closely associated with the crystals.[11,12] It is our understanding that cell debris, formed as a result of exposure to high concentration of Ox and CaOx crystals, collects with the crystals resulting in the formation of larger particles. Membrane lipids with properly aligned calcium binding head groups bridge crystals together and promote crystal aggregation.

5.4.5 Renal Cell Injury, Crystallization Modulators, Inflammation, and Fibrosis

When renal epithelial cells are exposed to oxalate ions and CaOx or CaP crystals, whether in vitro in cell culture or in vivo in animal models, there is an increase in gene expression and production of several urinary macromolecules (Table 5.2), which modulate the nucleation, growth, aggregation, and retention of crystals in the kidneys.[86] Some of them, such as OPN, have specific domains to interact with cell membranes, which may facilitate immobilization and promotion of crystal attachment. Almost all of the modulators are produced by the kidneys and excreted in the urine.[6] Many signaling molecules – such as protein kinase C (PKC), c-Jun N-terminal kinase (JNK), and p38 mitogen-activated protein kinase (MAPK), and transcription factors such as NF-κB and activated protein-1 (AP-1) – involved in the expression and production of macromolecules are activated by reactive oxygen species (ROS).[182–184] ROS are produced when renal epithelial cells are exposed to Ox and/or CaOx crystals. Exposure to excessive Ox and CaOx crystals produces more ROS than can be dealt with by endogenous antioxidant defenses, thus inducing oxidative stress in the kidneys resulting in renal injury, inflammation, and fibrosis.

5.4.5.1 Animal Model Studies

CaOx crystal deposition in the rat kidneys increases the expression of THP[185,186], OPN[148,178], IαI,[152,153] prothrombin fragment-1 (PT)[187], and heparan sulfate (HS)[105] as determined by immunocytochemical localization using specific antibodies (Table 5.2). Other studies, however, have shown either a decrease[188] or an increase[189] in THP expression and production. Production and urinary excretion of OPN[148,178], PT[187], various IαI-related proteins,[152,153], and HS[190] are substantially increased as determined by the detection of their specific mRNAs using in situ hybridization and/or reverse transcription polymerase chain reaction. The upregulated macromolecules play significant roles in inflammatory process.[191,192] HS regulates extracellular matrix production. Bikunin, a constituent of IαI, is a proteinase inhibitor. Acute inflammatory conditions are known to up- or downregulate transcription of IαI genes. Bikunin is associated with inflammation and stabilizes the extracellular matrix.[193,194] THP is seen in the renal interstitium in several forms of tubulointerstitial diseases. Interestingly, inactivating the THP gene in mouse embryonic stem cells results in spontaneous formation of calcium oxalate crystals in adult kidneys.[111] The administration of THP is shown to produce interstitial inflammation and scarring. It can activate alternate pathways, interact with neutrofils, and bind to certain cytokines. Prothrombin is the precursor of thrombin and fragments 1 and 2. Thrombin is involved in platelet aggregation and blood coagulation and plays a major role in the recruitment and activation of infiltrating immune cells.

Several studies have provided evidence for the activation of renin-angiotensin system (RAS) during the development of tubulointerstitial lesions of CaOx crystals.[159,160,195] Reduction of angiotensin production by inhibiting the angiotensin converting enzyme as well as blocking the angiotensin receptor reduced crystal deposition and ameliorated the associated inflammatory response. We have shown that CaOx crystal deposition in rat kidneys activates the (RAS, increases renin expression in the kidneys and serum, and regulates OPN production.[196]

As mentioned previously, renal CaOx crystal deposits are associated with tubulointerstitial inflammation not only in the patients with primary and enteric hyperoxaluria but also in hyperoxaluric rats.[191] Multinucleated giant cells and ED1 positive cells are seen in the renal interstitium of hyperoxaluric patients. We investigated the production of monocyte chemoattractant protein-1 (MCP-1) by the kidneys of hyperoxaluric rats using immunohistochemical staining with a rabbit anti-rat MCP-1 antibody. MCP-1 is a key regulator of the inflammatory response known to attract cells of the inflammatory cascade such as monocytes. Cells of crystal-containing tubules stained positive for MCP-1. In addition, after 8 weeks on a hyperoxaluric diet, male Sprague-Dawley rats excreted higher amounts of arachidonic acid and prostaglandin E2 than the normal controls. Metabolites of arachidonic acid such as prostaglandins are known chemical mediators of inflammation.

Osteopontin is not only a modulator of crystallization but also a monocyte chemoattractant, specifically for the renal interstitium, and upregulation of osteopontin precedes interstitial monocyte infiltration.[197,198] Osteopontin knockout studies demonstrated a reduced influx of macrophages into obstructed kidneys of knockout mice compared to wild-type mice at day 4 and 7 but not at day 14. It was concluded that osteopontin mediated early interstitial macrophage influx.[197] Ethylene glycol administration to OPN knockout mice resulted in intratubular deposition of CaOx while there was no deposition in the wild-type mice given the same treatment.[101]

CaOx crystals have been seen in the renal interstitium of hyperoxaluric rats inside the macrophages.[157] The interstitial crystals eventually disappear.[163] We have suggested that crystals formed in the renal tubules migrate to the renal interstitium by being endocytosed at the luminal side and exocytosed at the basolateral.[174] We have shown that both luminal as well as basolateral exposure to crystals leads to production and secretion of the chemottractants: OPN and MCP-1.[199] The macrophages engulf and break down the crystals.

5.4.5.2 Tissue Culture Studies

The response of renal epithelial cells to COM crystals is characterized by increased expression of specific genes that encode (1) transcriptional activator such as early growth response-1, c-*myc*, Nur-77, and c-*jun*; (2) regulator of the extracellular matrix composition, the fast-acting plasminogen activator inhibitor-1; and (3) growth factors that could stimulate fibroblast proliferation in a paracrine manner such as platelet-derived growth factor-A chain, a connective tissue growth factor.[200] Exposure to CaOx crystals increased osteopontin mRNA and stimulated MDCK and BSC-1 cells to produce osteopontin.[128] The bikunin gene was also expressed and bikunin produced when MDCK cells were exposed to oxalate.[201]

Since CaOx crystal deposition in human and rat kidneys is associated with the migration of monocytes/macrophages (M/M) into the interstitium, we hypothesized that, in response to crystal exposure, renal epithelial cells produce chemokines, which attract the M/M to the sites of crystal deposition.[202,203] We investigated the expression of MCP-1 mRNA and protein by NRK52E rat renal tubular epithelial cells exposed to CaOx crystals. Confluent cultures of NRK52E cells were exposed to CaOx at a concentration of 250 μg/mL (66.7 μg/cm^2). They were exposed for 1, 3, 6, 12, 24 and 48 h for isolation of mRNA and 24 h for ELISA to determine the secretion of protein into the culture medium. Because cells are known to produce free radicals on exposure to CaOx crystals, we also investigated the effect of free radical scavenger, catalase on the crystal-induced expression of MCP-1 mRNA and protein. Exposure of NRK52E cells to the crystals resulted in increased expression of MCP-1 mRNA and production of the chemoattractant.[202,203] Treatment with catalase had a negative effect on the increased expression of both MCP-1 mRNA and protein, which indicates the involvement of free radicals in upregulation of MCP-1 production. Results indicate that MCP-1, which is often associated with localized inflammation[203], may be one of the chemokine mediators associated with the deposition of various urinary crystals in the kidneys.

5.4.6 Shock Wave Lithotripsy and Cellular Dysfunction

Shock wave lithotripsy (SWL) is the treatment of choice for most kidney stones. However, from its inception treatment has been demonstrated to cause renal injury. Studies in humans[204–206] and animal models such as dog,[207–213] rat[23,214,215], rabbit[216–218], and pig[219–223] all have shown that treatment causes extensive renal damage, particularly to the blood vessels. Animal model studies have shown that damage to the renal tubules ranges from total tubular destruction to focal cellular fragmentation, necrosis, cell vacuolarization, and membrane blebbing.[212,218]

A likely cause for SWL-induced renal injury might be cavitation, the growth and collapse of bubbles in small blood vessels and tubules exposed to tensile stresses; and cavitation-generated free radicals.[224–226] Clinical as well as experimental studies have suggested that renal ischemia with free radical formation may be an important factor in SWL-induced renal injury; and that certain medications and antioxidants may protect the kidney from shock wave-induced renal damage, and that renal injury may be reduced by administration of free radical scavengers prior to SWL treatment.[115,224,225,227–233]

Even though morphological and functional damage is generally considered transient, results of a number of investigations suggest new onset hypertension and diabetes as long-term complications of the SWL treatment.[234–240] Other studies indicate that multiple lithotripsies may also exacerbate stone disease. Over the past 30 years there has been an increase in the number of calcium phosphate contents of the stones as well as the calcium phosphate stones.[211] In fact, calcium oxalate stone formers have transitioned into brushite stone formers.[241] An analysis of the clinical data showed that calcium phosphate stone formers received more SWL treatments than patients with other types of stones. It is suggested that SWL treatment may alter the normal physiology of collecting ducts resulting in increased urinary pH, calcium phosphate supersaturation, and crystallization of calcium phosphate rather than calcium oxalate.

5.5 Signaling Pathways

When CaOx or CaP crystals come in contact with renal epithelial cells their response is both morphological as well as biochemical. Cells send slender finger-like projections to probe the crystal surface (Fig. 5.5). These extensions are similar to microvilli but are much longer and more numerous than short stubby microvilli of the cells not in contact with the crystals.[199,242,243] Cilia present on the cell surfaces also appear to be involved. Interestingly, the primary cilium is considered a sensory organelle that relays information about extracellular environment.[244] After initial contact with the surface projections, cells grow over the crystals and/or endocytose them (Fig. 5.5). Crystals have been seen, inside the cells, in the intercellular spaces as well as under the basement membrane. These observations have been made both in vitro in cell culture as well as in vivo in animal models. The movement of crystals into the cells and interstitium is considered a protective cell response. Endocytosed crystals

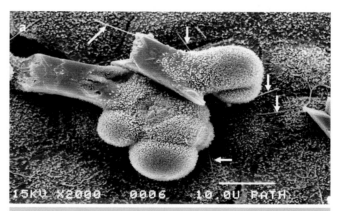
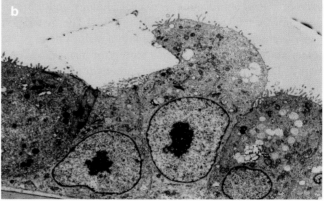

Fig. 5.5 Crystal–cell interaction in culture. *MDCK* cells were exposed in culture to *CaOx* monohydrate crystals and examined by scanning (*SEM*) and transmission electron microscopy (*TEM*). (**a**) SEM of MDCK cells exposed to CaOx monohydrate crystals. Crystals are being endocytosed. Slender projection and cilia appear in contact with the crystals (*arrows*). (**b**) TEM of MDCK cell endocytosing the CaOx crystal, which appears as crystal ghost (Modified from[156], p. S457)

are suggested to be degraded inside the lysosomes. Crystals pushed into the interstitium become surrounded with the macrophages, and have been seen inside the giant cells.[157] Long-term studies in animal models have also shown that experimentally induced renal crystals seen inside cells and interstitium eventually disappear.

Cell exposure to oxalate and/or CaOx or apatitic CaP crystals leads to increased gene expression and production of a variety of macromolecules involved in tissue remodeling, inflammation, and biomineralization. We have shown that renal tubular epithelial cells are stimulated by the exposures to produce prostaglandin E2 (PGE2), monocyte chemoattractant protein-1 (MCP-1), and osteopontin (OPN).[191,199] These molecules are involved in crystal-induced inflammation in various organs including kidneys. In experimentally induced CaOx crystal deposition in the kidneys, monocytes and macrophages move to the sites of crystal deposition. Osteopontin also plays a key role in biomineralization, including kidney stone formation where it modulates crystal nucleation, growth, aggregation, and retention within the renal tubules.[245,246] Exposure of NRK52E cells to the crystals results in increased expression of OPN as well as MCP-1 mRNA and production of the macromolecules.[202,203] Treatment with antioxidants and free radical scavengers significantly reduces the increased expression of both the mRNA and protein, indicating the involvement of reactive oxygen species in upregulation of OPN and MCP-1 production.

Interestingly, an exposure to high Ox and CaOx crystals is also injurious, and injury is associated with the development of oxidative stress, a condition in which either the endogenous antioxidant defenses are depleted or more reactive oxygen species (ROS) such as superoxide and H_2O_2 are produced than can be dealt with. This oxidative stress initiates a cascade of events culminating in renal pathology and the production of reactive oxygen species.[184,247–249] The generation of large amounts of free radicals plays a major role in tissue injury since ROS can damage a variety of macromolecules such as DNA, lipids, proteins, and carbohydrates.[182,250] There is, however, compelling evidence that under stress ROS-initiated signals activate protective and repair mechanisms. Furthermore, redox signaling is also considered a part of normal metabolism in non-stressed cells, and regulated generation of low concentrations of oxygen radicals, however, represent a second messenger system for generation of cytokines involved in tissue injury and repair in general.[154] We have proposed that oxygen radicals serve as a second messenger system for oxalate and crystal-induced activation of the genes.[251]

ROS activate signaling molecules such as protein kinase C (PKC), c-Jun N-terminal kinase (JNK), and p38 mitogen-activated protein kinase (MAPK), and transcription factors such as NF-κB and activated protein-1 (AP-1). Activation of these molecules leads to upregulation of genes and proteins such as MCP-1, OPN, fibronectin, and transforming growth factor (TGF)-β(beta)1. Recently, it has been shown that CaOx crystals selectively activate p38 MAPK signal transduction pathways.[252,253] In addition, p38 MAPK is essential for re-initiation of the induced DNA synthesis. Oxalate exposure also causes modest activation of JNK as determined by c-Jun phosphorylation. Apparently, the renal epithelial response to CaOx oxalate involves signal transduction via MAP kinases, similar to the cellular responses to many other challenges. Cytosolic phospholipase A_2 (cPLA$_2$) is released upon the activation of MAP kinases and translocated to the cell membrane. cPLA$_2$ preferentially hydrolyses arachidonoyl phospholipids generating a number of byproducts including arachidonic acid and lysophospholipids. Exposure of MDCK cells to oxalate produced a time- and concentration-dependent increase in cPLA$_2$ activity.[248] Inhibition of cPLA$_2$ activity blocked ceramide production and the oxalate-induced upregulation of Egr-1, c-jun, and c-myc genes. Exposure of MDCK cells to oxalate also increased the generation of ceramide, another signaling lipid, most probably through the activation of neutral sphingomyelinase.

Mitochondria have been shown to be a source of free radicals and ROS.[247–249] However, the possibility of other sources cannot be ruled out. NADPH oxidase is also a major source of ROS in the kidney[254,255] and may be involved in generation of ROS by renal epithelial cells exposed to CaOx crystals. We have shown a reduction in oxalate-induced injury of NRK52E cells in the presence of diphenyleneiodonium (DPI) chloride, an NADPH oxidase inhibitor.[256] NADPH oxidase is a major source of ROS in the presence of Angiotensin II.[257] Angiotensin II is implicated in causing oxidative stress by stimulating membrane bound NAD(P)H oxidase leading to increased generation of superoxide.[258] A significant reduction in hyperoxaluria-induced production of renal lipid peroxides after administration of AT 1 receptor blockers[160,196] or ACE inhibitors[159] was seen in hyperoxaluric rats. In addition, these treatments produced a reduction in TGF-β(beta) expression in the kidneys. TGF-β has been shown to participate in ROS production through the activation of NADPH oxidase. Similarly Ox-induced generation of ROS in LLC-PK1 cells was associated with increased production of TGF-β$_1$, which was significantly reduced by treatment with neutralizing TGF-β antibodies.[259] The catalytic core of NADPH oxidase is gp91[phox] that contains two hemes in the N-terminal transmembrane region and NADPH-binding and FAD-binding domains in the C-terminal cytoplasmic region. Electrons are transported from NADPH via FAD and two hemes to molecular oxygen. The gp95[phox] is complexed with p22[phox] to form a flavocytochrome b$_{558}$ complex, and constitutively generates superoxide. DPI targets flavin containing domain and is a commonly used inhibitor of NADPH oxidase activities. DPI is suggested to attenuate oxidase activity by withdrawing an electron from the oxidase, causing adduct formation with FAD and inhibiting superoxide formation. We have shown earlier that oxalate-induced injury of NRK52E cells was significantly reduced in the presence of DPI.[260] Prior incubation with10^{-6} M DPI resulted in a reduction of oxalate as well as CaOx and brushite crystal-induced LDH release, and production of H_2O_2 and 8-isoprostane. In addition, DPI reduced both CaOx and brushite crystal-induced gene expression and production of MCP-1. We have also demonstrated that DPI and catalase, a free radical scavenger, cause similar reductions in LDH release and production of H_2O_2 and 8-isoprostane as well as MCP-1 gene expression and protein production.

We have specifically shown that exposure to CaOx crystals results in increased expression of p47[phox], a NADPH oxidase subunit.[256] When exposed to CaOx crystals, renal epithelial cells in culture showed upregulated p47[phox] expression, which was associated with a significant increase in the production of superoxide as well as MCP-1 and OPN. Crystal-induced production of MCP-1 and OPN was significantly reduced following treatment with DPI. As mentioned earlier, NADPH oxidase consists of a number of subunits, cytosolic as well as membrane associated. Cytosolic units not only translocate to the membrane but also assemble with the cytochrome to activate the enzyme. In this study cytosolic p47[phox] was upregulated but exposure to DPI inhibited its assembly with the cytochrome resulting in reduced enzyme activity and superoxide production as well as MCP-1 and OPN synthesis and production. The results suggested that the calcium oxalate crystal-induced ROS production and MCP-1 and OPN synthesis occurs through activation of NADPH oxidase and that activation of NADPH oxidase may be one of the crucial mechanisms responsible for oxalate-induced production of ROS, which may be playing a significant role as second messengers for expression of molecules such as osteopontin and monocyte chemoattractant protein-1. Low level hyperoxaluria and passing crystals provoke a protective physiological response while long exposure to high oxalate levels and crystals leads to oxidative stress and renal pathology. The pathways involved may prove important in developing therapies for the recurrent stone formers.

Administration of angiotensin receptor-1 blocker (ARB) to hyperoxaluric rats results in reduction of oxidative stress, CaOx crystal deposition, and expression of OPN synthesis and production in the kidneys, suggesting involvement of renin angiotensin system involvement in coax nephrolithiasis. The kidney produces all components of (RAS; and intrarenal RAS plays a major role in renal disease progression. Kidneys produce both angiotensinogen and ACE and the juxtaglomerular apparatus is the main source of circulating renin. Renin catalyzes the production of angiotensin I, which is converted to angiotensin II by the actions of ACE. Angiotensin II acts through two receptors – types 1 (AT1) and 2 (AT2) – and mediates many effects of the RAS,

regulating numerous physiological reactions including salt and water balance, aldosterone release, and blood pressure. Oxidative stress plays a significant role in proinflammatory effects of angiotensin II. Angiotensin II is implicated in causing oxidative stress by stimulating membrane bound NADH/NADPH oxidase, which leads to an increased generation of superoxide.[257,258] ACE inhibitors and AT1 receptor blockers have been shown to provide protection against angiotensin II-induced fibrosis and oxidative stress.

Figure 5.6 illustrates signaling pathways active in the kidneys during CaOx nephrolithiasis. Kidneys are under oxidative stress when renal epithelial or interstitial cells are exposed to high oxalate or CaOx crystals and the mechanical stress associated with crystal deposition in the renal tubules. ROS are produced by the activation of NADPH oxidase located at the plasma membrane or by the activation of PLA-2 and neutral sphingomyelinase (N-Smase) with effect on mitochondria through lipid products, arachidonic acid, lysophosphatidylcholine (LysoPC), and ceramide. The production of ROS and cytochrome-C (Cyt-C) goes up. Mitochondrial membrane potential ($\Delta\psi$ [delta psi]) and glutathione (GSH) are reduced. ROS also activate the p38 MAPkinase signal transduction pathways influencing various transcription factors such as NF-κB and AP-1. There is an increase in expression of immediate early genes and production of various crystallization modulators such as osteopontin (OPN), bikunin (BK), and alpha(α)-1-microglobulin (α-1M) and chemoattractants such as monocyte chemoattractant protein-1 (MCP-1).

5.6 Formation of Stone Nidus and Development of Stone

Crystals can be retained at many sites in the kidneys through the size enhancing process of aggregation and by attachment to the renal epithelium. How do the crystals present inside the kidneys evolve into stones attached to the renal papillary surfaces? Obviously, crystals deposited in the renal cortical tubules or inside tubules of the renal papilla cannot become a nidus for the stone formation. Studies of Randall's plaques in human kidneys have shown interstitial CaP deposits and intraluminal CaOx deposits in stone formers kidneys. It has been suggested that in idiopathic stone formers, CaP deposits originate in the basement membrane of the loops of Henle and from there continuously grow outward reaching the papillary surface.[168] The CaP deposits on papillary surface then become focal points for the development of CaOx kidney stones. Randall's own studies, as well as of others, described the involvement of renal pathology in the development of the plaque. Both human and animal model studies have shown renal inflammation in association with crystal deposits[191],

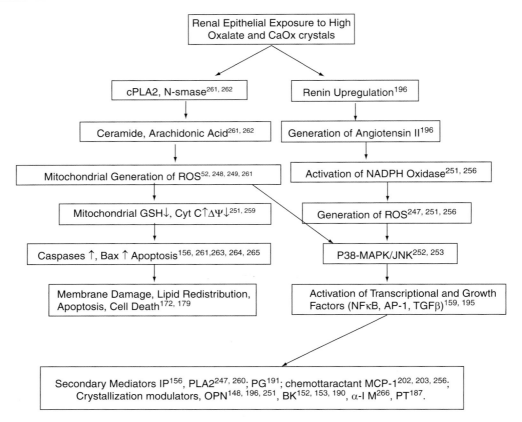

Fig. 5.6 Signalling pathways involved in cell response to oxalate and/or calcium oxalate crystals. Kidneys are under oxidative stress when renal epithelial or interstitial cells are exposed to high oxalate and/or CaOx crystals and the mechanical stress associated with crystal deposition in the renal tubules. Reactive oxygen species (*ROS*) are produced by the activation of NADPH oxidase located at the plasma membrane or by the activation of PLA-2 and neutral sphingomyelinase (*N-Smase*) with effect on mitochondria through lipid products, arachidonic acid, lysophosphatidylcholine (*LysoPC*), and ceramide. The production of ROS and cytochrome-C (*Cyt-C*) goes up. Mitochondrial membrane potential ($\Delta\psi$ – delta psi) and glutathione (GSH) are reduced. ROS also activate the p38 MAPkinase signal transduction pathways influencing various transcription factors and growth factors such as NF-κB, TGFβ(beta) and AP-1. There is an increase in expression of immediate early genes and production of various crystallization modulators such as osteopontin (*OPN*), bikunin (*BK*), and alpha-1-microglobulin (*α-1M*) and chemoattractants such as monocyte chemoattractant protein-1 (*MCP-1*)

which become surrounded by multinucleate giant cells, and ED-1 positive monocytes and macrophages. Exposure of renal epithelial cells to CaOx as well as CaP crystals induces the production of monocyte chemoattractant protein-1.[199,202,203]

The migration of macrophages to plaque site and development of inflammation are likely to play significant roles in ulceration of the subepithelial deposits to renal papillary surface leading to the formation of stone nidus. Cultured nontransformed macrophages release proinflammatory cytokines, tumor necrosis factor-alpha(α) (TNF-α) and interleukin-6 (IL-6) into the medium[120] in response to CaOx crystal binding and phagocytosis. TNF-α induces the transcription and expression of several matrix metalloproteinases (MMP). Activation of MMPs requires cleavage by proteases derived from inflammatory cells such as neutrophils and monocytes. Thus macrophages play a significant role in MMP gene expression and their subsequent activation. MMPs are the main matrix degrading enzymes and are considered to play a significant role in the erosion of atherosclerotic plaque and may play a similar role during stone formation in crystal erosion to renal papillary surface.

5.7 Conclusions

Intrinsic cellular dysfunctions that lead to hyperoxaluria, hypercalciuria, and hypocitarturia, individually or in combination, can lead to increased urinary CaP and/or CaOx supersaturation (Fig. 5.7). Mild supersaturation by itself, can, however, only produce small particle crystalluria. The crystals do not grow and aggregate, do not come in contact with the epithelial cells for long durations, are not retained inside the kidneys, and are excreted in the urine without causing any pathological changes and urolithiasis. Mild hyperoxaluria and hypercalciuria provoke protective responses. The exposed

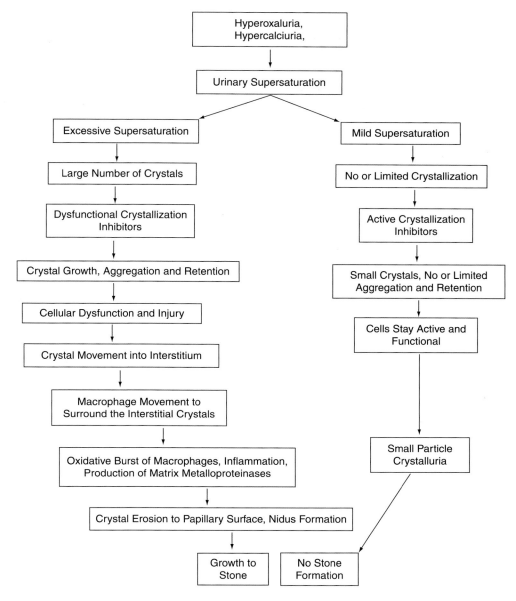

Fig. 5.7 Interaction between intrinsic factors causing hyperoxaluria, hypercalciuria, or hypocitraturia and extrinsic factors such as cell injury in the development of nephrolithiasis

cells respond by producing macromolecular crystallization inhibitors leading to reduced crystal nucleation, growth, and aggregation. Any crystals formed are excreted in the urine. If crystals come in contact with the cells, they are endocytosed and moved to lysosomes for removal. Other crystals are sent to the renal interstitium where macrophages become involved in crystal elimination.

Additional cellular dysfunctions that produce reduced or inefficient macromolecular inhibitors can, however, cause crystals to grow and aggregate or attach to renal epithelial cells and thus be retained inside the kidneys. In addition, CaP may crystallize in the renal interstitium and later evolve into a platform on papillary surface for the deposition of CaOx. In case of excessive urinary excretion of oxalate or calcium, such as in the primary or enteric hyperoxaluria secondary to bariatric surgery and distal renal tubular acidosis,

supersaturation can reach very high levels. A large number of crystals sufficient to slow down their movement through the tubular lumen are formed. Crystals may eventually plug the renal tubules. Slowing of the crystal movement and the blockage of renal tubules would result in prolonged interaction between crystals and renal epithelium leading to cellular dysfunction and degradation. Renal cells respond according to severity of the challenge. Response may be physiological, leading to the production of active crystallization inhibitors, or pathological, producing defective inhibitors promoting crystal aggregation and adherence. In addition damage to the cells can lead to both crystal nucleation and adherence. Crystallization modulators, both ionic and macromolecular, can affect supersaturation by binding calcium and/or oxalate. The most critical aspect of stone formation is the migration of interstitial crystal deposits to the papillary surfaces, which is most likely directed by inflammatory cells and the production of metalloproteinases.

Supersaturation is considered necessary for crystallization. Therefore, reduction of supersaturation is one of the major goals of most therapies. But supersaturation can only promote crystallization. That is why some non-stone formers have highly supersaturated urine but only produce crystalluria. An additional approach to prevent stone formation would be to stop retention of crystals and their migration to the papillary surface. Without these two processes there will be no kidney stones. As discussed previously, cellular damage promotes crystal retention through promotion of nucleation, aggregation, and attachment of crystals to the renal epithelium. In addition, an inflammatory response to the crystals may be necessary for the evolution of interstitial crystals into the stone nidus. Functional crystallization inhibitors are essential for the control of stone production. Damaged or dysfunctional state of the inhibitor producing cells may explain why stone formers produce insufficient and/or ineffective inhibitors. Since ROS appear responsible for cellular dysfunction/injury, control of renal oxidative stress may prove an effective therapy.

Acknowledgments Research supported by NIH grants # RO1DK065658 and RO1DK59765, and The University of Florida Center for the Study of Lithiasis.

References

1. Stamatelou KK, Francis MF, Jones CA, Curhan GC. Time trends in reported prevalence of kidney stones in the United States: 1976–1994. *Kidney Int.* 2003;63:1817–1823.
2. Butt AJ. Historical survey of etiologic factors in renal lithiasis. In: Butt AJ, ed. *Etiologic Factors in renal Lithiasis.* Springfield, IL: Charles C. Thomas; 1956:3–47.
3. Randall A. The etiology of primary renal calculus. *Intl Abst Surg.* 1940;71:209.
4. Kavanagh JP. Calcium oxalate crystallization *in vitro.* In: Khan SR, ed. *Calcium Oxalate in Biological Systems.* Boca Raton, FL: CRC Press; 1995:p1.
5. Robertson WG, Peacock M, Nordin BEC. Activity products in stone forming and non-stone forming urine. *Clin Sci.* 1968;34:579–594.
6. Khan SR, Kok DJ. Modulators of urinary stone formation. *Front Biosci.* 2004;9:1450–148.
7. Finlayson B, Reid S. The expectation of free or fixed particles in urinary stone disease. *Invest Urol.* 1978;15:442–448.
8. Kok DJ, Khan SR. Calcium oxalate nephrolithiasis, a free or fixed particle disease. *Kid Intl.* 1994;46:847–854.
9. Khan SR. Calcium oxalate crystal interaction with renal epithelium, mechanism of crystal adhesion and its impact on stone development. *Urol Res.* 1996;23:71–79.
10. Fasano JM, Khan SR. Intratubular crystallization of calcium oxalate in the presence of membrane vesicles: an in vitro study. *Kid Intl.* 2001;59:169–178.
11. Khan SR, Glenton PA, Backov R, Talham DR. Presence of lipids in urine, crystals and stones: Implications for the formation of kidney stones. *Kidney Int.* 2002;62:2062–2072.
12. Khan SR, Shevock PN, Hackett RL. Membrane-associated crystallization of calcium oxalate. *Calcif Tissue Intl.* 1990;46:116–120.
13. Khaskhali MH, Byer KJ, Khan SR. The effect of calcium on calcium oxalate monohydrate crystal induced renal epithelial injury. *Urol Res.* 2009;37(1):1–6.
14. Kaude JV, Williams CM, Millner MR, Scott KN, Finlayson B. Renal morphology and function immediately after extracorporeal shock-wave lithotripsy. *Am J Roentgenol.* 1985;145:305–313.
15. Vezzoli G, Soldati L, Gambaro G. Update on primary hypercalciuria from a genetic perspective. *J Urol.* 2008;179:1676–1682.
16. Geng W, Wang Z, Zhang J, Reed BY, Pak CY, Moe OW. Cloning and characterization of the human soluble adenylyl cyclase. *Am J Physiol Cell Physiol.* 2005;288:C1305-C1311.
17. Pastor-Soler N, Beaulieu V, Litvin TN, et al. Bicarbonate-regulated adenylyl cyclase (sAC) Is a sensor that regulates pH-dependent V-ATPase recycling. *J Biol Chem.* 2003;278:49523–49529.
18. Reed BY, Heller HJ, Gitomer WL, Pak CY. Mapping a gene defect in absorptive hypercalciuria to chromososme 1q23.3-q24. *J Clin Endocrinol Metab.* 1999;84:3907–3911.
19. Reed BY, Gitomer WL, Heller HJ, et al. Identification and characterization of a gene with base substitutions associated with the absorptive hypercalciuria phenotype and low spine bone density. *J Clin Endocrinol Metab.* 2002;87:1476–1481.
20. Rendina D, Mossetti G, Viceconti R, et al. Association between vitamin D receptor gene polymorphisms and fasting idiopathic hypercalciuria in recurrent stone-forming patients. *Urology.* 2004;64:838–842.
21. Bushinsky DA. Genetic hypercalciuric stone-forming rats. *Curr Opin Nephrol Hypertens.* 1999;8:479–489.
22. Khullar M, Relan V, Singh SK. VDR gene and urinary calcium excretion in nephrolithiasis. *Kidney Int.* 2006;69:943–951.
23. Recker F, Rubben H, Bex A, Constantinides C. Morphological changes following ESWL in the rat kidney. *Urol Res.* 1989;17:229–233.
24. Relan V, Khullar M, Singh SK, Sharma SK. Association of vitamin D receptor genotypes with calcium excretion in nephrolithiatic subjects in northern India. *Urol Res.* 2004;32:236–241.
25. Soylemezoglu O, Ozkaya O, Gonen S, Misirlioglu M, Kalman S, Buyan N. Vitamin D receptor gene polymorphism in hypercalciuric children. *Pediatr Nephrol.* 2004;19:724–730.
26. Bushinsky DA, Asplin JR, Grynpass MD, et al. Calcium oxalate stone formation in genetic hypercalciuric stone-forming rats. *Kidney Intl.* 2002;61:975–987.
27. Zerwekh JE, Hughes MR, Reed BY, et al. Evidence for normal vitamin D receptor messenger ribonucleic acid and genotype in absorptive hypercalciuria. *J Clin Endocrinol Metab.* 1995;80:2960–2965.
28. Scott P, Ouimet D, Valiquette L, et al. Suggestive evidence for a susceptibility gene near the vitamin D receptor locus in idiopathic calcium stone formation. *J Am Soc Nephrol.* 1999;10:1007–1013.
29. Muller D, Hoenderop JG, Vennekens R, et al. Epithelial Ca(2_) channel (ECAC1) in autosomal dominant idiopathic hypercalciuria. *Nephrol Dial Transplant.* 2002;17:1614–1621.
30. Bid HK, Kumar A, Kapoor R, Mittal RD. Association of vitamin D receptor- gene (*FokI*) polymorphism with calcium oxalate nephrolithiasis. *J Endourol.* 2005;19:111–115.
31. Chen W-C, Chen H-Y, Lu H-F, Hsu C-D, Tsai F-J. Association of the vitamin D receptor gene start codon Fok I polymorphism with calcium oxalate stone disease. *BJU Int.* 2001;87:168–174.
32. Nishijima S, Sugaya K, Naito A, Morozumi M, Hatano T, Ogawa Y. Association of vitamin D receptor gene polymorphism with urolithiasis. *J Urol.* 2002;167:2188–2195.

33. Ozkaya O, Soylemezoglu O, Misirlioglu M, Gonen S, Buyan N, Hasanoglu E. Polymorphisms in the vitamin D receptor gene and the risk of calcium nephrolithiasis in children. *Eur Urol*. 2003;44: 150–154.

34. Devuyst O, Pirson Y. Genetics of hypercalciuric stoen forming diseases. *Kidney Int*. 2007;72:1065–1072.

35. Tfelt-Hansen J, Brown EM. The calcium-sensing receptor in normal physiology and pathophysiology: a review. *Crit Rev Clin Lab Sci*. 2004;42:35–48.

36. Vezzoli G, Tanini A, Ferrucci L, et al. Influence of calcium-sensing receptor gene on urinary calcium excretion in stone-forming patients. *J Am Soc Nephrol*. 2002;13:2517–2125.

37. Vezzoli G, Terranegra A, Arcidiacono T, et al. R990G polymorphism of calcium-sensing receptor does produce a gain-of-function and predispose to primary hypercalciuria. *Kidney Int*. 2007;71: 1155–1163.

38. Hough TA, Bogani D, Cheeseman MT, et al. Activating calcium-sensing receptor mutation in the mouse is associated with cataracts and ectopic calcification. *Proc Natl Acad Sci USA*. 2004; 101:13566–13571.

39. Prie D, Huart V, Bakouh N, et al. Nephrolithiasis and osteoporosis caused by mutations in the type 2a sodium-phosphate cotransporter. *N Engl J Med*. 2002;347:983–988.

40. Lapointe Y, Tessier J, Paquette Y, et al. NPT2 gene variation in calcium nephrolithiasis with renal phosphate leak. *Kidney Int*. 2006;69:226–233.

41. Bergwitz C, Roslin NM, Tieder M, et al. SLC34A3 mutations in patients with hereditary hypophosphatemic rickets with hypercalciuria predict a key role for the sodium-phosphate cotransporter NaPi-Iic in maintaining phosphate homeostasis. *Am J Hum Genet*. 2006;78:179–192.

42. Tennenhouse HS. Regulation of phosphorus homeostasis by the type !!a Na/phosphate cotransporter. *Annu Rev Nutr*. 2005;25: 197–214.

43. Khan SR, Glenton PA. Calcium oxalate crystal deposition in kidneys of hypercalciuric mice with disrupted type IIa sodium-phosphate cotransporter. *Am J Physiol Renal Physiol*. 2008;294: F1109–1115.

44. Wrong OM, Norden AG, Feest TG. Dent's disease; a familial proximal renal tubular syndrome with low-molecularweight proteinuria, hypercalciuria, nephrocalcinosis, metabolic bone disease, progressive renal failure and a marked male predominance. *QJM*. 1994;87:473–493.

45. Christensen EI, Devuyst O, Dom G, et al. Loss of chloride channel ClC-5 impairs endocytosis by defective trafficking of megalin and cubilin in kidney proximal tubules. *Proc Natl Acad Sci USA*. 2003;100:8472–8479.

46. Devuyst O, Jouret F, Auzanneau C, Courtoy PJ. Chloride channels and endocytosis: new insights from Dent's disease and CIC-5 knockout mice. *Nephron Physiol*. 2005;99:69–73.

47. Piwon N, Gunther W, Schwake M, Bosl MR, Jentsch TJ. ClC-5 Cl- -channel disruption impairs endocytosis in a mouse model for Dent's disease. *Nature*. 2000;408:369–373.

48. Gunther W, Piwon N, Jentsch TJ. The ClC-5 chloride channel knock-out mouse—an animal model for Dent's disease. *Pflugers Arch*. 2003;445:456–462.

49. Loffing J, Loffing-Cueni D, Valderrabano V, et al. Distribution of transcellular calcium and sodium transport pathways along mouse distal nephron. *Am J Physiol Renal Physiol*. 2001;281:F1021–27.

50. Suzuki Y, Landowski CP, Hediger MA. Mechanisms and regulation of epithelial Ca absorption in health and disease. *Annu Rev Physiol*. 2008;70:257–271.

51. Hoenderop JG, van Leeuwen JP, van der Eerden BC, et al. Renal Ca2 wasting, hyperabsorption, and reduced bone thickness in mice lacking TRPV5. *J Clin Invest*. 2003;112:1906–1914.

52. Jiang Y, Ferguson WB, Peng JB. WNK4 enhances TRPV5-mediated calcium transport: potential role in hypercalciuria of familial hyperkalemic hypertension caused by gene mutation of WNK4. *Am J Physiol Renal Physiol*. 2007;292(2):F545–F554.

53. Colegio OR, Van Itallie CM, McCrea HJ, Rahner C, Anderson JM. Claudins create charge-selective channels in the paracellular pathway between epithelial cells. *Am J Physiol Cell Physiol*. 2002;283:C142-C147.

54. Konrad M, Schlingmann KP, Gudermann T. Insights into the molecular nature of magnesium homeostasis. *Am J Physiol Renal Physiol*. 2004;286:F599-F605.

55. Weber S, Schneider L, Peters M, et al. Novel paracellin-1 mutations in 25 families with familial hypomagnesemia with hypercalciuria and nephrocalcinosis. *J Am Soc Nephrol*. 2001;12: 1872–1881.

56. Muller D, Kausalya PJ, Claverie-Martin F, et al. A novel claudin 16 mutation associated with childhood hypercalciuria abolishes binding to ZO-1 and results in lysosomal mistargeting. *Am J Hum Genet*. 2003;73:1293–1301.

57. Arking DE. Association of human aging with a functional variant of klotho. *Proc Natl Acad Sci USA*. 2002;99:856–861.

58. Kuro-o M, Matsumora Y, Aizawa H, et al. mutation of the mouse klotho gene leads to a syndrome resembling aging. *Nature*. 1997;390:45–51.

59. Ogata N, Matsumura Y, Shiraki M, et al. Association of klotho gene polymorphism with bone density and spondylosis of the lumbar spine in postmenopausal women. *Bone*. 2002;31:37–41.

60. Tsuruoka S, Nishi K, Ioka T, et al. Defect in parathyroid hormone induced luminal calcium absorption in connecting tubuless of klotho mice. *Nephrol Dial Transplant*. 2006;21:2762–2767.

61. Chang Q, Hoefs S, ven der Kemp AW, Topala AW, Bindels RJ, Hoenderop JG. The beta glucoronidase klotho hydrolyzes and activates TRPV5 channel. *Science*. 2005;310:490–493.

62. Kurosu H, Ogawa Y, Miyoshi M, et al. Regulation of fibroblast growth factor-23 signaling by klotho. *J Biol Chem*. 2006;281:6120–3.

63. Medetognon-Benissan J, Tardivel S, Hennequin C, Daudon T, Drueke T, Lacour B. Inhibitory effect of bikunin on calcium oxalate crystallization *in vitro* and urinary bikunin decrease in renal stone formers. *Urol Res*. 1999;27:69–75.

64. Danpure CJ, Rumsby G. Enzymology and molecular genetics of primary hyperoxaluria type 1, consequences for clinical management. In: Khan SR, ed. *calcium Oxalate in Biological Systems*. Boca Raton, FL: CRC Press Inc; 1995:189–205.

65. Cramer SD, Ferree PM, Lin K, Milliner DS, Holmes RP. The gene encoding hydroxypyruvate reductase (GRHPR) is mutated in patients with primary hyperoxaluria type II. *Hum Mol Genet*. 1999;8:2063–2069.

66. Salido EC, Li XM, Yang Lu, et al. Alanine-glyoxylate aminotransferase-deficient mice, a model for primary hyperoxaluria that responds to adenoviral gene transfer. *Proc Natl Acad Sci USA*. 2006;103:18249–18254.

67. Alper SL. Diseases of mutations in the SLC4A1/AE1 (band 3) Cl⁻/HCO$_3^-$ exchanger. In: Broer S, Wagner CA, eds. *Membrane Transporter Diseases*. New York: Kluwer/Plenum Publishers; 2003:39–63.

68. Stehberger PA, Shmukler BE, Stuart-Tilley AK, Peters LL, Alper SL, Wagner CA. Distal renal tubular acidosis in mice lacking the AE1 (band3) Cl-/HCO3- exchanger (slc4a1). *J Am Soc Nephrol*. 2007; 18:1408–1418.

69. Knight J, Holmes RP, Assimos DG. Intestinal and renal handling of oxalate loads in normal individuals and stone formers. *Urol Res*. 2007;35:111–117.

70. Krishnamurthy M, Hruska KA, Chandhoke PS. The urinary response to an oral oxalate load in recurrent calcium stone formers. *J Urol*. 2003;169:2030–2035.

71. Hatch M, Freel RW. Intestinal transport of an obdurate anion: oxalate. *Urol Res.* 2005;33:1–16.

72. Mount DB, Romero MF. The *SLC26* gene family of multifunctional anion exchangers. *Pflugers Arch.* 2004;447:710–721.

73. Soleimani M. Expression, regulation and the role of SLC26 Cl–/HCO3– exchangers in kidney and gastrointestinal tract. *Novartis Found Symp.* 2006;273:91–102.

74. Soleimani M, Xu J. SLC26 chloride/nase exchangers in the kidney in health and disease. *Seminars in Nephrol.* 2006;26:375–385.

75. Xie Q, Welch R, Mercado A, Romero MF, Mount DB. Molecular characterization of the murine Slc26a6 anion exchanger: functional comparison with Slc26a1. *Am J Physiol Renal Physiol.* 2002;283:F826–F838.

76. Wang Z, Wang T, Petrovic S, et al. Renal and intestinal transport defects in Slc26a6-null mice. *Am J Physiol Cell Physiol.* 2005;288:C957-C965.

77. Freel RW, Hatch M, Green M, Soleimani M. Ileal oxalate absorption and urinary oxalate excretion are enhanced in Slc26a6 null mice. *Am J Physiol.* 2006;290:G719–G728.

78. Jiang Z, Asplin JR, Evan AP, et al. Calcium oxalate urolithiasis in mice lacking anion transporter Slc26a6. *Nat Genet.* 2006;38:474–478.

79. Parks JH, Ruml LA, Pak CYC. Hypocitraturia. In: Coe FL, Favus MJ, Pak CYC, Parks JH, Preminger GM, eds. *Kidney Stones: Medical and Surgical Management.* Philadelphia, PA: Lippincott-Raven; 1996:905–920.

80. Meyer JL, Smith LH. Growth of calcium oxalate crystals II: Inhibition by natural urinary crystal growth inhibitors. *Invest Urol.* 1975;13:36–39.

81. Pak CY, Nicar M, Northcutt C. The definition of the mechanism of hypercalciuria is necessary for the treatment of recurrent stone formers. *Contrib Nephrol.* 1982;33:136–151.

82. Shah O, Assimos DG, Holmes RP. Genetic and dietary factors in urinary citrate excretion. *J Endourol.* 2005;19:177–182.

83. Pak CY. Citrate and renal calculi. *Miner Electrolyte Metab.* 1987;13:257–266.

84. Hamm LL, Alpern RJ. Regulation of acid–base balance, citrate, and urine pH. In: Coe FL, Favus MJ, Pak CYC, Parks JH, Preminger GM, eds. *Kidney Stones: Medical and Surgical Management.* Philadelphia, PA: Lippincott-Raven; 1996:289–302.

85. Hamm LL, Hering-Smith KS. Pathophysiology of hypocitraturic nephrolithiasis. *Endocrinol Metab Clin North Am.* 2002;31:885–893.

86. Pajor AM. Conformationally sensitive residues in transmembrane domain 9 of the Na+/dicarboxylate co-transporter. *J Biol Chem.* 2001;276:29961–29968.

87. Okamoto N, Aruga S, Matsuzaki S, Takahashi S, Matsushita K, Kitamura T. Associations between renal sodium-citrate co-transporter (hNaDC-1) gene polymorphism and urinary citrate excretion in recurrent renal calcium stone formers and normal controls. *Int J Urol.* 2007;14:344–349.

88. He Y, Chen X, Yu Z, et al. Sodium dicarboxylate cotransporter-1 expression in renal tissues and its role in rat experimental nephrolithiasis. *J Nephrol.* 2004;17:34–42.

89. Kok DJ, Papapoulos SE, Blomen LMJ, Bijvoet OLM. Modulation of calcium-oxalate monohydrate crystallization kinetics in vitro. *Kidney Int.* 1988;34:346–350.

90. Ryall RL, Harnett RM, Marshall VR. The effect of urine, pyrophosphate, citrate, magnesium and glycosaminoglycans on the growth and aggregation of calcium oxalate crystals in vitro. *Clin Chim Acta.* 1988;112:349–356.

91. Schwille PO, Rumenapf G, Wolfel G, Kohler R. Urinary pyrophosphate in patients with recurrent urolithiasis and in healthy controls: a reevaluation. *J Urol.* 1988;140:239–245.

92. Sidhu H, Gupta R, Thind SK, Nath R. Inhibition of calcium oxalate monohydrate crystal growth. by pyrophosphate, citrate and rat urine. *Urol Res.* 1986;14:299–303.

93. Achilles W, Coors D, Reifenberger B, Sallis JD, Schalk CH. Natural and artificial substances as inhibitors of crystal growth of calcium oxalates in gel matrices. In: Vahlensieck, W., Gasser, G. Hesse A., Schoeneich G., eds. Urolithiasis, Proceedings 1st European Symposium on Urolithiasis, Bonn 1989. Excerpta Medica Amsterdam, ISBN 90 219 9865 3, 1989:65–67.

94. Grases F, Ramis M, Costa-Bauza A. Effects of phytate and pyrophosphate on brushite and hydroxyapatite crystallization - Comparison with the action of other polyphosphates. *Urol Res.* 2000;28:136–140.

95. Robertson WG. Factors affecting the precipitation of calcium phosphate in vitro. *Calcif Tissue Res.* 1973;11:311–322.

96. Laminski NA, Meyers AM, Sonnekus MI, Smyth AE. Prevalence of hypocitraturia and hypopyrophosphaturia in recurrent calcium stone formers: as isolated defects or associated with other metabolic abnormalities. *Nephron.* 1990;56:379–384.

97. Tsui HW, Inman RD, Paterson AD, Reveille JD, Tsui FW. ANKH varian is associated with ankylosing spondylitis: gender differences. *Arthritis Res Ther.* 2005;7:R513–525.

98. Korkmaz C, Ozcan A, Akcar N. Increased frequency of ultrasonographic findings suggestive of renal stone patients with ankolysing spondylitis. *Clin Exp Rheumatol.* 2005;23:389–392.

99. Min W, Sgiraga H, Chalko C, Goldfarb S, Krishna GG, Hoyer JR. Quantitative studies of human urinary excretion of uropontin. *Kidney Intl.* 1998;53:189–193.

100. Nishio S, Hatanaka M, Takeda H, Iseda T, Iwata H, Yokoyama M. Analysis of urinary concentrations of calcium phosphate crystal-associated proteins: alpha-2-HS-glycoprotein, prothrombin F1, and osteopontin. *J Am Soc Nephrol.* 1999;10:S394–S396.

101. Wesson JA, Johnson RJ, Mazzali M, et al. Osteopontin is acritical inhibitor of calcium oxalate crystal formation and retention in renal tubules. *J Am Soc Nephrol.* 2003;14:139–147.

102. Gao B, Yasui T, Itoh Y, et al. Association of osteopontin gene heplotypes with nephrolithiasis. *Kidney Intl.* 2007;72:592–598.

103. Fisher LW, Hawkins GR, Tuross N, Termine JD. Purification and partial characterization of small proteoglycans I and II, bone sialoproteins I and II, and osteonectin from the mineral compartment of developing human bone. *J Biol Chem.* 1987;262:9702–9708.

104. Singh K, DeVouge MW, Mukherjee BB. Physiological properties and differential glycosylation of phosphorylated and nonphosphorylated forms of osteopontin secreted by normal rat kidney cells. *J Biol Chem.* 1990;265:18696–18701.

105. Hunter GK, Kyle CL, Goldberg HA. Modulation of crystal formation by bone phosphoproteins; structural specificity of the osteopontin-mediated inhibition of hydroxyapatite formation. *Biochem J.* 1994;300:723–728.

106. Hoyer JR, Asplin JR, Otvos LJ. Phosphorylated osteopontin peptides suppress crystallization by inhibiting growth of calcium oxalate crystals. *Kidney Int.* 2001;60:77–82.

107. Atmani F, Glenton PA, Khan SR. Identification of proteins extracted from calcium oxalate and calcium phosphate crystals induced in the urine of healthy and stone forming subjects. *Urol Res.* 1998;26:201–207.

108. Glauser A, Horhreiter W, Jaeger P, Hess B. Determinants of urinary excretion of Tamm-Horsfall protein in non-selected kidney stone formers and healthy subjects. *Nephrol Dial Transplant.* 2000;15:158–1587.

109. Romero MC, Nocera S, Nesse AB. Decreased Tamm–Horsfall protein in lithiasis patients. *Clin Biochem.* 1997;30:63–67.

110. Schnierle P. A simple diagnostic method for the differentiation of Tamm-Horsfall glycoprotein from healthy probands and those from recurrent calcium oxalate renal stone formers. *Experimentia.* 1995;51:1068–1072.

111. Mo L, Huang H-Y, Zhu X-H, Shapiro E, Hasty DL, Wu X-Ru. Tamm–Horsfall protein is a critical renal defense factor protecting against calcium oxalate crystal formation. *Kidney Intl.* 2004;66:1159–1166.

112. Mo L, Liaw L, Evan AP, Sommer AJ, Lieske JC, Wu X-R. Renal calcinosis and stone formation in mice lacking osteopontin, Tamm-Horsfall protein, or both. *Am J Physiol Renal Physiol.* 2007;293: F1935–1943.

113. Bernascone I, Vavassori S, Di Pentima AD, et al. Defective intracellular trafficking of uromodulin mutant isoforms. *Traffic.* 2006;7:1567–1579.

114. Serafini-Cessi F, Maligolini N, Cavallone D. Tamm–Horsfall protein glycoprotein: biology and clinical relevance. *Am J Kidney Dis.* 2003;42:658–676.

115. Biri H, Ozturk HS, Buyukkocak KM, et al. Antioxidant defense potential of rabbit renal tissues after ESWL: protective effects of antioxidant vitamins. *Nephron.* 1998;79:181–185.

116. Atmani F, Lacour B, Jungers P, Drüeke T, Daudon M. Reduced inhibitory activity of uronic-acid-rich protein in urine of stone formers. *Urol Res.* 1994;22:257–260.

117. Suzuki S, Kobayashi H, Kageyama S, Shibata K, Fujie M, Terao T. Excretion of bikunin and its fragments in the urine of patients with renal stones. *J Urol.* 2001;166:268–274.

118. Atmani F, Khan SR. Role of urinary bikunin in the inhibition of calcium oxalate crystallization. *J Am Soc Nephrol.* 1999;10:S385–S390.

119. Atmani F, Mizon J, Khan SR. Identification of uronic-acid-rich protein as urinary bikunin, the light chain of inter-α-inhibitor. *Eur J Biochem.* 1996;236:984–990.

120. DeWater R, Leenen PJM, Noordermeer C, et al. Cytokine production induced by binding and processing of calcium oxalate crystals in cultured macrophages. *Am J Kidney Dis.* 2001;38:331.

121. Tardivel S, Medetognon J, Randoux C, et al. Alpha-1-microglobulin: inhibitory effect on calcium oxalate crystallization *in vitro* and decreased urinary concentration in calcium oxalate stone formers. *Urol Res.* 1999;27:243–249.

122. Coe FL, Parks JH. Pathophysiology of kidney stones and strategies for treatment. *Hosp Pract.* 1988;23:145–168.

123. Danpure CJ, Purdue PE. Primary hyperoxaluria. In: Scriver CR, Beaudet AL, Sly WS, Valle D, eds. *The Metabolic and Molecular Bases of Inherited Disease.* 7th ed. New York: McGraw-Hill; 1995:2385–2424.

124. Finlayson B. Physicochemical aspects of urolithiasis. *Kid Intl.* 1978;13:344–360.

125. Hatch M. Oxalate status in stone formers: Two distinct hyperoxaluric entities. *Urol Res.* 1993;21:55–59.

126. Osther PJ. Hyperoxaluria in idiopathic calcium nephrolithiasis, what are the limits? *Scand J Urol Nephrol.* 1999;33:368–371.

127. Robertson WG. Mild hyperoxaluria: a critical review and future outlook. In: Kidney Stones, Proceedings of the 8th European Symposium on Urolithiasis, Parma, Italy, June 9–12, 1999:33–42

128. Lieske JC, Hammes MS, Hoyer JR, Toback FG. Renal cell osteopontin production is stimulated by CaOx monohydrate crystals. *Kid Intl.* 1997;51:679–686.

129. Asplin JR, Coe FL. Hyperoxaluria in kiney stone formers treated with modern bariatric surgery. *J Urol.* 2007;177:565–569.

130. Canos HJ, Hogg GA, Jeffery JR. Oxalate nephropathy due to gastrointetsinal disorders. *Can Med Assoc J.* 1981;124:729–733.

131. Demaria EJ, Jamal MK. Surgical options for obesity. *Gastroenterol Clin North Am.* 2005;34:127–142.

132. Flegal KM, Carroll MD, Ogden CL, Johnson CL. Prevalence and trends in obesity among US adults. *JAMA.* 2002;288: 1723–1735.

133. Nelson WK, Houghton SG, Milliner DS, Lieske JC, Sarr MG. Enteric hyperoxaluria, nephrolithiasis, and oxalate nephropathy: potentially serious and unappreciated complications of Roux-en-Y gastric bypass. *Surg Obes Relat Dis.* 2005;1:481–485.

134. Nordenvall B, Backman L, Narsson L. Oxalate metabolism after intestinal bypass operation. *Scand J Gastroenterol.* 1981;16:395–399.

135. Roth J, Qiang X, Marban SL, Redelt H, Lowell BC. The obesity pandemic: where have we been and where are we going? *Obes Res.* 2004;12:88–94.

136. Shinogle JA, Owings MF, Kozak LJ. Gastric bypass as treatment for obesity, trends, characteristics, and complications. *Obes Res.* 2005;13:2202–2209.

137. Sinha MK, Collazo-Clavell ML, Milliner DS, et al. Hyperoxaluric nephrolithiasis is a complication of Roux-en-Y gastric bypass surgery. *Kidney Int.* 2007;72:8–10.

138. Gelbert DR, Brewer LL, Fajardo LF, Weinstein AB. Oxalosis and chronic renal failure after intestinal bypass. *Arch Int Med.* 1977;137:239–243.

139. Mandell I, Krauss E, Millan JC. Oxalate induced acute renal failure in Crohn's disease. *Am J Med.* 1980;69:628–632.

140. Wharton R, D'Agati V, Magun AM, Whitlock R, Kunis CL, Appel GB. Acute deterioration of renal function associated with enteric hyperoxaluria. *Clin Nephrol.* 1990;34:116–121.

141. Baggio B, Gambaro G, Ossi E, Favaro S, Borsatti A. Increased urinary excretion of renal enzymes in idiopathic calcium oxalate nephrolithiasis. *J Urol.* 1983;129:1161–1164.

142. Huang H-S, Ma M-C, Chen C-F, Chen J. Lipid peroxidation and its correlations with urinary levels of oxalate, citric acdi, and osteopontin in patients with renal calcium oxalate stones. *Urology.* 2003;62:1123–1128.

143. Tungsanga K, Sriboonlue P, Futrakul P, Yachantha C, Tosukhowong P. Renal tubular cell damage and oxidative stress in renal stone patients and the effect of potassium citrate treatment. *Urol Res.* 2005;33:65–9.

144. Khan SR. Experimental CaOx nephrolithiasis and the formation of human urinary stones. *Scann Microsc.* 1995;9:89–100.

145. Khan SR. Animal models of kidney stone formation: an analysis. *World J Urol.* 1997;15:236–243.

146. Khan SR, Finlayson B, Hackett RL. Experimental calcium oxalate nephrolithiasis in the rat, role of renal papilla. *Am J Pathol.* 1982;107:59–69.

147. Khan SR, Glenton PA, Byer KJ. Modeling of hyperoxaluric calcium oxalate nephrolithiasis: Experimental induction of hyperoxaluria by hydroxy-L-proline. *Kidney Int.* 2006;70:914–923.

148. Khan SR, Johnson JM, Peck AB, Cornelius JM, Glenton PA. Expression of osteopontin in rat kidneys: induction during ethylene glycol induced calcium oxalate nephrolithiasis. *J Urol.* 2002;168:1173–1181.

149. Khan SR, Shevock PN, Hackett R. Urinary enzymes and CaOx urolithiasis. *J Urol.* 1989;142:846–849.

150. Shevock KSR, PN HRL. Acute Hyperoxaluria, renal injury and calcium oxalate urolithiasis. *J Urol.* 1992;147:226–230.

151. Khan SR, Thamilselvan S. Nephrolithiasis: a consequence of renal epithelial cell exposure to oxalate and calcium oxalate crystals. *Mol Urol.* 2000;4:305–312.

152. Iida S, Peck AB, Johnson-Tardieu J, et al. Temporal changes in mRNA expression for bikunin in the kidneys of rats during CaOx nephrolithiasis. *J Am Soc Nephrol.* 1999;10:986–996.

153. Moriyama MT, Glenton PA, Khan SR. Expression of inter-α-inhibitor related proteins in kidneys and urine of hyperoxaluric rats. *J Urol.* 2001;165:1687–1692.

154. Thannickal VJ, Fanburg BL. Reactive oxygen species in cell signaling. *Am J Physiol Lung Cell Mol Physiol.* 2000;279: L1005–28.

155. Khan SR, Finlayson B, Hackett RL. Renal papillary changes in patient with calcium oxalate lithiasis. *Urology.* 1984;23: 194–199.

156. Khan SR, Byer KJ, Thamilselvan S, et al. Crystal-cell interaction and apoptosis in oxalate-associated injury of renal epithelial cells. *J Am Soc Nephrol.* 1999;10:S457-S463.

157. McKee MC, Nanci A, Khan SR. Ultrastructural immunodetection of osteopontin and osteocalcin as major matrix components of renal calculi. *J Bone Miner Res.* 1995;10:1913–1929.

158. De Bruijn WC, Boeve ER, van Run PR, et al. Etiology of CaOx nephrolithiasis in rats.I. Can this be a model for human stone formation? *Scann Microsc.* 1995;9:103–114.

159. Toblli JE, Ferder L, Stella I, Angerosa M, Inserra F. Protective role of enalapril for chronic tubulointerstitial lesions of hyperoxaluria. *J Urol.* 2001;166:275–280.

160. Toblli JE, Ferder L, Stella I, Angerosa M, Inserra F. Effects of angiotensin II subtype 1 receptor blockade by losartan on tubulointerstitial lesions caused by hyperoxaluria. *J Urol.* 2002;168:1550–1555.

161. Muller GA, Rodemann HP. Characterization of human renal fibroblasts in health and disease: immunophenotyping of cultural epithelial cells and fibroblasts derived from kidney with histologically proven interstitial fibrosis. *Am J Kid Dis.* 1991;17:680–683.

162. Nathan CF. Secretory products of macrophages. *J Clin Invest.* 1987;79:319–326.

163. Lieske JC, Deganello S. Nucleation, adhesion, and internalization of calcium-containing urinary crystals by renal cells. *J Am Soc Nephrol.* 1999;10:S422-S426.

164. Khan SR. Heterogeneous nucleation of calcium oxalate crystals in mammalian urine. *Scann Microsc.* 1995;9:597–616.

165. Khan SR, Whalen PO, Glenton PA. Heterogeneous nucleation of calcium oxalate crystals in the presence of membrane vesicles. *J Crystal Growth.* 1993;134:211–218.

166. Kirsch T. Determinants of pathologic mineralization. *Crit Rev Eukaryot Gene Expr.* 2008;18:1–9.

167. Khan SR, Shevock PN, Hackett RL. In vitro precipitation of calcium oxalate in the presence of whole matrix or lipid components of the urinary stones. *J Urol.* 1988;139:418–422.

168. Evan AP, Lingeman JE, Coe FL, et al. Randall's plaque of patients with nephrolithiasis begins in basement membranes of thin loops of Henle. *J Clin Invest.* 2003;111:607–617.

169. Hautmann R, Osswald H. Concentration profiles of calcium and oxalate in urine, tubular fluid and renal tissue-some theoretical considerations. *J Urol.* 1983;129:433.

170. Khan SR. Where do the renal stones form and how? *Int J Min Electr Metab.* 1996;10:75–81.

171. Khan SR, Cockrell CA, Finlayson B, Hackett RL. Crystal retention by injured urothelium of the urinary bladder. *J Urol.* 1984;132:153–157.

172. Riese RJ, Mandel NS, Wiessner JH, Mandel GS, Becker CJ, Kleinman JC. Cell polarity and CaOx crystal adherence to cultured collecting duct cells. *Am J Physiol.* 1992;262:F177-F183.

173. Verkoelen CF, van der Broom BG, Houtsmuller AB, Schroeder FH, Romijn JC. Increased CaOx monohydrate crystal binding to injured renal epithelial cells in culture. *Am J Physiol.* 1998;274:F958-F966.

174. Khan SR. Tubular cell surface events during nephrolithiasis. *Curr Opin Urol.* 1997;7:240–247.

175. Kumar V, Farell G, Deganello S, Lieske JC. Annexin II is present on renal epithelial cells and binmds calcium oxalate monohydrate crystals. *J Am Soc Nephrol.* 2003;14:289–297.

176. Sorokina EA, Wesson JA, Kleinman JG. An acidic peptide of nucleolin related protein can mediate the attachment of calcium oxalate to renal tubule cell. *J Am Soc Nephrol.* 2004;15:2057–2065.

177. Khan SR. Intercations between stone forming calcific crystals and macromolecules. *Urol Int.* 1997;59:59–71.

178. Verhulst A, Asselman M, Persy VP, et al. Crystal retention capacity of cells in the human nephron: involvement of CD 44 and its ligands hyaluronic acid and osetopontin in the transition from a crystal binding into a non adherent epithelium. *J Am Soc Nephrol.* 2003;13:107.

179. Wiessner JH, Hasegawa AT, Hung LY, Mandel NS. Oxalate-induced exposure of PS on surface of renal epithelial cells in culture. *J Am Soc Nephrol.* 1999;10:S441-S445.

180. Robertson WG. Kidney models of calcium oxalate stone formation. *Nephron Physiol.* 2004;98:21–26.

181. Robertson WG, Peacock M. Calcium oxalate crystalluria and inhibitors of crystallization in recurrent renal stone-formers. *Clin Sci.* 1972;43:499–505.

182. Brown SA. Oxidative stress and chronic kidney disease. *Vet Clin N Am: Small Anim Pract.* 2008;38:157–166.

183. Khan SR. Role of renal epithelial cells in the initiation of calcium oxalate stones. *Nephron Exp Nephrol.* 2004;98:e55-e60.

184. Khan SR. Hyperoxaluria-induced oxidative stress and antioxidants for renal protection. *Urol Res.* 2005;33:349–57.

185. Gokhale JA, Glenton PA, Khan SR. Immunocytochemical localization of Tamm-Horsfall protein and osteopontin in a rat nephrolithiasis model. *Nephron.* 1996;73:456–461.

186. Gokhale JA, Glenton PA, Khan SR. Characterization of Tamm-Horsfall protein in a rat nephrolithiasis model. *J Urol.* 2001;166:1492–1497.

187. Suzuki K, Tanaka T, Miyazawa K, et al. Gene expression of prothrombin in human and rat kidneys, basic and clinical approach. *J Am Soc Nephrol.* 1999;10:S408-S411.

188. Marengo SR, Chen DHC, Kaung HLC, Resnick MI, Yang L. Decreased renal xpression of the putative calcium oxalate inhibitor Tamm-Horsfall Protein in the ethylene glycol rat model of calcium oxalate urolithiasis. *J Urol.* 2002;167:2192–2197.

189. Katsuma S, Shiojima S, Hirasawa A, et al. Global analysis of differentially expressed genes during progression of calcium oxalate nephrolithiasis. *Biochem Biophys Res Commun.* 2002;296(3):544–552.

190. Iida S, Inoue M, Yoshi S, et al. Molecular detection of haparan sulfate proteoglycan mRNA in rat kidneys during CaOx nephrolithiasis. *J Am Soc Nephrol.* 1999;10:S412-S416.

191. Khan SR. Crystal-induced inflammation of the kidneys, results of human, animal model and tissue culture studies. *Clin Exp Nephrol.* 2004;8:75–88.

192. Lieske JC, Toback FG. Renal cell-urinary crystal interactions. *Curr Opin Nephrol Hypertens.* 2000;9:349–355.

193. Balduyck M, Albani D, Jourdain M, et al. Inflammation-induced systemic proteolysis of inter-alpha-ihibitor in plasma from patients with sepsis. *J Lab Clin Med.* 2000;135:188–198.

194. Fries E, Blom AM. Bikunin: not just a plasma proteinase inhibitor. *In J Biochem Cell Biol.* 2000;32:125–137.

195. Toblli JE, Cao G, Casas G, Stella I, Inserra F, Angerosa M. NF-kappaB and chemokine-cytokine expression in renal tubulointerstitium in experimental hyperoxaluria. Role of the renin-angiotensin system. *Urol Res.* 2005;33:358–67.

196. Umekawa T, Hatanaka Y, Kurita T, Khan SR. Effect of Angiotensin II Receptor blockage on Osteopontin Expression and Calcium Oxalate Crystal deposition in the Rat Kidneys. *J Am Soc Nephrol.* 2004;15:635–644.

197. Ophascharoensuk V, Giachelli CM, Gordon K, et al. Obstructive uropathy in the mouse: role of osteopontin in interstitial fibrosis and apoptosis. *Kid Intl.* 1999;56:571–580.

198. Young BA, Burdmann EA, Johnson RJ, et al. Cellular proliferation and macrophage influx precede interstitial fibrosis in cyclosporine nephrotoxicity. *Kid Intl.* 1995;48:439–448.

199. Escobar C, Byer KJ, Khaskheli H, Khan SR. Apatite induced renal epithelial injury: insight into the pathogenesis of kidney stones. *J Urol.* 2008;180:379–387.

200. Hammes MS, Lieske JC, Pawar S, Spargo BH, Toback FG. Calcium oxalate monohydrate crystals stimulate gene expreion in renal epithelial cells. *Kid Intl.* 1995;48:501–509.

201. Iida S, Peck AB, Byer KJ, Khan SR. Expression of bikunin mRNA in renal epithelial cells after oxalate exposure. *J Urol.* 1999;162:1480–1486.

202. Umekawa T, Chegini N, Khan SR. Oxalate ions and calcium oxalate crystals stimulate MCP-1 expression by renal epithelial cells. *Kid Intl.* 2002;61:105–112.

203. Umekawa T, Chegini N, Khan SR. Increased expression of monocyte chemoattractant protein-1 (MCP-1) by renal epithelial cells in culture on exposure to calcium oxalate, phosphate and uric acid crystals. *Nephrol Dial Transplant.* 2003;18:664–669.

204. Brewer SL, Atala AA, Ackerman DM, Steinbock GS. Shock wave lithotripsy damage in human cadaver kidneys. *J Endurol*. 1988;2: 333–339.

205. Rigatti P, Colombo R, Centemero A, et al. Histological and ultra-structural evaluation of extracorporeal shock wave lithotripsy-induced acute renal lesions: preliminary report. *Eur Urol*. 1989; 16:207–211.

206. Umekawa T, Kohri K, Yamate T, et al. Renal damage after extra-corporeal shock wave lithotripsy evaluated by Gd-DTPA-enhanced dynamic magnetic resonance imaging. *Urol Int*. 1992;48: 415–419.

207. Abrahams C, Lipson S, Ross L. Pathologic changes in the kidneys and other organs of dogs undergoing extracorporeal shock wave lithotripsy with a tubless lithotripter. *J Urol*. 1988;140:391–394.

208. Delius M, Enders G, Xuan Z, Liebich H, Brendel W. Biological effects of shock waves: kidney damage by shock waves in dogs—dose dependence. *Ultrasound Med Biol*. 1988;14:117–122.

209. Jaeger P, Redha F, Uhlschmid G, Hauri D. Morphological changes in canine kidneys following extra-corporeal shock wave treatment. *Urol Res*. 1988;16:161–166.

210. Karlsen SJ, Smevik B, Hovig T. Acute morphological changes in canine kidneys after exposure to extracorporeal shock waves. *Urol Res*. 1991;19:105–115.

211. Koga H, Matsuoka K, Noda S, Yamashita T. Cumulative renal damage in dogs by repeated treatment with extracorporeal shock waves. *Int J Urol*. 1996;3:134–140.

212. Newman R, Hackett R, Senior D, et al. Pathologic effects of ESWL on canine renal tissue. *Urology*. 1987;29:194–200.

213. Rassweiler J, Kohrmann KU, Back W, et al. Experimental basis of shockwave-induced renal trauma in the model of the canine kidney. *World J Urol*. 1993;11:43–53.

214. Neuerburg J, Daus HJ, Recker F, et al. Effects of lithotripsy on rat kidney: evaluation with MR imaging, histology, and electron microscopy. *J Comput Assist Tomogr*. 1989;13:82–89.

215. Weber C, Moran ME, Braun EJ, Drach GW. Injury of rat renal vessels following extracorporeal shock wave treatment. *J Urol*. 1992;147:476–481.

216. Fajardo LL, Hillman BJ, Weber C, Donovan JM, Drach GW. Microvascular changes in rabbit kidneys after extracorporeal shock wave treatment. *Invest Radiol*. 1990;25:664–669.

217. Kaji DM, Xie HW, Hardy BE, Sherrod A, Huffman JL. The effects of extracorporeal shock wave lithotripsy on renal growth, function and arterial blood pressure in an animal model. *J Urol*. 1991;146:544–547.

218. Karalezli G, Gogus O, Beduk Y, Kokuuslu C, Sarica K, Kutsal O. Histopathologic effects of extracorporeal shock wave lithotripsy on rabbit kidney. *Urol Res*. 1993;21:67–70.

219. Banner B, Ziesmer D, Collins LA. Proliferative lomerulopathy following extracorporeal shock wave lithotripsy in the pig. *J Urol*. 1991;146:1425–1428.

220. El-Damanhoury H, Schaub T, Stadtbaumer M, et al. Parameters influencing renal damage in extracorporeal shock wave lithotripsy: an experimental study in pigs. *J Endourol*. 1991;5:37–40.

221. Evan AP, Willis LR, Lingeman JE, McAteer JA. Renal trauma and the risk of long-term complications in shock wave lithotripsy. *Nephron*. 1998;78:1–8.

222. Connors BA, Evan AP, Willis LR, Blomgren PM, Lingemen JE, Fineberg NS. The effect of discharge voltage on renal injury and impairment caused by lithotripsy in the pig. *J Am Soc Nephrol*. 2000;11:310–318.

223. Shao Y, Connors BA, Evan AP, Willis LR, Lifshitz DA, Lingeman JE. Morphological changes induced in the pig kidney by extracor-poreal shock wave lithotripsy: nephron injury. *Anat Rec*. 2003;275A:979–289.

224. Munver R, Delvecchio C, Kuo RL, et al. In vivo assesment of free radical activity during shock wave lithotripsy using a microdialy-

225. Sarica K, Kosar A, Yaman O, et al. Detection of free oxygen radi-cal scavanger enzymes in renal parenchyma subjected to high-energy shock waves. *Urol Int*. 1996;57:221–223.

226. Suhr D, Brummer F, Hulser DF. Cavitation-generated free radicals during shock-wave exposure: investigations with cell free solu-tions and suspended cells. *Ultrasound Med Biol*. 1991;17: 761–768.

227. Benyi L, Weizheng Z, Puyun L. Protective effects of nefedipine and allopurinol on high energy shock wave induced acute changes of renal function. *J Urol*. 1995;153:596–598.

228. Delvecchio FC, Brizuela RM, Khan SR, et al. Citrate and vitamin E blunt the shock wave-induced free radical surge in an *in vitro* cell culture model. *Urol Res*. 2005;33:448–52.

229. Strohmaier WL, Pedro M, Wilbert DM, Bichler KH. Reduction of shock wave-induced tubular alteration by fosfomycin. *J Endourol*. 1991;5:57–60.

230. Strohmaier WL, Abelius A, Billes J, Grossmann T, Wilbert DM. Verapamil limits shock wave-induced renal tubular damage in vivo. *J Endourol*. 1994;8:269–273.

231. Strohmaier WL, Bichler KH, Koch J, Balk N, Wilbert DM. Protective effect of verapamil on shock wave induced renal tubular dysfunction. *J Urol*. 1993;150:27–29.

232. Strohmaier WL, Billes IC, Abelius A, Lahme S, Bichler KH. Selenium reduces high energy shock-induced renal injury in rats. *Urol Res*. 2002;30:31–34.

233. Strohmaier WL, Lahme S, Weidenbach PM, Bichler KH. Reduction of high-energy shock-wave-induced renal tubular injury by sele-nium. *Urol Res*. 1999;27:382–385.

234. Bataille P, Cardon G, Bouzernidji M, et al. Renal and hypertensive complications of extracorporeal shock wave lithotripsy: who is at risk? *Urol Int*. 1999;62:195–200.

235. Frauscher F, Hofle G, Janetschek G. Re A randomized controlled trial to assess the incidence of new onset hypertension in patients after shock wave lithotripsy for asymptomatic renal calculi [edi-torial]. *J Urol*. 1999;162(3):806.

236. Janetschek G, Frauscher F, Knapp R, Hofle G, Peschel R, Bartsch G. New onset hypertension after extracorporeal shock wave lithotripsy: age related incidence and prediction by intrarenal resistive index. *J Urol*. 1997;158:346–51.

237. Knapp R, Frauscher F, Helweg G, et al. Age-related changes in resistive index following extracorporeal shock wave lithotripsy. *J Urol*. 1995;154:955–958.

238. Knapp R, Frauscher F, Helweg G, et al. Blood pressure changes after extracorporeal shock wave nephrolithotripsy: Adverse effects of SWL 211 prediction by intrarenal resistive index. *Eur Radiol*. 1996;6:665–9.

239. Krambeck AE, Gettman MT, Rohlinger AL, Lohse CM, Patterson DE, Segura JW. Diabetes mellitus and hypertension associated with shock wave lithotripsy of renal and proximal ureteral stones at 19 years of followup. *J Urol*. 2006;175:1742–1747.

240. Williams CM, Kaude JV, Newman RC, Peterson JC, Thomas WC. Extracorporeal shock-wave lithotripsy: long-term complications. *AJR Am J Roentgenol*. 1988;150:311–315.

241. Mandel N, Mandel I, Fryjoff K, Rejniak T, Mandel G. Conversion of calcium oxalate to calcium phosphate with recurrent stone epi-sodes. *J Urol*. 2003;169:2026–2029.

242. Hackett RL, Shevock PN, Khan SR. Madin–Darby canine kidney cells are injured by exposure to oxalate and calcium oxalate crys-tals. *Urol Res*. 1994;22:197–204.

243. Hackett RL, Shevock PN, Khan SR. Alterations in MDCK and LLC-PK1 cells exposed to oxalate and calcium oxalate monohy-drate crystals. *Scann Microsc*. 1995;9:587–596.

244. Bisgrove BW, Yost HJ. The roles of cilia in developmental disorders and disease. *Development*. 2006;133:4131–4143.

245. Kleinman JG, Wesson JA, Hughes J. Osteopontin and calcium stone formation. *Nephron Physiol*. 2004;98:43–47.

246. Kumar V, Lieske JC. Protein regulation of intrarenal crystallization. *Curr Opin Nephrol Hypertens*. 2006;15:374–380.

247. Jonassen JA, Cao LC, Honeyman T, Scheid CR. Mechanisms mediating oxalate-induced alterations in renal cell functions. *Crt Rev in Eukar Gene Expr*. 2003;13:55–72.

248. Khand FD, Gordge MP, Robertson WG, Noronha-Dutra AA, Hothersall JS. Mitochondrial superoxide production during oxalate mediated oxidatve stress in renal epithelial cells. *Free Radic Biol Med*. 2002;32:1339–1350.

249. Meimaridou E, Lobos E, Hothersall JS. Renal oxidative vulnerability due to changes in mitochondrial-glutothione and energy homeostasis in a rat model of calcium oxalate urolithiasis. *Am J Physiol Renal Physiol*. 2006;291:731–740.

250. Linnane AW, Kios M, Vitetta L. Healthy aging: regulation of the metabolome by cellular redox modulation and prooxidant signaling system, the essential roles of superoxide anion and hydrogen peroxide. *Biogerontology*. 2007;8:445–467.

251. Umekawa T, Uemura H, Khan SR. Super oxide from NADPH oxidase as second messenger for expression of osteopontin and monocyte chemoattractant protein-1 in renal epithelial cells exposed to calcium oxalate crystals. *BJU Int*. 2009; 104(1):115–120.

252. Chaturvedi LS, Koul S, Sekhon A, Bhandari A, Menon M, Koul HK. Oxalate selectively activates the p38 mitoge-activated protein kinase and c-Jun N-terminal kinase signal transduction pathway in renal epithelial cells. *J Biol Chem*. 2002;277: 13321–13330.

253. Koul HK, Menon M, Chaturvedi LS, et al. COM crystals activate the p38 mitoge-activated protein kinase (MAPK) signal transduction pathway in renal epithelial cells. *J Biol Chem*. 2002;277:36845–36852.

254. Li N, Yi FX, Spurrier JL, Bobrowitz CA, Zou AP. Production of superoxide through NADH oxidase in thick ascending limb of the loop in rat kidney. *Am J Physiol*. 2002;282:F1111–F1119.

255. Shiose A, Kuroda J, Tsutuya K, et al. A novel superoxide-oroducing NAD(P)H oxidase in kidney. *J Biol Chem*. 2001;276: 1417–1423.

256. Umekawa T, Byer K, Uemura H, Khan SR. Diphenyleneiodium (DPI) reduces oxalate ion and calcium oxalate monohydrate and brushite crystal-induced upregulation of MCP-1 in NRK5E cells. *Nephrol Dial Transplant*. 2005;20:870–878.

257. Hanna IR, Taniyama Y, Szocs K, Rocic P, Griendling KK. NAD(P)H Oxidase-derived reactive oxygen species as mediators of angiotensin II signaling. *Antioxid Redox Signal*. 2002;4:899–913.

258. James EA, Galceran JM, Raij L. Angiotensin II induces superoxide anion production by mesangial cells. *Kidney Intl*. 1998;54:775–784.

259. Rashid T, Menon M, Thamilselvan S. Molecular mechanism of oxalate-induced free radical production and glutathione redox imbalance in renal epithelial cells: effect of antioxidants. *Am J Nephrol*. 2004;24:557–568.

260. Rovin BH, Phan LT. Chemotactic factors and renal inflammation. *Am J Kid Dis*. 1998;31:1065–1084.

261. Cao L-C, Honeyman T, Cooney R, Kennington L, Scheid CR, Jonassen JA. Mitochondrial dysfunction is a primary event in renal cell oxalate toxicity. *Kid Intl*. 2004;66:1890–1900.

262. Cao L-C, Honeyman T, Jonassen J, Scheid C. Oxalate-induced ceramide accumulation in Madin-Darby canine kidney and LLC-PK1 cells. *Kidney Intl*. 2000;57:2403–2411.

263. Jeong B-C, Kwak C, Cho KY, et al. Apoptosis induced by oxalate in human renal tubular epithelial HK-2 cells. *Urol Res*. 2005; 33(2):87–92.

264. Miller C, Kennington L, Cooney R, et al. Oxalate toxicity in renal epithelial cells: characteristics of apoptosis and necrosis. *Toxicology and Pharmacology*. 2000;162:132–141.

265. Miyazawa K, Suzuki K, Ikeda R, Moriyama MT, Ueda Y, Katsuda S. Apoptosis and its related genes in renal epithelial cells of the stone forming rat. *Urol Res*. 2005;33:31–38.

266. Grewal JS, Tsai JY, Khan SR. Oxalate-inducible AMBP gene and its regulatory mechanism in renal tubular epithelial cells. *Biochem J*. 2005;387:609–616.

Interaction of Stone Components with Cells and Tissues

Jack G. Kleinman

Abstract This chapter is a review of the interaction of stone-forming materials with cells and tissues. The evidence for intratubular and interstitial locations of calcium oxalate and calcium phosphate is examined; the latter mineral with particular reference to its appearance in Randall's plaques. The mechanisms of surface adherence and nucleation of crystals are discussed, as well as the evidence for internalization of crystals by renal tubular epithelium and their further processing. The cellular consequences of crystal–cell interaction, specifically stimulation of cell division and initiation of several varieties of cell damage or death, are reviewed. The specificity of crystal–cell interaction is also covered. This includes a discussion of the features of cultured cells responsible for the reported specificity and the molecules expressed on the cell surface responsible for crystal adherence, with particular emphasis on the case of calcium oxalate monohydrate (COM). The smaller amount of evidence regarding the above phenomena for other stone forming crystals – uric acid, brushite, and apatite is also reviewed. The issue of whether cell or tissue damage predisposes to stone formation is also covered; particularly the large amount of data on the toxic effects of oxalate, as well as the lesser amount of information available regarding hypercalciuria, hyperphosphaturia, and hyperuricosuria. The chapter concludes with a synthesis of the material into a comprehensive hypothesis for the initiation of stone disease through interaction of stone-forming constituents with cells and tissues.

6.1 Introduction

The symptoms of kidney stone disease require an interaction with renal tissue. Kidney stones are either passed spontaneously or produce pain due to obstruction of the urinary tract. However, crystalline material as originally formed appears to be of microscopic size. This chapter will cover the interaction of crystals or other solid amorphous material with renal tissues or cells. I will consider the sites of the attachment of such solids, the internalization of this material into cells and their transit through tissues, the cellular and tissue reactions to this process, and the mechanism of this adherence. Most of the material presented will derive from studies with calcium oxalate crystals. Where appropriate, similarities and differences between the other major stone crystals or solids,

uric acid, and the various calcium phosphates will be indicated. The limited amount of information available specifically regarding these other substances will be reviewed separately toward the end of the chapter. Finally, I will examine the evidence that oxalate, calcium, phosphate, and uric acid induces alterations in tubular cells that promote crystal adherence. The chapter closes with a synthesis of the material in the form of a hypothesis for stone formation.

6.2 Sites of Crystal Attachment

Precipitates of more or less ordered stone constituents may form in extracellular, interstitial sites by a mechanism yet to be described.[1] However, one can infer from the often striking presence of crystalluria that crystals almost certainly also form within tubular fluid. This may occur either spontaneously in free solution, in solution microenvironments, or on particulates in tubular fluid.[2,3] Crystal formation can also take place

J.G. Kleinman
Department of Nephrology, Veterans Affairs Medical Center and the Medical College of Wisconsin, Milwaukee, WI, USA
e-mail: kleinman@mcw.edu

P.N. Rao et al. (eds.), *Urinary Tract Stone Disease*,
DOI 10.1007/978-1-84800-362-0_6, © Springer-Verlag London Limited 2011

on surfaces that may be present in the tubule or bladder wall, whether of normal cells, abnormal cells, or areas denuded of cells due to pathologic processes.[4,5]

6.2.1 Interstitial Calcification and Randall's Plaques

Interstitial precipitation of calcium phosphate results in the phenomenon of Randall's plaques.[1] These structures have been proposed as platforms for the formation of idiopathic calcium oxalate stones; however, their evolution into clinical stones, at least on the basis of the microscopic analysis of the sites of stone attachment, does not primarily appear to involve a tissue interaction.[6] How the deposits of calcium phosphate form initially has not been addressed directly, but there are some notions of how this may be possible from considerations of calcification that occur in other sites. Calcium phosphate precipitation in interstitial sites occurs normally in bone and pathologically in both blood vessels and joints. Figure 6.1 shows hydroxyapatite deposition in Randall's plaques in the kidney, and similar deposits appear in atheromatous arteries.[7]

In all of these sites calcification has been associated with the presence of small membrane-bound structures referred to as matrix vesicles. These appear to function as the initiation sites for apatite crystallization. Investigators in this area have demonstrated that membrane-bound remnants similar, if not identical, to matrix vesicles were released by apoptotic vascular smooth muscle cells in vitro and appeared to act as nucleating structures for calcium crystal formation.[8] This same group has demonstrated that exposure to high calcium and inorganic phosphate concentrations induced vascular smooth muscle cell death and apoptotic body release as well as matrix vesicle release from living cells.[9]

In articular cartilage, calcium may precipitate within membrane bound structures.[10] These are referred to as matrix vesicles, and the calcium precipitates as pyrophosphate as a result of the generation of pyrophosphate mediated through the action of nucleoside triphosphate pyrophosphohydrolase, an enzyme enriched in the vesicles. Of course, pyrophosphate is a strong inhibitor of calcium phosphate and calcium oxalate nucleation.[11,12] Articular cartilage matrix vesicles can also produce hydroxyapatite.[13] Whether articular cartilage matrix vesicles calcify at all or produce calcium, either pyrophosphate or calcium phosphate, appears to depend on the pyrophosphate to phosphate ratio as well as the calcium to phospholipid ratios.[14] These ratios, in turn, may be determined by the relative activities of the inorganic phosphate-generating ectoenzyme tissue-nonspecific alkaline phosphatase versus pyrophosphate-generating pyrophosphatase phosphodiesterases and the vesicle content of annexins – a class of compounds that will come up later in connection with crystal adherence.[15] Stone formers may have low urinary excretion rates of pyrophosphate, suggesting that the balance may be shifted in favor of the alkaline phosphatase.[16]

Initially, the calcium phosphate is found within membrane-bound vesicles. These vesicles appear to coalesce and lose their membrane coat. The deposits then erode tissue, and evoke a biological response by interaction with the interstitium or a fluid-containing space.

6.2.2 Surface Adherence or Nucleation of Crystals

Crystals of several sorts can nucleate directly from supersaturated solutions, either on extracellular matrix constituents, on cellular debris, or on intact cells.

Gill utilized the catheterized bladder of the rat to study crystal formation on surfaces.[17] In the presence of supersaturated calcium oxalate solutions, he and his coworkers only observed adherent crystals in bladders that had been exposed to HCl or detergent. The question of which structure or structures had the attached crystals was not investigated in detail; polycrystalline masses were observed to be attached to a multiple-layered urothelium rather than to areas of bladder where the cells had been dislodged. Presciently, the investigators hypothesized that attachment may have either been mediated by loss of glycocalyx or the presence of an attachment factor or factors by the injured cells.

Khan and coworkers also performed similar studies.[18] In particular, they found that HCl or Triton-injured bladders showed increased calcium oxalate adherence to areas denuded of cells. The detergent-treated bladders showed strong staining for fibrin along the surface denuded of cells; staining was variable in the HCl-injured bladders. It seems fair to conclude from these studies, as well as the observations of Evan and coworkers discussed previously, that calcium oxalate crystals are able both to nucleate directly and to adhere to either cells or extracellular matrix.

Some components of extracellular matrix have been shown to adhere to crystals; either forming a component of their matrix or mediating attachment. I will elaborate below on the issue of whether these extracellular matrix components mediate attachment within the renal intertstitium, in association with tubular cell basement membranes, or to apical cell membranes (from which they are ordinarily excluded).

Using an innovative technique involving vapor diffusion of oxalic acid, Lieske and coworkers demonstrated direct nucleation followed by internalization of calcium oxalate crystals by a process that this group has also extensively investigated.[5]

Fig. 6.1 Randall's plaques and calcified matrix vesicles in atheromas. *Top 4 panels (A–D)* shows images of Randall's plaque in idiopathic calcium oxalate stone formers (Courtesy of A. Evan). Panel A shows an image of a papilla taken during a percutaneous nephrolithotomy. Several attached stones (*arrows*) are seen, which are surrounded by a large field of whitish, irregular suburothelial Randall's plaques (*arrowheads*). Panel B, a light-microscopic image of a papillary biopsy specimen, shows Yasue-positive sites of calcium deposits (*arrows*) in the interstitial space. Panel C shows single deposits (*arrows*) of varying size located in the basement membrane of the thin loops of Henle; panel D shows a single deposit as seen at a higher magnification to show the multilaminated nature of these structures. The electron dense layers are composed of matrix material while the electron lucent layers contain hydroxyapatite crystals. *Bottom 8 panels (A–H)* shows electron microscopy of calcified matrix vesicles in the fibrous cap of an atheromatous plaque. Deposits in both types of vesicles were identified as calcium phosphate (Reprinted from[7], with permission of Blackwell Publishing, Inc.)

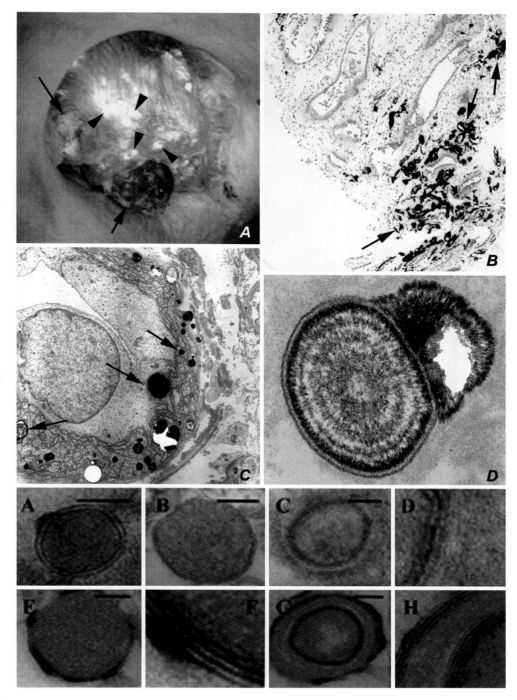

6.3 Consequences of Crystal Adherence

Stone constituent crystals may be washed off surfaces depending on the shear force applied, or they may adhere to surfaces for long periods. Crystals washing off the surfaces to which they adhered temporarily will end up in the urine and are generally of little consequence clinically. This, in fact, may be the fate of the majority of crystals formed in urine, as many relatives of stone formers as well as normal individuals demonstrate calcium oxalate or calcium phosphate crystalluria.[19,20] Crystals adhering for prolonged periods can presumably serve as the nidus for the development of clinical stones. As reviewed in the following sections, several groups have reported more complex interactions between crystals and cells, specifically, internalization, dissolution, and transcytosis.

Fig. 6.2 Internalization of calcium oxalate crystals. *Top panels* show internalization of calcium oxalate dihydrate by scanning electron microscopy (Reprinted with permission of Springer Science + Business Media from[21]. *Bottom panels* show internalization of *COM* into membrane-bound structures by transmission electron microscopy (Reprinted with permission from[22], copyright 1994 National Academy of Sciences, USA)

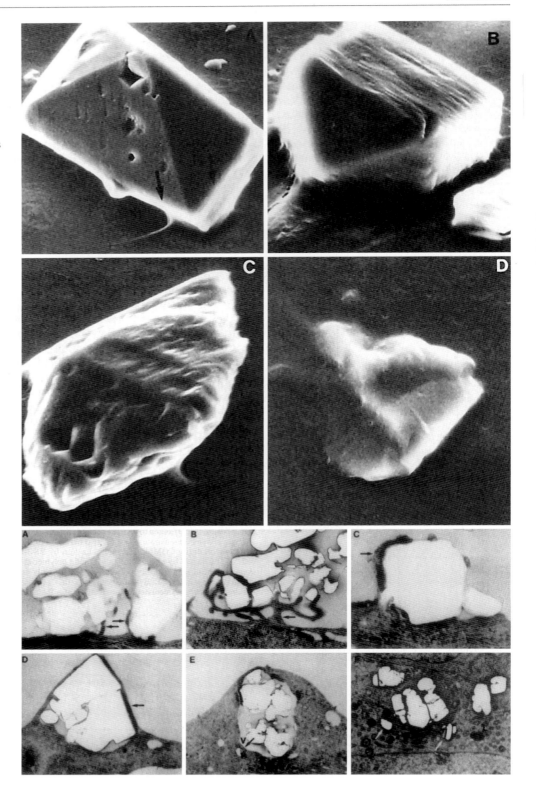

6.3.1 Crystal Internalization

Crystals can be internalized by interacting with cellular processes that become applied to certain crystal surfaces and then fully engulf the crystal so that by 24 h some crystals were observed beneath the plasma membrane of the cell

(Fig. 6.2).[21] In studies using scanning electron microscopy, crystals were shown to adhere first to apical microvilli.[22] These microvilli then migrate over the crystalline surface and appear to coalesce, resulting in migration of the crystal below the plasma membrane of the cell. By transmission electron microscopy, intracellular crystals were shown to

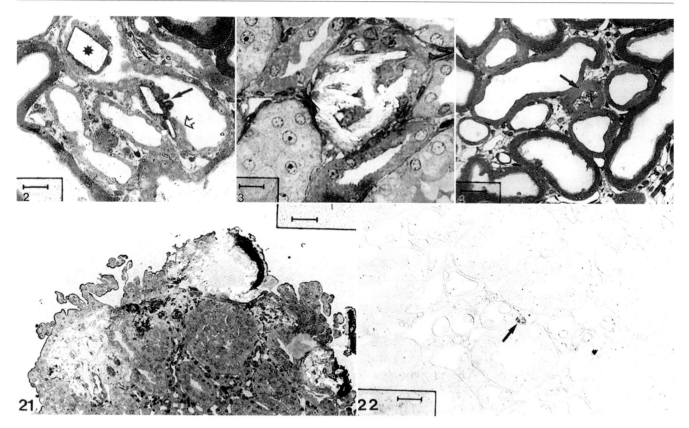

Fig. 6.3 Translocation of calcium oxalate crystals from tubule lumen to papillary surface. *Top panels* depicting calcium oxalate crystals at tubule cell surface, within cells and in the interstitium adjacent to tubules (Reprinted with permission of Scanning Microscopy Inc. from[25].)

Bottom panels showing masses of crystals at the papillary surface as well as clearance from the tubules and interstitium. Bars = 25 μm (micrometers) (Reprinted with permission of Scanning Microscopy Inc. from[26])

remain within membrane-bound vesicles. Factors reported to increase internalization were serum, exposure to low potassium medium, epidermal growth factor, and adenosine diphosphate.[23] Tamm–Horsfall glycoprotein, the tetrapeptide arginine-glycine-aspartic acid-serine, fibronectin, transforming growth factor-b2, and heparin all inhibited internalization of calcium oxalate.

In one of the few available studies in patients, this group has described internalization of calcium oxalate crystals in an individual with primary hyperoxaluria.[24]

6.3.2 Dissolution of Crystals and Transcytosis

As indicated in the next section, one of the things that can happen to the internalized crystals is that they can be dissolved. An additional fate has been proposed, however, that of transcytosis through the epithelial cell layer into the renal interstitium and migration to the surface of the renal papilla. Rats that have been made hyperoxaluric using ethylene glycol and ammonium chloride demonstrate what the investigators

called "exotubulosis," referring to free crystals or crystals surrounded by cells in the renal interstitium (Fig. 6.3).[25] Subsequent to the oxalate challenge, crystals were prominently observed in interstitial sites, at later time points in the papilla alone, under the epithelium covering the papillary surface or in the renal pelvis itself.[26,27] These authors suggest that the deposits of crystals under the epithelium covering the papilla could serve as the nidus for the development of calcium oxalate nephrolithiasis. Such deposits have been described in humans.[28] The Dutch investigators have suggested that macrophage-like cells could be responsible for the migration of crystals from intratubular sites to the papillary surface.

6.4 Cellular Consequences of Crystal–Cell Interaction

What happens to internalized crystals has been examined by several groups. In the case of synovial macrophage/monocytes or chondrocytes, internalization of crystals results in dissolution, increased cell calcium, and a number of cellular

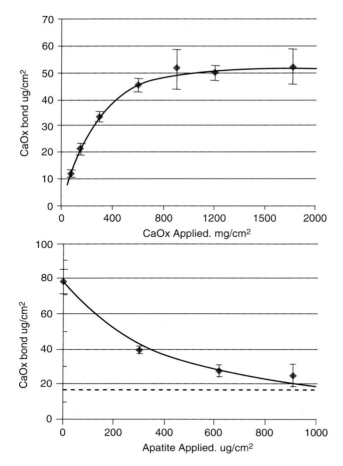

Fig. 6.4 Specificity of calcium oxalate adherence. *Upper panel* depicts saturation of *COM* crystal adherence to primary cultures of rat *IMCD* cells. *Lower panel* shows concentration-dependent inhibition of COM adherence with simultaneous incubation with apatite (Redrawn from data in[39], American Physiological Society)

kinase signaling cascade.[31] Even when overt changes in the state of the cells do not occur, signaling cascades may be initiated that affect processes external to the cells themselves, but whether such changes are due to exposure of cells to crystals, to oxalate, or to both is uncertain. In any event, such processes may, in fact, be an important component of the pathophysiology of both the acquired and the genetic forms of hyperoxaluria, which are characterized by inflammatory and fibrotic changes within the renal interstitium.[32,33] Reactive oxygen species (ROS) have been postulated to mediate some of these effects.[34]

6.5 Crystal Adherence Specificity

The structures involved in crystal–cell interactions have been investigated in cell culture systems by a number of investigators. In primary cultures of inner medullary collecting duct (IMCD) cells, exposure to preformed crystals of materials usually found in stones leads to their adhesion.[35–39] The process demonstrates some features of specificity, specifically a maximum capacity that is less than the total exposed cell surface and at least some degree of mutual inhibition (Fig. 6.5). All major types of crystals found in clinical kidney stones, hydroxyapatite, calcium oxalate, and uric acid can attach to various types of cultured cells demonstrating similar kinetic parameters.

6.5.1 Features Responsible for Specificity

The question of what features of cultured cells is responsible for the adhesion of crystals has been addressed in a number of ways. In primary cultures, calcium oxalate appears to attach to collections of cells that are beginning their organization into cord-like proto-tubules, thereby exposing to the crystals immunological epitopes usually confined to the basolateral cell surface (Fig. 6.5). Cultures "wounded" by scraping produce a population of cells whose polarity is lost during the process of division and migration to cover the deficit. These cells also exhibit enhanced crystal attachment capability (Fig. 6.5).

Cultured cells differ in their capacity to mediate cell adherence. In general, the more highly organized the cell monolayer is, the less capacity for crystal adherence there appears to be. Some cultured cell lines demonstrate significant capacity for crystal adherence (and engulfment) and some do not. In the primary IMCD cell cultures, lysing of intercellular junctions with EGTA was associated with increases in calcium oxalate adherence, which was restored to control levels with removal of EGTA and provision of calcium.[38]

signaling processes are initiated. These include stimulation of mitogenesis, activation of both cyclooxygenase and phospholipase C pathways, induction of c-fos and c-myc, increase secretion of matrix metalloproteinases, and decreased tissue metalloproteinase inhibitors.[29] These effects were linked to the demonstrated dissolution of the crystals.

As noted in the previous section, dissolution of crystals within renal tubule cells has also been described. Lieske, Toback, and coworkers described very slow dissolution of crystals in BSC-1 cells.[30] Mitogenesis was stimulated when crystals were internalized.

Interaction of calcium oxalate crystals with several types of cells leads to various changes in these cells. Lysis of membranes, mitogenesis, necrotic cell death, inflammatory changes, and apoptosis are some of the processes that have been reported to follow upon exposure of cells to these crystals. Exposure of a proximal tubule cell line to calcium oxalate crystal initiates DNA synthesis in cells made quiescent by serum starvation through a p38-dependent mitogen-activated protein (MAP)

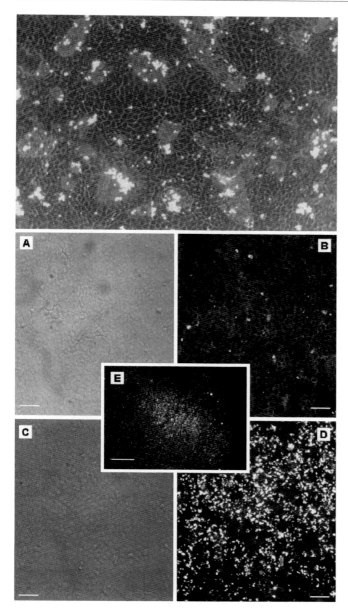

Fig. 6.5 Calcium oxalate adherence to structural features of cultured *IMCD* cells. Top panel shows calcium oxalate crystals adhering to aggregated cells in primary cultures. (Reprinted with permission of American Physiological Society from[39].) *Bottom panels* depict crystals adhering to cells repairing wound made by scraping of IMCD monolayers. Panels A and B show lack of crystals on quiescent areas of culture; Panels C and D show *COM* adherent to cells that have recently grown to cover defect. Panel E shows lower power view of wounded area and surrounding undisturbed culture (Reprinted with permission from[45])

It seems safe to conclude, therefore, that cells in the urinary tract are relatively resistant to interactions with crystals when they are organized into the well-differentiated monolayers or multilayers that are observed in tissues, specifically renal tubules, or distal urinary tract. As noted previously, in injured bladder, areas denuded of cells are those to which crystals were attached, apparently to masses of dead cells, cellular debris, and a fibrillar mesh that exhibits staining for fibrin.

This is analogous to the situation observed with stones that are attached to Randall's plaques. As elegantly illustrated by Evan and coworkers (Fig. 6.6), the stone appears to have been attached to an area of plaque over which the urothelium covering the renal papilla has become denuded.[6] The plaque itself (comprised of hydroxyapatite) appears to be firmly anchored within the intertstitium of the papilla rather than to cells themselves. At the periphery of the stone, there appear to be adherent urothelium, so direct crystal cell attachment also appears to take place. However, the major point of the attachment of the stone to the plaques appears to be mediated by matrix composed of urinary and perhaps cellular proteins. Osteopontin, of which more will be said later, appears to bridge the stone and the interstitium of the papilla.

The group of investigators mentioned previously contends that most, if not all, idiopathic calcium oxalate stone disease originates in Randall's plaques. However, a number of investigators have pointed out that calcifications of various types can be identified in almost all individuals if looked for carefully enough with the appropriate techniques.[28,97,98] Furthermore, only about 40% of passes stones that appeared to have been formed in the renal papilla showed evidence of having Randall plaque material.[99] Ryall has suggested that the failure of Evan and coworkers to find plaque in controls may be due to the small number of non-stone formers examined.[100] Thus, while the presence of Randall's plaques may be sufficient for stone formation, it may not be necessary. Even those who support the Randall's plaques initiation site of stone formation have reported some situations where free crystals are identified in the tubule lumens and attached to

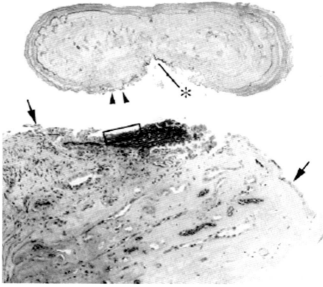

Fig. 6.6 Stone attached to Randall's plaques. The figure depicts a stone and underlying tissue removed from a patient, showing the site of attachment to a calcified plaque at the papillary surface from which the epithelium has become denuded (Reprinted from[6], with permission of Wiley)

the apical cell membranes of tubule cells. This has led investigators to study the mechanism of attachment of crystals to cells using in vitro systems.

6.5.2 Molecules Responsible for Crystal Adherence

Because of its preponderance in kidney stones, attachment of calcium oxalate, particularly calcium oxalate monohydrate (COM), has been studied most extensively of the stone crystallites. Enrichment of membrane phospholipid phosphatidylserine by incubation with phospholipid-containing liposomes was shown to enhance calcium oxalate crystal attachment.[40] In addition, these studies indicated that maneuvers that lessened membrane polarity, such as treatment with EGTA, as in studies alluded to previously, also increased phosphatidylserine-mediated COM attachment.

Glycosaminoglycans have also been implicated in crystal attachment to renal tubule cells. In proliferating subconfluent Madin–Darby canine kidney (MDCK) cells or in cells made to proliferate to cover a defect induced in confluent cultures, the binding of COM crystal was strongly correlated with the expression of hyaluronan and could be inhibited by treating susceptible cells with hyaluronidase.[41] In older, more indirect studies, several glycosaminoglycans were shown to strongly inhibit crystal attachment, suggesting that the cellular sites involved share features of these molecules.[41,42]

The membrane-associated proteins nucleolin was selectively depleted by COM from a preparation of biotinylated apical membrane proteins of cultured rat IMCD cells (Fig. 6.7). An otherwise unidentified 200 kDa band and the low-molecular-weight protein amphoterin also selectively adhere to COM[43], and are thus also candidate attachment molecules.[43] The role of these latter molecules as well as a 200 kDa(kilodalton)-sized membrane glycoprotein from culture medium of MDCK cells[44] has not, to my knowledge, been further evaluated.

Additional data is available regarding a proposed role for nucleolin in COM attachment.[45] Surface expression, both on apical and basolateral membranes, declined with time in culture, in a fashion similar to the decline in COM attachment. Cells stimulated to multiply to cover a defect induced by scraping of the cultures demonstrated increase apical surface nucleolin expression along with enhanced COM attachment. Furthermore, overexpression in the apical membranes of cells of a region of the molecule that contains a large amount of acidic amino acid residues leads to enhanced COM attachment, while the soluble acidic fragment competed with the membrane-bound form, preventing the increase in COM attachment.

COM affinity from a preparation of apical membrane of MDCK cells identified annexin II as a potential crystal adherence factor.[46] Annexin II was identified by

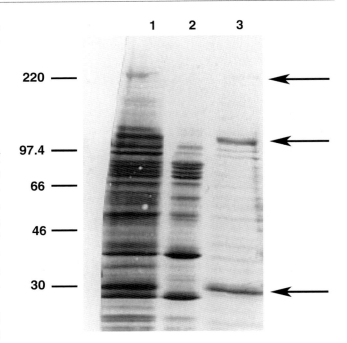

Fig. 6.7 Adsorption of specific proteins by *COM* crystals. Figure shows protein blots of solubilized apical membranes of *IMCD* cells before (lane 1) after (lane 2) incubation with COM crystals. *Arrows* mark bands at 220, 110 (nucleolin), and 26 kDa (amphoterin) depleted in supernatant (lane 2) and selectively adsorbed to crystals (lane 3) (Reprinted with permission from[43], American Society for Biochemistry and Molecular Biology)

immunofluorescence on the surface of the cultured cells, and a monoclonal anti-annexin II antibody significantly decreased COM adherence to the cells. Without identifying a specific membrane component, integral membrane glycoproteins appear to be able to mediate COM attachment based both on inhibition with soluble cations and, more significantly, inhibition of attachment with neuraminidase.[47]

Another urinary protein, osteopontin, has been associated with crystal binding in vitro.[48] Specifically, MDCK cells incubated with osteopontin demonstrated increased adhesion of calcium oxalate crystals, and incubation with thrombin – an inhibitor of osteopontin expression – led to decreased crystal adhesion. This same group has demonstrated that MDCK transfected with an antisense oligonucleotide against osteopontin demonstrated less calcium oxalate crystal adhesion.[49]

Against a role for osteopontin in mediating crystal adhesion is the observation that mice lacking the gene for this molecule were actually more susceptible to calcium oxalate crystal deposition after ethylene glycol feeding than were wild-type mice (Fig. 6.8).[50] In another study also shown in the figure, mice lacking the osteopontin gene developed spontaneous renal papillary interstitial calcifications that were identified as hydroxyapatite.[51] In addition, urine from osteopontin-deficient mice was less effective at inhibiting COM attachment to MDCK cells in vitro than was urine

Fig. 6.8 Enhanced susceptibility of osteopontin-deficient mice to intrarenal crystal formation. *Left two panels* shows calcium oxalate crystals in renal tubules in osteopontin-deficient mice after ethylene glycol feeding under condition when wild-type mice do not show crystals (Reprinted with permission from[50]). *Right panels* show interstitial hydroxyapatite crystals that developed spontaneously in osteopontin-deficient mice, top, and their absence in wild type, *bottom* (Courtesy of X.R. Wu)

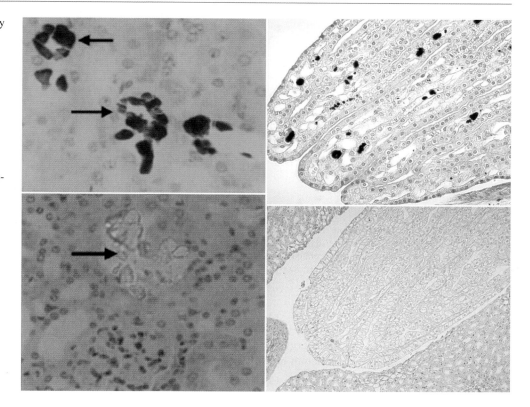

from wild-type animals. In unreported experiments from this author's laboratory, exogenous osteopontin did not adhere significantly to cultured rat IMCD cells, which is additional evidence against a role for this substance in crystal adherence, at least in vitro. Finally, the finding that the osteopontin-deficient mice were more susceptible than the wild type to calcium oxalate crystal deposition with induced hyperoxaluria also has been confirmed.[51]

To summarize to this point, it is clear that cells differ in their attraction for crystals found in stones. Cells deriving from distal nephron segments appear to manifest less affinity than other cell types. Affinity also appears to be related to damage to cells or the recovery from damage. Intercellular matrix appears to have considerable affinity for crystals. Thus it is likely that multiple components of tissue have features that can mediate crystal attachment. In the next section, we consider what features or components of the macromolecules comprising renal tissue may be responsible for the attachment of crystals.

6.5.3 Functional Group Requirements for Crystal–Cell Adherence

The common feature of most of the molecules listed is their acidic nature, provided by the carboxyl groups of amino acids, glucuronic acid, sulfated sugars, phosphorylated amino acids, or the terminal sialic acids of glycoprotein side chains. Various investigators have proposed that these acidic groups mediate crystal attachment by interacting with the partial cationic surface charges of some of the crystal surfaces of COM. Annexin II also has calcium-binding sites formed by coordination of peptide oxygen atoms, acidic amino acids, and water molecules. Spatial expression of some of these sites (hyaluronan and nucleolin) appears to correlate with crystal attachment[45,53], depletion of some sites (sialic acids)[47] has been shown to decrease crystal attachment, and overexpression of some purported acidic attachment sites correlates with increased attachment.[45] Although it is still not certain that binding to surface calcium atoms is totally responsible for calcium oxalate and, for that matter, calcium phosphate crystal attachment, it does appear that many compounds that block calcium-binding sites are effective blockers of calcium oxalate or other calcium-containing crystal attachment.

Atomic force microscopy (AFM) has been utilized to study the interaction between various functional groups and the surface of COM[53]. COM crystals were grown in a manner so as to maximize specific surfaces and were mounted in a fluid-filled chamber. The strength of adhesion of various chemical groups was examined by utilizing AFM tips functionalized with organosulfur molecules containing specific chemical groups. These tips were brought into contact with a particular COM crystal face and then retracted; the force of attraction was taken as the force required to detach the tip from the crystal

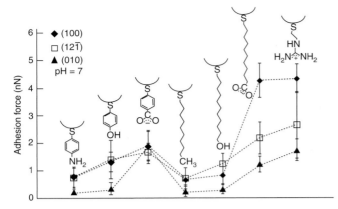

Fig. 6.9 Force of attraction of various functionalized *AFM* tips with specific faces of *COM* crystals. Figure depicts the strong interaction between both carboxyl and amidinium decorated tips and the (100) surface of COM (Reprinted with permission from[52], copyright 2005 National Academy of Sciences, USA)

surface. Figure 6.9 shows that both COO– and the amidinium groups strongly adhere to the (100) crystal face of COM, likely by binding to the ordered calcium atoms and oxalate groups on the crystal surface.

6.6 Uric Acid Attachment Sites

Our group was the first to describe uric acid attachment to cultured renal tubule cells[37]. Uric acid appeared to compete with COM for some of the same attachment sites, but no soluble inhibitors were studied. The only systematic study of uric acid attachment was performed on BSC-1 cells, a non-transformed cell line of uncertain tubular segment origin, and MDCK – a cell line derived from the distal nephron.[54] Urinary glycoproteins did not inhibit attachment, but other urinary and synthetic polyanions did. However, a number of cationic substances also demonstrated inhibition of attachment, apparently when they coated the cell surface. When crystals were preincubated with polycations, attachment was increased. The role of surface glycoproteins with terminal sialic acids in uric acid attachment is difficult to discern from these studies, as lectins that bind sialic acids were without effect, but neuraminidase treatment enhanced attachment. Although an attempt at a dose response was made, the relationship between the amount of inhibitor and the surface area of the uric acid crystals was not assessed.

The 200 kDa protein, alluded to previously, that is secreted into medium by MDCK cells, when coated on glass, promotes attachment of COM, calcium dihydrate, uric acid, and brushite, but not apatite.[44] The similarity in molecular mass of this protein to the surface glycoprotein that we have reported selectively adheres to COM[43] has been previously

remarked. Finally, in a genetically isolated population in Sardinia with a high incidence of uric acid stones, urinary excretion of glycosaminoglycans appeared to be decreased,[55] suggesting that these substances may act as endogenous inhibitors of stone formation, possibly by inhibiting crystal attachment.

6.7 Brushite and Apatite Attachment Sites

Both brushite and apatite adhere to cultured renal tubular cells of various types to a much lesser extent than does calcium oxalate.[39,56] However, attachment may be important, both for the relatively small number of patients who demonstrate predominantly calcium phosphate nephrolithiasis,[57] as well as for a purported role in the pathophysiology of calcium oxalate nephrolithiasis.[6,58] In the previous work, we reported that apatite appeared to share some of the same attachment sites as COM[39]. Others have provided evidence that apatite adheres to similar anionic sites as does calcium oxalate.[59] One study demonstrated brushite attachment to sulfur-rich sites on the surface of cultured human intestinal cells, presumably anionic sulfated mucins.[60] Studies, too numerous to cite, demonstrate effects of anionic molecules to inhibit apatite nucleation and growth.

6.8 Cell or Tissue Damage as a Prerequisite to Stone Formation

As already noted, the interaction of cells and tissues with crystals is characterized by responses that include cell division, inflammation, necrotic cell death, and apoptosis. As discussed previously, some of these cellular responses, by themselves, can make cells receptive to the adherence of crystals formed in renal tubules or could be responsible for interstitial calcification. In this section, I will examine the condition that may be present in stone formers that may induce the sorts of alterations in cell function that promote crystal nucleation or adhesion.

6.8.1 Hyperoxaluria

Oxalate, of course, is a primary constituent of most kidney stones. Oxalate excretion is normal in the majority of stone formers, but even in normal individuals oxalate concentrations can rise to fairly high levels under antidiuretic conditions and oxalate excretion can rise in response to oxalate or oxalate precursor-rich meals.[61,62] On the other hand, in our clinic, a fair proportion of stone formers exhibit mild hyperoxaluria, and hyperoxaluria of much larger degree can occur as a result of gastrointestinal disease or bowel resection.[63,64] In addition, individuals with genetic hyperoxaluria can demonstrate markedly increased oxalate excretion.[65] Hyperoxaluria associated with the conditions mentioned previously has been shown to confer a significant degree of risk for the development of stone disease, as well as kidney disease resulting in kidney failure.[66] A number of groups have examined the cellular effects of oxalate exposure.

Some evidence for oxalate-mediated cell injury derives from studies of human stone formers. Hyperoxaluric stone formers demonstrate markers of epithelial cell injury in blood, urine, or both.[67–69] Unfortunately, these findings may not be specific to stone formers nor is it possible to completely exclude an effect of stones themselves or treatments thereof on excretion of injury markers. As noted earlier some of the same effects of hyperoxaluria are induced by contact with calcium oxalate crystals.[31] Studies of hyperoxaluric non-stone formers who had been carefully screened for the presence of stones and other renal or cardiovascular diseases would be needed to resolve this issue.

Induction of hyperoxaluria in experimental animals using oxalate itself or physiologic oxalate precursors have been examined relatively infrequently. Most animal studies have been performed using ethylene glycol to induce hyperoxaluria, a maneuver that may induce cellular changes to other toxic metabolites. For example, acute peritoneal administration of sodium oxalate resulted in pathologic changes in the renal papillary tip; however, this maneuver also produced calcium oxalate crystal deposition, making it impossible to determine what the effects of oxalate ion alone were.[70]

In vitro exposure of cell cultures to oxalate is at least incontrovertible regarding toxicity of oxalate by itself. Exposure of a number of renal tubule cell types activates phospholipase A2, leading to release of arachidonic acid and lysophosphatidylcholine, and mitochondrial damage.[71] This effect, as well as other sources, such as through the activation of NADPH oxidase, likely contribute to the reactive oxygen species (ROS) observed in response to oxalate.[72] These studies lend support to the idea that the evidence of ROS in stone formers can be the result of elevated oxalate concentrations within renal tubules alone, not just the result of damage induced by stone deposition or interventions for stone treatment.

Signaling cascades associated with apoptosis have also been described with oxalate exposure in vitro. One of these is the redistribution of phosphatidylserine from the inner to outer cell membrane.[73,74] As indicated earlier in this chapter, phosphatidylserine can serve as an attachment site for COM.[40] Apoptotic cells may also demonstrate increased COM attachment, at least in vitro[4,75,*]; however, no increase

in crystal retention was observed when apoptosis was induced by an industrial toxin in experimental animals with mildly increased oxalate excretion.[76] These experiments do not rule out a more long-term effect of increased rates of apoptosis. Although, for this to be important in vivo, presumably the rate of production of apoptotic cells must be in excess of what can be easily cleared by the available mechanisms. Whether oxalate could induce limitations to clearance of apoptotic cells by macrophages has not been examined.

A number of renal cell lines demonstrate enhanced activity of p38 MAP kinase, consequently increased in DNA synthesis, and cell proliferation.[77,78] With higher concentrations of oxalate, usually in excess of what would be the expected exposure in vivo, cell damage and denudation of culture monolayers is observed.[79] As has been noted earlier, cells induced to divide by scraping of cultures demonstrate enhanced crystal attachment, so exposure to concentrations of oxalate that are too low to induce overt damage may still condition cells for crystal attachment if nucleation takes place. It should be noted, however, that cultured IMCD cells appear to be more resistant to the effects of oxalate than other cell types.[80] Consideration of the amounts of oxalate excreted in urine in both enteric hyperoxaluria and genetic hyperoxaluria of either type suggests that tubule cells in the IMCD could see the kind of concentrations observed to induce either proliferation or toxic effects. Whether they see concentrations of oxalate sufficient to induce these effects in the usual calcium oxalate stone former – even the significant proportion of them who demonstrate mild hyperoxaluria – has not been established. It does not seem that oxalate exposure due to intestinal bypass induces interstitial calcification with apatite.[1]

6.8.2 Hypercalciuria

While it is clear that acute hypercalciuria induces reversible changes in renal function, the more chronic effects on tubule structure and function are unclear. Probably the most informative data regarding this issue can be gleaned from considering the case of Dent's disease, where low molecular weight enzymuria and hypercalciuria are associated.[81] The former, however, appears to result from interference with proximal nephron endosomal function; the hypercalciuria appears to be a consequence of enhanced intestinal calcium absorption, at least in the CCL5-deficient mouse model.[82] While hypercalciuria may be responsible for crystal formation and deposition, with its attendant damage, it appears that hypercalciuria alone is not associated with changes in tissue that would promote urinary stone disease.[83]

---

*Plus unpublished observations

6.8.3 *Hyperphosphaturia*

Patients with stone disease often manifest high levels of urinary phosphate excretion, either as a result of excessive dietary intake or due to a renal phosphate leak as a component of the syndrome of absorptive hypercalciuria.[84] Renal injury as a result of phosphaturia has not been studied directly, as this condition is in clinical situations mostly associated with other abnormalities, such as the Fanconi Syndrome.[85] Patients with phosphaturia and nephrolithiasis due to mutations in the Na–phosphate cotransporter have been described.[86] These individuals were without overt evidence of renal damage. Individuals with mutations in the gene *PHEX*, who demonstrate x-linked hypophosphatemic rickets, also do not appear to have any abnormalities in renal structure or function unless nephrocalcinosis develops.[87] In rats, a diet containing 1% calcium and 2% elemental phosphorus has been reported to induce corticomedullary calcium phosphate deposition at least in females.[88,89] Once crystal deposition has occurred, however, it is impossible to say whether it was the phosphaturia or the crystal deposition that is producing renal injury, such as has been described in individuals with renal tubular acidosis.[90] In vascular tissue, however, phosphate exposure induces calcifications, some of which are reminiscent of that described in association with matrix vesicles.[91,92] Whether phosphate exposure could induce calcification in or around matrix vesicles that are produced constitutively by tubule cells in the inner medulla of the kidney, or whether, as a perhaps subtle form of damage, phosphate increases matrix vesicle production would be a fruitful area of future study.

6.8.4 *Hyperuricosuria*

Of course, uric acid crystals by themselves are very inflammatory. Consequently, deposition of such crystals would be expected to induce renal injury. Even mild hyperuricemia, however, appears to induce endothelial injury mediated by ROS, apparently through reduction of nitric oxide availability.[93] Whether renal tubules are susceptible in this way is unclear, however, as is well known, hyperuricosuria is a risk factor for calcium oxalate stone disease.[94] This has generally been attributed to several factors, including promotion of heterogeneous nucleation by uric acid or monosodium urate, blocking of some of the inhibitory effects of urine macromolecules on calcium oxalate crystal formation, or a lowering of the limit of metastability for calcium oxalate by uric acid.[95] However, exposure of renal tubule cells to either uric acid crystals or soluble uric acid also appears to enhance attachment of COM.[96]

6.9 Conclusions

The role of the interaction of crystals or other solid constituents of stones with cells or renal tissue is complex. At the sites at which stones are observed in the kidney or urinary tract, there ordinarily appears to be resistance to the fixation of this material, although they may adhere to and be taken up more readily by cells outside of the kidneys or urinary tracts. Even within the urinary tract, crystals or solids may adhere to and be taken up by proximal tubule cells rather than by those in the collecting duct or the urothelium. Crystalline material may also form within interstitial spaces. Whether by deposition and attachment from tubular fluid or formation outside of cells, some form of cell or tissue damage may be a prerequisite. While the crystals or solids themselves may induce cellular changes, other conditions such as hyperoxaluria may induce changes that facilitate crystal adherence. It appears that attachment is mediated by specific molecules that appear on the cell surface or are constituents of extracellular matrix when cell injury or tissue damage occurs. These molecules have functional groups that permit an interaction with molecular components of crystals. The best described of these is the interaction between carboxyl groups and the (100) face of COM.

Figure 6.10 illustrates the interaction of crystals or solids with renal tissue as the author of this chapter envisions its role in the pathophysiology of nephrolithiasis. The schematic drawing shows a representation of COM crystals that presumably formed within a tubule adhering either to intact cells (in the absence or presence of subtle alterations in function or injury, cells that have undergone apoptosis, or areas of the tubules that have become denuded of cells. These crystals would have formed by nucleation in tubular fluid supersaturated with stone constituents or, as has been proposed by Khan and coworkers, on cell fragments within tubules. Presumably, other types of crystals, such as uric acid or cystine, can also form in this way and become fixed to the tubule wall. The crystals that are adherent to tubule cells could grow by agglomeration of other crystals floating by or by secondary nucleation on their surfaces, eventually forming a clinical stone by erosion or extension to the papillary tip or surface. These crystals can also be engulfed by cells resulting in their movement to the interstitium. There they may be actively transported within monocytic cells to the papillary surface, where they erode and form the nidus for a clinical stone. Alternatively, calcification in the form of hydroxyapatite may occur in the basement membranes of loops of Henle, perhaps through calcification of apoptotic bodies or matrix vesicles shed from injured cells. As proposed by Evan and coworkers, these form the basis of the clinically observed Randall's plaques. The erosion of plaques through the papillary surface, in their view, provides the nidus for deposition of calcium oxalate.

Fig. 6.10 Interaction of calcium oxalate and hydroxapatite with renal tissue in the pathophysiology of nephrolithiasis. See text for description. Micrograph of calcified vesicles in Randall's plaques courtesy of A. Evan (Image of stone that was attached to renal papilla courtesy of Dr. Neil Mandel)

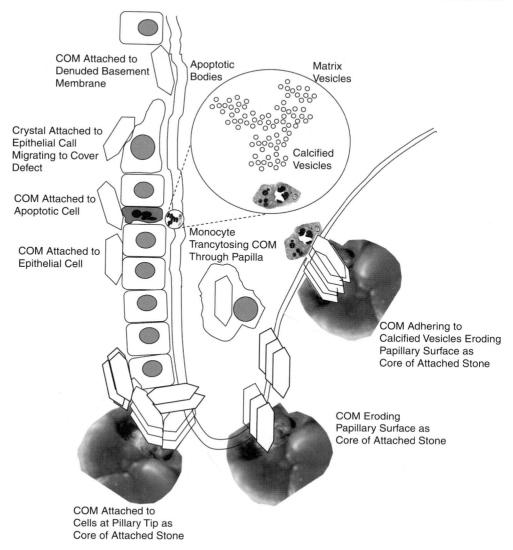

COM Attached to Denuded Basement Membrane

Apoptotic Bodies

Matrix Vesicles

Crystal Attached to Epithelial Call Migrating to Cover Defect

Calcified Vesicles

COM Attached to Apoptotic Cell

Monocyte Trancytosing COM Through Papilla

COM Attached to Epithelial Cell

COM Adhering to Calcified Vesicles Eroding Papillary Surface as Core of Attached Stone

COM Eroding Papillary Surface as Core of Attached Stone

COM Attached to Cells at Pillary Tip as Core of Attached Stone

References

1. Evan AP, Lingeman JE, Coe FL, et al. Randall's plaque of patients with nephrolithiasis begins in basement membranes of thin loops of Henle. *J Clin Invest.* 2003;111:607-616.
2. Olszta MJ, Odom DJ, Douglas EP, Gower LB. A new paradigm for biomineral formation: mineralization via an amorphous liquid-phase precursor. *Connect Tissue Res.* 2003;44(Suppl 1):326-334.
3. Khan SR. Heterogeneous nucleation of calcium oxalate crystals in mammalian urine [Review]. *Scan Microsc.* 1995;9:597-614.
4. Khan SR, Byer KJ, Thamilselvan S, et al. Crystal-cell interaction and apoptosis in oxalate-associated injury of renal epithelial cells. *J Am Soc Nephrol.* 199;10(Suppl 14):S457-S463.
5. Lieske JC, Toback FG, Deganello S. Direct nucleation of calcium oxalate dihydrate crystals onto the surface of living renal epithelial cells in culture. *Kidney Int.* 1998;54:796-803.
6. Evan AP, Coe FL, Lingeman JE, et al. Mechanism of formation of human calcium oxalate renal stones on Randall's plaque. *Anat Rec (Hoboken).* 2007;290:1315-1323.
7. Bobryshev YV, Killingsworth MC, Lord RS, Grabs AJ. Matrix vesicles in the fibrous cap of atherosclerotic plaque: Possible contribution to plaque rupture. *J Cell Mol Med.* 2008 Oct;12(5B):2073-82.

8. Reynolds JL, Joannides AJ, Skepper JN, et al. Human vascular smooth muscle cells undergo vesicle-mediated calcification in response to changes in extracellular calcium and phosphate concentrations: a potential mechanism for accelerated vascular calcification in ESRD. *J Am Soc Nephrol.* 2004;15:2857-2867.
9. Farzaneh-Far A, Shanahan CM. Biology of vascular calcification in renal disease. *Nephron Exp Nephrol.* 2005;101:e134-e138.
10. Derfus BA, Rachow JW, Mandel NS, et al. Articular cartilage vesicles generate calcium pyrophosphate dihydrate-like crystals in vitro. *Arthritis Rheum.* 1992;35:231-240.
11. Costa-Bauza A, Isern B, Perello J, Sanchis P, Grases F. Factors affecting the regrowth of renal stones in vitro: a contribution to the understanding of renal stone development. *Scand J Urol Nephrol.* 2005;39:194-199.
12. Costa-Bauza A, Perello J, Isern B, Sanchis P, Grases F. Factors affecting calcium oxalate dihydrate fragmented calculi regrowth. *BMC Urol.* 2006;6:16.
13. Derfus B, Kranendonk S, Camacho N, et al. Human osteoarthritic cartilage matrix vesicles generate both calcium pyrophosphate dihydrate and apatite in vitro. *Calcif Tissue Int.* 1998;63:258-262.
14. Thouverey C, Bechkoff G, Pikula S, Buchet R. Inorganic pyrophosphate as a regulator of hydroxyapatite or calcium pyrophosphate

dihydrate mineral deposition by matrix vesicles. *Osteoarthritis Cartilage*. 2009 Jan;17(1):64-72.

15. Vaingankar SM, Fitzpatrick TA, Johnson K, Goding JW, Maurice M, Terkeltaub R. Subcellular targeting and function of osteoblast nucleotide pyrophosphatase phosphodiesterase 1. *Am J Physiol Cell Physiol*. 2004;286:C1177-C1187.

16. Moochhala SH, Sayer JA, Carr G, Simmons NL. Renal calcium stones: insights from the control of bone mineralization. *Exp Physiol*. 2008;93:43-49.

17. Gill WB, Ruggiero K, Straus FH. Crystallization studies in a urothelial-lined living test tube (the catheterized female rat bladder). I. Calcium oxalate crystal adhesion to the chemically injured rat bladder. *Invest Urol*. 1979;17:257-261.

18. Khan SR, Cockrell CA, Finlayson B, Hackett RL. Crystal retention by injured urothelium of the rat urinary bladder. *J Urol*. 1984;132:153-157.

19. Hess B. Nutritional aspects of stone disease. *Endocrinol Metab Clin North Am*. 2002;31:1017-101x.

20. Rodgers AL, De Klerk DP. Crystalluria and urolithiasis in a relatively stone-free population. *Scan Electron Microsc*. 1986;0:1157-1167.

21. Lieske JC, Toback FG, Deganello S. Face-selective adhesion of calcium oxalate dihydrate crystals to renal epithelial cells. *Calcif Tissue Int*. 1996;58:195-200.

22. Lieske JC, Swift H, Martin T, Patterson B, Toback FG. Renal epithelial cells rapidly bind and internalize calcium oxalate monohydrate crystals. *Proc Natl Acad Sci USA*. 1994;91:6987-6991.

23. Lieske JC, Toback FG. Regulation of renal epithelial cell endocytosis of calcium oxalate monohydrate crystals. *Am J Physiol (Renal Fluid Electrolyte Physiol)*. 1993;264(33):F800-F807.

24. Lieske JC, Spargo BH, Toback FG. Endocytosis of calcium oxalate crystals and proliferation of renal tubular epithelial cells in a patient with type 1 primary hyperoxaluria. *J Urol*. 1992;148:1517-1519.

25. de Bruijn WC, Boeve ER, van Run PR, et al. Etiology of experimental calcium oxalate monohydrate nephrolithiasis in rats. *Scanning Microsc*. 1994;8:541-550.

26. de Bruijn WC, Boeve ER, van Run PR, et al. Etiology of calcium oxalate nephrolithiasis in rats. I. Can this be a model for human stone formation? *Scanning Microsc*. 1995;9:103-114.

27. de Bruijn WC, Boeve ER, van Run PRWA, et al. Etiology of calcium oxalate nephrolithiasis in rats. II. The role of the papilla in stone formation. *Scanning Microsc*. 1995;9:115-125.

28. Anderson L, McDonald JR. The origin, frequency, and significance of microscopic calculi in the kidney. *Surg Gynecol Obstet*. 1946; 82:275-282.

29. Cheung HS. Biologic effects of calcium-containing crystals. *Curr Opin Rheumatol*. 2005;17:336-340.

30. Lieske JC, Norris R, Swift H, Toback FG. Adhesion, internalization and metabolism of calcium oxalate monohydrate crystals by renal epithelial cells. *Kidney Int*. 1997;52:1291-1301.

31. Koul HK, Menon M, Chaturvedi LS, et al. COM crystals activate the p38 mitogen-activated protein kinase signal transduction pathway in renal epithelial cells. *J Biol Chem*. 2002;277: 36845-36852.

32. Drenick EJ, Stanley TM, Border WA, et al. Renal damage with intestinal bypass. *Ann Intern Med*. 1978;89:594-599.

33. Illum N, Lavard L, Danpure CJ, Horn T, AErenlund JH, Skovby F. Primary hyperoxaluria type 1: clinical manifestations in infancy and prenatal diagnosis. *Child Nephrol Urol*. 1992;12:225-227.

34. Khan SR. Crystal-induced inflammation of the kidneys: results from human studies, animal models, and tissue-culture studies. *Clin Exp Nephrol*. 2004;8:75-88.

35. Mandel N, Riese R. Crystal-cell interactions: crystal binding to rat renal papillary tip collecting duct cells in culture. *Am J Law Med*. 1991;17:402-406.

36. Riese RJ. "Adherence of kidney stone microcrystals to renal papillary collecting tubule cells in primary culture." Unpublished Ph.D. dissertation, Departments of Medicine and Biophysics, Medical College of Wisconsin, 1989; 0 edn, 1-141.

37. Riese RJ, Kleinman JG, Wiessner JH, Mandel GS, Mandel NS. Uric acid crystal binding to renal inner medullary collecting duct cells in primary culture. *J Am Soc Nephrol*. 1990;1:187-192.

38. Riese RJ, Mandel NS, Wiessner JH, Mandel GS, Becker CG, Kleinman JG. Cell polarity and calcium oxalate crystal adherence to cultured collecting duct cells. *Am J Physiol (Renal Fluid Electrolyte Physiol)*. 1992;262(31):F117-F184.

39. Riese RJ, Riese JW, Kleinman JG, Wiessner JH, Mandel GS, Mandel NS. Specificity in calcium oxalate adherence to papillary epithelial cells in cultures. *Am J Physiol*. 1988;255:F1025-F1032.

40. Bigelow MW, Wiessner JH, Kleinman JG, Mandel NS. Surface exposure of phosphatidylserine increases calcium oxalate crystal attachment to IMCD cells. *Am J Physiol (Renal Fluid Electrolyte Physiol)*. 1997;272:F55-F62.

41. Verkoelen CF, van der Boom BG, Romijn JC. Identification of hyaluronan as a crystal-binding moceule at the surface of migrating and proliferating MDCK cells. *Kidney Int*. 2000;58:1045-1054.

42. Lieske JC, Leonard R, Toback FG. Adhesion of calcium oxalate monohydrate crystals to renal epithelial cells is inhibited by specific anions. *Am J Physiol (Renal Fluid Electrolyte Physiol)*. 1995;268(37):F604-F612.

43. Sorokina EA, Kleinman JG. Cloning and preliminary characterization of a calcium-binding protein closely related to nucleolin on the apical surface of inner medullary collecting duct cells. *J Biol Chem*. 1999;274:27491-27496.

44. Yamaguchi S, Wiessner J, Hasegawa A, Hung L, Mandel G, Mandel N. Calcium oxalate monohydrate crystal binding substance produced from Madin-Darby canine kidney cells. *Int J Urol*. 2002;9:501-508.

45. Sorokina EA, Wesson JA, Kleinman JG. An acidic peptide sequence of nucleolin-related protein can mediate the attachment of calcium oxalate to renal tubule cells. *J Am Soc Nephrol*. 2004;15:2057-2065.

46. Kumar V, Farell G, Deganello S, Lieske JC. Annexin II is present on renal epithelial cells and binds calcium oxalate monohydrate crystals. *J Amer Soc Neph*. 2003;14:289-297.

47. Lieske JC, Leonard R, Swift H, Toback FG. Adhesion of calcium oxalate monohydrate crystals to anionic sites on the surface of renal epithelial cells. *Am J Physiol (Renal Fluid Electrolyte Physiol)*. 1996;270(39):F192-F199. Abstract.

48. Yamate T, Kohri K, Umekawa T, Amasaki N, Isikawa Y, Kurita T. The effect of osteopontin on the adhesion of calcium oxalate crystals to Madin-Darby canine kidney cells. *Eur Urol*. 1996;30:388-393.

49. Yamate T, Kohri K, Umekawa T, Iguchi M, Kurita T. Osteopontin antisense oligonucleotide inhibits adhesion of calcium oxalate crystals in Madin-Darby canine kidney cell. *J Urol*. 1998;160:1506-1512.

50. Wesson JA, Johnson RJMM, Beshensky AM, et al. Osteopontin is a critical inhibitor of calcium oxalate crystal formation and retention in renal tubules. *J Am Soc Nephrol*. 2003;14:139-147.

51. Mo L, Liaw L, Evan AP, Sommer AJ, Lieske JC, Wu XR. Renal calcinosis and stone formation in mice lacking osteopontin, Tamm-Horsfall protein, or both. *Am J Physiol Renal Physiol*. 2007;293: F1935-F1943.

52. Sheng X, Jung T, Wesson JA, Ward MD. Adhesion at calcium oxalate crystal surfaces and the effect of urinary constituents. *Proc Natl Acad Sci USA*. 2005;102:267-272.

53. Asselman M, Verhulst A, De Broe ME, Verkoelen CF. Calcium oxalate crystal adherence to hyaluronan-, osteopontin-, and CD44-expressing injured/regenerating tubular epithelial cells in rat kidneys. *J Am Soc Nephrol*. 2003;14:3155-3166.

54. Koka RM, Huang E, Lieske JC. Adhesion of uric acid crystals to the surface of renal epithelial cells. *Am J Physiol Renal Physiol*. 2000;278:F989-F998.

55. Ombra MN, Casula S, Biino G, et al. Urinary glycosaminoglycans as risk factors for uric acid nephrolithiasis: case control study in a Sardinian genetic isolate. *Urology*. 2003;62:416-420.

56. Lieske JC, Walsh-Reitz MM, Toback FG. Calcium oxalate monohydrate crystals are endocytosed by renal epithelial cells and induce proliferation. *Am J Physiol (Renal Fluid Electrolyte Physiol).* 1992;262(31):F622-F630.

57. Pak CY, Poindexter JR, Ms-Huet B, Pearle MS. Predictive value of kidney stone composition in the detection of metabolic abnormalities. *Am J Med.* 2003;115:26-32.

58. Pak CYC. Potential etiologic role of brushite in the formation of calcium (renal) stones. *J Cryst Growth.* 1981;53:202-208.

59. Lieske JC, Norris R, Toback FG. Adhesion of hydroxyapatite crystals to anionic sites on the surface of renal epithelial cells. *Am J Physiol.* 1997;273:F224-F233.

60. Mathoera RB, Kok DJ, Visser WJ, Verduin CM, Nijman RJ. Cellular membrane associated mucins in artificial urine as mediators of crystal adhesion: an in vitro enterocystoplasty model. *J Urol.* 2001;166:2329-2336.

61. Holmes RP, Assimos DG. The impact of dietary oxalate on kidney stone formation. *Urol Res.* 2204;32:311-316.

62. Levy FL, Adams-Huet B, Pak CY. Ambulatory evaluation of nephrolithiasis: an update of a 1980 protocol. *Am J Med.* 1995;98:50-59.

63. Bambach CP, Robertson WG, Peacock M, Hill GL. Effect of intestinal surgery on the risk of urinary stone formation. *Gut.* 1981;22:257-263.

64. McDonald GB, Earnest DL, Admirand WH. Hyperoxaluria correlates with fat malabsorption in patients with sprue. *Gut.* 1977;18:561-566.

65. Leumann E, Hoppe B. The primary hyperoxalurias. *J Am Soc Nephrol.* 2001;12:1986-1993.

66. Robertson WG, Hughes H. Importance of mild hyperoxaluria in the pathogenesis of urolithiasis—new evidence from studies in the Arabian peninsula. *Scanning Microsc.* 1993;7:391-401.

67. Huang HS, Ma MC, Chen CF, Chen J. Lipid peroxidation and its correlations with urinary levels of oxalate, citric acid, and osteopontin in patients with renal calcium oxalate stones. *Urology.* 2003;62:1123-1128.

68. Sumitra K, Pragasam V, Sakthivel R, Kalaiselvi P, Varalakshmi P. Beneficial effect of vitamin E supplementation on the biochemical and kinetic properties of Tamm-Horsfall glycoprotein in hypertensive and hyperoxaluric patients. *Nephrol Dial Transplant.* 2005;20:1407-1415.

69. Tungsanga K, Sriboonlue P, Futrakul P, Yachantha C, Tosukhowong P. Renal tubular cell damage and oxidative stress in renal stone patients and the effect of potassium citrate treatment. *Urol Res.* 2005;33:65-69.

70. Khan SR, Finlayson B, Hackett RL. Experimental calcium oxalate nephrolithiasis in the rat. Role of the renal papilla. *Am J Pathol.* 1982;107:59-69.

71. Jonassen JA, Kohjimoto Y, Scheid CR, Schmidt M. Oxalate toxicity in renal cells. *Urol Res.* 2005;33:329-339.

72. Khan SR. Role of renal epithelial cells in the initiation of calcium oxalate stones. *Nephron Exp Nephrol.* 2004;98:e55-e60.

73. Cao LC, Jonassen J, Honeyman TW, Scheid C. Oxalate-induced redistribution of phosphatidylserine in renal epithelial cells: implications for kidney stone disease. *Am J Nephrol.* 2001;21:69-77.

74. Wiessner JH, Hasegawa AT, Hung LY, Mandel GS, Mandel NS. Mechanisms of calcium oxalate crystal attachment to injured renal collecting duct cells. *Kidney Int.* 2001;59:637-644.

75. Wiessner JH, Hasegawa AT, Hung LY, Mandel NS. Oxalate-induced exposure of phosphatidylserine on the surface of renal epithelial cells in culture. *J Am Soc Nephrol.* 1999;10(Suppl 14):S441-S445.

76. Gambaro G, Valente ML, Zanetti E, et al. Mild tubular damage induces calcium oxalate crystalluria in a model of subtle hyperoxaluria: Evidence that a second hit is necessary for renal lithogenesis. *J Am Soc Nephrol.* 2006;17:2213-2219.

77. Greene EL, Farell G, Yu S, Matthews T, Kumar V, Lieske JC. Renal cell adaptation to oxalate. *Urol Res.* 2005;33:340-348.

78. Koul HK. Role of p38 MAP kinase signal transduction in apoptosis and survival of renal epithelial cells. *Ann NY Acad Sci.* 2003;1010:62-65.

79. Maroni PD, Koul S, Chandhoke PS, Meacham RB, Koul HK. Oxalate toxicity in cultured mouse inner medullary collecting duct cells. *J Urol.* 2005;174:757-760.

80. Maroni PD, Koul S, Meacham RB, Chandhoke PS, Koul HK. Effects of oxalate on IMCD cells: a line of mouse inner medullary collecting duct cells. *Ann NY Acad Sci.* 2004;1030:144-149.

81. Scheinman SJ, Cox JP, Lloyd SE, et al. Isolated hypercalciuria with mutation in CLCN5: relevance to idiopathic hypercalciuria. *Kidney Int.* 2000;57:232-239.

82. Luyckx VA, Leclercq B, Dowland LK, Yu AS. Diet-dependent hypercalciuria in transgenic mice with reduced CLC5 chloride channel expression. *Proc Natl Acad Sci USA.* 1999;96:12174-12179.

83. Sikora P, Glatz S, Beck BB, et al. Urinary NAG in children with urolithiasis, nephrocalcinosis, or risk of urolithiasis. *Pediatr Nephrol.* 2003;18:996-999.

84. Williams CP, Child DF, Hudson PR, et al. Inappropriate phosphate excretion in idiopathic hypercalciuria: the key to a common cause and future treatment? *J Clin Pathol.* 1996;49:881-888.

85. Laing CM, Toye AM, Capasso G, Unwin RJ. Renal tubular acidosis: developments in our understanding of the molecular basis. *Int J Biochem Cell Biol.* 2005;37:1151-1161.

86. Prie D, Huart V, Bakouh N, et al. Nephrolithiasis and osteoporosis associated with hypophosphatemia caused by mutations in the type 2a sodium-phosphate cotransporter. *N Engl J Med.* 2002;347:983-991.

87. Raeder H, Bjerknes R, Shaw N, Netelenbos C. A case of X-linked hypophosphatemic rickets (XLH): complications and the therapeutic use of cinacalcet. *Eur J Endocrinol.* 2008 Dec;159(Suppl 1):S101-5.

88. Chow FH, Taton GF, Boulay JP, Lewis LD, Remmenga EE, Hamar DW. Effect of dietary calcium, magnesium, and phosphorus on phosphate urolithiasis in rats. *Invest Urol.* 1980;17:273-276.

89. Khan SR, Glenton PA. Deposition of calcium phosphate and calcium oxalate crystals in the kidneys. *J Urol.* 1995;153:811-817.

90. Evan AP, Lingeman J, Coe F, et al. Renal histopathology of stone-forming patients with distal renal tubular acidosis. *Kidney Int.* 2007;71:795-801.

91. Chen NX, O'Neill KD, Duan D, Moe SM. Phosphorus and uremic serum up-regulate osteopontin expression in vascular smooth muscle cells. *Kidney Int.* 2002;62:1724-1731.

92. Wada T, McKee MD, Steitz S, Giachelli CM. Calcification of vascular smooth muscle cell cultures: inhibition by osteopontin. *Circ Res.* 1999;84:166-178.

93. Sanchez-Lozada LG, Soto V, Tapia E, et al. Role of oxidative stress in the renal abnormalities induced by experimental hyperuricemia. *Am J Physiol Renal Physiol.* 2008;295:F1134-F1141.

94. Favus MJ, Coe FL. Clinical characteristics and pathogenetic mechanisms in hyperuricosuric calcium oxalate renal stone disease. *Scand J Urol Nephrol.* 1980;53:171-177.

95. Grover PK, Marshall VR, Ryall RL. Dissolved urate salts out calcium oxalate in undiluted human urine in vitro: implications for calcium oxalate stone genesis. *Chem Biol.* 2003;10:271-278.

96. Farell G, Huang E, Kim SY, Horstkorte R, Lieske JC. Modulation of proliferating renal epithelial cell affinity for calcium oxalate monohydrate crystals. *J Am Soc Nephrol.* 2004;15:3052-3062.

97. Carr RJ. A new theory on the formation of renal calculi. *Br J Urol.* 1954;26:105-117.

98. Haggitt RC, Pitcock JA. Renal medullary calcifications: a light and electron microscopic study. *J Urol.* 1971;106:342-347.

99. Cifuentes D, Minon-Cifuentes J, Medina JA. New studies on papillary calculi. *J Urol.* 1987;137:1024-1029.

100. Ryall RL. The future of stone research: rummagings in the attic, Randall's plaque, nanobacteria, and lessons from phylogeny. *Urol Res.* 2008;36:77-97.

Randall's Plaques

7

Michel Daudon, Olivier Traxer, James C. Williams Jr, and Dominique C. Bazin

Abstract First described by Alexander Randall in the 1930s, carbapatite plaques formed in the interstitium of the inner medulla are now a major cause for calcium oxalate stone formation in western countries. At least 50% of all calcium stone formers (and even more than 75% of patients in the United States) exhibit such calcified deposits beneath and at the surface of the papillary epithelium as observed by endoscopic examination of kidney papillae. On the other hand, a majority of spontaneously passed calcium oxalate monohydrate stones exhibit a peculiar morphology suggestive of stone nucleation from a Randall's plaque. The stones developed from a papillary plaque are easily identified by microscopic examination due to the presence of a concave, depressed zone ("umbilication") at their surface, which corresponds to the attachment site at the tip of the papilla. The origin of the calcified deposits is the basement membrane of the deep thin Henle's loops. Calcium phosphate then spreads out through the interstitium of the inner medulla. The mechanisms involved in the formation of these plaques are not yet entirely clarified. Metabolic examination of urine suggests a predominant role of hypercalciuria in concordance with a high urine pH and a high phosphate concentration in the interstitium and a possible link with diet. Low diuresis is another factor often found in patients who exhibit stones developed from a Randall's plaque. As observed by electron microscopy from both tissue and stones, it appears that Randall's plaques may extend around the vasa recta and collecting ducts, which may be pulled out of the tissue when the stone breaks away from the papilla.

7.1 Historical Perspective

Seven decades ago, the American urologist Alexander Randall[1–3] first proposed that papillary pathology was at the origin of renal calculi. When examining kidneys from autopsy of 1,154 unselected subjects, he observed in 19.6% of them a peculiar lesion, in the form of whitish or cream-colored small flat areas near the tip of papillae, which he termed "plaques." Light microscopy revealed that these plaques were located beneath the epithelium of papillae in the interstitium of the inner medulla, and were not observed in tubular lumens. Chemical analysis showed that they were made of calcium phosphate deposits. Randall's hypothesis that such deposits would constitute a nidus for stone formation was confirmed by the finding of small calculi attached to plaque at the tip of

papillae in 65 kidneys; i.e., in 5.6% of renal units. Furthermore, he noted that interstitial plaques had lost their epithelial cover at the site of calculus anchorage, and that detached stones exhibited a concave, depressed zone at their surface, with traces of the same calcium phosphate material as plaques, thus likely to correspond to the attachment site to the papilla (Fig. 7.1).

In the same period, other authors confirmed the findings of Randall in autopsy studies. Rosenow[4] found plaques in 22.2% of 239 kidneys, whereas Anderson[5] observed plaques in 12% of kidneys in a series of 1,500 necropsies. In South Africa, Vermooten[6] examined 1,060 pairs of kidneys and found Randall's plaques in 17.2% of Caucasians and only 4.3% of Bantus – a finding in keeping with his observation of the lower incidence of calcium nephrolithiasis in the local population of African descent than Caucasian descent.

Papillary calcifications were seen in the subepithelial interstitial tissue together with collagen fibers, and were not found in the lumen of collecting ducts.[7] These seminal works were largely ignored during the four subsequent decades, but a renewed interest for Randall's plaques recently followed

M. Daudon (✉)
Department of Biochemistry, Stone Laboratory, Necker Hospital, Paris, France
e-mail: michel.daudon@nck.aphp.fr

P.N. Rao et al. (eds.), *Urinary Tract Stone Disease*,
DOI 10.1007/978-1-84800-362-0_7, © Springer-Verlag London Limited 2011

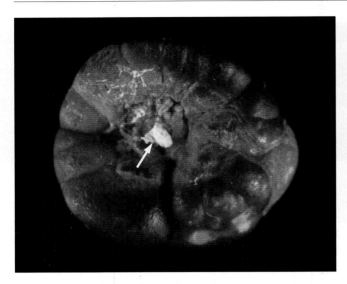

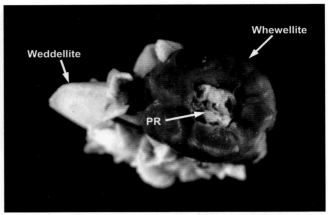

Fig. 7.2 Calcium oxalate stone in a hypercalciuric patient. The stone is made of both whewellite (calcium oxalate monohydrate) and weddellite (calcium oxalate dihydrate), the former being at the contact of the Randall's plaque (PR)

Fig. 7.1 Whewellite stone harboring a whitish Randall's plaque made of carbapatite (*white arrow*) in the depressed area ("umbilication")

the development of techniques allowing direct visualization of renal cavities by means of ureterorenoscopy.

7.2 Prevalence of Randall's Plaques and Umbilicated Calculi

Two decades ago, the Spanish urologist Cifuentes-Delatte and coworkers examining 500 consecutive calculi by means of scanning electron microscopy and X-ray diffraction coupled with infrared spectroscopy observed that 142 of the calculi (28.4%) exhibited a concavity characteristic of a papillary origin.[8] In 61 (43%) of these umbilicated calculi, plaques were typically made of apatite, some of them showing calcified collecting ducts.[9]

Among 45,774 calculi referred to the Necker hospital stone laboratory over the past 3 decades, morphologic examination coupled with Fourier transform infrared spectroscopy (FTIR) identified 8,916 (19.5%) umbilicated calculi,[10] most of which (92.5%) were made of calcium oxalate monohydrate (COM, whewellite) either pure (Fig. 7.1) or admixed with calcium oxalate dihydrate (COD, weddellite) as observed in Fig. 7.2.

Thus, stone examination in large series of patients shows a prevalence of about 20% of calculi harboring a typical umbilication characteristic of a papillary origin, with calcium phosphate (mainly carbapatite) being the major component of Randall's plaques in 90% of cases.[10] Of note, in the recent years, stones harboring an umbilication were found to be three times more frequent than at the beginning of the 1980s and patients were younger and younger.[11] In our experience, 39% of all spontaneously passed stones had a typical umbilication on their surface and 61% of passed COM stones were umbilicated and were developed from a Randall's plaque.

Direct evidence of the papillary origin of calcium oxalate stones in highly selected series of patients was recently provided by detailed endoscopic examination of renal papillae during percutaneous nephrolithotomy (PCNL) or ureteroscopic procedures. In 1997, Low and Stoller[12] observed the presence of Randall's plaques on one or more papillae in 74% of 57 stone formers treated with PCNL or ureteroscopy, the prevalence being 88% for calcium oxalate stones. Matlaga et al.[13] examined by digital imaging 172 renal papillae in 23 patients with idiopathic calcium oxalate nephrolithiasis undergoing PCNL. Virtually, all papillae (91%) were found to harbor plaques and half of papillae had attached calculi. Digital imaging provided undisputable evidence of stone attachment to plaque. Furthermore, the same group showed that patients with more stones also had a higher fraction of their papillae covered by plaques.[14] However, epidemiological differences in the occurrence of Randall's plaques may be observed according to the investigated population. Recent reports from European countries suggest that Randall's plaque could be less frequent in Europe than in the United States. In Italy, Ruggera et al. reported the occurrence of Randall's plaque in 44.4% of 27 stone formers who underwent ureterorenoscopy or percutaneous nephrolithotomy and renal papillae biopsy.[15]

In France, Traxer et al.* examined papillary morphology in 462 patients who underwent flexible ureterorenoscope either for kidney stone disease or for another pathologic condition (urothelial tumor, ureteral stenosis, or unexplained hematuria). They used only flexible ureterorenoscopy of new generation for an optimal observation of renal cavities (Flex-*X*2 Karl Storz, DUR-8E GYRUS-ACMI, URFP5 Olympus).

For this study, they describe four types of Randall's Plaques (Fig. 7.3) in comparison with the normal aspect of

---

*OT, personal unpublished data

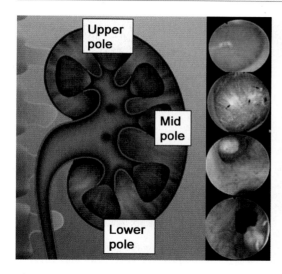

Fig. 7.3 Schematic classification of Randall's plaque related to the surface of the papilla covered by calcium phosphate deposits. All calices may be similarly affected by Randall's plaque

renal papillae. Type 1 represents very tiny calcifications on the surface of the renal papillae. Type 2 represents calcifications occupying less than one-third of the surface of the papillae. Type 3 represents calcifications occupying at least two-third of the surface of the papillae. Type 4 represents a stone fixed on the surface of renal papillae. Figure 7.4 illustrates an example of normal papilla and different degrees of Randall's plaques. In the case of wide plaque covering more than two-third of the surface of the papilla, a characteristic concavity may be observed (Fig. 7.4d). Using new generation ureterorenoscopes, it is now common to observe stones fixed on the plaque (Fig. 7.5).

Among the 289 stone formers, they found Randall's plaques in 57% (164 patients) corresponding to the presence of calcifications on one or more papillae. Sixty-four percent of patients with Randall's plaques were male. Randall's plaques were presented on all renal papillae in 54% of patients (upper, mid, and lower pole). According to their classification, 40% of patients had Randall's plaques type 1,

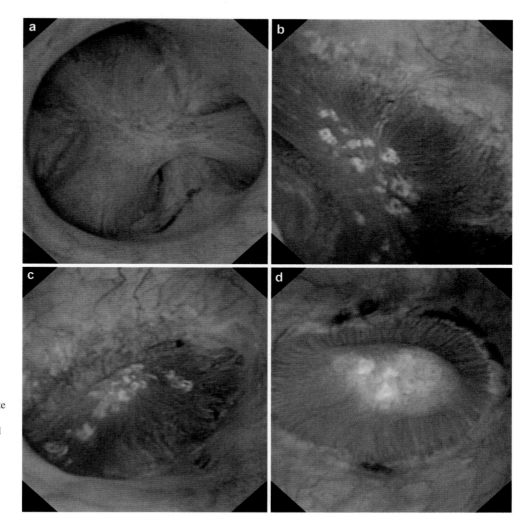

Fig. 7.4 (**a**) Normal papilla; (**b–d**): increasing amounts of surface plaque (white deposits) on papilla of three CaOx stone formers; (**b**) example of moderate calcium phosphate deposits scattered at the surface of a renal papilla; (**c**) more abundant deposits covering less than one-third of the papilla surface; (**d**) extensive Randall's plaque covering more than two-third of the surface area of a papilla

Fig. 7.5 Two examples of calcium stones anchored to a Randall's plaque. (**a**) small calcium stone fixed to a Randall's plaque (*arrow*). Note the presence of other calcium phosphate deposits on the right side (*arrowhead*). (**b**) Piece of a stone (*thick arrow*) that was anchored to the left side of an extensive Randall's plaque. The stone was broken during ureterorenoscopy procedure. Note the small tissue lesion (*red area*) corresponding to the anchorage of the stone (*thin arrow*) and the plaque that covers a large surface area of the papilla (*arrowheads*)

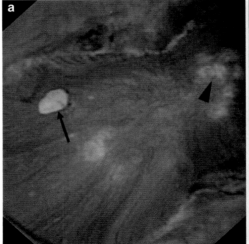 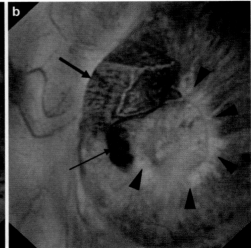

26% type 2, and 15% type 3. Presence of a stone fixed on renal papillae (Type 4) was observed in 19% of patients.

Such plaques were visible in only 27% (48 patients) of the 173 nonstone forming patients with the following repartition: 69% type 1, 10% type 2, 6% type 3, and 15% type 4. Randall's plaques were present on all renal papillae in 62% of these patients.

Thus ureterorenoscopic investigations provide evidence that Randall's plaques are frequent, mainly found in stone former patients, and are highly associated with stone formation.

Due to the new developments in terms of optics for flexible ureterorenoscopes (digital technology), exploration of renal cavities is more and more complete. These improvements allow the urologist today to describe precisely the intrarenal collecting system and particularly the Randall's plaques in terms of type and repartition, which could be a valuable help for assessing the risk of stone recurrence in a given patient.

All these studies validate and even reinforce the seminal concept of Randall that papillary plaques are at the origin of a substantial proportion of kidney stones.

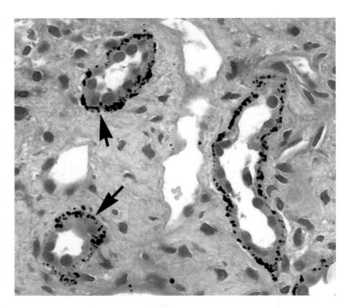

Fig. 7.6 Initial sites and size of calcium deposition in the papillary tissue of a CaOx patient as seen by light microscopy. Sites of crystalline material (*arrows*) are noted in the basement membranes, near the collagen of the thin loops of Henle. Calcium deposits may be seen also in the interstitium. Magnification × 1,000 (Reproduced with permission from[17])

7.3 Origin of Randall's Plaques

The initial site of plaques has been shown to be in the basement membrane of the thin loops of Henlé[16] in the form of small round particles in the nanometric range with concentric mineral and organic layers best seen by transmission electron microscopy (Figs. 7.6 and 7.7). These particles then spread into the surrounding interstitial space, associated with type 1 collagen (Fig. 7.8). Subsequently, particles fuse together with collagen in such a manner that the mineral phase is coated with organic matrix. Of note, plaques without stones remain covered by an intact epithelial layer, which itself is covered by a glycoprotein coat; whereas a plaque that has lost its epithelial layer indicates the site where a stone had been attached.

By high-resolution micro FTIR and electron diffraction, the mineral component of plaque particles was identified as calcium phosphate in the form of apatite.[16] In contrast, although calculi were made of calcium oxalate, oxalate crystals were never found either in the renal interstitium or in

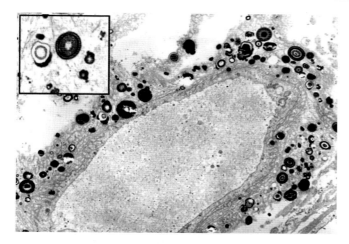

Fig. 7.7 Aspect of calcium deposits in the basement membranes of the thin loops of Henle as seen by transmission electron microscopy. Crystalline material appears as spherules composed of concentric alternate clear (mineral) and dark (organic material) layers. Magnification × 15,600. Inset, image confirmed that crystal site was associated with thin loops of Henle collagen. Magnification × 25,000 (Reproduced with permission from[17])

7.4 Mechanism of Plaque-Associated Stone Formation

The mechanisms by which calcium oxalate stones grow on apatite plaques have been elucidated by study of the ultrastructure of the plaque–stone interface in small calculi that could be extracted along with its underlying papillary tissue.[18] Papillary epithelium was disrupted at the attachment site. The denuded plaque was covered by ribbon-like layers of alternating lamina of apatite crystals and organic material, on the external face of which were found pure calcium oxalate crystals, as shown by FTIR. Immunohistochemistry revealed that osteopontin was present simultaneously in plaque, interface, and stone, whereas Tamm-Horsfall protein was present only on the urine side of the interface. Thus, the protein material present at the surface of plaques serves as the anchoring point for calcium oxalate crystals adhesion, followed by calcium oxalate crystals accretion and stone formation.[21,22]

This lithogenic mechanism, summarized in Fig. 7.9, appears to be unique to idiopathic calcium oxalate stones. Indeed, calcium oxalate stones formed in obese patients following bariatric procedures, or brushite stones formed in other patients, exhibited different histopathological findings.[17] Calcium stones developed in obese patients following bypass surgery had apatite crystals in lumens of collecting ducts with associated cell injury but not in the interstitium and had no visible papillary plaques.[16] Brushite stone formers had even more severe renal changes with both Randall's plaques and yellowish intraluminal apatite deposits in Bellini ducts,[23] as already reported by Randall as his type 2 form of plaques.[3] In addition, in patients with primary hyperparathyroidism and calcium phosphate stones, Evan et al.[24] recently reported abundant apatite deposits plugging dilated

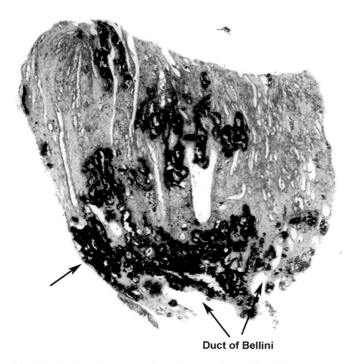

Duct of Bellini

Fig. 7.8 Papillary biopsy specimen from a patient with calcium oxalate calculi as seen by low power light microscopy. Calcium deposit sites (*arrows*) were stained black by Yasue metal substitution method for calcium histochemistry. Magnification × 100 (Reproduced with permission from[17])

plaques.[16,18] By immunochemistry, the organic component of plaques was shown to contain osteopontin[19] and interalphatrypsin inhibitor heavy chain 3.[20]

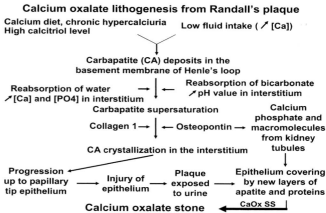

Fig. 7.9 Schematic representation of the successive steps for calcium oxalate stone formation from a Randall's plaque. [ ] designates the concentration of the corresponding solute; CaOx SS = calcium oxalate supersaturation

collecting ducts together with large interstitial deposits of Randall's plaques with attached stones, thus showing that these two patterns may coexist according to etiological factors.

Study of Randall's plaques present in the umbilication of papillary stones by means of scanning electron microscopy (SEM) coupled with FTIR analysis has allowed us to better characterize the structure of plaques at the mesoscopic scale. In particular, these techniques allow one to identify the various types of minerals involved in plaque composition, namely carbapatite, which is the commonest phase, and other calcium phosphates such as amorphous carbonated calcium phosphate, whitlockite, brushite; and sometimes purines such as sodium hydrogen urate or uric acid; and obviously COM and COD. These techniques also allow determining the respective localization of the components in the plaque. A total of 25 calcium oxalate kidney stones were examined by light microscopy, FTIR, and SEM. As shown in Fig. 7.10, the plaque anchored to the stone may be tiny, or in contrast bulkier, harboring calcified renal tubules.

Three main observations were made. First, as observed by SEM examination of Randall's plaques anchored to spontaneously passed calcium oxalate stones (Fig. 7.11), calcium phosphate deposits of carbapatite likely coming from the neighboring collecting ducts may cover the surface of the papillary epithelium. Second, the first mineral phase of calcium oxalate calculi (either made of COM or of COD as the main component) affixed onto the carbapatite is almost always COM. As observed in Fig. 7.12, large randomly oriented COM crystals are trapped on a phase made of carbapatite crystals embedded in proteins acting as a "glue." Even in stones made of an admixture of monohydrate and dihydrate, very large octahedral crystals of COD visually hang on COM crystal layers. Such size difference between carbapatite crystals and calcium oxalate crystals, together with the random distribution of COM or COD crystals inserted onto the carbapatite Randall's plaque make unlikely the hypothesis of epitaxial growth of calcium oxalate crystals on calcium phosphate crystals, in agreement with the observations made by other authors in crystallization studies.[25,26] Instead, they support the role of a protein interface between the two mineral phases, as suggested by Evan et al.[18] Third, several umbilicated calcium oxalate calculi exhibited a calcium phosphate plaque together with empty or filled cylindric channels (Fig. 7.11), which correspond both to calcified Bellini's ducts and vessels embedded in an extensive plaque, the former being either empty or filled with carbapatite. The latter situation suggests the intervention of a dual lithogenic mechanism, involving both interstitial and luminal calcium phosphate particles deposition, as shown in brushite stone formers.[23]

An interesting approach for examining stones with Randall's plaque is analysis of stones using micro CT.[27,28] This nondestructive technique offers the opportunity of

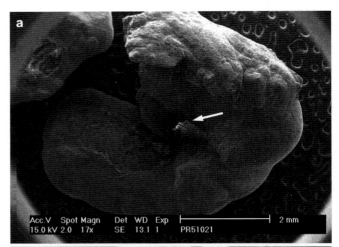

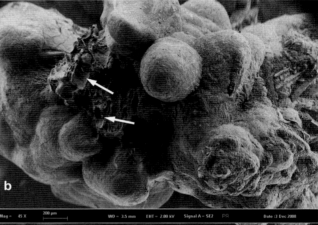

Fig. 7.10 Scanning electron micrographs showing two examples of calcium oxalate monohydrate stones developed from a Randall's plaque: (**a**) small plaque (*arrow*) observed at the surface of a spontaneously passed stone; (**b**) bulky plaque with calcified tubules (*arrows*) at the surface of a stone removed by ureteroscopy

visualizing the stone composition and the distribution of the components and provides very nice images of Randall's plaque, even when the plaque is coated by calcium oxalate layers. Based on 3D-reconstructions, the stone morphology may be accurately obtained as illustrated in Figs. 7.7 to 7.13. This figure shows several of the features already described for stones formed on Randall's plaques. The carbapatite region of the stone shows up distinctively because its calcium phosphate content makes it absorbs X-rays better than other stone minerals.[29] Note in panel A that the carbapatite region extends well into the stone, which is consistent with the addition of apatite from the urine, as described by Evan et al.[18] In panel B, it can be seen that this carbapatite region is exposed within a concave region of the stone, where the stone was attached to papillary plaque. It is not possible to tell (at least at the present time) which portion of this carbapatite region may be composed of Randall's plaque that pulled away from the renal

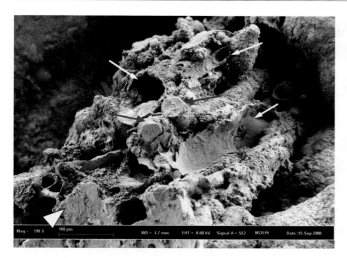

Fig. 7.11 Scanning electron micrograph of a Randall's plaque anchored to a calcium oxalate monohydrate stone. The plaque appears as a complex structure containing calcified tubules and vessels (*white arrows*), and tubules filled by carbapatite plugs (*red arrows*). The smooth part of the plaque (*white arrowhead*) suggests that a layer of carbapatite, probably issued from neighbouring tubules, has covered the papilla epithelium

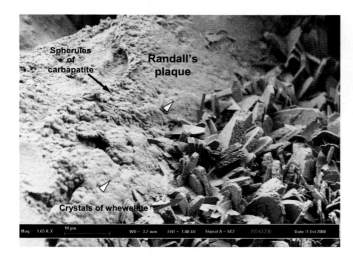

Fig. 7.12 Interface area between a Randall's plaque and a calcium oxalate monohydrate stone as seen by scanning electron microscopy. The micrograph shows randomly distributed calcium oxalate monohydrate crystals (*right*) trapped in the carbapatite of Randall's plaque (*left*). Note the presence of carbapatite spherules (*black thin arrow*) that appear joined by an unstructured material, identified as proteins by infrared spectroscopy (*white arrowheads*), which acts as a glue to fix CaOx crystals (*red thick arrows*)

tissue, and this small stone did not show evidence of calcified tubules in the carbapatite region (see below), which sometimes can be visualized using micro CT or other techniques such as scanning electron microscopy.

In the slice through the stone shown in panel A, it can also be seen that the first material laid down over the carbapatite

region was COM, which shows a slightly greater X-ray attenuation than does the COD, which composes the polyhedral crystals at the surface of the stone.

Indeed, scanning electron microscopy examination of Randall's plaque provides evidence that most plaques observed at the surface of calcium oxalate stones are the result of a triple mechanism:

- First, an interstitial deposit of carbapatite initiated in the basal membrane of the long Henle's loops, as showed by Evan et al.,[16] and secondarily spread out in the inner medulla toward the vasa recta, the renal tubules, and the papilla epithelium
- Second, after disruption of the epithelium, the deposit may be covered by laminates of new calcium phosphate deposits and macromolecules originated from the urine[18]
- Finally, as suggested by our SEM photographs and infrared analysis of Randall's plaque from umbilicated urinary COM calculi, the plaque may accumulate calcium phosphate deposits expelled from the lumen of local distal tubules and it may also be formed by plugs of carbapatite from neighboring distal tubules (Fig. 7.11)

Moreover, the photomicrographs suggest that most tubules covered by the Randall's plaque are surrounded by carbapatite deposits, which impair the exchanges between the tubule and the interstitium, probably making the tubule not functional. As it can be seen in Fig. 7.11, when the stone is breaking away from the papilla, it pulls out the calcified ends of the tubules, thus creating an irreversible damage of the tissue. These observations can help to explain why the carbonation rate of carbapatite in Randall's plaque is markedly variable, as observed by infrared analysis. Actually, among 416 umbilicated stones with carbapatite Randall's plaque, we found a high carbonation rate ($\geq 20\%$) of carbapatite in 47% of cases, a finding in agreement with the physicochemical conditions in the medulla, where the bicarbonate concentration is high. However, in 35% of cases, the carbonation rate was less than 15% and even less than 9% in 17% of cases. This low carbonate content suggests that the corresponding carbapatite, or at least a part of it, did not originate from the medullary interstitium but more probably from the urine discharged by the tubules.

7.5 Risk Factors for Randall's Plaque Formation

In their initial study of 15 patients with recurrent idiopathic, pure calcium oxalate nephrolithiasis, Evan et al.[16] observed that, compared with normal subjects, they had higher urine calcium levels and supersaturation with respect to calcium

Fig. 7.13 Micro-CT images of a calcium oxalate stone developed from a Randall's plaque

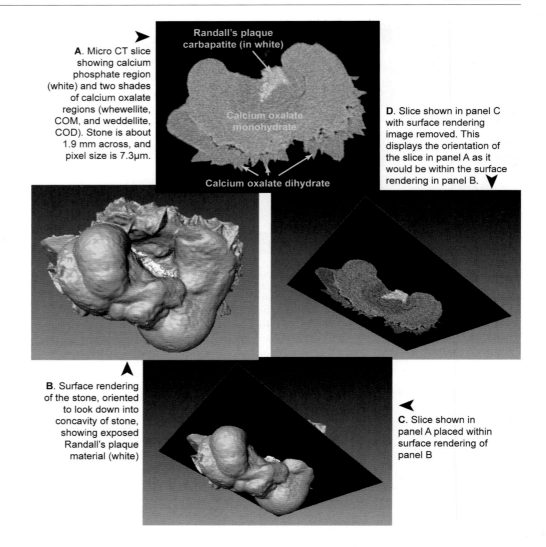

A. Micro CT slice showing calcium phosphate region (white) and two shades of calcium oxalate regions (whewellite, COM, and weddellite, COD). Stone is about 1.9 mm across, and pixel size is 7.3μm.

Randall's plaque carbapatite (in white)

Calcium oxalate monohydrate

Calcium oxalate dihydrate

D. Slice shown in panel C with surface rendering image removed. This displays the orientation of the slice in panel A as it would be within the surface rendering in panel B.

B. Surface rendering of the stone, oriented to look down into concavity of stone, showing exposed Randall's plaque material (white)

C. Slice shown in panel A placed within surface rendering of panel B

oxalate and calcium phosphate. In the same group, Kuo et al.[30] analyzed the correlation between the fraction of papillary surface occupied by plaques and urinary parameters in 14 idiopathic calcium oxalate stone formers and four controls. A low daily urine volume and a high daily calcium excretion were the only parameters significantly associated with increasing plaque coverage. Accordingly, Kim et al.[14] showed that stone formation is proportional to papillary surface coverage by Randall's plaques. This finding is in keeping with the high prevalence of idiopathic hypercalciuria in idiopathic calcium oxalate stone formers.[31] Moreover, Curhan et al.[32] identified daily urinary volume and calcium excretion as the only parameters significantly associated with stone incidence; and we identified a daily urine volume lower than 2 L and a urine calcium concentration higher than 3.8 mmol/L as the only parameters associated with calcium oxalate crystal formation and stone recurrence in idiopathic calcium oxalate stone formers.[33]

The physicochemical environment in the interstitium of the inner medulla favors calcium phosphate supersaturation around the tip of Henle's loops, especially in the presence of hypercalciuria and low urine output. Indeed, in conditions of antidiuresis, the pH increases in the inner medulla, together with calcium and phosphate concentration in the interstitium,[34,35] thus favoring the precipitation of calcium phosphate.[36] In addition, during antidiuresis, the hyaluronic acid content decreases in the inner medulla,[37] thus reducing its availability to act as an inhibitor of crystallization,[38,39] and results in increased concentration of solutes in the interstitium, due to its properties as a mechano-osmotic transducer.[40] In the absence of a suitable animal model of Randall's plaque,[21] the intimate molecular mechanism leading to deposition of small carbapatite particles in the basement membrane of thin loops of Henlé remains to be elucidated. Indeed, these particles closely resemble the so-called nanobacteria, which have recently been found to be self-propagating mineral complexes made of fetuin ("nanons") (and not living organisms), as recently shown by Raoult et al.,[41] and both fetuin and nanons were evidenced in human renal calculi.

Because fetuin plays a regulatory role in tissue mineralization, such finding suggests that formation of apatite particles in the epithelial cells of Henle's loops might represent an epithelial-to-mesenchymal transdifferentiation process in the kidneys, as already observed in arterial walls.[42] Factors inductive of such a process in stone formers remain to be elucidated.

7.6 Implications for Clinical Practice

The recent demonstration of an important role for Randall's plaques in the formation of calcium oxalate stones has implications for both a better understanding of the lithogenic process and for the clinical management of nephrolithiasis patients.

Direct visualization of renal papilla is available only if PCNL or ureteroscopy procedures are required for stone treatment, whereas nearly 80% of calcium oxalate stones are spontaneously passed. Therefore, morphologic examination of stones is a simple and reliable means for identifying umbilicated calculi, which reflect a papillary origin.[10,43,44] In addition, FTIR analysis of the plaque and other parts of the stone provides information about the composition of the plaque itself and surrounding parts of the stone.

In view of the close relationship between a high urine concentration of calcium and presence of Randall's plaques, finding of a carbapatite plaque in an umbilicated calcium oxalate calculus orients one toward the hypothesis of underlying hypercalciuria and/or low fluid intake (which by itself increases urinary concentration of both calcium and oxalate).

However, not all calcium oxalate stones formed by hypercalciuric patients harbor an umbilication. Therefore, other factors contributing to increase in interstitial pH, such as potassium depletion[36] should also be searched for.

7.7 Conclusions

In conclusion, there is renewed interest in Randall's plaques as initiating factors of calcium oxalate stone formation, in relation with hypercalciuria. Randall's plaques, made of carbapatite, extrude at the tip of papillae, onto which calcium oxalate monohydrate crystals adhere and grow. Accordingly, calcium oxalate stones developed on a Randall's plaque exhibit a characteristic depression ("umbilication") easily detected by morphologic examination of calculi. Such finding orients toward the search for hypercalciuria, in addition to hyperoxaluria, in calcium oxalate stone formers.

References

1. Randall A. An hypothesis for the origin of renal calculus. *N Engl J Med.* 1936;214:234-237.
2. Randall A. The origin and growth of renal calculi. *Ann Surg.* 1937;105:1009-1027.
3. Randall A. Papillary pathology as a precursor of primary renal calculus. *J Urol.* 1940;44:580-589.
4. Rosenow EC Jr. Renal calculi: study of papillary calcification. *J Urol.* 1940;44:19-23.
5. Anderson WAD. Renal calcification in adults. *J Urol.* 1940;44:29-34.
6. Vermooten V. The incidence and significance of the deposition of calcium plaques in the renal papilla as observed in the Caucasian and Bantu population in South Africa. *J Urol.* 1941;46:193-196.
7. Vermooten V. Origin and development in renal papilla of Randall's calcium plaques. *J Urol.* 1942;48:27-37.
8. Cifuentes Delatte L, Minon-Cifuentes JL, Medina JA. New studies on papillary calculi. *J Urol.* 1987;137:1024-1029.
9. Cifuentes Delatte L, Minon-Cifuentes JL, Medina JA. Papillary stones: calcified renal tubules in Randall's plaques. *J Urol.* 1985;133:490-494.
10. Daudon M, Traxer O, Jungers P, Bazin D. Stone morphology suggestive of Randall's plaque. In: Evan AP, Lingeman JE, Williams JC Jr, eds. *Renal Stone Disease.* Melville, NY: American Institute of Physics Conference Proceedings; 2007; 900:26-34.
11. Daudon M. Epidemiology of nephrolithiasis in France. *Ann Urol (Paris).* 2005;39:209-231.
12. Low RK, Stoller ML. Endoscopic mapping of renal papillae for Randall's plaques in patients with urinary stone disease. *J Urol.* 1997;158:2062-2064.
13. Matlaga BR, Williams JC Jr, Kim SC, et al. Endoscopic evidence of calculus attachment to Randall's plaque. *J Urol.* 2006;175:1720-1724.
14. Kim SC, Coe FL, Tinmouth WW, et al. Stone formation is proportional to papillary surface coverage by Randall's plaque. *J Urol.* 2005;173:117-119.
15. Ruggera L, Chiodini S, Gambaro G, et al. Does Randall's plaque represent a necessary condition in the pathogenesis of the idiopathic calcium oxalate stones? *Urol Res.* 2008;36:162-163 (A).
16. Evan AP, Lingeman JE, Coe FL, et al. Randall's plaque of patients with nephrolithiasis begins in basement membranes of thin loops of Henle. *J Clin Invest.* 2003;111:607-616.
17. Matlaga BR, Coe FL, Evan AP, et al. The role of Randall's plaques in the pathogenesis of calcium stones. *J Urol.* 2007;177:31-38.
18. Evan AP, Coe FL, Lingeman JE, et al. Mechanism of formation of human calcium oxalate renal stones on Randall's plaque. *Anat Rec (Hoboken).* 2007;290:1315-1323.
19. Evan AP, Coe FL, Rittling SR, et al. Apatite plaque particles in inner medulla of kidneys of calcium oxalate stone formers: osteopontin localization. *Kidney Int.* 2005;68:145-154.
20. Evan AP, Bledsoe S, Worcester EM, et al. Renal inter-alpha-trypsin inhibitor heavy chain 3 increases in calcium oxalate stone-forming patients. *Kidney Int.* 2007;72:1503-1511.
21. Evan A, Lingeman J, Coe FL, et al. Randall's plaque: pathogenesis and role in calcium oxalate nephrolithiasis. *Kidney Int.* 2006;69:1313-1318.
22. Evan AP, Lingeman JE, Coe FL, et al. Role of interstitial apatite plaque in the pathogenesis of the common calcium oxalate stone. *Semin Nephrol.* 2008;28:111-119.
23. Evan AP, Lingeman JE, Coe FL, et al. Crystal-associated nephropathy in patients with brushite nephrolithiasis. *Kidney Int.* 2005;67:576-581.
24. Evan AE, Lingeman JE, Coe FL, et al. Histopathology and surgical anatomy of patients with primary hyperparathyroidism and calcium phosphate stones. *Kidney Int.* 2008;74:223-229.

25. Meyer JL, Bergert JH, Smith LH. Epitaxial relationships in urolithiasis: the calcium oxalate monohydrate-hydroxyapatite system. *Clin Sci Mol Med*. 1975;49:369-374.

26. Khan SR. Calcium phosphate/calcium oxalate crystal association in urinary stones: implications for heterogeneous nucleation of calcium oxalate. *J Urol*. 1997;157:376-383.

27. Williams JC Jr, Matlaga BR, Kim SC, et al. Calcium oxalate calculi found attached to the renal papilla: Preliminary evidence for early mechanisms in stone formation. *J Endourol*. 2006;20: 885-890.

28. Zarse CA, Hameed TA, Jackson ME, et al. CT visible internal stone structure, but not Hounsfield unit value, of calcium oxalate monohydrate (COM) calculi predicts lithotripsy fragility in vitro. *Urol Res*. 2007;35:201-206.

29. Zarse CA, McAteer JA, Sommer AJ, et al. Nondestructive analysis of urinary calculi using micro computed tomography. *BMC Urol*. 2004;4:15.

30. Kuo RL, Lingeman JE, Evan AP, et al. Urine calcium and volume predict coverage of renal papilla by Randall's plaque. *Kidney Int*. 2003;64:2150-2154.

31. Coe FL, Evan A, Worcester E. Kidney stone disease. *J Clin Invest*. 2005;115:2598-2608.

32. Curhan GC, Willett WC, Speizer FE, Stampfer MJ. Twenty-four-hour urine chemistries and the risk of kidney stones among women and men. *Kidney Int*. 2001;59:2290-2298.

33. Daudon M, Hennequin C, Boujelben G, et al. Serial crystalluria determination and the risk of recurrence in calcium stone formers. *Kidney Int*. 2005;67:1934-1943.

34. Bushinsky DA. Nephrolithiasis: site of the initial solid phase. *J Clin Invest*. 2003;111:602-605.

35. Sepe V, Adamo G, La Fianza A, et al. Henle loop basement membrane as initial site for Randall plaque formation. *Am J Kidney Dis*. 2006;48:706-711.

36. Halperin ML, Cheema Dhadli S, Kamel KS. Physiology of acid-base balance: links with kidney stone prevention. *Semin Nephrol*. 2006;26:441-446.

37. Hansell P, Goransson V, Odlind C, Gerdin B, Hallgren R. Hyaluronan content in the kidney in different states of body hydration. *Kidney Int*. 2000;58:2061-2068.

38. Verkoelen CF. Crystal retention in renal stone disease: a crucial role for the glycosaminoglycan hyaluronan? *J Am Soc Nephrol*. 2006;17:1673-1687.

39. Verkoelen CF. Hyaluronan in tubular and interstitial nephrocalcinosis. In: Evan AP, Lingeman JE, Williams JC Jr, eds. *Renal Stone Disease*. Melville, NY: American Institute of Physics Conference Proceedings; 2007; 900:57-63.

40. Knepper MA, Saidel GM, Hascall VC, et al. Concentration of solutes in the renal inner medulla: interstitial hyaluronan as a mechano-osmotic transducer. *Am J Physiol Renal Physiol*. 2003;284:F433-446.

41. Raoult D, Drancourt M, Azza S, et al. Nanobacteria are mineralo fetuin complexes. *PLoS Pathog*. 2008;4:e41.

42. Gambaro G, D'Angelo A, Fabris A, et al. Crystals, Randall's plaques and renal stones: do bone and atherosclerosis teach us something? *J Nephrol*. 2004;17:774-777.

43. Daudon M, Bader CA, Jungers P. Urinary Calculi: Review of classification methods and correlations with etiology. *Scanning Microsc*. 1993;7:1081-1106.

44. Estépa L, Daudon M. Contribution of Fourier transform infrared spectroscopy to the identification of urinary stones and kidney crystal deposits. *Biospectroscopy*. 1997;3:347-369.

Dietary Factors

8

Roswitha Siener

Abstract Inappropriate dietary habits and overweight are suggested to promote the worldwide increasing incidence and prevalence of urolithiasis. Nutrition plays an important role in urinary stone formation, especially in calcium oxalate, uric acid, calcium phosphate, and cystine urolithiasis. Specific dietary factors can alter urinary composition and supersaturation, which can affect the process of crystallization and stone formation. Adequate dietary treatment can contribute to an effective prevention or reduction of stone recurrences and decrease the burden of invasive measures in patients with recurrent stone disease. The current knowledge of the impact of dietary factors on the risk of stone formation is presented.

8.1 Introduction

The prevalence and incidence of urinary stone disease in industrialized countries has markedly increased during the last decades. The prevalence of urolithiasis in the United States was estimated to be 5.2% during the years 1988–1994, compared to 3.8% from 1976 to 1980.[1] In Japan, the prevalence increased from 4.0% to 5.4% within 10 years, corresponding to a rise of 35%.[2] In Germany, a marked increase in the prevalence from 4.0% to 4.7% and a rise in the incidence of stone disease from 0.54% to 1.47% was observed between 1979 and 2001.[3] Because of its influence on hydration status and urine volume, global warming has been estimated to result in a further increase in kidney stone disease by 2050.[4]

Inappropriate dietary habits and overweight are suggested to promote the worldwide increasing incidence and prevalence of urolithiasis. Nutrition plays an important role in urinary stone formation. Specific dietary factors can alter urinary composition and supersaturation, which can affect the process of crystallization and stone formation. This chapter reviews the current knowledge of the impact of dietary factors on the risk of stone formation.

R. Siener
Department of Urology, University of Bonn, Bonn, Germany
e-mail: roswitha.siener@ukb.uni-bonn.de

8.2 Fluid Intake

One of the most important dietary measures for the prevention of stone recurrence is a sufficient urine dilution accomplished by an adequate fluid intake. A high fluid consumption increases urine volume and reduces the risk of stone formation by lowering the urinary activity product ratio (supersaturation) of stone-forming constituents.[5] Increased urine dilution might also exert its antilithogenic effect by reducing the renal intratubular transit time, thereby favoring the expulsion of the nuclei and inhibiting the formation of Randall's plaques.[6]

Thus, diminished urine dilution is an important risk factor for urinary stone formation. Low urine volume mainly results from inadequate fluid intake, increased respiratory-cutaneous water loss, or diarrhea. Any condition that brings on chronic dehydration like high ambient temperatures, high degree of physical activities, and insufficient replacement of water losses, increases the risk of stone formation. Inadequate fluid intake has been presumed to contribute to the high frequency of stone disease in areas with a hot climate.[7,8] In addition, certain types of work activity and physical exercise, which expose to excessive extrarenal fluid losses, are characterized by a higher risk of stone formation.[9–13]

Epidemiological studies have demonstrated that increased fluid intake reduces the risk of urinary stone formation. In a prospective study of a cohort of 45,619 men, who had no history of urolithiasis, an inverse association between fluid intake and the risk of stone formation was observed after 4 and 14 years of follow-up, respectively.[14,15] After adjustment

P.N. Rao et al. (eds.), *Urinary Tract Stone Disease*,
DOI 10.1007/978-1-84800-362-0_8, © Springer-Verlag London Limited 2011

for other potentially confounding variables in the multivariate analysis, the relative risk for the men in the highest (>2.5 L/day fluid intake) as compared with the lowest quintile group (<1.3 L/day fluid intake) was 0.71 – a 29% reduction in risk. These findings in men were consistent with results of two prospective studies among women.[16,17]

A prospective, randomized study in stone formers examined the impact of high fluid intake in preventing recurrence of stones.[18] Idiopathic first-time calcium oxalate stone formers were randomly assigned to two different groups. Patients in the intervention group were advised to increase fluid intake to at least 2 L/day, while patients in the control group received no specific instructions. During a 5-year follow-up, the patients in the intervention group with significantly higher urine volumes had a recurrence rate of 12% compared with 27% in the control group with no changes in fluid intake. Furthermore, the time interval before the onset of a recurrence was significantly longer in patients on a high water intake. Thus, observational and interventional trials confirm that high fluid intake is the initial therapy for the prevention of stone recurrences.

For the majority of stones, fluid intake should be adjusted to achieve a consistent urine volume of at least 2 L/24h. In patients with cystine stone disease, excessive urine dilution is necessary for a successful metaphylaxis. To remain below the critical limit of cystine solubility, urine volume should be at least 3.5 L/24h.[19]

Although a high fluid supply has been demonstrated to decrease the incidence of urolithiasis, data from observational and interventional studies on the effect of specific beverages on the risk of urinary stone formation are conflicting.

8.2.1 Citrus Juices

Citrus juices are rich sources of citric acid and potassium, which may enhance urinary pH and citrate excretion and thus reduce the risk of calcium oxalate, uric acid, and cystine stone formation. Ingested citrate is absorbed in the intestine and nearly completely metabolized to bicarbonate, providing an alkali load, which in turn increases urinary citrate excretion.[20] Orange, grapefruit, and lemon juices are among the most commonly consumed citrus juices.

Whereas two observational studies conducted by Curhan et al. (1996, 1998) revealed a positive association between grapefruit juice intake and risk of stone formation in men and women,[21,22] no changes in lithogenicity were observed by Goldfarb and Asplin (2001) in healthy men and women.[23] On the contrary, Hönow et al. (2003) found a reduction in the risk of calcium oxalate crystallization in healthy subjects, which was mainly due to a significant rise in urinary citrate excretion.[24] Grapefruit juice contains naringin, which is known to influence intestinal enzymes, but the mechanism for the

increased risk of stone formation observed in epidemiological studies is unknown.

Although orange juice has been demonstrated to increase urinary pH and citrate excretion, no significant decline in the calculated relative supersaturation for calcium oxalate was observed in interventional studies.[24–26] In accordance with these results, no association between the consumption of orange juice and the risk of stone formation was found in prospective cohort studies in men and women.[21,22]

Data from a prospective cohort study over 12 years suggested a positive association between the intake of orange juices and oranges, respectively, with the risk of gout in men.[27] However, interventional trials revealed a significant decrease in urinary undissociated uric acid levels and the relative supersaturation for uric acid.[24,26]

Of the most commonly consumed citrus juices, lemon juice appears to have the highest concentration of citric acid. The intake of lemon juice, with a nearly five times higher citrate concentration compared to orange juice, led to a twofold rise in urinary citrate levels in a short-term trial in patients with hypocitraturic calcium nephrolithiasis.[28] A retrospective evaluation of long-term lemonade therapy in patients with mild to moderate hypocitraturia confirmed these findings.[29] However, a randomized cross-over study in 21 stone-forming patients failed to detect significant improvements in urinary citrate excretion with lemonade use.[30]

The inconsistent results between the clinical trials could be explained by differences in the populations and the dosing of potassium and citric acid. Analysis of the citric acid concentration of various fruit juices revealed a higher citric acid content of lemon and lime juices, both from the fresh fruit and from juice concentrates, than orange juice from the fresh fruit and orange juice, grapefruit juice, and lemonade from ready-to-consume products.[31]

8.2.2 Other Fruit Juices

Besides citrus juices many other fruit juices – like apple, cranberry, and blackcurrant juices – contain considerable amounts of citric acid. In observational studies conducted by Curhan et al. (1996, 1998), a positive association between apple juice intake and the risk for stone formation has been shown in men but not in women.[21,22] Substituting 1 L apple juice for water in healthy female volunteers, Hönow et al. (2003) observed a significant increase in urinary pH, potassium, and citrate excretion, but failed to find a significant difference in the calculated supersaturation with calcium oxalate.[24]

The literature regarding the effect of cranberry juice on urinary stone risk factors has likewise yielded conflicting results. Urinary oxalate has been reported to be increased,[32] decreased,[33] or unchanged[34] in healthy subjects and to be increased in calcium oxalate stone formers.[34] Urinary citrate excretion has been shown to be unchanged[32,34] or increased[33] in healthy subjects and to be unchanged in stone formers.[34] Overall, the risk of calcium oxalate stone formation was reduced[33] or unaffected[32,34] by cranberry juice consumption in healthy subjects but increased in stone patients.[34]

On the contrary, cranberry juice is attributed a protective effect in the treatment of urinary tract infections.[35,36] The berries of *Vaccinium* species such as cranberries contain proanthocyanidins. By inhibiting the cellular expression of adhesion molecules, they inhibit bacterial adhesion to cellular surfaces.[36] Since studies on a controlled diet revealed an acidifying effect in healthy subjects and stone formers, cranberry juice could be suitable for the treatment of brushite and struvite stones as well as urinary tract infection.[32,34] However, the oxalate content of cranberry juice has to be taken into account.

The consumption of 330 mL/day of blackcurrant juice in healthy subjects on a controlled diet resulted in a significant increase in urinary pH and citrate excretion.[32] Despite favorable changes in urine composition, the relative supersaturation for calcium oxalate remained unchanged, probably due to the significant increase in urinary oxalate excretion. Since the blackcurrant juice used in the study contained a high amount of oxalate and ascorbic acid, it is suggested that the oxaluric effect of blackcurrant juice might have resulted from the oxalate load and conversion of ascorbic acid to oxalate in vivo.[37]

8.2.3 Coffee and Tea

Two cohort studies showed that each 240 mL serving of caffeinated coffee was associated with a 10% decrease in risk of stone formation in men and women.[21,22] An epidemiological trial by Goldfarb et al. (2005) supported the protective effect of coffee for stone disease.[38] Moreover, a large prospective study found that coffee consumption was inversely associated with risk of gout in men.[39]

In an interventional trial, Massey and Sutton (2004) examined the acute effect of caffeine consumption on urine composition and risk of stone formation in 39 normocalcemic patients with calcium stones and 48 control subjects.[40] The subjects received 6 mg caffeine/kg lean body mass in 180 mL of warm deionized water. The doses ranged from 250 to 400 mg caffeine, the equivalent of 11–17 ounces (330–510 mL) of brewed coffee. Caffeine loading resulted in an increased urinary calcium/creatinine ratio and an elevated Tiselius risk index. Since caffeine induces hypercalciuria, affects hydration, and may aggravate hypertension, patients should be recommended to consume caffeinated beverages in moderation and to drink water before or along with the coffee.

In prospective observational studies the risk of stone formation was found to be reduced by tea consumption.[21,22]

A limitation of these prospective studies is that no distinction was made between black tea and other types such as herbal tea, which are known to be lower in oxalate.[41] Although recent studies suggested a low to moderate bioavailability of oxalate from black tea in healthy subjects,[42,43] findings are not transferable to patients with intestinal hyperabsorption of oxalate.

8.2.4 Soft Drinks

Studies on the association between soda consumption and the risk of stone formation have likewise provided conflicting results. Assessing the data from two cohort trials and results from a case control study, the intake of soda (including sugared cola) was not associated with increased risk for stone formation,[21,22,44] while a randomized controlled trial in male stone patients suggested a strong association between the amount of soft drink consumption (acidified with phosphoric acid) and the recurrence of urinary stone formation in the course of a 3-year follow-up.[45] A cross-sectional study conducted by Soucie et al. (1996) confirmed the association between the consumption of soft drinks (including cola) and the history of urolithiasis.[46] An interventional trial in healthy subjects found that consumption of cola causes unfavorable changes in urinary risk factors associated with calcium oxalate stone formation.[47]

Although a limitation of most studies is that they did not adjust for other dietary factors in the analyses, thus limiting the interpretation of the results, it should be emphasized, that conventional soda contains a considerable amount of sugar, which contributes to energy surplus and can increase urinary calcium excretion.[48] In addition, phosphoric acid content of cola beverages increases dietary phosphate intake. Moreover, prospective cohort data indicate that consumption of sugar-sweetened soft drinks was strongly associated with an increased risk of gout in men.[27] Correspondingly, in a nationally representative sample of US adults, serum uric acid concentration increased with increasing intake of sugar-sweetened soft drinks.[49]

8.2.5 Alcoholic Beverages

In retrospective and prospective studies, beer and wine consumption were inversely associated with the risk for stone formation.[21,22,44] While the reduction in risk with wine compared with beer was even found to be higher in men and women, liquor was not associated with decreased risk.[21,22] However, alcohol consumption can promote urinary calcium excretion probably through a decreased reabsorption of calcium by the renal tubule, thus causing transient hypercalciuria.

Moreover, ethanol is suggested to increase uric acid production, a factor that is expected to increase the risk of stone formation.[50] Furthermore, beer is the only alcoholic beverage acknowledged to have a large purine content, which is predominantly guanosine.[51] In healthy subjects, the consumption of beer resulted in a reduction of urinary pH and an increase in urinary uric acid excretion.[25] Findings from a large prospective trial confirmed that alcohol intake is strongly associated with an increased risk of gout in men.[52]

8.2.6 Water

The results of retrospective trials on the relationship between drinking water hardness and urinary stone disease have been inconsistent. Whereas a higher incidence of urinary stones has been reported in soft-water areas in the U.S.A.,[53] no significant correlation between water hardness and urinary stone disease has been found after adjusting for other environmental factors.[54]

Although mineral water has been suggested to be a suitable beverage for urine dilution, the water composition has to be taken into account. The bicarbonate content of mineral water can replace alkalization therapy with potassium citrate and contribute to urine inhibitory power by increasing urinary citrate excretion.[25,55] The alkalizing effect due to the high bicarbonate content of mineral water is desired in the treatment of calcium oxalate, uric acid, and cystine stones, whereas it is contraindicated in struvite and calcium phosphate stones. The majority of the studies evaluating the effect of the calcium content of water on urine composition revealed significant increases in urinary calcium excretion both in normal subjects[56] and calcium stone formers[57–59] on a high calcium load with water. While this lithogenic effect was counterbalanced by a decrease in urinary oxalate excretion in some studies,[58,59] neither significant short-term[57] nor long-term reductions in urinary oxalate excretion were observed by others.[56] Further studies are necessary to evaluate whether the ingestion of calcium-rich water with, rather than between, meals may complex oxalate in the gut, thus limiting absorption and urinary excretion of calcium and oxalate.

The most important metaphylactic measure irrespective of stone composition is a sufficient urine dilution accomplished by an adequate fluid intake.[60] The type of beverage should be selected cautiously. Neutral beverages, i.e., fluids that dilute urine without affecting its composition, include tap water, mineral water with a low mineral content, fruit, and herbal teas. The administration of neutral beverages lowers the risk of urinary stone formation solely by urine dilution (Fig. 8.1). Alkalizing beverages, i.e., fluids that additionally increase urinary pH and citrate excretion, are bicarbonate-rich mineral

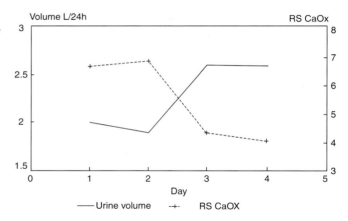

Fig. 8.1 Influence of urine volume on relative supersaturation for calcium oxalate (RS CaOx)

water and citrus juices. Neutral and alkalizing beverages are suitable for metaphylactic treatment of the majority of urinary stones, i.e., calcium oxalate, uric acid, and cystine. It needs to be emphasized that water is energy-free, a fact that has to be particularly considered by overweight patients.

8.3 Protein

Increasing dietary protein intake has been identified as a risk factor for the development of urinary stones for many years. A nationwide survey of vegetarians in the United Kingdom revealed the prevalence of urinary stone disease to be about half that found in the general population.[61] On the other hand, data from cohort studies on the association between animal protein consumption and new kidney stone formation are conflicting. A positive association between animal protein intake and risk of stone formation has been shown in men but not in women.[14,16,17]

A high consumption of animal protein has been consistently associated with an increase in urinary calcium excretion as well as a reduction of both urinary pH and citrate excretion, metabolic changes that are considered risk factors for stone formation.[62–64]

A high intake of animal protein may affect urinary calcium excretion by several different mechanisms. A high protein diet increases endogenous acid load that may require buffering from bone, thereby increasing calcium resorption.[65,66] Moreover, increasing dietary protein is related to increases in glomerular filtration rate[67] and decreases in renal reabsorption of calcium from distal tubular cells.[66] In normal subjects, every 25 g increment in dietary protein raises urinary calcium excretion by approximately 0.8 mmol.[68] In hypercalciuric patients, the calciuric effects of a high protein intake may be even greater.[69]

The rise in urinary pH, sulfate, and phosphate excretion, and the decrease in citrate excretion with increasing protein intake are mainly attributed to the acidifying effect of phosphoproteins and sulfur-containing amino-acids (methionine, cystine) that are in a higher proportion in animal than in vegetable protein. The high endogenous acid load generated by a protein-rich diet enhances citrate reabsorption in the proximal tubule, thus decreasing urinary excretion of citrate, a known inhibitor of calcium stone formation.[20] The associated mild metabolic acidosis results in a decrease in urinary pH that could promote uric acid and cystine lithiasis.

Studies on the effect of dietary protein on urinary oxalate excretion have provided conflicting results. Whereas some investigators reported that dietary protein increases urinary oxalate excretion[70–73] and that protein restriction reduces urinary oxalate,[69] others observed no relationship between protein intake and urinary oxalate excretion.[62,63,74] It has been suggested that elevated oxalate excretion with increasing protein consumption may be caused by an increase in generation of glycolate, a precursor of oxalate.[70] However, a limitation of the aforementioned studies is an inadequate control of dietary oxalate intake.

The food source of dietary protein may have different effects on urinary composition. Breslau et al. (1988) examined the effect of three diets with constant total protein intake (75 g/day) but differing protein sources, i.e., animal, vegetarian (soy-based), and ovo-vegetarian (soy-based with eggs), in healthy subjects.[62] While urinary oxalate excretion was lower, urinary calcium, sulfate, phosphate, uric acid, and net acid excretion were higher during the animal protein diet compared with the other phases. These differences can be explained by the different content of oxalate, sulfate, uric acid, and fiber of the diets. Siener and Hesse (2002) found similar effects.[75] Increasing buffering capacity by increasing fruit and vegetable intake with a balanced mixed or a vegetarian diet counteracts the acidity generated by the dietary protein, reduces calciuria, and consequently improves calcium balance. However, the oxalate content of a vegetarian diet should be taken into account.

There are only two randomized controlled trials that assessed the effects of a reduction in dietary protein on stone recurrence. Hiatt et al. (1996) reported a higher risk of recurrence after a 4.5-year follow-up in first-time calcium oxalate stone formers in the intervention group treated with a high-fiber and low-animal-protein diet than in the control group.[76] However, this trial had several limitations, including a higher fluid consumption in the control group, differences in dietary intake of fiber or patient compliance. A randomized trial by Borghi and colleagues (2002) compared a low-animal-protein, low-salt, and normal-calcium diet (intervention group) with a low-calcium diet (control group) in calcium oxalate stone formers with idiopathic hypercalciuria.[77] After 5 years, the risk of a recurrence was 50% lower in the intervention group as compared with the control group, but in this trial, it was not possible to distinguish the beneficial effect of the low-animal-protein intake from that of the lower salt and higher calcium intake.

8.4 Carbohydrates

Data from studies on the effect of carbohydrates on the risk of stone formation are conflicting. Whereas some investigators found a similar carbohydrate ingestion in stone formers compared to controls,[78,79] others have reported that intake of carbohydrates is higher in stone formers.[80–82] In prospective studies conducted by Curhan et al. (1993, 1997, 2004) and Taylor et al. (2004), a positive association between sucrose intake and the risk for stone formation has been shown in women but not in men.[14–17] A limitation of these studies is that they did not distinguish different types of carbohydrates, particularly glucose and fructose.

A rise in urinary calcium excretion has been observed after an acute glucose load both in normal subjects and calcium oxalate stone patients, which was more pronounced in the latter group.[48] The increase in urinary calcium has been ascribed to an increase in intestinal absorption and reduction in renal tubular reabsorption of calcium.[83–85] It is possible that this effect may be at least partially mediated by insulin.

A large prospective study reported a positive association between fructose intake and the risk of incident stone formation in men and women.[86] Fructose consumption has markedly increased over the past decades as many manufacturers use fructose instead of sucrose to sweeten beverages and foods. The mechanisms between fructose and the risk of calcium stone formation are unknown. The ingestion of a high fructose diet (20% of energy), in conjunction with lower dietary magnesium and higher phosphorus intake, resulted in higher urinary losses of calcium as a percentage of calcium intake versus starch in healthy men.[87] Furthermore, intravenous infusion of fructose increased urinary oxalate excretion compared to glucose infusion in healthy subjects.[88] On the contrary, an increase in urinary oxalate has been found in healthy subjects in the 3 h following oral glucose load but not in response to oral fructose load.[89]

Moreover, it has been suggested that fructose increases the risk of stone formation by effects on uric acid metabolism. Data from a prospective cohort study in men revealed a positive association between the risk of incident gout and fructose intake.[27] Large doses of oral fructose (>3 g/kg body weight/day) have been reported to increase serum and urinary uric acid levels.[90] This effect may be more pronounced in individuals with preexisting abnormalities of uric acid metabolism.[91] A study on the effects of moderate amounts of fructose (63–99 g/day) revealed no increase in serum and urinary uric acid over 2 weeks in healthy subjects.[92] Studies have demonstrated that large doses of fructose, especially when infused at rapid rates, deplete intrahepatic concentrations of ATP.[93] Fructose phosphorylation in the liver uses ATP, and the accompanying inorganic phosphate depletion inhibits the regeneration of ATP from ADP, which is subsequently metabolized to uric acid.[94]

8.5 Fat

The association between dietary fat intake and the risk of stone formation is unclear.[14–17] Whereas some studies found a similar total fat consumption in stone formers compared to controls,[78,79,81] others have reported that intake of fat is higher in stone patients.[80,82]

Several dietary fatty acids are suggested to influence calcium oxalate stone formation. An increased phospholipid arachidonic acid level, an n-6 fatty acid, may induce hyperoxaluria by activating the anion carrier and consequently the intestinal and renal transport of oxalate. Analyses of dietary records and 24-h urine samples of 58 idiopathic calcium oxalate stone formers revealed a positive correlation between the dietary content of arachidonic acid and urinary oxalate excretion.[95] Fish oil supplementation has been demonstrated to induce a reduction in the plasma arachidonic acid level in patients,[96] and to lower urinary calcium and oxalate excretion in idiopathic calcium oxalate stone formers.[96–98] However, a prospective cohort study based on data from a semiquantitative food-frequency questionnaire revealed no consistent association between fatty acid intake and the risk for stone formation.[99] Higher intake of arachidonic and linoleic acid did not increase the risk, and greater intake of n-3 fatty acids did not reduce the risk for incident kidney stones.

8.6 Oxalate

Urinary oxalate is predominantly derived from endogenous production of oxalate from ingested or metabolically generated precursors and from the diet. The impact of dietary oxalate in the pathogenesis of calcium oxalate stone formation is unclear. It has been suggested that dietary oxalate contributes up to 50% of urinary oxalate excretion.[100] However, a prospective study reported a modest positive association between oxalate intake and the risk for incident stone formation in men and older women.[101] Estimates of normal dietary oxalate intake are in the range of 50–200 mg daily.[75,101,102]

Although the impact of dietary oxalate in the pathogenesis of calcium oxalate stone formation is unclear, it is important to consider sources of excess dietary oxalate. Therefore, detailed knowledge of food oxalate content is essential for dietary treatment of recurrent calcium oxalate urolithiasis. So far, analysis of the oxalate content of diets has been limited by inaccurate or lacking data on food oxalate content. Analysis of the oxalate content of different foods by reliable methods revealed a considerable number of foods with high or extremely high oxalate concentrations. A selection of oxalate-rich foods is presented in Table 8.1.[41,103,104] Whereas most foodstuffs in a typical Western diet contain low or moderate concentrations of oxalate, a vegetarian diet may be associated with an increased oxalate intake.[41,75] The oxalate content of foods may vary according to growth conditions and preparation methods.[41,105]

The consumption of foodstuffs rich in oxalic acid can induce hyperoxaluria already in healthy individuals without disturbances in oxalate metabolism.[25] Intestinal hyperabsorption of oxalate can make a considerable contribution to urinary oxalate, even in the absence of gastrointestinal disorders. Data from studies on the effect of intestinal hyperabsorption of oxalate on urinary oxalate excretion using [^{14}C]oxalate are conflicting. Whereas some studies found increased oxalate absorption in stone formers,[106,107] others reported no differences between stone formers and healthy subjects.[108,109] A study using [^{13}C$_2$] oxalate reported an intestinal hyperabsorption, defined as an absorption exceeding 10%, in 46% of patients with calcium oxalate stone disease and in 28% of control subjects.[110] A deficiency of oxalate degradation by *Oxalobacter formigenes* in the intestine may additionally contribute to an increased absorption and urinary excretion of oxalate.[111,112] Moreover, a number

Table 8.1 Oxalate-rich foods (mg/100 g)[41,103,104]

Food	Oxalate (mg/100 g)	Portion (g)	Oxalate (mg)
Cereals and pseudocereals			
Bulgur	59	50	30
Couscous	65	50	33
Wheat flakes (whole grain)	76	50	38
Buckwheat	143	50	72
Quinoa	184	50	92
Wheat bran	457	30	137
Nuts			
Almond	383	100	383
Others			
Cocoa powder	567	50	284
Vegetables			
Beetroot	160	150	240
Mangold	874	150	1,311
Rhubarb	1,235	150	1,853
Sorrel	1,391	100	1,391
Spinach	1,959	150	2,939

of dietary factors may influence the excretion of oxalate, e.g., a decreased intake of calcium and magnesium or an increased consumption of ascorbic acid.

8.7 Calcium

Hypercalciuria carries a high risk for calcium oxalate stone formation.[77,113] Various nutritional factors are known to influence urinary calcium excretion, i.e., the dietary calcium, protein, and sodium ingestion. In healthy subjects, intestinal calcium absorption is approximately 25%.[114] However, most patients with hypercalciuria have intestinal hyperabsorption of calcium.[115]

Dietary calcium is suggested to be the most important factor to influence oxalate absorption. A low dietary intake reduces the concentration of calcium in the gastrointestinal lumen, which can increase intestinal absorption and urinary excretion of oxalate. Indeed, the inhibitory effect of calcium ingestion on urinary oxalate excretion has been demonstrated in oxalate loading studies.[116–118] Von Unruh et al. (2004) assessed the association between calcium intake and gastrointestinal oxalate absorption of healthy subjects with a standardized [$^{13}C_2$] oxalate absorption test.[118] Within the range of 200–1,200 mg calcium per day, oxalate absorption was clearly a linear function of the calcium intake. Additional calcium intake beyond 1,200 mg/day had only a minor effect on intestinal oxalate absorption. However, the increase in calcium intake resulted in a significant increase in urinary calcium excretion. Dietary calcium intake should therefore not exceed 1,200 mg daily.

Moreover, dietary calcium restriction can cause a negative calcium balance, leading in the long term to osteopenia. A study in 48 male calcium stone formers found a lower dietary calcium intake in patients with low bone density than in those with normal bone density.[119]

Prospective cohort studies revealed an inverse association between dietary calcium intake and the risk of stone formation in men and women.[14–17] The large follow-up studies confirm the general recommendation for an adequate dietary calcium intake of 1,000–1,200 mg/day. Moreover, a 5-year randomized prospective trial demonstrated that recurrences in male calcium oxalate stone patients with hypercalciuria are significantly less frequent on normal calcium intake (1,200 mg/day) combined with reduced intakes of salt and animal protein compared with patients on a low-calcium intake, accomplished by abolishing milk and dairy products.[77]

The effect of supplemental calcium appears to be different from dietary calcium. Supplemental calcium increased the risk of stone formation in older women, whereas no association between calcium supplementation and risk of stone disease was observed in younger women and men.[14,16,17]

The difference in the effect between dietary and supplemental calcium may be related to the timing of ingestion.

8.8 Magnesium

Magnesium is suggested to be an important inhibitor of calcium oxalate stone formation. Magnesium may reduce oxalate absorption and urinary excretion nearly as effectively as calcium by binding oxalate in the gut.[120] Moreover, a high urinary excretion and concentration of magnesium has been shown to decrease both nucleation and growth rates of calcium oxalate crystals, due to the higher solubility of magnesium oxalate compared with calcium oxalate.[121,122]

Data from prospective cohort studies found that magnesium intake was associated with a reduced risk of stone formation in men,[15] but not in women.[16,17] The high magnesium content of fruits, vegetables, and cereals is responsible for an increase in urinary magnesium excretion.[123,124] Related clinical investigations of supplemental magnesium have been conducted in both recurrent stone formers and normal subjects, but with little success. Indeed, magnesium supplementation resulted in an increase in urinary excretion, but this benefit was counteracted by an increase in urinary calcium excretion.[125,126]

8.9 Sodium

Increased sodium consumption has been linked to an increased risk of calcium stone formation, based on the propensity of sodium to increase urinary calcium excretion.[127] A high ingestion of sodium may promote urinary calcium excretion probably by inhibiting renal tubular reabsorption of calcium from sodium-induced expansion of extracellular fluid volume.[128] An association between sodium intake and stone formation was found in a large observational study,[16] but was not confirmed by others.[15,17] The discrepant results might reflect the difficulties in obtaining reliable estimates of dietary salt intake based on food questionnaires.[6]

From interventional studies, it has been estimated that urinary calcium excretion increases approximately 1 mmol for each 100 mmol increase in dietary sodium intake in normal adults.[129] In addition, hypercalciuric stone formers appear to be more sensitive to the calciuric effect of a sodium load.[130,131]

8.10 Ascorbic Acid

Ascorbate is a precursor of oxalate and the intake of high amounts of vitamin C is suggested to increase urinary oxalate levels. Approximately 35–50% of urinary oxalate is estimated to be derived from the conversion of ascorbic acid to oxalate in the organism.[132] Results from previous studies on the effect of ascorbic acid on urinary oxalate excretion are contradictory, in part because of difficulties in measuring urinary oxalate in the presence of ascorbate.[133]

A recent interventional trial demonstrated a significant increase in urinary oxalate excretion by 33% in calcium oxalate stone formers and by 20% in normal subjects, respectively, after ingestion of 2 g of supplemental ascorbic acid per day.[37] An observational study found a 40% higher risk of stone formation in men who consumed 1,000 mg or more per day of vitamin C compared to those who consumed less than 90 mg/day.[15] A case-control study in 186 calcium oxalate stone patients with and without hyperoxaluria yielded a positive association between urinary oxalate excretion and dietary ascorbate intake.[134] The dietary intake of vitamin C in the hyperoxaluric group exceeded the recommended dietary allowance by 80%. Based on the results of these studies, calcium oxalate stone formers should be advised to discontinue ascorbic acid supplementation.

8.11 Phytate

Dietary phytic acid, predominantly present in cereals, nuts, legumes, and oil seeds, is able to complex calcium and therefore to increase the absorption of dietary oxalate.[135] In contrast to its unfavorable effect in the gastrointestinal tract, urinary phytate has been demonstrated to exhibit a strong inhibitory effect on the crystallization of calcium salts. Grases et al. (2000) found a significantly lower urinary phytate excretion in calcium oxalate stone formers compared with healthy men (2.01 versus 3.27 mg/24h).[136] Data from two large observational studies revealed an inverse association of phytate intake with risk of stone formation in women, but not in men.[15,17]

8.12 Purines

Hyperuricosuria is a risk factor for the development of uric acid stones and may promote calcium oxalate stone formation. Uric acid is the end-product of purine metabolism in humans and is derived from endogenous production as well as from dietary sources.

A study in healthy subjects revealed the strongest decrease in urinary risk factors for uric acid stone formation on the intake of a balanced vegetarian diet compared to two omnivorous diets.[137] Although the balanced omnivorous and the vegetarian diet provided similar amounts of energy, purines, and protein, urinary uric acid excretion was lowest on the vegetarian diet. An epidemiological trial conducted by Choi et al. (2004) yielded an increased risk of gout among men with higher levels of meat and seafood consumption and a declined risk with a higher level of intake of dairy products.[138] The risk of gout remained unaffected by moderate intake of purine-rich vegetables. Findings from a nationally representative sample of men and women in the US suggest that increasing meat or seafood intake is associated with increasing serum levels of uric acid, whereas dairy consumption is inversely associated with the serum uric acid level.[139]

8.13 Dietary Habits

Overweight and associated dietary pattern are suggested to be significant risk factors for stone formation. A prospective cohort study demonstrated that body mass index (BMI), waist circumference, and weight gain are positively associated with an increased risk of nephrolithiasis in both men and women.[140]

Analysis of 527 idiopathic calcium oxalate stone formers with respect to their BMI yielded overweight or obesity in 44% of women and in 59% of men.[141] Multiple linear regression analysis of urinary parameters with reference to weight parameters revealed a significant positive relationship between BMI and urinary uric acid, sodium, ammonium, and phosphate excretion and a negative correlation between BMI and urinary pH. The risk of stone formation computed as relative supersaturation for calcium oxalate was higher in overweight and obese compared to normal weight patients (Fig. 8.2). Comparison of urinary stone risk factors from a group of overweight patients with those of a group of normal, nonstone formers confirmed that overweight might be associated with an elevated risk of stone formation owing to alterations in urine composition.[142] A trial in stone-forming and nonstone-forming individuals suggested that among other factors diet may contribute to changes in urinary composition with increasing BMI.[143]

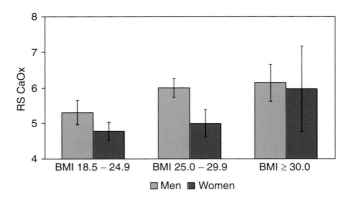

Fig. 8.2 Relative supersaturation for calcium oxalate (RS CaOx) according to BMI category in calcium oxalate stone patients (n = 527)[141]

An interventional study in 107 recurrent calcium oxalate stone patients confirmed that dietary pattern and urinary risk factors for stone formation are closely linked together.[144] The shift to a nutritionally balanced diet according to the recommendations significantly reduced the stone-forming potential of these patients.

8.14 Conclusions

Unfavourable dietary pattern and overweight are suggested to contribute markedly to the rise in the prevalence and incidence of urolithiasis over the past decades. A variety of dietary factors can affect crystallization and stone formation by altering the composition and supersaturation of urine. The results from clinical and epidemiological studies demonstrate the impact of dietary factors on the risk of stone formation. Appropriate dietary modifications and adequate fluid intake may considerably contribute to an effective prevention or reduction of stone recurrences and decrease the morbidity and costs associated with recurrent stone formation (see Chapter 59: Dietary assessment and advice).

References

1. Stamatelou KK, Francis ME, Jones CA, Nyberg LM, Curhan GC. Time trends in reported prevalence of kidney stones in the United States: 1976-1994. *Kidney Int.* 2003;63:1817-1823.

2. Yoshida O, Okada Y. Epidemiology of urolithiasis in Japan: a chronological and geographical study. *Urol Int.* 1990;45:104-111.

3. Hesse A, Brändle E, Wilbert D, Köhrmann KU, Alken P. Study on the prevalence and incidence of urolithiasis in Germany comparing the years 1979 vs 2000. *Eur Urol.* 2003;44:709-713.

4. Brikowski TH, Lotan Y, Pearle MS. Climate-related increase in the prevalence of urolithiasis in the United States. *Proc Nat Acad Sci USA.* 2008;105:9841-9846.

5. Pak CYC, Sakhaee K, Crowther C, Brinkley L. Evidence justifying a high fluid intake in treatment of nephrolithiasis. *Ann Intern Med.* 1980;93:36-39.

6. Borghi L, Meschi T, Maggiore U, Prati B. Dietary therapy in idiopathic nephrolithiasis. *Nutr Rev.* 2006;64:301-312.

7. Berlyne GM, Yagil R, Goodwin S, Morag M. Drinking habits and urine concentration of man in southern Israel. *Isr J Med Sci.* 1976;12:765-769.

8. Frank M, De Vries A, Atsmon A, Lazebnik J, Kochwa S. Epidemiological investigation of urolithiasis in Israel. *J Urol.* 1959;81:497-505.

9. Atan L, Andreoni C, Ortiz V, et al. High kidney stone risk in men working in steel industry at hot temperatures. *Urology.* 2005;65:858-861.

10. Borghi L, Meschi T, Amato F, Novarini A, Romanelli A, Cigala F. Hot occupation and nephrolithiasis. *J Urol.* 1993;150:1757-1760.

11. Irving RA, Noakes TD, Rogers AL, Swartz L. Crystalluria in marathon runners. 1. Standard marathon – males. *Urol Res.* 1986; 14:289-294.

12. Milvy P, Colt E, Thornton J. A high incidence of urolithiasis in male marathon runners. *J Sports Med.* 1981;21:295-298.

13. Sakhaee K, Nigam S, Snell P, Hsu MC, Pac CY. Assessment of the pathogenetic role of physical exercise in renal stone formation. *J Clin Endocr Metab.* 1987;65:974-979.

14. Curhan GC, Willett WC, Rimm EB, Stampfer MJ. A prospective study of dietary calcium and other nutrients and the risk of symptomatic kidney stones. *N Engl J Med.* 1993;328:833-838.

15. Taylor EN, Stampfer MJ, Curhan GC. Dietary factors and the risk of incident kidney stones in men: new insights after 14 years of follow-up. *J Am Soc Nephrol.* 2004;15:3225-3232.

16. Curhan GC, Willett WC, Speizer FE, Spiegelman D, Stampfer MJ. Comparison of dietary calcium with supplemental calcium and other nutrients as factors affecting the risk for kidney stones in women. *Ann Intern Med.* 1997;126:497-504.

17. Curhan GC, Willett WC, Knight EL, Stampfer MJ. Dietary factors and the risk of incident kidney stones in younger women. *Arch Intern Med.* 2004;164:885-891.

18. Borghi L, Meschi T, Amato F, Briganti A, Novarini A, Giannini A. Urinary volume, water and recurrences in idiopathic calcium nephrolithiasis: a 5-year randomized prospective study. *J Urol.* 1996;155:839-843.

19. Hesse A, Tiselius HG, Siener R, Hoppe B. *Urinary Stones. Diagnosis, Treatment, and Prevention of Recurrence.* Basel: Karger; 2009.

20. Simpson DP. Citrate excretion: a window on renal metabolism. *Am J Physiol.* 1983;244:F223-F234.

21. Curhan GC, Willett WC, Rimm EB, Spiegelman D, Stampfer MJ. Prospective study of beverage use and the risk of kidney stones. *Am J Epidemiol.* 1996;143:240-247.

22. Curhan GC, Willett WC, Speizer FE, Stampfer MJ. Beverage use and risk for kidney stones in women. *Ann Intern Med.* 1998;128:534-540.

23. Goldfarb DS, Asplin JR. Effect of grapefruit juice on urinary lithogenicity. *J Urol.* 2001;166:263-267.

24. Hönow R, Laube N, Schneider A, Keßler T, Hesse A. Influence of grapefruit-, orange- and apple-juice consumption on urinary variables and risk of crystallization. *Br J Nutr.* 2003;90:295-300.

25. Hesse A, Siener R, Heynck H, Jahnen A. The influence of dietary factors on the risk of urinary stone formation. *Scanning Microsc.* 1993;7:1119-1128.

26. Wabner CL, Pak CYC. Effect of orange juice consumption on urinary stone risk factors. *J Urol.* 1993;149:1405-1408.

27. Choi HK, Curhan G. Soft drinks, fructose consumption, and the risk of gout in men: prospective cohort study. *Br Med J.* 2008;336: 309-312.

28. Seltzer MA, Low RK, McDonald M, Shami GS, Stoller ML. Dietary manipulation with lemonade to treat hypocitraturic calcium nephrolithiasis. *J Urol.* 1996;156:907-909.

29. Kang DE, Sur RL, Haleblian GE, Fitzsimons NJ, Borawski KM, Preminger GM. Long-term lemonade based dietary manipulation in patients with hypocitraturic nephrolithiasis. *J Urol.* 2007;177: 1358-1362.

30. Koff SG, Paquette EL, Cullen J, Gancarczyk KK, Tucciarone PR, Schenkman NS. Comparison between lemonade and potassium citrate and impact on urine pH and 24-hour urine parameters in patients with kidney stone formation. *Urology.* 2007;69:1013-1016.

31. Penniston KL, Nakada SY, Holmes RP, Assimos DG. Quantitative assessment of citric acid in lemon juice, lime juice, and commercially-available fruit juice products. *J Endourol.* 2008;22:567-570.

32. Keßler T, Jansen B, Hesse A. Effect of blackcurrant-, cranberry- and plum juice consumption on risk factors associated with kidney stone formation. *Eur J Clin Nutr.* 2002;56:1020-1023.

33. McHarg T, Rodgers A, Charlton K. Influence of cranberry juice on the urinary risk factors for calcium oxalate kidney stone formation. *BJU Int.* 2003;92:765-768.

34. Gettman MT, Ogan K, Brinkley LJ, Adams-Huet B, Pak CYC, Pearle MS. Effect of cranberry juice consumption on urinary stone risk factors. *J Urol.* 2005;174:590-594.

35. Avorn J, Monane M, Gurwitz JH, Glynn RJ, Choodnovskiy I, Lipsitz LA. Reduction of bacteriuria and pyuria after ingestion of cranberry juice. *JAMA*. 1994;271:751-754.

36. Kontiokari T, Nuutinen M, Uhari M. Dietary factors affecting susceptibility to urinary tract infection. *Pediatr Nephrol*. 2004;19: 378-383.

37. Traxer O, Huet B, Poindexter J, Pak CYC, Pearle MS. Effect of ascorbic acid consumption on urinary stone risk factors. *J Urol*. 2003;170:397-401.

38. Goldfarb DS, Fischer ME, Keich Y, Goldberg J. A twin study of genetic and dietary influences on nephrolithiasis: a report from the Vietnam Era Twin (VET) registry. *Kidney Int*. 2005;67:1053-1061.

39. Choi HK, Willett W, Curhan G. Coffee consumption and risk of incident gout in men: a prospective study. *Arthritis Rheum*. 2007;56:2049-2055.

40. Massey LK, Sutton RAL. Acute caffeine effects on urine composition and calcium kidney stone risk in calcium stone formers. *J Urol*. 2004;172:555-558.

41. Hönow R, Hesse A. Comparison of extraction methods for the determination of soluble and total oxalate in foods by HPLC-enzyme-reactor. *Food Chem*. 2002;78:511-521.

42. Liebman M, Mulphy S. Low oxalate bioavailability from black tea. *Nutr Res*. 2007;27:273-278.

43. Savage GP, Charrier MJS, Vanhanen L. Bioavailability of soluble oxalate from tea and the effect of consuming milk with the tea. *Eur J Clin Nutr*. 2003;57:415-419.

44. Krieger JN, Kronmal RA, Coxon V, Wortley P, Thompson L, Sherrard DJ. Dietary and behavioral risk factors for urolithiasis: potential implications for prevention. *Am J Kidney Dis*. 1996;28: 195-201.

45. Shuster J, Jenkins A, Logan C, et al. Soft drink consumption and urinary stone recurrence: a randomized prevention trial. *J Clin Epidemiol*. 1992;45:911-916.

46. Soucie JM, Coates RJ, McClellan W, Austin H, Thun M. Relation between geographic variability in kidney stones prevalence and risk factors for stones. *Am J Epidemiol*. 1996;143:487-495.

47. Rodgers A. Effect of cola consumption on urinary biochemical and physicochemical risk factors associated with calcium oxalate urolithiasis. *Urol Res*. 1999;27:77-81.

48. Lemann J, Piering W, Lennon EJ. Possible role of carbohydrate-induced calciuria in calcium oxalate kidney-stone formation. *N Engl J Med*. 1969;280:232-237.

49. Choi JWJ, Ford ES, Gao X, Choi HK. Sugar-sweetened soft drinks, diet soft drinks, and serum uric acid level: the Third National Health and Nutrition Examination Survey. *Arthritis Rheum*. 2008;59:109-116.

50. Zechner O, Scheiber V. Alcohol as an epidemiological risk in urolithiasis. In: Smith LH, Robertson WG, Finlayson B, eds. *Urolithiasis Clinical and Basic Research*. New York: Plenum Press; 1981.

51. Gibson T, Rodgers AV, Simmonds HA, Toseland P. Beer drinking and its effect on uric acid. *Br J Rheumatol*. 1984;23:203-209.

52. Choi HK, Atkinson K, Karlson EW, Willett W, Curhan G. Alcohol intake and risk of incident gout in men: a prospective study. *Lancet*. 2004;363:1277-1281.

53. Sierakowski R, Finlayson B, Landes R. Stone incidence as related to water hardness in different geographical regions of the United States. *Urol Res*. 1979;7:157-160.

54. Shuster J, Finlayson B, Schaeffer R, Sierakowski R, Zoltek J, Dzegede S. Water hardness and urinary stone disease. *J Urol*. 1982;128:422-425.

55. Keßler T, Hesse A. Cross-over study of the influence of bicarbonate-rich mineral water on urinary composition in comparison with sodium potassium citrate in healthy male subjects. *Br J Nutr*. 2000;84:865-871.

56. Siener R, Jahnen A, Hesse A. Influence of a mineral water rich in calcium, magnesium and bicarbonate on urine composition and the risk of calcium oxalate crystallization. *Eur J Clin Nutr*. 2004;58:270-276.

57. Bellizzi V, De Nicola L, Minutolo R, et al. Effects of water hardness on urinary risk factors for kidney stones in patients with idiopathic nephrolithiasis. *Nephron*. 1999;81(suppl 1):66-70.

58. Caudarella R, Rizzoli E, Buffa A, Bottura A, Stefoni S. Comparative study of the influence of 3 types of mineral water in patients with idiopathic calcium lithiasis. *J Urol*. 1998;159:658-663.

59. Marangella M, Vitale C, Petrarulo M, Rovera L, Dutto F. Effects of mineral composition of drinking water on risk for stone formation and bone metabolism in idiopathic calcium nephrolithiasis. *Clin Sci*. 1996;91:313-318.

60. Hesse A, Siener R. Current aspects of epidemiology and nutrition in urinary stone disease. *World J Urol*. 1997;15:165-171.

61. Robertson WG, Peacock M, Marshall DH. Prevalence of urinary stone disease in vegetarians. *Eur Urol*. 1982;8:334-339.

62. Breslau NA, Brinkley L, Hill KD, Pak CYC. Relationship of animal protein-rich diet to kidney stone formation and calcium metabolism. *J Clin Endocrinol Metab*. 1988;66:140-146.

63. Kok DJ, Iestra JA, Doorenbos CJ, Papapoulos SE. The effects of dietary excesses in animal protein and in sodium on the composition and the crystallization kinetics of calcium oxalate monohydrate in urines of healthy men. *J Clin Endocrinol Metab*. 1990;71:861-867.

64. Reddy ST, Wang CY, Sakhaee K, Brinkley L, Pak CYC. Effect of low-carbohydrate high-protein diets on acid-base balance, stone-forming propensity, and calcium metabolism. *Am J Kidney Dis*. 2002;40:265-274.

65. Barzel US, Massey LK. Excess dietary protein can adversely affect bone. *J Nutr*. 1998;128:1051-1053.

66. Schuette SA, Hegsted M, Zemel MB, Linkswiler HM. Renal acid, urinary cyclic AMP, and hydroxyproline excretion as affected by level of protein, sulfur amino acid, and phosphorus intake. *J Nutr*. 1981;111:2106-2116.

67. Schuette SA, Zemel MB, Linkswiler HM. Studies on the mechanism of protein-induced hypercalciuria in older men and women. *J Nutr*. 1980;110:305-315.

68. Kerstetter JE, O'Brien KO, Insogna KL. Low protein intake: the impact on calcium and bone homeostasis in humans. *J Nutr*. 2003;133:855S-861S.

69. Giannini S, Nobile M, Sartori L, et al. Acute effects of moderate dietary protein restriction in patients with idiopathic hypercalciuria and calcium nephrolithiasis. *Am J Clin Nutr*. 1999;69:267-271.

70. Holmes RP, Goodman HO, Hart LJ, Assimos DG. Relationship of protein intake to urinary oxalate and glycolate excretion. *Kidney Int*. 1993;44:366-372.

71. Nguyen QV, Kälin A, Drouve U, Casez JP, Jaeger P. Sensitivity to meat protein intake and hyperoxaluria in idiopathic calcium stone formers. *Kidney Int*. 2001;59:2273-2281.

72. Robertson WG, Heyburn PJ, Peacock M, Hanes FA, Swaminathan R. The effect of high animal protein intake on the risk of calcium stone-formation in the urinary tract. *Clin Sci*. 1979;57:285-288.

73. Robertson WG, Peacock M, Heyburn PJ, et al. Should recurrent calcium oxalate stone formers become vegetarians? *Br J Urol*. 1979;51:427-431.

74. Marangella M, Bianco O, Martini C, Petrarulo M, Vitale C, Linari F. Effect of animal and vegetable protein intake on oxalate excretion in idiopathic calcium stone disease. *Br J Urol*. 1989;63:348-351.

75. Siener R, Hesse A. The effect of different diets on urine composition and the risk of calcium oxalate crystallisation in healthy subjects. *Eur Urol*. 2002;42:289-296.

76. Hiatt RA, Ettinger B, Caan B, Quesenberry CP, Duncan D, Citron JT. Randomized controlled trial of a low animal protein, high fiber diet in the prevention of recurrent calcium oxalate kidney stones. *Am J Epidemiol*. 1996;144:25-33.

77. Borghi L, Schianchi T, Meschi T, et al. Comparison of two diets for the prevention of recurrent stones in idiopathic hypercalciuria. *N Engl J Med.* 2002;346:77-84.

78. Fellström B, Danielson BG, Karlström B, Lithell H, Ljunghall S, Vessby B. Dietary habits in renal stone patients compared with healthy subjects. *Br J Urol.* 1989;63:575-580.

79. Power C, Barker DJP, Nelson M, Winter PD. Diet and renal stones: a case-control study. *Br J Urol.* 1984;56:456-459.

80. Al Zahrani H, Norman RW, Thompson C, Weerasinghe S. The dietary habits of idiopathic calcium stone-formers and normal control subjects. *BJU Int.* 2000;85:616-620.

81. Iguchi M, Umekawa T, Ishikawa Y, et al. Dietary intake and habits of Japanese renal stone patients. *J Urol.* 1990;143:1093-1095.

82. Trinchieri A, Mandressi A, Luongo P, Longo G, Pisani E. The influence of diet on urinary risk factors for stones in healthy subjects and idiopathic renal calcium stone formers. *Br J Urol.* 1991;67:230-236.

83. Barilla DE, Townsend J, Pak CYC. Exaggerated augmentation of renal calcium excretion after oral glucose ingestion in patients with renal hypercalciuria. *Invest Urol.* 1978;15:486-488.

84. Nguyen NU, Dumoulin G, Henriet MT, Regnard J. Effects of i.v. insulin bolus on urinary calcium and oxalate excretion in healthy subjects. *Horm Metab Res.* 1998;30:222-226.

85. Wood RJ, Gerhardt A, Rosenberg IH. Effects of glucose and glucose polymers on calcium absorption in healthy subjects. *Am J Clin Nutr.* 1987;46:699-701.

86. Taylor EN, Curhan GC. Fructose consumption and the risk of kidney stones. *Kidney Int.* 2008;73:207-212.

87. Milne DB, Nielsen FH. The interaction between dietary fructose and magnesium adversely affects macromineral homeostasis in men. *J Am Coll Nutr.* 2000;19:31-37.

88. Nguyen NU, Dumoulin G, Henriet MT, Regnard J. Increase in urinary calcium and oxalate after fructose infusion. *Horm Metab Res.* 1995;27:155-158.

89. Nguyen NU, Dumoulin G, Wolf JP, Berthelay S. Urinary calcium and oxalate excretion during oral fructose or glucose load in man. *Horm Metab Res.* 1989;21:96-99.

90. Emmerson BT. Effect of oral fructose on urate production. *Ann Rheum Dis.* 1974;33:276-280.

91. Stirpe F, Della Corte E, Bonetti E, Abbondanza A, Abati A, Stefano FD. Fructose-induced hyperuricaemia. *Lancet.* 1970;2:1310-1311.

92. Crapo PA, Kolterman OG. The metabolic effects of 2-week fructose feeding in normal subjects. *Am J Clin Nutr.* 1984;39: 525-534.

93. Raivio KO, Becker A, Meyer LJ, Greene ML, Nuki G, Seegmiller JE. Stimulation of human purine synthesis de novo by fructose infusion. *Metabolism.* 1975;24:861-869.

94. Fox IH, Palella TD, Kelley WN. Hyperuricemia: a marker for cell energy crisis. *N Engl J Med.* 1987;317:111-112.

95. Naya Y, Ito H, Masai M, Yamaguchi K. Association of dietary fatty acids with urinary oxalate excretion in calcium oxalate stone-formers in their fourth decade. *BJU Int.* 2002;89:842-846.

96. Baggio B, Budakovic A, Nassuato MA, et al. Plasma phospholipid arachidonic acid content and calcium metabolism in idiopathic calcium nephrolithiasis. *Kidney Int.* 2000;58:1278-1284.

97. Baggio B, Gambaro G, Zambon S, et al. Anomalous phospholipid n-6 polyunsaturated fatty acid composition in idiopathic calcium nephrolithiasis. *J Am Soc Nephrol.* 1996;7:613-620.

98. Buck AC, Davies RL, Harrison T. The protective role of eicosapentaenoic acid (EPA) in the pathogenesis of nephrolithiasis. *J Urol.* 1991;146:188-194.

99. Taylor EN, Stampfer MJ, Curhan GC. Fatty acid intake and incident nephrolithiasis. *Am J Kidney Dis.* 2005;45:267-274.

100. Holmes RP, Goodman HO, Assimos DG. Contribution of dietary oxalate to urinary oxalate excretion. *Kidney Int.* 2001;59: 270-276.

101. Taylor EN, Curhan GC. Oxalate intake and the risk for nephrolithiasis. *J Am Soc Nephrol.* 2007;18:2198-2204.

102. Holmes RP, Goodman HO, Assimos DG. Dietary oxalate and its intestinal absorption. *Scanning Microsc.* 1995;9:1109-1120.

103. Siener R, Hönow R, Seidler A, Voss S, Hesse A. Oxalate contents of species of the Polygonaceae, Amaranthaceae and Chenopodiaceae families. *Food Chem.* 2006;98:220-224.

104. Siener R, Hönow R, Voss S, Seidler A, Hesse A. Oxalate content of cereals and cereal products. *J Agr Food Chem.* 2006;54:3008-3011.

105. Chai W, Liebman M. Effect of different cooking methods on vegetable oxalate content. *J Agr Food Chem.* 2005;53:3027-3030.

106. Berg W, Haerting R, Bothor C, Meinig S, Eschholz A, Schulze HP. Assessing enteral oxalate absorption in patients with idiopathic recurrent calcium-oxalate urinary stone disease. *Urologe A.* 1990;29:148-151.

107. Lindsjö M, Danielson BG, Fellström B, Ljunghall S. Intestinal oxalate and calcium absorption in recurrent renal stone formers and healthy subjects. *Scand J Urol Nephrol.* 1989;23:55-59.

108. Marangella M, Fruttero B, Bruno M, Linari F. Hyperoxaluria in idiopathic calcium stone disease: Further evidence of intestinal hyperabsorption of oxalate. *Clin Sci.* 1982;63:381-385.

109. Tiselius HG, Ahlstrand C, Lundström B, Nilsson MA. [^{14}C]Oxalate absorption by normal persons, calcium oxalate stone formers, and patients with surgically disturbed intestinal function. *Clin Chem.* 1981;27:1682-1685.

110. Voss S, Hesse A, Zimmermann DJ, Sauerbruch T, von Unruh GE. Intestinal oxalate absorption is higher in idiopathic calcium oxalate stone formers than in healthy controls: measurements with the [$^{13}C_2$]oxalate absorption test. *J Urol.* 2006;175: 1711-1715.

111. Allison MJ, Cook HM, Milne DB, Gallagher S, Clayman RV. Oxalate degradation by gastrointestinal bacteria from humans. *J Nutr.* 1986;116:455-460.

112. Sidhu H, Schmidt ME, Cornelius JG, et al. Direct correlation between hyperoxaluria/oxalate stone disease and the absence of the gastrointestinal tract-dwelling bacterium Oxalobacter formigenes: Possible prevention by gut recolonization or enzyme replacement therapy. *J Am Soc Nephrol.* 1999;10:S334-S340.

113. Coe FL, Parks JH, Asplin JR. The pathogenesis and treatment of kidney stones. *N Engl J Med.* 1992;327:1141-1152.

114. Couzy F, Kastenmayer P, Vigo M, Clough J, Munoz-Box R, Barclay DV. Calcium bioavailability from a calcium- and sulfate-rich mineral water, compared with milk, in young adult women. *Am J Clin Nutr.* 1995;62:1239-1244.

115. Broadus AE, Insogna KL, Lang R, Ellison AF, Dreyer BE. Evidence for disordered control of 1, 25-dihydroxyvitamin D production in absorptive hypercalciuria. *N Engl J Med.* 1984;311:73-80.

116. Hess B, Jost C, Zipperle L, Takkinen R, Jaeger P. High-calcium intake abolishes hyperoxaluria and reduces urinary crystallization during a 20-fold normal oxalate load in humans. *Nephrol Dial Transplant.* 1998;13:2241-2247.

117. Liebman M, Chai W. Effect of dietary calcium on urinary oxalate excretion after oxalate loads. *Am J Clin Nutr.* 1997;65:1453-1459.

118. Von Unruh GE, Voss S, Sauerbruch T, Hesse A. Dependence of oxalate absorption on the daily calcium intake. *J Am Soc Nephrol.* 2004;15:1567-1573.

119. Trinchieri A, Nespoli R, Ostini F, Rovera F, Zanetti G, Pisani E. A study of dietary calcium and other nutrients in idiopathic renal calcium stone formers with low bone mineral content. *J Urol.* 1998;159:654-657.

120. Liebman M, Costa G. Effects of calcium and magnesium on urinary oxalate excretion after oxalate loads. *J Urol.* 2000;163: 1565-1569.

121. Kohri K, Garside J, Blacklock NJ. The role of magnesium in calcium oxalate urolithiasis. *Br J Urol.* 1988;61:107-115.

122. Li MK, Blacklock NJ, Garside J. Effects of magnesium on calcium oxalate crystallization. *J Urol.* 1985;133:123-125.

123. Meschi T, Maggiore U, Fiaccadori E, et al. The effect of fruits and vegetables on urinary stone risk factors. *Kidney Int.* 2004;66: 2402-2410.

124. Siener R, Hesse A. Influence of a mixed and a vegetarian diet on urinary magnesium excretion and concentration. *Br J Nutr.* 1995;73:783-790.

125. Fetner CD, Barilla DE, Townsend J, Pak CYC. Effects of magnesium oxide on the crystallization of calcium salts in urine in patients with recurrent nephrolithiasis. *J Urol.* 1978;120:399-401.

126. Tiselius HG, Ahlstrand C, Larsson L. Urine composition in patients with urolithiasis during treatment with magnesium oxide. *Urol Res.* 1980;8:197-200.

127. Muldowney FP, Freaney R, Moloney MF. Importance of dietary sodium in the hypercalciuria syndrome. *Kidney Int.* 1982;22: 292-296.

128. Sakhaee K, Harvey JA, Padalino PK, Whitson P, Pak CYC. The potential role of salt abuse on the risk for kidney stone formation. *J Urol.* 1993;150:310-312.

129. Massey LK, Whiting SJ. Dietary salt, urinary calcium, and kidney-stone risk. *Nutr Rev.* 1995;53:131-134.

130. Burtis WJ, Gay L, Insogna KL, Ellison A, Broadus AE. Dietary hypercalciuria in patients with calcium oxalate kidney stones. *Am J Clin Nutr.* 1994;60:424-429.

131. Wasserstein AG, Stolley PD, Soper KA, Goldfarb S, Maislin G, Agus Z. Case-control study of risk factors for idiopathic calcium nephrolithiasis. *Miner Electrolyte Metab.* 1987;13:85-95.

132. Williams HE, Wandzilak TR. Oxalate synthesis, transport and the hyperoxaluric syndromes. *J Urol.* 1989;141:742-747.

133. Wandzilak TR, D'Andre SD, Davis PA, Williams HE. Effect of high dose vitamin C on urinary oxalate levels. *J Urol.* 1994;151:834-837.

134. Siener R, Ebert D, Nicolay C, Hesse A. Dietary risk factors for hyperoxaluria in calcium oxalate stone formers. *Kidney Int.* 2003;63:1037-1043.

135. Siener R, Heynck H, Hesse A. Calcium-binding capacities of different brans under simulated gastrointestinal pH conditions. In vitro study with ^{45}Ca. *J Agr Food Chem.* 2001;49:4397-4401.

136. Grases F, March JG, Prieto RM, et al. Urinary phytate in calcium oxalate stone formers and healthy people. *Scand J Urol Nephrol.* 2000;34:162-164.

137. Siener R, Hesse A. The effect of a vegetarian and different omnivorous diets on urinary risk factors for uric acid stone formation. *Eur J Nutr.* 2003;42:332-337.

138. Choi HK, Atkinson K, Karlson EW, Willett W, Curhan G. Purine-rich foods, dairy and protein intake, and the risk of gout in men. *N Engl J Med.* 2004;350:1093-1103.

139. Choi HK, Liu SM, Curhan G. Intake of purine-rich foods, protein, and dairy products and relationship to serum levels of uric acid – The Third National Health and Nutrition Examination Survey. *Arthritis Rheum.* 2005;52:283-289.

140. Taylor EN, Stampfer MJ, Curhan GC. Obesity, weight gain, and the risk of kidney stones. *JAMA.* 2005;293:455-462.

141. Siener R, Glatz S, Nicolay C, Hesse A. The role of overweight and obesity in calcium oxalate stone formation. *Obes Res.* 2004;12: 106-113.

142. Sarica K, Altay B, Erturhan S. Effect of being overweight on stone-forming risk factors. *Urology.* 2008;71:771-775.

143. Taylor EN, Curhan GC. Body size and 24-hour urine composition. *Am J Kidney Dis.* 2006;48:905-915.

144. Siener R, Schade N, Nicolay C, von Unruh GE, Hesse A. The efficacy of dietary intervention on urinary risk factors for stone formation in recurrent calcium oxalate stone patients. *J Urol.* 2005;173:1601-1605.

Obesity, Metabolic Syndrome, and Stones

9

Bernhard Hess

Abstract Obesity (body mass index (BMI) above 30 kg/m^2) has become an epidemic condition that affects 10–27% of men and up to 38% of women in European countries. In the United States, more than 5% of the adult population are considered morbidly obese (BMI of 40 kg/m^2 or more). Worldwide, more than 300 million people are estimated to be obese. According to recent epidemiologic studies, greater BMI, greater weight, larger waist circumference, and heavy weight gain are independently associated with increased risk for renal stone formation. This appears to be related to two distinct metabolic conditions: (1) Abdominal obesity in the context of the so-called metabolic syndrome predisposes to insulin resistance, which at the renal level appears to cause reduced urinary ammonium excretion and low urine pH. The consequence is an increased risk for *uric acid stone formation*. (2) Bariatric surgery, more and more popular as the only intervention that facilitates significant weight loss in morbidly obese people, has been shown to increase the risk for *calcium oxalate nephrolithiasis*. The underlying pathophysiologic mechanisms may be enteric hyperoxaluria due to fat malabsorption or decreased intestinal colonization with oxalate-degrading bacteria.

9.1 Introduction

Obesity has become an epidemic condition around the world that affects 10–27% of men and up to 38% of women in European countries.[1,2] In the United States, the percentage of obese adults (defined as having a BMI above 30 kg/m^2) increased from 15% in 1995 to 24% in 2005,[1] and more than 5% of the US adult population are considered morbidly obese (BMI of 40 or more).[3] Worldwide, more than 300 million people are estimated to be obese.[1]

Most recently, it has become evident that greater BMI, greater weight, larger waist circumference, and heavy weight gain are independently associated with increased risk for renal stone formation.[4] Indeed, a study of nearly 6,000 renal stone formers demonstrated that subjects weighing more than 120 kg had significantly higher urinary excretion rates of calcium, oxalate, and uric acid – established risk factors for nephrolithiasis – than subjects weighing less than 100 kg.[5] However, when studying 2,176 male and female stone formers and

1,097 male and female healthy controls from the Health Professionals Follow-Up Study and the Nurses Health Studies I and II, Taylor and Curhan[6] found that the positive association between BMI and urinary calcium disappeared after adjustment for urinary sodium (an index of salt consumption) and phosphate (an index of protein consumption). Furthermore, urinary supersaturation of calcium oxalate, the main driving force for the most prevalent calcium oxalate stone formation, was not related to BMI.[6] On the other hand, urine pH was inversely related to BMI; i.e., more obese people had lower urinary pH values. A very similar finding was obtained when plotting urine pH against body weight in nearly 5,000 kidney stone formers from the United States; i.e., urine pH was inversely related to body weight.[7] Because urinary supersaturation of uric acid progressively rises with decreasing urinary pH,[8] it is of no surprise that Taylor and Curhan[6] found that urinary uric acid supersaturation was directly related to BMI. Their conclusion was that the greater incidences of renal stones that were observed more recently in the Unites States[9] as well as in Europe[10] may primarily be due to an increase in uric acid nephrolithiasis in obese people.[6]

Abdominal (central) obesity is the key feature of the so-called *metabolic syndrome*, as defined in Table 9.1. This cluster of cardiovascular risk factors in obese people is

B. Hess (✉)
Department of Internal Medicine & Nephrology/Hypertension,
Klinik Im Park, Zurich, Switzerland
e-mail: bernhard.hess@hirslanden.ch

P.N. Rao et al. (eds.), *Urinary Tract Stone Disease*,
DOI 10.1007/978-1-84800-362-0_9, © Springer-Verlag London Limited 2011

Table 9.1 Definition of the metabolic syndrome according to IDF (International Diabetes Federation). ATP III: Adult Treatment Panel III 2001

Metabolic syndrome – definition (IDF 2005)	
Central (abdomial) obesity – ethnicity-specific	
(Europeans: Waist circumference Men ≥94 cm, women ≥80 cm)	
(U.S. people: Waist circumference Men ≥102 cm, women ≥88 cm according to ATP III definition likely to be used, Ref.[12])	
Plus two out of the four following criteria constitute the syndrome:	
• Arterial hypertension	• Triglycerides >1.7 mmol/L *or* specific treatment
– Systolic≥130 mmHg	• HDL cholestrol
– Diastolic ≥85 mmHg	< 1.30 mmol/L (Women)
or treatment for diagnosed hypertension	<1.00 mmol/L (Men) *or* specific treatment
	• Plasma glucose ≥5.6 mmol/L *or* previously diagnosed type 2 diabetes

Adapted from[11]

increasingly prevalent around the world and affected 27% of the American population in 2000.[13] Recently, data from the Third National Health and Nutrition Examination Survey (NHANES III) have revealed that metabolic syndrome traits are significantly associated with a self-reported history of kidney stones: with zero traits of the metabolic syndrome, self-reported prevalence of kidney stones was 3% and increased to 7.5% with three traits and to 9.8% with five traits of the syndrome, respectively.[13]

The aim of the following paragraphs is to demonstrate that the increasing prevalence of obesity around the world may soon be followed by an epidemic of nephrolithiasis, mainly through two pathophysiologic mechanisms: (1) Increased prevalence of uric acid stone formation due to increasingly low urine pH values and (2) increased prevalence of calcium oxalate stones due to hyperoxaluria following bariatric surgery.

9.2 Obesity, Metabolic Syndrome, Low Urine pH, and Uric Acid Stone Formation

9.2.1 Pathophysiology

At low pH in human urine, uric acid is primarily present as poorly soluble undissociated uric acid (solubility 0.54 mmol/L).[8] Thus, abundant uric acid crystallization with subsequent stone formation can occur even if the urinary uric acid excretion rate is completely normal. Indeed, clinical experience tells that the main cause of uric acid stone formation is not hyperuricosuria, but *low urine pH*.[8] Since such abnormally low urine pH values are very often associated with primary gout, it was initially concluded that idiopathic uric acid nephrolithiasis may be a stone

manifestation of primary gout.[14] Subsequently, the reason for low urine pH in most normouricosuric uric acid stone formers was found to be reduced renal ammonium excretion in two independent studies.[15,16] In addition, Sakhaee et al.[16] found that the rise in urinary ammonium excretion following acid loading in uric acid stone formers was five- to sevenfold lower than in calcium stone formers or healthy controls.

9.2.2 Uric Acid Stones, Metabolic Syndrome, and Insulin Resistance

When studying the data of almost 5,000 stone patients in the United States, Maalouf et al.[7] found an inverse correlation between urine pH and sixtiles of body weight; i.e., more obese patients had significantly lower urine pH values. Furthermore, Sakhaee et al.[16] demonstrated that one-third of pure uric acid stone formers, but none of the calcium stone formers or healthy controls, were diabetic. Accordingly, Abate et al.[17] later found an increase in insulin resistance and significantly higher waist circumferences (i.e., abdominal obesity) in uric acid stone formers with reduced urinary ammonium excretion and low urinary pH values. However, laborious measures of insulin resistance appear not to be necessary in clinical routine,[18] since insulin resistance is highly correlated with abdominal (central) obesity[19]; i.e., abdominal obesity stands for insulin resistance.

In addition, Abate et al.[17] found that uric acid stone formers exhibited higher values for blood pressure, fasting blood glucose, and triglycerides as well as lower values for HDL cholesterol (Fig. 9.1a), all clinical key features of the so-called metabolic syndrome. The conclusion at that stage was that defective urinary ammonium excretion in uric acid stone formers could be linked to the insulin-resistant state.[17] Furthermore, Abate et al.[17] directly assessed insulin

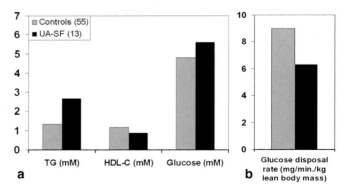

Fig. 9.1 (**a**) Fasting serum triglyceride, HDL cholesterol, and blood glucose in healthy controls and uric acid stone formers (UA-SF). mM: mmol/L. Values are means. (**b**) Glucose disposal rate as a measure of insulin sensitivity in healthy controls and uric acid stone formers (UA-SF). Values are means (Adapted from[17])

sensitivity by measuring glucose disposal rate during an euglycemic hyperinsulinemic clamp procedure, as originally described by DeFronzo et al.,[20] in 55 healthy controls and 13 selected pure uric acid stone formers. As depicted in Fig. 9.1b, glucose disposal rate as a surrogate for insulin sensitivity was significantly higher in healthy controls than in uric acid stone formers; i.e., uric acid stone formers exhibited increased insulin resistance. Furthermore, uric acid stone formers had a significantly lower ratio of urinary ammonium to net acid excretion and a lower urinary pH. A plot of urinary pH values against insulin sensitivity showed a positive correlation in healthy controls; i.e., higher urinary pH was associated with higher insulin sensitivity. Most likely due to the relatively low number of patients studied, this correlation could not be demonstrated in uric acid stone formers whose lower urinary pH values nevertheless tended to cluster in the area of lower insulin sensitivity (i.e., higher insulin resistance).[17] In summary, uric acid stone formers fulfilled the criteria for the diagnosis of metabolic syndrome and, in addition, were more insulin-resistant with lower urinary ammonium and pH values than healthy controls.

Table 9.2 summarizes important findings from animal studies, which have demonstrated that insulin is critical for ammoniagenesis as well as ammonium secretion in the proximal tubule. Based on this knowledge, the findings of Abate et al.[17] indicate that low urinary pH due to reduced urinary ammonium excretion may be a *novel renal manifestation of insulin resistance* in the context of *metabolic syndrome* with *central obesity* as its primary key feature. The consequence of this metabolic abnormality at the renal level is uric acid stone formation, which could be envisioned as a "renal bystander" in patients with the metabolic syndrome.

Treatment of uric acid stone in patients with the metabolic syndrome/abdominal obesity consists of treating the components of the syndrome as well as alkalinizing the urine to pH values between 6.2 and 6.8 throughout 24 h.

Table 9.2 Insulin actions in the proximal renal tubule (data from animal studies) and potential consequences in subjects with insulin resistance

Insulin and urinary NH_4^+ excretion – hypothesis based on in vitro studies
Insulin effect in proximal tubules
• Insulin stimulates renal genesis of ammonia from the substrate L-Glutamine
• Insulin stimulates Na^+/H^+-antiporter→critical for transport of NH_4^+(substites for H^+) into tubules
Consequences of insulin resistance at renal level
• ↓Ammoniagenesis
• ↓Ammonium transport into the tubular lumen
⇒ Low urine pH

Adapted from[17]

9.3 Bariatric Surgery and Calcium Oxalate Stone Formation

9.3.1 Epidemiologic Background

With at least 15 million of the US adult population meeting the criteria for obesity surgery (BMI ≥40 or BMI ≥35 with other conditions such as diabetes),[3] bariatric surgery has become more and more common as the only intervention that facilitates significant weight loss in the morbidly obese. *Restrictive* bariatric surgical procedures (gastric stapling, adjustable gastric banding, a combination of both, or vertical restrictive gastrectomy) limit caloric intake by creating a small gastric reservoir that delays emptying of the stomach, whereas *malabsorptive* procedures (biliopancreatic diversion, Roux-en-Y-gastric bypass) bypass varying portions of the small intestine where nutrients are absorbed.[1] Most recently, Roux-en-Y-gastric bypass (RYGB) has become the most common bariatric operation in the United States.[21] The RYGB procedure results in sustained weight loss as well as improvements in abnormal glucose homeostasis, insulin resistance, sleep apnea, hypertension, and cardiovascular risk factors.[21] Although consequences of malabsorption (i.e., osteoporosis and osteomalacia) have been recognized,[22,23] RYGB is generally felt to be safe, effective, and durable. As a consequence, the number of procedures has increased from an estimated 14,000 in 1998 to 108,000 in 2003.[24]

9.3.2 Renal Complications of Bariatric Surgery

Until most recently, little attention has been drawn on potential renal complications of bariatric surgical procedures. After a first small study reporting on hyperoxaluria, nephrolithiasis, and oxalate nephropathy as serious complications of the RYGB procedure,[25] two independent reports have now emphasized that one major complication of modern bariatric surgery may be *hyperoxaluric calcium oxalate nephrolithiasis*. As depicted in Fig. 9.2, Asplin et al.[26] reported in a retrospective study that in comparison with normal controls and "routine" kidney stone formers, 132 patients who had formed kidney stones after modern bariatric surgery excreted more than double amounts of urinary oxalate, not quite as high as patients who had been treated with jejunoileal bypass. In the smaller study from the Mayo Clinic,[21] an increasing number of patients developed calcium oxalate stones within a mean time of 2.9 years after RYGB bypass surgery. In the same study, a small cross-sectional analysis of patients before and after RYGB revealed hyperoxaluria and substantial increases in relative supersaturations of calcium oxalate in more than

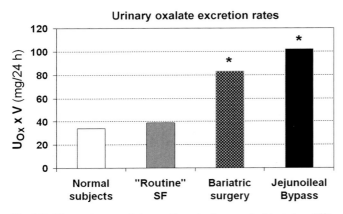

Fig. 9.2 Mean urinary oxalate excretion rates in normal subjects (n = 168), routine kidney stone formers (n = 2,048), patients having undergone modern bariatric surgery (n = 132), and patients after jejunoileal bypass (n = 27). *p < 0.001 versus normal subjects and versus routine kidney stone formers (Adapted from[26])

half of the preoperatively mostly normooxaluric patients after 12 months.[21] Most recently, the first prospective longitudinal study on 24 morbidly obese adults undergoing the RYGB procedure[27] reported considerable increases in urinary oxalate excretion rates and relative supersaturations of calcium oxalate. These changes occurred already 90 days after surgery, although the mean oxalate excretion rate was still below levels that indicate a clearly increased risk for the development of calcium oxalate stones.[27] However, the conclusion was that this early increase in urinary oxalate excretion could herald the onset of a clinically significant hyperoxaluric state.[27]

9.3.3 Pathogenesis of Hyperoxaluria After Bariatric Surgery

The pathogenesis of hyperoxaluria after RYGB is incompletely understood. Two possibilities have been discussed.[21,27] On the one hand, RYGB may induce an *enteric hyperoxaluric state* secondary to increased fatty acid, bile salt, and oxalate delivery to the intact colon, similar to what has been described in Crohn's disease and jejunoileal bypass. Due to fat malabsorption and binding of calcium to unabsorbed fatty acids, oxalates derived from the diet reach the colon uncomplexed with calcium and are then absorbed. It would appear logical that a longer common channel after RYGB surgery would predispose to more significant fat malabsorption. Indeed, studies in inflammatory bowel disease have suggested that the degree of hyperoxaluria corresponds with the degree of steatorrhea.[28]

On the other hand, disturbances in the intestinal flora after RYGB could play a role. *Oxalobacter formigenes*, a normal commensurate part of human intestinal microflora,

can metabolize oxalate as an energy source, and sufficient colonization with *O. formigenes* has a protective effect against increased oxalate absorption and excretion.[29] In patients who had undergone jenunoileal bypass surgery, decreased intestinal colonization with oxalate-degrading bacteria has been described.[30] Whether or not RYGB surgery also alters colonization with these bacteria is currently not known.

9.4 Conclusions

In conclusion, based on current knowledge, RYGB surgery may predispose to hyperoxaluria and calcium oxalate stone formation, either by causing enteric hyperoxaluria or decreasing intestinal colonization with oxalate-degrading bacteria.

References

1. DeMaria EJ. Bariatric surgery for morbid obesity. *N Engl J Med*. 2007;356:2176-2183.
2. James WPT, Van de Werf F. Obesity management: the cardiovascular benefits. *Eur Heart J*. 2005;7(Suppl L):L3-L4.
3. Flum DR, Khan TV, Dellinger EP. Toward the rational and equitable use of bariatric surgery. *JAMA*. 2007;298:1442. commentary.
4. Taylor EN, Stampfer MJ, Curhan GC. Obesity, weight gain, and the risk of kidney stones. *JAMA*. 2005;293:455-462.
5. Powell CR, Stoller ML, Schwartz BF, et al. Impact of body weight on urinary electrolytes in urinary stone formers. *Urology*. 2000;55:825-830.
6. Taylor EN, Curhan GC. Body size and 24-hour urine composition. *Am J Kidney Dis*. 2006;48:905-915.
7. Maalouf NM, Sakhaee K, Parks JH, Coe FL, Adams-Huet B, Pak CYC. Association of urinary pH with body weight in nephrolithiasis. *Kidney Int*. 2004;65:1422-1425.
8. Hess B. Acid-base metabolism: implications for kidney stone formation. *Urol Res*. 2006;34:134-138.
9. Stamatelou KK, Francis ME, Jones CA, Nyberg LM, Curhan GC. Time trends in reported prevalence of kidney stones in the United States: 1976–1994. *Kidney Int*. 2003;63:1817-1823.
10. Hesse A, Brändle E, Wilbert, Köhrmann K-U, Alken P. Study on the prevalence and incidence of urolithiasis in Germany comparing the years 1979 vs. 2000. *Eur Urol*. 2003;44:709-713.
11. Alberti KGMM, Zimmet P, Shaw J, for the IDF Epidemiology Task Force Consensus Group. The metabolic syndrome – a new worldwide definition. *Lancet*. 2005;366:1059-1062.
12. Ford ES, Giles WH, Dietz WH. Prevalence of the metabolic syndrome among US adults: findings from the third National Health and Nutrition Examination Survey. *JAMA*. 2002;287:356-359.
13. West B, Luke A, Durazo-Arvizu RA, Cao G, Shoham D, Kramer H. Metabolic syndrome and self-reported history of kidney stones: the National Health and Nutrition Examination Survey (NHANES III) 1988–1994. *Am J Kidney Dis*. 2008;51:741-747.
14. Pak CYC, Sakhaee K, Peterson RD, Poindexter JR, Frawley WH. Biochemical profile of idiopathic uric acid nephrolithiasis. *Kidney Int*. 2001;60:757-761.

15. Kamel KS, Cheema-Dhadli S, Halperin ML. Studies on the pathophysiology of the low urine pH in patients with uric acid stones. *Kidney Int.* 2002;61:988-994.

16. Sakhaee S, Adams-Huet B, Moe OW, Pak CYC. Pathophysiologic basis for normouricosuric uric acid nephrolithiasis. *Kidney Int.* 2002;62:971-979.

17. Abate N, Chandalia M, Cabo-Chan AV Jr, Moe OW, Sakhaee K. The metabolic syndrome and uric acid nephrolithiasis: novel features of renal manifestation of insulin resistance. *Kidney Int.* 2004;65:386-392.

18. Grundy SM, Cleeman JI, Daniels SR, et al. American Heart Association; National Heart, Lung, and Blood Institute, et al. Diagnosis and management of the metabolic syndrome: an American heart association/national heart, lung, and blood institute scientific statement. *Circulation.* 2005;112:2735-2752.

19. Carey DG, Jenkins AB, Campbell LV, Freund J, Chisholm DJ. Abdominal fat and insulin resistance in normal and overweight women: Direct measurements reveal a strong relationship in subjects at both low and high risk of NIDDM. *Diabetes.* 1996;45:633-638.

20. DeFronzo RE, Tobin JD, Andres R. Glucose clamp technique: a method for quantifying insulin secretion and resistance. *Am J Physiol.* 1979;233:E214-E223.

21. Sinha MK, Collazo-Clavell ML, Rule A, et al. Hyperoxaluric nephrolithiasis is a complication of Roux-en-Y-gastric bypass surgery. *Kindey Int.* 2007;71:100-107.

22. DePrisco C, Levine SN. Metabolic bone disease after gastric bypass surgery for obesity. *Am J Med Sci.* 2005;329:57-61.

23. Colazzo-Clavell ML, Jiminez A, Hodgson SF, Sarr MG. Osteomalacia after Roux-en-Y-gastric bypass. *Endocr Pract.* 2004;10:195-198.

24. Shinogle JA, Owings MF, Kozak LJ. Gastric bypass as treatment for obesity: trends, characteristics, and complications. *Obes Res.* 2005;13:2202-2209.

25. Nelson WK, Houghton SG, Milliner DS, Lieske JC, Sarr MG. Enteric hyperoxaluria, nephrolithiasis, and oxalate nephropathy: potentially serious and unappreciated complications of Roux-en-Y gastric bypass. *Surg Obes Relat Dis.* 2005;1:481-485.

26. Asplin JR, Coe FL. Hyperoxaluria in kidney stone formers treated with modern bariatric surgery. *J Urol.* 2007;177:565-569.

27. Duffey BG, Pedro RN, Mahklouf A, et al. Roux-en-Y gastric bypass is associated with early increased risk factors for development of caclium oxalate nephrolithiasis. *J Am Coll Surg.* 2008;206:1145-1153.

28. McLeod RS, Churchill DN. Urolithiasis complicating inflammatory bowel disease. *J Urol.* 1992;148:974-978.

29. Siener R, Ebert D, Hesse A. Urinary oaxalate excretion in female calcium oxalate stone formers with and without a history of recurrent urinary tract infections. *Urol Res.* 2001;29:245-248.

30. Allison MJ, Cook HM, Milne DB, et al. Oxalate degradation by gastrointestinal bacteria from humans. *J Nutr.* 1986;116:455-460.

Stone Disease in Animals

10

Doreen M. Houston, Andrew Moore, Denise A. Elliott, and Vincent C. Biourge

Abstract Uroliths have been reported in most animals, but their pathophysiology and management have been studied most in dogs and cats. In both species, urinary stones are responsible for 15–20% of cases of lower urinary tract disease. Despite common belief, stones are more frequent in dogs – especially small dogs – than in cats. Upper urinary tract stones are less common in dogs and cats than in humans. Dietary management has been definitively shown to modulate the occurrence of struvite and purine stones in both dogs and cats. The pathophysiology of calcium oxalate stones is likely to be multifactorial, and the exact roles of diet and urinary pH remain to be investigated. Pending this work, promotion of diuresis and urine dilution by feeding a moist and/or higher sodium diet could be beneficial in both dogs and cats. Prevalence of other stone types is very low in both dogs and cats and their treatment is a combination of surgical, dietary, and medical management.

10.1 Introduction

Uroliths have been reported in the urinary system of virtually all animals including dogs, cats, pigs, cattle, rabbits, horses, sheep, goats, birds, guinea pigs, monkeys, hamsters, camels, deer, turtles, otters, chinchillas, seals, mollusks, ferrets, minks, whales, sea lions, dolphins, kangaroos, raccoons, and gerbils.[1] Table 10.1 summarizes the types of uroliths most commonly found in some of them. Dogs and cats are most often presented to veterinary clinics, and the majority of information on animal urolithiasis comes from published literature on these two species. Consequently, this chapter will focus on urolithiasis in dogs and cats. Clinical signs of urolithiasis in dogs and cats are not specific for stone disease and a complete medical workup is required for diagnosis.[3,4] The major factors implicated in the etiology of urolithiasis in dogs and cats, either alone or in combination, are diet, genetics, urinary tract infection (UTI), metabolic disease, individual susceptibility, and ability to concentrate urine. The pathophysiologies of struvite and urate stones are reasonably well defined and

accepted in veterinary urology; however, other stone types (especially calcium oxalate [CaOx]) are still poorly understood and are the subject of controversy.[5]

10.2 Epidemiology

Worldwide, the incidence of urolithiasis in dogs and cats is believed to be <3%.[2,6] Contrary to what many people believe, stones are much more common in dogs, especially the small breeds, than in cats. From the opening of the Canadian Veterinary Urolith Centre (CVUC) in February 1998 to June 2008, 40,100 canine stones (including 23,700 stones from dogs weighing <10 kg) and only 11,200 feline stones were submitted for analysis.* In dogs, urolithiasis is the third most frequent (18%) lower urinary tract disorder (LUTD) after UTI and urinary incontinence[4] (Fig. 10.1). In cats aged 1–10 years, idiopathic cystitis is the most common cause of LUTD,[7–11] followed by urolithiasis (13–28%)[7,9,11,12] (Fig. 10.2).

Uroliths in dogs and cats are most frequently reported in the bladder (Figs. 10.3 and 10.4), the usual composition being struvite (magnesium ammonium phosphate hexahydrate [$Mg\,NH_4\,PO_4\,6H_2O$]) or CaOx.[2,13–25] The third most

V.C. Biourge (✉)
Health and Nutrition Scientific Director, Royal Canin,
Centre de Recherche, BP4, 650 Avenue de la Petite Camargue,
Aimargues, 30470, France
e-mail: biourge@royal-canin.fr

*(Andrew Moore, personal communication)

Table 10.1 Type of urinary stone in various animals

Stone type	Species
Calcium carbonate	Horse, donkey, cow, goat, llama, rabbit, guinea pig, dog, cat
Calcium phosphate	Horse, donkey, pig, sheep, guinea pig, dog, cat
Struvite	Cow, pig, sheep, goat, American mink, ferret, guinea pig, dog, cat
Calcium oxalate	Cow, pig, goat, deer, dog, cat
Silicate	Cow, sheep, llama, dog, cat
Uric acid	Birds, dog
Urates	Birds, tortoise, crocodile, snakes, sea lion, dog, cat
Cystine	Maned wolf, dog, cat

Modified from [2]

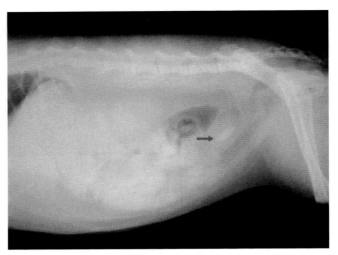

Fig. 10.3 Lateral radiograph of a cat showing radiodense urolith in the center of the bladder (Courtesy of D Houston)

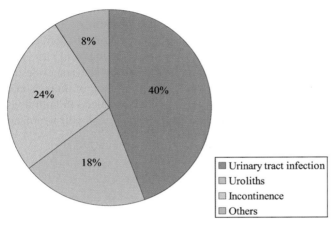

Fig. 10.1 Main conditions responsible for the clinical signs of lower urinary tract disease in dogs[4]

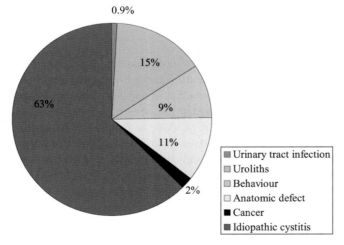

Fig. 10.2 Main conditions responsible for the clinical signs of non-obstructive feline lower urinary tract disease in cats 1–10 years of age[9]

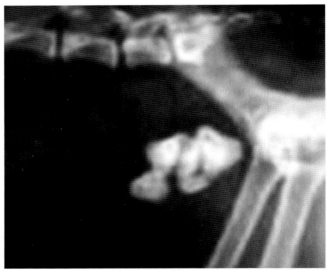

Fig. 10.4 Radiographic appearance of cystic calculi in a dog (Courtesy of CR Lamb)

Drug- and drug metabolite-containing uroliths are rare in dogs and cats.

Upper urinary tract (renal or ureteral) calculi are uncommon (<4% of all cases of urolithiasis in small animals) in dogs and relatively uncommon in cats (Fig. 10.5) compared with humans. An increasing number of nephroliths/ureteroliths have been reported in cats, especially in those with renal failure.[25–28] In one study, 47% of cats with chronic kidney disease had upper urinary tract nephroliths.[25] Nephroliths are typically composed of CaOx in cats and of CaOx or struvite in dogs.[28–31] Urethral stones are uncommon in dogs and cats (Fig. 10.6); they occur more often in males than females due to the longer length and decreased distensibility of the male urethra.

The prevalence of struvite and CaOx uroliths in dogs and cats has changed over the last 30 years. Although

common type of urolith reported worldwide in dogs and cats is urate/uric acid. Less frequently reported uroliths include cystine, silica, xanthine, calcium phosphate, pyrophosphate, and dried solidified blood calculi (DSBC).

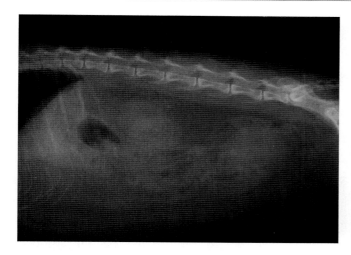

Fig. 10.5 Lateral radiograph showing an ureterolith and a nephrolith in a cat (Radiograph courtesy of Dr. C. Teed, Cat Clinic of Niagara, St. Catherines, Ontario, Canada)

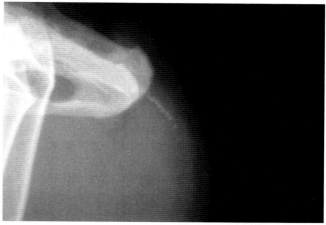

Fig. 10.6 Lateral radiograph showing numerous small, radiodense calculi in the urethra of a male cat presenting with obstructive lower urinary tract disease (Courtesy of Dr Brian Crabbe, Port Elgin, Ontario, Canada)

% submissions

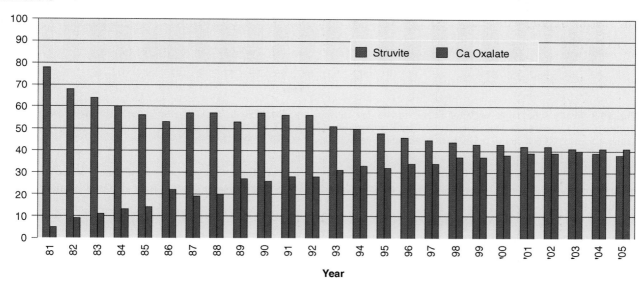

Fig. 10.7 Yearly submission, as percentage of canine struvite and calcium oxalate (CaOx) stones, to the Minnesota Urolith Center. Based on the quantitative analysis of approximately 93,000 stones (Modified from[32]). Note the continuous increase in CaOx over time

struvite predominated in the 1980s, there has been a progressive increase in the number of CaOx uroliths in dogs, reported in several studies around the world. In the USA, the prevalence of CaOx increased dramatically from 5% in 1981 to 41% in 2005 while struvite declined from 78% to 38% (Fig. 10.7).[4,14,16,22,32] In Canada (Table 10.2), Italy, the Czech Republic, Belgium, the Netherlands, and Luxembourg, CaOx surpassed struvite uroliths by 2002/2003.[19,21,24,33,34] In Germany and Spain, struvite, followed by cystine, were the most frequent in the 1980s and 1990s, but the prevalence of both have since declined.[2,35–38]

Feline struvite uroliths far outnumbered CaOx before the late 1980s in the USA.[23] By the mid 1980s, struvite submissions to the University of Minnesota Urolith Center began to

Table 10.2 The most common uroliths in dogs in Canada

Urolith type	% Canine urolith submissions, by year						
	1998	2000	2002	2003	2005	2006	2007
Struvite	52	42	40	42	39	32	30
Calcium oxalate	38	41	43	45	47	48	50
Urate	6	5	4	4	3	3	2

Data from the Canadian Veterinary Urolith Centre. Note that calcium oxalate submissions surpassed struvite in 2002[19,33]

% submissions

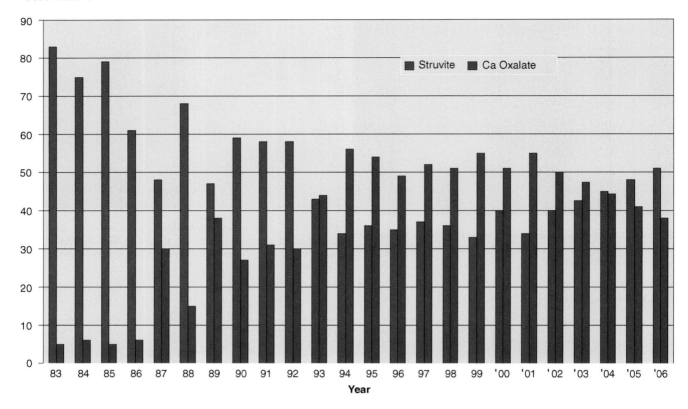

Fig. 10.8 Yearly submission, as % of feline struvite and calcium oxalate (CaOx) stones to the Minnesota Urolith Center, over the past 23 years; a total of 83,601 feline stones have been submitted over this period. Note the large increase in CaOx submissions starting in 1987, with CaOx the most prevalent stone until 2001; the reversal of this trend started in 2002 (Modified from[39,40])

decline, and, by the mid 1990s, CaOx became the most prevalent urolith in North America (Fig. 10.8), Canada (Table 10.3), and other parts of the world.[2,8,11,18,23,24,39,41] However, since 2002, feline struvite uroliths have been on the rise again and have surpassed CaOx as the number one urolith submission in the USA. In Canada, CaOx continues to be the most frequent submission to the CVUC.[41] In Hong Kong, Italy, and the UK in 1998–2000, struvite uroliths were most prevalent followed by CaOx.[34] In the Netherlands, CaOx was most frequent in the same time period, followed by struvite.[2,34] The geographical differences in the relative proportions of CaOx and struvite uroliths may be related to factors including climate and lifestyle.[34] For example, reported cases of urolithiasis increased following periods of inclement weather during which cats tended to remain indoors for prolonged periods of time.[42] Inactivity and foods with low moisture content may also play a role.[42]

10.3 Clinical Signs

The clinical presentation of a dog or cat with urolithiasis depends on the location, number, and physical characteristics of the urolith(s), and whether or not a UTI is present. In some cases, there are no clinical signs. In other cases, the animal may present with a history of LUTD signs including dysuria/stranguria, hematuria, pollakiuria, and inappropriate urination. Upper urinary tract signs include abdominal pain and hematuria, while systemic signs include anorexia and depression. In cases of pyelonephritis, fever may be present, while obstruction is indicated by inability to urinate and systemic signs of postrenal uremia (e.g., vomiting, depression). Some uroliths can be palpated in the bladder, but diagnosis often requires abdominal and pelvic radiography, or ultrasound examination. Double-contrast radiography may be required as some urolith types are not radioopaque. Based on the species, breed, sex, age, dietary history, medical history, and radiography, it is sometimes possible to accurately guess the nature of the urolith (e.g., a male Dalmatian is likely to have urate stones),

Table 10.3 The most common uroliths in cats in Canada

Urolith type	% Feline urolith submissions, by year							
	1998	2001	2002	2003	2004	2005	2006	2007
Struvite	48	39	39	42	43	45	41	43
Calcium oxalate	45	54	52	48	50	45	50	49
Urate	4	3	3	4	4	5	5	5

Data from the Canadian Veterinary Urolith Center[18,33]

but a definitive composition requires quantitative analysis; all uroliths – removed or voided – should be evaluated.

10.4 Dog and Cat Urine Composition

Cats are able to produce more concentrated urine (specific gravity of up to 1.095) than either humans or dogs.[43] However, frequency of meals and variation in dietary moisture, fiber, sodium, potassium, and protein content can result in a two- to threefold variation in urine volume (10–30 mL kg^{-1} day^{-1}).[44–47] Despite the higher dietary mineral intake of dogs and cats, their urinary calcium concentration is significantly lower than humans, whereas their oxalate concentration is significantly higher (Table 10.4).[43,48] The calcium:oxalate ratio is thus closer to one (slightly lower in cats, slightly higher in dogs) than in humans, and thus changes in either calcium or oxalate concentrations can affect supersaturation. Urinary pH is affected by diet, postprandial interval, stress, physiological status (e.g., growth), as well as equipment used to measure the pH. A urinary pH below 6.0 usually reflects some level of mild metabolic acidosis[44,49]; dogs can achieve a lower urinary pH (as low as 5.0) than cats (pH generally >5.5).

Artefactual struvite crystaluria is common in cat urine samples if the urine is concentrated, and the sample is allowed to cool down, or there is a delay before evaluation. The type of crystals in the urine does not necessarily reflect the nature of the stone present at the same time, although cystine crystals are pathognomonic for cystinuria.

10.5 Canine Uroliths

Small breeds – most noticeably the miniature schnauzer, bichon frise, shih tzu, lhasa apso, Yorkshire terrier, and miniature poodle – represent over 50% of canine uroliths submitted for analysis worldwide[4,14,17,19,21,22,34,50,51] (Table 10.5). The predisposition for smaller breeds may be related to their lower urine volume and fewer micturitions[20,52] (Fig. 10.9). Most forms of urolithiasis are more common in male dogs, whereas struvite urolithiasis has a higher incidence in female dogs. The average age for development of a urolith is middle age (mean 6 [range 1–8] years); calcium-containing uroliths (CaOx and phosphate) tend to be found in older (mean 8.5 [range 6–12] years) dogs. Other factors that help predict urolith composition are listed in Table 10.6.

Table 10.4 Comparison of urine composition between dogs and cats fed various diets[48]

Species	N	Units	Urinary concentrations					RSS		pH
			Calcium	Oxalate	Ammonia	Phosphate	Magnesium	Struvite	CaOx	
			mMol/L							
Dog (Dry)	317	Mean ± SD	1.94 ± 0.98	1.14 ± 0.75	96 ± 47	33 ± 23	3.61 ± 2.38	1.5 ± 6.0	10.0 ± 7.0	6.3 ± 0.8
		Range	0.32–7.21	0.12–4.38	5–357	1–119	0.17–15.32			
Cat (Dry)	2386	Mean ± SD	0.95 ± 0.58	1.66 ± 0.73	184 ± 63	84 ± 100	4.10 ± 2.30	1.3 ± 1.9	4.1 ± 2.4	6.4 ± 0.4
		Range	0.10–6.33	0.38–7.46	25–517	1–3593	0.04–15.47			
Cat (Wet)	178	Mean ± SD	0.64 ± 0.52	0.74 ± 0.48	97 ± 77	50 ± 27	2.39 ± 1.63	0.6 ± 0.5	2.2 ± 2.0	6.7 ± 0.5
		Range	0.02–3.31	0.17–2.67	14–372	15–130	0.33–9.51			

RSS relative supersaturation, *N* number of individual urine samples analyzed, *Dog (Dry)* dogs being fed various dry expanded food (<14% moisture), *Cat (Dry)* cats being fed various dry expanded diets, *Cat (Wet)* cats being fed various moist food (moisture >75%).

Table 10.5 Age, breed, and sex predispositions for urolithiasis in dogs

Urolith type	Commonly affected dogs		
	Age	Breed	Sex
Struvite	1–8 years (mean 6 years)	Miniature Schnauzer, Bichon Frisé, Shih Tzu, Miniature Poodle, Lhasa Apso	Female (>80%)
Calcium oxalate	6–12 years (mean 8.5 years)	Miniature Schnauzer, Lhasa Apso, Cairn Terrier, Yorkshire Terrier, Cocker Spaniel, Bichon Frisé, Shih Tzu, Miniature Poodle	Male (>70%)
Calcium phosphate	5–13 years	Yorkshire Terrier	Male (>70%)
Urate	Mean 3.5 years (mean <1 year with portosystemic shunt)	Dalmatian, English Bulldog. Miniature Schnauzer and Yorkshire Terrier with portosystemic shunt	Male (>85%)
Cystine	2–7 years (mean 5 years), but <1 year in Newfoundland	English Bulldog, Dachshund, Newfoundland	Male (>90%)
Silica	4–9 years	German Shepherd, Old English Sheepdog	Male (>90%)

Adapted from[14]

10.5.1 Struvite

10.5.1.1 Epidemiology

In all published reports, females significantly outnumber males in struvite stone submissions. Most struvite stones (Fig. 10.10) in dogs are infection-induced, and females are at greater risk. This is likely due, at least in part, to the anatomy of the female urethra (short and wide compared with the male).[14,53]

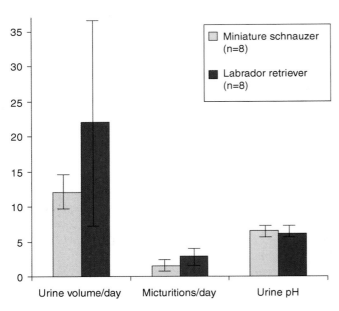

Fig. 10.9 Daily urine volume (mL/kg bodyweight$^{0.75}$), pH, and number of micturitions in Labrador retrievers and miniature schnauzers (Adapted from[20])

10.5.1.2 Pathophysiology

Ascending urea-splitting bacteria, such as *Staphylococcus* (and less commonly, *Proteus* and *Ureaplasma*), are implicated.[50,53] Urease hydrolyses urea, increasing urinary ammonium as well as pH, promoting the precipitation of struvite crystals.[53] Other conditions that promote struvite crystallization – such as foreign bodies in the bladder (Figs. 10.11 through 10.13), alkaline urine, diet, and genetic predisposition – may also be associated with urolith formation.[54–56] A significant number of infection-induced struvite uroliths have a small percentage of other minerals, most noticeably calcium phosphate, associated with them (Figs. 10.14 and 10.15). Recurrent struvite urocystolithiasis has been documented in three related English cocker spaniels.[56] Most dogs with struvite are middle-aged (typically 5–6 years of age) although older

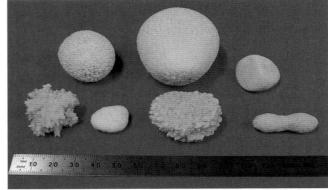

Fig. 10.10 Variability in the appearance of struvite uroliths in dogs (Courtesy of Andrew Moore, CVUC, Guelph, Ontario, Canada)

Table 10.6 Factors that help predict urolith composition in dogs and cats (see also Tables 10.5 and 10.7)

Breed, age, and sex		
Radiographic density of urolith	Calcium oxalate, calcium phosphate	++++
	Struvite, silica	++ to ++++
	Cystine	+ to ++
	Ammonium urate	0 to +
Urine pH	Struvite	Usually alkaline
	Calcium oxalate	No predisposition
	Ammonium urate, silica	Acid to neutral
	Cystine	Acid
Crystalluria	Cystine crystals are pathognomonic for cystinuria, which predisposes to cystine urolithiasis	
Presence of urinary tract infection (especially in dogs), and type of bacteria isolated from urine	Urease-producing bacteria (*Staphylococci, Proteus* spp, *Corynebacterium urealyticum*) suggests struvite urolithiasis (primary or secondary)	
Disease associations (serum chemistry evaluation)	Hypercalcemia may be associated with calcium-containing uroliths	
	Portosystemic shunts predispose to urate urolithiasis	
	Hyperchloremia, hypokalemia, and acidosis may be associated with distal renal tubular acidosis and calcium phosphate or struvite uroliths	
Urine chemistry evaluation	Urine relative supersaturation of various minerals included in the stone	
Family history of particular uroliths		
Quantitative analysis of uroliths passed during voiding, collected via catheter aspiration or by voiding urohydropulsion, or surgically removed		

Adapted from[12]

Labrador retrievers (6–10 years) and cocker spaniels (>10 years) were at risk compared with mixed-breed dogs in one study.[16] Infection-induced struvite is the most frequent type of urolith encountered in immature dogs.[14]

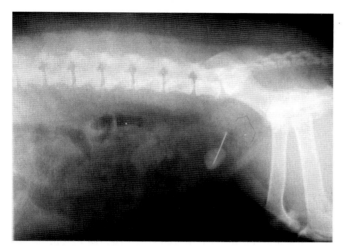

Fig. 10.11 Radiograph showing a sewing needle in the center of an infection-induced struvite bladder urolith in a mixed-breed female dog (Courtesy of Drs. Houston and Eaglesome)

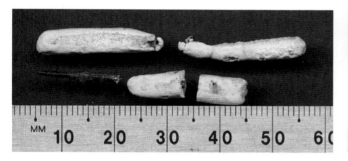

Fig. 10.12 Pine needles (plant material) in the center of infection-induced struvite stones in a dog (Courtesy of Andrew Moore, CVUC, Guelph, Ontario, Canada)

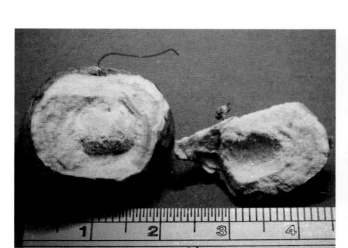

Fig. 10.13 Suture material in the center of a urolith in a dog (Courtesy of Andrew Moore, CVUC, Guelph, Ontario, Canada)

10.5.1.3 Treatment and Prevention

Medical dissolution of struvite uroliths is possible. In dogs, dietary protein restriction reduces the amount of urinary substrate (urea) available for urease-producing bacteria. The urine pH should be in the acidic range (5.8–6.5). Canine diets can be formulated to induce acidic urine by careful dosage of sulfur amino acids, acidifying mineral sources (calcium chloride, calcium sulfate), and acidifiers (phosphoric acid, ammonium chloride), at the same time minimizing the use of alkalinizing mineral sources (calcium carbonate). The efficacy of these so-called acidifying diets has been shown in clinical studies.[57,58] Antibiotics must be administered for as long as the uroliths are visible radiographically, and for one additional month. If a UTI persists despite appropriate antibiotic therapy, acetohydroxamic acid, an inhibitor of microbial urease, may be used[59]; adverse effects include anorexia, vomiting, and hemolytic anemia.[60]

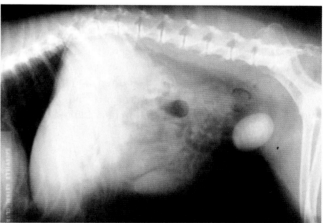

Fig. 10.14 Lateral radiograph showing concentric rings of calcium phosphate in an infection-induced struvite urolith from a female dog (Courtesy of Dr. Susan Purdy, Sackville Animal Hospital, Nova Scotia, Canada)

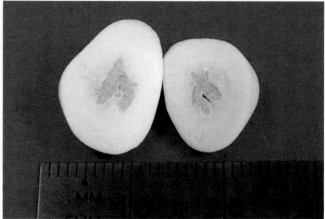

Fig. 10.15 Canine struvite stone with calcium oxalate nidus (Courtesy of Andrew Moore, CVUC, Guelph, Ontario, Canada)

On average, infection-induced struvite uroliths in dogs dissolve in approximately 3–4 months.[57] Following dissolution or mechanical removal of uroliths, a diet designed to help prevent recurrence is recommended. The diet should induce urine undersaturated for struvite (relative supersaturation [RSS] <1),[61] urine pH <6.5, and/or be high in moisture (canned, pouch, or tray product) or designed to encourage diuresis (enhanced with sodium chloride).

10.5.2 CaOx

10.5.2.1 Epidemiology

Males, small breeds (<10 kg), and older dogs are predisposed to CaOx uroliths (Fig. 10.16, Table 10.5).[14,19,34,50,51,62–65] Labrador retrievers, golden retrievers, and German shepherds appear to be at low risk for CaOx uroliths.[34,50,51] Although a genetic basis has not been established as a cause of CaOx formation in dogs, differences in mineral metabolism and urine composition may provide an explanation for such breed susceptibility.[20,64,65] For example, miniature schnauzers urinate significantly less often, and have a lower urine volume, significantly higher urine pH, and significantly higher urinary calcium concentration than Labrador retrievers[20] (Fig. 10.9).

10.5.2.2 Pathophysiology

The pathophysiology of CaOx uroliths is poorly understood. Compared with healthy individuals of the same breed, CaOx stone-formers have higher urinary concentrations of calcium and oxalate, but lower concentrations of potassium and phosphorus.[66,67] CaOx uroliths are rarely associated with UTI, and CaOx crystals can form at any physiological urine pH. A major risk factor for CaOx uroliths is urinary calcium and oxalate supersaturation. Intestinal hyperabsorption of calcium has been reported in stone-forming miniature schnauzers.[65] Other factors that have been suggested to promote CaOx supersaturation include excess dietary intake of calcium, vitamin D, or vitamin C; disorders contributing to hypercalcemia (e.g., lymphoma, primary hyperparathyroidism) or calcium mobilization (hyperadrenocorticism, chronic glucocorticoid treatment); and diets containing large quantities of oxalate (spinach, wheat germ, sweet potatoes).[4,51,62,68,69] Defective nephrocalcin or other natural inhibitors of CaOx uroliths have also been proposed. In epidemiological studies, dry diets – especially those resulting in increased acidification of urine – have been associated with a greater risk for CaOx uroliths.[68,69] Dietary factors associated with a decreased risk of CaOx urolithiasis in dogs include increased dietary water, protein, calcium, phosphorus, magnesium, sodium, potassium, and chloride and decreased carbohydrate content.[66–69]

10.5.2.3 Treatment and Prevention

Medical dissolution of CaOx uroliths is not possible; they require mechanical removal via surgery, voiding urohydropulsion, or lithotripsy, and basket retrieval of urolith fragments. Postsurgical recurrence rates are high (>50% within 3 years), and it is important to open the bladder fully and retrieve all uroliths, and to confirm this with postoperative radiography.[62,63,70,71] At the time of writing, only canine diets promoting diuresis by their high moisture and/or sodium content (around 1% on a dry matter basis) have been shown to reduce CaOx urine RSS in normal dogs, and return stone-formers to the metastable supersaturation range (Fig. 10.17).[66,67,72] Epidemiological studies have identified acidifying dry diets as a risk factor for CaOx; in contrast, a high moisture, high sodium diet reduces CaOx RSS in stone-forming dogs[67,68] (Fig. 10.18) and also has a preventive role.[68,69] The pathophysiology of CaOx uroliths is still poorly understood and the association with acidifying diet might be due to other confounding factors such as the increased lifespan of pets, or pet food formulation changes that have occurred over the same period.[5] The role of urinary pH remains controversial (see also section on **FELINE UROLITHS: CaOx**).[5,73] Hydrochlorothiazide diuretics may be used in dogs with recurring CaOx urolithiasis.[63]

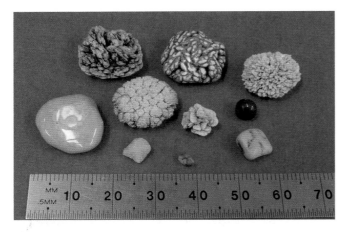

Fig. 10.16 Variability in appearance of calcium oxalate uroliths in dogs (Courtesy of Andrew Moore, CVUC, Guelph, Ontario, Canada)

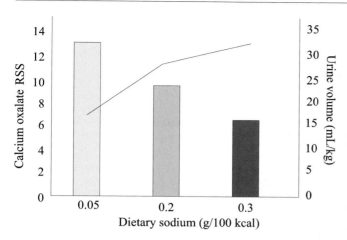

Fig. 10.17 The effect of dietary sodium content on calcium oxalate relative supersaturation (RSS) and urine volume in miniature schnauzers (Used with permission from[66])

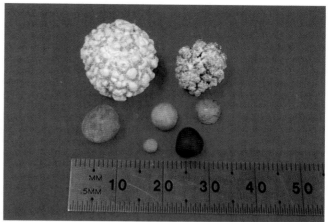

Fig. 10.19 Canine purine (ammonium urate) stones (Courtesy of Andrew Moore, CVUC, Guelph, Ontario, Canada)

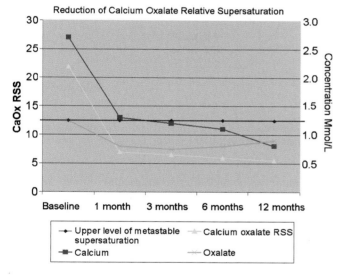

Fig. 10.18 Reduction of calcium oxalate relative supersaturation to within the metastable range (1–12) in stone-forming dogs (n = 17) after being fed a high moisture, high sodium (1% on a dry matter basis) diet for 1 year (Adapted from.[67])

10.5.3 Purine

10.5.3.1 Epidemiology

Purine uroliths (ammonium urate, sodium urate, calcium urate, uric acid, and xanthine; Fig. 10.19) account for 5–10% of uroliths submitted to stone laboratories and are the third most common urolith in dogs.[4,14,19,21,34,74,75] The most commonly affected breed is the Dalmatian; others include the English bulldog, miniature schnauzer, shih tzu, Yorkshire terrier, cocker spaniel, and black Russian terrier.[19,35,76] A familial tendency has been suggested for English bulldogs.[75]

10.5.3.2 Pathophysiology

All Dalmatians are genetically (autosomal recessive) at risk,[77–80] although not all suffer clinically, and males are significantly more affected than females.[19,21,74,75,77,81,82] Most females never show clinical signs, most likely due to the small size of the stones and the anatomical differences between the sexes.[77] Other factors may also modulate the phenotypic expression of the mutation – the urinary excretion of Tamm-Horsfall protein (THP) and glycosaminoglycans (GAGs) in hyperuricosuric, stone-forming Dalmatians is lower than in nonstone-formers.[83] Other susceptible breeds (black Russian terrier) have the same mutation.[77]

The molecular nature of this genetic disease has been determined. The mutation means that affected dogs are less efficient at metabolizing uric acid to allantoin in their liver, and urate is less efficiently reabsorbed in the renal proximal tubule because of a mutation in the gene $SLC2A9$ coding for the protein responsible for the transport of urate across the cell membrane of those tissues[77] (Fig. 10.20). Dalmatians convert only 30–40% of uric acid to allantoin and excrete 20-fold higher amounts (400–600 mg/day) of urate in their urine than normal dogs.[75] Hyperuricemia (1–2 mg/dL versus <0.5 mg/dL in normal dogs) is present in Dalmatians, but it does not induce gout (as it would in humans), probably due to a lower serum concentration (1–2 mg/dL versus 3–7 mg/dL, respectively). Hyperuricosuria predisposes affected dogs to forming urinary stones, LUTD signs, and obstruction.

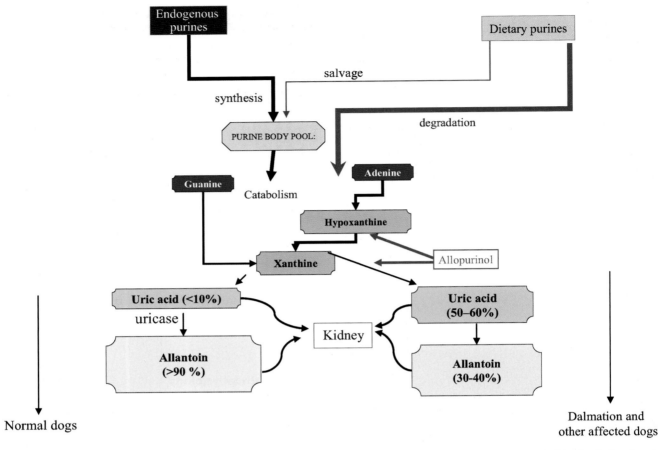

Fig. 10.20 Purine metabolism in normal and Dalmatian dogs (and other affected breeds). Because of a defect in the uric acid transport system in the hepatocytes and the proximal tubules of the kidney,

purine catabolism results in hyperuricosuria. Number in brackets is percentage excretion, in the urine, of purine as uric acid or allantoin

Younger animals with portosystemic vascular shunts are also at risk for purine stones,[75,79] and severe hepatic dysfunction (regardless of cause) may predispose any breed to urate uroliths.[4]

10.5.3.3 Treatment and Prevention

Surgical therapy is temporarily curative but medical therapy is required to minimize recurrence. Recurrence rates for urate uroliths are 33–50%, generally within 1 year, although in as little as 3–6 months in a high-risk dog without dietary/drug intervention.[75,82] Medical management consists of feeding a low purine, and low-to-moderate protein, diet as well as promoting diuresis.[75,84] A urinary pH of 6.5–7.0 is targeted. Urinary pH above 7.5 should be avoided as this increases the risk of calcium phosphate precipitation, while a more acidic pH promotes precipitation of uric acid.[4] It is possible to dissolve purine stones: a low purine diet, in combination with allopurinol and increased diuresis, is recommended.[75] The urine pH should be maintained at 6.5–7.0 to minimize levels of ammonia and ammonium ions, decreasing the risk of

ammonium urate urolithiasis. Potassium citrate may be needed to help maintain alkaline urine. Allopurinol, an inhibitor of xanthine oxidase (the enzyme responsible for catalyzing the conversion of xanthine and hypoxanthine to uric acid) is recommended to decrease urinary uric acid excretion in dogs. However, as when used for leishmaniasis, allopurinol treatment must be accompanied by a low purine diet to prevent the formation of xanthine stones.

Xanthine urolithiasis (Fig. 10.21) occurs naturally (although uncommonly) in some breeds (e.g., cavalier King Charles spaniel, dachshund).[2,85,86] Mechanical or surgical removal of xanthine uroliths is necessary as no medical dissolution protocol is available.

10.5.4 Cystine

10.5.4.1 Pathophysiology

Cystinuria is an inborn error of metabolism characterized by defective proximal tubular reabsorption of cystine and other

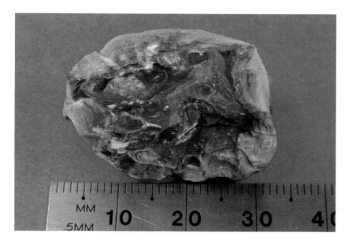

Fig. 10.21 Xanthine urolith from a dog (Courtesy of Andrew Moore, CVUC, Guelph, Ontario, Canada)

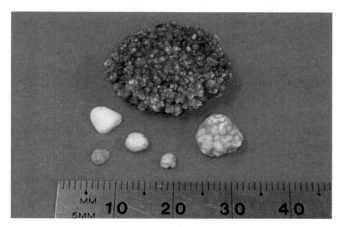

Fig. 10.22 Cystine calculi from a dog (Courtesy of Andrew Moore, CVUC, Guelph, Ontario, Canada)

amino acids (lysine, arginine, ornithine, citrulline, taurine, threonine, cystathionine, glutamine, and glutaminic acid).[87] Cystinuric dogs (Fig. 10.22) reabsorb a much smaller proportion of cystine than is filtered by the glomerulus, and some may even have net cystine secretion.[88] Not all cystinuric dogs form uroliths. In those that do, recurrence is common (38%), usually within a year.[89] Dogs with cystinuria can also have carnitinuria, with its associated increased risk of carnitine deficiency.[90]

Canine cystinuria is genetically heterogeneous; it has been recognized in more than 60 breeds worldwide with variable patterns of aminoaciduria.[88,89,91–95] A European study showed that cystine stones are most likely to affect Irish terriers, basset hounds and Munsterlanders, while, in Germany, dachshunds are most frequently affected, possibly due to their widespread popularity.[2] In North America, cystine stones are especially common in English bulldogs and Newfoundlands.[14,19]

The mode of inheritance has been documented in the Newfoundland to be a simple autosomal recessive pattern.[88,92] In French and English bulldogs, the genes *SLC3A1* and

SLC7A9 have been implicated.[96] Pedigrees from inbred lines of dachshunds, basset hounds, and Rottweilers suggest a sex-linked or autosomal recessive pattern of inheritance.[95]

10.5.4.2 Treatment and Prevention

For cystine dissolution, a low protein diet (25–50 g protein/1,000 kcal) is recommended, and this should be supplemented with carnitine (50–100 mg/kg orally, three times a day) and taurine (500 mg orally, twice a day).[90] Additional alkalinization may be needed with potassium citrate. N-(2-mercaptopropionyl)-glycine (2-MPG), a thiol-containing drug, is indicated for cystine urolith dissolution and prevention. These drugs react with cystine by a thiol disulfide exchange reaction, resulting in the formation of a complex that is more soluble in urine than cystine.[57]

10.5.5 Silica

Approximately 1% of submissions in North America are silica uroliths (Fig. 10.23).[4,19] They may occur in dogs with pica (i.e., eating soil) or in dogs eating diets high in cereal grains containing silicates (e.g., corn gluten and soybean hulls).[97] Silica crystals are not shed into the urine, and silica uroliths may be an incidental finding in some dogs. For prevention, a good quality dog food is recommended.

10.5.6 Calcium Phosphate

Calcium phosphate crystals are commonly found as a minor component within struvite and CaOx uroliths, and are more

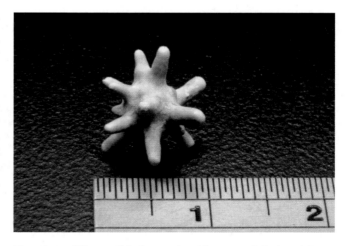

Fig. 10.23 Silica urolith from a dog (Courtesy of Andrew Moore, CVUC, Guelph, Ontario, Canada)

likely at high urine pH (>7.5).[4] Calcium phosphate uroliths occur in the same breeds as CaOx uroliths, and the risk factors are similar (including primary hyperparathyroidism, other hypercalcemia disorders, renal tubular acidosis, idiopathic hypercalciuria, and excessive dietary calcium and phosphorus ingestion).[98]

10.5.7 Pyrophosphate and DSBC

Pyrophosphate and DSBC are uncommon and, in dogs, little is known about them at this time. Further discussion on these urolith types is found in sections on feline **Potassium magnesium pyrophosphate** and **DSBC**.

10.5.8 Compound Uroliths

Compound uroliths consist of a nucleus of one mineral type and a shell of another mineral type (Figs. 10.14 and 10.15). They form because the factors promoting precipitation and formation of one type of urolith supersede earlier factors promoting the precipitation of another type. Some mineral types may also function as a nidus for deposition of another mineral; for example, all uroliths predispose to UTI, which may result in secondary struvite precipitation.[4]

10.5.9 Drug Metabolites Appearing as Urinary Stones

These are rare in dogs. First-generation sulphonamides, sulphadiazine, tetracycline, trimethoprim sulpha, enroflaxacin, and antacids have been implicated, with sulphonamide and sulphadiazine most frequently reported.[99]

10.6 Feline Uroliths

Uroliths are associated with around 20% of feline LUTD cases. Urethral obstruction is quite uncommon in cats with stones. Although most uroliths are found in the bladder, the prevalence of kidney and ureteral stones has increased, especially in cats with renal disease.[26] Age, breed, and sex predispositions have been reported in cats (Table 10.7). As in the dog, the composition of uroliths can also be predicted based on radiographic appearance, urine analysis and appearance of sediment, presence of UTI, and association with other diseases (Table 10.6), but all uroliths removed should be submitted for quantitative analysis.

10.6.1 Struvite

10.6.1.1 Epidemiology

Struvite (Fig. 10.24) is one of the most common minerals found in feline uroliths and urethral plugs. Himalayan, Persian, and mixed-breed domestic cats are commonly implicated, but they are also the most popular breeds. Rex, Burmese, Abyssinian, Russian blue, Birman, and Siamese cats appear to be at lower risk of developing struvite uroliths.[8,100–102] Some, but not all, authors have reported a higher incidence in females than males.[3,18] Although struvite can occur at any age, most occur in middle age (mean 7 ± standard deviation 3.5 years).[3,8,18]

10.6.1.2 Pathophysiology

In cats, the majority of struvite uroliths are sterile.[8,12,51,100,101,103] Infection with urease-splitting organisms is rare, except in kittens, elderly cats (>10 years of age), and those with concomitant disease (e.g., perineal urethrostomies, diabetes mellitus, hyperthyroidism, chronic

Table 10.7 Age, breed, and sex predispositions for urolithiasis in cats

Urolith type	Average age	Commonly affected breeds	Sex
Struvite	5.8 years	Domestic shorthair (mixed breed), Himalayan, Persian, Ragdoll, Chartreux	Relatively equal
Calcium oxalate	7.5 years	Himalayan, Persian, Ragdoll, domestic shorthair (mixed breed)	Male 1.5 times > female
Calcium phosphate	8 years	None	?
Urate	5 months to 15 years	Egyptian Mau, Siamese	Males slightly > females
Cystine	Middle age	None	Males slightly > females
Silica	?	None	Male

Adapted from[41]

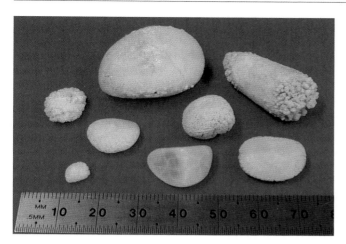

Fig. 10.24 Variability in appearance of struvite stones in cats. Note that although many struvite uroliths take on a wafer-shaped appearance like the urolith in the *bottom right hand corner*, there is wide variability in appearance (Courtesy of Andrew Moore, CVUC, Guelph, Ontario, Canada)

renal failure). The resistance of cats to ascending infection is due to the concentrated nature (specific gravity 1.025–1.090) and low pH (5.8–6.5) of their urine. The main cause of struvite uroliths in cats is urinary supersaturation with magnesium, ammonium, and phosphate; as well as elevated urinary pH (>6.5), because of poor diet formulation (see acidifying diets under *Treatment and Prevention*).

10.6.1.3 Urinary Plugs

A common cause of feline LUTD is the presence of gritty material, comprising large quantities of a proteinaceous matrix, which can aggregate in the urethra of male cats and form a urethral plug. In 16% of cases, urethral plugs are composed of the matrix alone, but 75.7% also contain struvite crystals; a minority (1.4%) comprises matrix and CaOx crystals.[104] Plugs are the most common cause of urethral obstruction and occur mostly in young (<4 years of age) male (97.4%) cats.[104] The pathophysiology underlying the formation of the proteinaceous matrix is still poorly understood but inflammation (of unknown origin) is the proposed hypothesis.[104]

10.6.1.4 Treatment and Prevention

Struvite crystal formation can be prevented, and struvite uroliths can be dissolved, by feeding a diet that induces a urine pH below 6.5 and contains moderate amounts of magnesium.[105–108] Urine pH is a much more important factor than dietary magnesium, however.[105] The ability of a diet to acidify

urine depends on the ingredients used and the addition of acidifiers such as methionine and phosphoric acid. Animal proteins, corn gluten, digests, and mineral salts such as calcium chloride or calcium sulfate promote acidic urine. Most vegetable proteins and mineral salts such as calcium carbonate promote alkaline urine. Urine acidification is not without potential toxicity. Excessive acid load (urine pH <6.0) can overwhelm the ability of the kidney to excrete protons and induce uncompensated metabolic acidosis. Chronic acidosis in cats increases urinary potassium loss and can lead to potassium deficiency. Excessive acidification may slow growth, increase calcium excretion, and promote bone demineralization. Urine dilution and increased urinary flow reduces the concentration of lithogenic substances and, by increasing the frequency of micturitions, reduces the time available for solutes to form crystals and stones. Diuresis can be stimulated by increased water intake, which can be achieved by feeding diets containing >75% moisture and by increasing the frequency of meals[46] (Fig. 10.25), and/or by a high dietary sodium content (2.5 g/1,000 kcal).[5,47,109,110]

The efficacy of magnesium-restricted, urine acidifying, canned[107,108] and dry[108,111] diets designed to dissolve feline struvite uroliths has been shown. Usually, struvite uroliths in cats dissolve in approximately 1 month. It is recommended that therapy should continue for 1 month after radiographic documentation of struvite dissolution. If the struvite stone is associated with a UTI, antibiotic therapy is required alongside the dietary management, and urine culture should be performed 1 month after complete dissolution of the stone. Following treatment for obstruction with a urethral plug associated with struvite crystals, it is recommended to feed lifelong an acidifying diet and to promote water consumption as long-term prophylaxis.[104]

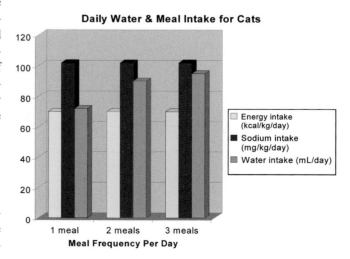

Fig. 10.25 Water consumption and daily frequency of meals in cats (Adapted from[46])

10.6.2 CaOx

10.6.2.1 Epidemiology

CaOx (Fig. 10.26) is the other common urolith found in cats. Most prevalent at the end of the 1990s, the latest surveys indicate that CaOx uroliths have subsequently declined, and are now slightly less frequent than struvite (Fig. 10.8).[2,23,40] Himalayans and Persians appear to be at risk for CaOx urolithiasis.[8,18] Indoor housing and older age (mean 10.6 ± 1.3 years) are also risk factors.[11,42,113]

10.6.2.2 Pathophysiology

Although not proven, the surge of CaOx submissions in the mid 1980s in North America (Fig. 10.8) and in the 1990s in Western Europe has been attributed to the widespread use of acidifying diets; as well as unmasking other causes of LUTD, these diets could promote CaOx formation.[3,9,40,73] Several retrospective case-controlled studies have found a positive association between the acidifying potential of commercial diets and the risk of CaOx uroliths.[101,112,113] Persistent aciduria may be associated with low-grade metabolic acidosis, resulting in increased urinary excretion of calcium (hypercalciuria).[13,20] In five cats with hypercalcemia and CaOx uroliths, discontinuation of acidifying diets or urinary acidifiers was associated with normalization of serum calcium concentration.[114] However, many cats are fed acidifying diets and yet few appear to develop hypercalcemia, metabolic acidosis, and CaOx urolithiasis. Also, the authors found that in normal cats, urinary pH was a rather poor predictor of CaOx RSS.[5,115] More work in stone-forming cats is necessary on this issue.

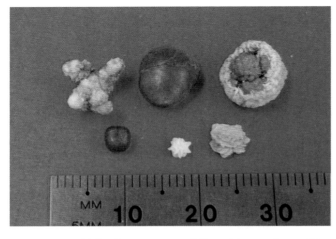

Fig. 10.26 Variability in appearance of feline calcium oxalate uroliths. Most often, calcium oxalate dihydrate has a speckled appearance as in *bottom right hand corner* of the figure; calcium oxalate monohydrate may appear *round* as in the *bottom left hand corner* (Courtesy of Andrew Moore, CVUC, Guelph, Ontario, Canada)

Other environmental factors might be involved. Case-controlled studies have found that aside from their moderate acidifying potential, diets with the highest levels of moisture, protein, sodium, and potassium, and with moderate levels of calcium, phosphorus, magnesium, fat, and carbohydrates, and low fiber contents were associated with a decreased risk for CaOx.[8,112] Excessive levels of vitamin D (>500 IU/1,000 kcal, because of its role in calcium absorption) and vitamin C (>50 mg/1,000 kcal, because it is a precursor of oxalic acid) should be avoided.[40] Experimentally induced vitamin B_6 deficiency, resulting in increased urinary oxalate concentrations and oxalate nephrocalcinosis, has been reported in kittens,[116] but a naturally occurring form of this syndrome is yet to be reported. Furthermore, supplementation with vitamin B_6 does not decrease urinary oxalic acid excretion compared with a diet containing adequate levels of vitamin B_6.[117] Both dietary magnesium restriction and supplementation have been associated with increased risk of CaOx urolithiasis in cats; consequently, diets should be neither severely restricted in, nor supplemented with, magnesium.[101]

Diets high in sodium (e.g., 1.75–5.2 g/1,000 kcal) and moisture (75–85%) are highly effective in stimulating water consumption and diuresis in cats (Fig. 10.27a, b, c),[5,47,109,110] and, as in dogs, reduce CaOx RSS.[72,110,118–121] Increased diuresis promotes urine dilution and increased frequency of micturition, providing insufficient time for the nucleation and aggregation of urine crystals.[44]

Higher salt intake has been associated with increased urinary calcium excretion in humans, dogs, and cats.[12,47] This led to the assumption that high salt diets could promote CaOx formation in both dogs and cats, and thus to the recommendation that diets designed for the management of LUTD should be low in sodium.[12] However, although increased sodium intake increases calcium excretion, urinary calcium concentration does not increase because of the concomitant increase in urine volume and significant decrease in CaOx RSS.[72,110,115,118–121] The levels of dietary salt that stimulate diuresis do not appear to affect blood pressure; this has been shown in healthy pets, in cats with early renal disease, as well as in feline models of renal failure.[122–124]

10.6.2.3 Treatment and Prevention

To date, no diet or treatment will promote the dissolution of CaOx uroliths. If they cannot be voided by urohydropropulsion, surgery is the only practical alternative. Hypercalcemia has been reported in up to 35% of cats with CaOx uroliths.[13,125,126] Serum calcium levels and urinary excretion should be checked and corrected if necessary. The use of hydrochlorothiazide has been suggested for use in cats, but its efficacy and safety have not been evaluated in those with CaOx uroliths. The recurrence rate for CaOx uroliths is 7.1%, occurring within a few years (mean 23 months).[127]

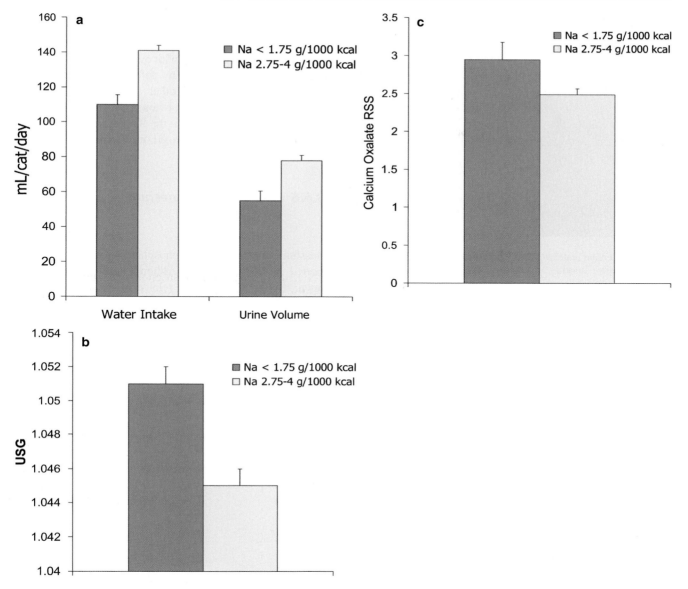

Fig. 10.27 Effect of dietary sodium on water balance, urine specific gravity (USG), and calcium oxalate (CaOx) relative supersaturation (RSS). (**a**) Cats fed diets containing a moderate sodium content (2.75–4.0 g/1,000 kcal) had significantly higher water intake and urine volume, and (**b**) significantly lower urine specific gravity, and (**c**) calcium oxalate RSS compared with cats fed lower sodium (<1.75 g/1,000 kcal) diets

Therefore, CaOx stone-forming cats should be fed a diet promoting diuresis and low CaOx RSS.

10.6.3 Purine

10.6.3.1 Epidemiology

Purine uroliths (Fig. 10.28) are the third most common type in cats. Ammonium urate is the most common, but sodium urate, sodium calcium urate, and potassium urate also occur; uric acid and xanthine uroliths are less frequent. Purine uroliths account for around 5–8% of stone submissions in cats[18,33,40,103] and this has not changed significantly in the last 2 decades (Table 10.3). In Canada, a significant number of urate submissions were from Egyptian Maus and further investigations in this breed are underway.[18,33] Xanthine uroliths are rare and may be due to an inborn error of purine metabolism or administration of allopurinol.[128] In most cases, no identifying risk factors are observed, and there is no apparent breed, age, or sex predisposition.[13,129,130] The risk of recurrence is high (within 3–12 months).[13,128–130]

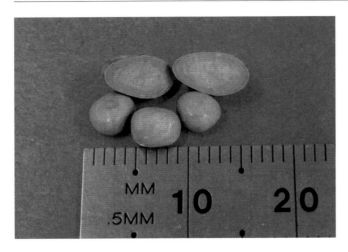

Fig. 10.28 Feline urate urolith (Courtesy of Andrew Moore, CVUC, Guelph, Ontario, Canada)

10.6.3.2 Pathophysiology

Urate uroliths may occur in cats with portosystemic shunts or any form of severe hepatic dysfunction. Other risk factors include UTI (leading to increased urinary ammonia), metabolic acidosis, highly acidic urine, and high dietary purine intake (e.g., liver or other organ meats).[17,129] The exact pathogenesis in most cats remains unknown.[102] Recurrence rates are 10.9% (mean 20 months). The recurrence rate is 1.8 times higher in females than in males.[127]

10.6.3.3 Treatment and Prevention

Diets low in purines and protein are recommended to help prevent these metabolic uroliths. The efficacy and potential toxicity of allopurinol in cats is unknown and, consequently, its use is not recommended.

10.6.4 Calcium Phosphate

Calcium phosphate uroliths are uncommon in cats. Hydroxyapatite and carbonate apatite are the most common forms; brushite (calcium hydrogen phosphate dihydrate) is less common. Pure calcium phosphate uroliths may be associated with primary hyperparathyroidism, disorders that predispose to hypercalciuria (hypercalcemia, vitamin D intoxication, systemic acidosis, excess dietary calcium), disorders that predispose to hyperphosphaturia (excess dietary phosphorus), decreased urine volume, highly alkaline urine, and, at least for nephroliths, the presence of blood clots.[13] They often occur as a minor component in struvite and CaOx stones.

10.6.5 Cystine

Cystine uroliths occur in cats with cystinuria, an inborn error of metabolism characterized by defective proximal tubular reabsorption of cystine and other amino acids (ornithine, lysine, arginine).[13,17,129,131] No obvious gender or other predisposition has been reported, but the Siamese breed may be at risk.[8,15] Most cats are middle-aged or older.[7]

10.6.6 Potassium Magnesium Pyrophosphate

Potassium magnesium pyrophosphate uroliths have been reported in Persian cats.[132] Although the etiology is not known, it is postulated to be related to some temporary or permanent enzymatic dysfunction, causing pyrophosphate supersaturation of the urine and leading to crystallization of the urolith.[132]

10.6.7 DSBC

Dried solidified blood calculi (DSBC) have been reported in North American cats.[133] The etiology is unknown. They generally contain no crystalline material, and are thought to be formed from organic material (Fig. 10.29). Many are radiolucent.

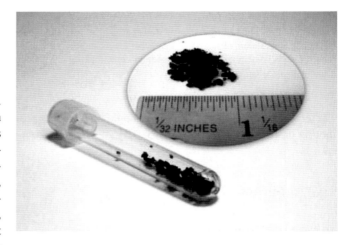

Fig. 10.29 Dried solidified blood calculi (Courtesy of Andrew Moore, CVUC, Guelph, Ontario, Canada)

10.6.8 Compound Uroliths and Drug Metabolite Containing Uroliths

Descriptions are found under the **CANINE UROLITHS** section.

10.7 Conclusions

In both dogs and cats, uroliths are common and represent one-fifth of cases of LUTD. Contrary to common belief, urinary stones are more common in dogs, especially small dogs than in cats. Upper urinary tract uroliths are less common than in humans, but their prevalence is increasing, especially in cats. Dietary management modulates the occurrence of struvite and purine stones in both dogs and cats. The pathophysiology of CaOx stones is probably multifactorial, and the exact roles of diet and urinary pH remain to be investigated. Pending this work, promotion of diuresis and urine dilution by feeding a moist and/or higher sodium diet could be beneficial in both dogs and cats. Prevalence of other stone types is low in both dogs and cats; their treatment is a combination of surgical, dietary, and medical management.

References

1. Robinson MR, Norris RD, Sur RL, et al. Urolithiasis: not just a 2-legged animal disease. *J Urol.* 2008;179:46-52.
2. Hesse A, Neiger R. *Harnsteine bei Kleintieren.* Stuttgart, Germany: Enke Verlag; 2008:1-192.
3. Osborne CA, Kruger JM, Lulich JP, et al. Feline lower urinary tract diseases. In: Ettinger SJ, Feldman EC, eds. *Textbook of Veterinary Internal Medicine.* 5th ed. Philadelphia, PA: WB Saunders; 2000:1710-1747.
4. Lulich JP, Osborne CA, Bartges JW, et al. Canine lower urinary tract disorders. In: Ettinger SJ, Feldman EC, eds. *Textbook of Veterinary Internal Medicine.* 5th ed. Philadelphia, PA: WB Saunders; 2000:1747-1781.
5. Biourge V, Kirk CA. Managing struvite/oxalate urolithiasis. Point/Counterpoint. Proceedings of The North American Veterinary Conference; January 7–11, 2006:749-752, Orlando, FL.
6. Bartges JW, Kirk C, Lane IF. Update: management of calcium oxalate uroliths in dogs and cats. *Vet Clin North Am Small Anim Pract.* 2004;34:969-987.
7. Kruger JM, Osborne CA, Goyal SM, et al. Clinical evaluation of cats with lower urinary tract disease. *J Am Vet Med Assoc.* 1991;199:211-216.
8. Lekcharoensuk C, Osborne CA, Lulich JP. Epidemiologic study of risk factors for lower urinary tract diseases in cats. *J Am Vet Med Assoc.* 2001;218:1429-1435.
9. Buffington CA, Chew DJ, Kendall MS, et al. Clinical evaluation of cats with nonobstructive lower urinary tract diseases. *J Am Vet Med Assoc.* 1997;210:46-50.
10. Chew DJ, Buffington CA. Advances in lower urinary tract diseases. Proceedings of the 23rd Waltham/OSU Symposium; Ohio; 1999:42-49.
11. Gerber B, Boretti FS, Kley S, et al. Evaluation of clinical signs and causes of lower urinary tract disease in European cats. *J Small Anim Pract.* 2005;46:571-577.
12. Osborne CA, Kruger JM, Lulich JP, et al. Feline lower urinary tract diseases. In: Ettinger SJ, Feldman EC, eds. *Textbook of Veterinary Internal Medicine.* 4th ed. Philadelphia, PA: WB Saunders; 1995:1805-1832.
13. Osborne CA, Lulich JP, Thumchai R, et al. Feline urolithiasis. Etiology and pathophysiology. *Vet Clin North Am Small Anim Pract.* 1996;26:217-232.
14. Osborne CA, Lulich JP, Polzin DJ, et al. Analysis of 77,000 canine uroliths. Perspectives from the Minnesota Urolith Center. *Vet Clin North Am Small Anim Pract.* 1999;29:17-38.
15. Ling GV, Franti CE, Ruby AL, et al. Epizootiologic evaluation and quantitative analysis of urinary calculi from 150 cats. *J Am Vet Med Assoc.* 1990;196:1459-1462.
16. Ling GV, Thurmond MC, Choi YK, et al. Changes in proportion of canine urinary calculi composed of calcium oxalate or struvite in specimens analyzed from 1981 through 2001. *J Vet Intern Med.* 2003;17:817-823.
17. Ling GV. Urinary stone disease. In: Ling GV, ed. *Lower Urinary Tract Diseases of Dogs and Cats.* Philadelphia, PA: Mosby Year Book; 1995:144-177.
18. Houston DM, Moore AEP, Favrin MG, et al. Feline urethral plugs and bladder uroliths: a review of 5484 submissions 1998–2003. *Can Vet J.* 2003;44:974-977.
19. Houston DM, Moore AEP, Favrin MG, et al. Canine urolithiasis: a look at over 16,000 urolith submissions to the Canadian Veterinary Urolith Center from February 1998 to April 2003. *Can Vet J.* 2004;45:225-230.
20. Stevenson AE, Markwell PJ. Comparison of urine composition of healthy Labrador retrievers and miniature schnauzers. *Am J Vet Res.* 2001;62:1782-1786.
21. Sosnar M, Bulkova T, Ruzicka M. Epidemiology of canine urolithiasis in the Czech Republic from 1997 to 2002. *J Small Anim Pract.* 2005;46:177-184.
22. Osborne CA. Improving management of urolithiasis: canine struvite uroliths. *DVM Mag.* April 1, 2004.
23. Cannon AB, Westropp JL, Ruby AL, et al. Evaluation of trends in urolith composition in cats: 5,230 cases (1985–2004). *J Am Vet Med Assoc.* 2007;231:570-576.
24. Picavet P, Detilleux J, Verschuren S, et al. Analysis of 4495 canine and feline uroliths in the Benelux. A retrospective study: 1994–2004. *J Anim Physiol Anim Nutr (Berl).* 2007;91:247-251.
25. Polzin DJ, Ross SJ, Osborne CA et al. Urolithiasis and feline renal failure part II. Proceedings of the 21st American College of Veterinary Internal Medicine Forum; North Carolina, USA; 2003:785-786.
26. Ross SJ, Osborne CA, Lekcharoensuk C, et al. A case-control study of the effects of nephrolithiasis in cats with chronic kidney disease. *J Am Vet Med Assoc.* 2007;230:1854-1859.
27. Lekcharoensuk C, Osborne CA, Lulich JP, et al. Trends in the frequency of calcium oxalate uroliths in the upper urinary tracts of cats. *J Am Anim Hosp Assoc.* 2005;4:39-46.
28. Cowgill LD. Ureteral obstruction: a new dilemma in feline nephrology. Proceedings of the 23rd forum of American College Veterinary Internal Medicine; Baltimore, MD; 2005:748-749.
29. Ling GV, Ruby AL, Johnson DL, et al. Renal calculi in dogs and cats: prevalence, mineral type, breed, age, and gender interrelationships (1981–1993). *J Vet Intern Med.* 1998;12:11-21.
30. Carter WO, Hawkins EC, Morrison WB. Feline nephrolithiasis: eight cases (1984–1989). *J Am Anim Hosp Assoc.* 1993;29:247-256.

31. Ross SJ, Osborne CA, Lulich JP, et al. Canine and feline nephro-lithiasis. Epidemiology, detection, and management. *Vet Clin North Am Small Anim Pract*. 1999;29:231-249.

32. Osborne CA, Lulich JP. Perspectives: Analysis of 27,500 uroliths. *DVM Mag*. July 1, 2006.

33. Houston DM, Moore AEP, Favrin MG, et al. Data on file, Canadian Veterinary Urolith Centre; 2008.

34. Stevenson AE. The incidence of urolithiasis in cats and dogs and the influence of diet in the formation and prevention of recurrence. PhD thesis, Institute of Urology and Nephrology, University College, London; 2001.

35. Hesse A. Canine urolithiasis: epidemiology and analysis of urinary calculi. *J Small Anim Pract*. 1990;31:599-604.

36. Hesse A, Steffes HJ, Graf C, et al. Current information on the composition and breed distribution of urinary stones in dogs. *Berl Münch Tierärztl Wochenschr*. 1997;110:436-439.

37. Escolar E, Bellanato J, Medina JA. Structure and composition of canine urinary calculi. *Res Vet Sci*. 1990;49:327-333.

38. Hicking W, Hesse A, Gebhardt M, et al. Analytical studies of urinary stones in mammals. *Prog Urol Nephrol*. 1981;17:40-49.

39. Forrester SD. Evidence-based nutritional management of feline lower urinary tract disease. Proceedings of the 24th American College of Veterinary Internal Medicine Forum; Louisville, Kentucky; 2006:510-512.

40. Bartges JW, Kirk CA. Nutrition and lower urinary tract disease in cats. *Vet Clin North Am Small Anim Pract*. 2006;36:1361-1376.

41. Houston DM. Epidemiology of feline urolithiasis. *Vet Focus*. 2007;17:4-9.

42. Jones BR, Sanson RL, Morris RS. Elucidating the risk factors of feline lower urinary tract disease. *NZ Vet J*. 1997;45:100-108.

43. Markwell PJ, Robertson WG, Stevenson AE, et al. Urolithiasis: a comparison of humans, dogs and cats. In: Rodgers AL, Hibbert BE, Hess B, eds. *Urolithiasis*. Cape Town: University of Cape Town; 2000:785-788.

44. Markwell PJ, Buffington CA. Feline lower urinary tract disease. In: Wills J, Simpson K, eds. *The Waltham Book of Clinical Nutrition of the Dog and Cat*. Oxford, UK: Elsevier Science Ltd; 1994:293-312.

45. Burger IH, Anderson RS, Holme DW. Nutritional factors affecting water balance in the dog. In: Anderson RS, ed. *Nutrition of the Dog and Cat*. Oxford, UK: Pergamon; 1980:145-156.

46. Kirschvink N, Lhoest E, Leemans J, et al. Effects of feeding frequency on water intake in cats. *J Vet Intern Med*. 2005;19:476.

47. Devois C, Biourge V, Morice G, et al. Influence of various amounts of dietary NaCl on urinary Na, Ca, and oxalate concentrations and excretions in adult cats. Proceedings of the 10th Congress of the European Society of Veterinary Internal Medicine; Neuchâtel, Switzerland; 2000:85 (abst).

48. Royal Canin. Data on file. 2008

49. Dumon H, Nguyen P, Martin L, et al. Influence of wet vs. dry food on cat urinary pH: preliminary study. *J Vet Intern Med*. 1999;13:726. abst.

50. Ling GV, Franti CE, Ruby AL, et al. Urolithiasis in dogs. II. Breed prevalence, and interrelations of breed, sex, age, and mineral composition. *Am J Vet Res*. 1998;59:630-642.

51. Lekcharoensuk C, Lulich JP, Osborne CA, et al. Patient and environmental factors associated with calcium oxalate urolithiasis in dogs. *J Am Vet Med Assoc*. 2000;217:515-519.

52. Ling GV, Franti CE, Ruby AL, et al. Urolithiasis in dogs. I. Mineral prevalence and interrelations of mineral composition, age, and sex. *Am J Vet Res*. 1998;59:624-629.

53. Seaman R, Bartges JW. Canine struvite urolithiasis. *Compend Contin Educ Pract Vet*. 2001;23:407-420.

54. Houston DM, Eaglesome H. Unusual case of foreign body-induced struvite urolithiasis in a dog. *Can Vet J*. 1999;40:125-126.

55. Klausner JS, Osborne CA, O'Leary TP, et al. Struvite urolithiasis in a litter of miniature Schnauzer dogs. *Am J Vet Res*. 1980;41:712-719.

56. Bartges JW, Osborne CA, Polzin DJ. Recurrent sterile struvite urocystolithiasis in three related cocker spaniels. *J Am Anim Hosp Assoc*. 1992;28:459-469.

57. Osborne CA, Lulich JP, Polzin DJ, et al. Medical sissolution and prevention of canine struvite urolithiasis. *Vet Clin North Am Small Anim Pract*. 1999;29:73-111.

58. Rinkardt NE, Houston DM. Dissolution of infection-induced struvite bladder stones using a non-calculolytic diet and antibiotic therapy. *Can Vet J*. 2004;45:838-840.

59. Krawiec D, Osborne CA, Leininger JR, et al. Effect of acetohydroxamic acid on dissolution of canine struvite uroliths. *Am J Vet Res*. 1984;45:1266-1275.

60. Plumb DC. *Veterinary Drug Handbook*. 4th ed. Ames, IA: Iowa State Press; 2002.

61. Robertson WG, Jones JS, Heaton MA, et al. Predicting the crystallization potential of urine from cats and dogs with respect to calcium oxalate and magnesium ammonium phosphate (struvite). *J Nutr*. 2002;132:1637S-1641S.

62. Lulich JP, Osborne CA, Thumchai R, et al. Epidemiology of canine calcium oxalate uroliths. Identifying risk factors. *Vet Clin North Am Small Anim Pract*. 1999;29:113-122.

63. Lulich JP, Osborne CA, Lekcharoensuk C, et al. Canine calcium oxalate urolithiasis. Case-based applications of therapeutic principles. *Vet Clin North Am Small Anim Pract*. 1999;29:123-139.

64. Lulich JP, Osborne CA, Unger LK, et al. Prevalence of calcium oxalate uroliths in Miniature Schnauzers. *Am J Vet Res*. 1991;52:1579-1582.

65. Lulich JP, Osborne CA, Nagode LA, et al. Evaluation of urine and serum metabolites in miniature Schnauzers with calcium oxalate urolithiasis. *Am J Vet Res*. 1991;52:1583-1590.

66. Stevenson AE, Robertson WG, Markwell P. Risk factor analysis and relative supersaturation as tools for identifying calcium oxalate stone-forming dogs. *J Small Anim Pract*. 2003;44:491-496.

67. Stevenson AE, Blackburn JM, Markwell PJ, et al. Nutrient intake and urine composition in calcium oxalate stone-forming dogs: comparison with healthy dogs and impact of dietary modification. *Vet Ther*. 2004;5:218-231.

68. Lekcharoensuk C, Osborne CA, Lulich JP, et al. Associations between dry dietary factors and canine calcium oxalate uroliths. *J Am Vet Res*. 2002;63:330-337.

69. Lekcharoensuk C, Osborne CA, Lulich JP, et al. Associations between dietary factors in canned food and formation of canine calcium oxalate uroliths in dogs. *J Am Vet Res*. 2002;63:163-169.

70. Lulich JP, Perrine L, Osborne CA, et al. Postsurgical recurrence of calcium oxalate uroliths in dogs. *J Vet Int Med*. 1992;6:119.

71. Lulich JP, Osborne CA, Polzin DJ, et al. Incomplete removal of canine and feline urocystoliths by cystotomy. Proceedings of the 11th American College of Veterinary Internal Medicine Forum; Washington, DC; 1993:397.

72. Lulich JP, Osborne CA, Sanderson SL. Effects of dietary supplementation with sodium chloride on urinary relative supersaturation with calcium oxalate in healthy dogs. *Am J Vet Res*. 2005;66:319-324.

73. Lulich JP, Osborne CA. Why study the past: Shifting urolith types. Proceedings of the 25th American College of Veterinary Internal Medicine Forum; Seattle, WA; 2007:463-464.

74. Wallerstrom BI, Wagberg TI. Canine urolithiasis in Sweden and Norway: retrospective study of prevalence and epidemiology. *J Small Anim Pract*. 1992;33:534-539.

75. Bartges JW, Osborne CA, Lulich JP, et al. Canine urate urolithiasis. Etiopathogenesis, diagnosis, and management. *Vet Clin North Am Small Anim Pract*. 1999;29:161-191.

76. Bende B, Németh T. High prevalence of urate urolithiasis in the Russian black terrier. *Vet Rec*. 2004;155:239-240.

77. Bannasch DL. The genetic and molecular basis of urate calculi formation in Dalmatians. Proceedings of the 26th American College of Veterinary Internal Medicine Forum; San Antonio, TX; 2008:475-477.

78. Bannasch DL, Ling GV, Bea J, et al. Inheritance of urinary calculi in the Dalmatian. *J Vet Intern Med.* 2004;18:483-487.

79. Sorenson JL, Ling GV. Diagnosis, prevention, and treatment of urate urolithiasis in Dalmatians. *J Am Vet Med Assoc.* 1993;203:863-869.

80. Safra N, Schaible RH, Bannasch DL. Linkage analysis with an interbreed backcross maps Dalmatian hyperuricosuria to CFA03. *Mamm Genome.* 2006;17:340-345.

81. Albasan H, Lulich JP, Osborne CA, et al. Evaluation of the association between sex and risk of forming urate uroliths in Dalmatians. *J Am Vet Med Assoc.* 2005;227:565-569.

82. Case LC, Ling GV, Ruby AL, et al. Urolithiasis in Dalmatians: 275 cases (1981–1990). *J Am Vet Med Assoc.* 1993;203:96-100.

83. Carvalho M, Lulich JP, Osborne CA, et al. Role of urinary inhibitors of crystallization in uric acid nephrolithiasis: Dalmatian dog model. *Urology.* 2003;62:566-570.

84. Malandain E, Caussé E, Tournier C, et al. Quantification of endproducts of purine catabolism in dogs fed diets varying in protein and purine content. Proceeding of the 26th ACVIM Forum; San Antonio, TX; June 4–7, 2008; 803-804.

85. Bartges JW, Osborne CA, Felice LJ. Canine xanthine uroliths: risk factor management. In: Kirk RW, Bonagura JD, eds. *Current Veterinary Therapy XI.* Philadelphia, PA: WB Saunders; 1992:900-905.

86. Van Zuilen CD, Nickel RF, Van Dijk TH, et al. Xanthinuria in a family of cavalier King Charles spaniels. *Vet Q.* 1997;19:172-174.

87. Hoppe A, Denneberg T, Jeppsson JO, et al. Urinary excretion of amino acids in normal and cystinuric dogs. *Br Vet J.* 1993;149:253-268.

88. Casal ML, Giger U, Bovee KC, et al. Inheritance of cystinuria and renal defect in Newfoundlands. *J Am Vet Med Assoc.* 1995;207: 1585-1589.

89. Hoppe A, Denneberg T. Cystinuria in the dog: clinical studies during 14 years of medical treatment. *J Vet Intern Med.* 2001;15:361-367.

90. Sanderson SL, Osborne CA, Lulich JP, et al. Evaluation of urinary carnitine and taurine excretion in 5 cystinuric dogs with carnitine and taurine deficiency. *J Vet Intern Med.* 2001;15:94-100.

91. Bartges JW, Osborne CA, Lulich JP, et al. Prevalence of cystine and urate uroliths in bulldogs and urate uroliths in Dalmatians. *J Am Vet Med Assoc.* 1994;204:1914-1918.

92. Henthorn PS, Liu J, Gidalevich T, et al. Canine cystinuria: polymorphism in the canine SLC3A1 gene and identification of a nonsense mutation in cystinuric Newfoundland dogs. *Hum Genet.* 2000;107:295-303.

93. Case LC, Ling GV, Franti CE, et al. Cystine-containing urinary calculi in dogs: 102 cases (1981–1989). *J Am Vet Med Assoc.* 1992;201:129-133.

94. Escolar E, Bellanato J, Rodriquez M. Study of cystine urinary calculi in dogs. *Can J Vet Res.* 1991;55:67-70.

95. Wallerstrom BI, Wagberg TI, Lagergren CH. Cystine calculi in the dog: an epidemiological retrospective study. *J Small Anim Pract.* 1992;33:78-84.

96. Harnevik L, Hoppe A, Sonderkvist P. SLC7A9 cDNA cloning and mutational analysis of SLC3A1 and SLC7A9 in canine cystinuria. *Mamm Genome.* 2006;17:769-776.

97. Aldrich J, Ling GV, Ruby AL, et al. Silica-containing urinary calculi in dogs (1981–1993). *J Vet Intern Med.* 1997;11:288-295.

98. Kruger JM, Osborne CA, Lulich JP. Calcium phosphate uroliths. Etiopathogenesis, diagnosis, and management. *Vet Clin North Am Small Anim Pract.* 1999;29:141-159.

99. Osborne CA, Lulich JP, Bartges JW, et al. Drug-induced urolithiasis. *Vet Clin North Am Small Anim Pract.* 1999;29:251-266.

100. Lekcharoensuk C, Lulich JP, Osborne CA, et al. Association between patient-related factors and risk of calcium oxalate and magnesium ammonium phosphate urolithiasis in cats. *J Am Vet Med Assoc.* 2000;217:520-525.

101. Lekcharoensuk C, Osborne CA, Lulich JP, et al. Association between dietary factors and calcium oxalate and magnesium ammonium phosphate urolithiasis in cats. *J Am Vet Med Assoc.* 2001;219:1228-1237.

102. Westropp JL, Cannon AB, Ruby AL. Trends in feline urolithiasis. Proceedings of the 24th ACVIM; Louisville, Kentucky; 2006: 478-480.

103. Westropp JL, Buffington CA, Chew DJ. Feline lower urinary tract disorders. In: Ettinger SJ, Feldman EC, eds. *Textbook of Veterinary Internal Medicine.* 6th ed. St. Louis, Missouri: Elsevier Saunders; 2005:1828-1850.

104. Osborne CA, Lulich JP, Kruger JM, et al. Feline urethral plugs. Etiology and pathophysiology. *Vet Clin North Am Small Anim Pract.* 1996;26:233-253.

105. Buffington CA, Rogers QR, Morris JG. Effect of diet on struvite activity product in feline urine. *Am J Vet Res.* 1990;51: 2025-2030.

106. Tarttelin MF. Feline struvite urolithiasis: factors affecting urine pH may be more important than magnesium levels in food. *Vet Rec.* 1987;121:227-230.

107. Osborne CA, Lulich JP, Kruger JM, et al. Medical dissolution of feline struvite urocystoliths. *J Am Vet Med Assoc.* 1990;196: 1053-1063.

108. Houston DM, Rinkardt NE, Hilton J. Evaluation of the efficacy of a commercial diet in the dissolution of feline struvite bladder uroliths. *Vet Ther.* 2004;5:187-201.

109. Devois C, Biourge V, Morice G, et al. Struvite and oxalate activity product ratios and crystalluria in cats fed acidifying diets. Urolithiasis 2000 Proceedings; Cape Town; 2000:821-823.

110. Xu H, Laflamme DP, Bartges JW, et al. Effect of dietary sodium on urine characteristics in healthy adult cats. *J Vet Intern Med.* 2006;20: 103. abst.

111. Tournier C, Malandain E, Abouhafs S, et al. Struvite relative supersaturation: a good predictor of struvite stone dissolution in vitro. Proceedings of the 26th American College of Veterinary Internal Medicine Forum; San Antonio, TX; June 4–7, 2008:803 (abst).

112. Kirk CA, Ling GV, Franti CE, et al. Evaluation of factors associated with development of calcium oxalate urolithiasis in cats. *J Am Vet Med Assoc.* 1995;207:1429-1434.

113. Thumchai R, Lulich JP, Osborne CA, et al. Epizootiologic evaluation of urolithiasis in cats: 3,498 cases (1982–1992). *J Am Vet Med Assoc.* 1996;208:547-551.

114. McClain HM, Barsanti JA, Bartges JW. Hypercalcemia and calcium oxalate urolithiasis in cats: a report of five cases. *J Am Anim Hosp Assoc.* 1999;35:297-301.

115. Tournier C, Aladenise S, Vialle S, et al. The effect of urinary pH on calcium oxalate relative supersaturation in healthy cats. Proceedings of the ESCVN; Nantes; October 5–7, 2006: 189 (abst).

116. Bai SC, Sampson DA, Morris JG, et al. Vitamin B-6 requirement of growing kittens. *J Nutr.* 1989;119:1020-1027.

117. Wrigglesworth DJ, Stevenson AE, Smith BHE, et al. Effect of pyridoxine hydrochloride on feline urine pH and urinary relative supersaturation of calcium oxalate Proceedings of the 42nd British Small Animal Veterinary Association Conference, Birmingham, UK; 1999:324 (abst).

118. Tournier C, Aladenise S, Vialle S, et al. The effect of dietary sodium on urine composition and calcium oxalate relative supersaturation in healthy cats. Proceedings of the 10th ESVCN Congress; Nantes; 2006:190 (abst).

119. Lulich JP, Osborne CA, Lekcharoensuk C, et al. Effects of diet on urine composition of cats with calcium oxalate urolithiasis. *J Am Anim Hosp Assoc.* 2004;40:185-191.

120. Hawthorne AJ, Markwell PJ. Dietary sodium promotes increased water intake and urine volume in cats. *J Nutr.* 2004;134: 2128S-2129S.

121. Biourge V, Devois C, Morice G, et al. Dietary NaCl significantly increases urine volume but does not increase urinary calcium oxalate supersaturation in healthy cats. *J Vet Intern Med.* 2001;15:866. abst.

122. Buranakarl C, Mathur S, Brown SA. Effects of dietary sodium chloride intake on renal function and blood pressure in cats with normal and reduced renal function. *Am J Vet Res.* 2004;65:620-627.

123. Luckschander N, Iben C, Hosgood G, et al. Dietary NaCl does not affect blood pressure in healthy cats. *J Vet Intern Med.* 2004;18: 463-467.

124. Cowgill LD, Sergev G, Bandt C, et al. Effects of dietary salt intake on body fluid volume and renal function in healthy cats. *J Vet Intern Med.* 2007;21:600. abst.

125. Savary KC, Price GS, Vaden SL. Hypercalcemia in cats: a retrospective study of 71 cases (1991–1997). *J Vet Intern Med.* 2000;14:184-189.

126. Midkiff AM, Chew DJ, Randolph JF, et al. Idiopathic hypercalcemia in cats. *J Vet Intern Med.* 2000;14:619-626.

127. Albasan H, Osborne CA, Lulich JP, et al. Urolith recurrence in cats. Proceedings of the 24th American College of Veteri-nary Internal Medicine Forum; Louisville, Kentucky; 2006: 280 (abst), 825.

128. Tsuchida S, Kagi A, Koyama H, et al. Xanthine urolithiasis in a cat: a case report and evaluation of a candidate gene for xanthine dehydrogenase. *J Feline Med Surg.* 2007;9:503-508.

129. Osborne CA, Lulich JP, Bartges JW, et al. Feline metabolic uroliths: risk factor management. In: Kirk RW, Bonagura JD, eds. *Current Veterinary Therapy XI.* Philadelphia, PA: WB Saunders; 1992:905-909.

130. White RN, Tick NT, White HL. Naturally occurring xanthine urolithiasis in a domestic shorthair cat. *J Small Anim Pract.* 1997;38: 299-301.

131. DiBartola SP, Chew DJ, Horton ML, et al. Cystinuria in a cat. *J Am Vet Med Assoc.* 1991;198:102-104.

132. Frank A, Norrestam R, Sjödin A. A new urolith in four cats and a dog: composition and crystal structure. *J Biol Inorg Chem.* 2002;7:437-444.

133. Westropp JL, Ruby AL, Bailiff NL, et al. Dried solidified blood calculi in the urinary tract of cats. *J Vet Intern Med.* 2006; 20:828-834.

Pathogenesis of Stones: Summary of Current Concepts

11

Allen Rodgers

Abstract Research involving the traditional factors that direct the pathogenesis of kidney stone disease – hypercalciuria, primary hyperparathyroidism, hyperoxaluria, hypocitraturia – has progressed gently during the past several years, but has not unveiled any new dramatic findings. However, meaningful results have emerged from sophisticated scientific studies in at least three other areas – oxalate-degrading bacteria, Randall's plaque, and genetic determinants. Both groups of pathogenic factors – traditional and other – are summarized in this review.

11.1 Introduction

The pathogenesis of kidney stone disease has been a topic of discussion among researchers for many years. Numerous general reviews have been published.[1-6] Because of the vastness of the topic and the complexities of the individual pathological conditions giving rise to the formation of stones, the literature also bounds with more esoteric type reviews that have focused on individual conditions rather than on the entire spectrum of disorders giving rise to different types of stone. These reviews have been compiled by highly respected scientists and clinicians, each of whom is an expert in their particular fields. The entire body of work comprises a superb and in-depth description of the evolving knowledge-base on the pathogenesis of stones. A glance through the titles of the articles that have been published reveals the repetition of phrases having a common theme – "New insights" (1997, 2000, 2004, 2008), "Update" (1997), "Recent progress" (2007). Scrutiny of these articles reveals a subtle increase in our fundamental understanding of the pathogenesis of stone disease over the years, rather than one in which our understanding is accelerating. Indeed, many of the aforementioned articles do not really describe dramatic breakthroughs. Generally, they repeat that which is widely known, but nevertheless describe a small incremental move forward, as is the nature of an evolving field. This is not intended to be a criticism from the present author, but rather

A. Rodgers (✉)
Department of Chemistry, University of Cape Town, Cape Town, Western Cape, South Africa
e-mail: allen.rodgers@uct.ac.za

a personal observation. To the contrary, the present author remains in awe of the depth of knowledge displayed by the writers of reviews on this topic and feels it is unnecessary to rehash in a repackaged format that which is already known and which has been elegantly reviewed and critiqued by the aforementioned authors. A better approach, and the one adopted for this chapter, is to provide an up-to-date *summary* of the current concepts relating to the main pathogenic stone factors, and to highlight those which have indeed opened up new and fresh insights during the past 5–10 years.

The principal pathogenic factors that have been substantiated in numerous studies are hypercalciuria, primary hyperparathyroidism, hyperoxaluria, hypocitraturia, and hyperuricosuria. These have all been extremely well described and characterized. These conditions will be summarized with a view to providing background to the "new" concepts that provide the main focus of this chapter.

Irrespective of the individual pathogenic etiologies of the aforementioned conditions, they culminate in a chemical milieu in urine that favors the crystallization of urinary salts and stone formation. This gives rise to a range of physico-chemical scenarios that have also been previously grouped under the general heading of "pathogenesis." Among these are included supersaturation and the inhibitor-promoter theory. These too will be described in this chapter.

So, what are the pathogenic factors that, in the view of the present author, have attracted a lot of attention during the past 5–10 years and which have provided the stone research community with genuinely "new insights"? They are (1) oxalate-degrading bacteria, (2) plaque, and (3) genetic factors.

11.2 Idiopathic Hypercalciura

This pathogenic factor has been fully described in several excellent general reviews[1,2,4,5,7] and most recently by an article dedicated solely to this condition.[8]

Idiopathic hypercalciuria is the most common metabolic abnormality in patients suffering from calcium urolithiasis.[8] It has been termed as a "syndrome of unexplained hypercalciuria".[1] Despite the substantial body of work that has been published on this condition, attention has been drawn to the fact that the term "idiopathic hypercalciuria" has generally been applied to a heterogeneous group of disorders and that a more pathophysiologically oriented classification distinguishes between defects in one or a combination of three organs: kidney (renal leak), bone (resorptive), and gut (absorptive).[5]

Systemic acidosis and protein load with some overlapping pathogenetic mechanisms are cited as two very important causes of hypercalciuria.[5] The role of the latter of these two mechanisms is more complicated and questions remain concerning the components in protein, besides acid, that cause hypercalciuria and the effects, if any, on intestinal absorption.

Worcester and Coe[8] suggest that idiopathic hypercalciuria is not a disease but rather a manifestation of the high end of a wide range of physiological calcium excretion rates.

11.3 Hyperparathyroidism

About 5% of stone patients have this disease.[2] It is distinguished from idiopathic hypercalciuria by virtue of the high blood calcium levels that occur in this condition, while *normal* levels occur in idiopathic hypercalciuria. Parathyroid hormone increases the synthesis of calcitrol, which increases the intestinal absorption of calcium, culminating in an increase in calciuria. Hyperparathyroidism will therefore lead to hypercalcaemia and hypercalciuria. Several reviews have devoted descriptions to this disorder.[1,2,9]

11.4 Hyperoxaluria

As with idiopathic hypercalciuria, this pathogenic factor has been dealt with in some detail in the same reviews as those listed previously for idiopathic hypercalciuria. Coe, Evan, and Worcester[4] differentiate between dietary, enteric, and primary hyperoxalurias. The first of these is associated with a low calcium or high protein or high oxalate diet, while the second arises in patients with small bowel disease, reaction, or bypass. The final pathology arises from a rare genetic disorder.

Holmes and Assimos[10] are not convinced that an increased intestinal absorption is a consequence of a low calcium diet, claiming that this has been difficult to demonstrate. They

suggest that a proportion of stone formers may hyperabsorb oxalate, but this remains to be determined.

11.5 Hypocitraturia

Numerous studies have demonstrated the prevalence of hypocitraturia in calcium oxalate urolithiasis patients, thereby providing convincing evidence in support of it being a critical pathogenic risk factor in this disease.[11,12] Empirical support for this notion has been provided by in vitro calcium oxalate precipitation experiments that have compellingly demonstrated that citrate is an effective inhibitor of the three principal mechanisms of crystallization, namely nucleation,[13] growth,[14] and aggregation.[15] Hypocitraturia is estimated to be present in 20–60% of stone formers.[16]

Despite this compelling clinical and scientific evidence of the role of hypocitraturia in stone formation, its pathogenesis does not appear to have been exhaustively explored, but may arise from increased tubule reabsorption rather than reduced filtered load.[2] Holmes and Assimos[7] point out that while dietary factors – such as excessive sodium and animal protein intakes – can influence citrate excretion, its precise role has not yet been fully defined. These authors speculate that genetic factors may play an influential role, but that research in this area is limited.

11.6 Hyperuricosuria

Early evidence in support of the notion that hyperuricosuria contributes to the formation of calcium oxalate stones was provided by a trial that demonstrated a decrease in stone formation with allopurinol relative to placebo.[17] Since then there appears to be general acceptance of a pathogenic link between the condition and the disease, but the nature of this relationship is yet to be resolved, despite the fact that several mechanisms have been proposed including heterogeneous nucleation and salting out.[2]

Although it might be tempting to consider hyperuricosuria as a risk factor for uric acid calculi, only a small fraction of patients who develop this type of stone have this urinary condition. Other risk factors such as low urinary volume and persistently low urinary pH are more important.[18]

11.7 Physicochemical Factors, Inhibitors, and Promoters

Ultimately, for a stone to develop, at least two of the following crystallization processes have to occur: nucleation, growth, and aggregation. These processes themselves are governed by the laws of physical chemistry that embrace, among other factors, solubility, saturation, equilibrium, thermodynamics, and kinetics. Any scenario in which the exquisite homeostasis of the system is disturbed could have dire consequences in terms of the crystallization mechanisms mentioned. The physical chemistry of a sophisticated chemical solution like urine is subtle and complex. Detailed descriptions of the physicochemical factors that contribute toward stone formation can be found in several seminal papers.[19–22] The principles that are fully described by these and other authors have been successfully invoked in stone formation by numerous researchers during the past 35 years. Interestingly, a relatively recent article proposed a radical new approach in which the concept of urinary supersaturation being the cause of stone formation was challenged.[23] This prompted a rebuttal in which the arguments were articulately refuted.[24]

The classic physicochemical risk factor model developed by Robertson and co-workers[25] has recently been refined.[26] It lists hypercalciuria, hyperoxaluria, hypocitraturia, hypomagnesuria, hypouricosuria, low volume, and variations in pH as the key urinary conditions associated with stone formation. It is important to recognize that these are not pathogenic factors per se but are rather pathogenic *conditions* arising from an inherent pathology. While intervention strategies to correct these lithogenic conditions are available, it is the underlying pathology that needs attention.

Among the chemical factors involved with controlling and normalizing the crystal-forming potential of the chemical milieu are a group of naturally occurring agents that have the ability to either inhibit (or modulate) crystallization processes or to promote them. Here there exists a substantial body of research studies that support this notion. In particular, the reviews by Worcester[27] and Ryall[28] cover this area of urolithiasis research very thoroughly. Attention is also drawn to another excellent review that deals with both the physical chemistry and inhibitor approaches to urolithiasis.[29]

As is well known, inhibitors fall into two groups: micromolecular (citrate, pyrophosphate, magnesium) and macromolecular (glycosaminoglycans, proteins). They exert their influence either by chelating the offending ion (generally achieved by the micromolecular group) or they coat the surface of physiological urinary crystals in a manner that prevents or retards growth or aggregation of these discrete entities (generally achieved by the macromolecular group). Another protective mechanism arising from the coating of crystals is to retard or prevent their adhesion to renal cells. Finally, there is evidence indicating that proteins may inhibit urolithiasis by facilitating the intracellular disintegration and dissolution of crystals attached to and internalized by renal epithelial cells.[30] Of importance, however, is the point made by Bergsland and co-workers[31] that although several studies have hypothesized or demonstrated that proteins in stone formers might suffer defects, deficiencies, or variations in their molecular structure, it remains unclear whether any of

these is a cause or a consequence of stones. Herein lies a crucial issue. If it turns out that these inadequacies, whatever they might be, are not secondary to stone formation, then this syndrome can indeed be appropriately classified as a pathogenic factor of stone disease. The challenge for stone researchers is to solve this dilemma.

11.8 Oxalate Degrading Bacteria

Since Allison and coworkers proposed for the first time that oxalic acid degradation by *Oxalobacter formigenes* (an obligate anaerobe) may influence absorption of oxalate from the intestine and thereby contribute to hyperoxaluria,[32] there has been much interest and excitement among urolithiasis researchers. This interest has been entirely justified and continues in current times. Studies have demonstrated that there is a direct correlation between hyperoxaluria (and concomitant calcium oxalate stone disease) and low colonization or absence of this bacterium.[33–35] Similarly, infrequency of colonization with *O. formigenes* has been demonstrated in patients with cystic fibrosis[36] and inflammatory bowel disease,[37] in whom hyperoxaluria and calcium oxalate renal stones are common. These findings have prompted clinicians to administer this bacterium orally; some success has been reported.[38]

An alternative approach has been to explore the possibility of reducing the urinary excretion of oxalate using other intestinal bacteria. Campieri and coworkers[39] achieved a decrease in a group of stone-forming patients by oral administration of a mixture of freeze-dried lactic acid bacteria (used in the dairy industry to modify the intestinal flora). Yet another approach has been to investigate the possible presence of other oxalate-degrading bacteria in the intestine. *Providencia rettgeri*[40] and *Lactobacillus gasseri*[41] are among the new oxalate-degrading bacteria that have been identified and which are regarded as potential role players in calcium oxalate kidney stone formation.

Notwithstanding these impressive results, a recent critique views the outcomes achieved with *O. formigenes* with some skepticism.[42] However, it remains the view of the present author that low colonization or absence of oxalate-degrading bacteria of any type in the gut is a potential pathogenic factor for calcium oxalate stone disease.

11.9 Randall's Plaque

In recent years, there have been several highly sophisticated endoscopic and histopathologic studies[43–46] focused on sites of interstitial calcium phosphate crystals (plaque), which were first described by Randall nearly 70 years ago.[47] These studies have provided convincing evidence in support of a pathogenic mechanism for stone formation in which an anchored nidus of urinary crystals could form as an overgrowth on the interstitial plaque, permitting a fixed stone to form and grow over a period of several years.[48–50] The fundamental tenet of this hypothesis is that the interstitial plaque constitutes the initiating site of stone formation. In their review article, Coe, Evan, and Worcester[4] summarize the various stages of stone formation commencing with the deposition of plaque (in the form of biological apatite) in the basement membrane of the thin loops of Henle. It then extends to the suburothelial space where calcium oxalate stones form over the apatite particles that have coalesced in an organic milieu. While supersaturation of calcium oxalate is the driving force for the crystal overgrowth step, the forces that direct plaque formation are not obvious. Various mechanisms are currently under consideration. These include the hypothesis that in some patients the pH in inner medullary collecting ducts increases (potentially for a variety of reasons), which together with water extraction and high concentrations of calcium culminate in apatite crystal formation.[48] If Randall's plaque is to be justifiably classified as a pathogenic factor in stone disease, it is crucial to identify and characterize the underlying processes giving rise to its formation.

11.10 Genetics

Several relatively recent publications have provided detailed reviews of this vast and highly complex aspect of the pathogenesis of urolithiasis.[51–53] In discussing "the genetics of kidney stone disease," it is important to recognize that each lithogenic pathology requires its own dedicated consideration.

11.10.1 Hypercalciuria

About half of patients with idiopathic hypercalciuria have a family history of kidney stones.[54,55] This condition is a consequence of interactions between environmental and genetic determinants.[5,8] The genetic aspects have recently been described in detail.[56] Idiopathic hypercalciuria is a complex trait involving several genes that themselves might differ widely from one patient to another.[8] Several candidate genes have been tested for their possible association with this disease, but as yet a conclusive linkage has not been established.[5,8]

The genetic factors underlying hypercalciuria remain elusive.[53] Nevertheless, a substantial body of work has provided evidence in support of a genetic association. Several studies have implicated the vitamin D receptor gene in hypercalciuric nephrolithiasis.[53] Polymorphic variants of the gene encoding the calcium-sensing receptor, which regulates PTH secretion

from parathyroid cells and calcium reabsorption in the distal convolute tubule, have also been implicated in the pathogenesis of hypercalciuria.[4,57]

11.10.2 Hyperoxaluria

There have been considerable advances in the understanding of primary (genetic) hyperoxalurias Types I and II[5] during recent years. Type I, an autosomal trait arises from molecular abnormalities in the gene that codes for the activity of hepatic peroxisomal alanine-glyoxylate aminotransferase, thereby increasing the availability of glyoxylate, which is irreversibly converted to oxalic acid.[1] Type II is caused by inactivating mutations in the genes that code for glyoxylate reductase and hydroxypyruvate reductase.[5]

11.10.3 Hypocitraturia

Although mutations in renal citrate transporters such as NaCT, SLC13A5 have not yet been identified, these transporters are regarded as being possible candidate genes for stone formation.[53]

11.10.4 Hyperurocosuria

Inactivating mutations in the gene coding for the anion exchanger URAT1, which has been identified as a urate transporter, have been found in patients with idiopathic renal hypouricaemia and nephrolithiasis.[5,53]

11.10.5 Cystinuria

Multiple inactivating mutations in the genes SLC3A1 and SLC7A9 are known, giving rise to high urinary cystine concentrations.[5,53] However, paradoxically, such concentrations can show great variability among patients. Moreover not all patients with these mutations form stones. Thus there are unresolved issues.

11.10.6 Experts' Comments

Sayer[53] is enthusiastic about stone research using genomic techniques as he believes these will help identify the heritable components of complex traits like hypercalciuria. Griffin[52] too is optimistic, stating that researchers are now making solid progress in separating the genetic complexities that will form the basis of an accurate genetic model of idiopathic urolithiasis. Moe[5] is a little more circumspect. He maintains that greater effort needs to be made to identify candidate loci and genes and that this will be extremely challenging.

11.11 Conclusions

It is apparent that the pathogenesis of kidney stone disease is a highly complex phenomenon involving multistep processes, all of which occur in an exquisite and orchestrated sequence of events. These processes are likely to involve physiological, physicochemical, biological, biochemical, and genetic principles, either individually or in synergy with one another. Attempting to unravel and characterize these presents huge challenges to researchers. Awareness of the difficulties is not new. The authors of the review articles cited in this chapter have all alluded to them. The fact that meaningful studies, many of them of a highly sophisticated scientific nature, continue to emerge is a great credit to the researchers in this field. Dogged perseverance and visionary insights are their hallmarks. These need to be sustained in the next era of stone research.

References

1. Coe FL, Parks JH, Asplin JR. The pathogenesis and treatment of kidney stones. *New Engl J Med*. 1992;327:1141-1152.
2. Coe FL, Parks JH. New insights into the pathophysiology and treatment of nephrolithiasis: new research venues. *J Bone Miner Res*. 1997;12:522-533.
3. Baggio B, Plebani M, Gambaro G. Pathogenesis of idiopathic calcium nephrolithiasis: update 1997. *Crit Rev Clin Lab Sci*. 1998;35(2):153-187.
4. Coe FL, Evan A, Worcester E. Kidney stone disease. *J Clin Invest*. 2005;115:2598-2608.
5. Moe O. Kidney stones: pathophysiology and medical management. *Lancet*. 2006;367:333-344.
6. Sakhaee K. Recent advances in the pathophysiology of nephrolithiasis. *Kidney Int*. 2009;75:585-595.
7. Holmes RP, Assimos DG. Pathophysiology associated with risk factors for calcium oxalate stone disease. In: Gohel MD, Au DT, eds. *Kidney Stones: Inside and Out*. Hong Kong: Hong Kong Polytechnic University; 2004:153-156.
8. Worcester EM, Coe FL. New insights into the pathogenesis of idiopathic hypercalciuria. *Semin Nephrol*. 2008;28(2):120-132.
9. Heller HJ, Pak CYC. Primary hyperparathyroidism. In: Coe FL, Favus MJ, eds. *Disorders of Bone and Mineral Metabolism*. Philadelphia: Lippincott Willliams and Wilkins; 2002:516-534.
10. Holmes RP, Assimos DG. The impact of dietary oxalate on kidney stone formation. *Urol Res*. 2004;32:311-316.
11. Laminski NA, Meyers AM, Sonnekus MI, Smyth AE. Prevalence of hypocitraturia and hypopyrophosphaturia in recurrent calcium stone formers: as isolated defects or associated with other metabolic abnormalities. *Nephron*. 1990;56:379-386.
12. Cupisti A, Morelli E, Lupetti S, Meola M, Barsotti G. Low urine citrate excretion as main risk factor for recurrent calcium oxalate nephrolithiasis in males. *Nephron*. 1992;61:73-76.
13. Schwille PO, Schmiedl A, Hermann U, et al. Magnesium, citrate, magnesium citrate and magnesium-alkali citrate as modulators of calcium oxalate crystallization in urine: observations in patients with recurrent idiopathic calcium urolithiasis. *Urol Res*. 1999;27:117-121.
14. Bek-Jensen H, Fornander A-M, Nilsson M-A, Tiselius H-G. Is citrate an inhibitor of calcium oxalate crystal growth in high concentrations of urine? *Urol Res*. 1996;24:67-71.
15. Tiselius H-G, Fornander A-M, Nilsson M-A. The effects of citrate and urine on calcium oxalate crystal aggregation. *Urol Res*. 1993;21:363-366.
16. Pak CYC. Citrate and renal calculi: new insights and future directions. *Am J Kidney Dis*. 1991;17:420-425.
17. Ettinger B, Tang A, Citron JT, Livermore B, Williams T. Randomized trial of allopurinol in the prevention of calcium oxalate calculi. *N Engl J Med*. 1986;315:1386-1389.
18. Ngo TC, Assimos DG. Uric acid nephrolithiasis: recent progress and future directions. *Rev Urol*. 2007;9(1):17-27.
19. Finlayson B. Renal lithiasis in review. *Urol Clin N Am*. 1974;1(2):181-211.
20. Finlayson B. Physicochemical aspects of urolithiasis. *Kidney Int*. 1978;13:344-360.
21. Robertson WG, Nordin BEC. Physico-chemical factors governing stone formation. In: Williams DI, Chisholm GD, eds. *Scientific Foundations of Urology*. London: William Heinemann Medical Books Ltd; 1982:254-267.
22. Hess B, Kok DJ. Nucleation, growth and aggregation of stone forming crystals. In: Coe FL, Favus MJ, Pak CYC, Parks JH, Preminger GM, eds. *Kidney Stones: Medical and Surgical Management*. Philadelphia: Lippincott-Raven; 1996:3-32.
23. Ashby R, Gyory Az. A thermodynamic equilibrium model for calcium salt urolithiasis: clinical application. *Exp Nephrol*. 1997;5:246-252.
24. Kavanagh J. A critical appraisal of the hypothesis that urine is a saturated equilibrium with respect to stone-forming calcium salts. *BJU Int*. 2001;87:589-598.
25. Robertson WG, Peacock M, Heyburn PJ, Marshall DH, Clark PB. Risk factors in calcium stone disease of the urinary tract. *Br J Urol*. 1978;50:449-454.
26. Robertson WG. A risk factor model of stone-formation. *Front Biosci*. 2003;8:1330-1338.
27. Worcester EM. Inhibitors of stone formation. *Sem Nephrol*. 1996;16(5):474-486.
28. Ryall RL. Urinary inhibitors of calcium oxalate crystallization and their potential role in stone formation. *World J Urol*. 1997;15:155-164.
29. Marangella M, Vitale C, Petrarulo M, Bagnis C, Bruno M, Ramello A. Renal stones: from metabolic to physiochemical abnormalities. How useful are inhibitors? *J Nephrol*. 2000;13:S51-S60.
30. Ryall RL, Chauvet MC, Grover PK. Intracrystalline proteins and urolithiasis: a comparison of the protein content and ultra structure of urinary calcium oxalate monohydrate and dihydrate crystals. *BJU Int*. 2005;96:654-663.
31. Bergsland KJ, Kelly JK, Coe BJ, Coe FL. Urine protein markers distinguishes stone-forming from non-stone-forming relatives of calcium stone formers. *Am J Renal Physiol*. 2006;291:F530-F536.
32. Allison M, Cook HM, Milne DB, Gallagher S, Clayman RV. Oxalate degradation by gastrointestinal bacteria for humans. *J Nutr*. 1986;116:455-460.
33. Sidhu H, Schmidt ME, Cornelius JG, et al. Direct correlation between hyperoxaluria/oxalate stone disease and the absence of the gastrointestinal tract-dwelling bacterium Oxalobacter formigenes: possible prevention by gut recolonization or enzyme replacement therapy. *J Am Soc Nephrol*. 1999;10(14):S334-S340.

34. Mikami K, Akakura K, Takei K, et al. Associations of absence of intestinal oxalate degrading bacteria with urinary calcium oxalate stone formation. *Int J Urol.* 2003;10:293-296.

35. Troxel SA, Sidhu H, Kaul P, Low RK. Intestinal Oxalobacter formigenes colonization in calcium oxalate stone formers and its relation to urinary oxalate. *J Endourol.* 2003;17(3):173-176.

36. Sidhu H, Hoppe B, Hesse A, Tenbrock K, Bromme S, Dietchel E. Absence of Oxalobacter formigenes in cystic fibrosis patients: a risk factor for hyperoxaluria. *Lancet.* 1998;352:1026-1029.

37. Kumar R, Ghoshal U, Singh G, Mittal RD. Infrequency of colonization with Oxalobacter formigenes in inflammatory bowel disease: possible role in renal stone formation. *J Gastroenterol Hepatol.* 2004;19:1403-1409.

38. Hoppe B, von Unruh G, Laube N, Hesse A, Sidhu H. Oxalate degrading bacteria: new treatment option for patients with primary and secondary hyperoxaluria? *Urol Res.* 2005;33:372-375.

39. Campieri C, Campieri M, Bertuzzi V, Swennen E, et al. Reduction of oxaluria after an oral course of lactic acid bacteria at high concentration. *Kidney Int.* 2001;60:1097-1105.

40. Hokama S, Toma C, Iwanaga M, Morozumi M, et al. Oxalate-degrading Providencia rettgeri isolated from human stools. *Int J Urol.* 2005;12:533-538.

41. Lewanika T, Reid SJ, Abratt VR, Macfarlane GT, Macfarlane S. Lactobacillus gasseri Gasser AM63 [T] degrades oxalate in a multistage continuous culture simulator of the human colonic microbiota. *FEMS Microbiol Ecol.* 2007;61:110-120.

42. Siva S, Barrack ER, Reddy GPV, et al. A critical analysis of the role of gut Oxalobacter formigenes in oxalate stone disease. *BJU Int.* 2008;103:18-21.

43. Kim SC, Coe FL, Tinmouth WW, et al. Stone formation is proportional to papillary surface coverage by Randall's plaque. *J Urol.* 2005;173:117-119.

44. Williams JC, Matlaga BR, Kim SC, et al. Calcium oxalate calculi found attached to the renal papilla: preliminary evidence for early mechanisms in stone formation. *J Endourol.* 2006;20(11):885-890.

45. Evan AP, Coe FL, Lingeman JE, et al. Mechanism of formation of human calcium oxalate renal stones on Randall's plaque. *Anat Rec.* 2007;290:1315-1323.

46. Miller NL, Gillen DL, Williams JC, et al. A formal test of the hypothesis that idiopathic calcium oxalate stones grow on Randall's plaque. *BJU Int.* 2009 Apr;103(7):966-971.

47. Randall A. The etiology of primary renal calculus. *Int Abstr Surg.* 1940;71:209-240.

48. Evan A, Lingeman J, Coe FL, Worcester E. Randall's plaque: pathogenesis and role in calcium oxalate nephrolithiasis. *Kidney Int.* 2006;69:1313-1316.

49. Matlaga BR, Coe FL, Evan AP, Lingeman JE. The role of Randall's plaque in the pathogenesis of calcium stones. *J Urol.* 2007;177:31-38.

50. Evan AP. Physiopathology and etiology of stone formation in the kidney and the urinary tract. *Pediatr Nephrol* 2009 Feb 7. [Epub ahead of print]

51. Gambarro G, Vezzoli G, Casari G, Rampoldi L, D'Angelo A, Borghi L. Genetics of hypercalciuria and calcium nephrolithiasis: from the rare monogenic to the common polygenic forms. *Am J Kidney Dis.* 2004;44:963-986.

52. Griffin DG. A review of the heritability of idiopathic nephrolithiasis. *J Clin Pathol.* 2004;57(8):793-796.

53. Sayer JA. The genetics of nephrolithiasis. *Nephron Exp Nephrol.* 2008;110(2):e37-e43.

54. Coe FL, Parks JH, Moore ES. Familial idiopathic hypercalciuria. *New Engl J Med.* 1979;300:337-340.

55. Curhan GC, Willett WC, Rimm EB, Stampfer MJ. (Family history and risk of kidney stones. *J Am Soc Nephrol.* 1997;8:1568-1573.

56. Stechman MJ, Loh NY, Thakker RV. Genetics of hypercalciuric nephrolithiasis. *Ann NY Acad Sci.* 2007;1116:461-484.

57. Corbetta S, Eller-Vainicher C, Frigerio M, Valaperta R, et al. Analysis of the 206M polymorphic variant of the SLC26A6 gene encoding a Cl⁻ oxalate transporter in patients with primary hyperparathyroidism. *Eur J Endocrin.* 2009;160:283-288.

Calcium Metabolism and Hypercalciuria

George E. Haleblian and Glenn M. Preminger

Abstract Calcium metabolism and homeostasis are highly regulated and maintained within a narrow physiologic range. An understanding of its metabolism and various disorders in absorption and excretion is essential to the understanding of nephrolithiasis. In this chapter, an overview of calcium metabolism in the nephron is presented. The role of diuretic effects on calcium transport is reviewed. Hormonal effects on calcium metabolism are discussed. Various medical treatment options for calcium nephrolithiasis are also presented along with guidelines for therapy.

12.1 Calcium Metabolism

Calcium metabolism and homeostasis are highly regulated and maintained within a narrow physiologic range. A total of 1–2 kg of calcium is present in the average adult. Calcium is found predominantly as a divalent cation (Ca^{2+}) in the body and is essential to intracellular and extracellular signal transduction as well as the major structural component of the skeleton and teeth in the adult. Ninety-nine percent of calcium found in the adult is in the bony skeleton and teeth. Of the calcium in circulation, 50% is found in the biologically active ionized form, 40% is bound to plasma proteins (predominantly albumin), and 10% travels with other anions (PO_4, citrate) to form a neutral complex. Normal plasma Ca^{2+} concentrations range from 8.8 to 10.3 mg/dL, while ionized calcium concentrations are regulated to between 1.05 and 1.23 μ(micro)M.

An average of 800–1,000 mg of calcium is ingested on a daily basis by adults, mostly in the form of dairy products (Table 12.1) with an increasing number of adults taking dietary supplements. In addition, approximately 200 mg of Ca^{2+} enters the gastrointestinal (GI) tract through bile and GI secretions. Approximately 25% of dietary Ca^{2+} is absorbed by the intestine with the remainder found in the stool. Balance between absorbed calcium, secreted calcium, and serum calcium is then maintained through complex interaction between calcitonin, 1,25-dihydroxycholecalciferol,

parathyroid hormone (PTH), and ionized calcium (iCa). Average renal excretion of calcium is 200 mg/day. See Fig. 12.1 for a summary of daily calcium intake and output.

Calcium homeostasis is maintained by the interactions of extracellular calcium, PTH, 1,25(OH)$_2$D, and calcitonin. Each of these compounds exerts its effect on either the kidneys, the parathyroid glands, or the intestinal tract. In instances of hypocalcemia, a number of events occur to correct the abnormality, starting with stimulation of PTH secretion from the parathyroid gland leading to stimulation of osteoclast-mediated bone reabsorption, stimulation of renal calcium reabsorption in the distal tubule, and stimulation of 25-hydroxyvitamin D-1α(alpha)-hydroxylase, which converts 25-hydroxyvitamin D to 1,25 (OH)$_2$D, which acts in the intestines to cause calcium absorption. Conversely, in instances of hypercalcemia, PTH expression is inhibited and resultant effects of PTH are inhibited. Moreover, elevated Ca^{2+} leads to calcitonin secretion from the thyroid leading to inhibition of osteoclast activity. In addition, direct effects of extracellular Ca^{2+} on renal tubular cells are thought to directly inhibit calcium reabsorption. A summary of calcium homeostasis is outlined in Fig. 12.2.

12.2 Calcium Transport in the Nephron

Renal handling of calcium is limited to forms of calcium that are ultrafiltered through the glomerulus (iCa^{2+} and complexed Ca^{2+}) as calcium bound to serum proteins are not filtered. Approximately 60–70% of the total plasma calcium concentration can be found in the ultrafiltrate and 98–99% of

G.E. Haleblian (✉)
Division of Urology, The Warren School of Brown University, Rhode Island Hospital, Providence, RI, USA
e-mail: ghaleblian@lifespan.org

Table 12.1 Average calcium concentrations of various dairy products

Food product	Serving size	Calcium (mg)
Milk	1 cup	300
Yogurt	¾ cup	200
Ice Cream	¾ cup	150
Pudding	½ cup	150
Salmon (with bones)	¼ cup	150
Broccoli	1 ½ cup	150
Cheese[a]	1 ounce	200
Cottage cheese[a]	1 cup	150

[a]These foods are high in sodium and may increase urinary calcium levels

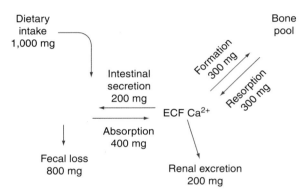

Fig. 12.1 Summary of calcium intake and output (Reprinted with permission from Brenner.[1])

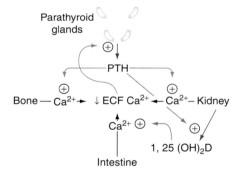

Fig. 12.2 Calcium homeostasis summary (Reprinted with permission from Brenner.[1])

the filtered Ca^{2+} is reabsorbed by the renal tubules with different segments performing differing degrees of reabsorption (Table 12.2).

The proximal tubule is responsible for the majority of Ca^{2+} reabsorption. Proximal tubule reabsorption occurs via passive permeability and diffusion via paracellular routes, both facilitated by a number of membrane proteins. Reabsorption is driven by slight concentration gradient effect and associated electrochemical gradient formed by transcellular Na^+ reabsorption, which promotes reabsorption of Ca^{2+}.[2-7]

Table 12.2 Calcium reabsorption by nephron segments

Nephron segment	(%) Reabsorption of Calcium
Proximal tubule	50–60
Thin descending and ascending limbs	0
Thick ascending limb	15
Distal convoluted tubule and connecting tubule	10–15
Collecting duct	?

The thick ascending limb of the loop of Henle is responsible for reabsorption of 15% of the filtered Ca^{2+} load. In vitro studies have shown that there is significant Ca^{2+} permeability in this segment and that reabsorption is directly dependent on the electrochemical gradient formed between the luminal and basal surface of the tubular cells.[7] This gradient is formed as a result of active reabsorption of NaCl via the Na-K-2Cl cotransporter. These findings suggest that the Ca^{2+} reabsorption in this segment is passive and paracellular in nature.

Within the distal convoluted tubule and connecting tubule, 10–15% of total Ca^{2+} reabsorption occurs. Reabsorption in this portion of the nephron occurs in a transcellular manner. Ca^{2+} enters the tubular cells via the TRPV5 epithelial Ca^{2+} channel, is bound by the intracellular transport protein calbindin-D28k, and is transported to the basal membrane where it exits via the plasma membrane Ca^{2+} pump (PMCA) or the Na–Ca exchange pump. Paracellular transport is not possible in this portion of the nephron due to membrane proteins that are impermeable to Ca^{2+}. Importantly, this active transport of calcium is dependent on the action of PTH as well as adenylate cyclase.[7-10] Since this portion of the nephron transports Ca^{2+} actively, manipulation of reabsorption in this segment of the nephron can have significant effects on the overall urinary calcium concentration. The ability of the collecting duct to reabsorb Ca^{2+} is controversial as some suggest that there is a mild ability to promote reabsorption in a mechanism similar to that of the distal tubule.[7]

12.3 Hormonal Effects on Calcium Reabsorption

12.3.1 PTH Effects on the Kidney

PTH and parathyroid-related peptide (PTHrP) play a major role in the handling of calcium in the renal tubule in all areas. These hormones work through secondary messenger systems using the adenylyl cyclase/protein kinase A pathway and the phospholipase C/protein kinase C pathway. In the glomerulus, PTH directly affects the filtered calcium load. In the proximal tubule, the secondary messenger pathways affect Na^+

and water reabsorption thereby affecting diffusion of Ca^{2+}. Effects in the remainder of the tubule, however, result in increased reabsorption of Ca^{2+}. The mechanism of action in the thick ascending limb is controversial.[9,11-13] The primary site for PTH action is in the distal tubule.[14] In this segment, the hormone works to significantly increase Ca^{2+} reabsorption in a transcellular active transport manner via the aforementioned secondary signal mechanisms.[9,10,14-16]

12.3.2 Role of Vitamin D

Evidence points to a minor role for vitamin D in the renal handling of Ca^{2+}. Studies have shown that vitamin D and related metabolites can play a role in increasing distal tubular reabsorption of Ca^{2+} by regulation of both luminal and basolateral transport channels.[17,18]

12.3.3 Calcitonin

Calcitonin has been shown to have a direct effect on Ca^+ reabsorption. In physiologic levels, increased reabsorption is seen. In supraphysiologic doses, however, a hypercalciuric effect is observed. Receptors have been found on the thick ascending limb of the loop of Henle, the distal convoluted tubule, as well as the cortical collecting duct.[19]

12.4 Diuretic Effects on Calcium Transport

12.4.1 Role of Loop Diuretics

Loop diuretics function by blocking the Na-K-2Cl transporter in the thick ascending limb of the loop of Henle. As discussed earlier, this active transport system generates an electrochemical gradient that allows for passive diffusion of Ca^{2+} from the luminal portion of the loop of Henle to the extraluminal portion of the loop. Blocking this channel therefore eliminates the electrochemical gradient and therefore eliminates the driving force for movement of Ca^{2+}.

12.4.2 Thiazide Diuretics

The action of thiazide diuretics can be divided into acute and chronic effects. In the acute setting, thiazides lead to natriuresis by inhibiting the NaCl cotransporter in the distal convoluted tubule and stimulate acute reabsorption of Ca^{2+}.[8,20-22]

In the chronic setting, thiazide effects are seen in the proximal tubule. Studies suggest that the mechanism of action is due to extracellular fluid contraction leading to increased Na^+ reabsorption in the proximal tubule. This action leads to increased reabsorption of Ca^{2+} by associated diffusion. Several studies have shown that thiazide diuretics use in a chronic setting has no effects on calcium absorption in the distal tubule.[21-23] Most importantly, the hypocalciuric effects of thiazides can be reversed by salt replacement.[24]

12.5 Hypercalciuria

Hypercalciuria is defined as the excretion of urinary calcium exceeding 200 mg/24-h collection (or an excess of 4 mg of calcium/kg/24 h). Some investigators use higher levels to define hypercalciuria in men (>250–300 mg/day) and women (>200–250 mg/day). The association of hypercalciuria with recurrent calcium nephrolithiasis has long been recognized, although the exact nature of this relationship continues to be debated. Nephrolithiasis resulting from hypercalciuria is heterogeneous in origin, and comprises several entities.[25] Figures 12.3a, b, c, and d summarize many of the causes of hypercalciuria.

12.5.1 Absorptive Hypercalciuria

The basic abnormality in absorptive hypercalciuria is the intestinal hyperabsorption of calcium. The consequent increase in the circulating concentration of calcium enhances the renal filtered load and suppresses parathyroid function. Hypercalciuria results from the combination of increased filtered load and reduced renal tubular reabsorption of calcium, caused by parathyroid suppression. The excessive renal loss of calcium compensates for the high calcium absorption from the intestinal tract and helps to maintain serum calcium in the normal range. Absorptive hypercalciuria Type I (AH-I) is considered a more severe form, whereas the Type II presentation (AH-II) is a mild-to-moderate form of this condition.

The exact cause for the hyperabsorption of calcium is not known. In most patients, it probably occurs by a vitamin D-independent process. In some patients with severe absorptive hypercalciuria, an enhanced renal synthesis of 1,25-$(OH)_2$ vitamin D (1,25-$(OH)_2$D) or an increase in vitamin D receptors may contribute to high intestinal absorption and renal excretion of calcium.[25-28]

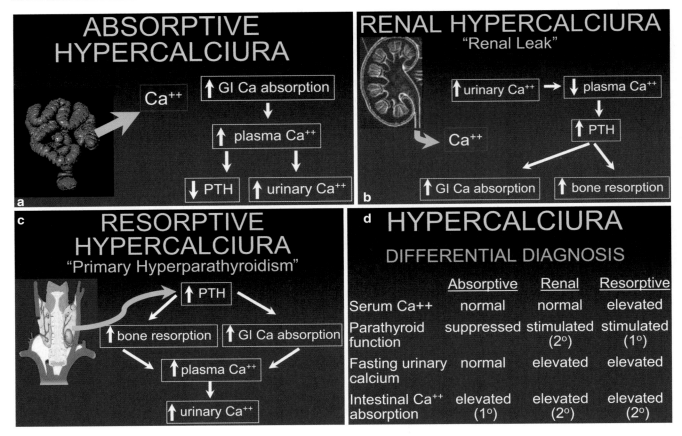

Fig. 12.3 Summary of forms of hypercalciuria. (**a**) Absorptive hypercalciuria. (**b**) Renal hypercalciuria. (**c**) Resorptive hypercalciuria. (**d**) Differential diagnosis

12.5.2 Renal Hypercalciuria

The primary abnormality in renal hypercalciuria is believed to be impairment in the renal tubular reabsorption of calcium. The resulting reduction in the serum calcium concentration stimulates parathyroid function. There may be excessive mobilization of calcium from bone and an enhanced intestinal absorption of calcium because of the PTH excess and the ensuing stimulation of the renal synthesis of 1,25-(OH)$_2$D. These effects increase the circulating concentration and the renal filtered load of calcium, often causing significant hypercalciuria. Unlike primary hyperparathyroidism, serum calcium is normal and the state of hyperparathyroidism is considered secondary.

12.5.3 Resorptive Hypercalciuria

Resorptive hypercalciuria is characterized by primary hyperparathyroidism. The initial event is the excessive resorption of bone resulting from hypersecretion of PTH. Intestinal absorption of calcium is frequently elevated because of the PTH-dependent stimulation of the renal synthesis of 1,25-(OH)$_2$D. These effects increase the circulating concentration and the renal filtered load of calcium, often causing significant hypercalciuria.

12.5.4 Other Forms of Hypercalciuria

Other causes of hypercalciuria, though poorly documented, include renal phosphate "leak," primary enhancement of 1,25-(OH)$_2$D synthesis, and excessive prostaglandin E$_2$ production.

Improved elucidation of pathophysiology and formulation of diagnostic criteria for different causes of nephrolithiasis have made feasible the adoption of selective treatment programs. Such programs should (a) reverse the underlying physicochemical and physiological derangements, (b) inhibit new stone formation, (c) overcome nonrenal complications of the disease process, and (d) be free of serious side effects. The rationale for the selection of certain treatment programs is the assumption that the particular physicochemical and physiological aberrations identified with the given disorder are etiologically important in the formation of renal stones, and that the correction of these disturbances would prevent stone formation. Moreover, it is assumed that such a selected treatment program would be more effective and safer than a "random" treatment. Despite a lack of conclusive experimental verification, these hypotheses appear reasonable and logical. For many pharmacologic treatment programs recommended for nephrolithiasis, sufficient information is now available to characterize their physicochemical and physiological actions.

12.6 Absorptive Hypercalciuria

12.6.1 Thiazides

Thiazide diuretics are not considered a selective therapy for absorptive hypercalciuria, since it does not decrease intestinal calcium absorption in this condition. However, this drug has been widely used to treat absorptive hypercalciuria, because of its hypocalciuric action and the high cost and inconvenience of alternative therapy (sodium cellulose phosphate).

Current studies indicate that thiazides may have a limited long-term effectiveness in absorptive hypercalciuria Type I. Despite an initial reduction in urinary calcium excretion, the intestinal calcium absorption remains persistently elevated. These studies suggest that the retained calcium may be accreted in bone at least during the first few years of therapy. Bone density, may increase during thiazide treatment in absorptive hypercalciuria. With continued treatment, however, the rise in bone density stabilizes and the hypocalciuric effect of thiazides becomes attenuated. The results suggest that thiazide treatment has caused a low turnover state of bone, which interferes with a continued calcium accretion in the skeleton. The "rejected" calcium would then be excreted in urine. In contrast, bone density is not significantly altered in renal hypercalciuria where thiazides cause a decline in intestinal calcium absorption commensurate with a reduction in urinary calcium.[21,29]

12.6.1.1 Thiazides in Absorptive Hypercalciuria Type I

Thiazide diuretics do not correct the basic, underlying physiologic defect in absorptive hypercalciuria. In patients with absorptive hypercalciuria Type I who may be at risk for bone disease (growing children, postmenopausal women), thiazide may be the first choice. When thiazides lose their hypocalciuric

action (after long-term treatment), a break in thiazide therapy must be given to allow the body to resensitize to the effects of thiazides. The medication can then be resumed.[22]

Potassium supplementation, preferably as potassium citrate, should be employed when using thiazide therapy in order to prevent hypokalemia and hypocitraturia. A typical treatment program might be trichlormethiazide 4 mg/day and potassium citrate 15–20 meq twice per day. Amiloride in combination with thiazide may be more effective than thiazides alone in reducing calcium excretion. However, it does not augment citrate excretion. Potassium supplementation should be used with caution in patients taking amiloride.[30]

In absorptive hypercalciuria Type II, no specific drug treatment may be necessary since the physiologic defect is not as severe as in absorptive hypercalciuria Type I. Moreover, many patients have extremely concentrated urine due to a disdain for drinking fluids. Therefore, a low calcium intake (400–600 mg/day) and high fluid intake (sufficient to achieve a minimum urine output of greater than 2 l/day) would seem ideally indicated, since normocalciuria could be restored by dietary calcium restriction alone, and increased urine volume has been shown to reduce urinary saturation of calcium oxalate.

12.6.2 Slow-Release Potassium Phosphate

The most common form of absorptive hypercalciuria is secondary to increased intestinal calcium absorption. Various theories exist regarding the exact pathophysiology of absorptive hypercalciuria including both vitamin D-dependent as well as vitamin D-independent absorptive hypercalciuria. It is believed that in a significant subset of patients, increased $1–25 (OH)_2$ D (vitamin D) levels may be responsible for enhanced intestinal calcium absorption in patients with absorptive hypercalciuria.[31] Previous studies have demonstrated that neutral phosphates may indeed be a useful preparation to reduce serum vitamin D levels as well as to inhibit urinary calcium excretion in patients with absorptive hypercalciuria. However, there are a number of problems with current forms of orthophosphate therapy. These preparations provide rapid release of neutral phosphate, which may cause GI upset and diarrhea from an increased osmotic load. In addition, many orthophosphate preparations provide an inadequate hypocalciuric response as compared to thiazide or sodium cellulose phosphate preparations due to the renal effect of sodium contained in most currently available orthophosphate preparations (see section on dietary sodium intake). Finally, previous studies have also demonstrated that orthophosphate preparations may increase the urinary saturation of calcium phosphate (brushite) due to a substantial rise in urinary pH, caused by the increased alkalinity of most available orthophosphate preparations.[32]

A new formulation of low-release, neutral potassium phosphate has been developed to obviate the aforementioned problems with currently available orthophosphate preparations. This potassium phosphate preparation (UroPhos-K) is carried out in a wax matrix to provide slow release of the orthophosphate. This restricted release limits the amount of GI upset found with most current orthophosphate preparations. In addition, UroPhos-K contains phosphate salts of potassium and does not contain sodium. Therefore, this preparation does not provide a sodium load that could offset the hypocalciuric action of the orthophosphate. Finally, this medication is designed to yield a pH of 7.0 as compared to 7.3 for some available orthophosphate preparations. Therefore, it is less likely that the crystallization of calcium phosphate may occur in the urine.[33]

Recently, a randomized prospective double-blind trial was performed in 21 patients with documented stone formation and absorptive hypercalciuria Type I. Patients received either UroPhos-K or placebo in a double-blinded fashion. No significant GI side effects were noted with the slow-release potassium phosphate preparation nor was there a significant increase in fasting serum potassium or phosphorus. However, the UroPhos-K treatment did significantly reduce urinary calcium from 288 to 171 mg/d without altering oxalate excretion. Moreover, the urinary saturation of calcium oxalate was significantly reduced without altering brushite saturation. Also noted was a significant increase of inhibitor activity secondary to increased urinary citrate and pyrophosphate, thereby inhibiting the potential crystallization of calcium oxalate in the urine.[31,33,34]

12.7 Renal Hypercalciuria

Thiazide diuretics are ideally indicated for the treatment of renal hypercalciuria. This diuretic has been shown to correct the renal leak of calcium by augmenting calcium reabsorption in the distal tubule and by causing extracellular volume depletion and stimulating proximal tubule reabsorption of calcium. The ensuing correction of secondary hyperparathyroidism restores normal serum $1,25\text{-}(OH)_2D$ and intestinal calcium absorption. Thiazides have been shown to provide a sustained correction of hypercalciuria commensurate with a restoration of normal serum $1,25\text{-}(OH)_2D$ and intestinal calcium absorption for up to 10 years of therapy. Physicochemically, the urinary environment becomes less saturated with respect to calcium oxalate and brushite during thiazide treatment, largely because of the reduced calcium excretion. Moreover, urinary inhibitor activity, as reflected in the limit of metastability, is increased by an unknown mechanism.

The above effects are shared by hydrochlorothiazide 50 mg twice/day, chlorthalidone 50 mg/day, or trichlormethiazide 4 mg/day. Potassium supplementation (approximately 60 meq/day) may sometimes be required to prevent hypokalemia and attendant hypocitraturia. Potassium citrate has been shown to be effective in averting hypokalemia and in increasing urinary citrate when administered to patients with calcium nephrolithiasis taking thiazides. Concurrent use of triamterene, a potassium-sparing agent, should be undertaken with caution because of recent reports of triamterene stone formation. Thiazides are contraindicated in primary hyperparathyroidism because of potential aggravation of hypercalcemia.[21,30,34-36]

12.8 Primary Hyperparathyroidism

Parathyroidectomy is the optimum treatment for nephrolithiasis of primary hyperparathyroidism. Following removal of abnormal parathyroid tissue, urinary calcium is restored to normal commensurate with a decline in serum concentration of calcium and intestinal absorption. The urinary environment becomes less saturated with respect to calcium oxalate and brushite and the limit of metastability (formation product ratio) for these calcium salts increases. There is typically a reduced rate of new stone formation, unless urinary tract infection is present. Parathyroidectomy is contraindicated in secondary hyperparathyroidism of renal hypercalciuria and in absorptive hypercalciuria.

There is no established medical treatment for the nephrolithiasis of primary hyperparathyroidism. Although orthophosphates have been recommended for the disease of mild-to-moderate severity, their safety or efficacy has not yet been proven. They should be used only when parathyroid surgery cannot be undertaken. Estrogen has been reported to be useful in reducing serum and urinary calcium in postmenopausal women with primary hyperparathyroidism.

12.9 Dietary Recommendations Related to Calcium Metabolism

12.9.1 Dietary Sodium

Hypercalciuria may be diet related with increased intestinal absorption of ingested calcium or secondary to a renal leak of calcium. Unfortunately, not enough emphasis has been placed on the role of dietary sodium and its impact on urinary calcium excretion. It has long been known that an increased intake of dietary sodium will result in increased urinary sodium excretion with the development of subsequent hypercalciuria. Moreover, increased urinary sodium excretion can also exacerbate nephrolithiasis since urinary sodium may block the action of thiazide diuretics administered to reduce urinary calcium excretion.

Recently, continued studies of the effect of dietary sodium in the stone forming population have demonstrated that high sodium intake not only increases calcium excretion, but may also increase urine pH and decrease urinary citrate excretion. These latter effects are probably due to sodium-induced bicarbonate excretion in the urine, a significant decrease in serum bicarbonate concentration. Along with these changes, the urinary saturation of calcium phosphate (brushite) and monosodium urate will increase and inhibitor activity against calcium oxalate crystallization will decrease. It is important to remember that the net effect of a high sodium diet can be an increased propensity for the crystallization of calcium salts in the urine.[38]

Therefore, in treating patients with hypercalciuric nephrolithiasis, not only is it important to identify the underlying cause of hypercalciuria, but to also have the patient avoid excessive intake of dairy products as well as salty foods. Urinary sodium should be maintained at a level less than 150 mEq/24 h. We therefore find it imperative to not only monitor 24-h urine calcium excretion, but also note urinary sodium values as well. All hypercalciuric patients should be placed on a sodium-restricted diet.

12.9.2 Dietary Calcium

Early recommendations suggested that a low calcium diet will decrease urinary calcium excretion, thereby reducing the risk for stone formation. However, a number of recent studies have suggested that a low calcium diet may pose a risk for recurrent stone formation as well as increasing the incidence of bone disease in those patients with nephrolithiasis.

Several studies have suggested that patients with idiopathic hypercalciuria may have low bone density, thought to be secondary to problems with intestinal calcium absorption as well as mobilization of calcium from the bone. These studies suggest that a low calcium diet may put certain hypercalciuric patients at risk for continued bone disease and subsequent osteoporosis.

Additional large-scale epidemiological studies have also demonstrated that a low calcium diet may increase one's risk for recurrent stone formation. In one study, 45,000 men ages 40–75 with no history of stones were followed for 4 years. This study found that calcium intake was inversely associated with stone formation and that a low calcium diet may increase the risk for renal stone formation. A second study of over 97,000 women ages 34–59 with no history of stones and 12 years of follow-up again found an inverse relationship between calcium intake and stone formation. In addition,

calcium supplementation appeared to be positively associated with the incidence of stone disease. This study concluded that high dietary calcium intake decreases the risk of stone formation.[25,27,39–41]

Both of these studies suggest that a low calcium intake increases intestinal oxalate absorption with a subsequent increase in urinary oxalate. The increased oxalate load will increase the risk for calcium oxalate stone formation. However, one should be aware that certain patients with hypercalciuria may be at risk for increased dietary calcium. Specifically, those patients with absorptive hypercalciuria will only increase their urinary calcium excretion on a high calcium diet. In addition, studies have demonstrated that a low calcium diet in patients with increased calcium absorption (absorptive hypercalciuria) does not routinely augment oxalate excretion. Therefore, our overall recommendation is to not put patients on a calcium-restricted diet, yet to recommend avoidance of an excessive intake of dairy products and salty foods.

12.9.3 Calcium Supplementation

Osteoporosis continues to be an increasing public health problem in the United States. As the "baby boomer" generation approaches menopause, the lay press has continued to emphasize osteoporosis and its prevention. Perhaps the most common method of preventing osteoporosis continues to be the use of calcium supplements. Yet, concern exists regarding the impact of calcium supplementation in stone forming patients, specifically with regard to the potential risks of hypercalciuria with subsequent stone disease induced from the excessive intake of calcium supplementation.

A number of over-the-counter calcium supplements are currently available and marketed under various brand names. Calcium carbonate and calcium phosphate continue to be some of the more widely advertised and subsequently utilized calcium supplements. However, studies have demonstrated that these calcium supplements may be poorly absorbed from the intestinal tract and can increase urinary calcium excretion and perhaps promote calcium oxalate or calcium phosphate stone disease.

An alternative calcium supplement has been formulated to provide increased intestinal absorption of calcium (to prevent osteoporosis) as well as to prevent concurrent supersaturation of the urine with regard to calcium-forming salts. Calcium citrate is an over-the-counter calcium preparation that provides 950 mg of calcium citrate and 200 mg of elemental calcium in each tablet. As with other available calcium supplements, calcium citrate will significantly increase urinary calcium excretion. Yet, this preparation offers the benefit of increasing urinary citrate excretion as well.

The concomitant increase in citraturia potentially offsets the lithogenic potential of calcium supplement-induced hypercalciuria and therefore provides a more "stone-friendly" calcium supplement.

Recently, a long-term clinical trial was completed that further studied the effects of long-term calcium citrate supplementation in premenopausal women. This study demonstrated that the urinary saturation of calcium oxalate and calcium phosphate (brushite) did not significantly change during calcium citrate therapy. It appears that the lack of calcium supplement-induced hypercalciuria was secondary to the down-regulation of intestinal calcium absorption, due to prolonged calcium supplementation and the inhibitory effects of citrate included in the calcium citrate preparation. The results of this long-term calcium citrate trial suggest that calcium supplementation using calcium citrate does not increase the propensity for crystallization of calcium salts within the urine. This protective effect is most likely due to an attenuated increase in urinary calcium excretion (from a decrease in fractional intestinal calcium absorption), a decrease in urinary phosphorus, and an increased citraturic response.[36,42-44]

Therefore, if calcium supplementation is to be considered in a patient who is concerned about the development of osteoporosis, calcium citrate preparations should be utilized due to their increased bioavailability as well as their reduced risk of calcium stone formation. In women who have a previous history of stone formation, one may institute calcium citrate supplementation, but then perform a 24-h urine collection to identify those patients who will become/remain hypercalciuric while on calcium supplementation. In the patients who are normocalciuric while receiving calcium citrate, no further intervention is necessary. However, in those patients who are found to be hypercalciuric, treatment with thiazide diuretics or perhaps slow-release potassium phosphate preparations are warranted.

12.10 Conclusions

Calcium metabolism is a complex interaction between the bony skeleton, thyroid/parathyroid function, the GI tract, and renal physiology. These interactions lead to calcium homeostasis within a very narrow physiological range. Daily urinary excretion of Ca^{2+} is 200 mg. Many disorders can lead to hypercalciuria and effective therapeutic modalities have been developed to control hypercalciuria in these patients.

Selective medical therapy of nephrolithiasis is effective in preventing new stone formation. A remission rate of greater than 80% and overall reduction in individual stone formation rate of greater than 90% can be obtained in patients with recurrent nephrolithiasis. In patients with mild-to-moderate severity of stone disease, a virtual total control of stone disease can be achieved as evidenced by remission rates of greater than 95%. The need for stone removal may be dramatically reduced by an effective prophylactic program.

References

1. Amasheh S, Meiri N, Gitter AH, et al. Claudin-2 expression induces cation-selective channels in tight junctions of epithelial cells. J Cell Sci. 2002;115:4969–4976.
2. Bourdeau J. Calcium transport across the pars recta of cortical segment 2 proximal tubules. *Am J Physiol.* 1986;251:F718-F724.
3. Brunette M, Aras M. A microinjection study of nephron permeability to calcium and magnesium. Am J Physiol. 1971;221:1442–1448.
4. Ng RC, Rouse D, Suki WN. Calcium transport in the rabbit superficial proximal convoluted tubule. *J Clin Invest.* 1984;74:834–842.
5. Rocha AS, Magaldi JB, Kokko JP. Calcium and phosphate transport in isolated segments of rabbit Henle's loop. *J Clin Invest.* 1977;59:975–983.
6. Yu A. Renal transport of calcium, magnesium, and phosphate. In: Brenner BM, ed. *Brenner and Rector's The Kidney.* Philadelphia: Saunders; 2004:535–572.
7. Costanzo LS, Windhager EE. Calcium and sodium transport by the distal convoluted tubule of the rat. *Am J Physiol (Renal Fluid Electrolyte Physiol).* 1978;235:F492-F506.
8. Imai M. Effects of parathyroid hormone and N6, O2¢-dibutyryl cyclic AMP on Ca2+ transport across the rabbit distal nephron segments perfused in vitro. *Pflügers Arch.* 1981;390:145–151.
9. Shareghi GR, Stoner LC. Calcium transport across segments of the rabbit distal nephron in vitro. *Am J Physiol.* 1978;235:F367-F375.
10. Bourdeau JE, Burg MB. Effect of PTH on calcium transport across the cortical thick ascending limb of Henle's loop. *Am J Physiol.* 1980;239:F121-F126.
11. Friedman P. Basal and hormone-activated calcium absorption in mouse renal thick ascending limbs. *Am J Physiol.* 1988;254:F62-F70.
12. Lee K, Brown D, Ureña P, et al. Localization of parathyroid hormone/parathyroid hormone-related peptide receptor mRNA in kidney. *Am J Physiol.* 1996;270:F186-F191.
13. Costanzo LS, Windhager EE. Effects of PTH, ADH, and cyclic AMP on distal tubular Ca and Na reabsorption. *Am J Physiol.* 1980;239:F478-F485.
14. Bacskai BJ, Friedman PA. Activation of latent Ca2+ channels in renal epithelial cells by parathyroid hormone. *Nature (London).* 1990;347:388–391.
15. Shimizu T, Yoshitomi K, Nakamura M, Imai M. Effects of PTH, calcitonin, and cAMP on calcium transport in rabbit distal nephron segments. *Am J Physiol.* 1990;259:F408-F414.
16. Bindels RJ, Hartog A, Timmermans J, Van Os CH. Active Ca2+ transport in primary cultures of rabbit kidney CCD: stimulation by 1,25-dihydroxyvitamin D3 and PTH. *Am J Physiol.* 1991;261:F779-F807.
17. Hoenderop JG, Dardenne O, Van Abel M, et al. Modulation of renal Ca2+ transport protein genes by dietary Ca2+ and 1,25-dihydroxyvitamin D3 in 25-hydroxyvitamin D3–1alpha-hydroxylase knockout mice. *FASEB J.* 2002;16:1398–1406.
18. Firsov D, Bellanger AC, Marsy S, Elalouf JM. Quantitative RT-PCR analysis of calcitonin receptor mRNAs in the rat nephron. *Am J Physiol.* 1995;269:F702-F709.
19. Eknoyan G, Suki WN, Martinez-Maldonado M. Effect of diuretics on urinary excretion of phosphate, calcium, and magnesium in thyroparathyroidectomized dogs. *J Lab Clin Med.* 1970;76:257–266.

20. Pak CY. Hydrochlorothiazide therapy in nephrolithiasis. Effect on the urinary activity product and formation product of brushite. *Clin Pharmacol Ther.* 1973;14(2):209–217.

21. Preminger GM, Pak CY. Eventual attenuation of hypocalciuric response to hydrochlorothiazide in absorptive hypercalciuria. *J Urol.* 1987;137(6):1104–1109.

22. Nijenhuis T, Vallon V, van der Kemp AW, Loffing J, Hoenderop JG, Bindels RJ. Enhanced passive Ca2+ reabsorption and reduced Mg2+ channel abundance explains thiazide-induced hypocalciuria and hypomagnesemia. *J Clin Invest.* 2005;115:1651–1658.

23. Brickman AS, Massry SG, Coburn JW. Changes in serum and urinary calcium during treatment with hydrochlorothiazide: studies on mechanisms. *J Clin Invest.* 1972;51:945–954.

24. Pak CY. Physiological basis for absorptive and renal hypercalciurias. *Am J Physiol.* 1979;237(6):F415-F423.

25. Breslau NA, McGuire JL, Zerwekh JE, Pak CY. The role of dietary sodium on renal excretion and intestinal absorption of calcium and on vitamin D metabolism. *J Clin Endocrinol Metab.* 1982;55(2):369–373.

26. Pak CY. Calcium metabolism. *J Am Coll Nutr.* 1989;8(Suppl):46S-53S.

27. Pak CY, Sakhaee K, Hwang TI, Preminger GM, Harvey JA. Nephrolithiasis from calcium supplementation. *J Urol.* 1987;137(6):1212–1213.

28. Reed BY, Heller HJ, Gitomer WL, Pak CY. Mapping a gene defect in absorptive hypercalciuria to chromosome 1q23.3-q24. *J Clin Endocrinol Metab.* 1999;84(11):3907–3913.

29. Odvina CV, Mason RP, Pak CY. Prevention of thiazide-induced hypokalemia without magnesium depletion by potassium-magnesium-citrate. *Am J Ther.* 2006;13(2):101–108.

30. Van Den Berg CJ, Kumar R, Wilson DM, Heath H 3rd, Smith LH. Orthophosphate therapy decreases urinary calcium excretion and serum 1, 25-dihydroxyvitamin D concentrations in idiopathic hypercalciuria. *J Clin Endocrinol Metab.* 1980;51(5):998–1001.

31. Insogna KL, Ellison AS, Burtis WJ, Sartori L, Lang RL, Broadus AE. Trichlormethiazide and oral phosphate therapy in patients with absorptive hypercalciuria. *J Urol.* 1989;141(2):269–274.

32. Breslau NA, Padalino P, Kok DJ, Kim YG, Pak CY. Physicochemical effects of a new slow-release potassium phosphate preparation (UroPhos-K) in absorptive hypercalciuria. *J Bone Miner Res.* 1995;10(3):394–400.

33. Pearle MS, Roehrborn CG, Pak CY. Meta-analysis of randomized trials for medical prevention of calcium oxalate nephrolithiasis. *J Endourol.* 1999;13(9):679–685.

34. Pak CY, Peterson R, Sakhaee K, Fuller C, Preminger G, Reisch J. Correction of hypocitraturia and prevention of stone formation by combined thiazide and potassium citrate therapy in thiazide-unresponsive hypercalciuric nephrolithiasis. *Am J Med.* 1985;79(3):284–288.

35. Pak CY, Sakhaee K, Fuller CJ. Physiological and physiochemical correction and prevention of calcium stone formation by potassium citrate therapy. *Trans Assoc Am Physicians.* 1983;96:294–305.

36. Sakhaee K, Zisman A, Poindexter JR, Zerwekh JE, Pak CY. Metabolic effects of thiazide and 1, 25-(OH)2 vitamin D in postmenopausal osteoporosis. *Osteoporos Int.* 1993;3(4):209–214.

37. Sakhaee K, Harvey JA, Padalino PK, Whitson P, Pak CY. The potential role of salt abuse on the risk for kidney stone formation. *J Urol.* 1993;150(2 Pt 1):310–312.

38. Pak CY, Moe OW, Sakhaee K, Peterson RD, Poindexter JR. Physicochemical metabolic characteristics for calcium oxalate stone formation in patients with gouty diathesis. *J Urol.* 2005;173(5):1606–1609.

39. Pak CY, Smith LH, Resnick MI, Weinerth JL. Dietary management of idiopathic calcium urolithiasis. *J Urol.* 1984;131(5):850–852.

40. Preminger GM, Pak CY. The practical evaluation and selective medical management of nephrolithiasis. *Semin Urol.* 1985;3(3):170–184.

41. Giannini S, Nobile M, Sartori L, et al. Bone density and skeletal metabolism are altered in idiopathic hypercalciuria. *Clin Nephrol.* 1998;50(2):94–100.

42. Levine BS, Rodman JS, Wienerman S, Bockman RS, Lane JM, Chapman DS. Effect of calcium citrate supplementation on urinary calcium oxalate saturation in female stone formers: implications for prevention of osteoporosis. *Am J Clin Nutr.* 1994;60(4):592–596.

43. Odvina CV, Poindexter JR, Peterson RD, Zerwekh JE, Pak CY. Intestinal hyperabsorption of calcium and low bone turnover in hypercalciuric postmenopausal osteoporosis. *Urol Res.* 2008;36(5):233–239.

44. Brenner B. *Brenner and Rector's The Kidney.* Vol 1, 8th ed. Saunders: Elsevier; 2007

Vitamin D Metabolism and Stones

13

Joseph E. Zerwekh

Abstract It has been nearly 90 years since the discovery of the antirachitic activity of vitamin D. During that period, vitamin D structure, metabolism, and mechanism of action at target tissues have been delineated. We now recognize that vitamin D acts as a steroid hormone to help maintain normal calcium and phosphate homeostasis. Many diseases characterized by deranged calcium and phosphate metabolism have been explained by dysregulated vitamin D production and/or action. Calcium-containing kidney stones are believed to result from excessive urinary calcium excretion due to increased intestinal absorption of calcium, increased bone resorption, and renal calcium loss. To try and explain the cause of this hypercalciuria, many studies have focused on the role of deranged vitamin D metabolism and action. Much of our understanding of how such derangements in vitamin D metabolism and action can contribute to the development of hypercalciuria and ultimately kidney stones has come from both clinical and basic approaches that are discussed in this chapter. However, some studies have failed to observe any alteration in vitamin D production or action, while others have implicated a role for increased $1,25(OH)_2D$ production or increased tissue sensitivity in the face of normal circulating $1,25(OH)_2D$ concentrations. Resolution of these discrepancies will require additional studies in hypercalciuric stone-forming patients that focus on the genetics of vitamin D metabolism and the cellular and molecular actions of vitamin D at its target tissues.

13.1 Introduction

It has been nearly 90 years since the discovery of the antirachitic activity of vitamin D. Today, it is known that this fat-soluble vitamin is, in actuality, a steroid hormone that is synthesized principally in the kidney with actions at a multitude of target organs. In the last 20 years, there has been increasing interest in vitamin D's potential role in the prevention of many chronic disease including cancer, diabetes, cardiovascular disease, and neurodegenerative disorders. Such studies have led to the suggestion that our current definition of vitamin D sufficiency may be too low, generating renewed interest in maintaining adequate vitamin D repletion. Despite

these new and emerging concepts regarding vitamin D action at nonclassical tissues, the majority of studies have focused on vitamin D's role in maintaining adequate calcium homeostasis and bone health. Hypercalcemia and hypercalciuria are well-known consequences of elevated circulating vitamin D concentration and increased action at the three principal target organs, gut, bone, and kidney. Since hypercalciuria is a frequent finding in patients with nephrolithiasis, a causality role for deranged vitamin D concentration and or action in stone-forming patients with hypercalciuria has been proposed. Although some studies have supported such a pathophysiologic role for vitamin D in hypercalciuric stone-forming patients, an equal number of studies have not been able to support these observations. This chapter considers the chemistry, metabolism, and action of vitamin D in regulating calcium and phosphorus homeostasis. With this background, a discussion of the studies, both pro and con, directed at delineating vitamin D's action in the development of nephrolithiasis is presented.

J.E. Zerwekh
University of Texas Southwestern Medical Center, Charles and Jane Pak Center for Mineral Metabolism and Clinical Research, Dallas, TX, USA
e-mail: joseph.zerwekh@utsouthwestern.edu

P.N. Rao et al. (eds.), *Urinary Tract Stone Disease*,
DOI 10.1007/978-1-84800-362-0_13, © Springer-Verlag London Limited 2011

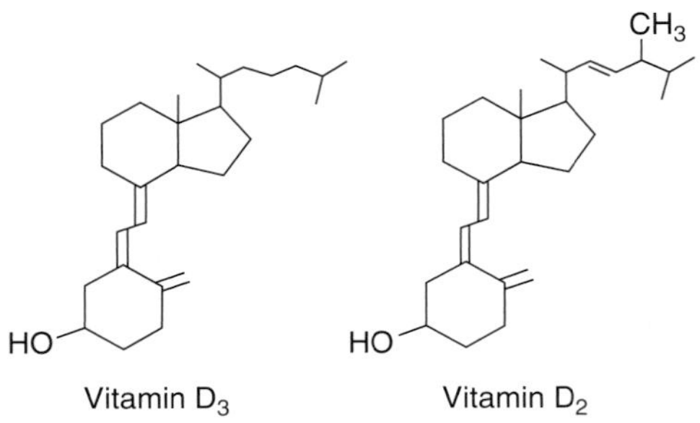

Fig. 13.1 Structures of the nutritional forms of vitamin D

13.2 Vitamin D Structure

The antirachitic activity of vitamin D was first described nearly a 90 years ago.[1] However, it was not until 1931 that the isolation and structure of vitamin D_2 was accomplished.[2] This was soon followed by the identification of vitamin D_3 by the Windaus group[3] and eventual syntheses of the vitamin D compounds confirming their structures. Today, vitamin D is classified as a secosteroid and the two best known examples of the nutritional forms of this vitamin are vitamin D_2, or ergocalciferol, and vitamin D_3, or cholecalciferol (Fig. 13.1). The rules of the International Union of Pure and Applied Chemists (IUPAC) for steroid nomenclature are used in naming the vitamin D compounds.[4] Since they are derived from cholesterol, they retain the numbering of that steroid. Thus the official name of vitamin D_3, based on the numbering of carbon atoms in cholesterol, is 9,10-seco(5Z,7E)-5,7,10(19) cholesta-triene-3β(beta)-ol, and the official name of vitamin D_2 is 9,10-seco(5Z,7E)-5,7,10(19), 22-ergostate-traene-3β(beta)-ol. In practice, it is simpler to refer to the two nutritional forms of vitamin D simply as vitamin D_2 and vitamin D_3. It should be made clear that for the remainder of this chapter the subscripts are included when discussing the specific forms of the vitamin while the term vitamin D implies either D_2 or D_3.

13.3 Vitamin D Manufacture

Both vitamin D_2 and vitamin D_3 are normally produced from their precursor molecules by the action of ultraviolet light. This mechanism explains the efficacy of exposure of rachitic children to sunlight or to ultraviolet light-irradiated food products.[5,6] When human skin is exposed to sunlight, solar photons with energies between 290 and 315 nm (UVB) promote the photolysis of 7-dehydrocholesterol (provitamin D_3) to previtamin D_3. Previtamin D_3 is thermodynamically unstable and undergoes a rapid rearrangement of double bonds to form vitamin D_3.[7] This conversion is rather efficient with about 50% of the previtamin D_3 being converted to vitamin D_3 within 2 h. Once formed in the membrane, the vitamin D_3

is rapidly extruded from the cell into the extracellular space where it is bound to the vitamin D binding protein (DBP) in the circulation. A similar mechanism operates to produce vitamin D_2 from ergosterol in plant products. With extended periods of sunlight exposure, nonisomerized vitamin D_3, as well as vitamin D_3 itself, can undergo isomerization to biologically inactive photoisomers.[8] This mechanism for vitamin D inactivation offers an explanation for the lack of reported cases of vitamin D intoxication-induced hypercalcemia from chronic excessive exposure to sunlight.

13.3.1 Factors Influencing the Cutaneous Production of Vitamin D_3

The cutaneous production of vitamin D_3 is responsible for supplying about 95% of the vitamin D_3 in human beings. Thus it is important to recognize the various environmental factors and social behaviors that can affect vitamin D_3 production. Any substance that can interfere with solar UVB radiation reaching the 7-dehydrocholesterol stores in the epidermis could potentially lead to vitamin D insufficiency. Sunscreen use has been popularized in recent years to prevent the damaging and aging effects of sunlight on the skin. Sunscreens with a sun protection factor (SPF) of eight or greater have been shown to effectively block any dermal production of vitamin D_3.[9] Likewise, melanin absorbs ultraviolet radiation and is believed to be the reason why African-Americans have reduced circulating concentrations of 25-hydroxyvitamin D_3 and are more prone to developing vitamin D deficiency.[10] In addition, environmental considerations such as latitude, season, and time of day can exert significant effects on dermal vitamin D_3 production. In general, there is greater synthesis of previtamin D_3 from its precursor during the summer months when solar radiation is most direct. There is also less previtamin D_3 production at northern latitudes compared to more southern locations and synthesis is greatest during the midday hours when the sun is at its zenith.[11]

13.4 Vitamin D Metabolism

Following the discovery and structural identification of vitamin D, it was believed that vitamin D was the active form and did not undergo further metabolic activation.[12] This concept was drastically altered in 1966 when chemical synthesis of radioactive vitamin D_3 of high specific activity disclosed the formation of biologically active metabolites.[13] By 1968, a more polar metabolite of radioactive vitamin D_3 was isolated, purified, and identified as 25-hydroxycholecalciferol (25OHD_3).[14] This metabolite was thought to be the active form of vitamin D_3, but another more polar peak of radioactivity, previously disregarded as an active metabolite of

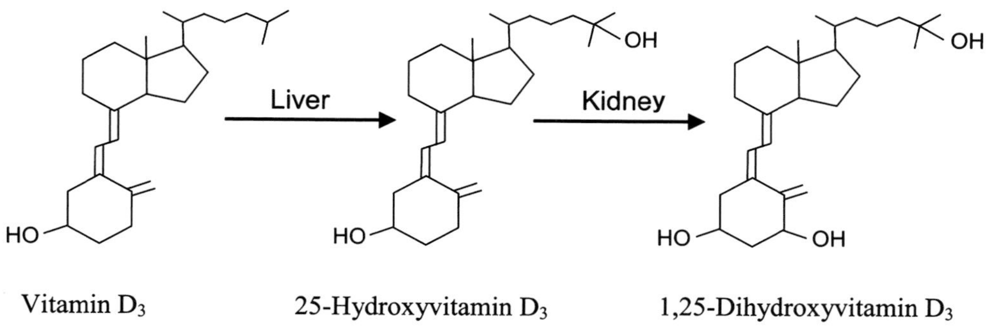

Fig. 13.2 Metabolic activation of the vitamin D molecule

Vitamin D_3 25-Hydroxyvitamin D_3 1,25-Dihydroxyvitamin D_3

vitamin D_3, was subsequently isolated from the intestines of 1,600 chickens given radiolabeled vitamin D_3. By means of mass spectrometric techniques and specific chemical reactions, the structure of the active form of vitamin D_3 in the intestine was unequivocally identified as 1,25-dihydroxycholecalciferol $(1,25(OH)_2D_3)$.[15] At about the same time, the kidney was demonstrated to be the site of synthesis of $1,25(OH)_2D_3$.[16] This observation was important in securing the identity of $1,25(OH)_2D_3$ as the active form of vitamin D_3. Anephric animals responded to $1,25(OH)_2D_3$ by increasing intestinal absorption of calcium and bone calcium mobilization, but animals receiving $25OHD_3$ at physiological doses did not.[17–19] The structures and metabolic activation of vitamin D_3 are summarized in Fig. 13.2.

13.4.1 Production of 25OHD

The 25-hydroxylation of vitamin D is the initial step in vitamin D activation. The 25-hydroxylase, the enzyme responsible for this step, is located in the liver. Determination of the subcellular localization of the vitamin D-25-hydroxylase was hampered by cross-contamination of microsomes and mitochondria, the numerous microsomal P450s in the liver, and instability of the 25-hydroxylase activity. After intensive studies, both mitochondria and microsomes were found to be responsible for the 25-hydroxylation of vitamin D, although the majority of the activity appears to reside in the mitochondria. In human beings, it is now known that the vitamin D hydroxylation is now catalyzed by CYP27A1 in mitochondria and CYP2R1 in microsomes.[20] Two additional hepatic cytochrome P450 enzymes have also been implicated in the production of 25OHD – namely CYP3A4 and CYP2J3. Irrespective of the enzyme(s) responsible for the hepatic production of 25OHD, it is well known that this step in the activation of vitamin D is not tightly regulated. An increase in either the cutaneous production of vitamin D_3 or ingestion of vitamin D from foods or from supplements will result in an increase in circulating concentrations of 25OHD.[21] Because of this fact and the relatively long half-life of 25OHD (about 3 weeks), its measurement in blood is used to determine whether a patient is vitamin D deficient, sufficient, or intoxicated. There have been very few reports of serum 25OHD concentration in the stone-forming patient. When examined, values have been within the normal range.

13.4.2 Production of $1,25(OH)_2D$

Following the identification of $1,25(OH)_2D$ as the physiologically active metabolite of vitamin D and its renal site of synthesis, many studies were undertaken to identify the P450 mixed function oxidase(s) responsible for its production. Early studies showed the enzymatic activity to be located in the inner mitochondrial membrane of the proximal convoluted tubule cells of the kidney.[22] The primary sequence of the 1α(alpha)-hydroxylase has been deduced from cloned cDNA from several mammalian species. Although purified preparations of the protein itself are not routinely obtained, the primary sequence of the P450 oxidase that catalyzes the 1-hydroxylation, as deduced from its cDNA sequence, reveals that it is structurally related to the mitochondrial sterol side chain hydroxylases and hence was given the systematic name of CYP27B1. In addition to the kidney, a wide variety of tissues and cells have been shown to have the capacity to produce $1,25(OH)_2D$ including activated macrophages, osteoblasts, keratinocytes, prostate, colon, and breast.[23] The placenta has also been shown to produce $1,25(OH)_2D$ during pregnancy.[24] It is unlikely that any of these extrarenal sites of $1,25(OH)_2D$ production significantly contribute to overall calcium economy since anephric patients have very low or undetectable blood concentrations of $1,25(OH)_2D$. One exception to this observation is found in patients with chronic granulomatous disorders such as sarcoidosis. In this condition, activated macrophages make and secrete $1,25(OH)_2D$ into the circulation. For such patients, the excess $1,25(OH)_2D$ can lead to hypercalcemia, hypercalciuria, and kidney stones.[25] The local production of $1,25(OH)_2D$ in tissues not associated with calcium homeostasis may be for the purpose of regulating a wide variety of emerging biological functions shown to be sensitive to the presence of $1,25(OH)_2D$. Such functions include cell growth, apoptosis, angiogenesis, differentiation, and regulation of the immune system.

13.4.3 Regulation of 1,25(OH)₂D Production

As mentioned earlier, the production of 25OHD does not appear to be tightly regulated since its production is directly dependent on the substrate (vitamin D) concentration. On the other hand, renal production of $1,25(OH)_2D$ is tightly regulated by the calcium needs of human beings. During conditions of reduced serum ionized calcium, the calcium-sensing receptors in the parathyroid gland respond by enhancing the release and synthesis of parathyroid hormone (PTH).[26] At the kidney, PTH not only enhances the reabsorption of calcium but also activates mitochondrial CYP27B1 in proximal tubular cells leading to an increase in $1,25(OH)_2D$ production. Through its action at the gut to increase the efficiency of intestinal calcium absorption and its concerted action with PTH on bone to increase osteoclast-mediated bone resorption, $1,25(OH)_2D$ helps promote a return of serum ionized calcium to normal. Excess phosphate liberated from bone during bone resorption and from increased intestinal absorption is lost in urine through PTH-dependent renal mechanisms. There is also experimental evidence that calcium deprivation can enhance 1-hydroxylase activity independent of secondary hyperparathyroidism.[27]

The production of $1,25(OH)_2D$ is also regulated by the prevailing serum phosphate concentration. Hypophosphatemia and hyperphosphatemia are associated with increased and decreased circulating concentration of $1,25(OH)_2D$, respectively.[28] It has recently been demonstrated that this effect is probably mediated by the phosphatonin, fibroblast growth factor 23 (FGF-23).[29,30] FGF-23 secretion from bone is increased following an increase in dietary phosphate intake. FGF-23 prevents serum phosphate concentration from becoming too high by initiating renal mechanisms to increase phosphate excretion and by decreasing the renal synthesis of $1,25(OH)_2D$, which reduces intestinal phosphate absorption (Fig. 13.3).

A number of other hormones and growth factors have also been shown to indirectly stimulate the production of $1,25(OH)_2D$. Many of these factors are associated with growth and development of the skeleton or calcium regulation including growth hormone and prolactin. Insulin-like growth factor-I (IGF-1) is also a potent stimulator of $1,25(OH)_2D$ production and may explain the strong correlation between growth velocity and serum $1,25(OH)_2D$ in children.[31]

13.4.4 Catabolism of 25OHD and 1,25(OH)₂D

Both 25OHD and $1,25(OH)_2D$ undergo 24-hydroxylation by the 25(OH)D-24-hydroxylase (CYP24A1) to form 24,25-dihydroxyvitamin D $(24,25(OH)_2D)$ and 1,24,25-trihydroxyvitamin D, respectively.[32] Regarded as the first step in

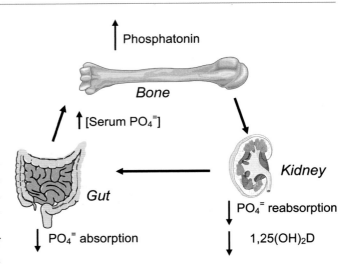

Fig. 13.3 Role of phosphatonins such as FGF23 in regulating phosphate homeostasis. During increased phosphate intake from the diet, FGF23 is elaborated from the bone. It then acts at the kidney to decrease the tubular reabsorption of phosphate and to suppress the renal synthesis of $1,25(OH)_2D$. The fall in $1,25(OH)_2D$ reduces the intestinal absorption of phosphate, and combined with the PTH-independent phosphaturia results in lowering of serum phosphate

the catabolism of 25OHD and $1,25(OH)_2D$, the 24-hydroxylase is upregulated by $1,25(OH)_2D$ by a vitamin D receptor (VDR)-mediated mechanism. Assessment of 24-hydroxylase activity is often used as a marker of $1,25(OH)_2D$ action through its receptor. This assessment has been previously used to assess VDR responsiveness to $1,25(OH)_2D$ in skin fibroblasts from hypercalciuric stone-forming patients[33] (see Sect. 13.6.3). To date, more than 50 different metabolites of vitamin D have been identified. However, only $1,25(OH)_2D$ is believed to be important for mediating the biological actions of vitamin D on calcium and bone metabolism.

13.5 Biologic Actions of Vitamin D in the Intestine and Bone

The major physiologic function of vitamin D is to maintain serum calcium within a physiologically acceptable range conducive to a wide variety of metabolic functions, signal transduction, and neuromuscular activity. It accomplishes this through genomic mechanisms after binding to its VDR in target tissues. In this respect, vitamin D is a steroid hormone and acts similar to estrogen and other steroid hormones in inducing its biological responses. The molecular biology of vitamin D action at its receptor has been examined in many tissues and systems. The major steps consist of binding to its cytoplasmic receptor, undergoing a conformational change to reorient the activation function 2 domain, permitting it to interact with other cytoplasmic proteins and coactivators. This action leads to its translocation to the nucleus where the VDR-1,25(OH)$_2$D complex binds with the retinoid X receptor (RXR) forming a heterodimeric complex that binds to the vitamin D response element (VDRE). This allows binding of several initiation factors and several other coactivators that initiate transcription of the vitamin D responsive gene.[34] It should also be mentioned that there is a growing body of evidence pointing to 1,25(OH)$_2$D-mediated nongenomic rapid responses in some target tissues including intestine, osteoblasts, pancreas, smooth muscle, and monocytes. Under this scenario, binding of 1,25(OH)$_2$D to a membrane surface receptor (e.g., caveolae) may result in the activation of one or more second messenger systems including phospholipase C, protein kinase C, G protein coupled receptors, and phosphatidyl-inositol-3-kinase (PI3). Some of the second messengers from this activation may engage in cross-talk with the nucleus to modulate gene expression.[35] Following its interaction with the VDR, 1,25(OH)$_2$D enhances calcium absorption by inducing the epithelial calcium channel TRPV6, a member of the vanillanoid receptor family,[36] calcium binding protein (calbindin D$_{9K}$), and a basal–lateral low affinity calcium ATPase. Activation of these channels and proteins facilitates the movement of calcium through the cytoplasm and entry into the circulation via the basal–lateral membrane calcium ATPase. 1,25(OH)$_2$D also enhances the absorption of dietary phosphorus through enhanced cellular brush border phosphate uptake. The uptake process is saturable with an affinity coefficient of 1.0 mM. Thus, the 1,25(OH)$_2$D – mediated transcellular mechanism is active only under conditions of low dietary phosphate. The net result is that there is an increase in the efficiency of intestinal calcium and phosphorus absorption. Under conditions of low dietary calcium intake, increased circulating 1,25(OH)$_2$D can also interact with the VDR in osteoblasts, resulting in signal transduction to induce RANKL expression, a cofactor necessary for the differentiation of preosteoclasts to fully mature osteoclasts that then resorb bone and liberate calcium and phosphorus into the extracellular space.

13.5.1 1,25(OH)$_2$D Action at the Parathyroid Gland

The parathyroid chief cell has a VDR and it responds to 1,25(OH)$_2$D by decreasing the expression of the PTH gene and decreasing PTH synthesis and secretion. Although it is uncertain whether this action of 1,25(OH)$_2$D plays any significant role in normal calcium homeostasis, it does have important implications in patients with renal failure and secondary or tertiary hyperparathyroidism. During long-standing secondary or tertiary hyperparathyroidism of the parathyroid gland, clusters of PTH secreting cells form that have little or no VDR. As might be expected, these cells are no longer responsive to the PTH lowering effects of 1,25(OH)$_2$D. In cases of mild to moderate secondary or tertiary hyperparathyroidism, PTH secretion can be suppressed by maintaining normal serum calcium by controlling for hyperphosphatemia. By lowering serum phosphate, the renal synthesis of 1,25(OH)$_2$D is stimulated, promoting increased intestinal calcium absorption and suppressing PTH secretion via its action at the parathyroid gland VDR. However, when serum phosphate is maintained in the normal range and PTH secretion continues to increase, the oral use of 1,25(OH)$_2$D or its less calcemic analogs to maintain serum calcium levels and suppress PTH synthesis is warranted. Analogs of 1,25(OH)$_2$D that have been used in this capacity are 19-nor-1,25-dihydroxyvitamin D$_2$, 1α(alpha)-hydroxyvitamin D$_3$, 1α(alpha)-hydroxyvitamin D$_2$, and 1,24-epi-dihydroxyvitamin D$_2$. This action of 1,25(OH)$_2$D at the parathyroid gland is directly applicable to patients with chronic renal failure, but not in stone-forming patients with hypercalciuria and normal or suppressed PTH.

13.6 The Role of Vitamin D in the Etiology of Stone Disease

From the foregoing discussion, it is clear that derangements in vitamin D metabolism and action might be responsible for the development of hypercalciuria and the attendant risk of forming a calcium-containing kidney stone. Because of the well-established action of vitamin D on intestinal calcium transport (see Sect. 13.5) and the recognition that increased intestinal calcium absorption is frequently encountered in hypercalciuric stone-forming patients, the pathogenetic role of vitamin D has been investigated. Despite this, it still remains controversial as to whether abnormalities in vitamin D action or metabolism exist in patients with kidney stones. The following discussion will consider these studies as they apply to the pathogenesis of urolithiasis.

13.6.1 Serum Vitamin D Metabolite Concentrations in Patients with Urolithiasis

With the availability of sensitive assays for measuring serum 1,25(OH)$_2$D, the majority of early reports indicated a mild increase in the serum concentration of this vitamin D metabolite for patients classified as having idiopathic hypercalciuria.

Table 13.1 Biochemical measurements from studies of stone-forming patients with intestinal hyperabsorption of calcium

Study	Ca_s (mmol/L)	P_s (mmol/L)	25OHD (nmol/L)	$1,25(OH)_2D$ (pmol/L)	Ca_u (mmol/d)	TmP	GI Ca absorp (%)	iPTH
Shen et al. 1977[37]								
Cont (n = 17)	2.50 ± 0.08^a	1.23 ± 0.10	ND	82 ± 17	4.5 ± 0.9	3.9 ± 0.3	27 ± 9	357 ± 78
IH $(n = 14)^b$	2.48 ± 0.08	$0.96 \pm 0.20^{**}$	ND	$130 \pm 46^{**}$	$8.6 \pm 1.8^{**}$	$2.7 \pm 0.6^{**}$	$40 \pm 9^{**}$	$238 \pm 55^{**}$
Gray et al. 1977[38]								
Cont (n = 48)	2.39 ± 0.08	1.25 ± 0.19	61 ± 20	87 ± 29	4.9 ± 1.9	ND	ND	6.5 ± 3.6
IH (n = 26)	2.40 ± 0.10	$1.10 \pm 0.18^{**}$	$45 \pm 21^*$	$150 \pm 74^{**}$	$8.0 \pm 2.5^{**}$	ND	ND	6.3 ± 2.1
Kaplan et al. 1977[39]								
Cont (n = 11)	2.43 ± 0.13	1.25 ± 0.23	ND	82 ± 22	2.5 ± 0.9	ND	48 ± 8	ND
AH (n = 21)	2.35 ± 0.08	1.23 ± 0.20	ND	$108 \pm 26^*$	$5.2 \pm 1.1^{**}$	ND	$73 \pm 7^{**}$	0.54 ± 0.21
Broadus et al. 1984[40]								
Cont (n = 25)	2.35 ± 0.08	1.17 ± 0.20	67 ± 23	113 ± 33	3.4 ± 1.3	3.6 ± 0.6	ND	ND
AH (n = 50)	2.38 ± 0.08	$1.06 \pm 0.13^{**}$	54 ± 19	$185 \pm 30^{**}$	$6.5 \pm 1.3^{**}$	$3.0 \pm 0.6^{**}$	ND	ND

^{a}All values presented as mean ± SD

^{b}Stone-forming patients were referred to as either idiopathic hypercalciuria (IH) or absorptive hypercalciuria (AH) despite the majority of patients demonstrating a phenotype consistent with intestinal hyperabsorption of calcium. iPTH was determined by different assays with differing units of expression. Abbreviations: Ca_s – serum calcium; P_s – serum phosphorus; Ca_u – urine calcium; GI Ca absorp – fractional intestinal calcium absorption; iPTH – immunoreactive parathyroid hormone; ND – not determined

*Significantly different from control at p<0.01

**Significantly different from control at p<0.001

Table 13.1 summarizes the pertinent laboratory values from these studies.[37–40] In all four of these studies, the majority of the stone-forming patients were of the absorptive variety as evidenced by direct assessment of intestinal calcium absorption[39,40] or from other laboratory values such as decreased immunoreactive PTH.[37] As can be seen, all four studies demonstrated a significantly higher mean serum $1,25(OH)_2D$ value in the hypercalciuric subjects as compared to the normal controls. Patients with frank elevations of serum $1,25(OH)_2D$ represented from 33% to 80% of the patient population studied. Another study indicated that the high circulating $1,25(OH)_2D$ in patients with absorptive hypercalciuria could be suppressed by increasing dietary calcium intake from 400 to 1,000 mg/d. However, with a longer dietary calcium challenge, there was an escape in which circulating $1,25(OH)_2D$ concentration rebounded toward its initial level providing evidence for disordered regulation of $1,25(OH)_2D$ production.[40] Elevations in the circulating concentration of $1,25(OH)_2D$ could result from increased production or decreased metabolic clearance. In order to discriminate between these two possibilities, Insogna et al.[41] used an infusion equilibrium technique to assess metabolic clearance and production rate in patients with absorptive hypercalciuria and compared the results to those from normal subjects. Although the absolute metabolic clearance values were nearly identical between normal subjects and stone-formers, a higher mean serum $1,25(OH)_2D$ concentration in the stone-formers yielded a significantly higher $1,25(OH)_2D$ production rate in the patients as compared to controls (3.4 ± 0.5 versus 2.2 ± 0.5 µg(micrograms)/d, p<0.001). In the few studies where serum 25OHD was measured, mean values were generally within normal limits.

13.6.2 Cause for Increased $1,25(OH)_2D$ Production

The cause for the exaggerated renal synthesis of $1,25(OH)_2D$ in patients with absorptive hypercalciuria has not been apparent since no perturbations in PTH have been observed. In patients with absorptive hypercalciuria, PTH tends to be normal to low normal. There has been considerable interest in the other known promoter of $1,25(OH)_2D$ production, namely serum phosphate. In three of the four studies cited in Table 13.1, serum phosphate in patients with absorptive hypercalciuria was significantly lower than that measured in controls. To explain this rise in serum $1,25(OH)_2D$, it was assumed that some absorptive hypercalciuric patients might have a primary renal phosphate leak. The ensuing hypophosphatemia would then stimulate the renal synthesis of $1,25(OH)_2D$ as discussed previously (see Sect. 13.4.3). Thus, the enhanced calcium absorption develops secondarily to the hypophosphatemia-induced synthesis of 1,25-dihydroxyvitamin D rather than as a primary event.[42] This proposed scheme is supported by studies showing that (1) serum phosphorus concentration and renal tubular threshold concentration for phosphate (TmP) are lower in absorptive hypercalciuria than in the control group[37,43]; (2) phosphate deprivation stimulates $1,25(OH)_2D$ production[44]; and (3) plasma concentration of $1,25(OH)_2D$ is inversely correlated with serum phosphorus concentration in a mixed group consisting of stone-formers, patients with primary hyperparathyroidism, and control subjects.[38]

However, there are substantial data that do not support the validity of this scheme, at least in the vast majority of patients with absorptive hypercalciuria. First, serum phosphorus concentration was not lower than in the control group if patients with absorptive hypercalciuria were evaluated under the same dietary regimen and study setting as the control subjects.[45,46] For unexplained reasons, serum phosphorus was found to be higher in an inpatient setting than in an ambulatory setting in both absorptive hypercalciuric and control subjects. When appropriately compared, hypophosphatemia and reduced TmP were found to be infrequent in absorptive hypercalciuria, occurring in only 3 of 56 patients.[45] Second, the serum concentration of $1,25(OH)_2D$ was not found to be correlated with serum phosphorus or TmP if only patients with absorptive hypercalciuria were considered. Third, the fractional intestinal absorption of calcium was not correlated with serum phosphorus or TmP. Finally, orthophosphate therapy failed to restore normal intestinal calcium absorption even though it reduced the serum concentration of $1,25(OH)_2D$. While attractive, there appears to be little experimental support for renal leak of phosphate stimulating $1,25(OH)_2D$ production in hypercalciuric stone-forming patients.

There also appears to be no association of urinary calcium excretion with the calcium sensing receptor or the 25OHD-1α(alpha)-hydroxylase as determined by linkage analysis.[47,48] These investigators studied 47 French-Canadian pedigrees with idiopathic hypercalciuria and calcium stone formation. While they found no linkage with either of these proteins, quantitative trait analysis of urinary calcium excretion revealed linkage to several markers near the vitamin D receptor locus.[49]

13.6.3 Role of the VDR in Patients with Hypercalciuria

From the preceding discussion, it appears that a majority of the hypercalciuric stone-forming patients do not have increased circulating $1,25(OH)_2D$ concentrations. Since intestinal calcium absorption is keenly sensitive to prevailing $1,25(OH)_2D$ concentrations, yet increased intestinal calcium absorption is present in many stone-forming patients in the face of normal circulating $1,25(OH)_2D$, it suggested that there might be an alteration in the half-life of the VDR or in its sensitivity to $1,25(OH)_2D$. With the advent of powerful new molecular biological approaches and the cloning of the VDR,[50] investigation of the role of vitamin D and its interaction with its receptor took on a new research direction in patients with urolithiasis. Early studies utilized peripheral blood mononuclear cells (PBMC) as a vitamin D target tissue to quantitate VDR in activated T-cells and resting monocytes from patients with absorptive hypercalciuria.[51] Scatchard analysis of binding was used to quantitate VDR number. Compared to normal subjects, absorptive hypercalciuric patients had a significantly higher mean value for

circulating $1,25(OH)_2D$ although it remained within the normal range. For the group, mean VDR concentration in resting (monocytes) and activated (T-lymphocytes) PBMC was not different between controls and absorptive hypercalciuric subjects. However, there were frank elevations in receptor number for six absorptive hypercalciuric patients compared to normals, suggesting that the disease may be heterogeneous with respect to VDR number. In four of these patients, serum $1,25(OH)_2D$ was determined to be normal, a finding similar to that observed for the genetic hypercalciuric stone-forming rat (see Sect. 13.6.4). While these studies failed to disclose any difference in VDR abundance between patients with absorptive hypercalciuria and age- and gender-matched normal subjects, patients with disorders characterized by hypercalcitriolemia demonstrated a significant elevation in VDR abundance compared to normal subjects and patients with absorptive hypercalciuria. This observation is consistent with the notion that increased $1,25(OH)_2D$ upregulated VDR protein and mRNA expression.[52] Although these studies were performed in vitro, assessment of peripheral blood mononuclear cell proliferation via ^{3}H-thymidine incorporation demonstrated a significant inverse relationship with the prevailing plasma $1,25(OH)_2D$ concentration at the time of blood draw for all patients. Since $1,25(OH)_2D$ is known to suppress peripheral blood mononuclear cell proliferation via interaction with its receptor,[53,54] it validates the experimental system utilized in this study.

A similar study utilizing PBMC from ten male IH calcium oxalate stone-formers was reported by Favus et al.[55] In that study, PBMC VDR was quantitated via Western blotting and was observed to be twofold greater in IH men as compared to age-matched men with no history of stone disease (49 ± 21 versus 20 ± 15 fmol/mg protein, $p < 0.008$). Despite this increase in VDR number for IH patients, serum $1,25(OH)_2D$ was not significantly different (48 ± 14 versus 39 ± 11 pg/ml). These results for VDR number are at variance with those obtained by Zerwekh et al.[51] and might be due to differences in the cell population utilized. Zerwekh et al. utilized a mixed cell population (monocytes and activated T-lymphocytes) while Favus et al. used a highly purified preparation of monocytes isolated via a monoclonal antibody to the CD14 plasma membrane antigen specific for monocytes. Although there were differences in the methodology employed to quantitate VDR number (i.e., Western blotting versus Scatchard analysis), VDR tissue and monocyte levels measured by Western blotting and saturation binding have been reported to have a high positive correlation in rats.[56] Therefore, VDR levels determined by saturation binding techniques would be expected to correlate with values obtained by Western blotting.

A follow-up study[33] took advantage of the expression of the VDR in human skin fibroblasts.[57] They measured VDR concentration and VDR mRNA levels in skin fibroblasts from 16 patients with absorptive hypercalciuria and 17 age-matched normal subjects before and following a 16-hour incubation with 10^{-8}M $1,25(OH)_2D$. There were no significant differences in VDR concentration between normal subjects and absorptive hypercalciuric patients in the basal state or following $1,25(OH)_2D$-mediated upregulation (Table 13.2) as measured by immunoblot methodology. Analysis of VDR mRNA/β(beta)-actin mRNA ratios demonstrated no significant differences between normal subjects and absorptive hypercalciuric patients prior to or following $1,25(OH)_2D$ exposure. As a measure of VDR bioactivity, the $1,25(OH)_2D$-mediated induction of the 25-hydroxyvitamin D_3-24-hydroxylase was quantitated. Again, no significant differences were observed between normal subjects and all patients. These findings indicated that there is neither an increase in VDR concentration in skin fibroblasts, a recognized vitamin D responsive cell, nor increased sensitivity to upregulation of VDR numbers by $1,25(OH)_2D$ in patients with absorptive hypercalciuria. The lack of change in the VDR mRNA levels, despite significant increases in VDR number following incubation with $1,25(OH)_2D$, is consistent with other reports that have demonstrated that $1,25(OH)_2D$-mediated upregulation of the VDR is not accomplished by increased transcription, but rather by increased VDR stability.[58–60]

Another approach to assess whether deranged $1,25(OH)_2D$ action might be a pathogenetic mechanism in absorptive hypercalciuria was performed by Zerwekh and colleagues.[61] This approach was undertaken on the basis of several observations. First, absorptive hypercalciuria is known to be inherited in an autosomal dominant fashion,[62,63] clearly implicating a genetic component to the disease. Second, Li et al.[64] reported increased VDR numbers in the intestine of normocalcemic, normal calcitriolemic genetic hypercalciuric rats (see Sect. 13.6.4). Because the hypercalciuria is passed on to subsequent generations, it again supports a genetic process, and more specifically, a possible defect in the molecular biology of the VDR. Third, it had been previously demonstrated that some patients with normal serum $1,25(OH)_2D$ concentration had significant increases in VDR numbers in activated lymphocytes (see previous). Finally, in a comparison of 62 patients with absorptive hypercalciuria and 31 nonhypercalciuric stone-forming patients, the lumbar bone density was lower (−10%) in the hypercalciuric group, with 74% of the

patients displaying values below the mean.[65] Although the mechanism for such bone loss in absorptive hypercalciuric patients is unknown, if $1,25(OH)_2D$ was increased or it exerted increased action at the skeleton, the bone loss could be the consequence of enhanced calcitriol-mediated bone resorption. In the face of normal serum $1,25(OH)_2D$ concentration, the bone loss could be the result of increased sensitivity of the skeleton to $1,25(OH)_2D$. One explanation for such increased sensitivity might reside in common allelic variation in the VDR as demonstrated for prediction of bone turnover and bone density.[66,67] In addition, the various VDR genotypes have been shown to be associated with differing levels of transcriptional expression.[67] Based on these observations, an examination of the VDR mRNA and genotype was performed in 33 patients with absorptive hypercalciuria and 36 normal volunteers. Sequence analysis of cDNA was performed for 11 unrelated patients with absorptive hypercalciuria and a strong family history of kidney stone disease. These samples were analyzed by chemical mismatch cleavage analysis and DNA sequencing. Both methods failed to demonstrate any point mutations, insertions, or deletions in the coding region of the VDR. Analysis of the restriction fragment length polymorphism (RFLP) *Bsm I* performed in all 33 absorptive hypercalciuric patients and 36 controls also failed to disclose any significant difference in the distribution of the various alleles between patients and controls. In addition, no significant differences were found between VDR genotype and serum or urine biochemical parameters. Although these studies failed to disclose an alteration in the VDR mRNA, they do not discount a potential increase in intestinal VDR number or action. Finally, the lack of a unique VDR genotype associated with the absorptive hypercalciuric phenotype does not eliminate from consideration an alteration in VDR gene expression since all patients studied were unrelated. Ideally, such a study should be undertaken in large kindreds wherein the absorptive hypercalciuric phenotype demonstrates an inherited pattern. RFLP analyses in such kindreds might demonstrate a VDR genotype common to all afflicted individuals that is distinct from that of unaffected relatives. Of course, the presence of a common VDR genotype in absorptive hypercalciuria would not provide

Table 13.2 VDR protein concentration, mRNA/β(beta)-actin mRNA, and 24-hydroxylase activity in skin fibroblasts from normal subjects and patients with absorptive hypercalciuria prior to and following incubation with $1,25(OH)_2D_3$

	Normal subjects		AH	
	$-1,25(OH)_2D_3$	$+1,25(OH)_2D_3$[a]	$-1,25(OH)_2D_3$	$+1,25(OH)_2D_3$
VDR protein, ng/mg protein	30 ± 11[b]	$43 \pm 18^*$	30 ± 15	$42 \pm 16^*$
VDR mRNA/β(beta)-actin mRNA	2.1 ± 1.7	2.7 ± 2.8	1.8 ± 2.4	1.9 ± 1.8
$25OHD_3$-24-hydroxylase, pmol/mg protein/30 min	–	2.1 ± 1.6	–	1.9 ± 1.6

[a]Sixteen hour incubation with 10^{-8} M $1,25(OH)_2D_3$

[b]Mean ± SD

*Significantly different from basal value at $p = 0.005$. Reprinted from Zerwekh et al.[33] with permission from S. Karger AG, Basel

evidence for a VDR defect per se, but could serve as a marker for the disease that could aid in the identification of a possible disease locus.

13.6.4 Role of the VDR in the Genetic Hypercalciuric Stone-Forming (GHS) Rat

Attempts to gain a cellular and molecular understanding of the role of deranged vitamin D metabolism and action in the pathophysiology of IH and increased intestinal hyperabsorption of calcium had been hampered by the lack of a suitable animal or cell model of the disease wherein such mechanisms might be explored. In 1988, Bushinsky and colleagues described the first animal model of IH.[68] This rat model of hypercalciuria was created by the selective breeding of the most hypercalciuric male and female rats from each progeny. It mimics many of the clinical and biochemical findings in stone-forming patients with absorptive hypercalciuria. These are represented by (1) marked hypercalciuria, (2) enhanced intestinal calcium absorption, (3) normal serum $1,25(OH)_2D$, (4) normocalcemia, and (5) both brushite and calcium oxalate stone formation.[69] Detailed studies in this animal model have demonstrated that the hypercalciuria is the result of dysregulation of calcium transport in all three calcium regulating organs, namely the gut, bone, and kidney. Thus, the hypercalciuria results from increased intestinal calcium absorption, increased bone resorption, and decreased renal calcium reabsorption. Because serum $1,25(OH)_2D$ is normal in these hypercalciuric rats, it suggested that there might be alteration of the VDR. It was subsequently shown that VDR number was increased in all three target organs compared to normocalciuric controls. The cause of the increased VDR number was shown not to be due to increases in VDR mRNA levels as measured by slot-blot analysis, suggesting that the altered regulation of the VDR occurs posttranscriptionally. As discussed earlier, similar findings were observed for PBMC and skin fibroblasts from patients with absorptive hypercalciuria. Further studies disclosed that duodenal VDR half-life was prolonged in GHS rats as compared to normal rats.[70] This finding supported the hypothesis that prolongation of VDR half-life increases VDR tissue levels and mediates increased VDR-regulated genes that result in hypercalciuria. At the gut, increased VDR number results in increased expression of calbindin D_{9K}. At the kidney, increased VDR number results in augmentation of the expression of calbindin D_{28K}. While calbindin D_{9K} is known to promote an increase in intestinal calcium transport across the duodenum, both calbindin D_{9K} and calbindin D_{28K} are believed to be involved in calcium transport across renal tubule epithelia.[71] However, increased renal calbindin D expression would be expected to decrease urinary calcium losses by driving more luminal calcium uptake, an effect opposite to that observed for the GHS rat.[72] This suggests that there may be defects at the other two sites of renal calcium transport, namely the epithelial calcium channel and the two basolateral calcium extruding pumps. Expression of the renal epithelial calcium channel (TrpV5) is known to be upregulated by $1,25(OH)_2D$.[73] However, examination of the expression level or primary sequence of TrpV5 failed to disclose any differences between the GHS and normal control rats.[69] At present, no such assessment of the basolateral sodium calcium exchanger or plasma membrane calcium ATPase has been performed in GHS rats. Thus, while it is clear that increased VDR number probably accounts for the increased intestinal calcium absorption and increased bone resorption observed in GHS rats, the role of vitamin D and the VDR in the renal mechanism of calcium loss is less clear.

13.7 Conclusions

There has been a renewed interest in vitamin D research in light of numerous recent epidemiological studies implicating a role for this steroid hormone in the development of many chronic diseases. Despite these investigations, there have been limited investigations into the role of deranged vitamin D metabolism and action in promoting hypercalciuria in patients with idiopathic hypercalciuria. While increased circulating 1,25-dihydroxyvitamin D concentrations have been found in up to one third of patients with idiopathic hypercalciuria (IH), the cause for the increased renal production of this active metabolite is not known.

The phosphate leak hypothesis and ensuing hypophosphatemia have been suggested as a mechanism for some patients with IH. To date, demonstration of a derangement in phosphate homeostasis has not been substantiated nor have alterations in immunoreactive PTH been observed. Furthermore, a limited number of genetic studies looking for derangements in the enzyme producing 1,25-dihydroxyvitamin D have been unfruitful. Thus, while increased circulating 1,25-dihydroxyvitamin D is an attractive explanation for hypercalciuria in calcium stone-formers, it remains speculative without a firm explanation for increased renal production.

On the other hand, studies have emerged supporting a role for increased end-organ sensitivity to vitamin D via increased vitamin D receptor numbers. Presumably, such an increase would result in increased intestinal calcium absorption and contribute to hypercalciuria. It should also increase the loss of calcium from bone due to increased vitamin D-mediated bone resorption. To date, such studies have been performed in an animal model of hypercalciuria or with nonclassical target organs in humans; e.g., skin fibroblasts, circulating monocytes.

Future research directions will require verification of increased vitamin D receptor number in classical target organs such as gut and bone of patients with IH. In addition, the role of increased vitamin D action at the kidney will also need in-depth evaluation, since calcium reabsorption at the distal convoluted tubule is increased in response to vitamin D – an effect that would act to decrease urinary calcium excretion. Clearly, the role of vitamin metabolism and action in promoting IH is far from complete.

References

1. Mellanby E. An experimental investigation on rickets. *Lancet.* 1919;1:407-412.
2. Askew FA, Bourdillon RB, Bruce HM, et al. The distillation of vitamin D. *Proc R Soc.* 1931;8107:76-90.
3. Windaus A, Schenk F, vonWerder F. Uber das antirachitisch wirksame Bestrahlungs-produkt aus 7-dehydrocholesterin. *Hoppe-Seylers Z Physiol Chem.* 1936;241:100-103.
4. International Union of Pure and Applied Chemists (IUPAC). IUPAC Commission on the nomenclature of organic chemistry and IUPAC-IUB commission on biochemical nomenclature. Revised tentative rules for nomenclature of steroids. *Biochem J.* 1969;113:5-28.
5. Huldshinsky K. Heilung von rachitis durch künstlich hohen-sonne. *Deut Med Wochenschr.* 1919;45:712-713.
6. Steenbock H, Black A. Fat soluble vitamins. XXIII. The induction of growth-promoting and calcifying properties in fats and their unsaponifiable constituents by exposure to light. *J Biol Chem.* 1925;64:263-298.
7. Holick MF, Tian XQ, Allen M. Evolutionary importance for the membrane enhancement of the production of vitamin D_3 in the skin of poikilothermic animals. *Proc Natl Acad Sci USA.* 1995;92:3124-3126.
8. Holick MF, MacLaughlin JA, Doppelt SH. Factors that influence the cutaneous photosynthesis of previtamin D_3. *Science.* 1981;211:590-593.
9. Matsuoka LY, Wortsman J, Hanifan N, Holick MF. Chronic sunscreen use decreases circulating concentrations of 25-hydroxyvitamin D: a preliminary study. *Arch Dermatol.* 1988;124:1802-1804.
10. Bell NH, Greene A, Epstein S, Oexmann MJ, Shaw W, Shary J. Evidence for alteration of the vitamin D endocrine system in Blacks. *J Pediatr.* 1985;76:470-473.
11. Webb AR, Kline L, Holick MF. Influence of season and latitude on the cutaneous synthesis of vitamin D_3;exposure to winter sunlight in Boston and Edmonton will not promote vitamin D_3 synthesis in human skin. *J Clin Endocrinol Metab.* 1988;67:373-378.
12. Kodicek E. The metabolism of vitamin D. In: Umbreit W, Molitor H, eds. *Proceedings of the Fourth International Congress of Biochemistry*, vol. 11. London: Pergamon; 1960.
13. Neville PF, DeLuca HF. The synthesis of [1, 2–3H]vitamin D3 and the tissue localization of a 0.25 mg (10 IU) dose per rat. *Biochemistry.* 1966;5:2201-2207.
14. Blunt JW, DeLuca HF, Schnoes HK. 25-Hydroxycholecalciferol. A biologically active metabolite of vitamin D_3. *Biochemistry.* 1968;7:3317-3322.
15. Holick MF, Schnoes HK, DeLuca HF, Suda T, Cousins RJ. Isolation and identification of 1, 25-dihydroxycholecalciferol A metabolite of vitamin D active in intestine. *Biochemistry.* 1971;10:2799-2804.
16. Fraser DR, Kodicek E. Unique biosynthesis by kidney of a biologically active vitamin D metabolite. *Nature.* 1970;228:764-766.
17. Boyle IT, Miravet L, Gray RW, Holick MF, DeLuca HF. The response of intestinal calcium transport to 25-hydroxy and 1, 25-dihydroxyvitamin D in nephrectomized rats. *Endocrinology.* 1972;90:605-608.
18. Holick MF, Garabedian M, DeLuca HF. 1, 25-Dihydroxy-cholecalciferol. Metabolite of vitamin D3 active on bone in anephric rats. *Science.* 1972;176:1146-1147.
19. Wong RG, Norman AW, Reddy CR, Coburn JW. Biologic effects of 1, 25-dihydroxycholecalciferol (a highly active vitamin D metabolite) in acutely uremic rats. *J Clin Invest.* 1972;51:1287-1291.
20. Cheng JB, Motola DL, Mangelsdorf DJ, Russell DW. De-orphanization of cytochrome P450 2R1: a microsomal vitamin D 25-hydroxilase. *J Biol Chem.* (2003);278
21. Hollis BW. Circulating 25-hydroxyvitamin D levels indicative of vitamin D insufficiency: implications for establishing a new effective dietary intake recommendation for vitamin D. *J Nutr.* 2005;135:317-322.
22. Paulson SK, DeLuca HF. Subcellular location and properties of rat renal 25-hydroxyvitamin D_3-1α-hydroxylase. *J Biol Chem.* 1985;260:11488-11492.
23. Bouillon R. Vitamin D: from photosynthesis, metabolism and action to clinical applications. In: Degroot LL, Jameson JL, eds. *Endocrinology. Vol 2.* 4th ed. Philadelphia, PA: Saunders; 2001.
24. Zerwekh JE, Breslau NA. Human placental production of 1α, 25-dihydroxyvitamin D3: biochemical characterization and production in normal subjects and patients with pseudohypoparathyroidism. *J Clin Endocrinol Metab.* 1986;62:192-196.
25. Sharma OP. Hypercalcemia in granulomatous disorders: a clinical review. *Curr Opin Pulmon Med.* 2000;6:442-447.
26. Diaz R, El-Hajj GF, Brown E. *Regulation of Parathyroid Function.* New York: Oxford University Press; 1998.
27. Mia D, He B, Lanske B, et al. Skeletal abnormalities in Pth-null mice are influenced by dietary calcium. *Endocrinology.* 2004;145:2046-2053.
28. Portale AA, Halloran BP, Morris RC Jr. Physiologic regulation of the serum concentration of 1, 25-dihydroxyvitamin D by phosphorus in normal men. *J Clin Invest.* 1989;83:1494-1499.
29. Shimada T, Kakitani M, Yamazaki Y, et al. Targeted ablation of Fgf23 demonstrates an essential physiological role of FGF23 in phosphate and vitamin D metabolism. *J Clin Invest.* 2004;113:561-568.
30. Liu S, Gupta A, Quarles LD. Emerging role of fibroblast growth factor 23 in a bone-kidney axis regulating systemic phosphate homeostasis and extracellular matrix mineralization. *Curr Opin Nephrol.* 2007;16:329-325.
31. Menna C, Vrtovsnik F, Friedlander G, Corvol M, Garabedian M. Insulin-like growth factor I, a unique calcium-dependent stimulator of 1, 25-dihydroxyvitamin D3 production. Studies in cultured mouse kidney cells. *J Biol Chem.* 1995;270:25461-25467.
32. Omdahl JL, Morris HA, May BK. Hydroxylase enzymes of the vitamin D pathway: expression, function, and regulation. *Annu Rev Nutr.* 2002;22:139-166.
33. Zerwekh JE, Reed BY, Heller HJ, Gonzalez GB, Haussler MR, Pak CYC. Normal vitamin D receptor concentration and responsiveness to 1, 25-dihydroxyvitamin D3 in skin fibroblasts from patients with absorptive hypercalciuria. *Min Elec Metab.* 1998;24:307-313.
34. Pike JW, Shevde NK. The vitamin D receptor. In: Feldman D, Pike JW, Glorieux FH, eds. *Vitamin D.* 2nd ed. New York: Elsevier; 2005.
35. Norman AW. 1α, 25(OH)2-vitamin D3-mediated rapid and genomic responses are dependent upon critical structure-function relationships for both the ligand and receptor(s). In: Feldman D, Pike JW, Glorieux FH, eds. *Vitamin D.* 2nd ed. New York: Elsevier; 2005.
36. Christakos S, Dhawan P, Liu Y, Peng X, Porta A. New insights into the mechanisms of vitamin D action. *J Cell Biochem.* 2003;88:695-705.

37. Shen FH, Baylink DJ, Nielsen RL, Sherrard DJ, Ivey JL, Haussler MR. Increased serum 1, 25-dihydroxyvitamin D in idiopathic hypercalciuria. *J Lab Clin Med.* 1977;90:955-962.
38. Gray RW, Wilz DR, Caldas AE, Lemann J Jr. The importance of phosphate in regulating plasma 1, 25-(OH)2-vitamin D levels in humans: studies in healthy subjects, in calcium stone-formers and in patients with primary hyperparathyroidism. *J Clin Endocrinol Metab.* 1977;45:299-306.
39. Kaplan RA, Haussler MR, Deftos LJ, Bone H, Pak CYC. The role of 1α, 25-dihydroxyvitamin D in the mediation of intestinal hyperabsorption of calcium in primary hyperparathyroidism and absorptive hypercalciuria. *J Clin Invest.* 1977;59:756-760.
40. Broadus AE, Insogna KI, Lang R, Ellison AF, Dreyer BE. Evidence for disordered control of 1, 25-dihydroxyvitamin D production in absorptive hypercalciuria. *N Eng J Med.* 1984;311:73-80.
41. Insogna KL, Broadus AE, Dreyer BE, Ellison AF, Gertner JM. Elevated production rate of 1, 25-dihydroxyvitamin D in patients with absorptive hypercalciuria. *J Clin Endocrinol Metab.* 1985;61:490-495.
42. Bordier P, Ryckewart A, Gueris J, Rasmussen H. On the pathogenesis of so-called idiopathic hypercalciuria. *Am J Med.* 1977;63: 398-409.
43. Lemann J Jr, Dominguez JH, Gray RW. Idiopathic hypercalciuria: a defect in phosphate and vitamin D metabolism. In: Finlayson B, Thomas WC Jr, eds. *Colloquium on Renal Lithiasis.* Gainesville, FL: University of Florida Press; 1976.
44. Dominguez JH, Gray RW, Lemann J. Dietary phosphate deprivation in women and men: effects on mineral and acid balances, parathyroid hormone, and the metabolism of 25-OH-vitamin D. *J Clin Endocrinol Metab.* 1976;43:1056-1068.
45. Barilla DE, Zerwekh JE, Pak CYC. A critical evaluation of the role of phosphate in the pathogenesis of absorptive hypercalciuria. *Min Elect Metab.* 1979;2:302-309.
46. Pak CYC, Fetner C, Townsend J, et al. Evaluation of calcium urolithiasis in ambulatory patients. Comparison of results with those of inpatient evaluation. *Am J Med.* 1978;64:979-987.
47. Scott P, Ouimet D, Proulx Y, et al. The 1 alpha-hydroxylase locus is not linked to calcium stone formation or calciuric phenotypes in French-Canadian families. *J Am Soc Nephrol.* 1998;9:425-432.
48. Petrucci M, Scott P, Ouimet D, et al. Evaluation of the calcium-sensing receptor gene in idiopathic hypercalciuria and calcium Nephrolithiasis. *Kidney Int.* 2000;58:38-42.
49. Scott P, Ouimet D, Valiquette L, et al. Suggestive evidence for a susceptibility gene near the vitamin D receptor locus in idiopathic calcium stone formation. *J Am Soc Nephrol.* 1999;105:1007-1013.
50. McDonnell DP, Mangelsdorf DJ, Pike JW, Haussler MR, O'Malley BW. Molecular cloning of complementary DNA encoding the avian receptor for vitamin D. *Science.* 1987;235:1214-1217.
51. Zerwekh JE, Yu X-P, Breslau NA, Manolagas S, Pak CYC. Vitamin D receptor quantitation in human blood mononuclear cells in health & disease. *Mol Cell Endocrinol.* 1993;96:1-6.
52. Mangelsdorf DJ, Pike JW, Haussler MR. Avian and mammalian receptors for 1, 25-dihydroxyvitamin D3: in vitro translation to characterize size and hormone-dependent regulation. *Proc Natl Acad Sci USA.* 1987;84:354-358.
53. Nun JD, Katz DR, Barker S, et al. Regulation of human tonsillar T-cell proliferation by the active metabolite of vitamin D₃. *Immunol.* 1986;59:479-484.
54. Rigby WF, Noelle RJ, Krause K, Fanger MW. The effects of 1, 25-dihydroxyvitamin D3 on human T lymphocyte activation and proliferation. *J Immunol.* 1985;135:2279-2286.
55. Favus MJ, Karnauskas AJ, Parks JH, Coe FL. Peripheral blood monocyte vitamin D receptor levels are elevated in patients with idiopathic hypercalciuria. *J Clin Endocrinol Metab.* 2004;89:4937-4943.
56. Sriussadaporn S, Wong M, Pike JW, Favus MJ. Tissue specificity and mechanism of vitamin D receptor up-regulation during dietary phosphorus restriction in the rat. *J Bone Min Res.* 1995;10:271-280.
57. Feldman D, Chen T, Hirst M, Colston K, Karasek M, Cone C. Demonstration of 1, 25-dihydroxyvitamin D3 receptors in human skin biopsies. *J Clin Endocrinol Metab.* 1980;51:1463-1465.
58. Wiese RJ, Uhland-Smith A, Ross TK, Prahl JM, DeLuca HF. Up-regulation of the vitamin D receptor in response to 1, 25-dihydroxyvitamin D3 results from ligand-induced stabilization. *J Biol Chem.* 1992;267:20082-20086.
59. Santiso-Mere D, Sore T, Hilliard GM IV, Pike JW, McDonnell DP. Positive regulation of the vitamin D receptor by its cognate ligand in heterologous expression systems. *Mol Endocrinol.* 1993;7:833-839.
60. Arbour NC, Prahl JM, DeLuca HF. Stabilization of the vitamin D receptor in rat osteosarcoma cells through the action of 1, 25-dihydroxyvitamin D3. *Mol Endocrinol.* 1993;7:1307-1312.
61. Zerwekh JE, Hughes MR, Reed BY, et al. Evidence for normal vitamin D receptor messenger ribonucleic acid and genotype in absorptive hypercalciuria. *J Clin Endocrinol Metab.* 1995;80:2960-2965.
62. Coe FL, Parks JA, Moore ES. Familial idiopathic hypercalciuria. *N Eng J Med.* 1979;300:337-340.
63. Pak CYC, McGuire L, Peterson R, Britton F, Harrod MJ. Familial absorptive hyper-calciuria in a large kindred. *J Urol.* 1981;126: 717-719.
64. Li X-Q, Tembe V, Horwitz GM, Bushinsky DA, Favus MJ. Increased intestinal vitamin D receptor in genetic hypercalciuric rats; a cause of intestinal calcium hyperabsorption. *J Clin Invest.* 1993;91:661-667.
65. Pietschmann F, Breslau NA, Pak CYC. Reduced vertebral bone density in hypercalciuric nephrolithiasis. *J Bone Min Res.* 1992;7: 661-667.
66. Morrison NA, Yeoman R, Kelly PJ, Eisman JA. Contribution of trans-acting alleles to normal physiological variability: vitamin D receptor gene polymorphisms and circulating osteocalcin. *Proc Natl Acad Sci USA.* 1992;89:6665-6669.
67. Morrison NA, Qi JC, Tokita A, et al. Prediction of bone density from vitamin D receptor alleles. *Nature.* 1994;367:284-287.
68. Bushinsky DA FMJ. Mechanism of hypercalciuria in genetic hypercalciuric rats: inherited defect in intestinal calcium transport. *J Clin Invest.* 1988;82:1585-1591.
69. Bushinsky DA, Frick KK, Nehrke K. Genetic hypercalciuric stone-forming rats. *Curr Opin Neph Hyperten.* 2006;15:403-418.
70. Karnauskas AJ, Van Leeuwen JPTM, van den Bemd G-J, et al. Mechanism and function of high vitamin D receptor levels in genetic hypercalciuric stone-forming rats. *J Bone Min Res.* 2005;20: 447-454.
71. Hoenderop JG, Nilius B, Bindels RJ. Molecular mechanism of active Ca²⁺ reabsorption in the distal nephron. *Annu Rev Physiol.* 2002;64: 529-549.
72. Tsuruoka S, Bushinsky DA, Schwartz GJ. Defective renal calcium reabsorption in genetic hypercalciuric rats. *Kidney Int.* 1997;51:1540-1547.
73. Hoenderop JG, Nilius B, Bindels RJ. Calcium absorption across epithelia. *Physiol Rev.* 2005;85:373-422.

Urinary Citrate and Citrate Metabolism

14

Bernhard Hess

Abstract Citrate is the most abundant organic anion in human urine. Its urinary excretion rate mainly depends on *acid–base status*: Alkalosis induces an increase in urinary citrate excretion, whereas acidosis has the opposite effect. It is important to note that citrate utilization by renal cells and urinary citrate excretion are mainly affected by *intracellular* changes in acid base homeostasis of proximal tubular cells. Even small acid loads such as meat protein-rich meals decrease urinary excretion of citrate. *Low urinary citrate (hypocitraturia)* is defined as daily urinary citrate excretion rates below 1.70 mmol (320 mg) in men and 1.90 mmol (350 mg) in women. Hypocitraturia occurs in 20–60% of calcium stone formers. Sufficient citrate in urine is important because citrate retards the crystallization of stone-forming calcium salts, mediates inhibitory effects of macromolecular modulators of calcium oxalate crystallization and – due to its alkalinizing effect – reduces rates of uric acid stone formation. Treatment with alkali citrate, usually in the form of potassium citrate or magnesium potassium citrate, is widely used to increase urinary citrate and reduce rates of stone formation in patients with hypocitraturic calcium nephrolithiasis as well as uric acid stone disease.

14.1 Introduction

The presence of citrate in human urine was first described by Amberg and McClure in 1917.[1] In 1931, it became evident that urinary excretion of citrate was closely linked to acid-base homeostasis: Alkalotic patients excreted more citrate in their urines than patients in metabolic acidosis.[2] Already a few years later, the association between low urinary citrate excretion and urinary stone formation was established.[3] At that time, however, it was concluded that low urinary citrate excretion in stone patients was caused by urinary tract infection, due to bacterial citrate consumption.[4,5] In 1962, it was claimed that overt hypocitraturia, defined as a urinary citrate excretion of less than 400 mg/day (2.1 mmol/day) in men and 200 mg/day in women, was only present in patients with urinary tract infection or renal failure.[6] The latter condition commonly goes along with hypocitraturia, because progressive metabolic acidosis with increasing renal failure causes a progressive decrease in urinary citrate excretion.[7] This points

again toward the close link between urinary citrate excretion and acid–base metabolism.

Citrate is a weak tricarboxylic acid with pK_a values of 2.91, 4.34 and 5.62.[8] At physiological pH values, it is primarily present in its dissociated trivalent form, citrate^{3-}, and thus has alkaline properties. Citrate can be endogenous or exogenous. Dietary citrate is nearly totally absorbed in the intestine and primarily used in the liver and kidneys.[9] When given orally, citrate is metabolized to bicarbonate in the liver and thus is a *provider of alkali*.[9] In whole blood, citrate mainly circulates unbound to larger molecules.[8] Plasma concentrations of citrate in humans are low and range between 0.05 and 0.3 mmol/l.[10] Plasma citrate can also derive from endogenous production in cells.[9] Intracellular citrate is a central component of the tricarboxylic acid cycle (Krebs' cycle) in which ATP is produced.[9]

14.2 Physiology and Pathophysiology of Urinary Citrate in Stone Disease

In the kidney, citrate is freely filtered in the glomeruli with 10–35% of the filtered citrate remaining in the urine.[9,10] Therefore, 65–90% is reabsorbed, mainly in the proximal

B. Hess
Department of Internal Medicine & Nephrology/Hypertension, Klinik
Im Park, Zurich, Switzerland
e-mail: bernhard.hass@hirslanden.ch

P.N. Rao et al. (eds.), *Urinary Tract Stone Disease*,
DOI 10.1007/978-1-84800-362-0_14, © Springer-Verlag London Limited 2011

convoluted tubule.[9–11] Citrate is the most abundant organic anion in human urine and an important substrate in the metabolism of renal cells.[8] Renal cells reabsorb about 6.6 μ(micro)mol citrate per minute from tubular fluid and remove another 1.5 μmol/min from peritubular blood, thus in total 8.1 μmol citrate is extracted per minute and enters renal cell metabolism.[12] Major parts of renal cell metabolism of citrate are oxidative processes in the Krebs citric acid or tricarboxylic acid cycle.[9,12]

The most important factor influencing urinary citrate excretion is *acid–base status*.[10,11] Alkalosis induces an increase in urinary citrate excretion, whereas acidosis has the opposite effect.[10,11] It is important to note that citrate utilization by renal cells and urinary citrate excretion are mainly affected by *intracellular* changes in acid base homeostasis of proximal tubular cells. Already under normal conditions, renal cortical citrate concentrations exceed plasma levels of citrate, indicating an active transport into tubular cells. Whereas citrate uptake across the basolateral membrane of proximal tubule cells appears to occur via a *tri*carboxylate transporter, a unique coupled sodium-dependent *di*carboxylic transporter is responsible for citrate reabsorption at the apical (luminal) membrane.[9,10] As depicted in Fig. 14.1, the transport at the apical membrane is electrogenic, because three sodium ions are transported for each citrate^{2-}. The preferred transport of the less abundant citrate^{2-} species is the major reason for the strong pH dependence of citrate transport at the apical membrane, because the divalent species becomes much more prevalent at lower pH values. Indeed, a threefold rise in citrate^{2-} concentration can be observed as pH decreases from 7.4 to 6.9.[9] This increases citrate reabsorption at the apical cell membrane. In addition, activity of citrate lyase rises in acidosis, which lowers intracellular citrate concentrations and further favors reabsorption from tubular fluid.[9] Moreover, the number of sodium-dependent citrate transporters is increased in acidosis.[9]

The combination of all these factors allows for a net increment in renal cell utilization and a decrease in urinary excretion of citrate even with rather small acid loads, such as a meat protein-rich meal. On the other hand, alkali loads raise intracellular pH, which inhibits mitochondrial citrate oxidation, causing cytosolic accumulation and reduction in cellular uptake of citrate.[10] Together with the reversal of the previously mentioned factors that affect citrate uptake in acidosis, this mechanism is responsible for an increase in urinary citrate excretion during alkali loads or alkalosis.

Sufficient citrate in urine is important because citrate retards the crystallization of stone-forming calcium salts,[12] mainly by formation of a pH-dependent calcium-citrate-phosphate complex,[13] and mediates inhibitory effects of macromolecular modulators of calcium oxalate crystallization.[14,15] In addition, due to its alkalinizing effect, citrate has successfully been used to raise urine pH and reduce rates of stone formation in patients with low urine pH and uric acid stones.[16] Moreover, initiation of urease-induced crystallization in urines of healthy volunteers taking oral potassium citrate is markedly delayed,[17] suggesting that alkali citrate treatment could also be beneficial in infection stone disease.

Low urinary citrate (hypocitraturia) is defined as daily urinary citrate excretion rates below 1.70 mmol (320 mg) in men and 1.90 mmol (350 mg) in women.[18] Hypocitraturia as a pathogenetically important risk factor occurs in 20–60% of calcium stone formers.[9] It is therefore mandatory to measure urinary citrate in idiopathic calcium stone formers and to know the relevant *risk factors for hypocitraturia*. The main conditions leading to intracellular acidosis as the common denominator of hypocitraturia are summarized in Table 14.1. Among those, the most prevalent is incomplete distal (or type 1) renal tubular acidosis (RTA); i.e., no systemic acidosis, but persistently high urine pH even after acid loading. It is due to a defect in net H$^+$ excretion by the collecting tubules[19] and has been found in up to 90% of "idiopathic" calcium stone formers with low urinary citrate.[20] Besides all

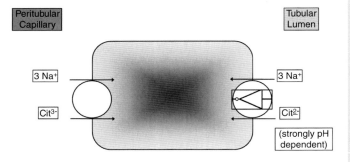

Fig. 14.1 Highly simplified model of citrate transport by renal proximal tubule cells (modified from[9]). For details, see text. The transport at the apical membrane is electrogenic; i.e., three sodium ions are transported for each citrate^{2-}

Table 14.1 List of conditions associated with hypocitraturia (Modified/updated from [19]

1. Due to intracellular acidosis
- **Systemic metabolic acidosis** (including acidosis in chronic renal failure)
- **Incomplete distal RTA**
- **Dietary acid loads** (exaggerated meat protein consumption)
- **Dietary salt loading** ($\rightarrow \downarrow$ Renin $\rightarrow \downarrow$ Angiotensin II $\rightarrow \downarrow$ activity of luminal Na$^+$-H$^+$-antiporter $\rightarrow \uparrow$ intracellular [H$^+$])
- **Carboanhydrase inhibitors**: Acetazolamide, Topiramate (anticonvulsant)
- **Malabsorption syndromes / chronic diarrhea** (HCO$_3^-$ loss)
- **Potassium depletion** (Thiazide diuretics!)

2. Due to other mechanisms
- $\downarrow$ **complex formation with cations** (relative shortage of urinary Ca and Mg)
- **bbTT polymorphism of the vitamin D receptor**

the conditions leading to intracellular acidosis, low urinary calcium or magnesium concentrations may also predispose to reduced urinary citrate excretion, since a relative shortage of these cations may result in reduced complex formation between citrate and the cations. Reduced complex formation would leave more citrate as free ions and thus increase citrate uptake by proximal tubular cells.[10] Finally, the bbTT polymorphism in the 3′ region of the vitamin D receptor gene has been described to be associated with hypocitraturia in hypercalciuric stone formers.[21]

Increases in urinary citrate are primarily associated with factors leading to intracellular alkalosis. Indeed, urinary citrate excretion is positively related to net gastrointestinal absorption of alkali.[12] In addition, increases in urinary citrate are associated with increases in urinary calcium and magnesium excretions due to more pronounced complex formation with subsequent reductions in cellular uptake of citrate.[9,10] This may even be seen as a protective mechanism against hypercalciuric renal stone formation. Finally, urinary citrate has been shown to increase during pregnancy.[9]

14.3 Citrate Treatment of Stone Disease

In calcium nephrolithiasis, treatment with alkali citrate, usually in the form of potassium citrate or magnesium potassium citrate, is widely used to increase urinary citrate and reduce rates of stone formation in patients with hypocitraturic calcium nephrolithiasis. When looking for "hard" scientific evidence of such a treatment, however, it appears that only four randomized controlled trials including 227 patients have been accomplished.[21] In our review, which was based on a true intention-to-treat analysis, these trials have revealed that 54% of alkali citrate-treated patients remained stone-free after at least 1 year of treatment, whereas a significantly lower fraction of 35% was stone-free on placebo treatment.[21] Of equal importance appear data from two randomized, placebo-controlled trials in a total of 104 stone patients.[22,23] With clearance or dissolution of preexisting (residual) stones as ultimate endpoint, 1 year of treatment left two thirds of alkali citrate-treated patients stone-free, again significantly more than on placebo (27.5%). It may be anticipated that more complete fragment clearance would be associated with a reduced likelihood of residual fragments becoming niduses for newly growing stones.

Alkali citrate treatment not only raises urinary citrate levels in patients with calcium nephrolithiasis, but also has a general alkalinizing effect, which is beneficial for patients with uric acid[16] as well as cystine stones.[24] Moreover, alkali citrate may even be beneficial for retarding growth of infection stones.[17] Therefore, alkali citrate could be a sort of *panacea* for almost any kind of kidney stone disease.

However, as obvious from studies as well as clinical experience, a more widespread use of alkali citrate preparations is limited due to the relatively low tolerability of available alkali citrate preparations. Overall, 17% of subjects on placebo, but almost one third on alkali citrate treatment for prevention of stone recurrences prematurely left the randomized trials.[21] It is noteworthy that the highest ever reported drop-out rate, almost half of the patients, was observed on treatment with potassium magnesium citrate,[25] which basically appears to be more efficient than potassium citrate in lowering the activity product of calcium oxalate.[26] Adverse effects that reduce treatment compliance have been noted mainly in the gastrointestinal tract and include eructation, bloating, or gaseousness in 26% and frank diarrhea in 12% of potassium magnesium citrate-treated patients.[25] Thus, the development of better tolerated alkali citrate preparations remains an important issue for the future.

The fact that any alkali would suffice to increase urinary pH and citrate excretion[9,19] could offer interesting alternatives for stone patients who do not tolerate currently available alkali citrate preparations. For instance, 1.2 l of orange juice per day cause increases in urine pH and citrate similar to conventional doses of potassium citrate,[27] and bicarbonate-rich mineral water appears equally effective to sodium potassium citrate in increasing urine pH and citrate as well as decreasing relative urinary supersaturations of calcium oxalate and uric acid.[28] Finally, equal stone size reductions over time have been reported in stone formers randomized to either sodium potassium citrate or a tea based on the herbal plant *Orthosiphus grandiflorus*, whereby patients treated with the herbal tea did not experience any adverse effects in comparison to 26% of sodium potassium citrate-treated patients.[29] It appears that many patients who do not tolerate currently available alkali citrate medications might profit from more "natural" sources of alkali in order to raise urinary citrate excretion.

14.4 Conclusions

Urinary excretion of citrate, the most abundant organic anion in human urine, highly depends on *acid–base status*. In proximal tubular cells, intracellular alkalosis induces an increase in urinary citrate excretion, whereas acidosis has the opposite effect. *Low urinary citrate (hypocitraturia)* is defined as daily urinary citrate excretion rates below 1.70 mmol (320 mg) in men and 1.90 mmol (350 mg) in women. It occurs in 20–60% of calcium stone formers and can be the consequence of a variety of conditions such as (incomplete) distal renal tubular acidosis, meat protein and/or salt overconsumption, potassium depletion, treatment with carboanhydrase inhibitors and malabsorption syndromes/chronic diarrhea.

Normal urinary citrate concentrations are required for retarding the crystallization of stone-forming calcium salts and enhancing inhibitory effects of certain macromolecular modulators of calcium oxalate crystallization. Furthermore, due to its alkalinizing effect, citrate reduces rates of uric acid stone formation. Treatment with alkali citrate, usually in the form of potassium citrate or magnesium potassium citrate, is always indicated in hypocitraturie calcium stone formers as well as in patients with low urine pH and uric acid stone disease.

References

1. Amberg S, McClure WB. Occurrence of citric acid in urine. *Am J Physiol*. 1917;44:453-462.
2. Östberg O. Studien über Zitronensäureausscheidung der Menschenniere in normalen und pathologischen Zuständen. *Scand Arch Physiol*. 1931;62:81-222.
3. Boothby WM, Adams M. Occurrence of citric acid in urine and body fluids. *Am J Physiol*. 1934;107:471-479.
4. Scott WW, Huggins C, Selman BC. Metabolism of citric acid in urolithiasis. *J Urol*. 1943;50:202-209.
5. Conway NW, Maitland ATK, Rennie JB. The urinary citrate excretion in patients with renal calculi. *Br J Urol*. 1949;21:30-38.
6. Hodgkinson A. Citric acid excretion in normal adults and in patients with renal calculus. *Clin Sci*. 1962;23:203-212.
7. Chen SM, Chung LC, Lee YH, Young TK. Renal excretion of citrate in patients with chronic renal failure or nephrolithiasis. *J Formos Med Assoc*. 1991;90:41-47.
8. Baruch SB, Burich RL, Eun CK, King VF. Renal metabolism of citrate. *Med Clin North Am*. 1975;59:569-582.
9. Hamm LL, Hering-Smith KS. Pathophysiology of hypocitraturic nephrolithiasis. *Endocrinol Metab Clin N Am*. 2002;31:885-893.
10. Unwin RJ, Capasso G, Shirley DG. An overview of divalent cation and citrate handling by the kidney. *Nephron*. 2004;98:15-20.
11. Simpson DP. Citrate excretion: a window on renal metabolism. *Am J Physiol*. 1983;244:F223-F234.
12. Pak CYC. Citrate and renal calculi: new insights and future directions. *Am J Kidney Dis*. 1991;17:420-425.
13. Rodgers A, Allie-Hamdulay S, Jackson G. Therapeutic action of citrate in urolithiasis explained by chemical speciation: increase in pH is the determinant factor. *Nephrol Dial Transplant*. 2006;21:361-369.
14. Erwin DT, Kok DJ, Alam J, et al. Calcium oxalate stone agglomeration reflects stone-forming activity: citrate inhi-bition depends on macxromolecules larger than 30 kilodalton. *Am J Kidney Dis*. 1994;24:893-900.

15. Hess B, Jordi S, Zipperle L, Ettinger E, Giovanoli R. Citrate determines calcium oxalate crystallization kinetics and crystal morphology – studies in presence of Tamm-Horsfall protein of a healthy subject and a severely recurrent calcium stone former. *Nephrol Dial Transplant*. 2000;15:366-374.
16. Moe OW, Abate N, Sakhaee K. Pathophysiology of uric acid nephrolithiasis. *Endocrinol Metab Clin N Am*. 2002;31:895-914.
17. Wang Y-H, Grenabo L, Hedelin H, Pettersson S. The effects of sodium citrate and oral potassium citrate on urease-induced crystallization. *Br J Urol*. 1994;74:409-415.
18. Hess B, Hasler-Strub U, Ackermann D, Jaeger Ph. Metabolic evaluation of patients with recurrent idiopathic calcium nephrolithiasis. *Nephrol Dial Transplant*. 1997;12:1362-1368.
19. Hess B. Acid-base metabolism: implications for kidney stone formation. *Urol Res*. 2006;34:134-138.
20. Hess B, Michel R, Takkinen R, Ackermann D, Jaeger Ph. Risk factors for low urinary citrate in calcium nephrolithiasis: low vegetable fibre intake and low urine volume to be added to the list. *Nephrol Dial Transplant*. 1994;9:642-649.
21. Mattle D, Hess B. Preventive treatment of nephrolithiais with alkai citrate – a critical review. *Urol Res*. 2005;33:73-79.
22. Cicerello E, Merlo F, Gambaro G, et al. Effect of alkaline citrate therapy on clearance of residual renal stone fragments after extracorporeal shock wave lithotripsy in sterile calcium and in-fection nephrolithiasis patients. *J Urol*. 1994;151:5-9.
23. Soygür T, Akbay A, Kupeli S. Effect of potassium citrate therapy on stone recurrence and residual fragments after shockwave lithotripsy in lower caliceal calcium oxalate urolithiasis: a randomized controlled trial. *J Endourol*. 2002;16:149-152.
24. Shekarriz B, Stoller ML. Cystinuria and other noncalcareous calculi. *Endocrinol Metab Clin N Am*. 2002;31:951-977.
25. Ettinger B, Pak CY, Citron JT, Thomas C, Adams-Huet B, Vangessel A. Potassium-magnesium citrate is an effective prophylaxis against recurrent calcium oxalate nephrolithiasis. *J Urol*. 1997;158:2069-2073.
26. Pak CY, Koenig K, Khan R, Haynes S, Padalino P. Physicochemical action of potassium-magnesium citrate in nephrolithiasis. *J Bone Miner Res*. 1992;7:281-285.
27. Wabner CL, Pak CY. Effect of orange juice consumption on urinary stone risk factors. *J Urol*. 1993;149:1405-1408.
28. Kessler T, Hesse A. Cross-over study of the influence of bicarbonate-rich mineral water on urinary composition in comparison with sodium potassium citrate in healthy subjects. *Br J Nutr*. 2000 Dec;84(6):865-871.
29. Premgamone A, Sriboonlue P, Disatapornjaroen W, Maskasem S, Sinsupan N, Apinives C. A long-term study on the efficacy of a herbal plant, ortho-siphon grandiflorus, and sodium potassium citrate in renal calculi treatment. *Southeast Asian J Trop Med Public Health*. 2001;32:654-660.

Abstract Uric acid nephrolithiasis comprises 8–10% of patients with kidney stone disease. However, this prevalence is higher in particular ethnic populations and in certain regions of the world. The major pathophysiologic mechanism for uric acid nephrolithiasis is unduly acidic urine. At a urinary pH below 5.5, the concentration of sparingly soluble uric acid increases and promotes the formation of uric acid stones. Unduly acidic urine is likely due to defective renal ammoniagenesis. Moreover, emerging studies suggest that increased endogenous acid production, in addition to defective urinary ammonium buffering, may also be responsible for the abnormally acidic urine in this population. The underlying mechanism of low urinary ammonium and increased endogenous acid production has been linked to the metabolic syndrome and may also be associated with renal fat accumulation in the kidney. Although low urinary pH is necessary, it alone is not sufficient for uric acid crystal precipitation. This implies the potential role of inhibitors and/or promoters of uric acid crystallization.

15.1 Introduction

Over the past decade, major progress has been made in our understanding of the pathophysiologic mechanisms of uric acid (UA) stone formation. A preliminary study initially described a high prevalence of UA stones among patients with type 2 diabetes (T2DM).[1] In studies following, a high prevalence of uric acid stones was also shown in obese patients.[2,3] Furthermore, it was later described that higher body mass index (BMI) and T2DM are independent risk factors for UA nephrolithiasis, and the prevalence of UA stones further rises with higher BMI in the presence of T2DM.[4] These observations were consistent with multiple large epidemiologic studies displaying a link between obesity, weight gain, T2DM, an aggregate of features that are characteristic of the metabolic syndrome (MS), and UA nephrolithiasis.[1–11]

15.2 Epidemiology of Uric Acid Nephrolithiasis

UA stones constitute 8–10% of all kidney stones.[12] The global prevalence of UA stones is heterogeneous, with its highest prevalence in the Middle East[13] and in certain parts of Europe.[14] In the Midwestern region of the United States, the prevalence of UA stone formation has been shown to be exceedingly high. This escalated prevalence is due to an increased Laotian Hmong immigrant population.[15] This abnormal tendency toward UA stone formation may be influenced by their specific dietary habits of consuming a large amount of purine with each meal and may also be due to consanguine marriages in this population (Table 15.1).

15.3 Uric Acid Metabolism

15.3.1 Uric Acid Homeostasis

The principle sources of UA production include de novo synthesis, tissue breakdown, and dietary sources. However, hepatic synthesis is the primary constituent in UA production.

K. Sakhaee
Department of Internal Medicine, University of Texas Southwestern Medical Center, Dallas, TX, USA
e-mail: khashayar.sakhaee@utsouthwestern.edu

P.N. Rao et al. (eds.), *Urinary Tract Stone Disease*,
DOI 10.1007/978-1-84800-362-0_15, © Springer-Verlag London Limited 2011

Table 15.1 Global distribution of UA nephrolithiasis

Region	Distribution percentage
United States	5–10% (50% Laotian Hmong population)
England	5–10%
Japan	10%
Germany	25%
Middle East	30%

Table 15.2 Uric acid homeostasis

Production	Excretion
Endogenous purine synthesis	Renal
Tissue nucleic acids	Intestinal
Dietary purines	

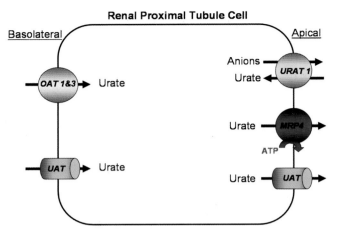

Fig. 15.1 Molecular mechanisms for urate transport. Urate is reabsorbed into the cell via URAT1 after stimulation by intracellular anions. Urate may also be taken up into the cell via OAT1, OAT3, or UAT. UAT is also present on the apical membrane and may be responsible for transcellular transport. MRP4 is found on the apical membrane, requires ATP, and may be responsible for apical urate secretion

This process involves the recycling of guanine and hypoxanthine nucleotides. In a state of excess these substrates are converted into xanthine, which, with the influence of the xanthine oxidase enzyme, is ultimately converted into UA.[16] In a steady state and under normal conditions, endogenous purine turnover does not change significantly.[17] However, in a diseased state – such as conditions with increased tissue catabolism, serum UA concentration, and urinary UA – excretion rises due to a substantial increase in purine turnover.[18] In general, approximately half of the daily urate burden is acquired from dietary sources while the remaining half is comprised of de novo UA synthesis and tissue breakdown. With the exception of overly high dietary purine consumption, the effect of dietary influences on serum UA concentration and urinary UA excretion is not significant.[19,20] UA excretion occurs in both the intestine and kidney, with 75% excreted in the urine and 25% excreted enterically.[21] (Table 15.2)

15.3.2 Renal Uric Acid Handling

15.3.2.1 Renal Tubular Uric Acid Reabsorption

The renal mechanism of urate handling is complex, consisting of glomerular filtration, tubular reabsorption, tubular secretion, and post-secretory reabsorption. Under normal conditions, 90% of filtered UA is reabsorbed by the proximal renal tubule. However, fractional urate excretion differs among the various mammalian species. It accounts for 40% in rats and 200% in pigs.[22,23]

In recent years, there has been major progress made in the discovery of various transporters regulating renal tubular UA reabsorption (Fig. 15.1). Specifically, the URAT1 transporter in the apical membrane of the proximal renal tubular cell encoded by Slc22A12 (solute carrier gene family 22,

member 12), has been shown to play a principle role in renal tubular UA reabsorption.[24,25] This apical urate-anion exchanger is found in all reabsorptive species including humans, primates, rats, and dogs. However, this transporter is inactivated in secretory species such as pigs and rabbits.[26,27] It has also been shown that certain organic anion transporters (OATs), such as lactate, nicotinate, and pyrazinamide, influence the activity of URAT1-mediated renal UA reabsorption.[24] Sodium-dependant apical entry of monovalent anions such as lactate, pyrizanimide, butyrate, and nicotinate are mediated through Slc5A8 and Slc5A12 co-transporters and enhance the apical urate reabsorption. This process occurs via the URAT1 anion exchanger.[28] Moreover, uricosuric agents including probenecid, benzbromarone, and nonsteroid anti-inflammatory agents have been identified to inhibit the activity of URAT1.

15.3.2.2 Renal Tubular Uric Acid Secretion

The exact mechanism for UA secretion has not been fully explored. It has been suggested that positive proximal renal tubular lumen potential stimulates urate secretion.[29] Recently, certain OATs have also been suggested to play a role in renal tubular UA secretion.[25,30,31] These transporters are expressed in the basolateral membrane, which may be a potential candidate that increases UA uptake into the renal proximal tubular cell and consequently increases its secretion.[25,30,31] Other candidate transporters playing a role in renal tubular urate secretion include urate transporter/channel 1 (UAT1),[32] voltage-driven organic anion transporter 1 (OATv1),[33] and multiresistant-associated protein 4 (MRP4).[34] However, the role of these transporters in human urate secretion has not been elucidated. Despite our progress in the knowledge and understanding of the molecular mechanism of apical urate entry, its exact exit pathway also remains unknown.

15.4 Physicochemical Properties of Uric Acid

UA is the end product of purine metabolism in higher mammals. Due to a lack of the hepatic enzyme, uricase, serum UA concentrations in these species are high. Uricase is known to transform UA to a more soluble compound, allantoin.[35] Urinary UA solubility is limited to 96 mg/L. Therefore, a urinary UA excretion in excess of 600 mg/day exceeds its limit of solubility and enhances the risk of UA precipitation.[16] Furthermore, urine pH also plays a key role in UA's solubility in the urinary environment. UA is a weak organic acid with an ionization constant (pKa) of 5.5.[36,37] With an unduly acidic urine (urinary pH ≤ 5.5), an invariable feature in subjects with UA stones, the urinary environment becomes supersaturated with respect to sparingly soluble undissociated UA.[38–40] In addition to increasing the tendency toward UA precipitation, this process also increases the propensity of mixed uric acid and calcium oxalate stone formation. The latter process involves the heterogeneous nucleation and epitaxial crystal growth.[41–44] UA solubility in the urine is also influenced by the urinary electrolyte composition. Urine enriched with monopotassium urate has been shown to have a higher solubility than in urine saturated with monosodium urate.[44,45] These differences in the physicochemical properties of various urate salts has been the principle factor in the development of potassium alkali treatment, an agent which has been shown to be superior to alkali treatment in UA stone forming subjects.[40]

In addition to the aforementioned factors, the potential roles of inhibitors and/or promoters have been suggested for the propensity of UA stone formation. Experimental evidence has shown that macromolecules may inhibit the adhesion of UA crystals to renal epithelial cells.[46] Moreover, reduced urinary excretion of glycosaminoglycans has been reported in UA stone formers compared to non-stone forming controls.[47]

15.5 Etiology of Uric Acid Stones

The major etiologic factors for the development of uric acid stones are low urine volume, hyper uricosuria, and unduly acidic urine (Fig. 15.2). Multiple etiologic mechanisms, including congenital, idiopathic, and acquired causes, are operative in UA stone formation.[48] Idiopathic UA nephrolithiasis (IUAN) is the most common cause of UA stone formation.[49] The pathogenesis of IUAN cannot be a result of an inborn error in metabolism,[48,50,51] disease states such as chronic diarrhea,[52] or environmental influences such as strenuous physical exercise or overindulgence in a high purine diet.[19,52]

15.6 Pathophysiology of Uric Acid Stones

15.6.1 Low Urine Volume

Low urine volume is known to increase the urinary supersaturation of stone forming constituents.[53] This mechanism is important in conditions such as a chronic diarrheal state or

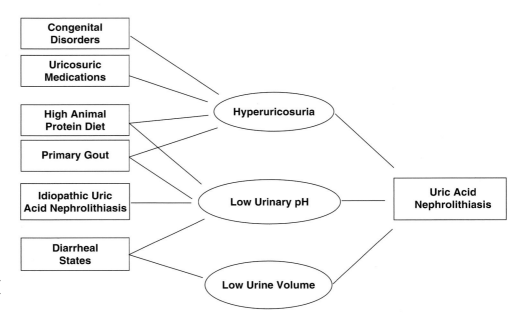

Fig. 15.2 Pathogenesis and etiologies (Reprinted with permission from Maalouf et al.[48])

following strenuous physical exercise, specifically when low urinary volume is accompanied by unduly acidic urine due to diarrheal alkali loss or excessive endogenous acid production commonly encountered with strenuous physical activity.[19,52]

15.6.2 Hyperuricosuria

Hyperuricosuria may occur due to genetic and/or dietary factors. One example is subjects with primary gout in which both dietary influences and endogenous UA production may contribute to hyperuricemia and consequent hyperuricosuria.[39,54] Hyperuricosuria invariably occurs in a few rare hereditary disorders with mutations in the enzymatic pathways responsible for UA production. These conditions include X-linked hypoxanthine guanine phosphoribosyl transferase deficiency, X-linked phosphoribosyl synthetase overactivity, and autosomal recessive glucose-6-phosphatase deficiency.[50] The clinical course of these disorders is accompanied by a significant risk of kidney stone formation, gout, and renal failure. Biochemically, these subjects present profound hyperuricemia and significantly elevated urinary UA excretion in excess of 10 mg/dl and 1,000 mg/day, respectively. These abnormalities commonly manifest during childhood, however, they may remain silent until puberty.[55]

Recently, a genetic mutation localized on chromosome 11q13 encoding URAT1 has been described as showing evidence of hyperuricosuria, hyperuricemia, increased UA kidney stone formation, and exercise-induced acute renal failure.[24] Moreover, in a Sardinian population, a putative gene locus localized on chromosome 10q122 has been linked to UA nephrolithiasis. A protein product identified and designated as zinc finger protein 365 (ZNF365) has also been linked to UA nephrolithiasis in this population. However, the function of this protein has not been fully elucidated.[56]

The escalated tissue breakdown encountered with malignancies and chemotherapy increases UA production and may also lead to hyperuricosuria.[18,57] Additionally, certain uricosuric drugs such as high-dose salicylates, probenecid, radiocontrast agents, and losartan have also been known to increase UA excretion, which thereby increase the risk of UA stone formation.[48,58] This complication specifically occurs after the initial institution of the drug and/or in combination with hyperuricemia.[16] Therefore, it is imperative not to recommend the use of these drugs in subjects with UA overproduction.[38]

15.6.3 Acidic Urine pH

Abnormally acidic urine (urinary pH ≤ 5.5) is an invariant feature in patients with IUAN.[39] (Fig. 15.3) Acidic urinary pH as

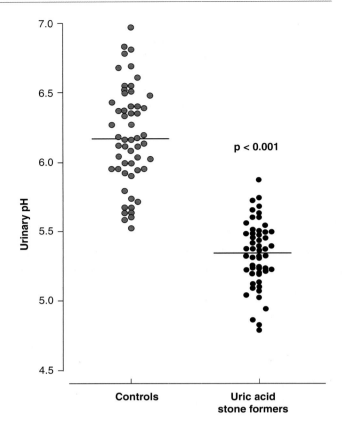

Fig. 15.3 Unduly acidic urine in UA stone formers (Reprinted with permission from Pak et al.[59])

a key factor in UA stone formation was originally described 4 decades ago and was attributed to defective urinary ammonium (NH_4^+) excretion.[60] This defective ammoniagenesis was first proposed to be a result of enzymatic disturbances in the conversion of glutamine to α(alpha)-ketoglutarate, which consequently lowered urinary NH_4^+ excretion.[61–64] However, the validity of this concept did not prevail. A major advance in our understanding of the pathophysiology of unduly acidic urine in IUAN has evolved over the past decade. Multiple cross-sectional clinical studies conducted in both kidney stone formers and normal subjects have shown an inverse relationship between urinary pH, body weight, and features of the MS.[65,66] Furthermore, careful metabolic studies have also displayed that unduly acidic urine may be due to a combination of lowered NH_4^+ excretion and increased endogenous acid production. These conditions are associated with obesity and T2DM and are responsible for fatty infiltration of the kidney.[67]

15.6.4 Impaired Ammonium Excretion

NH_4^+ excretion plays a key role in the regulation of acid base balances. Due to its high pKa of 9.3 (NH_3/NH_4^+ system), under normal circumstances NH_4^+ is able to effectively buffer the majority of secreted protons.[68] The residual protons are then buffered by titratable acid (TA), as a result of its favorable pKa of 6.8 and its relatively high concentration, in order to maintain a normal urinary pH.[68] However, in IUAN patients with defective NH_4^+ excretion, TA plays a key role in maintaining these acid base balances by buffering most of the secreted protons. The trade-off in this process is unduly acidic urine, which increases the propensity of UA precipitation and UA stone formation. A single metabolic study under a fixed metabolic diet recently displayed defective NH_4^+ excretion in IUAN subjects (Fig. 15.4).[39] The defective NH_4^+ excretion seen in these subjects was further unmasked by the administration of an acute acid load that was shown to exaggerate this ammoniagenic effect.[39] These results were consistent with an additional study, conducted on an ad-lib diet, showing a defective NH_4^+ excretion in both IUAN subjects and also in T2DM patients without kidney stones who shared the same phenotypic characteristics of MS.[55] Moreover, a study in normal subjects showed that urinary pH and NH_4^+ excretion progressively falls with increasing features of the MS.[69] These studies cumulatively suggest that renal ammoniagenesis and low urinary pH may not be specifically related to IUAN, but may be general features of the MS.

A pathophysiologic link between peripheral insulin resistance, urinary pH, and NH_4^+ excretion was first revealed in a metabolic study using the hyperinsulinemic euglycemic clamp technique in IUAN subjects.[70] This study further inferred the potential causal relationship between insulin resistance, defective urinary NH_4^+ excretion, and consequent

unduly acidic urine in this patient population. Several experimental studies have determined that insulin receptors are expressed in various segments of the kidney.[71,72] Furthermore, it has been demonstrated that insulin has a significant role in renal ammoniagenesis and renal NH_4^+ excretion.[70,73–75] NH_4^+ secretion is mediated by the sodium-hydrogen exchanger NHE3.[70] This transporter activity is regulated by insulin and it participates in the transport or trapping of NH_4^+ in the renal tubular lumen.[70] Therefore, it is plausible to suggest that renal insulin resistance may potentially influence NH_4^+ excretion. Another possible mechanism is the substitution of glutamine with circulating free fatty acids as a major fuel source of renal metabolism.[76] Circulating free fatty acids are known to increase with insulin resistance and, by the process of substrate competition, may reduce the proximal renal tubular cell utilization of glutamine, thereby reducing renal ammonia synthesis.[76]

15.6.5 Increased Endogenous Acid Production

Under normal conditions in a steady state, net acid production equals net acid excretion (NAE). High NAE can occur as a result of increased endogenous organic acid production or due to dietary factors such as high dietary acid consumption or low dietary alkali intake.[77] A metabolic study under a constant diet has shown that NAE is higher in IUAN patients compared to control subjects.[16] This study suggests that endogenous acid production is elevated in this population. Furthermore, another similar study determined that urinary NAE for any given level of urinary sulfate (a marker of acid intake) was higher in IUAN patients and also in T2DM subjects without kidney stones.[55] From these studies one may infer that the pathophysiologic mechanisms accounting for increased NAE may be linked to obesity and insulin resistance. These results were consistent with findings from other related studies, which demonstrated a correlation between increased organic acid excretion, higher body weight, and higher body surface area.[43,44] To date, the nature of these putative organic anions remains unknown. From the above circumstances, one may speculate that defective NH_4^+ excretion is the principle reason for the development of unduly acidic urine in IUAN. However, this defect alone is necessary but not sufficient for the development of persistently acidic urine. One can also speculate that high endogenous acid production may exacerbate the acidic urine caused by impaired NH_4^+ excretion. Moreover, a third mechanism involving a lack of inhibitors or the presence of promoters of UA stone formation may also participate in UA nephrolithiasis (Fig. 15.5).

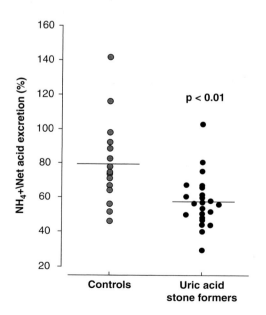

Fig. 15.4 Impaired urinary ammonium excretion in UA stone formers (Reprinted with permission from Sakhaee et al.[39])

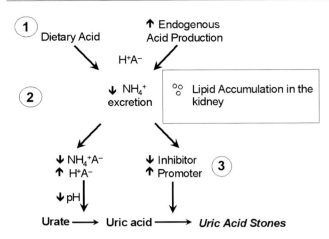

Fig. 15.5 Pathogenesis of uric acid stone formation

15.6.6 Role of Renal Lipotoxicity

A tight balance between caloric intake and caloric utilization, under normal conditions, is conducive to triglyceride accumulation in adipocytes.[78,79] The disequilibrium in this tight regulation leads to tissue redistribution of triglycerides within parancheymal liver cells, cardiac myocytes, skeletal muscle cells, and pancreatic β(beta)-cells.[79–84] The extra-adipocyte tissue fat deposition is termed lipotoxicity.[79] This process has been associated with impaired insulin sensitivity,[81] cardiac abnormalities,[83] and steatohepatitis.[80,85] This cellular injury has been attributed to the accumulation of nonesterified free fatty acids (NEFA) and their toxic byproducts, fatty acyl CoA, diacylglycerol, and ceramide.[78,86,87] There has been growing evidence that renal lipotoxicity plays a pathogenetic role in the development of renal disease. A pathophysiologic link between obesity, the MS, and the development of chronic kidney disease has been suggested in several recent studies.[79,88,89] To date, there is insufficient data available to suggest whether renal fat accumulation actually occurs, whether renal lipotoxicity contributes to endogenous acid production, or whether renal lipotoxicity causes defective NH_4^+ excretion (Fig. 15.5).

Several interventions, including caloric restriction, bariatric surgery, intestinal lipase blocker, thiazolidinediones (TZD), Metformin, and α(alpha)-lipoic acid, have been suggested to reverse tissue lipotoxicity in various organs.[90–100] TZD stimulates PPAR-γ in adipocytes and facilitates adipocyte differentiation. As a result, it diminishes renal lipotoxicity by redistributing lipids to adipocytes.[101,102] In humans, this intervention has been shown to reduce skeletal muscle and hepatic fat accumulation.[90,94,95] Currently, a double-blind study using magnetic resonance spectroscopy in IUAN subjects is underway to determine the effects of treatment with pioglitazone in the reversal of biochemical abnormalities and renal fat content. Additionally, an experimental animal model, the Zucher Diabetic Fatty rat (ZDF), is a rodent model

that shares phenotypic features of the MS[103] and biochemical characteristics similar to IUAN including acidic urine pH, defective NH_4^+ excretion, increased TA excretion, high renal triglyceride, and lower levels of brush border membrane NHE3 (a sodium-hydrogen exchanger that plays a principle role in ammonium excretion).[67] Another experimental rodent model, Sprague-Dawley rats, display a transient reduction of urinary NH_4^+ excretion and pH following a high fat feeding. These abnormalities are resolved, however, upon feeding with a normal fat content diet.[67] These findings suggest that renal fat accumulation may potentially affect renal NH_4^+ excretion by reducing NHE3 activity.

15.7 Conclusions

The primary abnormality responsible for UA stone formation is unduly acidic urine as a result of defective NH_4^+ excretion. However, in addition to this defect, IUAN subjects present a secondary defect in which they produce high amounts of endogenous organic acid. This abnormality further exaggerates urinary acidity, increases the risk of UA precipitation, and consequently increases UA stone formation. Based on our current knowledge from both human and animal studies, one may speculate that renal steatosis from obesity and T2DM may impair the capacity of the kidney to excrete NH_4^+. In addition, one may also speculate that fat deposition in multiple organs may lead to increased endogenous organic acid production. The combined effect of these conditions would lead to abnormally acidic urine, which increases the propensity for UA nephrolithiasis. Furthermore, the risk of UA stone formation may also be affected by the presence of urinary promoters and/or the absence of urinary inhibitors of UA crystallization. Our understanding of the pathogenic link between UA stone formation and the MS, and its connection to renal lipotoxicity, can potentially lead to the development of novel drugs to reverse the basic metabolic abnormalities and reduce the risk of stone formation.

Acknowledgments The author would like to acknowledge the editorial support of Ms. Hadley Armstrong.

The author was supported by the National Institutes of Health Grant R01-DK081423-01A1.

References

1. Pak CY, Sakhaee K, Moe O, et al. Biochemical profile of stone-forming patients with diabetes mellitus. *Urology.* 2003;61(3): 523-527.
2. Ekeruo WO, Tan YH, Young MD, et al. Metabolic risk factors and the impact of medical therapy on the management of nephrolithiasis in obese patients. *J Urol.* 2004;172(1):159-163.

3. Daudon M, Lacour B, Jungers P. Influence of body size on urinary stone composition in men and women. *Urol Res.* 2006;34(3): 193-199.

4. Daudon M, Traxer O, Conort P, Lacour B, Jungers P. Type 2 diabetes increases the risk for uric acid stones. *J Am Soc Nephrol.* 2006;17(7):2026-2033.

5. Executive Summary of The Third Report of The National Cholesterol Education Program (NCEP) Expert Panel on Detection, Evaluation, And Treatment of High Blood Cholesterol In Adults (Adult Treatment Panel III). JAMA 2001; 285(19):2486-2497.

6. Alberti KG, Zimmet PZ. Definition, diagnosis and classification of diabetes mellitus and its complications. Part 1: diagnosis and classification of diabetes mellitus provisional report of a WHO consultation. *Diabet Med.* 1998;15(7):539-553.

7. Eckel RH, Grundy SM, Zimmet PZ. The metabolic syndrome. *Lancet.* 2005;365(9468):1415-1428.

8. Reaven GM. The kidney: an unwilling accomplice in syndrome X. *Am J Kidney Dis.* 1997;30(6):928-931.

9. Taylor EN, Stampfer MJ, Curhan GC. Obesity, weight gain, and the risk of kidney stones. *JAMA.* 2005;293(4):455-462.

10. Taylor EN, Stampfer MJ, Curhan GC. Diabetes mellitus and the risk of nephrolithiasis. *Kidney Int.* 2005;68(3):1230-1235.

11. Daudon M, Lacour B, Jungers P. High prevalence of uric acid calculi in diabetic stone formers. *Nephrol Dial Transplant.* 2005;20(2): 468-469.

12. Mandel NS, Mandel GS. Urinary tract stone disease in the United States veteran population II. Geographical analysis of variations in composition. *J Urol.* 1989;142(6):1516-1521.

13. Atsmon A, DeVries A, Frank M. *Uric Acid Lithiasis.* Amsterdam: Elsevier; 1963.

14. Hesse A, Schneider HJ, Berg W, Hienzsch E. Uric acid dihydrate as urinary calculus component. *Invest Urol.* 1975;12(5): 405-409.

15. Portis AJ, Hermans K, Culhane-Pera KA, Curhan GC. Stone disease in the Hmong of Minnesota: initial description of a high-risk population. *J Endourol.* 2004;18(9):853-857.

16. Asplin JR. Uric acid stones. *Semin Nephrol.* 1996;16(5):412-424.

17. Cameron MA, Sakhaee K. Uric acid nephrolithiasis. *Urol Clin North Am.* 2007;34(3):335-346.

18. Sorensen L. Extrarenal disposal of uric acid. In: Kelley W, Weiner I, eds. *Uric Acid.* New York: Springer; 1978:325-336.

19. Sakhaee K, Nigam S, Snell P, Hsu MC, Pak CY. Assessment of the pathogenetic role of physical exercise in renal stone formation. *J Clin Endocrinol Metab.* 1987;65(5):974-979.

20. Fellstrom B, Danielson BG, Karlstrom B, Lithell H, Ljunghall S, Vessby B. The influence of a high dietary intake of purine-rich animal protein on urinary urate excretion and supersaturation in renal stone disease. *Clin Sci (Lond).* 1983;64(4):399-405.

21. Sorensen LB. Role of the intestinal tract in the elimination of uric acid. *Arthritis Rheum.* 1965;8(5):694-706.

22. Roch-Ramel F, Diezi-Chomety F, De Rougemont D, Tellier M, Widmer J, Peters G. Renal excretion of uric acid in the rat: a micropuncture and microperfusion study. *Am J Physiol.* 1976;230(3): 768-776.

23. Simmonds HA, Hatfield PJ, Cameron JS, Cadenhead A. Uric acid excretion by the pig kidney. *Am J Physiol.* 1976;230(6): 1654-1661.

24. Enomoto A, Kimura H, Chairoungdua A, et al. Molecular identification of a renal urate anion exchanger that regulates blood urate levels. *Nature.* 2002;417(6887):447-452.

25. Hediger MA, Johnson RJ, Miyazaki H, Endou H. Molecular physiology of urate transport. *Physiology (Bethesda).* 2005;20:125-133.

26. Guggino SE, Martin GJ, Aronson PS. Specificity and modes of the anion exchanger in dog renal microvillus membranes. *Am J Physiol.* 1983;244(6):F612-F621.

27. Martinez F, Manganel M, Montrose-Rafizadeh C, Werner D, Roch-Ramel F. Transport of urate and p-aminohippurate in rabbit renal brush-border membranes. *Am J Physiol.* 1990;258(5 Pt 2): F1145-F1153.

28. Mount DB, Kwon CY, Zandi-Nejad K. Renal urate transport. *Rheum Dis Clin North Am.* 2006;32(2):313-331. vi.

29. Roch-Ramel F, Werner D, Guisan B. Urate transport in brush-border membrane of human kidney. *Am J Physiol.* 1994;266(5 Pt 2): F797-F805.

30. Sekine T, Watanabe N, Hosoyamada M, Kanai Y, Endou H. Expression cloning and characterization of a novel multispecific organic anion transporter. *J Biol Chem.* 1997;272(30):18526-18529.

31. Cha SH, Sekine T, Fukushima JI, et al. Identification and characterization of human organic anion transporter 3 expressing predominantly in the kidney. *Mol Pharmacol.* 2001;59(5):1277-1286.

32. Lipkowitz MS, Leal-Pinto E, Rappoport JZ, Najfeld V, Abramson RG. Functional reconstitution, membrane targeting, genomic structure, and chromosomal localization of a human urate transporter. *J Clin Invest.* 2001;107(9):1103-1115.

33. Jutabha P, Kanai Y, Hosoyamada M, et al. Identification of a novel voltage-driven organic anion transporter present at apical membrane of renal proximal tubule. *J Biol Chem.* 2003;278(30):27930-27938.

34. Van Aubel RA, Smeets PH, van den Heuvel JJ, Russel FG. Human organic anion transporter MRP4 (ABCC4) is an efflux pump for the purine end metabolite urate with multiple allosteric substrate binding sites. *Am J Physiol Renal Physiol.* 2005;288(2):F327-F333.

35. Rafey MA, Lipkowitz MS, Leal-Pinto E, Abramson RG. Uric acid transport. *Curr Opin Nephrol Hypertens.* 2003;12(5):511-516.

36. Coe FL, Strauss AL, Tembe V, Le Dun S. Uric acid saturation in calcium nephrolithiasis. *Kidney Int.* 1980;17(5):662-668.

37. Finlayson B, Smith L. Stability of first dissociable proton of uric acid. *J Chem Engl Data.* 1974;19:94-97.

38. Riese RJ, Sakhaee K. Uric acid nephrolithiasis: pathogenesis and treatment. *J Urol.* 1992;148(3):765-771.

39. Sakhaee K, Adams-Huet B, Moe OW, Pak CY. Pathophysiologic basis for normouricosuric uric acid nephrolithiasis. *Kidney Int.* 2002;62(3):971-979.

40. Sakhaee K, Nicar M, Hill K, Pak CY. Contrasting effects of potassium citrate and sodium citrate therapies on urinary chemistries and crystallization of stone-forming salts. *Kidney Int.* 1983;24(3):348-352.

41. Coe FL, Kavalach AG. Hypercalciuria and hyperuricosuria in patients with calcium nephrolithiasis. *N Engl J Med.* 1974;291(25): 1344-1350.

42. Pak CY, Arnold LH. Heterogeneous nucleation of calcium oxalate by seeds of monosodium urate. *Proc Soc Exp Biol Med.* 1975;149(4): 930-932.

43. Pak CY, Hayashi Y, Arnold LH. Heterogeneous nucleation with urate, calcium phosphate and calcium oxalate. *Proc Soc Exp Biol Med.* 1976;153(1):83-87.

44. Pak CY, Waters O, Arnold L, Holt K, Cox C, Barilla D. Mechanism for calcium urolithiasis among patients with hyperuricosuria: supersaturation of urine with respect to monosodium urate. *J Clin Invest.* 1977;59(3):426-431.

45. Wilcox WR, Khalaf A, Weinberger A, Kippen I, Klinenberg JR. Solubility of uric acid and monosodium urate. *Med Biol Eng.* 1972;10(4):522-531.

46. Koka RM, Huang E, Lieske JC. Adhesion of uric acid crystals to the surface of renal epithelial cells. *Am J Physiol Renal Physiol.* 2000;278(6):F989-F998.

47. Ombra MN, Casula S, Biino G, et al. Urinary glycosaminoglycans as risk factors for uric acid nephrolithiasis: case control study in a Sardinian genetic isolate. *Urology.* 2003;62(3):416-420.

48. Maalouf NM, Cameron MA, Moe OW, Sakhaee K. Novel insights into the pathogenesis of uric acid nephrolithiasis. *Curr Opin Nephrol Hypertens.* 2004;13(2):181-189.

49. Pak CY. Medical management of nephrolithiasis in Dallas: update 1987. *J Urol.* 1988;140(3):461-467.

50. Moe OW, Abate N, Sakhaee K. Pathophysiology of uric acid nephrolithiasis. *Endocrinol Metab Clin North Am.* 2002;31(4):895-914.

51. Mineo I, Kono N, Hara N, et al. Myogenic hyperuricemia. A common pathophysiologic feature of glycogenosis types III, V, and VII. *N Engl J Med.* 1987;317(2):75-80.

52. Grossman MS, Nugent FW. Urolithiasis as a complication of chronic diarrheal disease. *Am J Dig Dis.* 1967;12(5):491-498.

53. Pak CY, Skurla C, Harvey J. Graphic display of urinary risk factors for renal stone formation. *J Urol.* 1985;134(5):867-870.

54. Alvarez-Nemegyei J, Medina-Escobedo M, Villanueva-Jorge S, Vazquez-Mellado J. Prevalence and risk factors for urolithiasis in primary gout: is a reappraisal needed? *J Rheumatol.* 2005;32(11):2189-2191.

55. Cameron MA, Maalouf NM, Adams-Huet B, Moe OW, Sakhaee K. Urine composition in type 2 diabetes: predisposition to uric acid nephrolithiasis. *J Am Soc Nephrol.* 2006;17(5):1422-1428.

56. Gianfrancesco F, Esposito T, Ombra MN, et al. Identification of a novel gene and a common variant associated with uric acid nephrolithiasis in a Sardinian genetic isolate. *Am J Hum Genet.* 2003;72(6):1479-1491.

57. Yu T, Weinreb N, Wittman R, Wasserman LR. Secondary gout associated with chronic myeloproliferative disorders. *Semin Arthritis Rheum.* 1976;5(3):247-256.

58. Shahinfar S, Simpson RL, Carides AD, et al. Safety of losartan in hypertensive patients with thiazide-induced hyperuricemia. *Kidney Int.* 1999;56(5):1879-1885.

59. Pak CY, Sakhaee K, Peterson RD, Poindexter JR, Frawley WH. Biochemical profile of idiopathic uric acid nephrolithiasis. *Kidney Int.* 2001;60(2):757-761.

60. Henneman PH, Wallach S, Dempsey EF. The metabolism defect responsible for uric acid stone formation. *J Clin Invest.* 1962;41:537-542.

61. Gutman AB, Yue TF. An abnormality of glutamine metabolism in primary gout. *Am J Med.* 1963;35:820-831.

62. Pollak VE, Mattenheimer H. Glutaminase activity in the kidney in gout. *J Lab Clin Med.* 1965;66(4):564-570.

63. Pagliara AS, Goodman AD. Elevation of plasma glutamate in gout. Its possible role in the pathogenesis of hyperuricemia. *N Engl J Med.* 1969;281(14):767-770.

64. Sperling O, Wyngaarden JB, Starmer CF. The kinetics of intramolecular distribution of 15N in uric acid after administration of (15N) glycine. A reappraisal of the significance of preferential labeling of N-(3+9) of uric acid in primary gout. *J Clin Invest.* 1973;52(10):2468-2485.

65. Maalouf NM, Sakhaee K, Parks JH, Coe FL, Adams-Huet B, Pak CY. Association of urinary pH with body weight in nephrolithiasis. *Kidney Int.* 2004;65(4):1422-1425.

66. Maalouf NM, Cameron MA, Moe OW, Adams-Huet B, Sakhaee K. Low urine pH: a novel feature of the metabolic syndrome. *Clin J Am Soc Nephrol.* 2007;2(5):883-888.

67. Bobulescu IA, Dubree M, Zhang J, McLeroy P, Moe OW. Effect of renal lipid accumulation on proximal tubule Na+/H+ exchange and ammonium secretion. *Am J Physiol Renal Physiol.* 2008;294(6):F1315-F1322.

68. DuBose TD Jr, Good DW, Hamm LL, Wall SM. Ammonium transport in the kidney: new physiological concepts and their clinical implications. *J Am Soc Nephrol.* 1991;1(11):1193-1203.

69. McCarron DA, Pingree PA, Rubin RJ, Gaucher SM, Molitch M, Krutzik S. Enhanced parathyroid function in essential hypertension: a homeostatic response to a urinary calcium leak. *Hypertension.* 1980;2(2):162-168.

70. Nagami GT. Luminal secretion of ammonia in the mouse proximal tubule perfused in vitro. *J Clin Invest.* 1988;81(1):159-164.

71. Meezan E, Freychet P. Specific insulin receptors in rat renal glomeruli. *Ren Physiol.* 1980;3(1–6):72-78.

72. Nakamura R, Emmanouel DS, Katz AI. Insulin binding sites in various segments of the rabbit nephron. *J Clin Invest.* 1983;72(1):388-392.

73. Krivosikova Z, Spustova V, Dzurik R. Participation of P-dependent and P-independent glutaminases in rat kidney ammoniagenesis and their modulation by metabolic acidosis, hippurate and insulin. *Physiol Res.* 1998;47(3):177-183.

74. Chobanian MC, Hammerman MR. Insulin stimulates ammoniagenesis in canine renal proximal tubular segments. *Am J Physiol.* 1987;253(6 Pt 2):F1171-F1177.

75. Klisic J, Hu MC, Nief V, et al. Insulin activates Na(+)/H(+) exchanger 3: biphasic response and glucocorticoid dependence. *Am J Physiol Renal Physiol.* 2002;283(3):F532-F539.

76. Vinay P, Lemieux G, Cartier P, Ahmad M. Effect of fatty acids on renal ammoniagenesis in in vivo and in vitro studies. *Am J Physiol.* 1976;231(3):880-887.

77. Remer T. Influence of diet on acid-base balance. *Semin Dial.* 2000;13(4):221-226.

78. Unger RH. Lipotoxic diseases. *Annu Rev Med.* 2002;53:319-336.

79. Lee Y, Hirose H, Ohneda M, Johnson JH, McGarry JD, Unger RH. Beta-cell lipotoxicity in the pathogenesis of non-insulin-dependent diabetes mellitus of obese rats: impairment in adipocyte-beta-cell relationships. *Proc Natl Acad Sci U S A.* 1994;91(23):10878-10882.

80. Szczepaniak LS, Nurenberg P, Leonard D, et al. Magnetic resonance spectroscopy to measure hepatic triglyceride content: prevalence of hepatic steatosis in the general population. *Am J Physiol Endocrinol Metab.* 2005;288(2):E462-E468.

81. Bachmann OP, Dahl DB, Brechtel K, et al. Effects of intravenous and dietary lipid challenge on intramyocellular lipid content and the relation with insulin sensitivity in humans. *Diabetes.* 2001;50(11):2579-2584.

82. McGavock JM, Victor RG, Unger RH, Szczepaniak LS. Adiposity of the heart, revisited. *Ann Intern Med.* 2006;144(7):517-524.

83. Szczepaniak LS, Dobbins RL, Metzger GJ, et al. Myocardial triglycerides and systolic function in humans: in vivo evaluation by localized proton spectroscopy and cardiac imaging. *Magn Reson Med.* 2003;49(3):417-423.

84. McGarry JD. Banting lecture 2001: dysregulation of fatty acid metabolism in the etiology of type 2 diabetes. *Diabetes.* 2002;51(1):7-18.

85. Browning JD, Szczepaniak LS, Dobbins R, et al. Prevalence of hepatic steatosis in an urban population in the United States: impact of ethnicity. *Hepatology.* 2004;40(6):1387-1395.

86. Weinberg JM. Lipotoxicity. *Kidney Int.* 2006;70(9):1560-1566.

87. Schaffer JE. Lipotoxicity: when tissues overeat. *Curr Opin Lipidol.* 2003;14(3):281-287.

88. Bagby SP. Obesity-initiated metabolic syndrome and the kidney: a recipe for chronic kidney disease? *J Am Soc Nephrol.* 2004;15(11):2775-2791.

89. Wahba IM, Mak RH. Obesity and obesity-initiated metabolic syndrome: mechanistic links to chronic kidney disease. *Clin J Am Soc Nephrol.* 2007;2(3):550-562.

90. Tiikkainen M, Hakkinen AM, Korsheninnikova E, Nyman T, Makimattila S, Yki-Jarvinen H. Effects of rosiglitazone and metformin on liver fat content, hepatic insulin resistance, insulin clearance, and gene expression in adipose tissue in patients with type 2 diabetes. *Diabetes.* 2004;53(8):2169-2176.

91. Gekle M. Renal tubule albumin transport. *Annu Rev Physiol.* 2005;67:573-594.

92. Russo LM, Sandoval RM, McKee M, et al. The normal kidney filters nephrotic levels of albumin retrieved by proximal tubule cells: retrieval is disrupted in nephrotic states. *Kidney Int.* 2007;71(6):504-513.

93. Iglesias J, Levine JS. Albuminuria and renal injury–beware of proteins bearing gifts. *Nephrol Dial Transplant.* 2001;16(2):215-218.

94. Belfort R, Harrison SA, Brown K, et al. A placebo-controlled trial of pioglitazone in subjects with nonalcoholic steatohepatitis. *N Engl J Med.* 2006;355(22):2297-2307.

95. Rasouli N, Raue U, Miles LM, et al. Pioglitazone improves insulin sensitivity through reduction in muscle lipid and redistribution of lipid into adipose tissue. *Am J Physiol Endocrinol Metab.* 2005; 288(5):E930-E934.

96. Ueno T, Sugawara H, Sujaku K, et al. Therapeutic effects of restricted diet and exercise in obese patients with fatty liver. *J Hepatol.* 1997;27(1):103-107.

97. Uygun A, Kadayifci A, Isik AT, et al. Metformin in the treatment of patients with non-alcoholic steatohepatitis. *Aliment Pharmacol Ther.* 2004;19(5):537-544.

98. Harrison SA, Fincke C, Helinski D, Torgerson S, Hayashi P. A pilot study of orlistat treatment in obese, non-alcoholic steatohepatitis patients. *Aliment Pharmacol Ther.* 2004;20(6): 623-628.

99. Lee Y, Naseem RH, Park BH, et al. Alpha-lipoic acid prevents lipotoxic cardiomyopathy in acyl CoA-synthase transgenic mice. *Biochem Biophys Res Commun.* 2006;344(1): 446-452.

100. Dixon JB. Surgical treatment for obesity and its impact on non-alcoholic steatohepatitis. *Clin Liver Dis.* 2007;11(1): 141-14x.

101. Shulman GI. Cellular mechanisms of insulin resistance. *J Clin Invest.* 2000;106(2):171-176.

102. Yki-Jarvinen H. Thiazolidinediones. *N Engl J Med.* 2004;351(11): 1106-1118.

103. Clark JB, Palmer CJ, Shaw WN. The diabetic Zucker fatty rat. *Proc Soc Exp Biol Med.* 1983;173(1):68-75.

Christopher J. Danpure

Abstract The primary hyperoxalurias are a group of rare hereditary calcium oxalate kidney stone diseases, the best characterized of which are primary hyperoxaluria type 1 (PH1) and type 2 (PH2). Deficiencies of alanine:glyoxylate aminotransferase (AGT) in PH1 and glyoxylate/hydroxypyruvate reductase (GR/HPR) in PH2 lead to the increased synthesis and excretion of the metabolic end product, oxalate. Insoluble calcium oxalate crystallizes out in the kidney and urinary tract, leading to kidney dysfunction and eventually complete organ failure. More than 100 mutations have been found in PH1, but less than 20 in PH2. The crystal structures of both AGT and GR/HPR have been solved, enabling rationalization of the untoward effects of at least some of the mutations, as well as how in PH1 some of the mutations interact synergistically with the common Pro11Leu polymorphism. A wide variety of enzyme phenotypes are found in PH1, but perhaps the most spectacular is the unparalleled peroxisome-to-mitochondrion AGT mistargeting caused by a combination of the Pro11Leu polymorphism and Gly170Arg mutation. Although remaining catalytically active in this location, mitochondrial AGT is metabolically ineffective. Classic stone treatments, such as hydration and crystallization inhibitors, are applicable to PH1 and PH2. However, some treatments such as pyridoxine therapy and liver transplantation (enzyme replacement therapy) are restricted to PH1.

16.1 Introduction

In humans, oxalate is a metabolic end product of no known use. In fact, it can be detrimental to the health of complex physiological life forms due to the low solubility of its calcium salt. The solubility product of calcium oxalate (CaOx) is readily exceeded, leading to the formation of microscopic crystals that can aggregate into macroscopic agglomerations. As oxalate, once formed, can only be removed from the body to any significant extent by renal excretion, it is the kidney that frequently suffers the consequences of low CaOx solubility. In extreme circumstances, deposition of CaOx in the kidney can result in complete organ failure.

Despite having been studied for many years, the sources of urinary oxalate are still not well established. Its origins can be conveniently divided into either exogenous (i.e., dietary) or endogenous (i.e., metabolic). However, even many of the endogenous metabolic sources of oxalate are indirectly dietary, insofar as they derive originally from dietary oxalate precursors. How much of the urinary oxalate is dietary or metabolic in origin is still a matter for conjecture. Estimates for a direct dietary origin of urinary oxalate have ranged from as little as 5% to as much as 50%, depending not only on the dietary composition, but also on the level of gastrointestinal integrity, renal function, and endogenous synthesis.[1] It is clear that dietary oxalate is not very efficiently absorbed, particularly when it is complexed with calcium.

A wide range of metabolites can act as precursors of oxalate, including amino acids, such as glycine and hydroxyproline, and carbohydrates and their derivatives, such as glycolate.[2–8] However, whatever the precursor, most are probably converted to oxalate via the glyoxylate metabolic bottleneck (see Fig. 16.1).

The great majority of oxalate consumed in the diet arises from plant-based foodstuffs (http://www.ohf.org/docs/Oxalate2008.pdf).[9,10] Very little is found in meat. Some of the dietary oxalate precursors, such as glycolate, which is a

C.J. Danpure
Department of Cell and Developmental Biology, University College London, London, UK
e-mail: c.danpure@ucl.ac.uk

P.N. Rao et al. (eds.), *Urinary Tract Stone Disease*,
DOI 10.1007/978-1-84800-362-0_16, © Springer-Verlag London Limited 2011

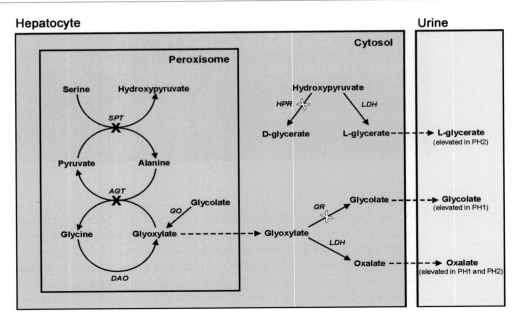

Fig. 16.1 Some of the hepatocyte metabolic pathways important in primary hyperoxaluria.Enzymes: *AGT* alanine:glyoxylate aminotransferase, *DAO* D-amino acid oxidase, *GO* glycolate oxidase, *GR* glyoxylate reductase, *HPR* hydroxypyruvate reductase, *LDH* lactate dehydrogenase, *SPT* serine:pyruvate aminotransferase. AGT and SPT are the same enzyme, as are GR and HPR. AGT & SPT are deficient in PH1, and GR & HPR are deficient in PH2. *Solid arrows*, metabolic conversions; *dashed arrows*, membrane transport/diffusion. Although only the exodus of glyoxylate from the peroxisome is shown, it is likely that the peroxisomal membrane is permeable to most of the metabolites shown. *Solid cross*, deficiency in PH1; *open cross*, deficiency in PH2

product of photorespiration, are also found mainly in plants, whereas others, such as hydroxyproline, which is a major component of collagen, are found almost exclusively in animals.

Because of the low solubility of CaOx, together with the high content of oxalate and its metabolic precursors in at least some foodstuffs, it is not surprising that the solubility product of CaOx is frequently exceeded. It is, therefore, equally unsurprising that CaOx kidney stones are common. Although the causes of "idiopathic" CaOx kidney stone disease are for the most part unknown, elevated urinary excretion of calcium (hypercalciuria) and oxalate (hyperoxaluria) are well-recognized risk factors. Whatever the causes are, they are likely to be multifactorial in nature, with both environmental and genetic components. On rare occasions, hyperoxaluria-associated CaOx kidney stone diseases have clearly established monogenic origins. These are the primary hyperoxalurias.

16.2 Primary Hyperoxaluria

Primary hyperoxaluria (PH) is a collective term that encompasses an unknown number of inherited disorders, of which only two are well characterized, namely primary hyperoxaluria type 1 (PH1, MIM259900) and primary hyperoxaluria type 2 (PH2, MIM260000).[11–15] There are other rather poorly characterized primary hyperoxalurias that are neither PH1 nor

PH2, based on current diagnostic criteria; these are sometimes grouped together as "atypical" primary hyperoxaluria.[†]

16.2.1 Pathophysiology

Although PH1 and PH2 have different genetic causes (see Sect. 16.2.2), their pathophysiology is very similar. They are both characterized by marked increase in synthesis and urinary excretion of oxalate, and the deposition of insoluble CaOx in the kidney and urinary tract. Most, but not all, PH1 and PH2 patients also have increased synthesis and urinary excretion of glycolate or L-glycerate, respectively. The presence or absence of hyperglycolic aciduria or hyper-L-glyceric aciduria appears to be of no pathological consequence, as it is the oxalate that causes all the problems in both diseases due to the low solubility of CaOx (see previous). CaOx deposition can take a number of different forms—stones/calculi in the kidney (nephrolithiasis) or urinary tract (urolithiasis), or as more diffuse crystalline deposits in the renal parenchyma (nephrocalcinosis).

[†]It has recently been found that one form of atypical primary hyperoxaluria, now called primary hyperoxaluria type 3, is due to mutations in the gene encoding the mitochondrial enzyme 4-hydroxy-2-oxoglutarate aldolase (Belototsky R et al, Am J Hum Genet. 2010; 87, 1-8.

The severity of PH1 and PH2, as manifested by age of onset, rate of progression, and response to different forms of treatment (see Sect. 16.2.4), is highly variable. Although most patients experience their first symptoms, often renal colic or haematuria, in early childhood, they can occur from as early as the first few months of life to as late as the fifth or sixth decade. Although there is not a clear-cut distinction, the infantile form of PH1, in particular, tends to be characterized by nephrocalcinosis and a rapid rate of progression, whereas the later onset childhood form is more likely to be characterized by nephro/urolithiasis and a slower rate of progression. In most cases, patients with PH1 will succumb eventually to chronic kidney failure, after which the increased synthesis of oxalate is exacerbated by the failure to remove it, leading to the deposition of CaOx throughout the body (systemic oxalosis). Although PH2 is generally thought to be a somewhat milder disease than PH1, kidney failure in PH2 can still be the long-term consequence of CaOx deposition.

16.2.2 Molecular Etiology

16.2.2.1 Enzyme and Metabolic Defects

Despite the similar pathophysiology of PH1 and PH2, they have completely different causes. PH1 is caused by a deficiency of the enzyme alanine:glyoxylate aminotransferase (AGT, EC 2.6.1.44),[16,17] whereas PH2 is caused by a deficiency of the enzyme glyoxylate reductase (GR, EC 1.1.1.26).[18] AGT is a liver-specific pyridoxal phosphate (PLP)-dependent enzyme located in hepatocyte peroxisomes[19,20] (http://symatlas.gnf.org/SymAtlas/symquery?q=AGXT). Although GR is more widely distributed than AGT, it has greatest activity in the liver hepatocytes, where it is located mainly in the cytosol but in a small amount in the mitochondria[18,21,22] (http://symatlas.gnf.org/SymAtlas/symquery?q=GRHPR).

AGT is a homodimeric enzyme of ~86 kDa, which catalyzes the transamination of glyoxylate to glycine, using alanine as the amino donor. The failure of this reaction in PH1 allows glyoxylate to diffuse through the peroxisomal membrane into the cytosol where it is oxidized to oxalate, catalyzed by LDH, and reduced to glycolate, catalyzed by GR (Fig. 16.1). AGT also catalyzes the transamination of pyruvate to alanine, using serine as the amino donor. The deficiency of this reaction has no obvious clinical implications in PH1, but nevertheless has resulted in some confusion having given rise to an alternative name for AGT (i.e., serine:pyruvate aminotransferase, SPT).

GR is a homodimeric enzyme of ~73 kDa, which catalyzes the reduction of glyoxylate to glycolate using either NADPH or NADH. Similar to the situation in PH1, the absence of GR in PH2 allows the glyoxylate to be oxidized to oxalate, again catalyzed by cytosolic LDH (Fig. 16.1). GR also catalyzes

another reaction, namely the reduction of hydroxypyruvate to D-glycerate. Again this reaction is of no pathophysiological significance in PH2, except that the resulting increased synthesis of L-glycerate, caused by the reduction of the hydroxypyruvate catalyzed by LDH, can be used in some patients to support a differential diagnosis of PH2. This dual action of GR leads many authors to call the enzyme glyoxylate reductase/hydroxypyruvate reductase (GR/HPR).

16.2.2.2 Crystal Structures of AGT and GR/HPR

Understanding the mechanistic basis of the normal functioning of AGT and GR/HPR, and how it goes wrong in PH1 and PH2, respectively, has been greatly enhanced by the solution of their crystal structures.

The crystal structure of normal human AGT (PDB: 1H0C)[23] shows it to have a similar overall architecture to other PLP-dependent transferases. It crystallizes as an intimate dimer (Fig. 16.2), each subunit of which can be divided into two main structural domains: a larger N-terminal domain of 282 amino acids that contains most of the active site and most of the dimerization interface, and a small C-terminal domain of 110 amino acids that contains the atypical C-terminal type 1 peroxisomal-targeting sequence (PTS1)[24] and an internal ancillary peroxisomal-targeting sequence (PTS1A).[25] The first 20 or so amino acids of the N-terminal domain make up an N-terminal extension that wraps over the surface of the opposing subunit. The large dimerization interface explains the high stability of dimeric AGT. Although it has been suggested that the unusual N-terminal extension might play a role in the dimerization process, it is unlikely to contribute much to the overall stability of the dimer once formed. Confirming previous biochemical studies,[26–28] the crystal structure shows that each subunit contains one functionally independent PLP biding site on Lys209.

The crystal structure of GR/HPR (PDB: 2GCG)[29] includes views of both the ternary (enzyme-NADPH-reduced substrate) and binary (enzyme-NADPH) complexes. Although this has been less useful in terms of rationalizing the effects of mutations than has the crystal structure of AGT (see Sect. 16.2.2.4), it has provided significant insights into its rather unusual substrate specificity. For example, it explains why, although GR/HPR is a typical D-2-hydroxyacid dehydrogenase, it can use glyoxylate and hydroxypyruvate as substrates, but not the closely related pyruvate.

16.2.2.3 Genes, Mutations, and Polymorphisms

The gene encoding AGT (i.e., AGXT) is located on chromosome 2q37.3 and consists of 11 exons spanning ~10 kb.[30] The open reading frame encodes a polypeptide of 392 amino acids.[31] The gene encoding GR/HPR (i.e., GRHPR) is located

Fig. 16.2 Crystal structure of normal human AGT (PDB 1H0C). *Yellow*, pyridoxal phosphate; *blue*, the locations of the residue 11 and 340 polymorphisms described in text; *red*, the locations of the residue 41, 82, 170, 205, and 244 mutations described in text. The N-terminal extensions, which form the polymorphic MTSs, are indicated. The PTS1s are located at the C-termini (Cα[alpha] and Cβ[beta])

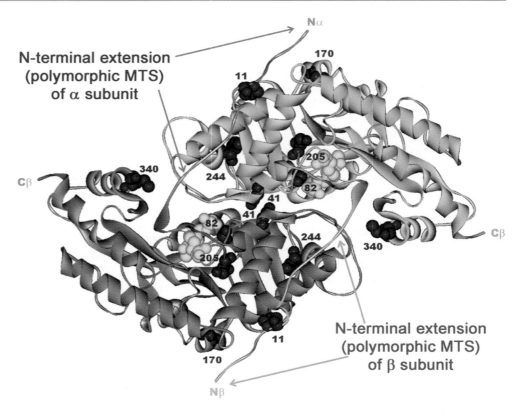

in the pericentromeric region of chromosome 9 and consists of 9 exons spanning ~9 kb.[32–34] The open reading frame of GRHPR encodes a polypeptide of 328 amino acids.

Two important polymorphic variants of AGXT have been identified called the "major" and "minor" alleles, with allelic frequencies in European and North American populations of 80–85% and 15–20%, respectively.[35,36] The minor AGXT allele differs from the major allele in three respects: (1) a C32>T base change that leads to a Pro11Leu amino acid replacement, (2) a A1020>G base change that leads to a Ile340Met amino acid replacement, and (3) a 74bp duplication in intron 1.[37] In addition, the frequencies of an intron 4 VNTR vary between the major and minor alleles.[38] Of all these differences, the only one known to have any significant effects on the properties of AGT is the Pro11Leu amino acid replacement (see Sect. 16.2.2.4).

About one hundred mutations have been found so far in the AGXT gene, including a wide variety of missense and nonsense mutations, small and large insertions and deletions, and splice-site mutations (for a review of some of them see[39]). Most mutations in AGXT are family specific, or fairly rare, but a few are quite common. By far the most common, at least in European and North American populations is a G508>A base change, which causes a Gly170Arg amino acid replacement[36] (Table 16.1). This has an allelic frequency of ~30% in PH1 patients. This is followed by a small frame-shifting insertion (33–34 insC) (~12%)[40] and a T731>C base change that results in a Ile244Thr amino acid replacement

(~9%).[41] The minor allele, in particular the Pro11Leu polymorphism, is much more common in PH1 than in the normal population with an allelic frequency of ~50%.[42] This is a consequence of the fact that many of the mutations in AGT in PH1, including some of the most common (e.g., Gly170Arg and Ile244Thr), segregate with the minor allele.

Most of the PH1 patients analyzed to date have come from European and North American backgrounds. Therefore, there is no reason to believe that the allelic frequencies of mutations and polymorphisms previously indicated would necessarily apply across the globe. In fact, there is strong evidence that the frequencies are very different in different genetic populations.[35,43] A good example of this is the founder-effect dominance of the Ile244Thr mutation in the Canary Islands.[44]

Far fewer mutations have been identified in the GRHPR gene, simply due to the smaller number of patients analyzed.[13] Therefore, it is impossible to draw any sensible conclusions about relative frequencies, either globally or in specific populations.

16.2.2.4 Relationships Between Genotype and Enzyme Phenotype in PH1

Many of the missense mutations in AGT are associated with very specific enzyme phenotypes. In addition, many of those that segregate with the minor allele functionally interact with

Table 16.1 Some of the better-studied missense mutations and polymorphisms, and their effects on the properties of AGT

Amino acid replacement	Allelic frequency in PH1 patients[f]	Overt enzyme phenotype (normal = +++)		Effect on the properties of AGT	
		Catalytic activity	Immunore-activity	On the background of the major allele[g]	On the background of the minor allele[h]
Pro11Leu[a]	50%	+++	+++	---	Delays dimerization, decreases catalytic activity, redirects 5–10% to mitochondria, sensitizes AGT to the effects of many PH1-specific mutations
Gly41Arg[b]	<1%	–	±	Markedly decrease catalytic activity	Abolishes catalytic activity, aggregates into intraperoxisomal cores
Gly82Glu[c]	<1%	–	+++	Interferes with PLP binding & abolishes catalytic activity	Unknown[i]
Gly170Arg[d]	30%	++	++	None known	Inhibition of dimerisation, redirects 90–95% to mitochondria
Ser205Pro[c]	<1%	–	–	Accelerated degradation	Unknown[i]
Ile244Thr[c]	9%	±	±	None known	Aggregation and accelerated degradation
Ile340Met[a]	50%	+++	+++	---	None

[a]Components of the normal minor allele
[b]Found on both the major and minor alleles
[c]Found only on the major allele
[d]Found only on the minor allele
[e]Found mainly on the minor allele
[f]Approximate allelic frequency in European and North American PH1 patients
[g]Residue 11 = Pro
[h]Residue 11 = Leu
[i]Probably the same effect as on the major allele

the Pro11Leu polymorphism.[27,45] Some of the better-studied enzymatic consequences of amino acid replacements in AGT are described as follows.

Pro11Leu – The normal Pro11Leu replacement characteristic of the minor allele is remarkable because, unlike most other polymorphisms in most other genes that tend to be neutral, it has significant effects on the properties of AGT. Not only does it sensitize AGT to the untoward effects of many mutations, such as Gly170Arg, Ile244Thr and Gly41Arg (see below), but also in a number of cases, it has more of an effect than does the mutation. For example, Pro11Leu on its own interferes with AGT dimerization, particularly at high temperatures. It decreases specific catalytic activity of purified recombinant AGT by two-thirds.[27] And finally, when expressed homozygously, it redirects 5–10% of the enzyme away from the peroxisomes toward the mitochondria in human hepatocytes in situ.[36] The Pro11Leu replacement generates an N-terminal mitochondrial targeting sequence (MTS), partly because it replaces a helix-breaking amino acid with a helix-forming one.[36,46] This makes it more likely that the N-terminus of AGT might fold into a α(alpha)-helical conformation, compatible with the optimal requirements for an MTS, in the right intracellular environment. Also, the newly generated Leu-X-X-Leu-Leu motif matches more closely with the optimum consensus

motif for interaction with the mitochondrial import receptor TOM20.[47,48] Although the Pro11Leu-generated MTS is very effective when attached to reporter proteins, such as green fluorescent protein, it is functionally weak when attached to AGT.[49] This is demonstrated by its ability to target only a small proportion of AGT to mitochondria, even when the PTS1 is removed. Residue 11 sits right in the middle to the N-terminal extension[23] (see Fig. 16.2). Even though the polymorphic N-terminal 20 amino acids have the potential to form an MTS and target AGT to mitochondria, they are prevented from doing so efficiently, probably because the N-terminus is trapped by binding to the surface of the opposing subunit. This would make it unavailable for interaction with TOM20. In addition, even polymorphic AGT rapidly dimerizes into a stable conformation not compatible with mitochondrial import. Rapid, almost irreversible, dimerization does not interfere with the peroxisomal import of AGT because these organelles can take up fully folded, multimerized, cofactor-bound proteins.[50,51] On the other hand, the mitochondrial import machinery can only deal with unfolded, or loosely folded polypeptides.[52,53]

Gly170Arg – Because of its high frequency in PH1, it is not surprising that Gly170Arg was the first disease-specific mutation to be identified in PH1.[36] However, what was surprising was the finding that patients homozygous for

Gly170Arg + Pro11Leu were only relatively mildly depleted in AGT catalytic activity and immunoreactivity. Typically, such patients have 10–30% of the normal levels,[54] but it can go as high as 72%.[45] This would not in itself be enough to explain the disease, particularly as some asymptomatic carriers can have AGT levels as low as 21% of the mean normal level.[54] Instead, PH1 in these patients is due to an unparalleled protein trafficking defect in which normally peroxisomal AGT is mistargeted to the mitochondria.[55] Mistargeted AGT remains catalytically active in the mitochondria but is metabolically inefficient, presumably because the majority of its substrate (i.e., glyoxylate) is synthesized in the peroxisomes rather than the mitochondria (see Fig. 16.1). Various in vitro biochemical experiments indicate that the contribution of the Pro11Leu replacement to the overall AGT trafficking defect is much greater than that of the Gly170Arg replacement, so much so that the latter appears to be completely innocuous in the absence of the former, at least in vitro.[27] The Gly170Arg replacement provides no further mitochondrial targeting information beyond that provided by the Pro11Leu polymorphism. In addition, it does not directly interfere with peroxisomal targeting. The increased functional efficiency of the polymorphic MTS, due to the extra presence of Gly170Arg, seems to be related to their combined effect on AGT dimerization, the rate of which is markedly decreased, even at normal temperatures.[56]

The exact effect of the Gly170Arg replacement is unclear. On its own, it has a relatively small effect on the structure of AGT (see PDB 1J04). It does not obviously affect folding or dimerization. However, it does interact synergistically with the Pro11Leu polymorphism to inhibit dimerization. One possible explanation for this is that the two replacements together decrease the affinity with which the N-terminal extension binds to the surface of the opposing subunit, with Pro11Leu altering the conformation of the extension and Gly170Arg disrupting the surface binding sites.[23] This "double whammy" would effectively prevent the N-terminal extension from binding, with the dual effect of exposing the MTS and inhibiting dimerization, both of which would encourage mitochondrial import.

Ile244Thr – Ile244Thr is the second most common missense mutation in PH1.[39] Like Gly170Arg, it too segregates with the minor allele and functionally interacts with the Pro11Leu polymorphism. Unlike Gly170Arg, however, it has been found, albeit rarely, on the background of the major allele.[45] When expressed in eukaryotic or prokaryotic expression systems, AGT containing Ile244Thr + Pro11Leu is unstable and readily aggregates.[27,44] In the livers of PH1 patients, it is associated with a complete loss or low levels of AGT catalytic activity and immunoreactivity.

Analysis of the crystal structure of AGT (see Fig. 16.2) suggests that the replacement of Ile244 by Thr would only generate a small defect in helix packing. However, it might

indirectly affect the inter-subunit binding of the N-terminal clamp, as suggested for Gly170Arg. This could destabilize AGT enough to aggregate and be rapidly degraded.

Gly41Arg – Gly41Arg is a rare mutation associated with complete loss of AGT catalytic activity and marked reduction of AGT immunoreactivity. Gly41Arg has been found in three compound heterozygote patients on the background on the minor AGXT allele.[57] In addition, there has been at least one case reported in the literature of this mutation being present in the homozygous state on the background of the major AGXT allele.[40] At least in the former situation, Gly41Arg results in the aggregation of AGT into core-like structures in the peroxisomal matrix. When expressed in *E. coli*, AGT containing both mutation and the Pro11Leu polymorphism aggregates into inclusion bodies. However, when expressed with the mutation alone, the protein is partially soluble, although its specific catalytic activity is markedly reduced.[27] This partial functional linkage between Gly41Arg and Pro11Leu is compatible with the findings, admittedly in a very small number of cases, that patients with Gly41Arg alone are more mildly affected than those in which both Gly41Arg and Pro11Leu are present.

Analysis of the crystal structure of AGT shows that Gly41 sits right in the middle of the dimerization interface and interacts with its counterpart in the other subunit (see Fig. 16.2). Replacement of the smallest amino acid (i.e., Gly) with one of the largest (i.e., Arg) amino acid would prevent the formation of the interface and prevent dimerization. This would inevitably destabilize AGT, leading to its aggregation and accelerated degradation. This again fits exactly with the enzymatic phenotype associated with the Gly41Arg mutation (i.e., loss of catalytic activity, very low immunoreactivity, and intraperoxisomal aggregation).

Gly82Glu – Unlike the previous mutations, Gly82Glu segregates with the major, rather than minor, allele.[58] It is associated with complete loss of AGT catalytic activity, but normal levels of peroxisomal AGT immunoreactivity.[17,19] Purified recombinant AGT containing Gly82Glu is perfectly stable and correctly targeted, but it fails to bind the cofactor PLP, thereby explaining its loss of activity.[27] However, recent work has shown that, although PLP binding is greatly reduced, the main effect of Gly82Glu is to prevent the efficient transaldimination of the PLP form of the enzyme as well as the efficient conversion of AGT-PMP into AGT-PLP.[59]

The crystal structure of AGT shows that Gly82 is situated right in the middle of the catalytic site where it makes hydrogen bond contact with the cofactor. Its replacement by the much larger amino acid Glu would certainly be expected to interfere with PLP and PMP binding, as well as interfering with transaldimination, etc.

Ser205Pro – Ser205Pro is a rare mutation identified in Japanese PH1 patients.[60] It has also been found only on the major allele. AGT containing Ser205Pro is highly unstable and prematurely degraded,[61] a finding that is compatible with the absence of both AGT immunoreactivity and catalytic activity in homozygous PH1 patients. The crystal structure (see Fig. 16.2) shows that the replacement of Ser205 by Pro would necessitate a large conformational change in the backbone of one of the β(beta)-strands of AGT that would completely disrupt the main chain hydrogen bonding of the central β(beta)-sheet. This would disrupt AGT folding and lead to accelerated degradation.

Other mutations – Most of the other missense mutations found in PH1 have not be studied in as much detail as those previously described. Nevertheless, it seems that the highly significant contribution made by the Pro11Leu polymorphism to the disease process is widespread. For example, a recent study analyzed the catalytic activities of 13 different recombinant AGTs, each containing a different newly discovered missense mutation.[45] Out of the eight AGTs containing mutations associated with the minor allele, six had much lower catalytic activities when expressed on the minor compared to the major allele. However, in none of the AGTs containing the five missense mutations associated with the major allele did the background allele make any difference.

16.2.2.5 Relationships Between Genotype and Clinical Phenotype in PH1

Although the relationship between genotype and enzyme phenotype in PH1 is in many cases well understood, the same cannot be said of the relationship between genotype and clinical phenotype. Patients with identical mutations can have completely different disease characteristics, as manifested by severity and rate of progression.[62] Notwithstanding this, there is a tendency for patients with the Gly170Arg mutation (and of course the Pro11Leu polymorphism) to have a milder disease on average than other PH1 patients. However, this might simply be due to the fact that these patients are more likely to be pyridoxine responsive (see Sect. 16.2.4). Although PH1 is clearly a monogenic disease, its clinical phenotype is presumably influenced by other factors, probably both genetic and environmental.

16.2.3 Diagnosis

Prior to the discovery of the enzyme defects, formal diagnosis of PH1 and PH2 was dependent on the presence of concomitant hyperoxaluria and hyperglycolic aciduria, in the case of PH1, or hyperoxaluria and hyper-L-glyceric aciduria, in the case of PH2.[12] This caused problems for two main reasons. Firstly, urinary metabolite analysis is rendered meaningless with approaching renal failure. Secondly, not all PH1 and PH2 patients, respectively, have elevated excretion of

glycolate[63] or L-glycerate.[64] In fact, not all patients with concomitant hyperoxaluria and hyperglycolic aciduria turn out to have PH1.[65] Diagnosis based on isolated hyperoxaluria requires more detailed clinical analysis of the extent and nature of the CaOx deposition, as well as exclusion of other causes for the elevated oxalate excretion, such as enteric hyperabsorption. Knowing that AGT and GR/HPR dysfunction are responsible for PH has enabled much better diagnostic procedures to be introduced. Enzyme analysis of samples obtained by liver biopsy can diagnose all forms of PH1[66,67] and PH2[22, 68] currently recognized, irrespective of the state of kidney function. Recently, it has even been shown that PH2 can be diagnosed by measuring GR/HPR activity in peripheral blood leukocytes.[69]

In families already known to carry PH1 or PH2, and in whom the disease-causing mutations are known, disease in further family members can more often than not also be diagnosed by mutational analysis of DNA isolated from peripheral blood leukocytes. Recently, it has been estimated that, even without prior family information, complete gene sequencing, or limited exon-specific sequencing, is a practical proposition for PH1 diagnosis.[45,70,71]

Prenatal diagnosis of PH1 was first carried out successfully in the late 1980s by AGT assay following fetal liver biopsy in the second trimester.[72,73] Although this procedure had the potential to identify all forms of PH1, it has now been supplanted by DNA (mutation and/or linkage) analysis in the first trimester.[74]

16.2.4 Treatment

The classic treatments for PH1 and PH2 are similar to those of other CaOx kidney stone diseases, such as good hydration while kidney function is good, and the use of CaOx crystallization inhibitors, such as citrate and magnesium salts[14,15] (see Fig. 16.3). Following kidney failure, patients have to be dialyzed and, when available, the kidney has to be transplanted. Neither of these are long-term solutions. Unfortunately, the inefficiency of dialysis means that the problems associated with excessive oxalate synthesis are exacerbated by the failure of its efficient removal.[75] This can lead to the deposition of CaOx throughout the body. Although under the right circumstances, the transplanted kidney can last several years, it will inevitably succumb to CaOx deposition as did the original kidney. This is because the basic defect is not in the kidney, but in the liver (particularly in the case of PH1).

It has been known for many years that a proportion of PH1, but not PH2, patients responds well to the administration of pharmacological doses of pyridoxine (vitamin B6)[76] (see Fig. 16.3). Pyridoxine is metabolized to PLP,

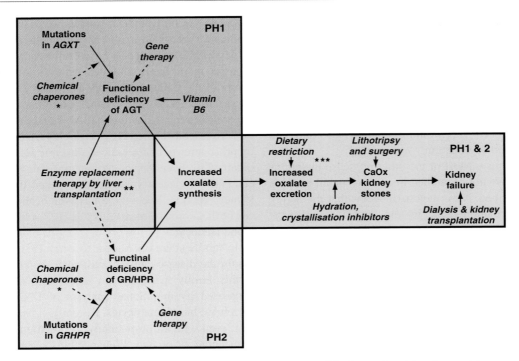

Fig. 16.3 Current treatments for PH and potential treatments for the future. The color coding is as follows: *pink* – those treatments applicable only to PH1; cyan – only PH2; *green* – both PH1 and PH2; *mauve* – mainly PH1 but possibly also PH2. *Solid large arrows* – causal pathways in the molecular etiology and pathophysiology of PH; *solid small arrows* – treatments currently used in PH; *dashed small arrows* – potential

treatments of the future. *Asterisks* – * potential treatments (discussed in Sect. 16.2.5), chemical chaperones will have to be enzyme specific or even mutation specific; ** hepatocyte transplantation is equivalent to liver transplantation; *** *O. formigenes* would work similarly to dietary restriction, except that it might have a direct effect on the mucosal oxalate exporter

the essential cofactor for AGT. Although it is likely that the latter fact explains the efficacy of pyridoxine in some patients, the exact mechanism is unclear. It has been known since the early 1990s that the success of pyridoxine was related to the presence of residual levels of AGT catalytic activity and immunoreactivity.[63] Significant residual AGT is mainly found in PH1 patients in whom the enzyme is mistargeted from the peroxisomes to the mitochondria. The association between AGT mistargeting and pyridoxine responsiveness has been more formally established recently due to the finding that the latter is related to the presence of the Gly170Arg mutation.[77,78] Why these patients in particular should be responsive is unclear. However, it may be related to increased AGT stability, correction of AGT compartmentalization, or increased transport of pyridoxine/pyridoxal phosphate into the mitochondria, thereby shifting the equilibrium from the inactive apoenzyme to the active holoenzyme. There are also reports that patients expressing other mutations, such as Phe152Ile, are also pyridoxine responsive.[79] Interestingly, like Gly170Arg, Phe152Ile also segregates on the minor allele and has been implicated in partial mistargeting of AGT to the mitochondria.[57]

The discovery that PH1 was caused by a deficiency of AGT, and that AGT was expressed mainly in hepatocytes, opened up the possibility that liver transplantation could be

used as a rather specialized form of enzyme replacement therapy (ERT) (see Fig. 16.3). In this context, liver transplantation is an almost perfect form of ERT because it can supply the body's total requirement for AGT in the correct cell (hepatocyte), the correct subcellular location (peroxisomes), and in the correct relationship with its substrate (glyoxylate).[80] Several hundred liver transplantations have been carried out for PH1 worldwide.[81–84] Because most PH1 patients receiving liver transplants are suffering from renal failure, more often than not the kidneys are transplanted as well. Although it is clear that liver transplantation can provide a "cure" for PH1, at least in metabolic terms, it can take a long time for this cure to be realized, especially in terms of urinary oxalate excretion. This is thought to be due to the remobilization of CaOx deposited throughout the body, particularly the bones, during periods of compromised renal function and extended periods of dialysis.

Although liver transplantation in PH1 can be more readily understood as a specialized form of ERT, it might better be considered as a rather specialized form of gene therapy. The long-term success of the procedure results not from the AGT enzyme reintroduced with the transplanted liver, which will be turned over with a half life of 1–3 days, but rather from the introduction of a normal AGXT gene, which will continue to produce normal AGT hopefully for years.

16.2.5 Treatments of the Future?

The importance attached to the design of new strategies for the treatment of PH was clearly demonstrated at the 8th International Primary Hyperoxaluria Workshop held in June 2007 at the Institute of Child Health, University College London.[85] Half of the meeting was devoted to this area of research. Three main topics were covered: chemical chaperones, hepatocyte transplantation, and *Oxalobacter formigenes* (see Fig. 16.3).

16.2.5.1 Chemical Chaperones

The realization that most missense mutations in protein-encoding genes cause their effects by destabilizing the gene product has led to a completely new way of thinking about the treatment of genetic diseases by pharmacological means.[86] If a mutant protein could be stabilized, by a chemical or pharmacological chaperone for example, then the function of that protein, albeit still containing the mutation, should be able to be restored. Proof of principle that this can work in PH1 has been demonstrated in transfected tissue culture cell lines using nonspecific protein-stabilizing agents for two of the most common missense mutations. Thus, lowering the temperature or the addition of glycerol can completely normalize the targeting of AGT containing Gly170Arg + Pro11Leu,[87] whereas betaine and a number of other small molecules can protect AGT containing Ile244The + Pro11Leu from aggregation and proteolysis.[44]

16.2.5.2 Hepatocyte Transplantation

Whether it is a specialized form of ERT or gene therapy (see previous), liver transplantation has the potential to cure PH1, at least at the metabolic level. However, it is far from ideal because of the expense of the procedure, the scarcity of the organs, the significant acute morbidity, and the possible adverse consequences of long-term immunosuppression. Partial liver transplantation from a living related donor might be able to get over some of these problems, but is strongly discouraged because of the interfering negative effect of the diseased liver remaining in situ.[80] Hepatocyte transplantation could offer a solution, especially if the transplanted cells were obtained from the patient's own liver and then virally transduced ex vivo to express normal AGT.[88–90] Notwithstanding any worries about the safety of the adenoviral vectors etc., this approach has great potential as long as the AGT-expressing transduced hepatocytes are given a proliferative advantage over the patient's nontransduced AGT-negative cells. Any remaining AGT-negative hepatocytes would continue the disease process due to the continued excessive production of oxalate, exactly as would happen after partial liver transplantation.

16.2.5.3 Oxalobacter Formigenes

Oxalobacter formigenes is an anaerobic enteric bacterium that requires oxalate as its sole nutritional carbon source. It is found in the guts of a wide range of mammals, including humans.[91,92] Not all people are colonized and the determinants of colonization are not understood. It has been proposed that the presence of *O. formigenes* is a good thing insofar as it should lower the gut oxalate levels and therefore diminish oxalate uptake from the diet.[93] Whether this actually decreases the corporeal load of oxalate is unclear and presumably depends on how much is in the diet, what form it is in (i.e., whether it is complexed with calcium), and how much oxalate is actually transported across the mucosal wall into the body. It has been suggested that *O. formigenes* might be a possible treatment for PH,[94] despite the fact that only a small proportion of urinary oxalate in PH patients actually comes directly from the diet. Logic would indicate that *O. formigenes* colonization could not have any significant effect on urinary oxalate excretion in PH were it not for a recent exciting observation that there may be a transporter in the gut wall that can actually excrete oxalate from the body back into the intestine.[95,96] It has always been assumed that almost all the body's oxalate was removed by renal excretion, but it is possible that the gut might provide another route of disposal, particularly in the terminal phases of PH during which renal function can markedly deteriorate. There is still the problem, however, of how decreasing intestinal oxalate could have any major effect on its excretion from the body into the gut. This potential problem has been countered by another suggestion, as yet unproven, that *O. formigenes* might adhere to the mucosal wall and interact with the mucosal oxalate transporter directly.[95]

16.3 Conclusions

Although the past twenty years have seen enormous increases in our understanding of the molecular etiology and pathophysiology of PH, there remain a number of significant gaps in our knowledge. One of the unknowns is the molecular basis of atypical PH. Although a number of theories have been advanced about its causes, they still remain speculative.[97,98] There is currently no reason to believe that it is a single entity at all. Because it is defined negatively, atypical PH could be a collection of different diseases. Another possibility is that it could be a metabolic "disorder of normality." For example, there may be a number of key enzyme activities that are within, but at the extreme ends of, their normal ranges. For example, the rate of oxalate synthesis and excretion in an individual with AGT and GR activities at the bottom of, but within, the normal range, and GO activity at the top of, but within, the normal range might be expected to be significantly higher than an individual with activities in the middle of the normal ranges, or even more so than someone with activities at the opposite ends of the ranges.

At first glance, there may appear to be more differences than similarities between PH and idiopathic CaOx kidney stone disease. For example, PH is a group of rare monogenic diseases, in most cases with well-established molecular etiologies, and, in the absence of disease-specific therapies, potentially life threatening. Idiopathic CaOx stone disease, on the other hand, is a group of common, multifactorial diseases, with poorly understood molecular etiologies, and usually not life threatening. However, the one very important thing they have in common is the risk associated with elevated urinary oxalate excretion. PH1 and PH2 demonstrate clearly that AGT and GR/HPR are two of the most important enzymatic determinants of endogenous oxalate synthesis and excretion. So what are the chances that one or other of these enzymes might be involved in idiopathic CaOx stone disease? This is really a rhetorical question because we do not know the answer. Nevertheless, the important role of the Pro11Leu polymorphism in the molecular etiology of PH1 (see Sect. 16.2.2.4), and its high frequency in some "normal" populations, might suggest that it has a role in human disease outside the confines of PH. Studies on the evolution of AGT intracellular trafficking[99] have demonstrated that the relationship between diet and AGT compartmentalization is an important one. As far as humans are concerned, it has been suggested that the presence of the Pro11Leu polymorphism might be an advantage if the diet contains a lot of meat, but a disadvantage if it does not. Population studies on its frequency give circumstantial support for such an idea.[35] The most likely consequence of inappropriate AGT distribution or reduced catalytic activity would be hyperoxlauria and CaOx kidney stones. Whether there is any substance in the speculation that the Pro11Leu polymorphism might contribute to the pathophysiological spectrum of idiopathic CaOx stone disease remains to be seen.

References

1. Holmes RP, Goodman HO, Assimos DG. Contribution of dietary oxalate to urinary oxalate excretion. *Kidney Int.* 2001;59:270-276.
2. Crawhall JC, de Mowbray RR, Scowen EF, Watts RW. Conversion of glycine to oxalate in a normal subject. *Lancet.* 1959;2:810.
3. Knight J, Holmes RP. Mitochondrial hydroxyproline metabolism: implications for primary hyperoxaluria. *Am J Nephrol.* 2005;25:171-175.
4. Knight J, Jiang J, Assimos DG, Holmes RP. Hydroxyproline ingestion and urinary oxalate and glycolate excretion. *Kidney Int.* 2006;70:1929-1934.
5. Noguchi T. Amino acid metabolism in animal peroxisomes. In: Fahimi HD, Sies H, eds. *Peroxisomes in Biology and Medicine.* Berlin: Springer-Verlag; 1987:234-243.
6. Rofe AM, Chalmers AH, Edwards JB. (14C)oxalate synthesis from (U-14C)glyoxylate and (1–14C)glycollate in isolated rat hepatocytes. *Biochem Med.* 1976;16:277-283.
7. Rofe AM, James HM, Bais R, Edwards JB, Conyers RA. The production of [14C] oxalate during the metabolism of [14C] carbohydrates in isolated rat hepatocytes. *Aust J Exp Biol Med Sci.* 1980;58:103-116.
8. Takayama T, Fujita K, Suzuki K, et al. Control of oxalate formation from L-hydroxyproline in liver mitochondria. *J Am Soc Nephrol.* 2003;14:939-946.
9. Holmes RP, Kennedy M. Estimation of the oxalate content of foods and daily oxalate intake. *Kidney Int.* 2000;57:1662-1667.
10. Massey LK, Roman-Smith H, Sutton RA. Effect of dietary oxalate and calcium on urinary oxalate and risk of formation of calcium oxalate kidney stones. *J Am Diet Assoc.* 1993;93:901-906.
11. Barratt TM, Danpure CJ. Hyperoxaluria. In: Barratt TM, Avner ED, Harmon WE, eds. *Pediatric Nephrology.* Baltimore, MD: Williams & Wilkins; 1999:609-619.
12. Danpure CJ. Primary hyperoxaluria. In: Scriver CR, Beaudet AL, Sly WS, Valle D, Childs B, Kinzler KW, Vogelstein B, eds. *The Metabolic and Molecular Bases of Inherited Disease,* vol. II. New York: McGraw-Hill; 2001:3323-3367.
13. Danpure CJ, Rumsby G. Molecular aetiology of primary hyperoxaluria and its implications for clinical management. *Expert Rev Mol Med.* 2004;2004:1-16.
14. Danpure CJ, Smith LH. The primary hyperoxalurias. In: Coe FL, Favus MJ, Pak CY, Parks JH, Preminger GM, eds. *Kidney Stones: Medical and Surgical Management.* Philadelphia: Lippincott-Raven; 1996:859-881.
15. Danpure CJ, Milliner DS. Hereditary disorders of oxalate metabolism – the primary hyperoxalurias. In Warrell DA, Cox TM, Firth JD, eds. *Oxford Textbook of Medicine,* 5th edition, Oxford: OUP; 2010:1730-1737.
16. Danpure CJ, Jennings PR. Peroxisomal alanine:glyoxylate aminotransferase deficiency in primary hyperoxaluria type I. *FEBS Lett.* 1986;201:20-24.
17. Danpure CJ, Jennings PR. Further studies on the activity and subcellular distribution of alanine:glyoxylate aminotransferase in the livers of patients with primary hyperoxaluria type 1. *Clin Sci (Lond).* 1988;75:315-322.
18. Mistry J, Danpure CJ, Chalmers RA. Hepatic D-glycerate dehydrogenase and glyoxylate reductase deficiency in primary hyperoxaluria type 2. *Biochem Soc Trans.* 1988;16:626-627.
19. Cooper PJ, Danpure CJ, Wise PJ, Guttridge KM. Immunocytochemical localization of human hepatic alanine: glyoxylate aminotransferase in control subjects and patients with primary hyperoxaluria type 1. *J Histochem Cytochem.* 1988;36:1285-1294.
20. Kamoda N, Minatogawa Y, Nakamura M, Nakanishi J, Okuno E, Kido R. The organ distribution of human alanine-2-oxoglutarate aminotransferase and alanine-glyoxylate aminotransferase. *Biochem Med.* 1980;23:25-34.
21. Cregeen DP, Williams EL, Hulton S, Rumsby G. Molecular analysis of the glyoxylate reductase (GRHPR) gene and description of mutations underlying primary hyperoxaluria type 2. *Hum Mutat.* 2003;22:497.
22. Giafi CF, Rumsby G. Kinetic analysis and tissue distribution of human D-glycerate dehydrogenase/glyoxylare reductase and its relevance to the diagnosis of primary hyperoxaluria type 2. *Ann Clin Biochem.* 1998;35:104-109.
23. Zhang X, Roe SM, Hou Y, et al. Crystal structure of alanine:glyoxylate aminotransferase and the relationship between genotype and

enzymatic phenotype in primary hyperoxaluria type 1. *J Mol Biol.* 2003;331:643-652.

24. Motley A, Lumb MJ, Oatey PB, et al. Mammalian alanine/glyoxylate aminotransferase 1 is imported into peroxisomes via the PTS1 translocation pathway. Increased degeneracy and context specificity of the mammalian PTS1 motif and implications for the peroxisome-to-mitochondrion mistargeting of AGT in primary hyperoxaluria type 1. *J Cell Biol.* 1995;131:95-109.

25. Huber PA, Birdsey GM, Lumb MJ, et al. Peroxisomal import of human alanine:glyoxylate aminotransferase requires ancillary targeting information remote from its C terminus. *J Biol Chem.* 2005;280:27111-27120.

26. Ishikawa K, Kaneko E, Ichiyama A. Pyridoxal 5'-phosphate binding of a recombinant rat serine: pyruvate/alanine:glyoxylate aminotransferase. *J Biochem (Tokyo).* 1996;119:970-978.

27. Lumb MJ, Danpure CJ. Functional synergism between the most common polymorphism in human alanine:glyoxylate aminotransferase and four of the most common disease-causing mutations. *J Biol Chem.* 2000;275:36415-36422.

28. Oda T, Miyajima H, Suzuki Y, Ichiyama A. Nucleotide sequence of the cDNA encoding the precursor for mitochondrial serine:pyruvate aminotransferase of rat liver. *Eur J Biochem.* 1987;168:537-542.

29. Booth MP, Conners R, Rumsby G, Brady RL. Structural basis of substrate specificity in human glyoxylate reductase/hydroxypyruvate reductase. *J Mol Biol.* 2006;360:178-189.

30. Purdue PE, Lumb MJ, Fox M, et al. Characterization and chromosomal mapping of a genomic clone encoding human alanine:glyoxylate aminotransferase. *Genomics.* 1991;10:34-42.

31. Takada Y, Kaneko N, Esumi H, Purdue PE, Danpure CJ. Human peroxisomal L-alanine: glyoxylate aminotransferase Evolutionary loss of a mitochondrial targeting signal by point mutation of the initiation codon. *Biochem J.* 1990;268:517-520.

32. Cramer SD, Ferree PM, Lin K, Milliner DS, Holmes RP. The gene encoding hydroxypyruvate reductase (GRHPR) is mutated in patients with primary hyperoxaluria type II. *Hum Mol Genet.* 1999;8:2063-2069.

33. Rumsby G, Cregeen DP. Identification and expression of a cDNA for human hydroxypyruvate/glyoxylate reductase. *Biochim Biophys Acta.* 1999;1446:383-388.

34. Webster KE, Ferree PM, Holmes RP, Cramer SD. Identification of missense, nonsense and deletion mutations in the GRHPR gene in patients with primary hyperoxaluria type II (PH2). *Hum Genet.* 2000;107:176-185.

35. Caldwell EF, Mayor LR, Thomas MG, Danpure CJ. Diet and the frequency of the alanine:glyoxylate aminotransferase Pro11Leu polymorphism in different human populations. *Hum Genet.* 2004;115:504-509.

36. Purdue PE, Takada Y, Danpure CJ. Identification of mutations associated with peroxisome-to-mitochondrion mistargeting of alanine/glyoxylate aminotransferase in primary hyperoxaluria type 1. *J Cell Biol.* 1990;111:2341-2351.

37. Purdue PE, Lumb MJ, Allsop J, Danpure CJ. An intronic duplication in the alanine: glyoxylate aminotransferase gene facilitates identification of mutations in compound heterozygote patients with primary hyperoxaluria type 1. *Hum Genet.* 1991;87:394-396.

38. Danpure CJ, Birdsey GM, Rumsby G, Lumb MJ, Purdue PE, Allsop J. Molecular characterization and clinical use of a polymorphic tandem repeat in an intron of the human alanine:glyoxylate aminotransferase gene. *Hum Genet.* 1994;94:55-64.

39. Coulter-Mackie MB, Rumsby G. Genetic heterogeneity in primary hyperoxaluria type 1: impact on diagnosis. *Mol Genet Metab.* 2004;83:38-46.

40. Pirulli D, Puzzer D, Ferri L, et al. Molecular analysis of hyperoxaluria type 1 in Italian patients reveals eight new mutations in the alanine: glyoxylate aminotransferase gene. *Hum Genet.* 1999;104: 523-525.

41. von Schnakenburg C, Rumsby G. Primary hyperoxaluria type 1: a cluster of new mutations in exon 7 of the AGXT gene. *J Med Genet.* 1997;34:489-492.

42. Tarn AC, von Schnakenburg C, Rumsby G. Primary hyperoxaluria type 1: diagnostic relevance of mutations and polymorphisms in the alanine:glyoxylate aminotransferase gene (AGXT). *J Inherit Metab Dis.* 1997;20:689-696.

43. Coulter-Mackie MB. Preliminary evidence for ethnic differences in primary hyperoxaluria type 1 genotype. *Am J Nephrol.* 2005;25:264-268.

44. Santana A, Salido E, Torres A, Shapiro LJ. Primary hyperoxaluria type 1 in the Canary Islands: a conformational disease due to I244T mutation in the P11L-containing alanine:glyoxylate aminotransferase. *Proc Natl Acad Sci USA.* 2003;100:7277-7282.

45. Williams E, Rumsby G. Selected Exonic Sequencing of the AGXT Gene Provides a Genetic Diagnosis in 50% of Patients with Primary Hyperoxaluria Type 1. *Clin Chem.* 2007;53:1216-1221.

46. Purdue PE, Allsop J, Isaya G, Rosenberg LE, Danpure CJ. Mistargeting of peroxisomal L-alanine:glyoxylate aminotransferase to mitochondria in primary hyperoxaluria patients depends upon activation of a cryptic mitochondrial targeting sequence by a point mutation. *Proc Natl Acad Sci USA.* 1991;88:10900-10904.

47. Abe Y, Shodai T, Muto T, et al. Structural basis of presequence recognition by the mitochondrial protein import receptor Tom20. *Cell.* 2000;100:551-560.

48. Muto T, Obita T, Abe Y, Shodai T, Endo T, Kohda D. NMR identification of the Tom20 binding segment in mitochondrial presequences. *J Mol Biol.* 2001;306:137-143.

49. Lumb MJ, Drake AF, Danpure CJ. Effect of N-terminal alpha-helix formation on the dimerization and intracellular targeting of alanine:glyoxylate aminotransferase. *J Biol Chem.* 1999;274:20587-20596.

50. Glover JR, Andrews DW, Rachubinski RA. Saccharomyces cerevisiae peroxisomal thiolase is imported as a dimer. *Proc Natl Acad Sci USA.* 1994;91:10541-10545.

51. McNew JA, Goodman JM. An oligomeric protein is imported into peroxisomes in vivo. *J Cell Biol.* 1994;127:1245-1257.

52. Chen WJ, Douglas MG. The role of protein structure in the mitochondrial import pathway Unfolding of mitochondrially bound precursors is required for membrane translocation. *J Biol Chem.* 1987;262:15605-15609.

53. Eilers M, Schatz G. Protein unfolding and the energetics of protein translocation across biological membranes. *Cell.* 1988;52:481-483.

54. Danpure CJ, Jennings PR, Fryer P, Purdue PE, Allsop J. Primary hyperoxaluria type 1: genotypic and phenotypic heterogeneity. *J Inherit Metab Dis.* 1994;17:487-499.

55. Danpure CJ, Cooper PJ, Wise PJ, Jennings PR. An enzyme trafficking defect in two patients with primary hyperoxaluria type 1: peroxisomal alanine/glyoxylate aminotransferase rerouted to mitochondria. *J Cell Biol.* 1989;108:1345-1352.

56. Leiper JM, Oatey PB, Danpure CJ. Inhibition of alanine:glyoxylate aminotransferase 1 dimerization is a prerequisite for its peroxisome-to-mitochondrion mistargeting in primary hyperoxaluria type 1. *J Cell Biol.* 1996;135:939-951.

57. Danpure CJ, Purdue PE, Fryer P, et al. Enzymological and mutational analysis of a complex primary hyperoxaluria type 1 phenotype involving alanine:glyoxylate aminotransferase peroxisome-to-mitochondrion mistargeting and intraperoxisomal aggregation. *Am J Hum Genet.* 1993;53:417-432.

58. Purdue PE, Lumb MJ, Allsop J, Minatogawa Y, Danpure CJ. A glycine-to-glutamate substitution abolishes alanine:glyoxylate aminotransferase catalytic activity in a subset of patients with primary hyperoxaluria type 1. *Genomics.* 1992;13:215-218.

59. Cellini B, Bertoldi M, Montioli R, Paiardini A, Borri VC. Human wild-type alanine:glyoxylate aminotransferase and its naturally occurring G82E variant: functional properties and physiological implications. *Biochem J.* 2007;408:39-50.

60. Nishiyama K, Funai T, Katafuchi R, Hattori F, Onoyama K, Ichiyama A. Primary hyperoxaluria type I due to a point mutation of T to C in the coding region of the serine:pyruvate aminotransferase gene. *Biochem Biophys Res Commun.* 1991;176:1093-1099.

61. Nishiyama K, Funai T, Yokota S, Ichiyama A. ATP-dependent degradation of a mutant serine: pyruvate/alanine:glyoxylate aminotransferase in a primary hyperoxaluria type 1 case. *J Cell Biol.* 1993;123:1237-1248.

62. Hoppe B, Danpure CJ, Rumsby G, et al. A vertical (pseudodominant) pattern of inheritance in the autosomal recessive disease primary hyperoxaluria type 1: lack of relationship between genotype, enzymic phenotype, and disease severity. *Am J Kidney Dis.* 1997;29:36-44.

63. Danpure CJ. Molecular and clinical heterogeneity in primary hyperoxaluria type 1. *Am J Kidney Dis.* 1991;17:366-369.

64. Rumsby G, Sharma A, Cregeen DP, Solomon LR. Primary hyperoxaluria type 2 without L-glycericaciduria: is the disease underdiagnosed? *Nephrol Dial Transplant.* 2001;16:1697-1699.

65. Van Acker KJ, Eyskens FJ, Espeel MF, et al. Hyperoxaluria with hyperglycoluria not due to alanine:glyoxylate aminotransferase defect: a novel type of primary hyperoxaluria. *Kidney Int.* 1996;50: 1747-1752.

66. Danpure CJ, Jennings PR, Watts RW. Enzymological diagnosis of primary hyperoxaluria type 1 by measurement of hepatic alanine: glyoxylate aminotransferase activity. *Lancet.* 1987;1:289-291.

67. Rumsby G, Weir T, Samuell CT. A semiautomated alanine:glyoxylate aminotransferase assay for the tissue diagnosis of primary hyperoxaluria type 1. *Ann Clin Biochem.* 1997;34(Pt 4):400-404.

68. Rumsby G. Is liver analysis still required for the diagnosis of primary hyperoxaluria type 2? *Nephrol Dial Transplant.* 2006;21:2063-2064.

69. Knight J, Holmes RP, Milliner DS, Monico CG, Cramer SD. Glyoxylate reductase activity in blood mononuclear cells and the diagnosis of primary hyperoxaluria type 2. *Nephrol Dial Transplant.* 2006;21:2292-2295.

70. Monico CG, Rossetti S, Schwanz HA, et al. Comprehensive Mutation Screening in 55 Probands with Type 1 Primary Hyperoxaluria Shows Feasibility of a Gene-Based Diagnosis. *J Am Soc Nephrol.* 2007;18:1905-1914.

71. Rumsby G. An overview of the role of genotyping in the diagnosis of the primary hyperoxalurias. *Urol Res.* 2005;33:318-320.

72. Danpure CJ, Jennings PR, Penketh RJ, Wise PJ, Cooper PJ, Rodeck CH. Fetal liver alanine: glyoxylate aminotransferase and the prenatal diagnosis of primary hyperoxaluria type 1. *Prenat Diagn.* 1989;9: 271-281.

73. Danpure CJ, Jennings PR, Penketh RJ, Wise PJ, Rodeck CH. Prenatal exclusion of primary hyperoxaluria type 1. *Lancet.* 1988;1:367.

74. Danpure CJ, Rumsby G. Strategies for the prenatal diagnosis of primary hyperoxaluria type 1. *Prenat Diagn.* 1996;16:587-598.

75. Watts RW, Veall N, Purkiss P. Oxalate dynamics and removal rates during haemodialysis and peritoneal dialysis in patients with primary hyperoxaluria and severe renal failure. *Clin Sci.* 1984;66:591-597.

76. Gibbs DA, Watts RW. The action of pyridoxine in primary hyperoxaluria. *Clin Sci.* 1970;38:277-286.

77. Monico CG, Olson JB, Milliner DS. Implications of genotype and enzyme phenotype in pyridoxine response of patients with type I primary hyperoxaluria. *Am J Nephrol.* 2005;25:183-188.

78. Monico CG, Rossetti S, Olson JB, Milliner DS. Pyridoxine effect in type I primary hyperoxaluria is associated with the most common mutant allele. *Kidney Int.* 2005;67:1704-1709.

79. van Woerden CS, Groothoff JW, Wijburg FA, Annink C, Wanders RJ, Waterham HR. Clinical implications of mutation analysis in primary hyperoxaluria type 1. *Kidney Int.* 2004;66:746-752.

80. Danpure CJ. Scientific rationale for hepatorenal transplantation in primary hyperoxaluria type 1. In: Touraine JL, ed. *Transplantation and Clinical Immunology,* vol. 22. Amsterdam: Excerpta Medica; 1991:91-98.

81. de Pauw L, Gelin M, Danpure CJ, et al. Combined liver-kidney transplantation in primary hyperoxaluria type 1. *Transplantation.* 1990;50:886-887.

82. Watts RW, Calne RY, Rolles K, et al. Successful treatment of primary hyperoxaluria type I by combined hepatic and renal transplantation. *Lancet.* 1987;2:474-475.

83. Watts RW, Danpure CJ, de Pauw L, Toussaint. Combined liver-kidney and isolated liver transplantations for primary hyperoxaluria type 1: the European experience. The European Study Group on Transplantation in Hyperoxaluria Type 1. *Nephrol Dial Transplant.* 1991;6:502-511.

84. Watts RW, Morgan SH, Danpure CJ, et al. Combined hepatic and renal transplantation in primary hyperoxaluria type I: clinical report of nine cases. *Am J Med.* 1991;90:179-188.

85. Danpure CJ, Rumsby G. Proceedings of the 8th International Primary Hyperoxaluria Workshop, UCL-Institute of Child Health, 29–30 June 2007. *Urol Res* 2007;35:253–254.

86. Morello JP, Petaja-Repo UE, Bichet DG, Bouvier M. Pharmacological chaperones: a new twist on receptor folding. *Trends Pharmacol Sci.* 2000;21:466-469.

87. Lumb MJ, Birdsey GM, Danpure CJ. Correction of an enzyme trafficking defect in hereditary kidney stone disease in vitro. *Biochem J.* 2003;374:79-87.

88. Guha C, Yamanouchi K, Jiang J, et al. Feasibility of hepatocyte transplantation-based therapies for primary hyperoxalurias. *Am J Nephrol.* 2005;25:161-170.

89. Jiang J, Salido EC, Guha C, et al. Correction of hyperoxaluria by liver repopulation with hepatocytes in a mouse model of primary hyperoxaluria type-1. *Transplantation.* 2008;85:1253-1260.

90. Salido EC, Li XM, Lu Y, et al. Alanine-glyoxylate aminotransferase-deficient mice, a model for primary hyperoxaluria that responds to adenoviral gene transfer. *Proc Natl Acad Sci USA.* 2006;103:18249-18254.

91. Allison MJ, Cook HM, Milne DB, Gallagher S, Clayman RV. Oxalate degradation by gastrointestinal bacteria from humans. *J Nutr.* 1986;116:455-460.

92. Allison MJ, Dawson KA, Mayberry WR, Foss JG. Oxalobacter formigenes gen. nov., sp. nov.: oxalate-degrading anaerobes that inhabit the gastrointestinal tract. *Arch Microbiol.* 1985;141:1-7.

93. Duncan SH, Richardson AJ, Kaul P, Holmes RP, Allison MJ, Stewart CS. Oxalobacter formigenes and its potential role in human health. *Appl Environ Microbiol.* 2002;68:3841-3847.

94. Hoppe B, Beck B, Gatter N, von UG, Tischer A, Hesse A, Laube N, Kaul P, Sidhu H. Oxalobacter formigenes: a potential tool for the treatment of primary hyperoxaluria type 1. Kidney Int 2006;70: 1305–1311.

95. Hatch M, Cornelius J, Allison M, Sidhu H, Peck A, Freel RW. Oxalobacter sp. reduces urinary oxalate excretion by promoting enteric oxalate secretion. *Kidney Int.* 2006;69:691-698.

96. Hatch M, Freel RW. The roles and mechanisms of intestinal oxalate transport in oxalate homeostasis. *Semin Nephrol.* 2008;28: 143-151.

97. Monico CG, Milliner DS. Hyperoxaluria and urolithiasis in young children: an atypical presentation. *J Endourol.* 1999;13:633-636.

98. Monico CG, Persson M, Ford GC, Rumsby G, Milliner DS. Potential mechanisms of marked hyperoxaluria not due to primary hyperoxaluria I or II. *Kidney Int.* 2002;62:392-400.

99. Birdsey GM, Lewin J, Holbrook JD, Simpson VR, Cunningham AA, Danpure CJ. A comparative analysis of the evolutionary relationship between diet and enzyme targeting in bats, marsupials and other mammals. *Proc R Soc B.* 2005;272:833-840.

Cystinuria and Cystine Stones

17

Patrick Krombach, Gunnar Wendt-Nordahl, and Thomas Knoll

Abstract Cystinuria is responsible for up to 2% of all renal stones, and up to 10% of childhood stone disease. Patients affected by this inherited disease suffer from recurrent stone formation, leading to repeated surgical/endoscopic interventions, consecutive renal impairment, and, consequently, a significant impairment of life quality. The responsible genes causing cystinuria were first described in 1994. Unfortunately, the rarity of the disease accounts for the absence of large clinical series. The establishment of the International Cystinuria Consortium attempts to combine small single-center series, which already has led to a better genetic understanding and a recently revised classification.

17.1 Introduction

Cystinuria is responsible for up to 2% of all renal stones, and up to 10% of childhood stone disease.[1] Patients affected by this inherited disease suffer from recurrent stone formation, leading to repeated surgical/endoscopic interventions, consecutive renal impairment, and, consequently, a significant impairment of life quality. The responsible genes causing cystinuria were first described in 1994.[2,3]

Unfortunately, the rarity of the disease accounts for the absence of large clinical series. An attempt to combine small single center series was the establishment of the International Cystinuria Consortium, which already has led to a better genetic understanding and a recently revised classification.[4]

17.2 Epidemiology

The prevalence of cystinuria is regionally variable (Table 17.1). Since regular screening programs are very rare, all numbers are approximate. Some of the data was derived from routine newborn urine screening. However, since maturation of SLC3A1 gene expression between mid-gestation and 4.5 years postnatal age may account for transient neonatal cystinuria,[15] such newborn screenings may have resulted in false high incidences.

17.3 Pathophysiology and Classification

17.3.1 Pathophysiology

Cystinuria is an autosomal-recessive genetic disorder with a complex pattern of inheritance. Two genes, each one coding for a subunit of a heterodimeric amino acid transporter situated at the brush border of the proximal tubule and in the gastrointestinal tract, are proven to be implicated: SLC3A1 situated on chromosome 2 (gene loci 2p16.3) codes for the heavy rBAT subunit. SLC7A9 situated on chromosome 19 (gene loci 19q12–13) codes for the light b0,+AT subunit (Fig. 17.1). The hydrophobic light subunit (~50 kDa) with 12 transmembrane domains and the heavy subunit (~80 kDa) with a large extracellular part and one transmembrane domain are linked by a disulfide bridge.[16]

A disorder of this transporter results in an impairment of reabsorption of the dibasic amino acids cystine, ornithine, lysine, and arginine (COLA) in the kidney and the small intestine. Usually about 98–99% of the filtered load of those amino acids is reabsorbed in the proximal tubule.[5] The defect of the transporter causes a dramatic increase in urinary concentration of these substances while serum concentration is reported to just drop by 20–30%.[16] Although all of these amino acids reach high concentrations within the urine, only cystine is insoluble enough to form stones.[1]

P. Krombach (✉)
Urologische Klinik, Universitätsmedizin Mannheim,
Mannheim, Germany
e-mail: patrick.krombach@umm.de

P.N. Rao et al. (eds.), *Urinary Tract Stone Disease*,
DOI 10.1007/978-1-84800-362-0_17, © Springer-Verlag London Limited 2011

Table 17.1 Prevalence of cystinuria in different regions

Average	1 : 7,000[5]
Libyan Jews	1 : 2,500[6]
USA and Europe	1 : 1,000–20,000[1,6]
Sweden	1: 100,000[1]
Mediterranean East Coast	1 : 1,887[7]
Turkey	1 : 772–1,000[8,9]
Czech Republic	1 : 5,600[10]
Japan	1 : 16,000–50,000[11,12]
Australia	1 : 4,000[13]
Quebec	1 : 7,200[14]

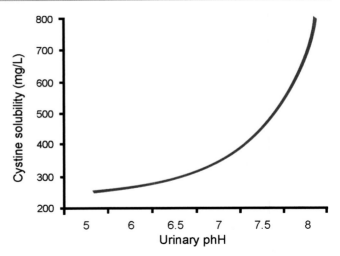

Fig. 17.2 Solubility of cystine at different urinary pH values[17]

Cystine is poorly soluble at physiological urine pH values between 5 and 7, and stones are formed especially at concentrations exceeding 240–300 mg/L (1.33–1.66 mmol/L). Higher pH values >8 lead to a threefold increase of cystine solubility (Fig. 17.2).[17] Other known and yet unknown factors seem to play a role since the effect of pH on cystine solubility varies among patients.[18–20] Factors known to influence cystine excretion are dietary salt and animal protein intake. Both increase cystine excretion, yet no prospective studies have demonstrated changes in stone activity as a result of sodium restricted diets.[18] As for protein intake, just one study demonstrated that lowering intake of cystine's dietary precursor methionine reduces urinary cystine excretion.[21]

Today more than 145 mutations are identified for both genes (>80 for SLC3A1, >65 for SLC7A9).[4,16,22–31] A genotype–phenotype correlation is strongly suspected.[4,16,24,32,33] Mutations of the heavy rBAT subunit (SLC3A1) are transmitted in a recessive way. Transmission for the light subunit b0,+AT (SLC7A9) is supposed to be autosomal dominant with incomplete penetrance.[4] Also, additional heavy subunits, that still remain to be identified, are suspected to play a role.[34,35]

17.3.2 Classification

The first classification created by Rosenberg et al. in 1966[36] was based on clinical features and divided the disease into three subgroups: type I, type II, and type III (the two latter ones being referred to as non-type-I). New insights into the genetic and functional characteristics of the disease led to a new classification in 2002 by the International Cystinuria Consortium.[37] Based on the type of mutation, the disease is

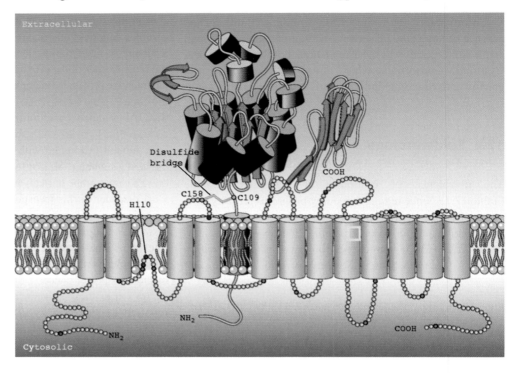

Fig. 17.1 Heterodimeric amino acid transporter. The heavy subunit (*pink*) and the light subunit (*blue*) are linked by a disulfide bridge (*yellow*)[16] (Illustration used with permission of the American Physiology Society and M. Palacín)

Table 17.2 Overview of clinical and genetic classification of cystinuria

Classification	Type A	Type B		Type AB
Frequency	45%	53%		2%
Gene locus	Chromosome 2 (SLC3A1)	Chromosome 9 (SLC7A9)		Chromosomes 2 and 9 (SLC3A1/SLC7A9)
Subunit affected	rBAT (heavy subunit)	$b^{0,+}AT$ (light subunit)		rBAT/ $b^{0,+}AT$
Former classification	Type I	Type non-I		
		Type II	Type III	
Urinary excretion of cystine in heterozygotes (in µmol/g creat.)	Normal	Elevated	Moderately elevated	Normal
	0–100	990–1,740	100–600	(Rare, mild phenotype)

divided into type A, type B, and type AB, respectively. An overview is presented in Table 17.2. In contrast to former assumptions, there seem to be no clinical differences between the distinct types.[37]

In heterozygote patients, urinary excretion of cystine is type dependent. In type A (former type I) heterozygotes excretion is normal, whereas in type B heterozygotes (former non-type I) excretion is mildly (former type III) to seriously elevated (former type II). This indicates an autosomal recessive transmission mode for type A cystinuria where the heavy subunit rBAT is affected. The inheritance mode for type B cystinuria is suspected to be autosomal dominant with incomplete penetrance, depending on the type of mutation.[4] This hypothesis is further supported by the fact that reconstitution in liposomes show that the light subunit b0,+AT is fully functional in the absence of the heavy subunit rBAT.[38]

17.4 Natural Course

If generally stones may be formed in every age, more than 80% of the patients develop their first stone within the first two decades.[37,39,40] Male patients seem to have a more severe evolution and an earlier onset of symptoms.[37] In 2003, Purohit published his data on 34 patients and found that 15% had their first stone after the age of 30, 6% even after the age of 50 years.[41] On a patient cohort of 224 cystinuric patients Dello Strologo found, in 2002, an average onset of disease of 13 years and 11 years for type I and non-I, respectively.[37] In their cohort of 34 cystinuric patients, Purohit and Stoller found 30% patients with just unilateral stone formation without any anatomical explanation.[42]

Incidence of stone formation in the affected population varies between 0.2 and 0.8 stone events/year.[43,44] A 5-year recurrence rate of 73%, independent of the amount of urinary cystine, type of intervention, or presence of residual calculi, has been described by Chow and Steem in 1996.[44] The repeated stone formation leading to repeated interventions may lead to renal impairment in up to 70%. End stage renal disease may occur in up to 5%, unilateral nephrectomy in up to 15%.[45–47]

The role of stone prevention remains controversial. If some authors report frustrating results[41,44,48] others report a reduced incidence of stone formation and/or interventions under therapy.[20,49–51] Limitations of the prophylactic measures are largely due to compliance problems. Regular follow-up seems to have a positive effect on compliance.[50] The positive effect of preventive measures on long-term renal function has never been demonstrated but is strongly suspected.

The natural course of disease in cystinuric patients is paved with stone recurrences. There may be several factors influencing the natural course of the disease. This theory is supported by the following facts[16]:

- The factors triggering these recurrences are partly unknown as some cystinuric patients tend to have periods with high frequency relapses without any medical explanation.[41]
- Thirty percent unilaterality of the disease.[42]
- Siblings sharing the same mutation and environment may have very different clinical outcomes.[6,52]
- Male patients have a more severe form of the disease.[37]
- Lithiasic (50%) and nonlithiasic (50%) SLC7A9 knockout mice hyperexcrete the same levels of cystine.[53]

17.5 Diagnostics and Definition

In the past the diagnosis of cystinuria was only possible after stone expulsion. Nowadays an earlier detection of the disease is theoretically possible. Specific analyses can be made in relatives of a cystinuric family member. Cystine stones should be expected in every younger stone-forming patient, especially in cases with known family history.

17.5.1 Clinical Appearance of Stones

Cystine stones have an amber color and a waxy appearance (Fig. 17.3). As they grow rapidly they often present as staghorn stones at first diagnosis.

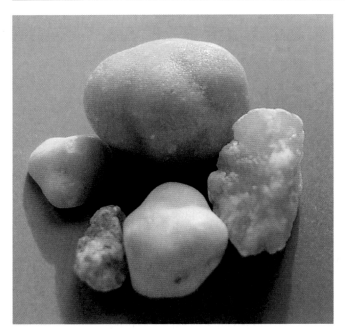

Fig. 17.3 Cystine stones (Image courtesy of Dieter Hannak, Institute for Clinical Chemistry, University Hospital, Mannheim, Germany)

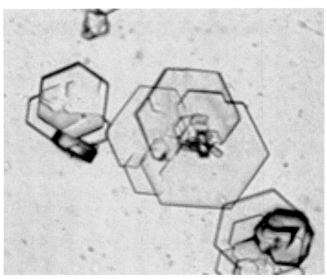

Fig. 17.4 Cystine crystals in urine (160×)

17.5.2 Radiological Appearance

On radiography, cystine stones can be suspected if the stone material appears poorly radiopaque. Nevertheless they may appear radiopaque in case of a large stone mass or a mixed stone composition (e.g., with calcium oxalate).

In computed tomography (CT) scans, cystine stones appear poorly attenuated. In vivo studies on 27 cystine stones in 1999 revealed that CT-collimation and stone size influence the attenuation. Nevertheless, accurate prediction of stone nature was possible with a mean attenuation for cystine stones at 1 mm collimation of 860 ± 26 Hounsfield units.[54] In an experimental ex vivo study, cystine stone morphology (void regions/homogenous stones) on micro-CT data positively predicted stone sensibility to shock wave lithotripsy.[55]

17.5.3 Urine Microscopy

Microscopic morning urine examination may reveal typical hexagonal cystine crystals (Fig. 17.4) that confirm the diagnosis and may be a risk factor for stone formation in cystinurics. However, as such, crystals are detectable only in 20–39% of urine specimens, the diagnosis cannot be excluded by their absence.[1,56]

17.5.4 24-h Urine

Quantitative cystine excretion is determined by acid chromatography from collection urine. Twenty-four-hour urine collection should be performed regularly to monitor the current treatment and to decide about further treatment (although the urine collection might be difficult in children). This is not only important for proper determination of daily cystine excretion but also for analyzing the presence of other stone-promoting conditions such as hypercalciuria, hyperuricosuria, and hypocitraturia that can be found in up to 45% of cystinuric patients.[57]

For a proper cystine determination in the 24-h-urine specimen, sodium bicarbonate has to be added until pH values exceed 7.5 in order to promote cystine dissolution and, thus, avoiding false low cystine values. Patients excreting 1,300 μ(micro)mol/g creatinine (150 mmol/mmol creatinine) cystine or more are supposed to be homozygote and need further evaluation and treatment.[24]

The cyanid-nitroprusside test allows fast qualitative diagnosis of cystinuria and was propagated as a screening method for homozygous patients. However, as several potential sources of error exist, this method is not in use anymore.[1]

17.5.5 Definition

In 2006 Dello Strologo et al. proposed a definition of cystinuria[6]:

• Demonstration of a cystine stone in a patient, AND
• Increased urinary excretion of COLA, OR

Table 17.3 Definition of cystinuria with stones in the upper urinary tract

Demonstration of a cystine stone in a patient AND	
Increased urinary excretion of	Identification of mutations on both alleles of one of the two genes involved
Cystine	
Ornithine OR	
Lysine	
Arginine	

Table 17.4 Definition of cystinuria without present cystine stones

	μmol/g creatinine	mmol/mmol creatinine
$[\text{cystine}]_{24\text{-h urine}}$	>1,300	>150
$[\text{cystine} + \text{ornithine} + \text{lysine} + \text{arginine}]_{24\text{-h urine}}$	>5,900	>670

- Identification of mutations on both alleles of one of the two genes involved (Tables 17.3 and 17.4)

A patient can be considered having cystinuria in the absence of a urinary stone if urine cystine excretion exceeds 1,300 μ(micro)mol/g creatinine (150 mmol/mmol creatinine) or the sum of COLA excretion via the urine exceeds 5,900 μ(micro)mol/g creatinine (670 mmol/mmol creatinine).

While determination of cystine excretion in heterozygotes is still the method of choice for classification,[58] it remains unclear whether genetic determination will play a leading role in the future. Since a wide variability in daily cystine excretion of the same patient has been clearly demonstrated[52] this method could lose its importance.

Furthermore, a correlation between stone formation and urine cystine concentration has never been demonstrated.[18]

New methods of direct urine supersaturation in cystine measurements could afford a more reliable way of therapy control and risk assessment.[19,59] Direct measurement of cystine crystal volume in the urine of cystinurics has also been reported to be a reliable indicator for stone formation.[56]

17.6 Cystine Stone Prevention

The primary goal of conservative treatment is the improvement of the solubility of urinary cystine. Several approaches are possible: (a) dietary measures, (b) measures leading to a decrease of urinary cystine concentration, and (c) drugs leading to reduction of cystine to the more soluble cysteine. For all patients, first-line treatment includes increased fluids, low salt diet, and appropriate urinary alkalinization. Other medical approaches are reserved for those patients who do not sufficiently respond to these measures (Fig. 17.5).

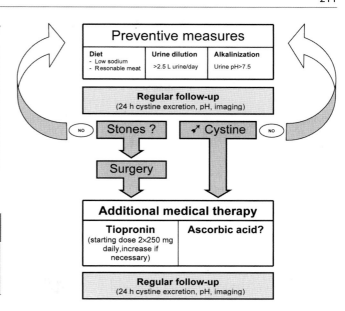

Fig. 17.5 Treatment algorithm for the management of cystinuria

17.6.1 Diet

Methionine is metabolized to cystine within the organism. Reduction of methionine intake – which is abundant in protein-rich food like meat, fish, eggs, soy, and wheat – could therefore lead to reduced urinary cystine excretion. However, such restrictions to the menu are poorly accepted by most patients with the result of low patient compliance. Furthermore, protein restriction is not recommended in children.[60] Adolescents and adults should follow a mixed commonsense diet with relatively low protein (<0.8 g protein/day). Reduction of sodium chloride has been shown to reduce cystine excretion, so sodium chloride intake should be limited to 2 g/day for adolescents and grown-ups.[61] Rodriguez et al. could demonstrate a low salt diet being effective in reducing urinary cystine concentration in children as well (by reduction of natriuresis from 6 to 1.5 mmol/kg day).[62] This can be achieved effectively when avoiding repeated salting and by the reduction of salty meals. However, long-term compliance even for modest salt restriction is often poor.

17.6.2 Urine Dilution

High liquid intake remains the most important procedure to reduce urinary cystine concentration. Fluid intake should reach at least 3 L/day in children and approximately 4–5 L in adults, resulting in a urine volume of >2.5 L/day. In theory, one liter of water per mmol cystine excretion should be ingested. It is important that the patient does not only drink throughout the day but also assures sufficient overnight diuresis. To guarantee nocturia, the patient has to drink before going to bed as well as during the night after micturition.[63,64] Urine neutral and alkalizing beverages like mineral water, herbal teas, and citrus juices are recommended.

17.6.3 Urine Alkalinization

Urine alkalinization with alkali citrates to pH values of at least >7.5 is an important measure to guarantee sufficient cystine solubility. Sodium bicarbonate is only recommended in cases with severe renal insufficiency as sodium increases urinary cystine excretion. Potassium citrate, given in 2–4 single doses of 3–10 mmol, allows adequate urine alkalinization.[65] Especially in children, treatment starts with the lowest dose and is checked by regular urine pH determination at least three times a day. Dosage should be adapted carefully until reaching therapeutic pH values. Very high urine alkalization has to be avoided as it comes with the risk of calcium phosphate stone formation or urinary tract infections. Alkalinization can be supported by drinking citrus juices containing potassium citrate.

17.6.4 Medical Reduction of Cystine

In case of failure of other measures, application of chelating agents is recommended if cystine excretion exceeds 3 mmol/day. Substances most widely used are D-penicillamine (DP) and a-mercaptopropionylglycine (MPG, thiopronin).[44,66] Both drugs are equally effective in cleaving the disulfide bond of cystine into cysteine, which is 50 times more soluble.[20,66] MPG dosage for children is 20–40 mg/kg given in two doses, which is important as cystine excretion is higher during the night.[63] Dosage should be adjusted by measuring the urine free-cystine level and keeping it under 100 μ(micro) mol/mmol creatinine.[50] MPG seems to have significantly less side effects compared to DP, so it is preferred by most physicians.[20] However, side effects occur in 20–50% of cases and limit treatment success. Typical side effects of MPG are rash, arthralgia, exanthem, pemphigus, thrombozytopenia, polymyositis, proteinuria, and nephritic syndrome. DP can induce pyridoxine depletion that requires supplementation.[60]

Captopril, a first-generation angiotensin-converting-enzyme inhibitor, contains free sulfhydryl groups. Some groups reported a positive effect of captopril application at dosages of 75–150 mg/day on cystine stone formation.[67,68] However, others could not confirm these findings.[44,69] In 1993 ascorbic acid had been reported to reduce cystine into cysteine when given in very high doses.[70] However, the positive effect on cystine stone formation might be explained by the presence of sodium bicarbonate in the fizzy tablets used. In vitro tests on cystinuric mouse models could not demonstrate any reduction of cystine excretion under ascorbic acid.[71]

Many patients do not only form pure cystine stones but also stones of mixed composition.[72] Hypercalcuria, hyperuricosuria, hyperoxaluria, and hypocitraturia or infections might accompany cystinuria.[57] These parameter also have to be determined during follow-up and treated if necessary.

17.7 Urological Interventions

Most cystinuria patients require multiple urological interventions during their lifetime despite preventive measures. However, the urological intervention rate seems to be decreased in patients with high medical compliance.[73] The chosen technique does not influence stone recurrence, but after being completely stone free, the time interval until stone recurrence is longer.[74]

While all methods of stone extraction are possible, minimally invasive procedures should be preferred. Some particularities will be discussed in the following paragraphs.

17.7.1 Shockwave Lithotripsy

Because of its low morbidity, shockwave lithotripsy (SWL) is the method of choice for all patients with a cystine stone within the upper urinary tract with a maximal diameter up to 1.5 cm.[75,76] Although cystine stones respond worse to SWL than calcium stones, in children the stone-free rate after SWL, even for large cystine stones, is significantly higher than in adults with matching stone size.[77,78] The pediatric ureter seems to be at least as efficient as the adult's for transporting stone fragments after SWL. Thus, SWL can be offered as a first-line treatment for most ureter or kidney stones in children.

17.7.2 Ureteroscopy

With the development of new small rigid and flexible scopes, ureteroscopy (URS) for upper urinary stones is safe and effective even in prepubertal children.[79] Furthermore, URS offers a good treatment opportunity for fragments refractory to prior SWL treatment.[80] While the neodymium:YAG laser was ineffective in cystine stones, the holmium:YAG laser now offers a very potent tool for cystine stone fragmentation.

17.7.3 PNL

For stone sizes exceeding 1.5–2 cm, percutaneous nephrolithotomy (PNL) is recommended. Monotherapy with PNL is safe and effective in the management of staghorn and complex renal calculi in one single hospital stay and may be combined with SWL or URS if necessary.[81] The introduction of new instruments (so-called Mini-PERC) with small diameter access shafts has optimized PNL treatment in children.[82]

17.7.4 Open Surgery

Open surgery should be reserved for special situations. It could be considered for cases with complex staghorn stones, difficult anatomy (e.g., dystopic or horseshoe kidney), and if simultaneous abnormalities like ureteropelvic junction (UPJ) obstruction have to be corrected.[81,83] To preserve kidney function, open nephrolithotomy should be performed under conditions of renal ischemia and hypothermia.[84] Ileal pyclovesicostomies can be considered in therapy refractory cystinuric stone formers to facilitate the spontaneous passage of large stones.

17.8 Conclusions

Cystinuria is a major challenge for the physician. It is a rare hereditary disease resulting in recurrent stone formation and, consequently, the need for recurrent stone treatment. With two identified genes being responsible for the disease, gene therapy may become a future therapy. However, today dealing with cystinuria remains difficult, as successful management requires lifelong patient compliance, regular follow-up examinations and, if necessary, state-of-the-art urological therapy. As medical treatment in particular requires great experience of the disease, the patient is probably best treated by an interdisciplinary approach (urology, nephrology, pediatrics). Greater vigilance in complicated, recurrent stone former is required to achieve successful prophylactic management. Furthermore, not only physicians but also patients require more information about the disease to improve compliance.

References

1. Knoll T, Zöllner A, Wendt-Nordahl G, Michel MS, Alken P. Cystinuria in childhood and adolescence: recommendations for diagnosis, treatment, and follow-up. *Pediatr Nephrol.* 2005; 20(1):19-24.

2. Pras E, Arber N, Aksentijevich I, et al. Localization of a gene causing cystinuria to chromosome 2p. *Nat Genet.* 1994;6(4): 415-419.

3. Wright EM. Cystinuria defect expresses itself. *Nat Genet.* 1994;6(4):328-329.

4. Font MA, Feliubadaló L, Estivill X, et al. Functional analysis of mutations in SLC7A9, and genotype-phenotype correlation in non-Type I cystinuria. *Hum Mol Genet.* 2001;10(4):305-316.

5. Goodyer P. The molecular basis of cystinuria. *Nephron Exp Nephrol.* 2004;98(2):45-49.

6. Dello Strologo L, Rizzoni G. Cystinuria. *Acta Paediatr Suppl.* 2006;95(452):31-33.

7. Cabello-Tomás ML, García-Gómez AM, Guillén-Domínguez ML. Pilot screening programme for cystinuria in the Valencian Community. *Eur J Epidemiol.* 1999;15:681-684.

8. Ozalp I, Coskun T, Tokol S, Demircin G, Mönch E. Inherited metabolic disorders in Turkey. *J Inherit Metab Dis.* 1990;13(5): 732-738.

9. Tanzer F, Ozgur A, Bardakci F. Type I cystinuria and its genetic basis in a population of Turkish school children. *Int J Urol.* 2007;14(10):914-917.

10. Hyánek J. Cystinurie. In: *Dedicné metabolické poruchy.* Praha: Avicenum; 1991:53-58.

11. Ito H, Murakami M, Miyauchi T, et al. The incidence of cystinuria in Japan. *J Urol.* 1983;129(5):1012-1014.

12. Segal S, Thier S. Cystinuria. In: Scriver CR, Beaudet AL, Sly WS, Valle D, eds. *The Molecular and Metabolic Basis of Inherited Disease, B.A.* New York: McGraw-Hill; 1995:3581-3601.

13. Turner B, Brown DA. Amino acid excretion in infancy and early childhood. A survey of 200,000 infants. *Med J Aust.* 1972;1(2): 62-65.

14. Scriver CR, Clow CL, Reade TM, et al. Ontogeny modifies manifestations of cystinuria genes: implications for counseling. *J Pediatr.* 1985;106(3):411-416.

15. Boutros M, Vicanek C, Rozen R, Goodyer P. Transient neonatal cystinuria. *Kidney Int.* 2005;67(2):443-448.

16. Palacín M, Nunes V, Font-Llitjós M, et al. The genetics of heteromeric amino acid transporters. *Physiology (Bethesda).* 2005;20: 112-24.

17. Dent CE, Senior B. Studies on the treatment of cystinuria. *Br J Urol.* 1955;27(4):317-332.

18. Goldfarb DS, Coe FL, Asplin JR. Urinary cystine excretion and capacity inpatients with cystinuria. *Kidney Int.* 2006;69(6):1041-1047.

19. Nakagawa Y, Asplin JR, Goldfarb DS, Parks JH, Coe FL. Clinical use of cystine supersaturation measurements. *J Urol.* 2000;164(5): 1481-1485.

20. Pak CY, Fuller C, Sakhaee K, Zerwekh JE, Adams BV. Management of cystine nephrolithiasis with alphamercaptopropionylglycine. *J Urol.* 1986;136(5):1003-1008.

21. Rodman JS, Blackburn P, Williams JJ, Brown A, Pospischil MA, Peterson CM. The effect of dietary protein on cystine excretion in patients with cystinuria. *Clin Nephrol.* 1984;22(6):273-278.

22. Botzenhart E, Vester U, Schmidt C, et al. Cystinuria in children: distribution and frequencies of mutationsin the SLC3A1 and SLC7A9 genes. *Kidney Int.* 2002;62(4):1136-1142.

23. Egoshi KI, Akakura K, Kodama T, Ito H. Identification of five novel SLC3A1 (rBAT) gene mutations in Japanese cystinuria. *Kidney Int.* 2000;57(1):25-32.

24. Guillén M, Corella D, Cabello ML, et al. Identification of novel SLC3A1 gene mutations in Spanish cystinuria families and association with clinical phenotypes. *Clin Genet.* 2005;67:240-251.

25. Ito H, Egoshi K, Mizoguchi K, Akakura K. Advances in genetic aspects of cystinuria. *Mol Urol.* 2000;4(4):4038.

26. Lahme S, Bichler KH, Eggermann T, Lang F. Genomic and functional investigations of mutations of the SLC3A1 gene in cystinuria. *Urol Int.* 2002;69(3):207-211.

27. Leclerc D, Boutros M, Suh D, et al. SLC7A9 mutations in all three cystinuria subtypes. *Kidney Int.* 2002;62(5):1550-1559.

28. Schmidt C, Albers A, Tomiuk J, et al. Analysis of the genes SLC7A9 and SLC3A1 in unclassified cystinurics: mutation detection rates and association between variants in SLC7A9 and the disease. *Clin Nephrol.* 2002;57(5):342-348.

29. Schmidt C, Tomiuk J, Botzenhart E, et al. Genetic variations of the SLC7A9 gene: allele distribution of 13 polymorphic sites in German cystinuria patients and controls. *Clin Nephrol.* 2003;59(5):353-359.

30. Schmidt C, Vester U, Hesse A, et al. The population-specific distribution and frequencies of genomic variants in the SLC3A1 and SLC7A9 genes and their application in molecular genetic testing of cystinuria. *Urol Res.* 2004;32(2):75-78.

31. Shigeta Y, Kanai Y, Chairoungdua A, et al. A novel missense mutation of SLC7A9 frequent in Japanese cystinuria cases affecting the C-terminus of the transporter. *Kidney Int.* 2006;69(7):1198-1206.

32. Brauers E, Schmidt C, Zerres K, Eggermann T. Functional characterization of SLC7A9 polymorphisms assumed to influence the cystinuria phenotype. *Clin Nephrol.* 2006;65(4):262-266.

33. Chatzikyriakidou A, Sofikitis N, Kalfakakou V, Siamopoulos K, Georgiou I. Evidence for association of SLC7A9 gene haplotypes with cystinuria manifestation in SLC7A9 mutation carriers. *Urol Res.* 2006;34(5):299303.

34. Chairoungdua A, Kanai Y, Matsuo H, Inatomi J, Kim DK, Endou H. Identification and characterization of a novel member of the heterodimeric amino acid transporter family presumed to be associated with an unknown heavy chain. *J Biol Chem.* 2001;276(52):49390-49399.

35. Matsuo H, Kanai Y, Kim JY, et al. Identification of a novel Na+-independent acidic amino acid transporter with structural similarity to the member of a heterodimeric amino acid transporter family associated with unknown heavy chains. *J Biol Chem.* 2002;277(23):21017-21026.

36. Rosenberg LE, Downing S, Durant JL, Segal S. Cystinuria: biochemical evidence for three genetically distinctdiseases. *J Clin Invest.* 1966;45(3):365-371.

37. Dello Strologo L, Pras E, Pontesilli C, et al. Comparison between SLC3A1 and SLC7A9 cystinuria patients and carriers: a need for a new classification. *J Am Soc Nephrol.* 2002;13(10):2547-2553.

38. Reig N, Chillarón J, Bartoccioni P, et al. The light subunit of system b(o,+) is fully functional in the absence of the heavy subunit. *EMBO J.* 2002;21(18):4906-4914.

39. Fjellstedt E, Harnevik L, Jeppsson JO, Tiselius HG, Söderkvist P, Denneberg T. Urinary excretion of total cystine and the dibasic amino acids arginine, lysine and ornithine in relation to genetic findings in patients with cystinuria treated with sulfhydryl compounds. *Urol Res.* 2003;31(6):417-425.

40. Leusmann DB, Blaschke R, Schmandt W. Results of 5, 035 stone analyses: a contribution to epidemiology of urinary stone disease. *Scand J Urol Nephrol.* 1990;24(3):205-210.

41. Purohit RS, Stoller ML. Stone clustering of patients with cystine urinary stone formation. *Urology.* 2004;63(4):630-634. discussion 634–5.

42. Purohit RS, Stoller ML. Laterality of symptomatic cystine calculi. *Urology.* 2003;62(3):421-424.

43. Akakura K, Egoshi K, Ueda T, et al. The long-term outcome of cystinuria in Japan. *Urol Int.* 1998;61(2):86-89.

44. Chow GK, Streem SB. Medical treatment of cystinuria: results of contemporary clinical practice. *J Urol.* 1996;156(5):1576-1578.

45. Gambaro G, Favaro S, D'Angelo A. Risk for renal failure in nephrolithiasis. *Am J Kidney Dis.* 2001;37(2):233-243.

46. Jungers P, Joly D, Barbey F, Choukroun G, Daudon M. ESRD caused by nephrolithiasis: prevalence, mechanisms, and prevention. *Am J Kidney Dis.* 2004;44(5):799-805.

47. Lindell A, Denneberg T, Granerus G. Studies on renal function in patients with cystinuria. *Nephron.* 1997;77(1):76-85.

48. Pietrow PK, Auge BK, Weizer AZ, et al. Durability of the medical management of cystinuria. *J Urol.* 2003;169(1):68-70.

49. Barbey F, Joly D, Rieu P, Méjean A, Daudon M, Jungers P. Medical treatment of cystinuria: critical reappraisal of long-term results. *J Urol.* 2000;163(5):1419-1423.

50. Dello Strologo L, Laurenzi C, Legato A, Pastore A. Cystinuria in children and young adults: success of monitoring free-cystine urine levels. *Pediatr Nephrol.* 2007;22(11):1869-1873.

51. Worcester EM, Coe FL, Evan AP, Parks JH. Reduced renal function and benefits of treatment in cystinuria vs other forms of nephrolithiasis. *BJU Int.* 2006;97(6):1285-1290.

52. Langen H, von Kietzell D, Byrd D, et al. Renal polyamine excretion, tubular amino acid reabsorption andmolecular genetics in cystinuria. *Pediatr Nephrol.* 2000;14(5):376-384.

53. Feliubadaló L, Arbonés ML, Mañas S, et al. Slc7a9-deficient mice develop cystinuria non-I and cystine urolithiasis. *Hum Mol Genet.* 2003;12(17):2097-2108.

54. Saw KC, McAteer JA, Monga AG, Chua GT, Lingeman JE, Williams JC Jr. Helical CT of urinary calculi: effect of stone composition, stone size, and scan collimation. *AJR Am J Roentgenol.* 2000;175(2):329-332.

55. Kim SC, Burns EK, Lingeman JE, Paterson RF, McAteer JA, Williams JC Jr. Cystine calculi: correlation of CT-visible structure, CT number, and stone morphology with fragmentation by shock wave lithotripsy. *Urol Res.* 2007;35(6):319-324.

56. Daudon M, Cohen-Solal F, Barbey F, Gagnadoux MF, Knebelmann B, Jungers P. Cystine crystal volume determination: a useful tool in the management of cystinuric patients. *Urol Res.* 2003;31(3):207-211.

57. Sakhaee K, Poindexter JR, Pak CY. The spectrum of metabolic abnormalitiesin patients with cystine nephrolithiasis. *J Urol.* 1989;141(4):819-821.

58. Goodyer PR, Clow C, Reade T, Girardin C. Prospective analysis and classification of patients with cystinuria identified in a newborn screening program. *J Pediatr.* 1993;122(4):56872.

59. Coe FL, Clark C, Parks JH, Asplin JR. Solid phase assay of urine cystine supersaturation in the presence of cystine binding drugs. *J Urol.* 2001;166(2):688-693.

60. Sakhee KS. RAL, Cystinuria. 1st ed; 1996.

61. Jaeger P, Portmann L, Saunders A, Rosenberg LE, Thier SO. Anticystinuric effects of glutamine and of dietary sodium restriction. *N Engl J Med.* 1986;315(18):1120-3.

62. Rodríguez LM, Santos F, Málaga S, Martínez V. Effect of a low sodium diet on urinary elimination of cystine in cystinuric children. *Nephron.* 1995;71(4):416-418.

63. Fjellstedt E, Denneberg T, Jeppsson JO, Christensson A, Tiselius HG. Cystine analyses of separate day and night urine as a basis for the management of patients with homozygous cystinuria. *Urol Res.* 2001;29(5):30310.

64. Monnens LA, Noordam K, Trijbels F. Necessary practical treatment of cystinuria at night. *Pediatr Nephrol.* 2000;14(12):1148-1149.

65. Fjellstedt E, Denneberg T, Jeppsson JO, Tiselius HG. A comparison of the effects of potassium citrate and sodium bicarbonate in the alkalinization of urine in homozygous cystinuria. *Urol Res.* 2001;29(5):295-302.

66. Harbar JA, Cusworth DC, Lawes LC, Wrong OM. Comparison of 2-mercaptopropionylglycine and D-penicillamine in the treatment of cystinuria. *J Urol.* 1986;136(1):146-149.

67. Cohen TD, Streem SB, Hall P. Clinical effect of captopril on the formation and growth of cystine calculi. *J Urol.* 1995;154(1):164-166.

68. Perazella MA, Buller GK. Successful treatment of cystinuria with captopril. *Am J Kidney Dis.* 1993;21(5):504-507.

69. Michelakakis H, Delis D, Anastasiadou V, Bartsocas C. Ineffectiveness of captopril in reducing cystine excretion incystinuric children. *J Inherit Metab Dis.* 1993;16(6):1042-1043.

70. Lux B, May P. Long-term observation of young cystinuric patients under ascorbic acid therapy. *Urol Int.* 1983;38(2):91-94.

71. Sagi S, Wendt-Nordahl G, Krombach P, Häcker A, Alken P, Knoll T. Long-term evaluation of captopril and ascorbic acid therapy in cystinuria mouse model. *J Urol.* 2007;177(4):543.

72. Evans WP, Resnick MI, Boyce WH. Homozygous cystinuria–evaluation of 35 patients. *J Urol.* 1982;127(4):707-709.

73. Pareek G, Steele TH, Nakada SY. Urological intervention in patients with cystinuria is decreased with medical compliance. *J Urol.* 2005;174(6):2250-2252. discussion 2252.

74. Chow GK, Streem SB. Contemporary urological intervention for cystinuricpatients: immediate and long-term impact and implications. *J Urol.* 1998;160(2):341-344. discussion 344-5.

75. Brinkmann OA, Griehl A, Kuwertz-Bröking E, Bulla M, Hertle L. Extracorporeal shock wave lithotripsy in children. Efficacy, complications and long-term follow-up. *Eur Urol.* 2001;39(5):591-597.

76. Kachel TA, Vijan SR, Dretler SP. Endourological experience with cystine calculi and a treatment algorithm. *J Urol.* 1991;145(1):25-28.

77. Gofrit ON, Pode D, Meretyk S, et al. Is the pediatric ureter as efficient as the adult ureter in transporting fragments following extracorporeal shock wave lithotripsy for renal calculi larger than 10 mm.? *J Urol.* 2001;166(5):1862-1864.

78. Katz G, Lencovsky Z, Pode D, Shapiro A, Caine M. Place of extracorporeal shock-wave lithotripsy (ESWL) in management of cystine calculi. *Urology.* 1990;36(2):124-128.

79. Desai M. Endoscopic management of stones in children. *Curr Opin Urol.* 2005;15(2):107-112.

80. Delakas D, Daskalopoulos G, Metaxari M, Triantafyllou T, Cranidis A. Management of ureteral stones in pediatric patients. *J Endourol.* 2001;15(7):675-680.

81. Tiselius HG, Ackermann D, Alken P, et al. Guidelines on urolithiasis. European Association of Urology Guidelines. 2006: European Association of Urology; 2006.

82. Jackman SV, Hedican SP, Peters CA, Docimo SG. Percutaneous nephrolithotomy in infants and preschool age children: experience with a new technique. *Urology.* 1998;52(4):697-701.

83. Paik ML, Wainstein MA, Spirnak JP, Hampel N, Resnick MI. Current indications for open stone surgery in the treatment of renal and ureteral calculi. *J Urol.* 1998;159(2):374-378. discussion 378-9.

84. Choong S, Whitfield H, Duffy P, et al. The management of paediatric urolithiasis. *BJU Int.* 2000;86(7):857-860.

Urinary Infection and Struvite Stones

18

Sean P. Stroup and Brian K. Auge

Abstract Struvite stones, also known as infection stones, have a chemical composition of magnesium ammonium phosphate, with or without calcium carbonate. They are named "infection stones" due to their association with urea-splitting bacteria, which degrade urea into ammonium and carbon dioxide, thus providing a major substrate for the development of a large, branched renal calculus. The most important urease producers include *Proteus*, *Pseudomonas*, *Klebsiella*, and *Staphylococcus* species. Moreover, bacterial endotoxins produced by many of these organisms contribute to the formation of a biofilm, which can entrap cations and promote crystallization. Staghorn calculi have been known to grow rapidly, in some instances as quick as 4–6 weeks. In addition to urea breakdown, urinary stasis may also contribute to calculus formation as seen in patients with urinary diversion, ureteropelvic junction (UPJ) obstruction, bladder outlet obstruction, or neurogenic voiding dysfunction. The management of infection stones includes antibiotic administration and complete stone removal. Retained fragments have a propensity to be associated with regrowth of renal stones in the vast majority of patients, demonstrating the necessity for an aggressive therapeutic approach.

18.1 Introduction: Infection Stones

Struvite calculi have plagued humanity since the beginning of civilization, dating back approximately 7,000 years ago to the era of the ancient Egyptians.[1] In 1901, G. Elliot Smith discovered a bladder calculus, found within a prehistoric tomb at Al Amrah near Abydos in present day Egypt that was dated to about 4800 BCE. It was found among the bones in the grave of a 16-year-old boy. The stone was yellow, with a uric acid nucleus and concentric laminations of calcium oxalate and ammonium magnesium phosphate. It was first described by Shattock in 1905 and placed in the Museum at the Royal College of Surgeons in London. The stone had been broken by the excavating workman's pick but was estimated to have been 6.5 cm in diameter. It was later destroyed when the museum received direct bomb hits in 1941.[2] In 387 BCE, Hippocrates first documented an association between urinary tract infections, urinary stones, and groin abscesses.[3] More than 2,000 years later, in 1817, Marcet reported on the

association of phosphate calculi with infection, ammonia, and alkaline urine. In 1901 Brown proposed that urea-splitting bacteria were responsible for urinary ammonia, alkalinity, and ultimately stone formation.[4]

Struvite was first discovered by a Swedish geologist named Ulex in 1845 after studying bat guano. He named it after his friend and mentor, the nineteenth century Russian diplomat and naturalist Baron von Struve (1772–1851). Struvite, a crystalline substance, is composed of magnesium ammonium phosphate ($MgNH_4PO_4 \cdot 6H_2O$).[5] Von Struve had published one of the earliest scholarly geological works in 1807 entitled "Mineralogical Memoirs."

Struvite urinary stones have also been referred to as "infection stones" and "triple phosphate" stones. Early chemical analyses of these stones demonstrated the presence of calcium, magnesium, ammonium, and phosphate, a total of three cations and one anion. Carbonate ions were also commonly identified; they were assumed to be associated with calcium as calcium carbonate ($CaCO_3$). Other terms for infection calculi include magnesium ammonium phosphate ($MgNH_4PO_4 \cdot 6H_2O$), calcium carbophosphate, carbonate apatite ($Ca_{10}[PO_4]_6 - CO_3$), and urease. Modern crystallographic analyses have shown that human "struvite" stones are a mixture of struvite ($MgNH_4PO_4 \cdot 6H_2O$) and

S.P. Stroup (✉)
Department of Urology, Naval Medical Center San Diego,
San Diego, CA, USA
e-mail: spstroup@gmail.com

P.N. Rao et al. (eds.), *Urinary Tract Stone Disease*,
DOI 10.1007/978-1-84800-362-0_18, © Springer-Verlag London Limited 2011

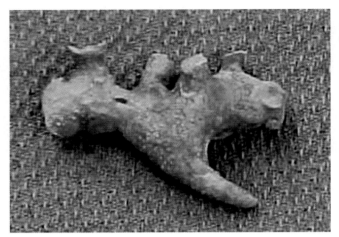

Fig. 18.1 An example of a staghorn calculus removed en bloc from a patient with a nonfunctioning kidney secondary to xanthogranulomatous pyelonephritis

Table 18.1 Urease producing organisms

Urease producing organisms	Usually	Occasionally
Gram-negative	*Bacteroides corrodens*	*Aeromonas hydrophila*
	Bordetella pertussis	*Bordetella bronchiseptica*
	Brucella species	*Haemophilus parainfluenzae*
	Haemophilus influenzae	*Klebsiella pneumoniae*
	Proteus mirabilis	*Klebsiella oxytoca*
	Proteus morganii	*Pseudomonas aeruginosa*
	Proteus rettgeri	*Pasteurella species*
	Proteus vulgaris	*Serratia marcescens*
	Providencia stuartii	
	Yersinia enterocolitica	
Gram-positive	*Corynebacterium hofmannii*	*Bacillus* species
	Corynebacterium ovis	*Clostridium tetani*
	Corynebacterium renale	*Corynebacterium equi*
	Corynebacterium ulcerans	*Corynebacterium murium*
	Micrococcus	*Mycobacterium rhodochrous* group
	Flavobacterium species	*Peptococcus asaccharolyticus*
	Staphylococcus aureus	*Staphylococcus epidermidis*
Mycoplasma	T-strain *Mycoplasma*	
	Ureaplasma urealyticum	
Yeasts	*Cryptococcus*	
	Rhodotorula	
	Sporobolomyces	
	Candida humicola	
	Trichosporon cutaneum	

Organisms that usually produce urease do so in >90% of isolates, whereas, occasional producers have urease detected in 5–30% of isolates

carbonate-apatite ($Ca_{10}[PO_4]_6$–CO_3). In some stones, struvite may be more abundant, whereas in other stones apatite may predominate. Evidence links the formation of struvite and carbonate-apatite stones to urinary infection.

The American Urological Association (AUA) 2005 Guidelines define staghorn calculi as those "branched stones that occupy a large portion of the collecting system, and typically, fill the renal pelvis and branch into several or all of the calices"[6] (Fig. 18.1). Although all types of urinary stones can potentially form staghorn calculi, approximately 75% are composed of a struvite-carbonate-apatite matrix. Interestingly, an article investigating the structural analysis of renal calculi in northern India reported that 90% of staghorn stones were composed of oxalates.[7] Other less common staghorn calculi can be composed of mixtures of calcium oxalate and calcium phosphate, cystine, or pure uric acid. The term "staghorn" refers to a description of configuration (i.e., a deer's antlers) rather than composition.

18.2 Bacteriology

Struvite calculi are typically referred to as infection stones because of their association with urinary tract infections with urease-producing bacteria. The most important urease producers include *Proteus, Pseudomonas, Klebsiella,* and *Staphylococcus* species and are listed in Table 18.1.[8] *Escherichia coli*, the most common uropathogen, however, rarely produce urease and thus is an infrequent cause of staghorn calculi.[9]

Proteus species are motile gram-negative bacteria belonging to the *Enterobacteriacae* family that cause urinary tract infections primarily in patients with long-term urinary catheters in place or structural abnormalities of the urinary tract.[10] Proteus infections are known to be persistent and difficult to treat and can lead to several complications such as acute or chronic pyelonephritis. They are the most common bacilli associated with the formation of bacteria-induced bladder and kidney stones (about 70% of all bacteria isolated from such urinary calculi).[11–13]

Urease is the essential virulence factor of these bacteria involved in stone formation. Ammonia, produced by the enzymic hydrolysis of urea, elevates urine pH, causing supersaturation and crystallization of magnesium and calcium ions as struvite ($MgNH_4PO_4.6H_2O$) and carbonate apatite [$Ca_{10}(PO_4)_6.CO_3$].[14,15] In addition to urease activity, bacterial exopolysaccharides contribute to stone formation. Nickel and colleagues have demonstrated bacterial cells growing as microcolonies together with bacterial biofilms within extensive organic matrices.[16] This matrix, or glycocalyx, which is produced by the bacteria, harbors the organisms and protects them from antibiotic therapy. Moreover, matrix may also contribute to stone formation by adherence of urine components onto its surface acting as a nidus for stone growth.[17]

Proteus bacilli have capsular polysaccharide (CPS) and lipopolysaccharide (LPS, endotoxin) on their surfaces. CPS is the most external surface component of these bacteria, but detailed studies have shown that only a few strains can synthesize a capsule antigen, and its structure is identical to the O-specific chain of their LPS.[17–19] LPS is the main component of the outer membrane and one of the major virulence factors of these bacteria. It consists of a polysaccharide part, containing an O-specific chain (O-antigen, O-PS), and a core region, as well as a lipophilic region, termed lipid A, which anchors the LPS to the bacterial outer membrane. It has been well documented that *Proteus* is an antigenically heterogeneous genus, principally because of structural differences in the O-specific polysaccharide chain of LPS. In most *Proteus* strains, O-specific polysaccharides have been found to be acidic due to the presence of uronic acids and various noncarbohydrate acidic components, including phosphate groups.[17]

The role of acidic polysaccharides in the pathogenicity of *Proteus*, especially in urinary tract infections, is controversial. The negatively charged polysaccharides are important barriers against the bactericidal action of the complement system.[20] Yet the acidic character of *Proteus* extracellular polysaccharides may play a crucial role in stone formation within the urinary tract.[21,22] Clapham et al. had previously hypothesized that anionic groups found on bacterial polysaccharides influence struvite and carbonate apatite formation because they enable these macromolecules to bind cations (Ca^{2+}, Mg^{2+}) via electrostatic interactions that accelerate supersaturation and crystallization of these ions.[21] Torzewska et al. showed that the polysaccharide of *Proteus vulgaris* O12 bound magnesium and calcium ions weakly but increased the crystallization rate, whereas *Proteus mirabilis* O28 and *P. vulgaris* O47 cells were able to bind large amounts of the cations but inhibited the process of crystallization in vitro.[23] The aim of this work was to show that negatively charged polysaccharide, being a part of the *Proteus* LPS, may bind the cations present in urine. Such binding leads to the accumulation of cations around bacterial cells and increases the crystallization rate and formation of urinary tract stones. The polysaccharide part of *Proteus* LPS may either enhance or inhibit the process of crystal formation, depending on the chemical composition of the molecule and its affinity for cations.

Bacterial endotoxin is present not only as a component of glycocalyx in biofilms, but also as free molecules originating from dead cells or released from urinary stones during their surgical removal, which causes serious health problems.[24,25] Hence, it is possible that the same polysaccharide, through its cation affinity, may increase or inhibit the process of crystallization, depending on its location. Free endotoxin molecules with a high affinity for cations may act as crystallization inhibitors, since cations bound to such macromolecules would be washed out by the flow of urine. Conversely, in the biofilm, local accumulation of ions by anchored endotoxin would lead to stimulation of the crystallization process. It is obvious that the development of infectious urolithiasis is multifactorial, and despite long-term clinical and experimental investigation, some of the specific mechanisms responsible for urinary calculi formation remain a mystery.

18.3 Mineral Composition

Infection stones are composed primarily of magnesium ammonium phosphate hexahydrate ($MgNH_4PO_4 \bullet 6H_2O$) but may, in addition, contain calcium phosphate in the form of carbonate apatite ($Ca_{10}[PO_4]_6 \bullet CO_3$).[26] Urease is not constitutively produced or present in sterile human urine, therefore, infection with urease-producing bacteria is a requirement for the formation of infection stones. Infection stones are formed following a series of chemical reactions that generate conditions conducive to the formation of stones. Urea, which is concentrated in the urine, is first hydrolyzed to ammonia and carbon dioxide in the presence of bacterial urease. The lysis of urea provides an alkaline urine environment and adequate concentrations of carbonate and ammonia to drive the formation of infection stones.

The conversions of urea to ammonia, ammonia to ammonium, and acidification from carbon dioxide are as follows:

$$\left(NH_2\right)_2 CO + H_2O \rightarrow 2NH_3 + CO_2$$

The reaction is then driven to the left in the presence of alkaline urine (pH 7.2–8.0) and favors the formation of ammonium hydroxide:

$$NH_3 + H_2O \leftrightarrow NH_4^+ + OH^- pK = 9.0$$

In the typical physiologic setting, as this reaction moves forward to produce ammonium, the alkaline urine would prevent generation of further ammonium. However, in the presence of urease, the reaction continues to produce ammonia, further increasing urinary pH. The alkaline environment also promotes the hydration of carbon dioxide to carbonic acid, which then dissociates into HCO^{-3} and H^+. Further dissociation of HCO^{-3} yields a carbonate anion and two hydrogen cations:

$$CO_2 + H_2O \rightarrow H_2CO_3 \, pK = 4.5$$

$$H_2CO_3 \rightarrow H^+ + HCO_3^- \, pK = 6.3$$

$$HCO_3^- \rightarrow H^+ + CO_3^{2-} \, pK = 10.2$$

Hydrogen phosphate then dissociates under alkaline conditions and generates free phosphate, and creates the end products necessary for infection stone formation:

$$H_2PO_4^- \rightarrow H^+ + HPO_4^{2-} \, pK = 7.2$$

$$HPO_4^{2-} \rightarrow H^+ + PO_4^{3-} \, pK = 12.4$$

This chemical cascade, along with physiologic concentrations of magnesium, provides the constituents necessary for precipitation of struvite. In addition, the concentrations of calcium, phosphate, and carbonate allow precipitation of carbonate apatite and hydroxyapatite, thereby comprising the components of infection stones. Citrate normally forms complexes with calcium and magnesium to inhibit stone formation, but this protective effect is lost in infective conditions due to the metabolic activity of the bacteria on citrate.[27]

In contrast to struvite stones, calcium phosphate stones consist of either apatite or brushite ($CaHPO_4 \cdot 2H_2O$). Apatite stones are associated with formation in an alkaline environment with a pH greater than 6.6 and are considered "infection-related" stones. Brushite calculi develop in more acidic settings with a urinary pH less than 6.6 as in type I (distal) renal tubular acidosis. In these cases, they are not associated with infection or urease-producing bacteria.

18.4 Mechanism of Calculogenesis of Struvite Stones

Infection stones are characterized by their large size and exceptionally rapid growth. In fact, 4–6 weeks may be sufficient time for an infection stone to form and subsequently develop into a staghorn stone that involves the entire renal pelvis and calices.[28] Most commonly, staghorn stones are composed of a mixture of struvite (magnesium ammonium phosphate) and calcium carbonate apatite. Normal urine is undersaturated with ammonium phosphate, and struvite stones only form when ammonia production is elevated and urine pH is increased, thereby decreasing the solubility of phosphate.[29]

Brown first theorized that bacteria split urea, thereby setting up the condition for stone formation; and, indeed, he later isolated *P. vulgaris* from a stone.[4] Sumner in 1926 isolated urease from *Canavalia ensiformis*. It is now well established that struvite stones (magnesium ammonium phosphate) occur only in association with urinary infection by urea-splitting bacteria.[28] First, bacteria-produced urease breaks down urinary urea into ammonia plus carbon dioxide, which then hydrolyzes to ammonium ions and bicarbonate. Binding to available cations then produces carbonate apatite and magnesium ammonium phosphate. Carbonate apatite begins to crystallize at a urine pH greater than or equal to 6.8 while struvite precipitates only at a pH greater than or equal to 7.2. Two conditions must coexist for the formation of crystals and subsequently struvite calculi. These are (1) alkaline urine (pH >7.2) and (2) the presence of ammonia in the urine. However, equally important is the formation of the biofilm, which contributes to the formation of the matrix within which the bacteria may adhere and reside. The biofilm becomes the nidus for crystal aggregation and stone growth via a gel growth mechanism within the biofilm itself.[29]

18.5 Bacteria within the Stone and Its Significance

Cultures of "infection stone" fragments obtained from both the surface and inside of the stone have demonstrated that bacteria reside within the stone, thereby causing the stone itself to be infected, in contrast to stones made of other substances where the stones remain sterile inside.[3] Repeated urinary tract infections with urea-splitting organisms may result in stone formation, and once an "infection stone" is present, infections tend to recur.

"Struvite–apatite dust" is formed around the bacteria and facilitates crystal growth. Crystallization may occur both intra- and peribacterially. Apatite crystals grow inside the bacteria, and, after bacteriolysis, microliths formed may serve as a nidus for stone formation. Crystals growing peribacterially may settle on the bacteria and form a phosphate cover, and bacteria enclosed within the stone serve as a source of recurrent infections. Stone propagation occurs extremely quickly because of the constant supply of reactants and the alkaline milieu, in which struvite and apatite are poorly soluble.[30]

Bacteria may be involved in stone formation by damaging the mucosal layer of the urinary tract, resulting in both increased bacterial colonization and crystal adherence.[31,32] It has been proposed that ammonium, generated as a result of urealysis, may alter the glycosaminoglycan (GAG) layer present on the surface of the transitional cell layer and significantly increase bacterial adherence to normal bladder mucosa, further exacerbating infection risk.[32] In addition, a study in rats found that injury to the bladder mucosa increased crystal adherence to the bladder wall, a process that was potentiated by the presence of common bacteria such as *Proteus, E. coli, Enterococcus,* and *Ureaplasma urealyticum.*[31]

Another potential mechanism for increased stone formation in the presence of bacteria is the finding that particular bacteria, such as *E. coli* and *Proteus,* may alter the activity of urokinase and sialidase, whereas organisms not typically associated with infection stones do not.[33] This altered enzymatic activity may explain the frequent association of *E. coli* with stone formation despite lacking urease activity.[34]

18.6   Urease and Its Role

Struvite/calcium carbonate apatite stones also are referred to as "infection stones" because of their strong association with urinary tract infection caused by specific organisms that produce the enzyme urease that catalyzes the hydrolysis of urea into ammonia and carbon dioxide.[35,36] Urea was the first organic compound to be artificially synthesized from inorganic starting materials in 1828 by Friedrich Wöhler, who prepared it by the reaction of potassium cyanate with ammonium sulfate. The isolation of urease, the first enzyme ever purified, earned Sumner the Nobel Prize for Chemistry in 1946.[37] Urease is found in bacteria, yeast, and several higher plants.

The alkaline urinary environment and high ammonia concentration produced as a result of urea hydrolysis, along with abundant phosphate and magnesium in urine, promote crystallization of magnesium ammonium phosphate (struvite), thereby leading to formation of large, branched stones. Other factors play a role, including the formation of an exopolysaccharide biofilm and the incorporation of mucoproteins and other organic compounds into this matrix:

$$\underset{\text{UREA}}{H_2N - \overset{\overset{\textstyle O}{\|}}{C} - NH_2}$$

Bacterial urease can be detected by the Urea-Rapid Test, a urea-indole medium from Bio-Merieux, Inc. (Durham, NC).[38]

18.7   Matrix in Struvite Stones and Its Role

Matrix appears to play a major role in the formation of struvite stone and is composed of mineralized, gelatinous organic material and an exopolysaccharide biofilm secreted by the bacteria.[39] Inflammation also leads to increased mucus secretion, which can be absorbed onto crystal surfaces, which in turn adds to the matrix for crystal aggregation. Glycosaminoglycan within the cell walls of the urothelial cells – in the form of chondroitin sulfate, heparin sulfate, hyaluronic acid, and keratin sulfate – may positively or negatively impact crystal adherence and subsequent stone growth as different GAG species have affinities for different stone crystals. By complexing with crystals, they can inhibit stone growth. However, adherence can also create accumulation within the stone, thereby propagating stone formation.[40] Finally, ammonia induces damage to the surrounding protective urothelial glycosaminoglycan layer and thus increases bacterial adherence to the transitional epithelium.[41] The proportion of matrix is greater in struvite stones than in other types of calcium-based stones and is thought to protect the bacteria from antimicrobials.

18.8   Role of Urinary Stasis

Although infection stones are a direct result of persistent or recurrent infection with urease-producing bacteria, they may also be associated with or exacerbated by urinary obstruction or stasis as seen in patients with urinary diversion, ureteropelvic junction (UPJ) obstruction, bladder outlet obstruction, or neurogenic voiding dysfunction.[38] It must be noted, however, that the development of calculi within an obstructed system is a complex multifactorial event. Patients not only have stasis, but also are predisposed to infection due to bacterial adherence and virulence factors and may have a urinary milieu within the obstructed system with metabolic derangements influencing stone development.[42,43] In addition, it is unclear whether patients with UPJ obstruction presenting with stones had developed the stone first or the obstruction first. Although studies have demonstrated the changes in muscular and collagenous composition of the UPJ in those with obstruction, it remains unclear whether that may predispose one to calculogenesis.[44–47] Certainly, patients with chronically impacted stones at the UPJ are subjected to inflammatory changes that may lead to edema, fibrosis, and/or necrosis with subsequent obstruction. Stasis is not the only mitigating factor for stone development in pediatric patients with UPJ obstruction. Only 1–5% of these patients are found to have concomitant stones, supporting the concept that metabolic abnormalities and infection are primary stimuli for stone formation.[42,43]

Intestinal segments are used in urological surgery to replace the bladder, either as a conduit to drain urine to the abdominal wall as a urinary stoma or refashioned to form a substitute bladder. Not uncommonly, stones develop within the diversion segments in the postoperative period. Many factors contribute to stone formation in this patient population, the most important being urinary stasis, mucus production, the presence of a foreign body, and bacteriuria. Metabolic changes induced by exposure of segments of the alimentary tract to urine promote struvite, calcium oxalate, and calcium phosphate stone formation.[48]

18.9 Clinical Manifestations

18.9.1 Epidemiology

Infection stones comprise 5–15% of all stones.[49] However, struvite/carbonate apatite was the most common stone composition among a population of African-American stone formers in Ohio, accounting for a third of stones in males and nearly half the females in this population.[50] Similarly, struvite stones comprise up to 30% of all stone compositions worldwide. Because infection stones occur most commonly in those prone to frequent urinary tract infections, struvite stones occur more often in women than men by a ratio of 2:1.[51] Other populations at risk of recurrent infection include the elderly; premature infants or infants born with congenital urinary tract malformation; diabetics; and those with urinary stasis as a result of urinary tract obstruction, urinary diversion, or neurologic disorders. Spinal cord injured patients are at particular risk for both infection and metabolic stones owing to neurogenic urinary tract dysfunction and hypercalciuria related to immobility. Patients with a functionally complete cord transection are at highest risk of developing a staghorn calculus.[52]

18.9.2 Clinical Presentation

The clinical presentation of patients with struvite stones can be variable. Infection stones typically grow insidiously over a period of weeks to months, and, if left untreated, will eventually grow into the typical staghorn calculus. They rarely produce typical symptoms of acute colic from an obstructing ureteral stone as would be the case in patients with calcium-based or uric acid stones. Instead, patients may not realize they have a stone until investigated for recurrent infections, or obtain abdominal cross-sectional imaging for another indication. Gross hematuria, mild abdominal pain, renal dysfunction, fever, or urosepsis may also prompt clinicians to investigate for the possibility of infection stones. Concomitant urinary obstruction and hydronephrosis may be present and can result in nausea or vomiting.

In institutionalized patients susceptible to infection stones, the ability to elicit symptoms may be limited; sepsis may be the only evidence of an underlying struvite staghorn calculus. Note that patients with struvite calculi can be asymptomatic,

even when calculi occupy the entire renal collecting system. Even with progression to xanthogranulomatous pyelonephritis, 25% of patients may remain completely free of symptoms. Systemic manifestations of large struvite stones and associated chronic infection include generalized fatigue, malaise, and weight loss. Urinalysis will demonstrate an alkaline pH (>7.2) and may reveal magnesium ammonium phosphate crystals (Fig. 18.2).

Staghorn stones are easily detected on plain film imaging (Fig. 18.3). Computed tomography (CT) scan has emerged as the imaging modality of choice for stones of all chemical

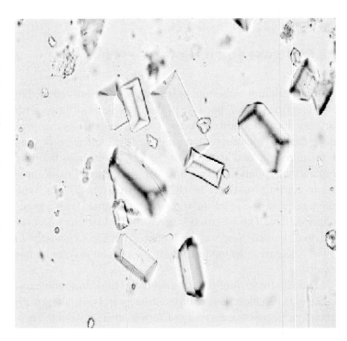

Fig. 18.2 Image of magnesium ammonium phosphate crystals. Note the classic "coffin lid" appearance (Reprinted with permission from[53] copyright Elsevier 2001)

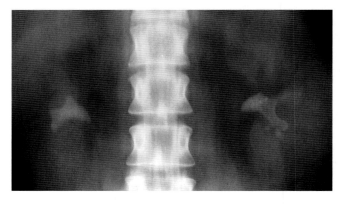

Fig. 18.3 Plain tomogram of a patient with bilateral staghorn calculi. This patient underwent bilateral percutaneous nephrolithotomies to completely clear both kidneys of all stone material. Stone composition was struvite

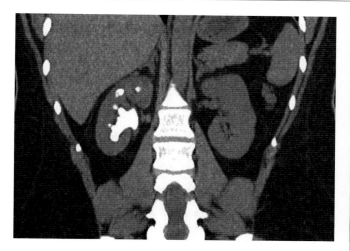

Fig. 18.4 CT scan coronal reconstruction of a right staghorn stone

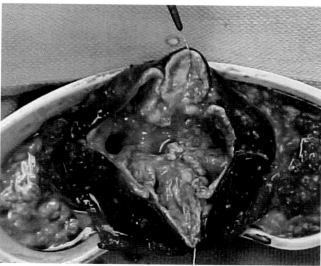

Fig. 18.5 Xanthogranulomatous pyelonephritis status post-nephrectomy. In this gross specimen, incised longitudinally along the lateral aspect of the kidney, note the abundance of purulent fluid within the basin, thinned renal cortex, and markedly dilated collecting system

compositions, and especially for preoperative planning for staghorn calculus removal (Fig. 18.4) and postoperative follow-up to ensure complete resolution. Renal scintigraphy may be indicated to assess differential renal function in those patients with chronic pyelonephritis and/or obstruction.

Disclosure The views of this manuscript are those of the authors and are in no way to be construed as the views of the US Department of the Navy, US Department of Defense, or the US Government.

18.10 Conclusions

The natural history of staghorn calculus disease is one of progressive morbidity and mortality; thus the rationale for an aggressive therapeutic approach has long been recognized. The presence of an active, untreated urinary tract infection is a contraindication to stone removal. Patients with struvite stones have chronic bacteriuria, and their urine is never sterilized by antibiotics alone; however, appropriate antibiotics should be administered prior to surgical intervention in an attempt to minimize the potential for sepsis during treatment. Similarly, if concomitant urinary obstruction and purulent infection exist (i.e., pyonephrosis), percutaneous drainage and antibiotics are necessary before further manipulation of the stone and urinary tract.

In 2005, the AUA Nephrolithiasis Guidelines Panel published a critical meta-analysis of the existing literature to determine the optimal management for staghorn calculi. They identified risk factors for patients developing staghorn stones, and potential outcomes for those undergoing treatment and those electing observation. Clearly, if left untreated, a staghorn/infection stone will destroy the kidney (Fig. 18.5), and has a significant chance of causing death in affected patients.[6] Complete surgical removal of the stone is recommended as recurrence rates for the redevelopment of a staghorn calculus in those with residual fragments approach 100%.[54]

References

1. Ahlmen J. Incidence of chronic renal insufficiency: a study of the incidence and pattern of renal insufficiency in adults during 1966-1971 in Gothenberg. *Acta Med Scand Suppl.* 1975;582:3.
2. Haddad CT. Highlights on the history of medicine in the Middle East. *Turkiye Klinikleri J Med Ethics.* 2002;10:243-257.
3. Andersen JA. Benurestat: a urease inhibitor for the therapy of infected ureolysis. *Invest Urol.* 1975;12:381.
4. Brown TR. On the relation between the variety of microorganisms and the composition of stone in Calculous Pyelonephritis. *JAMA.* 1901;36:1394-13947.
5. Gleeson MJ, Griffith DP. Infection stones. In: Resnick MI, Pak CYC, eds. *Urolithiasis: A Medical and Surgical Reference.* Philadelphia, PA: WB Saunders; 1990:134-136.
6. Preminger GM, Assimos DG, Lingemen JE, Nakada SY, Pearle MS, Wolf JS. Chapter 1: AUA guideline on management of staghorn calculi: Diagnosis and treatment recommendations. *J Urol.* 2005;173:1991-2000.
7. Ansari MS, Gupta NP, Hemal AK, et al. Spectrum of stone composition: structural analysis of 1050 upper urinary tract calculi from northern India. *Int J Urol.* 2005;12(1):12-6.
8. Heimbach D, Jacobs D, Muller SC, et al. Chemolitholysis and lithotripsy of infectious urinary stones – an in vitro study. *Urol Int.* 2002;69:212-218.
9. Rahman NU, Meng MV, Stoller ML. Infections and urinary stone disease. *Curr Pharm Des.* 2003;9:975-981.
10. Warren JW. Clinical presentations and epidemiology of urinary tract infections. In: Mobley HLT, Warren JW, eds. *Urinary tract infection: Molecular pathogenesis and clinical management.* Washington, DC: American Society for Microbiology; 1996:3-27.

11. Lerner SP, Gleeson MJ, Griffith DP. Infection stones. *J Urol.* 1989;141:753-758.

12. Rodman JS. Struvite stones. *Nephron.* 1999;81(suppl 1):50-59.

13. Coker C, Poore CA, Li X, Mobley HLT. Pathogenesis of *Proteus mirabilis* urinary tract infection. *Microbes Infect.* 2000;2: 1497-1505.

14. Griffith DP, Musher DM, Urease IC. The primary cause of infection-induced urinary stones. *Invest Urol.* 1976;13:346-350.

15. Kramer G, Klingler HC, Steiner GE. Role of bacteria in the development of kidney stones. *Curr Opin Urol.* 2000;10:35-38.

16. Nickel JC, Eintage J, Costerton JW. Ultrastructural microbial ecology of infection-induced urinary stones. *J Urol.* 1985;133:622-27.

17. McLean RJC, Nickel JC, Beveridge TJ, Costerton JW. Observations of the ultrastructure of infected kidney stones. *J Med Microbiol.* 1989;29:1-7.

18. Benyon LM, Dumanski AJ, McLean RJ, MacLean LL, Richards JC, Perry MB. Capsule structure of Proteus mirabilis (ATCC 49565). *J Bacteriol.* 1992;174(7):2172-7.

19. Perry MB, MacLean LL. The structure of the polysaccharide produced by Proteus vulgaris (ATCC 49990). *Carbohydr Res.* 1994; 253:257-63.

20. Kaca W, Literaka E, Sjoholm AG, Weintraub A. Complement activation by Proteus mirabilis negatively charged lipopolysaccharides. *J Endotoxin Res.* 2000;6(3):223-234.

21. McLean RJ, Downey J, Clapham L, Nickel JC. Influence of chondroitin sulfate, heparin sulfate, and citrate on Proteus mirabilis-induced struvite crystallization in vitro. *J Urol.* 1990;144(5):1267-71.

22. McLean RJ, Downey J, Clapham L, Nickel JC. A simple technique for studying struvite crystal growth in vitro. *Urol Res.* 1990;18(1): 39-43.

23. Torzewska A, Staczek P, Rózalski A. Crystallization of urine mineral components may depend on the chemical nature of *Proteus* endotoxin polysaccharides. *J Med Microbiol.* 2003;52:471-477.

24. Boelke E, Jehle PM, Storck M, Orth K, Schams S, Abendroth D. Urinary endotoxin excretion and urinary tract infection following kidney transplantation. *Transpl Int.* 2001;14(5):307-10.

25. McAleer IM, Kaplan GW, Bradley JS, Carroll SF. Staghorn calculus endotoxin expression in sepsis. *Urology.* 2002;59(4):601.

26. Bichler KH, Eipper E, Naberk, et al. Urinary infection stones. *Int J Antimicrob Agents.* 2002;19:488-98.

27. Hesse A, Heimbach D. Causes of phosphate stone formation and the importance of metaphylaxis by urinary acidification: a review. *World J Urol.* 1999;17:308-315.

28. Asplin JR, Mandel NS, Coe FK. Evidence of calcium phosphate supersaturation in the loop of Henle. *Am J Physiol.* 1996;270:604.

29. Clapham L, McLean RJC, Nickel JC, Downey J, Costerton JW. The influence of bacteria on struvite crystal habit and its importance in urinary stone formation. *J Crystal Growth.* 1990;104(2): 475-484.

30. Healy KA, Ogan K. Pathophysiology and management of infectious staghorn calculi. *Urol Clin North Am.* 2007;34(3): 363-374.

31. Grenabo L, Hedelin H, Hugosson J, Pettersson S. Adherence of urease-induced crystals to rat bladder epithelium following acute infection with different uropathogenic microorganisms. *J Urol.* 1988;140(2):428-430.

32. Parsons CL, Stauffer C, Mulholland SG, Griffith DP. Effect of ammonium on bacterial adherence to bladder transitional epithelium. *J Urol.* 1984;132(2):365-6.

33. du Toit PJ, van Aswegen CH, Steyn PL, Pois A. do Plessis DJ. Effects of bacteria involvedwith the pathogenesis of infection-induced urolithiasison the urokinase and sialidase (neuramidase) activity. *Urol Res.* 1992;20(6)):393-397.

34. Holmgren K, Danielson BG, Fellstrom B, Ljunghall S, Niklasson F, Wikstrom B. The relation between urinary tract infections and stone composition in renal stone formers. *Scand J Urol Nephrol.* 1989;23(2):131-136.

35. Griffith DP, Musher DM, Campbell JW. Inhibition of bacterial urease. *Invest Urol.* 1973;11(3):234-238.

36. Griffith DP, Osborne CA. Infection (urease) stones. *Miner Electrolyte Metab.* 1987;13(4):278-285.

37. Sumner JB. The isolation and crystallization of the enzyme urease. *J Biol Chem.* 1926;69:435-441.

38. Bichler KH, Eipper E, Naber K, Braun V, Zimmermann R, Lahme S. Urinary infection stones. *Int J Antimicrob Agents.* 2002; 19(6):488-498.

39. Choong S, Whitfield H. Biofolms and their role in infections in urology. *BJU Int.* 2000;86(8):935-941.

40. Roberts SD, Resnick MI. Glycosaminoglycans content of stone matrix. *J Urol.* 1986;135(5):1078-1083.

41. Rahman NU, Meng MV, Stoller ML. Infections and urinary stone disease. *Curr Pharm Des.* 2003;9(12):975-981.

42. Husmann DA, Milliner DS, Segura JW. Ureteropelvic junction obstruction with concurrent renal pelvic calculi in the pediatric patient: a long-term followup. *J Urol.* 1966;156:741-743.

43. Husmann DA, Milliner DS, Segura JW. Ureteropelvic junction obstruction with a simultaneous renal calculus: long-term followup. *J Urol.* 1995;153:1399-1402.

44. Hanley HG. Hydronephrosis. *Lancet.* 1960;2:664.

45. Hanna MK. Some observations of congenital ureteropelvic junction obstruction. *Urology.* 1978;12:151-159.

46. Koff S. Pathophysiology of uerteropelvic junction obstruction. *Urol Clin North Am.* 1990;17:263-272.

47. Notley RG. Electron microscopy of the upper ureter and pelvi-ureteric junction. *Br J Urol.* 1968;40:37.

48. Drach GW. Secondary and miscellaneous urolithiasis. *Urol Clin North Am.* 2000;27(2):269-273.

49. Levy AR, McGregor M. How has extracorporeal shock-wave lithotripsy changed the treatment of urinary stones in Quebec? *CMAJ.* 1995;153(12):1729-1736.

50. Sarmina I, Spirnak JP, Resnick MI. Urinary lithiasis in the black population: an epidemiological study and review of the literature. *J Urol.* 1987;138(1):14-17.

51. Resnick MI. Evaluation and management of infection stones. *Urol Clin North Am.* 1981;8(2):265-76.

52. DeVivo MJ, Fine PR, Cutter GR, Meatz HM. The risk of renal calculi in soinal cord injury patients. *J Urol.* 1984;131(5):857-860.

53. Raskin RE, Meyer D, eds. *Atlas of Canine and Feline Cytology.* Philadelphia, PA: WB Saunders; 2001.

54. Beck EM, Riehle RA Jr. The fate of residual fragments after extracorporeal shock wave lithotripsy monotherapy of infection stones. *J Urol.* 1991;145(1):6-9.

Drug-Induced Renal Stones

19

Michel Daudon and Paul Jungers

Abstract Drug-induced stones represent about 1% of all renal stones. They involve two main mechanisms. The first one includes stones made of the drug and/or its metabolites identified by X-ray diffraction or infrared spectroscopy on the basis of their specific diagrams. Nowadays, the most commonly observed ones are antiproteases (such as indinavir) used in HIV-infected patients, high-dose sulfadiazine used for the treatment of cerebral toxoplasmosis, and abuse of ephedrine/guaifenesin-containing preparations, whereas triamterene, formerly the most often involved drug, is less frequently observed. The second one includes stones of common composition, induced by the metabolic effects of the drug on urinary pH and excretion of calcium, oxalate, phosphate, citrate, uric acid, or other purines. The most frequent causes are unsupervised calcium/vitamin D supplementation and carbonic anhydrase inhibitors, including anticonvulsants (such as topiramate). Incidence of metabolically induced stones is probably underestimated, because they are of apparently usual composition and may reveal long after drug withdrawal. Formation of iatrogenic calculi is favored by high-dose or long-lasting treatments, high renal excretion and low solubility of the drug or its metabolites, low urine output or inadequate urine pH, and is especially frequent in patients with a history of stones. Better awareness of potentially lithogenic drugs may allow more efficient prevention and reduce the incidence of drug-induced nephrolithiasis.

19.1 Introduction

Drug-induced stones currently account for about 1% of urinary stones.[1] Sulfonamides were the first drugs associated with the formation of renal calculi soon after their introduction in the early 1940s.[2] Thereafter, only sparse reports appeared in the following four decades, until Ettinger et al.[3] reported the frequent occurrence of stones in patients treated with triamterene. This led to the proposal of the innovative concept of drug-induced nephrolithiasis.[4,5] Subsequently, a number of reports appeared about a variety of drugs, involving different mechanisms and risk factors, leading to the additional concept that drug-induced stone formation involves two distinct mechanisms.[1,6]

19.2 Mechanisms of Drug-Induced Stone Formation

Analysis of a large number of stones in drug-exposed patients allows the identification of two main types of drug-induced stones:

1. Stones made, in majority or partly, of the drug itself, or its metabolites. In such cases, diagnosis is easily made by X-ray diffraction[7] or Fourier transform infrared spectroscopy (FTIR),[8] which identify the presence of a foreign compound together with its location and amount in the stone.
2. Stones made of calcium oxalate, calcium phosphate, uric acid or ammonium urate resulting from the metabolic effects of the drug, through alteration of urine pH and/or of urinary excretion of calcium, oxalate, phosphate, uric acid, or electrolytes. Here, the diagnosis is more difficult because stones have a common composition. It relies on the patient's history and comorbidity, and recording of drugs currently or formerly used by the patient.[1,6,9]

M. Daudon (✉)
Department of Biochemistry, Stone Laboratory, Necker Hospital, Paris, France
e-mail: michel.daudon@nck.aphp.fr

P.N. Rao et al. (eds.), *Urinary Tract Stone Disease*,
DOI 10.1007/978-1-84800-362-0_19, © Springer-Verlag London Limited 2011

Of note, in both cases, iatrogenic calculi often develop on a preexisting stone, thus leading to a stone of mixed composition, as revealed by thorough morphologic examination and sequential analysis of stones.[10]

19.3 Risk Factors Favoring Drug-Induced Stone Formation

Formation of drug-induced stones is not universal with all drugs. Drugs having a propensity for inducing crystalluria, and stone formation have common characteristics, several of which may be simultaneously involved: high daily dose of the drug (in the order of several hundreds milligrams or few grams); long-lasting prescription; high urinary excretion of the drug and/or its metabolites; urinary concentration peaks (short half-lived drugs); poor solubility of the drug and/or metabolites; peculiar characteristics of drug crystals (size and morphology); or concomitant administration of a drug altering pharmacokinetics or metabolism of the drug. On the other hand, only a very limited proportion of the large number of patients treated with potentially lithogenic drugs develop crystalluria or stones. This indicates that risk factors specific to individuals may favor stone formation. The most important factor is a history of nephrolithiasis, which is found in a high proportion of affected patients. Other favoring factors are urinary stasis (malformative uropathy, prostatic hypertrophy); underlying latent lithogenic metabolic abnormality (such as idiopathic hypercalciuria, hyperuricosuria, hyperoxaluria, or hypocitraturia); individual pattern of drug-detoxification; abnormally low or high urinary pH; urinary tract infection; low urine output; or excessive urine concentration (dehydration episodes, hot climate, etc.).

19.4 Epidemiology of Drug-Induced Stones

Incidence of drug-induced stones is likely to be underestimated. Indeed, most published studies report only on calculi containing a drug or its metabolites, identifiable by X-ray diffraction of FTIR, whereas stones of common composition without presence of a foreign component are usually not identified as drug-induced.[1]

The first large-scale epidemiological study of drug-induced nephrolithiasis was presented in 1980 by Ettinger et al.,[3] who reported that 0.4% of 50,000 renal calculi in the US contained triamterene. Asper[7] reported a prevalence of 0.1% of drug-containing calculi in a series of 14,165 calculi analyzed by X-ray diffraction between 1982 and 1985 in Switzerland, whereas Rapado et al.[9] in Spain observed the presence of a drug in 0.8% of 1,500 calculi. During the decade 1975–1985, Réveillaud and Daudon identified the presence of a drug in 58 (1.4%) of 4,000 calculi.[11] Triamterene was the most frequently involved drug.

More recently, new drugs used in the treatment of human immunodeficiency virus (HIV) infected patients, namely indinavir and sulfadiazine, became the most prevalent, whereas the incidence of triamterene-containing stones declined, as shown in a survey of the distribution of drug-containing calculi among urinary stones examined at our laboratory over the period 1977–2002.[1] Of note, stones induced by the metabolic effects of drugs were nearly as frequent as drug-containing ones. Among 45,000 stones analyzed at CRISTAL Laboratory between 1977 and 2006, 0.95% contained a drug or metabolites, whereas 0.65% resulted from metabolic drug induction.

19.5 Drug-Containing Renal Stones

About 20 different drugs have been found in calculi (Table 19.1).

19.5.1 Triamterene

The potassium-sparing diuretic triamterene was commonly prescribed in the past decades to hypertensive patients. It was associated to thiazide diuretics in order to prevent hypokalemia. A popular pill in the US was Dyazide®, which contained 25 mg hydrochlorothiazide and 50 mg triamterene per tablet.

In the first case reported by Ettinger et al.,[12] a 52-year-old female patient who passed nearly 50 mustard-color calculi was taking 300 mg/day triamterene. Subsequently, a number of reports appeared (reviewed in Daudon and Jungers[1]). Most affected patients received 150–200 mg triamterene per day. Triamterene-containing stones (Fig. 19.1a) were more frequent in patients with a history of stones than in those without it and especially in cases where a calculus was still present, providing a physical support for the deposition of triamterene or its metabolites.[3,13]

As shown by FTIR, only one-third of triamterene-associated calculi were made mainly of triamterene, whereas in most cases, minor amounts of triamterene were associated with variable amounts of common components such as calcium oxalate or uric acid.[1,3] However, in our experience, triamterene was present in the nucleus of 70% of calculi, thus indicating its initiating role in the lithogenic process, whereas in 30% of cases triamterene coated a preexisting calculus.[1]

Chromatographic analysis revealed that triamterene calculi contain, in variable proportions, both triamterene and its metabolites, hydroxy-4'-triamterene in its free form or, most frequently, as hydroxy-4'-triamterene sulphate, with the sulphate metabolite often being the major component.[14] Other insoluble metabolites were also reported in stones.[15]

Despite the fact that urinary crystals of triamterene metabolites appear in about half of patients treated with this drug,[16]

Table 19.1 Drugs found in calculi

Drug	Components of Stones
Antibacterial agents	
Sulfamides	
Sulfadiazine	N-acetylsulfadiazine, sulfadiazine
Sulfaguanidine	N-acetylsulfaguanidine, N, N-diacetylsulfaguanidine
Sulfamethoxazole	N-acetylsulfamethoxazole chlorhydrate
Sulfaperine	N-acetylsulfaperine
Sulfasalazine et sulfapyridine	N-acetylsulfapyridine
Sulfisoxazole	N-acetylsufisoxazole
Aminopenicillins	
Amoxicillin	Amoxicillin trihydrate
Ampicillin	Ampicillin trihydrate
Cephalosporins	
Ceftriaxone	Calcium ceftriaxonate
Quinolones	
Flumequine	Flumequine
Oxolinic acid	Oxolinic acid
Ciprofloxacin	Ciprofloxacin, magnesium salt
Norfloxacin	Norfloxacin, magnesium salt
Furanes	
Nitrofurantoine	Nitrofurantoine
Pyridines	
Phenazopyridine	Hydroxyphenazopyridine sulfate and other metabolites
Proteases inhibitors	
Indinavir sulfate	Indinavir monohydrate
Atazanavir	Atazanavir
Nelfinavir	Nelfinavir
Antinucleosidic drugs	
Efavirenz	Efavirenz metabolites
Analgesics	
Amino-4-quinoleines	
Glafenine	Free glafenic and hydroxyglafenic acids
Antrafenine	Free antrafenic acid
Floctafenine	Floctafenic acid glucuronide
Antihypertensive drug	
Pteridine	
Triamterene	Triamterene, hydroxy-4′-triamterene sulfate, hydroxy-4′-triamterene and glucuronide metabolites
Others	
Silicium derivatives	
Magnesium trisilicate	Amorphous silica (opale)
Hydrated silica	Amorphous silica (opale)

(continued)

Table 19.1 continued

Drug	Components of Stones
Cough and stimulant preparations	
Guaifenesine	Bêta-(2-methoxyphenoxy) lactic acid, calcium salt
Ephedrine	Ephedrine
Hypouricemic drug	
Allopurinol	Oxypurinol
Oxypurinol	Oxypurinol

less than 1 of 1,000 triamterene-treated patients develop stones. This clearly suggests the role of favoring factors. Besides excessive daily dose of the drug (150–200 mg/day), a low urine pH is also a risk factor. Moreover, because a low urine pH simultaneously favors the formation of uric acid stones,[17,18] often, triamterene-containing calculi also contain uric acid, as observed by Ettinger et al.[3] and in our patients.

The incidence of triamterene-induced renal calculi markedly declined in recent years, due to better awareness of the lithogenic risk of triamterene[19] and to the availability of new antihypertensive drugs, including other potassium-sparing drugs devoid of lithogenic effects, such as amiloride.[20] In any case, triamterene therapy should be avoided in patients with a history of nephrolithiasis, especially uric acid nephrolithiasis.

19.5.2 Protease Inhibitors

Shortly after its introduction in the tritherapy of HIV infection in 1995, indinavir rapidly became the commonest cause of drug-induced stones in the past decade. Subsequently, other protease inhibitors have been reported to induce crystalluria and stones, although less frequently than indinavir because of their much lower daily dose.

Incidence of stones in indinavir-treated patients is as high as 10–20%[21–23] or even 40%.[24,25] Indinavir-associated stones present with typical renal colic, or only loin pain or dysuria.[26–28] Pure indinavir calculi are totally radiolucent on kidneys, ureters, and bladder (KUB), and also on computed tomography (CT), unless CT scan is contrast-enhanced.[29] Indinavir-containing stones are rather small (2–6 mm in diameter) with a beige, rough surface; they are composed of large rods with a radiating organization of the crystals (Fig. 19.1b). FTIR and mass spectroscopy showed indinavir in stones in the form of indinavir monohydrate, the unchanged form, admixed with variable amounts of proteins in about 70% of cases, and with calcium oxalate or phosphate in 30% of cases.[1]

Most indinavir-containing stones are passed spontaneously. However, stone extraction may require intervention of the urologist, preferably by means of ureteroscopy or ureteral stenting, because extracorporeal shock wave lithotripsy (ESWL) is often ineffective due to the high protein content

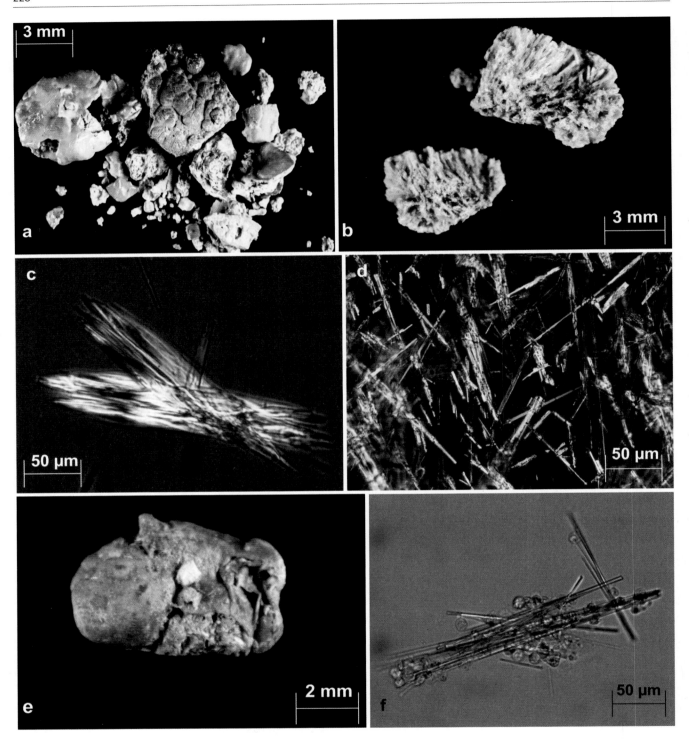

Fig. 19.1 (**a**) Stone fragments composed of triamterene and metabolites. (**b**) Stone fragments composed of indinavir monohydrate crystals mixed with proteins. (**c**) Indinavir monohydrate crystals observed in urine using polarized light microscopy. (**d**) Acyclovir crystals observed in urine using polarized light microscopy. (**e**) Atazanavir stone. (**f**) Atazanavir crystals observed in urine using polarized light microscopy

and loose structure of indinavir calculi.[30,31] Often, a transient increase in serum creatinine is observed during stone episodes.[28,32] In some cases, impaired renal function persisted despite relief of obstruction and discontinuation of the drug.[33]

In addition to stones, several cases of acute renal failure have been reported, associated with heavy indinavir crystalluria.[34] In such cases, FTIR of kidney biopsy showed multiple indinavir crystals in collecting ducts.[34]

The frequent development of stones in indinavir-treated patients reflects the very frequent induction of crystalluria, in as much as indinavir crystals (Fig. 19.1c) are especially large (100–500 μm) and needle-shaped,[35] and therefore are prone to obstruct renal tubules. Indinavir crystalluria results from the high amounts of indinavir excreted by renal route, and its very weak solubility in urine at its usual pH. Indeed, the standard schedule consists of three oral doses of 800 mg per day, of which 20% are excreted via renal route within 24 h, with an excretion peak in the 3 h following each daily administration.[21,36] Therefore, urinary indinavir concentration in the 3 h following a 800 mg dose may be as high as 200–300 mg/L when a daily urine output is about 1,500 ml,[21] whereas indinavir solubility is only 35 mg/L at urine pH 6.0 and reaches 300 mg/L or more only when urine pH is below 5.0.[37] It results that indinavir crystalluria is a very frequent finding in indinavir-treated patients.[23,26,38,39] We found indinavir crystals in 34% of urine samples taken within 3 h of the first indinavir morning dose of 800 mg, with a clear influence of urine pH.[35]

Additional risk factors for stone formation are episodes of dehydration, such as those provoked by severe diarrhea, a frequent symptom in acquired immunodeficiency syndrome (AIDS) patients,[39] concomitant administration of other antiviral drugs such as acyclovir[28] or cotrimoxazole,[22] which may also crystallize in the kidney (Fig. 19.1d), coinfection with hepatitis B or C virus,[40] or excessive dosing of indinavir in patients with a low body mass.[41]

Prevention of indinavir-induced stones relies on simple, easily implemented measures: ingestion of 150 ml water when taking each dose of the drug and hourly in the following 2 h[21] and preferred use of acidifying beverages such as colas, either regular or diet, which contain phosphoric acid. Therapeutic protocols for HIV with reduced doses of indinavir in association with ritonavir, another antiprotease with much less crystalluria risk,[42] may be used as an alternative.

Other antiproteases are less frequently involved in stone formation. Nelfinavir[43] and tenofovir[44] have been reported as the cause of stones. More recently, several cases of crystal nephropathy[45] or of nephrolithiasis[46,47] have been reported in HIV-positive patients treated with atazanavir (Fig. 19.1e and f). Incidence of this cause of drug-induced stones is increasing in our experience.

Efavirenz, an antinucleosidic molecule used in the treatment of HIV-positive patients, was described as metabolites in urinary stones.[48,49]

19.5.3 Sulfonamides

First-generation sulfonamides were early shown to provoke drug-induced stones,[50,51] or acute renal failure episodes caused by massive crystal precipitation.[2,52] Indeed, sulfonamides are excreted by the kidneys mainly in the form of N-acetyl metabolites,[2] all of which are poorly soluble. Subsequently, new antibacterial agents were developed, thus resulting in decreased use of sulfonamides. However, in the recent decade, a resurgence of sulfonamide-induced stones took place with the widespread use of sulfadiazine for the treatment of encephalic toxoplasmosis, a common localization of this opportunistic infection in HIV-positive patients, because the drug readily crosses the blood-brain barrier. In this indication, sulfadiazine is used at very large doses (4–8 g/day), thus resulting in heavy crystalluria, especially if urine pH and urine output are low.[53–55] Stones formed in sulfadiazine-treated patients are mostly made of N-acetyl-sulfadiazine (Fig. 19.2a), present in the nucleus of 93% of stones in our patients.[1] Of note, N-acetyl-sulfadiazine crystals are needle-shaped and form large aggregates that are likely to form calculi or obstruct tubular lumens (Fig. 19.2b).

Other sulfonamides used in other indications are less lithogenic. Sulfasalazin, used in patients with Crohn's disease and ulcerative colitis at doses of 4–8 g/day, has caused stones[56] or acute renal failure[57] in some patients.

Sulfamethoxazole, a component of the antibacterial agent cotrimoxazole, induces frequent crystalluria but infrequently results in nephrolithiasis.[53,58] In the study by Albala et al., N-acetylsulfamethoxazole was the main component of such stones. Crystals of N-acetylsulfamethoxazole are of small size and of round or losangic shape, and are thus easily passed in urine.[53] This likely explains why stone formation is infrequent despite the wide use of this antibacterial agent.[1]

Fortunately, sulfonamides are highly soluble in alkaline urine. Thus, active alkalinization is the cornerstone of curative and preventive therapy, in association with high urine output.

19.5.4 Other Antibacterial Agents

A number of antibacterial agents (listed in Table 19.1) have been reported to cause nephrolithiasis. They include quinolones such as flumequine,[59] oxolinic acid,[60] ciprofloxacin[61] and norfloxacin,[1] aminopenicillins such as amoxicillin and ampicillin,[6,62] cephalosporins such as ceftriaxone (especially in children),[63–65] phenazopyridine,[66] or nitrofurantoin.[67] However, such cases are very infrequent and occurrence of stones in these patients suggests the intervention of favoring factors, such as unusually high daily dose, prolonged administration, and low urine pH, except with regard to fluoroquinolones such as ciprofloxacin or norfloxacin, which rather crystallize in alkaline urine.[68]

Crystals of quinolones and aminopenicillins are large and needle-shaped, thus favoring crystal aggregation and stone formation (Fig. 19.2c and d).

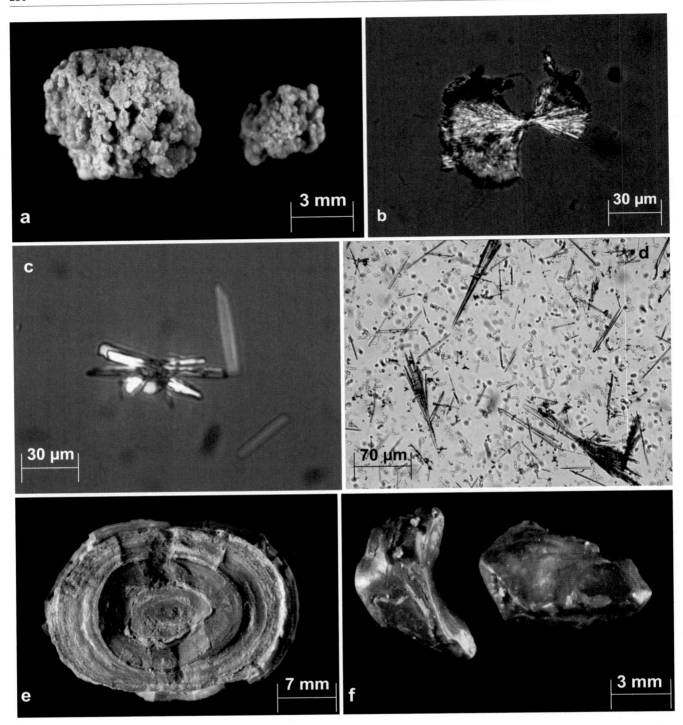

Fig. 19.2 (**a**) N-acetylsulfadiazine stones spontaneously passed. (**b**) N-acetylsulfadiazine crystals observed in urine using polarized light microscopy. (**c**) Ciprofloxacin crystals (magnesium salt) observed in urine using polarized light microscopy. (**d**) Amoxicillin trihydrate crystals observed in urine using light microscopy. (**e**) Section of an ammonium hydrogen urate stone induced by laxative abuse. (**f**) Renal stones composed of a mixture of xanthine and oxypurinol in a child treated with allopurinol for Lesch-Nyhan syndrome

19.5.5 Other Drugs

A variety of drugs occasionally induce drug-containing stones (reviewed by Daudon and Jungers[1]).

19.5.5.1 Magnesium Trisilicate

Magnesium trisilicate, component of a number of antacid preparations, when administered for long periods, has been reported to cause the formation of stones made of pure amorphous silicon dioxide, with about 30 cases reported worldwide.[69,70] Several cases of calculi have been observed in babies receiving colloid silica (Gelopectose®) in their feeding bottle as a milk thickener to prevent esophageal regurgitation.[71] Opaline silica was found in the core of all calculi.[1,71,72] In Japan, silicate calculi observed in adult subjects, as well as in an infant, were attributed to the consumption of silicate-rich water.[73]

19.5.5.2 Glafenine

Glafenine, an amino-4-quinoleine derivative widely used as an analgesic in some European countries in the past decades, was responsible for about 40 cases of nephrolithiasis until its withdrawal in 1992.[1,11]

19.5.5.3 Oxypurinol, Allopurinol, and Xanthine

Calculi made of oxypurinol admixed with allopurinol or xanthine may develop in children treated with high doses of allopurinol for the Lesch-Nyhan syndrome.[8,74,75] Oxypurinol stones developed in a patient treated for recurrent uric acid nephrolithiasis complicating ileostomy.[76]

19.5.5.4 Guaifenesin, Ephedrine, and Other Stimulants

Guaifenesin, a popular over-the-counter expectorant and cough-suppressant drug, has been reported as a cause of calculi following its excessive consumption as a stimulant, most often in preparations also containing ephedrine as decongestant.[77] Stones contain metabolites of guaifenesin.[78] Severe complications resulting from overdosing in infants and young children have been reported.[79]

Ephedrine, a naturally occurring alkaloid, is associated with guaifenesin in a number of antitussives and expectorants. It is also the active component of the popular Chinese herbal product Ma-huang (*Ephedra sinica*)[80] used for weight loss, energy, sexual enhancement, and euphoria. This preparation has been responsible for multiple adverse effects, including hepatic and cardiovascular, some of which have been fatal. Hundreds of cases of nephrolithiasis have been reported in the US. Stones contain ephedrine, norephedrine, and pseudoephedrine. In a patient, dissolution of such stones could be obtained by alkalinization.[81] Abuse of ephedrine and guafenesin taken individually or in combination results in nearly 35% of drug-induced stones, and accounts for 0.1% of all urinary stones in the US.[82]

19.6 Metabolically Induced Renal Stones

Drugs shown to induce formation of stones as a result of their metabolic effects are summarized in Table 19.2. These stones may be categorized into two main types:

* Stones made of calcium oxalate or phosphate
* Radiolucent stones made of purine derivatives

19.6.1 Calcium-Containing Stones

19.6.1.1 Calcium and Vitamin D Supplementation

Calcium and even more vitamin D supplementation may induce hypercalciuria and calcium oxalate stone formation, especially in patients having underlying idiopathic hypercalciuria.[83–85] In a randomized study including 36,282 postmenopausal women, participants assigned to receive daily 1,000 mg of calcium plus 400 IU of vitamin D had, as expected, a lower incidence of hip fractures than women who received the placebo, but the risk of renal calculi was 17% higher.[86] This observation is of clinical relevance, because combined calcium and vitamin D supplementation appears to be increasingly prescribed to prevent osteoporosis in postmenopausal women, due to the growing reluctance to use hormonal substitutive treatment. Unsupervised vitamin D supplementation is also frequently given to children and adolescents, with an increased risk of calcium oxalate dihydrate stone formation. We observed in the recent years an increasing number of weddellite stones (indicative of hypercalciuria) in young adults and in postmenopausal women.[87] In order to prevent this complication, urinary calcium excretion should be measured before initiation of such therapy and monitored while under treatment. In patients with hypercalciuria, calcium-vitamin D supplementation should be preferably avoided or discontinued, or combined with a thiazide diuretic, which reduces urinary excretion of calcium.[83]

Some patients on maintenance hemodialysis or peritoneal dialysis formed calculi made of calcium oxalate monohydrate admixed with a large proportion of proteins after vitamin D supplementation aimed at preventing hypocalcemia.[88,89] In these patients, the vitamin D-induced increase in urinary calcium concentration, in the face of a high oxalate concentration, resulted in calcium oxalate supersaturation and formation of whewellite stones.[90]

Table 19.2 Drug-induced metabolic stones

Drugs	Stone composition
Radioopaque stones	
Calcium/vitamin D supplements	
– In patients with normal kidney function	Mixtures of calcium oxalates and phosphates
– In end-stage renal disease	Whewellite mixed with proteins
Carbonic anhydrase inhibitors: acetazolamide, methazolamide, dorzolamide, dichlorphenamide, zonisamide, topiramate…	Calcium phosphates with or without calcium oxalates
Piridoxilate	Whewellite and calcium oxalate trihydrate
Furosemide	Calcium oxalates with or without calcium phosphates
Carbonate or hydrogenocarbonate-containing drugs (high doses)	Calcite mixed with calcium phosphates
Corticosteroids	Mixtures of calcium oxalates and calcium phosphates
Ascorbic acid	Calcium oxalates
Naftidrofuryl oxalate	Calcium oxalates, mainly whewellite
Nimesulide	Calcium oxalates
Antibiotics (long treatments)	Calcium oxalates
Alkalizing drugs: sodium or potassium hydrogenocarbonate, other carbonates	Calcium phosphates
Radiolucent stones	
Laxatives	Ammonium hydrogen urate ± uric acid ± calcium oxalates
Uricosuric drugs	Uric acids
Allopurinol	Xanthine (+ oxypurinol)
Alkalizing drugs	Sodium hydrogen urate, sodium and potassium urate, potassium hydrogen urate, ammonium hydrogen urate…
Acidifying drugs: ammonium chloride, phosphoric acid…	Uric acids

19.6.1.2 Carbonic Anhydrase Inhibitors

Carbonic anhydrase inhibitors are widely used in the treatment of glaucoma, and of epilepsy either in monotherapy or as an adjunct to other anticonvulsants.[91] In patients with glaucoma, treatments with acetazolamide[92–94] and its analogues, methazolamide[95] or dorzolamide[96] are complicated by nephrolithiasis in about 10% of cases. Stones are predominantly made of calcium phosphate.[1,97] This composition is in keeping with the biochemical changes induced by these drugs. Indeed, carbonic anhydrase inhibitors block the reabsorption of bicarbonate ions in the proximal convoluted tubule and inhibit the excretion of hydrogen ions, thus inducing intracellular acidosis with increased tubular citrate reabsorption and hypocitraturia. Patients treated with carbonic anhydrase inhibitors exhibit decreased plasma bicarbonate, marked hypocitraturia and hypercalciuria, and elevated urine pH,[98–100] all conditions which favor the precipitation of calcium phosphate, mainly in the form of carbapatite.[1] Patients with a history of nephrolithiasis or with underlying idiopathic hypercalciuria are especially susceptible to this complication. Prevention of stone recurrence is difficult if maintaining the drug is necessary. Fortunately, alternative treatments are now available.

Topiramate and zonisamide are newer neuromodulatory agents, widely used in the treatment of epilepsy.[101–103] Topiramate has been shown to induce the frequent formation of calcium phosphate stones,[104–106] whereas incidence of stones in patients treated with zonisamide seems to be lower.[107] Topiramate inhibits the activity of carbonic anhydrase enzymes in the kidney. Patients treated with the drug exhibit reduced serum bicarbonate level, hypocitraturia, hypercalciuria, and high urine pH, with increased saturation ratio for brushite.[106,108–110] Therefore, patients treated with these drugs should have regular urine biochemistry surveillance.[106,110] If renal stones occur, drug discontinuation should be the preferred measure.[104]

19.6.1.3 Furosemide

Furosemide used in premature neonates or in infants with congestive heart failure may induce nephrocalcinosis and formation of stones made of calcium oxalate, either pure or admixed with calcium phosphate,[111,112] with a strikingly increased calcium excretion. ESWL with adapted technology has been successfully used in small infants with persistent stones.[113] Medullary nephrocalcinosis has been reported in

18 women who had long-term furosemide abuse for the purpose of slimming.[114] However, no cases of calcium nephrolithiasis have been reported in hypertensive patients treated with furosemide.

19.6.1.4 Antibacterial Agents in Cystic Fibrosis

Repeated, long-standing antibacterial treatments in patients with cystic fibrosis provoke decolonization of *Oxalobacter formigenes*, a gut commensal that degrades oxalate ions in the colon lumen, thus resulting in overabsorption of oxalate and hyperoxaluria. This factor may explain, at least in part, the frequent occurrence of calcium oxalate stones (or nephrocalcinosis) in cystic fibrosis patients.[115,116] Most patients with cystic fibrosis exhibit hyperoxaluria and hypocitraturia, these anomalies being more marked in those affected by stone formation or nephrocalcinosis.[117–120] Absence of *Oxalobacter formigenes* in the gut may also be a favoring lithogenic factor in idiopathic calcium stone formers.[115,121]

19.6.1.5 Other Drugs

Antacid preparations in prolonged use as self-medication before the era of gastric proton-pump inhibitors induced the formation of stones,[122] made of mixtures of calcium carbonate and calcium phosphate.[1]

Corticosteroid therapy induces hypercalciuria and hyperphosphaturia, although formation of urinary calculi is infrequent.[123,124]

Ascorbic acid (vitamin C) overdosing increases urinary oxalate excretion[125,126] and therefore may result in calcium oxalate nephrolithiasis.[127] However, epidemiological studies failed to observe an association between high vitamin C ingestion and incidence of stones, both in men[128] and in women.[129] Traxer et al.[126] found a greater increase in urinary oxalate excretion following oral intake of 2 g/day vitamin C or more in stone formers. This suggests that certain people have a peculiar susceptibility to the metabolic effects of ascorbic acid.

Naftidrofuryl oxalate has been shown to induce hyperoxaluria and formation of calcium oxalate stones after long-term oral therapy, especially in elderly patients.[130] One may mention that piridoxilate, a vasodilatory drug made of an equimolar combination of glyoxylate and pyridoxine, widely used in some European countries in the 1970s and 1980s for the treatment of coronary and peripheral artery disease, was responsible for more than 100 cases of calcium oxalate nephrolithiasis[131] or even

nephrocalcinosis.[132] These untoward effects led to the withdrawal of this drug.

19.6.2 Purine-Containing Stones

19.6.2.1 Laxative Abuse

Laxative abuse as self-medication in anorectic women may provoke the formation of radiolucent calculi made of ammonium urate.[1,133,134] Such stone composition with peculiar morphologic characteristics (Fig. 19.2e) should alert to the hypothesis of laxative abuse, often associated with diuretic abuse.

19.6.2.2 Uricosuric Drugs

Uricosuric drugs such as benziodarone, benzbromarone, probenecid, or tienilic acid (ticrynafen) reduce hyperuricemia by enhancing urinary urate excretion, and thus entail the risk of uric acid nephrolithiasis in patients who already had uricosuria.[135] Use of xanthine oxidase inhibitors, such as allopurinol, oxypurinol, or febuxostat[136] should be preferred in patients with hyperuricosuria, a history of stones, or concomitant use of diuretics.[135]

19.6.2.3 Allopurinol

Allopurinol has been reported to induce the formation of xanthine calculi in patients with massive hyperuricaemia and hyperuricosuria, as in the Lesch-Nyhan syndrome, when treated with high doses.[74,75,137,138] Indeed, all stones resulting from treatment of Lesch-Nyhan syndrome with allopurinol contain xanthine mixed with oxypurinol (Fig. 19.2f).

19.6.2.4 Urine pH Modifiers

Urinary acidification by means of ammonium chloride or phosphoric acid may induce formation of uric acid calculi when the urine pH is consistently maintained below 5.2.[1] Conversely, alkalinization used in the treatment of uric acid nephrolithiasis sometimes results in the coating of uric acid calculi by poorly soluble urate salts such as sodium urate monohydrate, sodium potassium urate, calcium urate hexahydrate, or ammonium urate, especially in patients with uricosuria and a low diuresis or a high urinary concentration of sodium, potassium, or other cations.[1]

Table 19.3 Pathological conditions susceptible of leading to drug-induced nephrolithiasis

Pathological condition	Potentially lithogenic therapy	Stone composition
Acute or chronic infections	Sulfonamides	DC[a] (N-acetyl derivatives)
	Aminopenicillins	DC[a] (native drug)
	Quinolones	DC[a] (native drug or magnesium salt)
Specific diseases		
HIV infection	Antiproteases	DC[a] (indinavir, atazanavir, other)
Efavirenz	Antinucleosidic drugs	DC[a] (metabolites)
CNS toxoplasmosis	Sulfadiazine	DC[a] (N-acetylsulfadiazine)
Cystic fibrosis	Decolonisation of Oxalobacter formigenes (multiple antibacterial courses)	DI (calcium oxalate)
Hypertension	Triamterene	DC[a] (triamterene and metabolites)
Glaucoma	Acetazolamide, methazolamide, dorsolamide, dichlorphenamide, other	DI (calcium phosphate)
Epilepsy	Topiramate, zonisamide	DI (calcium phosphate)
Osteoporosis	Calcium, Vitamin D	DI (calcium oxalate ± calcium phosphate)
Constipation, laxative abuse	Laxatives	DI (ammonium urate)
Cough and cold preparations	Guaifenesin	DC[a] (calcium salt of a metabolite)
Stimulant abuse	Guaifenesin/Ephedrine	DC[a] (calcium salt of a metabolite/ephedrine)
Preterm born babies	Furosemide	DI (calcium oxalate ± calcium phosphate)
Congestive heart failure in infants	Furosemide	DI (calcium oxalate ± calcium phosphate)
Diuretic abuse	Furosemide	DI (calcium oxalate ± calcium phosphate)
Gouthy diathesis	Uricosuric drugs	DI (uric acids)

DC drug-containing stones, *DI* metabolically drug-induced stones

[a]Specific diagram at FTIR or X-ray diffraction

19.7 Diagnosis and Prevention

Incidence of drug-induced calculi is probably underestimated. As mentioned earlier, diagnosis is obvious whenever X-ray diffraction or FTIR analysis of a stone reveals a foreign component identified as a drug or its metabolites. In the case of metabolically induced calculi, the iatrogenic origin of stones is much less apparent. History of the patient, including record of all prescribed or self-administered drugs taken in the period preceding onset of stones, is the only way to identify the drug-induced origin of a stone of common composition and apparent idiopathic nature. In this situation, diagnosis should be oriented by the clinical context. For instance, a patient suffering from epilepsy should be asked if he (or she) received in the past, or is currently treated with, drugs such as topiramate.

Table 19.3 presents a tentative list of various diseases or conditions that may lead to therapy with drugs having a lithogenic potential, which may serve as a check-list for use in clinical practice.

19.8 Conclusions

Drug-induced calculi, although they represent less than 2% of renal stones, merit consideration because they are frequently underdiagnosed and will provoke relentless stone formation until the lithogenic drug has been discontinued.

The nature of drugs responsible for iatrogenic stones evolved with time. Three decades ago, triamterene was the leading cause. Nowadays, treatments of HIV infection/AIDS and associated cerebral toxoplasmosis are the most frequent causes of drug-containing calculi. Worthy to mention, abuse of over-the-counter preparations containing ephedrine or guaifenesin is also currently a frequent cause of undue stones. Infrared spectroscopy is the most efficient method to identify drug-containing calculi. However, only careful clinical inquiry may diagnose stones of common composition resulting from the metabolic effects of drugs. Better awareness of potentially lithogenic drugs and careful surveillance of patients on long-term treatments with such drugs will allow early diagnosis of iatrogenic stones and prevention of this complication.

References

1. Daudon M, Jungers P. Drug-induced renal calculi: epidemiology, prevention and management. *Drugs*. 2004;64:245-275.
2. Barnes RW, Kawaichi GK. Factors influencing the formation of sulfonamide urinary concretions. *J Urol*. 1943;49:324-330.
3. Ettinger B, Oldroyd NO, Sorgel F. Triamterene nephrolithiasis. *JAMA*. 1980;244:2443-2445.
4. Curtis JR. Drug-induced renal disease. *Drugs*. 1979;18:377-391.
5. Réveillaud RJ, Daudon M. Drug-induced urinary lithiasis (in French). *Presse Méd*. 1983;12:2389-2392.
6. Daudon M, Estepa L. Drug induced lithiases (in French). *Presse Méd*. 1998;27:675-683.

7. Asper R. Iatrogenic urinary calculi. Detection and identification by X-ray diffraction. *Clin Chem.* 1986;24:767-768.

8. Nguyen Quy D, Daudon M. *Infrared and Raman Spectra of Calculi.* Paris: Elsevier; 1997.

9. Rapado A, Traba ML, Caycho C, et al. Drug-induced renal stones: incidence, clinical expression and stone analysis. *Contrib Nephrol.* 1987;58:25-29.

10. Daudon M, Jungers P. Clinical value of crystalluria and quantitative morphoconstitutional analysis of urinary calculi. *Nephron Physiol.* 2004;98:31-36.

11. Réveillaud RJ, Daudon M. Les lithiases urinaires médicamenteuses. *Sémin Uro-Néphrol.* 1986;12:14-39.

12. Ettinger B, Weil E, Mandel NS, et al. Triamterene-induced nephrolithiasis. *Ann Intern Med.* 1979;91:745-746.

13. Carey RA, Beg MM, McNally CF, et al. Triamterene and renal lithiasis: a review. *Clin Ther.* 1984;6:302-309.

14. Sorgel F, Ettinger B, Benet LZ. The true composition of kidney stones passed during triamterene therapy. *J Urol.* 1985;134: 871-873.

15. Sabot JF, Bernard P, Pinatel H, et al. Analysis of urinary calculi containing triamterene. Presence of a glucuronic metabolite. *Anal Lett.* 1996;29:1319-1327.

16. Fairley KF, Birch DF, Haines I. Abnormal urinary sediment in patients on triamterene. *Lancet.* 1983;i:421-422.

17. Sakhaee K, Adams-Huet B, Moe OW, Pak CYC. Pathophysiologic basis for normouricosuric uric acid nephrolithiasis. *Kidney Int.* 2002;62:971-979.

18. Daudon M, Traxer O, Conort P, Lacour B, Jungers P. Type 2 diabetes increases the risk for uric acid stones. *J Am Soc Nephrol.* 2006;17:2026-2033.

19. Carr MC, Prien EL Jr, Babayan RK. Triamterene nephrolithiasis: renewed attention is warranted. *J Urol.* 1990;144:1339-1340.

20. Spence JD, Wong DG, Lindsay RM. Effects of triamterene and amiloride on urinary sediment in hypertensive patients taking hydrochlorothiazide. *Lancet.* 1985;8446:73-75.

21. Daudon M, Estepa L, Viard JP, et al. Urinary stones in HIV-1-positive patients treated with indinavir. *Lancet.* 1997;9061:1294-1295.

22. Boubaker K, Sudre P, Bally F, et al. Changes in renal function associated with indinavir. *AIDS.* 1998;12:F249-F254.

23. Reiter WJ, Schon-Pernerstorfer H, Dorfinger K, et al. Frequency of urolithiasis in individuals seropositive for human immunodeficiency virus treated with indinavir is higher than previously assumed. *J Urol.* 1999;161:1082-1084.

24. Gulick RM, Mellors JW, Havlir D, et al. 3-year suppression of HIV viremia with indinavir, zidovudine, and lamivudine. *Ann Intern Med.* 2000;133:35-39.

25. Saltel E, Angel JB, Futter NG, et al. Increased prevalence and analysis of risk factors for indinavir nephrolithiasis. *J Urol.* 2000;164:1895-1897.

26. Kopp JB, Miller KD, Mican JA, et al. Crystalluria and urinary tract abnormalities associated with indinavir. *Ann Intern Med.* 1997; 127:119-125.

27. Hermieu JF, Prevot MH, Ravery V, et al. Nephritic colic due to indinavir (in French). *Presse Méd.* 1998;27:465-467.

28. Herman JS, Ives NJ, Nelson M, et al. Incidence and risk factors for the development of indinavir-associated renal complications. *J Antimicrob Chemother.* 2001;48:355-360.

29. Schwartz BF, Schenkman N, Armenakas NA, et al. Imaging characteristics of indinavir calculi. *J Urol.* 1999;161:1085-1087.

30. Gentle DL, Stoller ML, Jarrett TW, et al. Protease inhibitor-induced urolithiasis. *Urology.* 1997;50:508-511.

31. Kohan AD, Armenakas NA, Fracchia JA. Indinavir urolithiasis: an emerging cause of renal colic in patients with human immunodeficiency virus. *J Urol.* 1999;161:1765-1768.

32. Kopp JB, Falloon J, Fili A, et al. Indinavir-associated with interstitial nephritis and urothelial inflammation: clinical and cytologic findings. *Clin Infect Dis.* 2002;34:1122-1128.

33. Tashima KT, Horowitz J, Rosen S. Indinavir nephropathy. *N Engl J Med.* 1997;336:138-140.

34. Martinez F, Mommeja-Marin H, Estepa-Maurice L, et al. Indinavir crystal deposits associated with tubulointerstitial nephropathy. *Nephrol Dial Transplant.* 1998;13:750-753.

35. Daudon M, Estepa L, Viard JP, et al. Épidémiologie et facteurs de risque des complications lithiasiques de l'indinavir. *Feuill Biol.* 2001;42(242):31-34.

36. Balani SH, Arison BH, Mathai L, et al. Metabolites of L-735, 524, a potent HIV-1 protease inhibitor, in human urine. *Drug Metab Dispos.* 1995;23:266-270.

37. Chen IW, Vastag KJ, Lin JH. High-performance liquid chromatographic determination of a potent and selective HIV protease inhibitor (L-735, 524) in rat, dog and monkey plasma. *J Chromatogr B.* 1995;672:111-117.

38. Gagnon RF, Tecimer SN, Watters AK, et al. Prospective study of urinalysis abnormalities in HIV-positive individuals treated with indinavir. *Am J Kidney Dis.* 2000;36:507-515.

39. Famularo G, Di Toro S, Moretti S, et al. Symptomatic crystalluria associated with indinavir. *Ann Pharmacother.* 2000;34:1414-1418.

40. Malavaud B, Dinh B, Bonnet E, et al. Increased incidence of indinavir nephrolithiasis in patients with hepatitis B or C virus infection. *Antivir Ther.* 2000;5:3-5.

41. Dieleman JP, Sturkenboom MC, Jambroes M, et al. Risk factors for urological symptoms in a cohort of users of the HIV protease inhibitor indinavir sulfate: the ATHENA cohort. *Arch Intern Med.* 2002;162:1493-1501.

42. Burger DM, Hugen PW, Aamoutse RE, et al. A retrospective, cohort-based survey of patients using twice-daily indinavir + ritonavir combinations: pharmacokinetics, safety, and efficacy. *J Acquir Immune Defic Syndr.* 2001;26:218-224.

43. Engeler DS, John H, Rentsch KM, et al. Nelfinavir urinary stones. *J Urol.* 2002;167:1384-1385.

44. Cicconi P, Bongiovanni M, Melzi S, Tordato F, d'Arminio Monforte A, Bini T. Nephrolithiasis and hydronephrosis in an HIV-infected man receiving tenofovir. *Int J Antimicrob Agents.* 2004;24:284-285.

45. Izzedine H, M'Rad MB, Bardier A, Daudon M, Salmon D. Atazanavir crystal nephropathy. *AIDS.* 2007;21:2357-2358.

46. Chang HR, Pella PM. Atazanavir urolithiasis. *N Engl J Med.* 2006;355:2158-2159.

47. Couzigou C, Daudon M, Meynard JL, et al. Urolithiasis in HIV-positive patients treated with atazanavir. *Clin Infect Dis.* 2007;45:e105-e108.

48. Wirth GJ, Teuscher J, Graf JD. Iselin CE (2006) Efavirenz-induced urolithiasis. *Urol Res.* 2006;34:288-289.

49. Izzedine H, Valantin MA, Daudon M, Ait Mohand H, Caby F, Katlama C. Efavirenz urolithiasis. *AIDS.* 2007;21:1992. letter.

50. Antopol W, Robinson H. Urolithiasis and renal pathology after administration of sulfapyridine. *Proc Soc Exp Biol Med.* 1939;40: 428-439.

51. Newman HR, Shleser IH. Sulfonamide renal calculus. *J Urol.* 1942;47:258-259.

52. Schreiner GE, Maher JF. Toxic nephropathy. *Am J Med.* 1965;38:409-449.

53. Albala DM, Prien EL Jr, Galal HA. Urolithiasis as a hazard of sulfonamide therapy. *J Endourol.* 1994;8:401-403.

54. Potter JL, Kofron WG. Sulfadiazine/N4-acetylsulfadiazine crystalluria in a patient with the acquired immune deficiency syndrome (AIDS). *Clin Chim Acta.* 1994;230:221-224.

55. Catalano-Pons C, Bargy S, Schlecht D, et al. Sulfadiazine-induced nephrolithiasis in children. *Pediatr Nephrol.* 2004;19:928-931.

56. Erturk E, Casemento JB, Guertin KR, et al. Bilateral acetylsulfapyridine nephrolithiasis associated with chronic sulfasalazine therapy. *J Urol*. 1994;151:1605-1606.

57. Saito M, Takahashi C, Ishida G, Kadowaki H, Hirakawa S, Miyagawa I. Acute renal failure associated with sulfur calculi. *J Urol*. 2001;165:1985-1986.

58. Siegel WH. Unusual complication of therapy with sulfamethoxazole-trimethoprim. *J Urol*. 1977;117:397.

59. Rincé C, Daudon M, Moesch C, et al. Identification of flumequine in a urinary calculus. *J Clin Chem Clin Biochem*. 1987;25: 313-314.

60. Daudon M, Réveillaud RJ, Laurence C, et al. Drug-induced oxolinic acid crystalluria and nephrolithiasis. *Clin Nephrol*. 1987;28:156.

61. Chopra N, Fine PL, Price B, et al. Bilateral hydronephrosis from ciprofloxacin induced crystalluria and stone formation. *J Urol*. 2000;164:438.

62. Najjar MF, Rammah M, Oueslati A, et al. Apport de la spectrophotométrie infrarouge dans l'analyse des calculs urinaires. *Le Biologiste*. 1988;22:215-220.

63. Cochat P, Cochat N, Jouvenet M, et al. Ceftriaxone-associated nephrolithiasis. *Nephrol Dial Transplant*. 1990;5(11):974-976.

64. de Moor RA, Egberts AC, Schroder CH. Ceftriaxone-associated nephrolithiasis and biliary pseudolithiasis. *Eur J Pediatr*. 1999;158:975-977.

65. Avci Z, Koktener A, Uras N, et al. Nephrolithiasis associated with ceftriaxone therapy: a prospective study in 51 children. *Arch Dis Child*. 2004;89:1069-1072.

66. Crawford ED, Mulvaney WP. Rapid increase in calculous size: a possible hazard of phenazopyridine hydrochloride therapy in the presence of already formed stones. *J Urol*. 1978;119:280-281.

67. MacDonald JB, MacDonald ET. Nitrofurantoin crystalluria. *Br Med J*. 1976;ii:1044-1045.

68. Thorsteinsson SB, Bergan T, Oddsdottir S, et al. Crystalluria and ciprofloxacin, influence of urinary pH and hydration. *Chemotherapy*. 1986;32:408-417.

69. Herman JR, Goldberg AS. New type of urinary calculus caused by antacid therapy. *JAMA*. 1960;174:1206-1207.

70. Lagergren C. Development of silica calculi after oral administration of magnesium trisilicate. *J Urol*. 1962;87:994-996.

71. Augusti M, Mikaelian JC, Monsaint JC, Brin D, Daudon M. Un calcul urinaire de silice secondaire à l'absorption de Gélopectose chez un enfant. *Prog Urol*. 1993;3:812-815.

72. Ulinski T, Sabot JF, Bourlon I, Cochat P. Bilateral urinary calculi after treatment with a silicate-containing milk thickener. *Eur J Pediatr*. 2004;163:239-240.

73. Nishizono T, Eta S, Enokida H, Nishiyama K, Kawahara M, Nakagawa M. Renal silica calculi in an infant. *Int J Urol*. 2004;11:119-121.

74. Greene ML, Fujimoto WY, Seegmiller JE. Urinary xanthine stones: a rare complication of allopurinol therapy. *N Engl J Med*. 1969;280:426-427.

75. Kranen S, Keough D, Gordon RB, et al. Xanthine-containing calculi during allopurinol therapy. *J Urol*. 1985;133:658-659.

76. Stote RM, Smith LH, Dubb JW, et al. Oxypurinol nephrolithiasis in regional enteritis secondary to allopurinol therapy. *Ann Intern Med*. 1980;92:384-385.

77. Assimos DG, Langenstroer P, Leinbach RF, et al. Guaifenesin- and ephedrine-induced stones. *J Endourol*. 1999;13:665-667.

78. Pickens CL, Milliron AR, Fussner AL, et al. Abuse of guaifenesin-containing medications generates an excess of a carboxylate salt of beta-(2-methoxyphenoxy)-lactic acid, a guaifenesin metabolite, and results in urolithiasis. *Urology*. 1999;54:23-27.

79. Sharfstein JM, North M, Serwint JR. Over the counter but no longer under the radar–pediatric cough and cold medications. *N Engl J Med*. 2007;357:2321-2324.

80. Powell T, Hsu FF, Turk J, et al. Ma-Huang strikes again: ephedrine nephrolithiasis. *Am J Kidney Dis*. 1998;32:153-159.

81. Hoffman N, McGee SM, Hulbert JC. Resolution of ephedrine stones with dissolution therapy. *Urology*. 2003;61:1035.

82. Bennett S, Hoffman N, Monga M. Ephedrine- and guaifenesin-induced nephrolithiasis. *J Altern Complement Med*. 2004;10: 967-969.

83. Pak CYC. Nephrolithiasis from calcium supplementation. *J Urol*. 1987;137:1212-1213.

84. Jones G, Hogan DB, Yent DB, et al. Prevention and management of osteoporosis: consensus statements from scientific Advisory Board of the Osteoporosis Society of Canada. 8. Vitamin D metabolites and analogs in the treatment of osteoporosis. *Can Med Assoc J*. 1996;155:955-961.

85. Domrongkitchaiporn S, Ongphiphadhanakul B, Stitchantrakul W, et al. Risk of calcium oxalate nephrolithiasis after calcium or combined calcium and calcitriol supplementation in postmenopausal women. *Osteoporos Int*. 2000;11:486-492.

86. Jackson RD, LaCroix AZ, Gass M, et al. Calcium plus vitamin D supplementation and the risk of fractures. *N Engl J Med*. 2006;354: 669-683.

87. Daudon M. Épidémiologie actuelle de la lithiase rénale en France. *Ann Urol*. 2005;39:209-231.

88. Caralps A, Lloveras J, Andreu J, et al. Urinary calculi in chronic dialysis patients. *Lancet*. 1979;2(8150):1024-1025.

89. Oreopoulos DG, Silverberg S. Calcium oxalate urinary-tract stones in patients on maintenance dialysis. *N Engl J Med*. 1974;290:1438-1439.

90. Daudon M, Lacour B, Jungers P, et al. Urolithiasis in patients with end-stage renal failure. *J Urol*. 1992;147:977-980.

91. Katayama F, Miura H, Takanashi S. Long-term effectiveness and side effects of acetazolamide as an adjunct to other anticonvulsants in the treatment of refractory epilepsies. *Brain Dev*. 2002;24:150-154.

92. Persky L, Chambers D, Potts A. Calculus formation and ureteral colic following acetazolamide therapy. *JAMA*. 1956;161:1625-1626.

93. Kass M, Kolker AE, Gordon M, et al. Acetazolamide and urolithiasis. *Ophtalmology*. 1981;88:261-265.

94. Tawil R, Moxley RT 3rd, Griggs RC. Acetazolamide-induced nephrolithiasis: implications for treatment of neuromuscular disorders. *Neurology*. 1993;43:1105-1106.

95. Ellis PP. Urinary calculi with methazolamide therapy. *Doc Ophtalmol*. 1973;34:137-142.

96. Carlsen J, Durcan J, Zabriskie N, et al. Nephrolithiasis with dorzolamide. *Arch Ophthalmol*. 1999;117:1087-1088.

97. Paisley KE, Tomson CR. Calcium phosphate stones during long-term acetazolamide treatment for epilepsy. *Postgrad Med J*. 1999;75:427-428.

98. Ahlstrand C, Tiselius HG. Urine composition and stone formation during treatment with acetazolamide. *Scand J Urol Nephrol*. 1987;21:225-228.

99. Higashihara E, Nutahara K, Takeuchi T, Shoji N, Araie M, Aso Y. Calcium metabolism in acidotic patients induced by carbonic anhydrase inhibitors: responses to citrate. *J Urol*. 1991;145: 942-948.

100. Barbey F, Nseir G, Ferrier C, Burnier M, Daudon M. Inhibiteurs de l'anhydrase carbonique et lithiase urinaire phosphocalcique. *Néphrologie*. 2004;25:169-172.

101. Perucca E. A pharmacological and clinical review on topiramate, a new antiepileptic drug. *Pharmacol Res*. 1997;35:241-256.

102. Natsch S, Hekster YA, Keyser A, et al. Newer anticonvulsant drugs: role of pharmacology, drug interactions and adverse reactions in drug choice. *Drug Saf*. 1997;17:228-240.

103. Saito Y, Yanagaki S, Oguni H, et al. Urolithiasis induced by combined ACTH and zonisamide treatment in a patient with startle induced epilepsy. *No To Hattatsu*. 2002;34:415-420.

104. Kossoff EH, Pyzik PL, Furth SL, Hladky HD, Freeman JM, Vining EP. Kidney stones, carbonic anhydrase inhibitors, and the ketogenic diet. *Epilepsia.* 2002;43:1168-1171.

105. Kuo RL, Moran ME, Kim DH, Abrahams HM, White MD, Lingeman JE. Topiramate-induced nephrolithiasis. *J Endourol.* 2002;16:229-231.

106. Vega D, Maalouf NM, Sakhaee K. Increased propensity for calcium phosphate kidney stones with topiramate use. *Expert Opin Drug Saf.* 2007;6:547-557.

107. Wroe S. Zonisamide and renal calculi in patients with epilepsy: how big an issue? *Curr Med Res Opin.* 2007;23:1765-1773.

108. Lamb EJ, Stevens PE, Nashef L. Topiramate increases biochemical risk of nephrolithiasis. *Ann Clin Biochem.* 2004;41:166-169.

109. Welch BJ, Graybeal D, Moe OW, Maalouf NM, Sakhaee K. Biochemical and stone-risk profiles with topiramate treatment. *Am J Kidney Dis.* 2006;48:555-563.

110. Sheth RD. Metabolic concerns associated with antiepileptic medications. *Neurology.* 2004;63:S24-S29.

111. Noe HN, Bryant JF, Roy S 3rd, et al. Urolithiasis in pre-term neonates associated with furosemide therapy. *J Urol.* 1984;132:93-94.

112. Alon US. Nephrocalcinosis. *Curr Opin Pediatr.* 1997;9:160-165.

113. Shukla AR, Hoover DL, Homsy YL, Perlman S, Schurman S, Reisman EM. Urolithiasis in the low birth weight infant: the role and efficacy of extracorporeal shock wave lithotripsy. *J Urol.* 2001;165:2320-2323.

114. Kim YG, Kim B, Kim MK, et al. Medullary nephrocalcinosis associated with long-term furosemide abuse in adults. *Nephrol Dial Transplant.* 2001;16:2303-2309.

115. Sidhu H, Schmidt ME, Cornelius JG, et al. Direct correlation between hyperoxaluria/oxalate stone disease and the absence of the gastrointestinal tract-dwelling bacterium Oxalobacter formigenes: possible prevention by gut recolonization or enzyme replacement therapy. *J Am Soc Nephrol.* 1999;10(Suppl 14):S334-S340.

116. Gibney EM, Goldfarb DS. The association of nephrolithiasis with cystic fibrosis. *Am J Kidney Dis.* 2003;42:1-11.

117. Böhles H, Gebhardt B, Beeg T, Sewell AC, Solem E, Posselt G. Antibiotic treatment-induced tubular dysfunction as a risk factor for renal stone formation in cystic fibrosis. *J Pediatr.* 2002;140:103-109.

118. Perez-Brayfield MR, Caplan D, Gatti JM, Smith EA, Kirsch AJ. Metabolic risk factors for stone formation in patients with cystic fibrosis. *J Urol.* 2002;167:480-484.

119. Hoppe B, von Unruh GE, Blank G, et al. Absorptive hyperoxaluria leads to an increased risk for urolithiasis or nephrocalcinosis in cystic fibrosis. *Am J Kidney Dis.* 2005;46:440-445.

120. Terribile M, Capuano M, Cangiano G, et al. Factors increasing the risk for stone formation in adult patients with cystic fibrosis. *Nephrol Dial Transplant.* 2006;21:1870-1875.

121. Troxel SA, Sidhu H, Kaul P, Low RK. Intestinal Oxalobacter formigenes colonization in calcium oxalate stone formers and its relation to urinary oxalate. *J Endourol.* 2003;17:173-176.

122. Robson RH, Heading RC. Obsolete but dangerous antacid preparations. *Postgrad Med J.* 1978;54:36-37.

123. Howard SC, Kaplan SD, Razzouk BI, et al. Urolithiasis in pediatric patients with acute lymphoblastic leukemia. *Leukemia.* 2003;17:541-546.

124. Kamitsuka MD, Williams MA, Nyberg DA, et al. Renal calcification: a complication of dexamethasone therapy in preterm infants with bronchopulmonary dysplasia. *J Perinatal.* 1995;15:359-363.

125. Urivetzky M, Kessaris D, Smith AD. Ascorbic acid overdosing: a risk factor for calcium oxalate nephrolithiasis. *J Urol.* 1992;147:1215-1218.

126. Traxer O, Huet B, Poindexter J, Pak CY, Pearle MS. Effect of ascorbic acid consumption on urinary stone risk factors. *J Urol.* 2003;170:397-401.

127. Smith LH. Risk of oxalate stone from large doses of vitamin C. *N Engl J Med.* 1978;298:856.

128. Curhan GC, Willett WC, Rimm EB, et al. A prospective study of the intake of vitamins C and B6, and the risk of kidney stones in men. *J Urol.* 1996;155:1847-1851.

129. Curhan GC, Willett WC, Speizer FE, et al. Intake of vitamins B6 and C and the risk of kidney stones in women. *J Am Soc Nephrol.* 1999;10:840-845.

130. Moesch C, Charmes JP, Bouthier F, et al. Calcium oxalate crystalluria in elderly patients and treatment with naftidrofuryl oxalate. *Age Ageing.* 1995;24:464-467.

131. Daudon M, Reveillaud RJ, Jungers P. Piridoxilate-associated calcium oxalate urinary calculi: a new metabolic drug-induced nephrolithiasis. *Lancet.* 1985;8441:1338.

132. Vigeral P, Kenouch S, Chauveau D, et al. Piridoxilate-associated nephrocalcinosis: a new form of chronic oxalate nephropathy. *Nephrol Dial Transplant.* 1987;2:275-278.

133. Dick WH, Lingeman JE, Preminger GM, et al. Laxative abuse as a cause for ammonium urate renal calculi. *J Urol.* 1990;143:244-247.

134. Soble JJ, Hamilton BD, Streem SB. Ammonium acid urate calculi: a reevaluation of risk factors. *J Urol.* 1999;161:869-873.

135. Schlesinger N. Management of acute and chronic gouty arthritis: present state-of-the-art. *Drugs.* 2004;64:2399-2416.

136. Becker MA, Schumacher HR Jr, Wortmann RL, et al. Febuxostat compared with allopurinol in patients with hyperuricemia and gout. *N Engl J Med.* 2005;353:2450-2461.

137. Sperling O, Brosh S, Boer P, et al. Urinary xanthine stones in an allopurinol-treated gouty patient with partial deficiency of hypoxanthine-guanine phosphoribosyltransferase. *Isr J Med Sci.* 1978;14:288-292.

138. Brock WA, Golden J, Kaplan GW. Xanthine calculi in the Lesch-Nyhan syndrome. *J Urol.* 1983;130:157-159.

Endemic Bladder Stones

20

Narmada P. Gupta and Anup Kumar

Abstract The bladder is the most commonly affected site for stone formation in the lower urinary tract. The incidence of vesical calculi has declined significantly in the last 50 years in developed countries due to improvements in nutrition and diet. Bladder calculi can be classified as primary idiopathic/endemic, migrant, and secondary calculi. Primary idiopathic/endemic bladder calculi are those calculi that form typically in children, in absence of bladder outlet obstruction/neurogenic bladder leading to urinary stasis, urinary tract infection, or foreign body.

20.1 Introduction

Bladder calculi have affected mankind for many centuries. The bladder is the most commonly affected site for stone formation in the lower urinary tract. The incidence of vesical calculi has declined significantly in the last 50 years in developed countries due to improvements in nutrition and diet. Presently, bladder calculi account for 5% of all urinary tract calculi in adults.[1-4]

Bladder calculi can be classified, according to underlying etiology, as primary idiopathic/endemic, migrant, and secondary calculi. Migrant bladder calculi develop in the upper urinary tract, migrate into the bladder, and are subsequently retained in the bladder. The primary etiology of these stones is due to metabolic factors associated with formation of renal stones. The secondary calculi form due to urinary stasis, recurrent urinary tract infection due to bladder outlet obstruction/neurogenic bladder, and foreign bodies. The primary idiopathic/endemic bladder calculi are those calculi that form typically in children, in absence of bladder outlet obstruction/neurogenic bladder leading to urinary stasis, urinary tract infection, or foreign body.

20.2 Epidemiology

Endemic bladder calculi virtually disappeared from Northern Europe during the late nineteenth century[5] and from Southern Europe by 1970.[6] The endemic bladder calculi have become rare in developed countries due to industrialization and improvement in nutrition and diet. The incidence of these stones is very low in Central and South America, and Central and South Africa. However, these stones remain an important cause of morbidity in an endemic belt extending from the Middle East across India and Thailand to Indonesia, including North Africa, whose economies are primarily dependent on agriculture. This belt includes Algeria, Sub-Saharan Africa, Rwanda, Ethiopia, Sudan, and Egypt, through Iraq, Iran, Afghanistan, India, Southeast Asia, and Indonesia. The stones are more common in India in the northern and western regions as compared to southern and eastern regions. The incidence of endemic bladder calculi was high in children living in rural areas of India until 1980. However, this incidence has decreased in the last few years due to better nutrition and diet. There is a simultaneous increase in upper urinary tract stones.[7-12] The incidence has decreased in the Philippines, Taiwan, and Singapore.[13-15] However, these stones have also been found in the western Australian region, especially in aboriginal children.[16] These stones are typically found in infants and children of lower socioeconomic status. Children younger than 10 years are most commonly affected, with a peak incidence around 3 years. The male-to-female ratio is 10:1.[8,9,17]

N.P. Gupta (✉)
Department of Urology, All India Institute of Medical Sciences, New Delhi, India
e-mail: narmadagupta@gmail.com

P.N. Rao et al. (eds.), *Urinary Tract Stone Disease*,
DOI 10.1007/978-1-84800-362-0_20, © Springer-Verlag London Limited 2011

20.3 Etiopathogenesis

The composition of endemic bladder calculi includes most commonly ammonium acid urate alone, or in combination with calcium oxalate, but may also contain calcium phosphate. These stones form mainly due to dietary and nutritional deficiencies in these children, who are fed with a cereal-based diet (low protein, high carbohydrate diet), lacking in animal proteins.[17-24] The cereals commonly used are whole wheat flour, millet, and rice. The animal proteins constitute less than 25% of total protein intake in these children. Endemic bladder calculi are more prevalent at low levels of animal protein intake, as compared to upper urinary tract stones in adults.[23] A study has related hospitalization rates due to bladder stones to average protein intake of the respective country. There is an increasing incidence of bladder calculi in children, as animal protein intake falls below 40 g/day. As animal protein intake increases to more than 40 g/day, incidence of bladder stones decreases; however, incidence of upper tract stones increases in adults worldwide.[18]

Human breast milk and cereals are deficient in phosphorus, as compared to cow's milk. Therefore, a high cereal/low animal protein diet is acidogenic and low in phosphate. This causes a decrease in urinary phosphate concentration, which is insufficient to buffer relative high excretion of hydrogen ions. Therefore renal ammonia production increases. The other contributing factors include: decrease in urinary volume due to chronic diarrhea/poor water supply/high ambient temperature; increased urinary uric acid concentration due to rapid tissue turnover in children (which falls back to normal adult concentration by the age of 10 years); deficiencies in vitamin A, B1, B6, and magnesium. All these factors result in supersaturation of urine by ammonium acid urate, leading to risk of crystalluria. These crystals aggregate in the bladder forming ammonium acid urate stones, instead of the upper urinary tract, because urinary stasis occurs in the bladder for some time. Also, a diet low in calcium, such as rice, little or no milk, and soft water, would cause hypocalciuria, leading to precipitation of ammonium acid urate in vitro.[25] Additionally, high intake of green leafy vegetables containing high levels of oxalate causes increases in urinary oxalate concentration. Therefore, these children have crystalluria of both ammonium acid urate and calcium oxalate, leading to formation of mixed ammonium acid urate and calcium oxalate stones.[17-26]

The predisposing risk factors are listed in Table 20.1, and the etiopathogenesis is summarized in Fig. 20.1.

Endemic bladder calculi are more prevalent in boys as compared to girls. Boys have a longer urethra that is more tortuous, containing narrow regions, therefore less likely to pass any crystals and aggregates formed in the bladder. Therefore, boys are more predisposed to bladder stones

Table 20.1 Predisposing risk factors

1. Hot climate
2. Chronic diarrhea/dehydration states
3. Cereal-based diet: low phosphate, acidogenic
4. Decreased animal milk intake (less than 25% of total protein intake): low phosphate, calcium
5. Increased oxalate consumption (green leafy vegetables)
6. Nutritional deficiency of vitamin A, B_1, B_6, and magnesium
7. Male sex: longer, tortuous urethra
8. Increased tissue turnover in children younger than 10 years

formation. However, girls have a short, non-tortuous urethra, therefore more likely to pass crystals formed in the bladder.[8,9,17]

20.4 Clinical Presentation

Endemic bladder stones are commonly found in infants and children of less than 10 years of age, with a male-to-female predisposition of 10:1. The clinical presentation may be in the form of passage of cloudy, sandy urine, indicating early stages of stone formation. The symptoms may be relieved by making a recumbent position. Other presenting features include interruption of urinary stream intermittently, with increase in terminal dysuria, caused due to impaction of stone at the bladder neck. Other clinical features include lower abdominal pain referring to tip of penis, scrotum, perineum, or hip; pain may be of varying intensity, increasing by sudden movements; pulling and rubbing of penis; frequency, intermittent dysuria, hematuria, and dribbling of urine. The smaller calculi may pass spontaneously; however, larger stones may cause acute urinary retention (although rare). The repeated straining during voiding can give rise to rectal prolapse and conjunctival hemorrhages. The symptoms may be present from a few days to several years.[1,2,9,17]

20.5 Diagnosis

Endemic bladder calculi are usually solitary.[9,17] A detailed clinical history including the dietary history will help in identifying predisposing risk factors (listed in Table 20.1), as well as ruling out underlying pathology; e.g., neurogenic bladder, posterior urethral valves, urinary tract infection. The clinical symptoms may simulate a urinary tract infection/inflammatory pathology. Urine routine microscopy and culture sensitivity should be done to rule out urinary infection, and also to detect urine pH, presence of red blood cells, and crystals. A plain X-ray KUB (kidney, ureter, and bladder) region (after adequate bowel preparation) can detect a radio-opaque

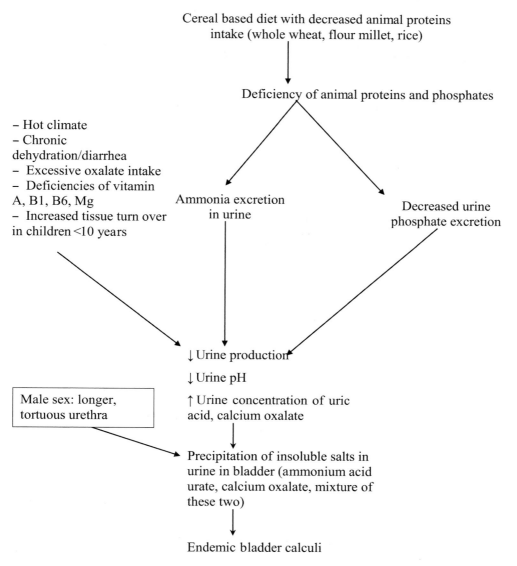

Fig. 20.1 Pathophysiology of endemic bladder stones

bladder calculus. However, some stones can be missed due to their radiolucent nature and poor bowel preparation with overlying gas shadows. A pure ammonium acid urate calculus is radiolucent. However, calcium oxalate stones or mixed ammonium acid urate and calcium oxalate calculi are radio-opaque. These stones can also be diagnosed using an ultrasound of the KUB region, which can also help in ruling out causes of secondary bladder stones. However, this is operator dependent. An intravenous urogram can detect a radiolucent calculus as a filling defect in a partially filled bladder. Non-contrast computed tomography (NCCT) of the KUB region can detect both radiolucent and radio-opaque bladder calculi. It can also predict the composition of bladder stone depending on the Hounsefield unit value of stone density. Cystoscopy

is considered to be the most accurate examination to diagnose a bladder stone.[1,2,9,17]

20.6 Treatment

Endemic calculi have a unique feature that they rarely recur after removal. The optimal treatment modality can be decided based on the following considerations: size and composition of stone, previous surgery on the lower urinary tract, patient morphology, compliance and follow-up risk, cost, available instrumentation, experience of the surgeon, along with risks and complications involved with a particular procedure for the patient.[1,2,9,17]

Small calculi may pass spontaneously with adequate hydration, antispasmodic drugs, and analgesics. The patients are advised to eat a mixed cereal diet, along with milk protein supplements (animal protein >25% of total protein intake). The majority of cases require surgical intervention.[1,2]

Shockwave lithotripsy (SWL) can be considered in those children who are unfit for surgery due to coexisting comorbidities, and if parents refuse surgery. Multiple treatment sessions of SWL may be required to achieve stone-free status. The use of piezoelectric lithotripters and larger bladder calculi have shown lower success rates with SWL.[1,2,27]

Endemic bladder calculi of less than 1 cm can be managed safely by transurethral cystolithotripsy. The small caliber penile urethra and concerns about iatrogenic urethral stricture make this procedure more difficult. However, the availability of newer, small-sized pediatric rigid/flexible cystoscopes, along with small-sized probes of pneumatic lithoclast and holmium: YAG laser for lithotripsy (200/365 μm), has made this procedure safer and easier.[1,2]

Percutaneous cystolithotripsy (PCCLT) is a safer alternative with low morbidity and complication rates for large bladder calculi up to 5 cm in size. A suprapubic puncture is made under cystoscopic guidance. The tract is subsequently dilated sequentially with amplatz fascial dilators. Using a 30 Fr amplatz sheath, a 26 Fr nephroscope can be passed into the bladder without urethral injury. The large and hard stones can be broken and removed in large fragments, thus decreasing the operating time. PCCLT has advantages of shorter hospital stay, better cosmesis, and decreased morbidity and wound infection as compared to open surgery.[28–32]

Open cystolithotomy is recommended for multiple bladder calculi, large bladder calculus >5 cm, and solitary bladder stone of any size where PCCLT is not available. The poor socioeconomic status favors cost, and an assured stone-free status makes open surgery more popular in developing countries, rather than giving importance to incision-free surgery. Moreover, the healing is much faster and less complicated in children, as compared to adults, leading to a shorter convalescence period. Open cystolithotomy has the problems of a long scar, prolonged catheterization, risk of infection, and increased hospitalization, as compared to PCCLT. It is still the main modality of treatment in developing countries, in spite of development of miniature endoscopes.[1,33–35] A study comparing the efficacy of open cystolithotomy and cystolitholapaxy in pediatric patients with primary bladder calculi concluded that endourological procedures have a shorter hospital stay, similar operating time, but significantly more complications, as compared to open surgery.[34]

20.7 Conclusions

A mixed cereal diet supplemented with animal milk/animal proteins, along with correction of dehydration/diarrhea, and avoiding excess oxalate consumption (green leafy vegetables) can decrease the incidence of endemic bladder stones.[8,9,17]

References

1. Athanasios GP, Ioannis V, Athanasios D, Deliveliotis C. Bladder lithiasis: From open surgery to lithotripsy. *Urol Res.* 2006;34(3): 163-167.
2. Schwartz BF, Stoller ML. The vesical calculus. *Urol Clin North Am.* 2000;27(2):333-346.
3. Takasaki E, Murahashi I, Nagata M. A 4 year retrospective study of urolithiasis. *Dokkyo J Med Sci.* 1979;6:120.
4. Yoshida O. A chronological and geographical study of urolithiasis in Japan. *Jpn J Endourol ESWL.* 1990;3:5.
5. Ellis H. *A History of Bladder Stone.* Oxford: Blackwell; 1969.
6. Pavone-Maculuso M, Miano L. Epidemiology of urolithiasis in Italy. In 18th Congress de la Societe Internationale d'Urology, Paris, July 1979, pp. 113-137.
7. Robertson WG. The changing pattern of urolithiasis in UK and its causes. In: Kok DJ, Romijn HC, Verhagen PCMS, et al., eds. *Eurolithiasis.* Maastricht: Shaker; 2001:9-11.
8. Robertson WG. Renal stones in the tropics. *Semin Nephrol.* 2003;23(1):77-87.
9. Halstead SB. Studies on the epidemiology of idiopathic bladder stone disease. In: Van Reen R, ed. *Proceedings of WHO Regional Symposium on Vesical calculus Disease.* Washington: US Department of Health, Education and Welfare; 1977:121-134.
10. Kamardi T, Soemanto M, Rizal A, et al. Epidemiology of bladder stones in West Sumatra. In: Brockis JG, Finlayson B, eds. *Urinary Calculus.* Littleton: PSG; 1981:195-203.
11. Bakane BC, Nagtilak SB, Patil B. Urolithiasis: a tribal scenario. *Indian J Pediatr.* 1999;66:863-865.
12. Rahman MA, Van Reen R. Current investigations of vesical calculus disease in Pakistan. In: Van Reen R, ed. *Proceedings of WHO Regional Symposium on Vesical calculus Disease.* Washington: US Department of Health, Education and Welfare; 1977:57-67.
13. Hsu T-C. Petrographic studies on urinary calculi. *J Formos Med Assoc.* 1962;61:937-941.
14. Tambyah JA, Murugasu JJ, Tan IK, et al. Urinary calculi in Singapore – a study of 254 patients. *Singapore Med J.* 1972;13:269-272.
15. Navarro MD, Guevara BQ. An analytical study by infra-red spectroscopy of the constituents of urinary calculi found among Philippine residents. *J Philipp Med Assoc.* 1974;50:185-214.
16. Jones TW, Henderson TR. Urinary calculi in children in Western Australia. *Aust Paediatr.* 1989;25:93-95.
17. Teotia M, Teotia SP. Endemic vesical stone: nutritional factors. *Indian Pediatr.* 1987;24(2):1117-1121.
18. Robertson WG. Urolithiasis: epidemiology and pathogenesis. In: Husain I, ed. *Tropical Urology and Renal Disease.* London: Heinemann; 1982:267-278.
19. Ansari MS, Gupta NP. Impact of socio-economic status in etiology and management of urinary stone disease. *Urol Int.* 2003;70(4): 255-261.

20. Brockis JG, Bowyer RC, McCulloch RK, et al. Physiopathology of endemic bladder stones. In: Brockis JG, Finlayson B, eds. *Urinary Calculus*. Littleton: PSG; 1981:225-236.

21. Anasuya A, Narasinga Rao BS. Studies on the role of nutritional factors in urinary lithiasis. *Invest Urol.* 1973;10:426-428.

22. Valyasevi A, Halstead SB, Dhanamitta S. Studies of bladder stone disease in Thailand.VI. Urinary studies in children, 2–10 years old, resident in a hypo and hyper-endemic area. *Am J Clin Nutr.* 1967;20:1362-1368.

23. Anderson DA. History of bladder stone disease. In: Van Reen R, ed. *Proceedings of WHO Regional Symposium on Vesical Calculus Disease*. Washington: US Department of Health, Education and Welfare; 1977:1-16.

24. Valyasevi A, Halstead SB, Dhanamitta S. Studies of bladder stone disease in Thailand. IV. Dietary habits, nutritional intake and infant feeding practices among residents of a hypo and hyper-endemic area. *Am J Clin Nutr.* 1967;20:1340-1351.

25. Bowyer RC, Brockis JG, McCulloch RK. The role of common urinary constituents in the precipitation of ammonium acid urate. *Clin Chem Acta.* 1979;99:221-227.

26. Brockis JG, Bowyer RC, Ryan G, Taylor TA, Kamardi T, Rizal A. Endemic bladder stones in Indonesia. In: Smith LH, Robertson WG, Finlayson PB, eds. *Urolithiasis. Clinical and basic research*. London: Plenum; 1981:329-332.

27. Kostakopoulos A, Stavropoulos NJ, Makrichortis C, et al. Extracorporeal shock wave lithotripsy monotherapy for bladder stones. *Int Urol Nephrol.* 1996;28:157.

28. Salah MA, Holman E, Khan AM, Toth C. Percutaneous cystolithotomy for pediatric endemic bladder stone: experience with 155 cases from 2 developing countries. *Pediatr Surg.* 2005;40(10): 1628-1631.

29. Agrawal MS, Aron M, Goyal J, Elhence IP, Asopa HS. Percutaneous suprapubic cystolithotomy for vesical calculi in children. *J Endourol.* 1999;13:173-175.

30. Maheshwari PN, Oswal AT, Bansal M. Percutaneous cystolithotomy for vesical calculi: a better approach. *Tech Urol.* 1999;5:40-42.

31. Demirel F, Cakan M, Yalcinkaya F, Demirel AC, Aygun A, Altug UU. Percutaneous suprapubic cystolithotomy approach: for whom? Why? *J Endourol.* 2006;20:429-431.

32. Salah MA, Holman E, Toth C. Percutaneous suprapubic cystolithotomy for pediatric bladder stones in a developing country. *Eur Urol.* 2001;39:466-470.

33. Paik ML, Resnick MI. Is there a role for open stone surgery? *Urol Clin North Am.* 2000;27:323-331.

34. Mahran MR, Dawaba MS. Cystolitholapaxy versus cystolithotomy in children. *J Endourol.* 2000;14:423-426.

35. Zargooshi J. Open stone surgery in children: is it justified in the era of minimally invasive therapies? *BJU Int.* 2001;88:928-931.

Economic Implications of Medical and Surgical Management

21

Walter Ludwig Strohmaier

Abstract Urolithiasis is a considerable economic burden for the health systems, especially in industrialized countries where the incidence of stone disease increased continuously during the last decades, and probably will further increase for several reasons. The costs for surgical and medical treatment, as well as for diagnosis of stones, vary tremendously between the different health care systems. Several calculation models showed that metaphylaxis is not only medically but also economically effective when used in a rational way. Rational metaphylaxis does mean that not every stone former is evaluated metabolically and given specific metaphylaxis. This is restricted to patients with a high risk for recurrence (brushite, uric acid, cystine and infected stones, patients with residual fragments after stone treatment, and recurrent calcium oxalate stone formers). For these patients, metaphylaxis is cost-effective in almost all health care systems, the amount of savings however being different. The savings increase even more when adding the economic loss by avoiding the missed days of work due to treatment of recurrent stones.

21.1 Introduction

In industrial countries, the incidence of urolithiasis increased significantly during the last decades.[1] In the USA, the expenses for the treatment of stone disease increased between 1994 and 2000 by 50%.[2] This is an enormous burden for health care systems. There are several reasons for this development.

Extracorporeal shock wave lithotripsy (ESWL) has revolutionized the therapy of urolithiasis. It is a noninvasive treatment with only a few side effects.[3] During the last decades, endoscopic stone therapy evolved into a very effective, only minimally invasive treatment with a low complication rate as well.

Regarding the ease of these therapies, many urologists have challenged the role of metabolic evaluation and metaphylaxis in renal stone disease.[4] Why should we bother our patients with cumbersome dietary restrictions and medical treatment and not treat the recurrent stone when it occurs?

A number of medical reasons speak well for stone metaphylaxis: The recurrence rate is probably higher following

ESWL.[5,6] ESWL is not without side effects.[3,7] Twenty percent of all recurrent calcium stone formers eventually develop renal insufficiency.[8] Urolithiasis increases the risk for arterial hypertension.[9] Apart from medical arguments for metaphylaxis, the economic standpoint plays an ever-increasing role in developing therapeutic strategies.

21.2 Costs for Stone Removal (Surgical Management)

Although its role is declining due to increasingly sophisticated endoscopic treatment modalities, ESWL is still the treatment used most frequently. Originally, it was assumed that ESWL could save 40–140 million DM (i.e., 20–60 million €) in Germany. In 1986, however, it has already caused an increase in cost of 42 million DM (21 million €).[10] So far, there were only few data on the actual cost for stone removal. Most of these were estimations.

In 1995 (USA), the costs for the treatment of a ureter and a renal stone were estimated at 2,500 and 3,000 € respectively.[11] Between 1994 and 2000, the total annual expenditure for stone treatment in the USA increased by 50%. In 2000, the total

W.L. Strohmaier (✉)
Professor, Head, Department of Urology and Paediatric, RegioMed, Klinikum Coburg, Coburg, Bayern, Germany
e-mail: walter.strohmaier@klinikum-coburg.de

P.N. Rao et al. (eds.), *Urinary Tract Stone Disease*,
DOI 10.1007/978-1-84800-362-0_21, © Springer-Verlag London Limited 2011

costs were estimated at \$2.1 billion annually.[2] By far the most of this was spent for surgical treatment (stone removal). Due to climate change, an increase in the prevalence of urolithiasis is predicted (about 4% per °C). Annual stone-related health care costs will increase by 25% in 2050 when compared to the present-day costs.[12]

For Sweden (1991), the average cost for renal/ureteral stone therapy was valued 2,900 € per episode.[13]

For Great Britain, another publication[6] assessed the average cost at 3,520 €.

For the first time in Germany, some years ago we could obtain actual figures on the cost for stone treatment. In a district of a German social health care insurance company with 150,000 insured people, in 1997 the actual cost for inpatient renal and ureteral stone therapy was 5,907 € per case. In 1997, there were 426 patients off work in this district due to urolithiasis (N 20, ICD 10). This was about 300 urolithiasis cases per 100,000 people. Of 426 patients, 293 (68.9%) with renal stone disease were hospitalized; the others were treated on an outpatient basis. This is in accordance with a previous estimation of 75% of patients requiring hospitalization.[14]

In the USA, the number of stone patients per year is estimated at 485 of 100,000 people, a number that is in accordance to that found in Germany. In the USA, however, only 140 admissions to hospital of 100,000 people were estimated (29%).[11] In Sweden, during the early 1980s, 140 stone formers of 100,000 people were seen – 38% requiring hospitalization.[15]

In Germany, the new reimbursement system with the introduction of diagnosis related groups (DRG) changed the situation when compared to our calculation model mentioned previously. The costs now are related to stone location and treatment modality. For our hospital, the Klinikum Coburg, the reimbursement for ESWL is 1,394 €; percutaneous nephrolithotomy (PCNL) 3,107 €; ureterorenoscopy (URS) in kidney stones 1,532 €; and URS for ureteral stones 1,632 €. The figures for PCNL and URS for ureteral stones can go up to 4,487 and 2,771 € in complicated cases. Repeated treatments for the same stone will be reimbursed again when done 2 weeks after the end of the first treatment. It is a paradox that reimbursement for the more complicated cases with flexible URS for kidney stones with expensive scopes and ancillary instruments is worse than for a standard rigid ureteroscopy for ureteral stones (concerning costs for flexible URS see below).

The reimbursement, however, is different from hospital to hospital due to the individual "base rate." This "base rate" is dependent on the budget for the year 1995. For many hospitals, the reimbursement for these treatments is about 15–20% higher than ours. In 2009, however, the "base rates" will be the same for all hospitals in one federal state.

These different data clearly demonstrate that figures from one cannot be taken for calculation models in another health care system. Structures and expenses in the different health care systems vary considerably. This also applies to one and the same health care system when the rules for reimbursement are changed.

Concerning the cost-effectiveness of the different treatment modalities, only some data exist. For large stag horn stones, PCNL has been shown to be more cost-effective than ESWL.[16] For smaller stones (<1 cm), however, ESWL was better.[17] When regarding the cost-effectiveness, it should, however, be considered that the third-generation lithotripters most commonly used today, are less powerful than the first-generation machines.

The progress in endoscopic stone therapy by using flexible scopes undoubtedly has increased success rates and lowered morbidity. On the other hand, the expenses for flexible ureteroscopes and even more for disposable instrumentation are considerable. Collins et al.,[18] calculated 52.000 £ for 100 procedures (520 £ = 780 €), only for the scope and the ancillary instruments.

21.3 Costs for Metabolic Evaluation and Metaphylaxis (Medical Management)

Parks and Coe[19] calculated the cost-effectiveness of metaphylaxis for patients attending their stone clinic: They found a reduction of about 2,800 € in costs for stone removal per patient.

The Bonn group[20] showed that an effective metabolic evaluation and metaphylaxis lowered the recurrence rate by 46%. This was achieved by an extensive metabolic evaluation program in every stone former. The costs for such a screening are 250–350 €[6,19] while the costs for drug treatment were estimated at 130 €, 350 €, and 13 € per patient per year.[6,19,21]

The benefit of such extensive programs, however, is questionable. First, the overall recurrence rate in stone disease is 50%. More than 50% of recurrent stone formers have only one recurrence during their life. Only less than 10% of recurrent stone patients have more than three recurrences.[22,23] The figure of six or more recurrences over 30 years for one stone former[6,19] are derived from patients attending special referring centers that are not representative for the average stone patient.

Second, metabolic evaluation is not a good predictor for the risk of recurrence.[15,24–26]

Third, from the therapeutic standpoint, such extensive programs are abundant. Many parameters do not result in consequences for therapy. In patients with a low risk for recurrence, the motivation to keep on a strict metaphylaxis regimen is low.

Therefore, a more rational approach for metabolic evaluation and metaphylaxis[14,27,28] is reasonable. This approach should be oriented to the stone composition, recurrence rate, therapeutic consequences and expenses. It is the base for our following calculation model.

21.4 Calculation Models: Comparison of Costs for Stone Removal Versus Metabolic Evaluation/Metaphylaxis

The epidemiology of urolithiasis and costs for stone removal, metabolic evaluation, and metaphylaxis vary from country to country. Therefore, as shown by Chandhoke,[29] cost-effectiveness of metaphylaxis is dependent not only on stone frequency but also on the costs for the different treatment modalities, which can vary considerably between the national health care systems.

Some years ago, we developed a calculation model that was based not only on estimations but on actual figures from a German social health care insurance company.[30] The principles of the following calculation model, however, are applicable to every health care system. Therefore it is reported here in more detail.

21.4.1 Calculation Model: Comparison of Costs for Stone Removal Versus Metabolic Evaluation/Metaphylaxis in Germany

21.4.1.1 Costs for Stone Removal

The calculation model of the cost-effectiveness of metabolic evaluation and metaphylaxis (i.e., annual cost for stone removal vs. metabolic evaluation and metaphylaxis) is presented with figures from Germany. Our model uses representative figures for epidemiology and recurrence rates that are not derived from selected patients attending specialized referring centers.

In Germany, the number of stone recurrence is about 200,000 per year.[23,31] According to figures from the previously mentioned district of the German social health care insurance company (hospitalization rate 68.9%), the annual costs were 0.815 billion €. To avoid being blamed for taking the part for metaphylaxis, a hospitalization rate of only 50% is assumed for this calculation model. Thus, the annual costs for inpatient stone removal in recurrent stone formers are 0.59 billion € in Germany.

The actual costs for outpatient stone removal can hardly be calculated due to the structures of the Kassenärztliche Vereinigungen (i.e., associations of office physicians). According to the "EBM" (list of medical fees in the German social health care insurance system) it may be estimated, however, that the diagnosis of a stone episode and conservative treatment aiming in spontaneous stone passage cost about 85 € and 8 € respectively. Thus, outpatient treatment of recurrent stone formers (i.e., 100,000 cases annually) costs about 9 million €. Expenses for active outpatient stone removal (e.g., ESWL, URS) are not considered. The number of such procedures is, however, low when compared to active stone removal on an inpatient base.

21.4.1.2 Costs for Metabolic Evaluation/Metaphylaxis

The rational and cost-effective metabolic evaluation and metaphylaxis program as outlined previously is oriented to stone analysis, recurrence rates, and risk factors with therapeutic implications.

Special metaphylaxis seems to be justified in patients with the following types of stone disease: cystine, uric acid, calcium phosphate, and infected stones. In calcium oxalate stone disease, a special metaphylaxis program should be performed only in recurrent cases, since the recurrence rate is quite low. It is assumed that this program reduces recurrence by 40%, a figure somewhat less than that reported by Nolde et al.[20]

In Germany, 335,000 stone episodes occur per year.[23,31] Assuming 70% are calcium oxalate stones,[22] there are 234,000 calcium oxalate stone episodes annually. Assuming a high recurrence rate of 50% (in order not to take the part for metaphylaxis, the calculation model uses this high figure for calcium oxalate stone recurrence rate), there are 117,000 recurrent calcium oxalate stone formers per year.

According to epidemiological data,[22] the following estimations are made for the other types of calculi: calcium phosphate stones 30,000; infected stones 20,000; uric acid stones 20,000; and cystine stones 1,000 annually.

The rational evaluation program examines only the risk factors relevant for the respective type of stone disease (Tables 21.1–21.5). The costs for this evaluation are also given there. The expenses are calculated according to the EBM. The value of one point can vary; an average value

Table 21.1 Cost for risk factor-oriented evaluation in cystine stone patients according to the EBM

Parameter	Points (EBM)
Ordinations- u.	330
Konsultationsgebühr (fee for medical history, physical examination and counseling)	
Stone analysis	300
Cystine (urine)	200
pH (urine)	–
Creatinine (serum/urine)[a]	25
Total	855

[a]For plausibility control of urine collection

Table 21.2 Cost for risk factor-oriented evaluation in uric acid stone patients according to the EBM

Parameter	Points (EBM)
Ordinations- u.	330
Konsultationsgebühr	
Stone analysis	300
Uric acid (serum/urine)	50
pH (urine)	–
Creatinine (serum/urine)	25
Total	705

Table 21.3 Cost for risk factor-oriented evaluation in infected stone patients according to the EBM

Parameter	Points (EBM)
Ordinations- u.	330
Konsultationsgebühr	
Stone analysis	300
Bact. culture	240
Susceptibility testing	250
Creatinine (serum)	25
Total	1,145

Table 21.4 Cost for risk factor-oriented evaluation in calcium phosphate stone patients according to the EBM

Parameter	Points (EBM)
Ordinations- u.	330
Konsultationsgebühr	
Stone analysis	300
Ion.Ca (serum)/	50
Ca (urine)	
pH (urine)	–
Creatinine (serum/urine)[a]	25
Citrate (urine)	225
Total	955

[a]For plausibility control of urine collection

Table 21.5 Cost for risk factor-oriented evaluation in calcium oxalate stone patients according to the EBM

Parameter	Points (EBM)
Ordinations- u.	330
Konsultationsgebühr	
Stone analysis	300
Ion.Ca (serum)/	50
Oxalic/uric acid (urine)	275
Citrate (urine)/	
Creatinine (serum/urine)	275
Total	1,230

Table 21.6 Daily cost for drug therapy in stone metaphylaxis. Prices on the German market

Drug	Prices (€)
Hydrochlorothiazide (50 mg)	0.20
Alkali citrate (three tablets)	1.05
Orthophosphate (six tablets)	0.65
Allopurinol (300 mg)	0.10
Tiopronin (1,000 mg)	
Antibiotics	2.00
L-methionine	1.05

of 0.04 € per point is used. Since two 24-h urine specimens should be analyzed due to the considerable day-to-day variation,[32] the costs for these programs are calculated twice per patient.

Therefore, the annual costs for 188,000 patients undergoing metabolic evaluation are 16.1 million €.

To calculate the annual expenses for drug treatment, the rate of patients treated with drugs was estimated at a high level: all recurrent calcium oxalate stone formers (50% alkali citrate, 30% orthophosphate, 20% thiazides); 30% of calcium phosphate stone patients (10% citrate, 20% thiazides); all infected stone formers (100% antibiotics and L-methionine for 100 days); all uric acid stone patients (100% alkali citrate, 50% allopurinol); and all cystinurics (100% alkali citrate and tiopronine). The daily costs for these drugs in Germany are shown in Table 21.6.

Under these premises, special metaphylaxis for 188,000 patients costs 52.7 million € per year.

21.4.1.3 Comparison of Annual Costs for Stone Removal Versus Metabolic Evaluation and Metaphylaxis

As outlined previously, the annual savings for stone removal due to effective metaphylaxis is 240 million €. The annual expenses for metabolic evaluation and metaphylaxis are 16.1 and 52.7 million €, respectively. Thus, the net annual savings due to rational metabolic evaluation and metaphylaxis is

171.2 million €. For the new German reimbursement system (DRG), so far no calculations are available.

21.4.2 Calculation Models: Comparison of Costs for Stone Removal Versus Metabolic Evaluation/Metaphylaxis in Other Countries

Robertson[33] and Tiselius[34] calculated for their countries (UK and Sweden respectively) that medical prophylaxis is cost-effective as well. However, as already mentioned, cost-effectiveness is dependent on the costs for stone removal versus metaphylaxis, which can differ considerably from country to country.

Lotan et al.,[35] compared the cost-effectiveness of medical management strategies for urolithiasis in several countries. Their model was based on the international cost survey published by Chandhoke.[29] The following measures were included: dietary measures, potassium citrate, thiazides, and allopurinol. They showed that conservative therapy (i.e., diet) is the most costly treatment strategy in all countries but the United Kingdom. Drug therapy was more costly. In most countries, stone frequency must exceed one stone/patient/year before medical therapy is more cost-effective than dietary measures. However, drug therapy produces a good control. On the other hand, compliance is an important factor. First stone formers and patients with a low stone frequency/low risk for recurrence will hardly keep on drug therapy for a longer period. Therefore, specific metaphylaxis should be restricted to patients with a substantial risk for recurrence (rational metaphylaxis,[14,27,28,36] see also *Costs for Metabolic Evaluation/ Metaphylaxis*).

21.5 Off Work due to Stone Disease

In the previously mentioned district of a German social health care insurance company, there were 426 of 150,000 insured people off work due to urolithiasis (N20, ICD 10). The mean duration of being off work was 96.6 days! Most of the patients were off work for a remarkably shorter period (up to 14 days for 307 patients, up to 42 days for 94 patients). Due to long-term off work patients (up to 180 days for 19 cases, longer than 180 days for six cases), a high mean duration of being off work resulted.

Compared to other countries such as the USA, these figures look very high. In the USA, a time span of being off work for 5 days in hospitalized and 2 days in outpatient stone patients is estimated.[11] For the United Kingdom, only 30% of employed persons with the diagnosis urolithiasis missed days of work (mean 19 h annually).[2]

Although these figures are only estimates, they clearly show the striking differences between the national health care systems. One of the most important reasons for the long time being off work in Germany is the fact that socially insured people receive the full wages for up to 42 days being not fit for work. The long duration of being off work due to urinary stone disease is not so surprising when regarding the fact that 40.9% of all days off work in Germany result from diseases with duration of more than 6 weeks (statistics from the Scientific Institute of Regional Social Health Care Insurance Companies Bonn, 1997). For all Germany, a rational metaphylaxis (lowering the recurrence rate by 40%) could avoid 60,000 cases and 5.8 million days off work due to stone disease per year. These figures clearly demonstrate the enormous economic implications of an effective stone metaphylaxis.

21.6 Conclusions

As shown with our calculation model for Germany, metabolic evaluation and metaphylaxis in stone formers can lower health care cost significantly. Although health care conditions may vary from country to country, the principles of this calculation model are applicable to every health care system. Only the amount of savings may be different. Today ESWL is the most frequently used treatment modality for urolithiasis. Regarding the potentially increased recurrence rate following ESWL[5,6] due to "clinically insignificant" residual fragments as foci for regrowth and new stone formation, rational metabolic evaluation and metaphylaxis is not only a medical, but – being more and more important – an economic must. First results on such metaphylaxis programs following ESWL are promising.[37]

Rational metaphylaxis does not mean that every stone former needs a thorough metabolic evaluation and a special metaphylaxis program. Rational metaphylaxis is oriented to the recurrence rate.[14,28,36] Patients with the first episode of a calcium oxalate stone without risk factors are no candidates for special metaphylaxis. Only in stone formers with a substantial risk for recurrence are such programs justified and – as shown by Chandhoke[29] – cost-effective.

References

1. Hesse A. Reliable data from diverse regions of the world exist to show that there has been a steady increase in the prevalence of urolithiasis. *World J Urol.* 2005;23:302-3303.
2. Pearle MS, Calhoun EA, Curhan GC. Urologic diseases in America project: urolithiasis. *J Urol.* 2005;173:848-857.

3. Strohmaier WL. Potential deleterious effects of shock wave lithotripsy. *Curr Opinion Urol.* 1995;5:198-201.

4. Tiselius HG. Rational evaluation of the stone forming patient. In: Bichler KH, Strohmaier WL, Mattauch W, eds. *Urolithiasis.* Tübingen: Attempto; 1995.

5. Carr LK, Honey RJD, Jewett MAS, Ibanez D, Ryan M, Bombardier C. New stone formation: a comparison of extracorporeal shock wave lithotripsy and percutaneous nephrolithotomy. *J Urol.* 1996; 155:1565-567.

6. Robertson WG. Medical management of urinary stone disease. *Eur Urol Update Ser.* 1998;7:139-144.

7. Strohmaier WL, Bichler KH, Koch J, Balk N, Wilbert DM. Protective effect of verapamil on shock wave induced renal tubular dysfunction. *J Urol.* 1993;153:148-154.

8. Marangella M, Bruno M, Vitalo C, Cosseddu D, Trincieri A, Linari F. The occurence of chronic renal insufficiency in calcium nephrolithiasis. In: Vahlensieck W, Gasser G, Schöneich G, eds. *Urolithiasis.* Amsterdam: Excerpta Medica; 1990.

9. Madore F, Stampfer MJ, Rimm EB, Curhan GC. Nephrolithiasis and the risk of hypertension. *Am J Hypertens.* 1998;11:46-53.

10. Bruckenberger E. Beispiel nierenlithotriptor: ursachen des kostenbooms. *Dtsch Ärztebl.* 1988;85:383-394.

11. Resnick MI, Persky L. Summary of the National Institutes of Arthritis, Diabetes, Digestive and Kidney Diseases conference on urolithiasis: state of the art and further needs. *J Urol.* 1995; 153:4-9.

12. Pearle MS, Lotan Y, Brikowski T. Predicted climate-related increase in the prevalence and cost of nephrolithaisis in the U.S. *J Urol.* 2008;179:481-482A.

13. Grabe M. The estimated cost of treatment of urinary tract stones in a Swedish municipal hospital, 1991 – 1993. In: Tiselius HG, ed. *Renal Stones – Proceedings of the 6th European Symposium Urolith.* Edsbruk: Akademitryck AB; 1996.

14. Strohmaier WL. Is there a place for stone metaphylaxis in the era of shock wave lithotripsy? – the economic standpoint. In: Chaussy C, Eisenberger F, Jocham D, Wilbert D, eds. *High energy Shock Waves in Medicine.* Stuttgart New York: Thieme; 1997.

15. Ahlstrand C, Tiselius HG. Renal stone disease in a Swedish district during one year. *Scand J Urol Nephrol.* 1981;15:143-146.

16. Chandhoke PS. Cost-effectiveness of different treatment options for staghorn calculi. *J Urol.* 1996;156:1567-1571.

17. May DJ, Chandhoke PS. Efficacy of cost-effectiveness of extracorporeal shockwave lithotripsy for solitary lower pole renal calculi. *J Urol.* 1998;159:24-27.

18. Collins JW, Keeley FX, Timoney A. Cost analysis of flexible ureterorenoscopy. *BJU Int.* 2004;93:1023-126.

19. Parks JH, Coe FL. The financial effects of kidney stone prevention. *Kidney Int.* 1996;50:1706-1712.

20. Nolde A, Hesse A, Scharrel O, Vahlensieck W. Modellprogramm zur nachsorge bei rezidivierenden harnsteinpatienten. *Urologe B.* 1993;33:148-154.

21. Hesse A, Nolde A, Scharrel O. Qualitätssicherung mit diagnostikstandards und wirtschaftliche aspekte der nachsorge bei urolithiasis. *Urol B.* 1993;33:155-159.

22. Schneider HJ. Epidemiology of urolithiasis. In: Schneider HJ, ed. *Urolithiasis: Etiology and Diagnosis.* Berlin: Springer; 1985.

23. Vahlensieck W, Hesse A. Nephrolithiasis. *Urologe B.* 1993;33:73.

24. Ljunghall S, Danielson BG. A prospective study of renal stone recurrences. *Brit J Urol.* 1984;56:122-124.

25. Marshall V, White RH, Chaput de Saintonge M, Tresidder GC, Blandy JP. The natural history of renal and ureteric calculi. *Brit J Urol.* 1975;47:117-124.

26. Strohmaier WL, Kellner T, Lahme S, Bichler KH (1999) Calcium oxalate urolithiasis – course of the disease in first stone formers without metaphylaxis. Abstracts of the 8th European Symposium on Urolith Parma, Italy

27. Bichler KH, Strohmaier WL, Wilbert DM, Mittermüller B, Eipper E. Harnsteinmetaphylaxe – heute noch aktuell ? *TW Urol Nephrol.* 1996;8:44-52.

28. Strohmaier WL. Harnsteingenese. *Urologe B.* 1993;33:S6-S9.

29. Chandhoke PS. When is medical prophylaxis cost-effective for recurrent calcium stones? *J Urol.* 2002;168:937-940.

30. Strohmaier WL, Hörmann M. Economic aspects of urolithiasis (U) and metaphylaxis (M) in Germany. In: Rodgers AL, Hibbert BE, Hess B, Khan SR, Preminger GM, eds. *Urolithiasis 2000.* Capetown: University of Cape Town Press; 2000.

31. Vahlensieck W, Hesse A, Bach D. Zur prävalenz des harnsteinleidens in der Bundesrepublik Deutschland. *Urologe B.* 1980;20:272-276.

32. Strohmaier WL, Hölz KJ, Bichler KH. Spot urine samples for the metabolic evaluation of urolithiasis patients. *Eur Urol.* 1997;32:294-300.

33. Robertson WG. The economic case for the biochemical screening of stone patients. In: Rodgers AL, Hibbert BE, Hess B, Khan SR, Preminger GM, eds. *Urolithiasis 2000.* Capetown: University of Cape Town Press; 2000.

34. Tiselius HG. Comprehensive metabolic evaluation of stone formers is cost-effective. In: Rodgers AL, Hibbert BE, Hess B, Khan SR, Preminger GM, eds. *Urolithiasis 2000.* Capetown: University of Cape Town Press; 2000.

35. Lotan Y, Cadeddu JA, Pearle MS. International comparison of cost effectiveness of medical management strategies for nephrolithiasis. *Urol Res.* 2005;33:223-230.

36. Bichler KH, Strohmaier WL, Eipper E, Lahme S. *Das Harnsteinleiden.* Berlin: Lehmanns Media – LOB; 2007.

37. Nomura K, Ito H, Masai M, Akakura K, Shimazaki J. Reduction of urinary stone recurrence by dietary counseling after SWL. *J Endourol.* 1995;9:305-311.

What Are Shock Waves?

22

Achim M. Loske

Abstract Extracorporeal shock wave lithotripsy (SWL) has become the primary, noninvasive treatment modality for patients with stones in the kidney or ureter. Given this, it is essentially mandatory for all urologists to have basic knowledge of shock waves so that they may perform safer and more efficient SWL treatments. Unfortunately, most of the literature on shock wave physics is highly specialized. With this in mind, the aim of this chapter is to provide an easy to follow description of what lithotripter shock waves are. This chapter may also serve as a guide for physicians working on non-urological shock wave lithotripsy or other clinical and experimental applications of shock waves to medicine. The physics behind shock wave lithotripsy is quite a large subject, so a special effort has been made here to focus the discussion on an understanding of what shock waves are.

22.1 Introduction

Motivated by the success of extracorporeal shock wave lithotripsy (SWL), underwater shock waves have been the subject of considerable research in the last 25 years. The study of shock waves belongs to the field of acoustics, which is an interesting and broad field having applications in physics, engineering, biology, medicine, architecture, aeronautics, music, noise control, and many other topics. In general, the literature describing the physics of shock waves is highly specialized and difficult to follow by readers without a solid background in physics.[1] The objective of this chapter is to provide a useful and easy to understand description of shock waves and their applications in medical fields.

This chapter may also be useful to physicians working on other clinical and experimental applications of shock waves to medicine, like non-urological SWL,[2–4] orthopedic application of shock waves,[5,6] treatment of refractory angina pectoris, the possible treatment of Peyronie's disease,[7,8] cell transfection, tumor therapy,[9–12] thrombus ablation,[13] and inactivation of bacteria with shock waves.[14–16]

A.M. Loske
Centro de Física Aplicada y Tecnología Avanzada, Universidad Nacional Autónoma de México, Querétaro, México
e-mail: loske@fata.unam.mx

22.2 Waves

It is important to distinguish between two main types of waves: *mechanical* waves and *electromagnetic* waves. Electromagnetic waves – such as light, laser waves, radio and television signals, microwaves, and X-rays – do not require a medium to propagate. In this case, so-called "electric fields" and "magnetic fields" oscillate in a plane perpendicular to the direction of wave propagation. Since shock waves do not belong in this category no more information on electromagnetic waves will be given in this chapter.

22.2.1 Mechanical Waves

All mechanical waves are generated by a source, which causes a disturbance in the medium. It is this disturbance traveling through a medium that is called a "wave" (Fig. 22.1). Unlike electromagnetic waves, mechanical waves require a medium for propagation and cannot travel through a vacuum. This is essentially because mechanical waves are made up of vibrations of the molecules that make up the medium. These vibrations spread throughout the medium and energy is transferred from one molecule to the next. It is important to note that waves carry energy – not matter – over large distances. Individual particles (molecules) oscillate a small

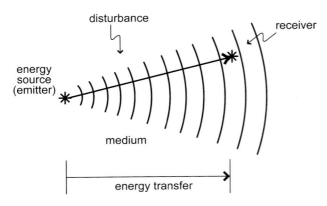

Fig. 22.1 Schematic of a mechanical disturbance traveling through a medium. The wave transports energy from the source to the receiver

distance, but do not travel along with the wave. In addition, as the wave moves through the medium, there is a loss of energy due to friction. In general, the pressure "amplitude" of the wave decreases as the distance traveled increases.

Examples of mechanical waves are shock waves, sound, vibration, seismic waves, water waves, and ultrasound. Mechanical waves can be regarded as useful or useless. Very useful mechanical waves are speech and music, while generally useless sound waves in air are called "noise." Many vibrations are also considered useless or even dangerous. In most situations, both useful and useless waves will be present.

22.2.2 Transverse Waves

Mechanical waves are further divided into two groups by the type of motion that the molecules execute: *transverse waves* and *longitudinal waves*. In transverse waves, the motion of the particles is perpendicular to the propagation of the wave. This is easily visualized, by imagining a floating object, while a so-called "surface" wave passes by (Fig. 22.2). Another example is the case of waves that propagate on a string. Transverse waves are sometimes referred to as *shear waves*.

22.2.3 Longitudinal Waves

In a longitudinal wave, all particles oscillate parallel to the direction of propagation. They are also called *compressional waves*. A well-known example is the compression (and *rarefaction*) of the segments of a spring as a wave travels along its length. Sound, which is produced by variations in the density of air, is also a longitudinal wave (Fig. 22.3). At a particular point in space, "sound" is a rapid variation in the pressure of a medium around a steady-state value. This steady-state pressure can be, for example, the atmospheric pressure or a hydrostatic pressure (the pressure caused by the height of a liquid above a certain point of reference). Since all states of matter can be compressed, longitudinal waves propagate through solids, liquids, and gases. It is important to remember that the individual particles of the medium are only displaced locally; the only thing that travels all the way from the source to the receiver is the wave itself. The wave's speed, referred to as the *speed of sound* or *speed of wave propagation,* depends on the density, the elasticity, and the temperature of the medium. The speed of propagation is much higher in a solid medium than in a liquid medium as the restoring force between individual molecules is much higher in a solid. Furthermore, at higher temperatures, molecules move faster and collide with each other more often. One therefore finds that mechanical waves propagate faster as the temperature of the medium is increased. For instance, the speed of sound in pure water at 0°C is approximately 1,400 m/s while its speed at 30°C is about 1,510 m/s.

22.2.4 A Few Definitions

There are several definitions used in physics to describe the properties of a wave. It is important for any physician to distinguish clearly between these definitions as they may frequently appear in treatment protocols, equipment specifications, and scientific articles.

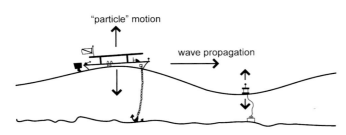

Fig. 22.2 A boat floating on the ocean with the engine turned off moves perpendicular to a passing wave. Particles always move perpendicular to the propagation of transversal waves

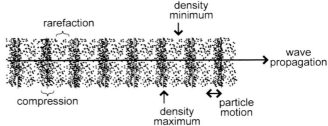

Fig. 22.3 A longitudinal wave is characterized by the propagation of rarefactions and compressions of the medium. Particles oscillate parallel to the direction of the wave propagation and are not transported from the emitter to the receiver

If a small spherical object is dropped into a pool, circular ripples travel outward from the spot where the object hit the water. All points on a specific ripple that are in the same state of motion are on a surface called a *wavefront*. One may imagine lines drawn perpendicularly to the wavefronts; these are called *rays* and are often used to show the path of a wave as it propagates (Fig. 22.4). Waves can spread in one, two, and three dimensions. For medical applications, the study of three-dimensional wave propagation is the most important. In three dimensions, one may imagine wavefronts with a spherical shape, with associated rays being radial lines.

The *wavelength* is defined as the distance between two successive peaks or two successive troughs (Fig. 22.4). The time interval between the passage of two successive peaks or troughs is called the *period*. Some textbooks also define the period as the time it takes a wave to complete a *cycle* (Fig. 22.5). The *amplitude* is defined as the *height* of the wave, generally measured from the baseline to the highest (or lowest) value. The amplitude may refer to the actual height of a water wave

above the water's still height or to the *pressure amplitude* (that is, the difference between the pressure in highly compressed regions and some specified baseline pressure).

A well-known parameter used to describe a wave is its *frequency* – this is the number of cycles that pass by a certain position in 1 s – which is measured in hertz (Hz). In other words, the frequency gives information on how many wavelengths happen in 1 s. A concept that may be somewhat more difficult to imagine is that of a *frequency spectrum*. The fact is that all waves, even non-periodic waves, can be built up by the superposition of a series of *harmonic* waves of different frequencies and amplitudes (Fig. 22.6). A mathematical technique, called *Fourier analysis,* is used to calculate the

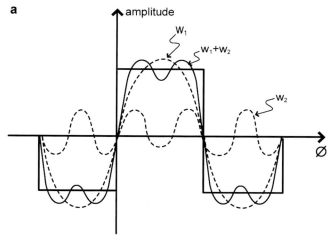

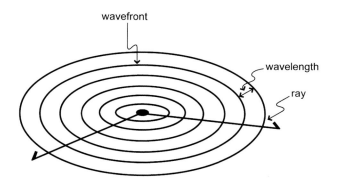

Fig. 22.4 Schematic of a circumferential surface-wave propagating through a liquid. Each circle corresponds to a crest. The wavelength can be determined by measuring the distance between two consecutive crests. Rays are imaginary lines that indicate the direction of propagation. They are drawn perpendicular to the wavefronts. In this figure, rays are directed radially, away from the source

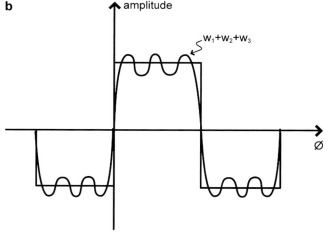

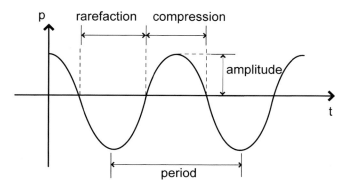

Fig. 22.5 Graph of pressure as a function of time, showing how the pressure changes as a longitudinal wave passes a certain point in space. The sinusoidal shape of this pressure variation should not be confused with a transversal wave moving through space. This plot gives information on how the pressure varies *in time*

Fig. 22.6 Any wave can be imagined as the superposition of a certain number of harmonic waves (w_1, w_2, w_3...) with specific frequencies and amplitudes. The sum of only two harmonic waves ($w_1 + w_2$) is a bad representation of the square wave shown in (**a**). Adding one more harmonic wave ($w_1 + w_2 + w_3$) improves the result (**b**). The similarity between the original profile and the sum of harmonic waves increases as the number of harmonic waves increases. It would be necessary to draw the sum of a large number of harmonic waves with the adequate amplitude and wavelength to represent the square wave adequately

frequencies, amplitudes, and phases of the harmonic waves (w_1, w_2, w_3...) that have to be added to synthesize the desired waveform. The number of harmonic waves needed to describe a non-periodic wave depends on the profile of the wave. A sinusoidal wave is periodic (and harmonic) and has only one fundamental frequency associated to it. A lithotripter shock wave, which is a single high-pressure peak with a steep onset and a gradual decline into a pressure trough, is non-periodic and can be imagined as consisting of a large number of waves of different frequencies.

The *power* of a wave, measured in watts (W), is defined as the energy transported by the wave during a certain time interval. Furthermore, the power delivered by a wave per unit area (i.e., per square meter) is called the *intensity*. The standard units of intensity are watts per square meter (W/m²). Since the energy emitted from a point source spreads out in all directions, its intensity will decrease with radial distance from the source. The intensity of a wave is proportional to the square of its amplitude. As the measured values of sound intensity have an expansive range, a logarithmic scale is typically used. Sound intensities are normally given with respect to a reference, the threshold of hearing: $I_o = 10^{-12}$ W/m². The *sound level* is defined as 10 log (I/I_0), where I is the intensity in W/m² to which the sound level corresponds. Sound levels are expressed in *decibels* (dB).

Shock waves undergo *refraction* and *reflection* when passing from one medium to another. Refraction occurs as shock waves enter the patient's body. An important definition related to the reflection of acoustic waves is the *specific acoustic impedance*, or simply the *acoustic impedance,* of a medium. The acoustic impedance measures the ease with which the wave propagates through a certain material. For a *plane wave*, the impedance is just the product of the density of the medium and the wave speed.

22.3 Shock Waves

In general, the word *sound* is used to describe waves in the frequency and intensity range that our auditory system is capable to detect (about 20 Hz–20 kHz). The science of acoustics, however, also includes the study of waves that we cannot hear (Fig. 22.7). Acoustic waves having a frequency below the frequency limit of our ears are called *infrasound*. *Ultrasound* refers to waves with frequencies above our range of hearing. Shock waves are sometimes referred to as ultrasound or *explosive ultrasound* waves because they share some properties with ultrasound. Though similarities exist, one should not confuse shock waves with the type of ultrasound used in diagnostic imaging systems or therapeutic applications (such as high intensity focused ultrasound and focused ultrasound surgery). For instance, the pressure

amplitude generated by a lithotripter shock wave can have up to 75 times the pressure amplitude of the waves used in diagnostic ultrasound.

Shock waves are transient pressure changes that propagate

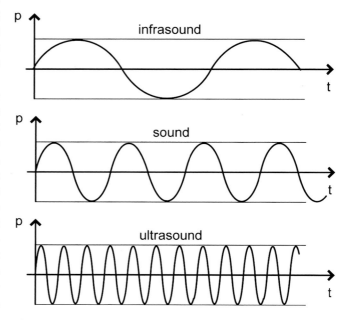

Fig. 22.7 Graphs of pressure as a function of time for harmonic waves. According to their frequency, acoustic waves are classified as infrasound, sound, or ultrasound

through three-dimensional space. They result from a very fast release of a large amount of energy in a relatively small space. Shock or *blast waves* differ from acoustic waves (which consist exclusively of small pressure changes) in that they may propagate in a manner entirely different from that of ordinary acoustic waves. An example is the acoustic boom following a lightning bolt during a thunderstorm. The initial shock wave pressure decays as the wave expands until it degenerates into a sound wave. This is inevitable as a fixed amount of energy has to be spread out over an ever-increasing volume. The detonation of an explosive and the passage of supersonic aircraft are also well-known examples of shock wave generation (Fig. 22.8). Shock waves can be produced in all states of matter. It is not usually possible to see a shock wave; however, shock waves can be made visible with suitable optical instrumentation.

22.3.1 Lithotripter Shock Waves

22.3.1.1 Shock Wave Generators

Extracorporeal shock wave lithotripters consist of a shock wave head (shock wave source), a treatment table, and a localization system (a coaxial or lateral ultrasound imaging

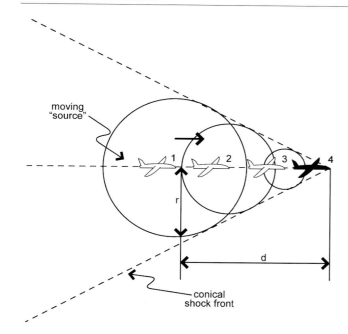

Fig. 22.8 Schematic of the shock front produced by a supersonic aircraft moving at a speed greater than the speed of sound. The aircraft traveled a distance d (from point 1 to point 4) in the same time needed for the wave, generated at point 1, to travel the distance r. The envelope of the three-dimensional pressure waves produced is a three-dimensional cone. Its angle depends on the speed of the aircraft

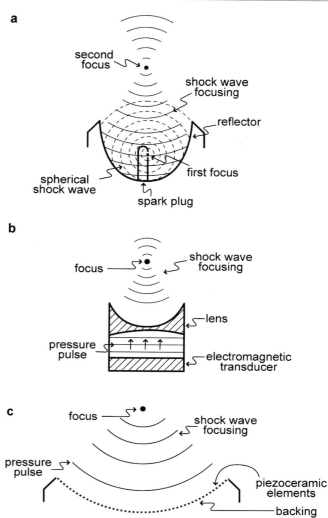

Fig. 22.9 Schematic of three different shock wave generation principles. (**a**) Electrohydraulic lithotripters produce shock waves by electrical breakdown of water at the first focus of a metallic ellipsoidal reflector. Part of the spherical shock front is reflected off of the reflector and focused at the second focus. (**b**) Electromagnetic lithotripters generate pressure pulses by moving a metal diaphragm, located at the base of a water-filled shock tube. Magnetic forces cause the membrane to be repelled, transmitting mechanical energy to the water. The flat pressure wave induced by the sudden movement of the membrane is focused by an acoustical lens. Shock waves are formed only *after* passage through the lens. (**c**) Piezoelectric lithotripters consist of a set of piezoelectric crystals mounted on a hemispherical bowl-shaped aluminum backing. A high-voltage pulse applied to all crystals at the same time causes their rapid expansion, producing a pressure wave in the water. A shock wave arrives at the focus after superposition of the pressure wave formed by each crystal

system and/or an isocentric C-arm fluoroscope). It is not the purpose of this chapter to describe the details of shock wave generators; however, having some information on their working principles is useful to better understand what lithotripter shock waves are. More information on extracorporeal lithotripters can be found in the literature.[17–19]

Nowadays, there are three main shock wave generation techniques on the market: electrohydraulic, piezoelectric, and electromagnetic (Fig. 22.9). All release large amounts of energy inside a transducer and generate shock waves outside the patient's body. To prevent shock waves from losing energy, focusing devices like lenses or reflectors are needed. In electrohydraulic lithotripters, shock waves are generated by an underwater high-voltage spark that is discharged between two electrodes (the arc is localized in the first focus of an ellipsoidal reflector, see Fig. 22.9a). The fast expansion of the *plasma* bubble at the first focus generates a shock wave, which propagates spherically outward and reflects off of the metallic reflector. The shock front gets focused toward the second focal point. Shock waves reflect off of the reflector of an electrohydraulic lithotripter in a manner similar to that found in optical waves. This is because under certain circumstances the same law of reflection is followed by both sound and light. The low-energy unfocused part of the primary spherical shock wave will always propagate through the patient. The first spark-gap lithotripters were manufactured by Dornier Medizintechnik GmbH in Germering, Germany.

Three different electromagnetic systems are in use. The classical shock wave head, designed by Siemens GmbH in Erlangen, Germany, generates pressure pulses by moving a circular metal diaphragm that is placed in a water-filled shock tube (Fig. 22.9b). A high voltage pulse is sent through a coil, placed behind the diaphragm, so that it is repelled. A lens focuses the pulse, forcing its pressure profile to steepen, quickly transforming the pulse into a shock wave. Coupling of the shock wave to the patient is done using a water-filled cushion. The second type of electromagnetic shock wave generator (not shown in Fig. 22.9), uses a cylindrical coil to produce a cylindrical wave that is reflected by a parabolic reflector and transformed into a spherically focused shock wave. This shock wave generator, manufactured by Storz Medical AG in Kreuzlingen, Switzerland, has also been very successful.[20,21] Using this shock wave generation principle, the manufacturer has also developed a shock wave head that allows the user to change the focal size, even during treatment. The third type of electromagnetic shock wave generator, manufactured by XiXin Medical Instruments Co. Ltd (not shown in Fig. 22.9), is a self-focusing design; it does not use a lens or a reflector to concentrate shock wave energy. Analogous to a piezoelectric lithotripter, this generator uses a spiral coil mounted on a spherical backing.[22]

Piezoelectric shock wave generators as manufactured by Richard Wolf GmbH are called self-focusing. These generators produce shock waves in water by exciting piezoceramic crystals. The crystals are arranged on the concave surface of a spherical metallic dish and expand suddenly when they are exposed to an electric discharge (Fig. 22.9c). The sudden displacement of the crystals produces a pressure wave with most of the energy focused toward the center of the generator. Relatively small piezoelectric shock wave heads, with two layers of piezoelectric elements, have become available.[19,23]

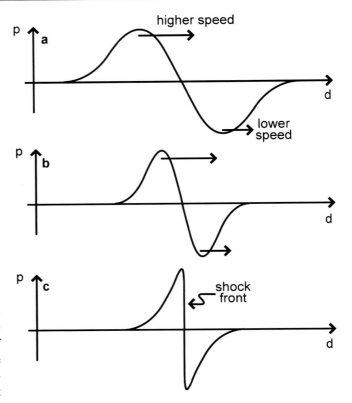

Fig. 22.10 Simplified graphs of pressure as a function of distance, explaining shock formation. If an acoustic wave, having high pressure propagates through a medium then the higher pressure parts travel faster than the lower pressure parts (**a**), distorting the shape of the wave (**b**). After traveling certain distance, a shock front is formed (**c**)

22.3.1.2 Shock Wave Formation

Spark gap generated shock waves are formed almost immediately after the electrical energy is released. In contrast, electromagnetic and piezoelectric lithotripters produce strong compressions that degenerate into a shock wave as they travel trough liquid. In piezoelectric lithotripters, the shock wave develops while the pressure pulse, generated by the piezoelectric transducer, travels toward the focus. In electromagnetic systems, the shock front develops after passing through the lens. At low-energy settings, some lithotripters do not produce shock waves at all (though any extracorporeal lithotripter pulses are typically called shock waves to denote the high amplitude of the pulse).

Recall that the speed of a mechanical wave increases as the density of the medium increases. As shock waves propagate, they transiently cause the medium to become denser. For small pressure amplitudes, each part of an acoustic wave travels at the same speed – the propagation speed; however, if the pressure differences are large, the sound speed is not the same for all points. In an extracorporeal lithotripter, a large positive pressure pulse is initially formed due to a sudden compression of the fluid contained inside the shock wave head. This compression pulse gets distorted as it travels through the

medium. This is because high-pressure parts of the wave travel faster than the low-pressure parts. As the high-pressure parts travel faster, they increase the pressure at the wave front, pushing the wave profile forward. As this continues, a steep front, called a *shock front*, is formed. A compression pulse is fully transformed into a shock wave when the pressure profile ceases to pile up any further (Fig. 22.10). At this stage, the pressure and density along the shock front vary wildly in a very short region. The wavefront of a lithotripter shock front has a thickness less than 1 mm. Normally the entire pressure profile is called a shock wave; however, the word *shock* should only be used for the first fast pressure rise. Formally it is only the sharp positive pressure jump that is shocked. Shock fronts can have different amplitudes and widths. The steepness of the shock profile depends on the particular lithotripter.

22.3.1.3 Parameters Describing a Lithotripter Shock Wave

There is an international consensus that the most important parameters describing a shock wave for medical application are (Fig. 22.11): positive maximum pressure (p^+), negative

Fig. 22.11 Graph of pressure as a function of time, showing the most important parameters defining a lithotripter shock wave: *FWHM* full-width-half-maximum, t_r = rise time, t_e = time used to calculate the "total energy" of the shock wave, p^+ = positive maximum pressure, p^- = negative maximum pressure

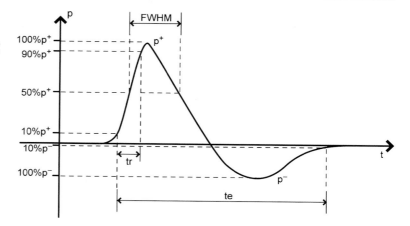

maximum pressure (p^-), rise time (t_r), full-width-half-maximum (FWHM), energy flux density (EFD), and focal energy.[24]

The *positive maximum pressure* (p^+) is defined as the pressure difference between the maximum positive pressure of the shock wave and the ambient pressure. In an analogous manner, the *negative maximum pressure* (p^-) is the maximum negative pressure found in the tensile phase of the shock wave. The amplitude of p^- may be as much as 20% of p^+.

The time needed for the pressure to rise from 10% to 90% of p^+ is defined as the *rise time* (t_r). For lithotripter shock waves, t_r has the unbelievable value of less than 5 ns (five billionths of a second). The time interval between the instant when the pressure first reaches 50% of p^+, and the first time it falls under 50% (Fig. 22.11), is the so-called *full-width-half-maximum* (FWHM). This duration varies between about 0.2 and 0.5 μs.

The *dynamic focus, focal region*, or *−6 dB focal zone* of a lithotripter is defined as the volume in which, at any point, the positive pressure peak amplitude is equal to or higher than 50% of p^+. The size of this volume depends on the shock wave generation and focusing mechanism, as well as on the voltage setting. It is called the −6 dB focal zone, because −6 dB is equivalent to 50%. This definition is widely used among manufacturers; however, it typically does not give enough information for medical applications. One does not know enough about the energy contained in the focal volume and, as a consequence, one does not know enough about the stone disintegration efficiency of a lithotripter. Given this, a more convenient parameter to describe the performance of a shock wave generator has been defined: the *treatment zone* or the *5 MPa focus*. As shown in Fig. 22.12, the treatment zone is the volume inside which any point has a pressure equal to or larger than 5 MPa.[17] The 5 MPa figure is used as it has been identified (by the German Society of Shock Wave Lithotripsy) as the lowest pressure that is medically effective. Both of the focal volumes mentioned previously have the shape of an elliptical cigar. A noteworthy difference is that the −6 dB focal zone depends on relative pressure measurements, while calibrated (i.e., absolute) measurements must be used to set the limits of the 5 MPa focus.

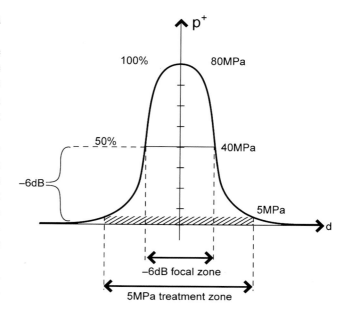

Fig. 22.12 Graph of pressure as a function of distance in the neighborhood of the focus of an extracorporeal lithotripter. The −6 dB focus and the 5 MPa treatment zone are compared

Another definition that will prove useful in SWL applications is the *energy density* or *energy flux density* (EFD). This is defined as the amount of energy transmitted through an area of 1 mm², per shock wave. It should not be confused with the *total acoustical energy* per released shock wave, which is the sum of all energy densities across the beam profile multiplied by the area of the beam profile. If only the positive phase of the shock wave is considered in calculating the energy density, the EFD is referred to as the *positive EFD*.

22.3.1.4 Shock Wave Pressure Profile

At the focal zone, extracorporeal lithotripters generate a strong acoustic field with extremely fast pressure variation. It is not easy to accurately record such a field (Fig. 22.13). Taking accurate pressure measurements of a shock wave that

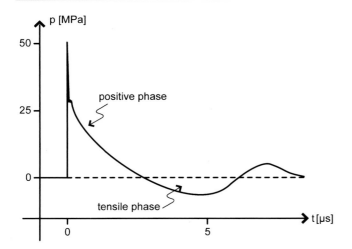

Fig. 22.13 Typical pressure profile recorded using a fiber-optic hydrophone (FOPH 2000, RP Acoustics) at the focus of an extracorporeal lithotripter. An extremely short positive pressure rise is followed by a fast pressure decrease and a pressure trough

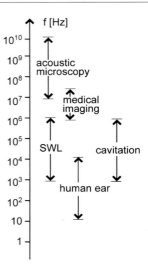

Fig. 22.14 Frequency spectrum showing the range of human hearing and extracorporeal shock wave lithotripsy (SWL) compared to other acoustical phenomena

lasts 1 μs or less and has a rise time of about 5 ns requires a pressure gauge with an extraordinarily fast response. Nowadays, the most convenient instruments to perform pressure measurements in SWL are the fiber-optic hydrophone,[25] and the light spot hydrophone.[26] Fiber-optic hydrophones were recommended as a measurement standard in 1998.

The pressure pulse in the focal region of a lithotripter consists of a short compression pulse with a peak pressure between 30 and 150 MPa, and a subsequent decompression pulse, sometimes referred to as the *negative* pressure peak or *tensile phase*. The tensile phase will typically have a tensile peak of up to −20 MPa and a phase duration of 2–20 μs. Lithotripter shock waves can be created over a broad range of frequencies, in about the 16 kHz range to about the 20 MHz range. The therapeutically effective components for SWL are above 200 kHz (Fig. 22.14). Most energy is between about 100 kHz and 1 MHz, with a peak at about 300 kHz. *Total pulse energies* are in the range of about 10–100 mJ[27] and *energy densities* are between about 0.2 and 2.0 mJ/mm². Time durations (i.e., the time between the positive peak and the negative peak) are similar in all lithotripters.

During SWL, stones fracture mainly due to spalling, cavitation, circumferential squeezing, superfocusing, and fatigue.[28,29] Most of these mechanisms act synergistically, rather than independently. For many years, other shock wave profiles have been proposed in order to improve calculi fragmentation with the least amount of tissue damage. The use of composite reflectors[30] or two confocal electrohydraulic lithotripters with a controlled delay between their pulses have been tested.[31] Results indicate that stone comminution can be enhanced, or tissue damage reduced, by controlling the delay between shock wave emissions. Another well-known example is that of tandem shock waves (Fig. 22.15). In order to understand the basics of this alternate pressure profile, it is

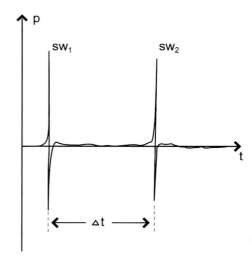

Fig. 22.15 Graph of pressure as a function of time at the focus of a piezoelectric tandem lithotripter, showing to similar shock waves (sw_1 and sw_2), arriving with a time delay Δt (delta t)

helpful to recall the physics of acoustic cavitation.[32] During SWL, bubbles contained in the fluid near a calculus are compressed by the positive peak of each shock wave. As the tensile phase reaches these micro-bubbles, their volume increases significantly. After a few hundred microseconds, the bubbles collapse violently, generating secondary shock waves and high-speed microjets.[33,34] Comparison between the effects of cavitation induced by two different pressure–time shock waveform pulses was studied by Cathignol.[35]

Several authors showed that the energy of collapsing cavitation bubbles can be intensified if a second shock wave appears shortly after their stable phase.[36,37] The time delay between the first and second shock wave should correspond to the collapse time of the bubble cluster formed by the first shock wave. This type of lithotripsy, called tandem SWL, is still under research. No clinical results have been reported so far.

Tandem SWL should not be confused with *dual-head* SWL. Dual-head lithotripters, sometimes called dual-pulse lithotripters, have two separate shock wave generators. From the theoretical standpoint, dual-head lithotripters have interesting advantages but, nevertheless, they are not tandem lithotripters because they generate two pulses with a delay that is too long to enhance bubble collapse.

22.3.1.5 Shock Wave Attenuation

Experiments that attempt to use ultrasound for SWL have failed, as these waves are highly attenuated in tissue and pose some risk of thermal injury to the tissue.[38] Shock waves undergo less attenuation than ultrasound waves when propagating through tissue. This is because, in a biological medium, high frequency waves are absorbed more than low frequency waves. Since shock waves have lower frequencies than ultrasound waves, they have a higher penetration power.

Absorption in tissue is higher than in water. Since the shock front contains high frequencies, it is absorbed faster than other parts of the shock wave profile. After traveling a few centimeters through tissue, the amplitude of the shock wave reduces and its rise time increases. Despite this, the negative phase of the shock wave will remain almost unaltered.

Some studies have revealed that stone to skin distance may predict SWL outcome.[39] The amount of acoustic energy that is actually transformed into mechanical energy (energy that can be used to fracture a renal stone) depends on both the acoustic impedance of the media and on the angle of arrival of the shock wave. Peak-pressure attenuation of shock waves in water is about 10–20% for a distance of 100 mm while the energy attenuation due to passage of a shock wave through the membrane of a lithotripter water cushion is about 20%. Furthermore, poor coupling between patient skin and water cushion may increase shock wave attenuation up to 50% or more.

22.4 Conclusions

Intensive research has been carried out worldwide in order to find improvements in SWL technology that increase fragmentation efficiency while reducing renal damage. Stone location, composition, and the existence of a fluid-filled expansion chamber influence SWL outcome. Shock wave energy, the pressure profile, and the shape of the focal zone, as well as patient positioning and coupling are also crucial. As technology develops, it becomes more and more important for a physician to have basic knowledge in physics. Extensive training by certified technicians should be required in all lithotripsy centers to guarantee good results and to prevent overtreating.

What are shock waves? To imagine an event lasting a tenth of a second or even a hundredth of a second might be possible for most people. However, to visualize an event occurring in a millionth of a second is far beyond our capacity. As a lithotripter shock wave passes through water or tissue at a speed of more than 1,500 m/s, the pressure rises in one to five billionths of a second and returns to its original value in a few millionths of a second. In a time of five billionths of a second, the bullet of a firearm having a speed of 800 m/s only travels about four thousandths of a millimeter – a distance so small that a microscope is needed to see it! Shock waves are an incredible phenomenon, quite impossible to conceive with our senses.

Acknowledgments The author acknowledges Francisco Fernández, Ulises Mora, and Arturo Méndez for support. All figures were designed by Gabriela Trucco.

References

1. Rossing TD. *Springer Handbook of Acoustics*. New York: Springer Verlag; 2007.
2. van der Hul R, Plaisier P, Jeekel J, Terpstra O, den Toom R, Bruinning H. Extracorporeal shockwave lithotripsy of pancreatic duct stones: Immediate and long-term results. *Endoscopy*. 1994;26:573.
3. Capaccio P, Ottaviani F, Manzo R, Schindler A, Cesana B. Extracorporeal lithotripsy for salivary calculi: a long-term clinical experience. *Laryngoscope*. 2004;114:1069-1073.
4. Kim HG. Role of extracorporeal shockwave lithotripsy for the treatment of pancreatic duct stone. *Korean J Gastroenterol*. 2005;46: 418-22.
5. Schleberger R, Senge T. Non-invasive treatment of long bone pseudarthrosis by shock waves (ESWL). *Archiv Orthop Trauma Surg*. 1992;111:224-227.
6. Haupt G. Use of extracorporeal shock waves in the treatment of pseudarthrosis, tendinopathy and other orthopedic diseases. *J Urol*. 1997;158:4-11.
7. Lebret T, Loison G, Herve JM, et al. Extracorporeal shock wave therapy in the treatment of Peyronie's disease: experience with standard lithotriptor (Siemens-Multiline). *Urol*. 2002;59:657-661.
8. Hauck EW, Hauptmann A, Bschleipfer T, Schmelz HU, Altinkilic BM, Weidner W. Questionable efficacy of extracorporeal shock wave therapy for Peyronie's disease: results of a prospective approach. *J Urol*. 2004;171:296-299.
9. Steinbach P, Hofstädter H, Nicolai H, Rössler W, Wieland W. In vitro investigations on cellular damage induced by high energy shock waves. *Ultrasound Med Biol*. 1992;18:691-699.
10. Oosterhof GON, Cornel EB, Smits GAHJ, Debruyne FM, Schalken JA. The influence of high-energy shock waves on the development of metastases. *Ultrasound Med Biol*. 1996;22:339-344.
11. Lauer U, Bürgelt E, Squire Z, et al. Shock Wave permeabilization as a new gene transfer method. *Gene Ther*. 1997;4:710-715.
12. Armenta E, Varela A, Escalera G, Loske AM. Transfección de la línea celular Hela derivada de un tumor cervico-uterino por medio de ondas de choque in vitro. *Rev Mex Fis*. 2006;52:352-358.

13. Kodama T, Tatsuno M, Sugimoto S, Uenohara H, Yoshimoto T, Takayama K. Liquid jets, accelerated thrombolysis: a study for revascularization of cerebral embolism. *Ultrasound Med Biol.* 1999;25:977-983.

14. von Eiff C, Overbeck J, Haupts G, et al. Bactericidal effect of extracorporeal shock waves on Staphylococcus aureus. *J Med Microbiol.* 2000;49:709-712.

15. Álvarez UM, Loske AM, Castaño-Tostado E, Prieto FE. Inactivation of *Escherichia coli* O157:H7, *Salmonella* Typhimurium and *Listeria monocytogenes* by underwater shock waves. *Innov Food Sci Emerg Technol.* 2004;5:459-463.

16. Álvarez UM, Ramírez A, Fernández F, Méndez A, Loske AM. The influence of single-pulse and tandem shock waves on bacteria. *Shock Waves.* 2008;17:441-447.

17. Cleveland RO, McAteer JA. The physics of shock wave lithotripsy. In: Smith AD, Badlani GH, Bagley DH, et al., eds. *Smith's Textbook on Endourology.* Ontario, Canada: BC Decker Inc.; 2007.

18. Lingeman JE. Lithotripsy systems. In: Smith AD, Badlani GH, Bagley DH, et al., eds. *Smith's Textbook on Endourology.* Ontario, Canada: BC Decker Inc; 2007.

19. Loske AM. *Shock Wave Lithotripsy Physics for Urologists.* Querétaro, México: Centro de Física Aplicada y Tecnología Avanzada, UNAM; 2007.

20. Wess O, Marlinghaus EH, Katona J. A new design of an optimal acoustic source for extracorporeal lithotripsy. In: Burhenne J, ed. *Billiary Lithotripsy II.* Chicago, Illinois: Year Book Medical Publishers, Inc.; 1990.

21. Köhrmann KU, Rassweiller JJ, Manning M, et al. The clinical introduction of a third generation lithotripter: Modulith SL 20. *J Urol.* 1995;153:1379-1383.

22. Eisenmenger W, Du X, Tang C, et al. The first clinical results of wide-focus and low-pressure ESWL. *Ultrasound Med Biol.* 2002; 28:769-774.

23. Riedlinger R, Dreyer T, Krauss W. Small aperture piezo sources for lithotripsy. In: Bettucci A (ed). Proceedings of the 17th International Congress on Acoustics Vol. IV, Rome, 2002.

24. Wess O, Ueberle F, Dührssen RN, et al. Working group technical developments – consensus report. In: Chaussy Ch, Eisenberger F, Jocham D, Wilbert D, eds. *High Energy Schock Waves in Medicine.* Stuttgart: Thieme Verlag; 1997.

25. Staudenraus J, Eisenmenger W. Fibre-optic hydrophone for ultrasonic and shock wave measurements in water. *Ultrasonics.* 1993;31:267-273.

26. Granz B, Nank R, Fere J. Light spot hydrophone, innovation in lithotripsy. *Med Solut.* 2004;6:86-87.

27. Folberth W, Köhler G, Rohwedder A, Matura E. Pressure distribution and energy flow in the focal region of two different electromagnetic shock wave sources. *J Lithotr Stone Dis.* 1992;4:1-7.

28. Lokhandwalla M, Sturtevant B. Fracture mechanics model of stone comminution in ESWL and implications for tissue damage. *Phys Med Biol.* 2000;45:1923-1949.

29. Eisenmenger W. The mechanism of stone fragmentation in ESWL. *Ultrasound Med Biol.* 2001;27:683-693.

30. Prieto FE, Loske AM. Bifocal reflector for electrohydraulic lithotripters. *J Endourol.* 1999;13:65-75.

31. Sokolov DL, Bailey MR, Crum LA. Use of a dual-pulse lithotripter to generate a localized and intensified cavitation field. *J Acoust Soc Am.* 2001;110:1685-1695.

32. Bailey MR, Pishchalnikov YA, Sapozhnikov OA, et al. Cavitation detection during shock-wave lithotripsy. *Ultrasound Med Biol.* 2005;31:1245-1256.

33. Crum LA. Cavitation microjets as a contributory mechanism for renal calculi disintegration in ESWL. *J Urol.* 1988;140:1587-1590.

34. Brennen CE. *Cavitation Bubble Dynamics.* New York: Oxford University Press; 1995.

35. Cathignol D. Comparison between the effects of cavitation induced by two different pressure-time shock waveform pulses. *IEEE Trans Ultrason, Ferroel Freq Control.* 1998;45:788-799.

36. Zhong P, Xi X, Zhu S, Cocks F, Preminger GM. Recent developments in ESWL physics research. *J Endourol.* 1999;13:611-617.

37. Loske AM, Fernández F, Zendejas H, Paredes M, Castaño-Tostado E. Dual-pulse shock wave lithotripsy: in vitro and in vivo study. *J Urol.* 2005;174:2388-2392.

38. Mulvaney WP. Attempted disintegration of calculi by ultrasonic vibrations. *J Urol.* 1953;70:704-707.

39. Pareek G, Hedigan SP, Lee FT, Nakada SY. Shock wave lithotripsy success determined by skin-to-stone distance on computed tomography. *Urol.* 2005;66:941-944.

Extracorporeal Shock Wave Lithotriptors

23

Kai Uwe Köhrmann and Jens Rassweiler

Abstract After clinical introduction in 1980, extracorporeal shock wave lithotripsy (ESWL) became the primary choice of treatment for most urinary stones within less than 10 years. Stone disintegration and passage of fragments are influenced by technical demands on the lithotripter and clinical prerequisites on behalf of the patient and surgeon. There are no standardized parameters to characterize shock waves physically or to define their optimal configuration. Primarily there is the discussion about the size of focal zone and the energy flux within it. Actually, there is a trend to use smaller focal sizes for ureter stones and larger for renal stones without proof by relevant studies. The shock waves disintegrate the calculi in a sequential process by different mechanisms, for example, spallation, squeezing, cavitation induced by microbubbles, and dynamic fatigue. The propagation of the shock wave from the generator through the patient to the stone has to be ensured by optimal acoustic coupling of the waves. The stones have to be positioned precisely in the focal point imaged by fluoroscopy or sonography. Prospective randomized trials proofed that pulse rate should not exceed 90 pulses/min and shock wave energy should be ramped along ESWL session from low to high level up to the limit of applicable shock wave dose (shot number and energy) to improve stone fragmentation and reduce the risk of kidney trauma. After treatment, including retreatment in some cases, the diagnostic tools of radiology and ultrasound define if the stone is "completely" disintegrated and passage of fragments can be expected. In case of incomplete fragmentation, alternative endoscopic treatments have to be respected. The efficiency of lithotripters can be estimated by calculating quotients including stone-free rate, number of retreatments, auxiliary and alternative treatments. This is a nonstandardized possibility to compare different lithotripters additionally to the possibility of in vitro studies and the rare prospective randomized trials.

Meanwhile the number of ESWL-treatments decrease progressively since efficacy and invasiveness of endourological procedures (e.g., ureterorenoscopy and percutaneous litholapaxy) improves more and more. Since the development of new lithotripters did not reach higher success rates in the last 25 years and optimal fragmentation is achieved by ESWL applying high energy in general anesthesia the endoscopic procedures are reasonable alternatives with a higher immediate stone-free rate in even more cases.

23.1 Introduction

Within a very short time period after the first clinical treatment of a patient with a kidney stone in February 1980 using the prototype lithotripter Dornier HM1 (Fig. 23.1), the first serial-type HM3 was installed in Germany (in 1983) and thereafter distributed all over the world. The revolution of the shock wave lithotripter (SWL) was so successful that this treatment option quickly was accepted as a reasonable alternative to surgical procedures[1,2] Already 5 years after its introduction, SWL was the first choice treatment for nearly all calculi located in the upper urinary tract. Despite the necessity of general anesthesia, the low morbidity for the patient with this noninvasive procedure justified retreatment when the stone was not completely disintegrated by the first session.

K.U. Köhrmann (✉)
Department of Urology, Theresienkrankenhaus, Mannheim, Germany
e-mail: kai.uwe.koehrmann@theresienkrankenhaus.de

P.N. Rao et al. (eds.), *Urinary Tract Stone Disease*,
DOI 10.1007/978-1-84800-362-0_23, © Springer-Verlag London Limited 2011

Fig. 23.1 First lithotripter for clinical use – the Dornier HM 1

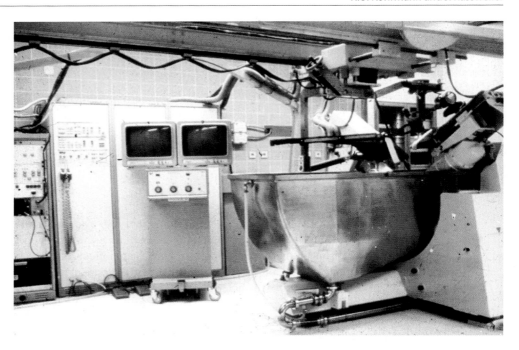

Therefore SWL was applied for almost all renal and ureteral stones, excepting staghorn stones, diverticular stones, asymptomatic stones, and nephrocalcinosis. Certainly, the short learning curve for SWL compared to endoscopic procedures has been an important reason for the fast spread of shock wave lithotripters. The application of shock waves was possible after a short training period for young urologists and has sometimes been performed successfully by medical technicians. This is explained by the low risk of severe complications in SWL, even when it is mishandled.

In the first phase of its introduction, SWL seemed to cause no adverse side effects[1] but with time and the arrival of computed tomography (CT) and magnetic resonance imaging (MRI), the risk for the kidney became apparent.[3,4] The rate of hematoma has been calculated to be around 0.5%.

The further development of lithotripters was intended to improve stone disintegration and to reduce side effects.[5] Concerning the side effects, on the one hand, the trauma to the kidney and adjacent organs should be reduced. On the other hand, pain during shock wave application had to be reduced to avoid general anesthesia. Both effects were thought to be reached by concentrating the shock wave energy to a smaller focal area. Under this intention the electrohydraulic shock wave generator has been modified, but also electromagnetic and piezoelectric sources were developed. The development was successful since pain was limited and SWL without anesthesia became possible.[6]

Improvement of the disintegrative efficacy was not so prosperous. Some in vitro and ex vivo studies seemed to prove an advantage in stone comminution by the modern shock wave machines. But no clinical, prospective randomized trial could confirm a benefit compared with the unmodified Dornier HM3. Nevertheless, some further improvements were gained:

Stone localization by X-ray and/or sonography enabled the treatment of stones with weak or no radiodensity. Additionally, ultrasound localization reduced X-ray exposure to the patient. But sonographic localization did not became widely accepted since this procedure is more time-consuming and ureteral stones usually are not detectable by ultrasound. In the US, urologists usually are not so experienced using sonography. All this has argued against the expensive addition of ultrasound.

The optimal medium for transmission of acoustic shock waves is degassed water. In the Dornier HM3, the patient was immersed in a large water basin. This was also technically elaborate and costly. Therefore the basin was reduced to a water cushion to be coupled by a membrane and jelly between the water and the skin surface. On the downside, it has been shown that this coupling method reduces shock wave energy and can impair disintegration efficacy significantly.

The upgrading of lithotripters to a multifunctional workstation or the integration of the shock wave generator into a urological workstation necessitated compromises. But this was driven by economic demands to enable the acquisition of a lithotripter by smaller hospitals. Therefore modular systems were developed with the possibility to use different parts of the workstation (e.g., the C-arm) separately from the lithotripsy system or to upgrade a urologic table by addition of a shock wave generator.

Today there is a large variety of lithotripter systems (Table 23.1), from expensive high-end devices down to low-budget machines. In a lot of cases, financial limits influence the choice of the lithotripter significantly. Beyond that, there are no hard criteria for selecting the "best" lithotripter.

Table 23.1 Characteristics of recently introduced lithotripters

Machine	SW Generation	Aperture (mm)	Localization		Clinical Application
			X-ray	Ultrasound	
Dornier					
Compact Sigma	Electromagnetic (flat coil, EMSE 140f)	140	Parallel isocentric X-ray C-arm and Isocentric C-arm of shock wave source	Lateral ultrasound	2003
Compact Delta	Electromagnetic (flat coil, EMSE 140f)	140	Parallel Isocentric X-ray C-arm and isocentric C-arm of shock wave source,	Lateral ultrasound	1997
Lithotripter S	Electromagnetic (flat coil, EMSE 220f EMSE 220f-XXP)	220	Isocentric X-ray C-arm	Lateral ultrasound	1997
Lithotripter S II	Electromagnetic (flat coil, EMSE 220f EMSE 220f-XXP)	220	Isocentric X-ray C-arm	Lateral ultrasound	2003
Siemens					
Multiline	Electromagnetic (flat coil, System M)	145	In-line fluoroscopy	In-line ultrasound (optional)	1994
Modularis	Electromagnetic (flat coil, System C/Cplus)	130	Isocentric C-arm	Lateral ultrasound	1998
Lithoskop	Electromagnetic (flat coil, System Pulso)	168	Parallel isocentric in-line fluoroscopy C-arm (double C)	In-line ultrasound	2003
Storz Medical					
Modulith SLX	Electromagnetic (cylinder)	300	In-line fluoroscopy	In-line ultrasound	1995
Modulith SLK	Electromagnetic	178	Off-line fluoroscopy (Lithotrack-navigation)	In-line ultrasound	1998
Modulith SLX-F2	Electromagnetic (dual focus)	300	In-line fluoroscopy	In-line ultrasound	2004
Xinin					
Compact CS	Electromagnetic (self-focusing)	120	–	Lateral ultrasound	2001
Richard Wolf					
Piezolith 3000	Piezoelectric (double layer)	360	Isocentric C-arm	Coaxial ultrasound	2000
Edap-Technomed					
LT02–X	Piezoelectric	500	In-line C-arm	Coaxial ultrasound	1997
Vision	Electrohydraulic (Diatron III)	220	Isocentric C-arm	Lateral ultrasound	2001
Sonolith I-sys	Electroconductive	290	Isocentric C-arm	Lateral ultrasound	2004
Medstone					
Mestone STS-T	Electrohydraulic	150	Isocentric C-arm	Lateral ultrasound (very optional)	1999
Direx					
Nova Ultima	Electrohydraulic (Trigen-technology, turnable)	150	Isocentric-C-arm	Lateral ultrasound (very optional)	2000
Duet	Two electrohydraulic Sources (!)	150	Isocentric C-arm	Lateral ultrasound	2001
Integra	Electromagentic (trapezoid, hollow)	220	In-line fluoroscopy	Lateral ultrasound	2004
HMT Healthtronics					
LithoDiamond	Electrohydraulic (10.000 SW/electrode)	200	Isocentric C-arm		2002
AST					
LithoSpace	Electrohydraulic		External C-arm	External ultrasound	2007

Fig. 23.2 Essential parts of a lithotripter (Wolf Piezolith 3000): 1 = Shock wave generator with coupling cushion; 2 = Localization system (2a = fluoroscopic C-arm; 2b = ultrasound system); 3 = Table for stable patient positioning; 4 = Control unit (Modified with permission from Richard Wolf GmbH)

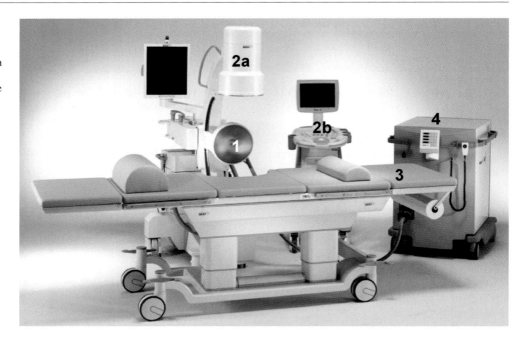

In the following, some essential details of lithotripters (Fig. 23.2) are discussed from the present point of view as a basis for developing optimized units for the future.

The task to characterize extracorporeal shock wave lithotriptors is burdened with severe problems: There are multiple known attributes that influence the lithotripters quality. For many of these, there is no consented definition. These known features are not sufficient enough to predict extracorporeal shock wave lithotripsy (ESWL) success; therefore, some unidentified characteristics have to be assumed. So we cannot judge about the best lithotripter on the market. Therefore this chapter does not add a further description of the current generators, but reflects the actual discussion on this research. In the following some principle factors are given, which should be respected when lithotripters are characterized and compared.

23.2 Modality of Lithotripter Function

In Chapter 22 (Basic Sciences III) Loske describes perfectly the principles of shock wave generation by the different generator systems and the pressure profiles of waves. Based on this, in this chapter the resulting energy with its mechanisms to fragment the stone is described.

23.2.1 Acoustic Energy of Shock Waves

There is consensus that the classical focal zone definition (±6 dB) has only a minor relevance to describe the energy output respectively of the disintegrative efficacy of a shock wave source, whereas it mainly depends on the applied energy with a minimal pressure of about 30 MPa.

The focal size corresponds to the location where the peak pressure decreases to 50 MPa. The energy flux density (ED) includes the positive and negative temporary pressure of the shock wave in the focal plane. In a rotational shock wave field the energy flux density ED is determined by the integral.

Stone fragmentation correlates with the shock wave energy delivered into the focal zone.[7, 8] The acoustic energy of a shock wave pulse should be determined within an area corresponding to an average stone; that is, 12 mm. Outside of this area, the pressure and energy density of the shock wave pulse are usually below the threshold where stone disintegration or shock wave induced side effects are probable. The effective energy (E_{eff}) (12 mm) is calculated by integrating the energy flux density ED in the focal plane over the time.

In accordance with Eisenmenger,[9] the peak pressure may play only a minor role for stone disintegration as long as the threshold of 10–30 Mpa is exceeded. Further experiments confirmed the early findings of Granz[7] that the focal shock wave energy represents the most important physical parameter for stone fragmentation. The energy dose (E_{dose}) (12 mm) is defined as:

$$E_{dose}(12\ mm) = nE_{eff}(12\ mm)$$

Where n is the number of applied shocks and E_{eff} (12 mm) is the effective energy; that is, the acoustic energy per shock wave delivered to an area of 12 mm diameter in the focal plane.

In case intensity settings are changed, the energy dose is calculated by

$$E_{dose}(12\ mm) = n_1 E_{eff1} + n_2 E_{eff2} + n_3 E_{eff3} + \cdots$$

This accumulated energy dose is shown on the display of the Dornier Lithotripter S together with the number of shocks waves.

This Dornier Lithotripter S allows a comparison of the efficiency of different shock wave sources. In clinical studies with the different electromagnetic generators EMSE 220F and EMSE 220F-XP, an energy dose of 152–164 J for ureteral stones and 138–164 J for renal stones was used.[10,11] In Tailly's studies the energy dose was 228 J (EMSE 220F) and 307 (EMSE 220F-XP) for ureteral stones.[10] From the data of Sorensen,[11] an energy dose used for disintegration is about 110 J for a stone smaller than 10 mm and 140 J for a stone between 10 and 20 mm. These results recommend the energy doses for the clinical application: E_{dose} (12 mm) = 100–130 J for renal stones and 150–200 J for ureteral stones.

23.2.2 Shaping the Shock Wave Focus

The temporal and spatial pressure distribution of the shock wave determines its disintegrative efficacy on the stone and its traumatizing capacity in the tissue. The induction of cavitation plays a crucial role for both effects.[12–14] But, there may be a conformation of the shock wave that can allow both results; that is, it has been hypothesized that stone disintegration can be improved while tissue trauma is diminished by manipulating the dynamic of cavitation activity.[15,16] In this context, the definition of the focal zone may become an important parameter. Following the trend to increase the peak pressure of the shock wave source, novel research programs of the different lithotripter manufacturers aimed at an increase respectively in an adaptation of the focal zone to clinical requirement. Since the possibilities are limited for changing the relevant parameters specifically using a single source, studies have also been performed by combining different generators. One of the first devices used clinically was a "Twin-Head" lithotripter (FMD, Lorton, Virginia, USA, Fig. 23.3). In this design, two identical electrohydraulic sources are integrated to have the same focal point but the shockwave axes are perpendicular to each other. The bidirectional synchronous application of the Twin-head lithotripter can also modify the focal area. This device seems to be superior concerning the stone fragmentation and less traumatic compared to the solitary shock wave head of the Dornier Lithotripter S.[17]

Direx presented another electromagnetic lithotripter with trapezoid cone-shaped cylinder and a paraboloid reflector (Integra), offering a variable focal area selectable from 6 to 18 mm.

The double-layer arrangement of the piezoelectric elements of the Wolf device lead to a reduction of the aperture from 50 to 30 cm associated with a significant increase of focal zone (Fig. 23.4). The degree of synchronization of the traveling two shock waves realized by special thyristores allows the variation of delay and pulse forming resulting in three different focal zones[18] (Wolf Piezolith 3000, Fig. 23.2).

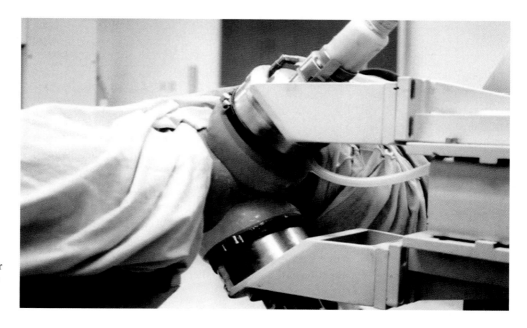

Fig. 23.3 Twin-Head Lithotripter (FMD): simultaneous application of two perpendicularly arranged generators

Fig. 23.4 Principle of piecoelectric double-layer technology: Superposing the front and back pulse of the shock wave source, the same amount of radiated energy can be focused with less up to high energy to provide 2, 4, and 8 mm focus ("triple focus")

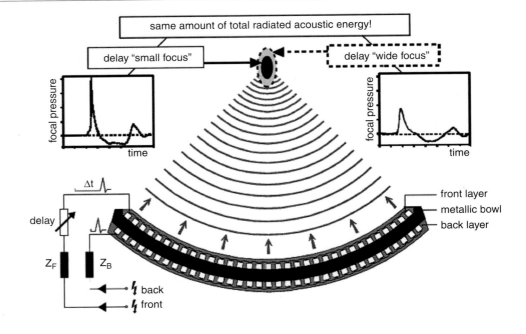

Fig. 23.5 Storz Medical Modulith SLX-F2 (Courtesy of Storz Medical AG, Switzerland)

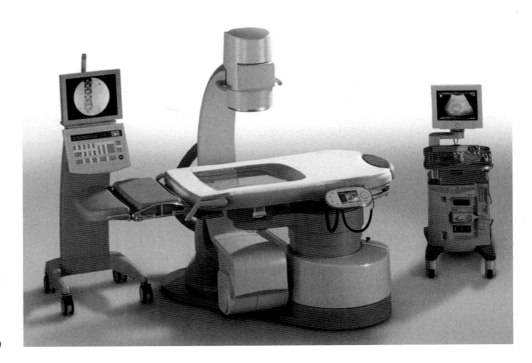

The use of two different focal sizes in the Storz Modulith SL-X2F (Fig. 23.5) is realized by two different rise times of the shock wave using the same generator and paraboloid reflector. Actually, the manufacturer recommends the larger focal zone (50×9 mm^2) for renal calculi and the smaller focal zone (28×6 mm^2) for ureteral stones.

Siemens and Dornier achieved a larger focal zone in their recent devices (Siemens Lithoskop, Fig. 23.6; Dornier Lithotripter S) by significantly prolonged duration of the shock wave pulse, but both manufacturers do not offer different focal sizes. The largest focal size of clinically used lithotripters provides the Xi Xin-Eisenmenger device (XX-ES, Xi Xin

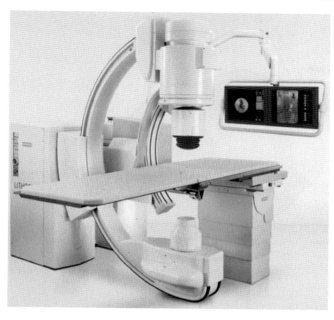

Fig. 23.6 Siemens Lithoskop (Siemens Pressephoto, courtesy of Siemens AG, Germany)

Medical Instruments, Suzhou, China) with a −6 dB width of 18 mm compared to 8 mm of the HM3.[19,20] Interestingly the disintegrative efficiency of this source was superior to the HM3 (634 vs 831 SW).

A very new and promising unit is the combination of an electrohydraulic with a piezoelectric generator. With this design, a variety of parameters can be controlled specifically to evaluate the ideal pulse profile and shock wave sequence. For in vitro application the optimization was successful, but this has to be confirmed in vivo and in the clinical setting.[8,21]

In summary, various companies realized different focal sizes. There is the trend to use the smaller focal sizes for ureteral calculi, but until now, there is no study proofing any advantage of the adaptation of the focus. Moreover, it is clear that the energy output will remain unchanged.

23.3 Physical Mechanisms of Fragmentation

To this date, the perfect design of a lithotripter generator cannot be defined, since the mechanisms of the shock wave to destroy stones and tissue are not elucidated sufficiently. None of the specific mechanisms – spallation, squeezing, or cavitation—alone completely describes stone fragmentation.

The initial stone fracture is similar to fracture of any brittle object and can be considered as a process whereby cracks form as a result of internal stresses generated by extracorporeally applied shock waves. Cracks are presumed to initiate at locations where the shock wave induced stress exceeds a critical value. The further stone disintegration is based on the growth and coalescence of these cracks under repetitive loading and unloading in a process described as dynamic fatigue.[8,22]

23.3.1 Spallation

In spallation, the distal surface of the stone represents an acoustically soft interface, therefore generating a reflected tensile wave from the initially compressive focused shock wave pulse that enters and propagates through the calculus (Fig. 23.7). The degree of reflection depends on the surface of the stone. Thus, spherical shock wave fronts contribute to compression-induced tensile cracks. In translucent oval calculi (i.e., ellipsoid type), it could be demonstrated by Zhong et al.,[23] that this maximum tension occurs close to the distal end of the stone, resulting in a fracture about two-thirds from the proximal end of the stone. The same could be demonstrated when using cylindric stones.[24]

23.3.2 Squeezing

In squeezing, the shock wave is assumed to be broader than the stone and travels in liquid along the side surface of the stone, thereby creating circumferential stress on the calculus. The positive part of the pressure wave acts on the stone by quasi-static squeezing inducing a binary fragmentation with first cleavage surfaces that are either parallel or perpendicular to the wave propagation (Fig. 23.8). Eisenmenger[9] supposed that the wave velocity in the surrounding fluid is much lower than the elastic wave velocities in the stone; that is, the longitudinal wave moves through the stone leaving the "thin shock wave" in the fluid encircling and squeezing the stone in a quasi-static manner. The mechanism of squeezing suggests for high stone fragmentation efficiency focal diameters up to 20 mm (to be larger than the stone) with pulse durations up to 2 μs, but not necessarily a steep shock front. The focal positive pressure could be reduced to the lower pressure range of 10–30 MPa, because this is completely sufficient to overcome the breaking threshold of maximum 2 MPa for human and artificial stones. This theory stimulated the discussion about the importance of a large focal size and a lower focal pressure (i.e., in the HM3) compared to the small focal size with high pressure due to the large aperture in these systems.

Fig. 23.7 Tear and shear forces and cavitation

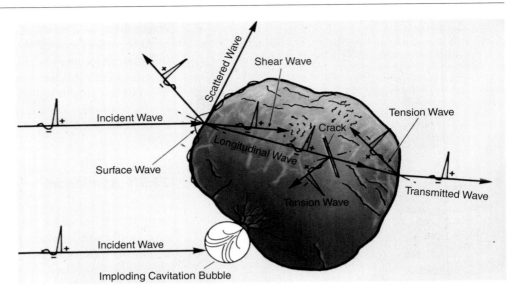

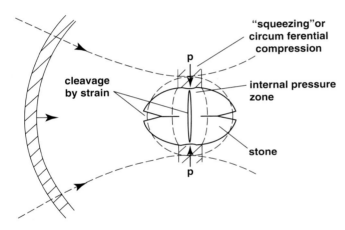

Fig. 23.8 Quasistatic squeezing (Reprinted from[9] with permission from Elsevier)

23.3.2.1 Dynamic Squeezing

Dynamic squeezing describes the phenomenon of shear waves, which are reinforced by squeezing from the lateral borders of the stone. Hereby, the shear wave initiated by the corners of the stone and driven by the squeezing wave along the stone leads to the greatest stress, whereas the reflection of the longitudinal wave at the posterior surface is of minor importance.[25] This theory is based on the parallel travelling of longitudinal waves propagating inside the stone and the shock wave front outside the stone in the liquid. As a result, all acoustic phenomena such as deflection, absorption, diffraction, or the shear and tear waves are considered as well as the phenomenon of reinforcing the longitudinal waves inside the stone by the waves travelling alongside the calculus.

Beside the direct action on the stone, the negative pressure wave causes *cavitation* in the water surrounding the stone, and also within the water in the microcracks and cleavage interfaces of the fragmenting calculus. Cavitation plays an increasing role in particular when fragments become smaller after initial spelling. Using in vitro stone models, the erosion by cavitation is especially observed at the anterior and posterior side of artificial stones in vitro.[26, 27] Cavitation may lead to fragmentation of materials being resistant to tear and shear waves (i.e., cystine, cholesterol). The substantial contribution of fragmentation by cavitation is proved by the observation that suppression of cavitation by highly viscous media surrounding the stone or hyperpressure significantly reduces the disintegrative efficacy of shockwaves. For two reasons of high clinical significance cavitation has to be respected: it causes air bubbles, attenuating the subsequent shock wave, and seems to be an important factor of shock wave induced tissue injury[28]; that is, vascular lesions.

23.3.2.2 Dynamic Fatigue

Dynamic fatigue has been proposed as a general theory for stone comminution and tissue injury in SWL.[22] The theory is based on the observation that stone fragmentation inflicted by the lithotripter shock waves accumulates during the course of the treatment, leading to eventual destruction of the stone configuration. The stone fracture process is therefore characterized as an evolutional process consisting of three phases: initiation (i.e., based on dynamic squeezing), propagation (associated by cavitation), and coalescence (due to the increasing fragility). Finally, microcracks are produced by the mechanical stresses associated with the lithotripter shock waves that may result in a sudden break off of the calculus once the molecular structure of the stone is completely destroyed. The theory relates the physical properties of the stone (i.e., fracture toughness, acoustic speed, density, and void dimensions) to the shock wave parameters (i.e., peak pressure, pulse width, pulse profile, and number of shocks for fragmentation).

23.4 Clinical Factors Influencing the Efficacy of Shock Waves

Between generation of the shock wave and its disintegrating effect on the stone, some essential prerequisites are to be provided by the lithotripter:

- Propagation and coupling of the shock wave from the generator to the patient
- Localization of the stone
- Stone positioning in the shock wave focus
- Control of shock wave dose
- Avoidance of tissue trauma

23.4.1 Propagation and Coupling

Any kind of air bubbles may attenuate the effect of shock wave propagation. Cavitation bubbles induced by the shock wave during its path decrease the energy by scattering and absorption of the following impulse.[29,30] Additionally, air bubbles may be created by mechanical release of oxygen within the water. Such air bubbles may have a much longer lifetime than cavitation bubbles. This can be monitored by real-time ultrasound (i.e., during treatment of distal ureteral stones).

Ideal coupling was realized in the Dornier HM3 using the water tank. Mainly due to cost reduction, modular, and multifunctional use, all manufacturers provide a shock wave source with a coupling cushion. Therefore, the quality of coupling has become one of the key factors of success and has been studied recently in several experimental models.[29,31] It has been shown that even the method of gel application has impact on disintegration. By far the best values were achieved by mound application from the stock container compared to hand or zigzag application from a squeeze bottle. Finally, the quality of the water cushion can be important. The membrane can be injured by the gel or cleaning substances. As a conclusion, the following recommendations assure high coupling quality: shaving the skin if necessary, not shaking the ultrasound gel before application, high amount of warm gel from a container with large opening (not from a squeeze bottle with narrow cone), and checking homogeneous and air bubble free coupling visually or by in-line ultrasound.

23.4.2 Stone Localization

The imaging system for stone localization has to be integrated together with the generator in the limited space in the lithotripter and has to provide identification of all kinds of stones.

There is still the debate over which imaging system fulfills best these demands.[8,16,32] Fluoroscopy is the predominantly used system in clinical routine. Stone localization using this system can identify stones in the whole upper urinary tract, allows fast handling with short learning curve but cannot detect radiolucent and sometimes small stones and is burdened by X-ray exposure to the patient and the physician.

Ultrasound has the advantage of targeting even radiolucent stones without radiation exposure and continuous real-time observation of stone positioning and disintegration process is possible. But calculi in the ureter are usually not detected sonographically (except in the very proximal and intramural part). Due to acoustic deviation, lateral ultrasound may differ from coaxial ultrasound by some millimeters. Theoretically, in-line ultrasound is the best imaging method, because the sound waves and shock waves travel similarly through the body to the stone. With the continuously improving ultrasound technology, sonographic localization has gained popularity. But its limitation lets fluoroscopy remain mandatory to ensure treatment of the broad spectrum of stone situations. Optimal, and realized in the high-end lithotripters, is the combination of both imaging systems. The geometry of the shock wave source sometimes limits their use (alternatively but not simultaneously). Dornier even implemented two ultrasound systems plus isocentric fluoroscopy in their Tri-mode system. In addition, the imaging system plays a crucial part in identifying fragmentation and complete disintegration (see later). Therefore this is, besides the shock wave generator, the most important component of a lithotripter.

The computer-aided system Lithotrack (Storz-Medical, Fig. 23.9) should help to reduce the radiation exposure of the patient. The system applies optical triangulation for 3-D navigation. Because the shock wave head is arranged geometrically in-line with the isocentric fluoroscopic C-arm, the correct position of the SW-source can be controlled by virtual reality without the need of continuous fluoroscopy. The SuperVision system (AST, Fig. 23.10) of the Lithospace uses an optical tracking system, which can be adapted to several ultrasonic devices as well as to fluoroscopic C-arms.

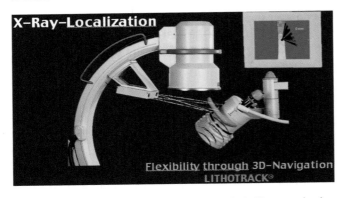

Fig. 23.9 Lithotrack for three-dimensional (3D) X-ray navigation (Storz Modulith SLK, courtesy of Storz Medical AG, Switzerland)

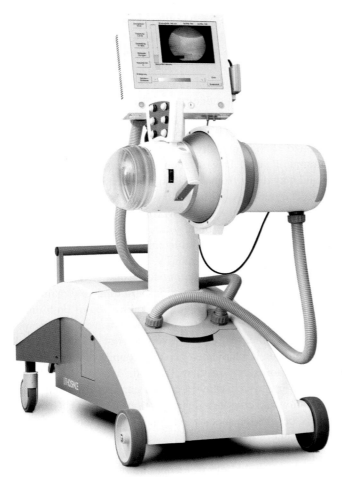

Fig. 23.10 LithoSpace AST (Courtesy of AST GmbH, Germany)

In the Sonolith I-sys (EDAP TMS, Fig. 23.11) the shock wave focus is automatically positioned after marking the stone position on the fluoroscopic or ultrasound screen.

23.4.3 Stone Positioning

A precise positioning and fixation of the stone in the focal point of the shock wave is aspired to; however, respiratory movement may dislodge the calculus considerably and will reduce disintegration. Immobilization of the stone by high-frequent ventilatory respiration and respiratory belts with triggering of SW-impulses were clinically effective but turned out to be too invasive or time consuming. A larger focal zone has the advantage of reducing the rate of incorrect hitting impulses. If lithotripters with smaller focal zones are used, real-time coaxial ultrasound localization may be the optimal alternative to guarantee adequate coupling and localization of the stone.[8]

23.4.4 Control of Shock Wave Dose

In the clinical ESWL session, the applied shock wave dose is controlled only by three parameters: rate (pulse/minute), generator voltage (energy level of the specific lithotripter), and the total number of shots.

23.4.4.1 Pulse Rate

A variety of experimental and clinical studies have been performed to evaluate the influence of shock wave rate on disintegration and side effects of ESWL. By increasing the shock wave rate over 60 or 90 pulses/min, the fragmentation efficacy decreases and tissue trauma can be more pronounced. An explanation is the boosted occurrence of cavitation, when consecutive shock waves are applied before the cavitation bubbles induced by the previous shot are not yet collapsed. A recent metaanalysis including 589 patients in four randomized controlled trials suggests that patients treated at a rate of 60 shocks/min have a significantly greater likelihood of a successful treatment outcome than patients treated at a rate of 120 shocks/min.[33] Based on these findings, the pulse rate should not exceed 60 pulses/min (1 Hz) and in critical patients (i.e., with solitary kidneys, previous anticoagulants) the shocks even work at lower rates.[34] In the clinical reality, however, such low PRF prolongs the treatment time significantly and may lead to inconvenience for the patient who may not maintain a stable position for such a long time.[13,21,34–38]

23.4.4.2 Process of Generator Voltage Along ESWL Session

According to several experimental in vitro and in vivo studies, the slow increase of the generator voltage ("ramping") was

Fig. 23.11 Sonolith® i-sys
Electroconductive lithotripter –
EDAP TMS (Courtesy of EDAP
TMS, France)

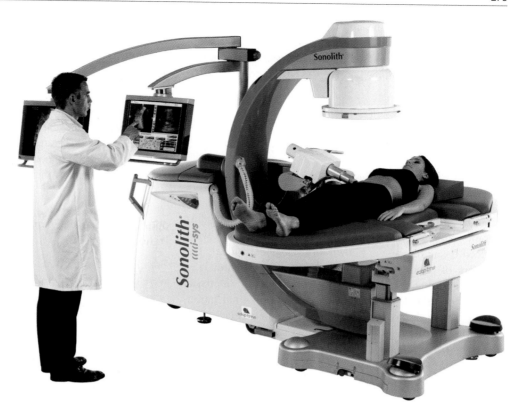

recommended.[39] The stress waves can initiate fragmentation at low output voltages, but higher-energy shockwaves are required to produce greater cavitation activity and overcome the attenuation and scattering effect created by the collection of stone fragments. In the later part of SWL therapy, increased output voltages compensate for attenuation created by the collection of small particles surrounding the larger residual stone fragments and also enhance the cavitation activity. Moreover in this manner the initial atraumatic low energy induces vasoconstriction to protect the kidney when the energy is raised.[40]

23.4.4.3 Defining Endpoint of Shock Wave Application

ESWL application in the clinical routine case is terminated either when the maximal shock wave number is reached or the stone is completely disintegrated. The number of applied shock waves has to be restricted due to increasing risk for tissue trauma (see later). This number depends on the applied shock wave energy. It is defined by experimental and clinical studies for each specific lithotripter and indicated by the manufacturer.

To define the endpoint of comminution of the particular stone is much more difficult for the physician. The prediction

of success, and fragmentation of stones in particular, is a multifactorial problem including attributes of the stone (e.g., composition, size, impaction), properties of shock wave (e.g., focus configuration, energy), application (e.g., shock wave rate, number, "ramping"), coupling, precision of stone localization (e.g., three-dimensional positioning in the focal area, tracking due to stone movement during breathing, patient repositioning), and patient's condition (obesity, acoustic window limited by bone and air-filled bowel).

Since the necessary shock wave doses cannot be predicted, it is essential to monitor the progress of fragmentation and to proof the "complete" disintegration (required maximal fragment size actually not defined!). This depends on the diagnostic principle and its quality during or after the treatment (e.g., fluoroscopy, digital plain film, CT-scan ultrasound). Actually, we have to concede that all imaging modalities (in particular those that are integrated in the lithotripters) do not allow the detection of complete disintegration, as far as the stone can be localized anyway. To stop the shock wave application before reaching the maximal allowed limit (unless stone cannot be localized anymore) implies the risk of incomplete treatment. This disadvantage of the noninvasive ESWL, compared to endoscopic procedures with the advantage of direct inspection, has to be considered and accepted.

The definition of comminution endpoint within one ESWL session or after retreatment is one of the most critical unsolved problems in the application of lithotripters. Here we have to consider that the personal operating experience is an essential predictive factor for success. According to "evidence-based medicine" this has to be integrated into the decision making.[41]

23.4.5 Avoidance of Tissue Trauma

Extracorporeal shock wave lithotripsy still can be dangerous and life threatening.[42] The incidence of gastrointestinal injury secondary to ESWL has been estimated at 1.8%,[43] including colonic perforation or duodenal erosions.[44] Shock wave induced tissue damage is known to be dose dependent. The numbers of shocks in relation to the energy output (i.e., generator voltage) contribute to mechanisms of tissue damage.[45–48] Shock wave induced damage of renal parenchyma primarily occurs at vessels and tubular cells. Depending mainly on the energy output (generator voltage), first, venules are damaged in the medulla followed by rupture of arterioles in the cortex. The main physical reasons for this are cavitation (i.e., for ecchymosis) and tear and shear forces depending on sudden changes (leaps) of impedance in the tissue penetrated by the shock wave; nuclei of cavitation in the parenchyma, blood, urine or bile; and the elasticity and resistance of the tissue exposed to shock waves. In the porcine model, there is a potential for unfocussed shockwaves to damage blood vessels outside the focal zone when the vasculature is seeded with cavitation nuclei.[49] The wide distribution of damage in this study suggests that the acoustic field of a lithotripter delivers negative pressure that exceeds the cavitation threshold far off the acoustic axis underscoring that conditions permissive for cavitation can lead to dramatic sequelae following ESWL.

There is still the controversy whether the energy flux density is the most important parameter for shock wave induced tissue damage.[20] If that will be proved, this would strongly support the theory of a larger focal zone providing similar energy output (correlated to stone fragmentation), but significantly less energy density (resulting in less trauma). Shock wave energy ramping along the ESWL session by pretreatment with low energy can additionally reduce the risk for renal damage.[40]

23.5 Comparison of Lithotripters

Numerous efforts have been made to define and compare efficacy of the different devices by experimental studies and clinical evaluations. But to this date no standards exist for this issue.

23.5.1 In Vitro Studies

Different centers used artificial or natural stones[50] to compare the different shock wave sources. Electrohydraulic and electromagnetic generators provided the highest disintegrative capacity and could destroy the hardest of the natural urinary stones. Within these findings, electromagnetic sources provided the widest range of energy from very low to very high energy levels. In contrast, piezoelectric generators need more shots to destroy the stones.

23.5.2 Clinical Efficacy Quotient

For clinical comparison, the essential parameters of efficacy were calculated to the efficacy quotient (EQ):

$$EQ\% = \frac{\text{rate of stonefree patients after 3 months}}{100\% + \text{rate of re - ESWL} + \text{rate of auxiliary procedures}}$$

The highest efficacy was provided by the lithotripter, which reached the highest rate of stone-free patients with the lowest number of retreatments and lowest rate of auxiliary procedures (to treat complications or to complete disintegration).

The highest EQ was calculated for the very first commercial lithotripter – the unmodified Dornier HM3. Few other generators reached this high efficacy level (Table 23.2). Due to the higher retreatment rate, usually piezoelectric lithotripters had a tendency to a lower efficacy quotient.

23.5.3 Clinical Trials

Retrospective evaluations show a wide range of efficacy for particular lithotripters and sometimes conflicting results.

It has to be mentioned that studies providing the highest scientific evidence – like multicenter, prospective randomized studies are missing. Single-center randomized trials[51–54] confirmed the superior efficacy of the classical Dornier HM3 compared to third-generation (Siemens Lithostar Plus) or fourth-generation (Storz Medical Modulith SLX) electromagnetic machines.[53] Hereby the different anesthetic

Table 23.2 Efficacy quotient (EQ) for different lithotripters according to a literature review by Teichmann[50]

	Generator System	No. of Patients	EQ
Dornier HM3	Electohydraulic	4,242	0.64–0.67
Modulith SL20	Electromagnetic	1,049	0.57–0.67
Lithostar C	Electromagnetic	23,559	0.56–0.64
Medstone STS	Electrohydraulic	3,015	0.60–0.67
Econolith	Electrohydraulic	500	0.56
Dornier Doli	Electromagnetic	103	0.36

regimens have to be respected: epidural anesthesia for HM3 and Lithostar compared to analgosedation for Modulith.

23.5.4 Clinical Classification of Lithotripters

Additional facilities of the lithotripter define the treatment comfort for the patient and the medical staff as well as the possibility for multiple and interdisciplinary use. The valuable equipment of fluoroscopic and sonographic imaging systems and treatment tables can be designed to be used for general diagnostic procedures as well as endourological and other interventional measures. For these issues the patient has to be positioned stable on the table. The table has to be movable in all three dimensions and optional to be tilted in Trendelenburg position. A comfortable access for the surgeon to perform transurethral or percutaneous procedures should be enabled. For a smooth work flow, a narrow arrangement using fixed integrated lithotripter components are optimally integrated in the high-end lithotripter for a urological workstation, with capital costs of about 300,000–350,000 €.

In the modular system, the components, for example, localization system (most frequently fluoroscopic C-arc) and operating table, can be used separately from the shock wave source. Usually these systems, with capital costs of 250,000–300.000 €, need more space and working time to be composed and adjusted for the ESWL session.

The low-budget lithotripter consists of a mobile shock wave source with limited efficacy, an integrated ultrasound localization system that is coupled by a water cushion to a patient, who is positioned on a common stretcher. The capital costs for such an "economy class" model is 150–250.000 €.

For the comprehensive clinical classification, additional parameters (e.g., adverse side effects) should be respected. With this respect, the most effective HM3 device usually requires general anesthesia; in contrast, the less effective piezoelectric lithotripters can be applied without any analgesia. In most institutions, those lithotripters are preferred that can be used in analgosedation (modified HM3, other electrohydraulic and electromagnetic lithotripters, high-energy piezoelectric lithotripter). Therefore, a correlation between disintegrative efficacy and pain/need for anesthesia can be assumed.

23.6 Treatment Philosophy: SWL Versus Endourology

For most of the calculi in the upper urinary tract, different options are offered as reasonable and successful treatments. The physician's experience is the next essential factor. However, the final decision is set by the patient's preference.

In general, patients have to decide among three different strategies (Table 23.3).

In Europe, the advantage of SWL being able to be used without anesthesia is highly appreciated.[55] Therefore, the second-generation lithotripters were favored even if they had limited efficacy compared to the HM3 under analgesia. In contrast, in the USA the application of general or spinal anesthesia for a comfortable shock wave treatment is not assessed as a disadvantage. Under anesthesia, maximal energy can be applied with the intention to reach the highest rate of stone disintegration independently of the induced pain. The solitary limit is the tissue trauma.

The difference in using anesthesia has resulted in a bias in the competition for the nomination of the "gold standard" lithotripter. Until now the unmodified Dornier HM3 is seen to provide the highest disintegrative efficacy and is usually run under anesthesia. The high-end second- or third-generation lithotripters (Storz Modulith, Siemens Lithostar, Wolf Piezolith, etc.) did not exceed this, but treatment usually was applied under analgesia-sedation.[53] Studies should be conducted to compare all these machines (including the flexible focal zones of the latest machines) under the same conditions (general anesthesia) with respect to disintegration and trauma. The results would then provide a basis for the next comparison against the endoscopic procedures.

Table 23.3 The three strategies for treating stones in the upper urinary tract

Strategy	Advantage	Disadvantage
SWL without anesthesia	• No anesthesia	• Lower stone clearance rate
	• Low complication rate by procedure	• Longer follow-up to stone clearance
	• Low treatment costs	• Risk of complication during passage of residual fragments
	• No drainage (stent, PCNL)	• Higher costs in follow-up
SWL under anesthesia	• Better disintegration rate	• Moderate duration up to stone clearance
	• Low complication rate by procedure	• Risk of complication during passage of residual fragments
	• Moderate treatment costs	• Moderate costs in follow-up
	• No drainage (stent, PCNL)	
Endourology under anesthesia	• Highest immediate stone clearance rate	• Risk for severe complications
	• Shortest treatment time	• Anesthesia
	• Shortest and least expensive follow-up	• Drainage (stent, PCNL) re-intervention for removal of drainage

23.7 Future of Shock Wave Lithotripsy

Epidemiology of urolithiasis and the tendency not to await spontaneous passage results in an increasing need for active stone removal.

Concerning their efficiency, lithotripter development seems to have reached a peak level in recent years. A further increase is not to be expected. But attention should be paid to the advance in our knowledge about shock wave physics, control parameters, and modes of action on the stones. A breakthrough with significantly improved clinical results by using new generator concepts is not foreseeable.

For most stone situations there will remain a reasonable choice between SWL versus endoscopic procedures. The evolution of tools for endoscopic stone removal is proceeding. Adverse side effects of both treatment concepts are minimized.

Patients can expect a nearly 100% success rate. Additionally they expect more and more a very comfortable treatment. Therefore, the tendency is to be treated under general anesthesia even for SWL to ensure pain-free and rapid (by using highly effective shock waves) therapy.

In conclusion, SWL will continue to play an established, if slightly reduced, role in stone treatment in the future.

23.8 Conclusions

Shock wave physics, mechanism of stone destruction, and developing the optimal shock wave source are not completely understood. Therefore, improvement of ESWL cannot be foreseeable up to now. Endourological procedures are the competitors. But due to the increasing need for stone intervention due to patients' demands for early stone removal and increasing stone incidence, ESWL will retain an established role in stone treatment.

Acknowledgments This chapter includes the results of two consensus meetings of the German Society of Shock Wave Lithotripsy in 2005[8] and 2009.[56] The aim of these meetings was to exchange knowledge and to reach a consensus with respect to the physics, technical issues, and applications of ESWL. This unique panel consisted of urological experts as well as representatives of lithotripter manufacturers and incorporated an extensive review of the current literature.

Besides the authors, the following experts were part of the panel:

Thorsten Bergsdorf, Christian Chaussy Department of Urology, Stadtkrankenhaus München-Harlaching, University of Munich, Germany

Christian Bohris, Bernd Forssmann, Department of Research, Dornier MedTech Systems, D 82234 Wesseling, Germany

Michael Burkhardt, Peter Vallon; Department of Research, Richard Wolf, D75434 Knittlingen, Germany

Leandro Burnes, Christian Meinert, R&D Urology, Siemens Medical Solutions, D91052 Erlangen, Germany

Paul Partheymüller; Department of Clinical Application, EDAP TMS GmbH, D24937 Flensburg, Germany

Othmar Wess; Department of Research, Storz-Medical, CH8280 Kreuzlingen, Switzerland

Jürgen Williger; AST GmbH, D07745 Jena, Germany

Dieter Jocham; Department Of Urology, University of Schleswig-Holstein (UKSH) Campus Lubeck Medica, Lübeck, Germany

Gerald Haupt; Department of Urology, St.-Vincentius-Krankenhauses, Speyer, Germany

Dirk Wilbert, Department of Urology, Kantonales Spital, CH-8730 Uznach, Switzerland

References

1. Chaussy C, Schmiedt E. Extracorporeal shock wave lithotripsy (ESWL) for kidney stones. An alternative to surgery? *UrolRadiol.* 1984;6:80–87.
2. Chaussy CG, Fuchs GJ. Current state and future developments of noninvasive treatment of human urinary stones with extracorporeal shock wave lithotripsy. *JUrol.* 1989;141:782–789.
3. Kaude JV, Williams CM, Millner MR, Scott KN, Finlayson B. Renal morphology and function immediately after extracorporeal shock-wave lithotripsy. *AJR AmJRoentgenol.* 1985;145:305–313.
4. Rubin JI, Arger PH, Pollack HM, et al. Kidney changes after extracorporeal shock wave lithotripsy: CT evaluation. *Radiology.* 1987;162:21–24.
5. Chow GK, Streem SB. Extracorporeal lithotripsy. Update on technology. *UrolClinNorth Am.* 2000;27:315–322.
6. Rassweiler J, Schmidt A, Gumpinger R, Mayer R, Eisenberger F. ESWL for ureteral calculi. Using the Dornier HM 3, HM 3+ and Wolf Piezolith 2,200. *JUrol(Paris).* 1990;96:149–153.
7. Granz B, Kohler G. What makes a shock wave efficient in lithotripsy? *JStoneDis.* 1992;4:123–128.
8. Rassweiler JJ, Bergsdorf T, Ginter S, et al. Progress in Lithotripter technology. In: Chaussy C, Haupt G, Jocham D, Köhrmann KU, Wilbert D, eds. *Therapeutic Energy Applications in Urology. Standards and recent developments.* Stuttgart – Nex York: Thieme; 2005:3–15.
9. Eisenmenger W. The mechanisms of stone fragmentation in ESWL. *Ultrasound Med Biol.* 2001;27:683–693.
10. Tailly GG. In situ SWL of ureteral stones: comparison between an electrohydraulic and an electromagnetic shockwave source. *JEndourol.* 2002;16:209–214.
11. Sorensen C, Chandhoke P, Moore M, Wolf C, Sarram A. Comparison of intravenous sedation versus general anesthesia on the efficacy of the Doli 50 lithotriptor. *JUrol.* 2002;168:35–37.
12. Jain A, Shah TK. Effect of air bubbles in the coupling medium on efficacy of extracorporeal shock wave lithotripsy. *EurUrol.* 2007;51:1680–1686.
13. Pishchalnikov YA, McAteer JA, Williams JC Jr, Pishchalnikova IV, VonDerHaar RJ. Why stones break better at slow shockwave rates than at fast rates: in vitro study with a research electrohydraulic lithotripter. *JEndourol.* 2006a;20:537–541.
14. Zeman RK, Davros WJ, Goldberg JA, et al. Cavitation effects during lithotripsy. Part II. Clinical observations. *Radiology.* 1990b;177:163–166.
15. Cleveland RO, Anglade R, Babayan RK. Effect of stone motion on in vitro comminution efficiency of Storz Modulith SLX. *JEndourol.* 2004;18:629–633.
16. Lingeman JE, Cleveland RO, Evan AP, et al. Stone technology: shock wave and intracorporeal lithotripsy. In: Denstedt J, Khoury S, eds. *Stone Disease. 2nd International Consulation on Stone Disease.* 21st ed. Paris: Health Publications; 2008:85–135.

17. Sheir KZ, Elhalwagy SM, Abo-Elghar ME, et al. Evaluation of a synchronous twin-pulse technique for shock wave lithotripsy: a prospective randomized study of effectiveness and safety in comparison to standard single-pulse technique. *BJU Int.* 2008;101:1420–1426.

18. Wang R, Faerber GJ, Roberts WW, Morris DS, Wolf JS Jr. Single-center North American experience with Wolf Piezolith 3000 in Management of Urinary Calculi. *Urology.* 2009;73(5):958–963.

19. Eisenmenger W, Du XX, Tang C, et al. The first clinical results of "wide-focus and low-pressure" ESWL. *Ultrasound MedBiol.* 2002;28:769–774.

20. Evan AP, McAteer JA, Connors BA, et al. Independent assessment of a wide-focus, low-pressure electromagnetic lithotripter: absence of renal bioeffects in the pig. *BJUInt.* 2008b;101:382–388.

21. Talic RF, Rabah DM. Effect of modification of shock-wave delivery on stone fragmentation. *CurrOpinUrol.* 2006b;16:83–87.

22. Lokhandwalla M, Sturtevant B. Fracture mechanics model of stone comminution in ESWL and implications for tissue damage. *PhysMedBiol.* 2000a;45:1923–1940.

23. Zhong P, Preminger GM. Mechanisms of differing stone fragility in extracorporeal shockwave lithotripsy. *J Endourol.* 1994;8:263–68.

24. Sapozhnikov OA, Maxwell AD, MacConaghy B, Bailey MR. A mechanistic analysis of stone fracture in lithotripsy. *JAcoustSocAm.* 2007a;121:1190–1202.

25. Sapozhnikov OA, Maxwell AD, MacConaghy B, Bailey MR. A mechanistic analysis of stone fracture in lithotripsy. *JAcoustSocAm.* 2007b;121:1190–1202.

26. Crum LA. Cavitation microjets as a contributory mechanism for renal calculi disintegration in ESWL. *JUrol.* 1988;140:1587–1590.

27. Sass W, Dreyer HP, Kettermann S, Seifert J. The role of cavitational activity in fragmentation processes by lithotripters. *JStoneDis.* 1992;4:193–207.

28. Seemann O, Rassweiler J, Chvapil M, Alken P, Drach GW. The effect of single shock waves on the vascular system of artificially perfused rabbit kidneys. *JStoneDis.* 1993;5:172–178.

29. Pishchalnikov YA, Neucks JS, VonDerHaar RJ, Pishchalnikova IV, Williams JC Jr, McAteer JA. Air pockets trapped during routine coupling in dry head lithotripsy can significantly decrease the delivery of shock wave energy. *JUrol.* 2006c;176:2706–2710.

30. Zeman RK, Davros WJ, Garra BS, Horii SC. Cavitation effects during lithotripsy. Part I. Results of in vitro experiments. *Radiology.* 1990a;177:157–161.

31. Neucks JS, Pishchalnikov YA, Zancanaro AJ, VonDerHaar JN, Williams JC Jr, McAteer JA. Improved acoustic coupling for shock wave lithotripsy. *UrolRes.* 2008;36:61–66.

32. Auge BK, Preminger GM. Update on shock wave lithotripsy technology. *CurrOpinUrol.* 2002;12:287–290.

33. Semins MJ, Trock BJ, Matlaga BR. The effect of shock wave rate on the outcome of shock wave lithotripsy: a meta-analysis. *JUrol.* 2008;179:194–197.

34. Paterson RF, Lifshitz DA, Lingeman JE, et al. Stone fragmentation during shock wave lithotripsy is improved by slowing the shock wave rate: studies with a new animal model. *JUrol.* 2002a;168:2211–2215.

35. Madbouly K, El Tiraifi AM, Seida M, El Faqih SR, Atassi R, Talic RF. Slow versus fast shock wave lithotripsy rate for urolithiasis: a prospective randomized study. *JUrol.* 2005;173:127–130.

36. McAteer JA, Evan AP, Williams JC Jr, Lingeman JE. Treatment protocols to reduce renal injury during shock wave lithotripsy. *CurrOpinUrol.* 2009;19:192–195.

37. Pace KT, Ghiculete D, Harju M, Honey RJ. Shock wave lithotripsy at 60 or 120 shocks per minute: a randomized, double-blind trial. *JUrol.* 2005;174:595–599.

38. Yilmaz E, Batislam E, Basar M, Tuglu D, Mert C, Basar H. Optimal frequency in extracorporeal shock wave lithotripsy: prospective randomized study:. *Urology.* 2005;66:1160–1164.

39. Pishchalnikov YA, McAteer JA, Williams JC Jr. Effect of firing rate on the performance of shock wave lithotriptors. *BJUInt.* 2008;102:1681–1686.

40. Handa RK, Bailey MR, Paun M, et al. Pretreatment with low-energy shock waves induces renal vasoconstriction during standard shock wave lithotripsy (SWL): a treatment protocol known to reduce SWL-induced renal injury. *BJU Int.* 2009;103(9): 1270–1274.

41. Sackett DL, Rosenberg WM, Gray JA, Haynes RB, Richardson WS. Evidence based medicine: what it is and what it isn't:. *BMJ.* 1996;312:71–72.

42. McAteer JA, Evan AP. The acute and long-term adverse effects of shock wave lithotripsy. *SeminNephrol.* 2008;28:200–213.

43. Williams AR, Delius M, Miller DL, Schwarze W. Investigation of cavitation in flowing media by lithotripter shock waves both in vitro and in vivo. *Ultrasound MedBiol.* 1989;15:53–60.

44. Kurz W, Klein B, Rumstadt B. Colonic perforation after extracorporeal shock wave lithotripsy. *DtschMedWochenschr.* 2009;134: 401–403.

45. Bergsdorf T, Thuroff S, Chaussy C. The isolated perfused kidney: an in vitro test system for evaluation of renal tissue damage induced by high-energy shockwaves sources. *JEndourol.* 2005;19: 883–888.

46. Evan AP, McAteer JA, Connors BA, Blomgren PM, Lingeman JE. Renal injury during shock wave lithotripsy is significantly reduced by slowing the rate of shock wave delivery. *BJUInt.* 2007;100: 624–627.

47. Kohrmann KU, Back W, Bensemann J, et al. The isolated perfused kidney of the pig: new model to evaluate shock wave-induced lesions. *JEndourol.* 1994;8:105–110.

48. Rassweiler J, Kohrmann KU, Back W, et al. Experimental basis of shockwave-induced renal trauma in the model of the canine kidney. *World JUrol.* 1993;11:43–53.

49. Matlaga BR, McAteer JA, Connors BA, et al. Potential for cavitation-mediated tissue damage in shockwave lithotripsy. *J Endourol.* 2008 Jan;22(1):121–6.

50. Teichman JM, Portis AJ, Cecconi PP, et al. In vitro comparison of shock wave lithotripsy machines. *JUrol.* 2000;164:1259–1264.

51. Chan SL, Stothers L, Rowley A, Perler Z, Taylor W, Sullivan LD. A prospective trial comparing the efficacy and complications of the modified Dornier HM3 and MFL 5000 lithotriptors for solitary renal calculi. *JUrol.* 1995;153:1794–1797.

52. Francesca F, Grasso M, Da Pozzo L, Bertini R, Nava L, Rigatti P. Ureteral lithiasis: in situ piezoelectric versus in situ spark gap lithotripsy. A randomized study. *ArchEspUrol.* 1995;48: 760–763.

53. Gerber R, Studer UE, Danuser H. Is newer always better? A comparative study of 3 lithotriptor generations. *JUrol.* 2005;173:2 013–2016.

54. Sheir KZ, Madbouly K, Elsobky E. Prospective randomized comparative study of the effectiveness and safety of electrohydraulic and electromagnetic extracorporeal shock wave lithotriptors. *JUrol.* 2003;170:389–392.

55. Tiselius HG. Removal of ureteral stones with extracorporeal shock wave lithotripsy and ureteroscopic procedures. What can we learn from the literature in terms of results and treatment efforts? *UrolRes.* 2005;33:185–190.

56. Rassweiler, JJ, Bergsdorf,T, Bohris,C, et al. Shock wave technology and application – state of the art in 2009. In: Chaussy C, Haupt G, Jocham D, Köhrmann KU, Wilbert D (eds.) Update in Therapeutic Energy Application in Urology. Thieme Stuttgart – New York, 2009:In press

Biological Effects Produced by High-Energy Shock Waves

24

Yifei Xing, Eric C. Pua, W. Neal Simmons, F. Hadley Cocks, Michael Ferrandino, Glenn M. Preminger, and Pei Zhong

Abstract High-energy shock waves are known to produce a wide range of bioeffects associated with their clinical applications. In shock wave lithotripsy (SWL), which is the most successful application of shock waves in clinical medicine for noninvasive disintegration of kidney and upper urinary stones, transient hematuria, hematoma, and temporary deterioration of renal function may be produced. These short-term side effects in the kidney usually disappear in a few days or weeks without leading to serious long-term complications. However, there are continued efforts to investigate and understand the relationship between shock wave exposure and potential chronic adverse effects, such as new onset of hypertension and diabetes mellitus (DM). In particular, it has been advocated that high-energy shock waves should be administered judiciously to elderly and pediatric patients who are at higher risk for shock-wave-induced adverse effects than are young adult patients. Besides SWL, bioeffects produced by high-energy shock waves have been harnessed and exploited for the treatment of a variety of non-urological diseases. Shock wave therapy has been used extensively to promote bone fracture healing, pain alleviation for conditions such as epicondylitis, and the healing of chronic ulcers. Although the effectiveness and efficacy of these treatments still need to be fully validated, numerous studies have suggested that shock waves can stimulate healing through promotion of both osteogenic and angiogenic pathways. In addition, new avenues of applications are emerging as the feasibility of using shock waves for transient permeabilization of cell membrane has been demonstrated, suggesting the possibility of shock wave-targeted, noninvasive drug and gene delivery to internal organs.

24.1 Introduction

Although the widespread use of shock wave lithotripsy (SWL) has proven effective for the management of urinary tract calculi, the adverse biological effects resulting from exposure of patients to high-energy shock waves are still not completely known. Acute and chronic injury produced by SWL remains a clinical concern and has been a topic of debate for more than 20 years. Furthermore, efforts to understand the bioeffects produced by high-energy shock waves is complicated by the evolution and diversity of technologies used in clinical lithotripters. Particular advances in methods of shock wave generation,

focusing, coupling, and stone localization confound investigations of bioeffects. As SWL enters its third decade of clinical use, a growing body of literature from laboratory and clinical studies has accumulated concerning the acute and chronic injuries associated with high-energy shock wave exposure.

Besides the adverse effects produced by shock wave–tissue interaction, numerous studies have explored the potentially beneficial bioeffects of high-energy shock waves that may be harnessed for therapeutic applications. Perhaps the most well-known therapeutic application outside SWL is in the field of orthopedics, where shock waves have been used to treat a number of conditions, including lateral epicondylitis, plantar fasciitis, and fracture healing. Moreover, therapeutic use of shock waves is not limited to the musculoskeletal system; angiogenic effects have been exploited to treat soft tissue in chronic lower extremity ulcers and ischemic myocardium. New applications of high-energy shock waves are emerging in the fields of targeted drug and gene delivery.

M. Ferrandino (✉)
Division of Urology and Department of Surgery,
Duke University Medical Center, Zootrent Drive, DUMC 2803,
Durham, North Carolina, 27713, USA
e-mail: michael.ferrandino@duke.edu

P.N. Rao et al. (eds.), *Urinary Tract Stone Disease*,
DOI 10.1007/978-1-84800-362-0_24, © Springer-Verlag London Limited 2011

In this chapter, we discuss the biological effects produced by high-energy shock waves, including acute and chronic side effects of SWL. The first section of this chapter focuses on shock wave treatment of urolithiasis along with its potential acute and chronic complications (renal and extrarenal). The second section of this chapter discusses additional existing and potential therapeutic applications of shock wave–tissue interactions, including the emerging fields of ultrasound-mediated gene transfer and drug delivery.

24.2 Adverse Bioeffects of SWL

24.2.1 Renal Complications

24.2.1.1 Acute Effects

Observations from animal studies and clinical treatment have demonstrated that shock waves can cause injury to the kidney. Pathological examination of human and animal kidneys have shown endothelial cell damage to midsized arteries and veins, as well as glomerular capillaries immediately following SWL.[1,2] Thin-walled arcuate veins in the corticomedullary junction are especially vulnerable to shock wave exposure and are related to hematuria and hematoma.[1] Injury to arteries is commonly limited to the level of the interlobular to afferent arterioles.[1] SWL-induced vascular injury includes disruption of the vessel wall, especially the endothelium, resulting in extravasation of blood cells into the surrounding tissue and clot formation at the site of the rupture.[3] Electron microscopy has revealed distinct sites of endothelial rupture, with significant changes observed in the peritubular capillaries, where complete breaks are seen to pass through the cell and its basement membrane.[1,4] This type of damage is not observed in other forms of renal trauma and may be unique to SWL.[5]

Hematuria is a commonly observed acute adverse effect of SWL, with most cases presenting as gross hematuria. In addition, SWL-targeted kidneys frequently exhibit hemorrhage of varying degrees in one or more areas, including the perirenal fat, the subcapsular tissue, and the tubular parenchyma.[5] Clinically, symptomatic intrarenal, subcapsular, or perirenal fluid collections and hematomas occur at a rate of 0.2–1.5% of patients undergoing SWL.[6–10] However, when computerized tomography or magnetic resonance imaging (MRI) is performed routinely post-SWL, the hematoma rate may increase to 20–25%.[11–13] While the number and energy level of the shock waves play a critical role in hematoma formation,[14] several additional risk factors have been identified, including bleeding diseases, diathesis, hypertension, obesity, diabetes mellitus (DM), and administration of antiplatelet activity medicine. Presentation of hematoma has also been shown to increase significantly with patient age.[15]

SWL-induced hematuria is often self-limited, typically not requiring intervention. Treatment is conservative in most cases. The most common outcome of hematoma formation is spontaneous radiographic resolution of the hematoma within a mean of 13 months without clinically evident adverse effects on blood pressure or renal function.[16]

24.2.1.2 Functional Alteration

Although the extent of acute alterations in renal function induced by shock wave treatment is not fully elucidated, several functional alterations are observed. Paraaminohippurate acid (PAH) clearance and extraction levels have been used pre-and post-SWL to evaluate renal function alterations after shock wave treatment. A change in PAH clearance indicates an alteration in renal blood flow, altered tubular function, or both. Animal studies have demonstrated that PAH clearance levels decreased significantly after SWL but returned to baseline levels within a few days.[17,18] Other blood and urine markers that serve as indicators of renal injury, such as rennin, creatinine, N-acetyl-b-D-glucosaminidase (NAG), β(beta)-galactosidase (β-Gal), β(beta)-2-microglobulin (β2M), were found to be altered immediately after SWL, implying deterioration of renal function by shock wave exposure.[14] However, similar to PAH, these biochemical markers return to near-normal levels within a few days, thereby negating their utility in determination of long-term bioeffects.[14]

An immediate decrease in effective plasma flow, as measured by renal scan, was reported in 30% of kidneys treated with SWL.[11] Nonobstructed kidneys were found to have partial delay to complete loss of contrast excretion after SWL.[11,19] The decrease in renal function has been linked to the number of shocks administered. Although the underlying mechanism is still unknown, preexisting renal diseases, urinary tract infection, and solitary kidneys have been found to correlate with more severe renal function alterations.

On the cellular level, SWL has been found to have an apoptotic effect on renal tubular cells that can be detected up to 4 weeks after the treatment, while, in contrast, no apoptotic effects on glomerular cells have been observed.[20] Treatment with SWL also attenuates the proliferative indices of both tubular and glomerular cells.[20] Animal studies have documented that the calcium channel blocker, verapamil, has a protective effect on histopathologic features at 24 h and 3 months following SWL.[21] Nifedipine, another calcium channel blocker, given pre-SWL has shown a significant reduction in urinary markers of acute tissue injury.[22] Based on these findings it has been suggested that some preventive medications, such as calcium channel antagonists, might be a reasonable option in patients who are at high risk for more severe renal lesions after SWL.[20]

Although the mechanisms for SWL-induced renal injury are believed to be mechanical in nature (from cavitation[23] and shear stresses[24,25]), several studies have indicated that free radical formation may also play a role in renal damage during SWL. Antioxidants such as vitamin C and E, as well as caffeic acid, phenethyl ester, and allopurinol, have been reported to reduce shock-wave-induced renal tubular oxidative stress, providing significant protection against radical damage or prevent free radical formation in animal models and patients.[26-29] Nifedipine, a calcium antagonist, was also found to significantly decrease the protein markers associated with impaired renal function in patients.[28] The potential mechanisms of calcium antagonists on renal function include inhibition of pathologically increased influx of calcium ions, restoration of impaired effective renal plasma flow by vasodilation, and prevention of renal parenchyma ischemia.[30-32]

24.2.1.3 Chronic Effects

During the past decade, a number of studies have been carried out to determine the link between SWL and renal failure, hypertension, and diabetes mellitus. Despite the concerns for potential long-term adverse effects, the correlation between SWL-induced injury and long-term complications have yet to be clearly determined.

Acute vascular lesions produced by shock wave treatment have been observed to progress to scar formation and may subsequently result in chronic loss of nephrons and functional renal mass. Renal fibrosis has been found in experimental canines 1 month following treatment by the Dornier HM3 lithotripter, with the severity of scarring dependent on the dose of shock waves.[33,34] It is believed that the inner medulla of the kidney may be particularly susceptible to damage from shock waves, but both tubules and glomeruli may also be affected. Necrotic atrophy of renal papillae at 3 months post-SWL has been reported,[35] with scar formation spanning throughout the thickness of the kidney.[35] Single-photon emission computed tomography (SPECT) has shown some loss of renal function and scarring persisting 1 month after treatment.[36]

The association of acute onset hypertension with SWL has been a controversial subject since it was first reported in the late 1980s.[37] A prospective study showed an increase in intrarenal resistive index in patients 60 years of age and older.[38] This finding implies that SW treatment of elderly patients may be associated with serious, long-term adverse effects, and that age is a risk factor.[39] However, despite these indications of a link between SWL and hypertension, a direct association is unclear and is the subject of considerable debate.[5,38-44] Concerns of the potential link between SWL and diabetes mellitus (DM) have been highlighted by a recent study from the Mayo Clinic. In a retrospective 19-year follow-up, it was found that patients who underwent SWL for the treatment of kidney stones in 1986 were at higher risk of

developing DM compared to the control group without shock wave treatment.[40] The development of diabetes mellitus in the SWL group was associated with the number of shocks administered and the total acoustic energy delivered during the treatment.[40] However, several drawbacks in the study design have been noted.[45,46] For example, the control cohort included patients who received conservative treatment for urinary stones. Additionally, stone disease in the SWL group was typically more severe than in the control group. Moreover, differences in stone size were not controlled in multivariate analysis, and therefore, the severity of urolithiasis may have been different between the SWL and control groups. These discrepancies might affect the new onset of diabetes mellitus, which is considered to be independently associated with the development of urinary stones.[47] Family history, a known risk factor for the development of diabetes mellitus, was not reported for either cohort. Furthermore, the data for the SWL group were collected via self-report questionnaire, whereas the data for controls were determined through chart review, potentially introducing collection bias.

In contrast to the findings of the Mayo Clinic study, Sato et al. compared the new onset of DM after SWL in renal and ureteral stone groups and did not find significant differences in the BMI, preoperative prevalence of hypertension, or DM as metabolic parameters.[44] Their data showed no significant difference in the new onset of DM between the renal (and ureteropelvic junction [UPJ]) and ureteral stone groups.[44] However, several limitations of this study have also been identified.[48] First, matched comparison between treatment groups was not performed and length of follow-up was not consistent for all patients. Second, although both groups required surgical intervention, stone size was significantly larger in the renal group compared with the ureteral group. Finally, the survey response rate was low (30%).[48] It should also be noted that there is significant difference in the shock wave dose and energy levels administered in these two studies. Significantly lower shock wave exposure was used in patients in Japan compared to their counterparts in the USA.[25,31] Therefore, it is fair to conclude that the Mayo Clinic report should be viewed as a warning of possible long-term adverse consequences of SWL, which should be applied more judiciously. Clearly, further clinical and basic research is warranted to determine the threshold and potential causal effect between SWL and DM.

Multiple SWL treatments may also exacerbate stone disease. In the past 3 decades, there has been a clear rise in the occurrence of calcium phosphate (CaP) stones and a transition from calcium oxalate (CaOx) stones to CaP stones.[49] A striking positive correlation between the percentage of CaP stones and the number of lithotripsy sessions per patient has been observed.[50] The number of SWL procedures was higher for CaP stone formers than for CaOx stone formers and was highest for patients with brushite stones.[50]

24.2.2 Effect of SWL in Pediatric Patients

Shock wave lithotripsy has been used for the treatment of renal stones in pediatric patients since the mid-1980s.[51] To date, there are conflicting reports in the literature regarding the potential detrimental effects of high-energy shock wave treatment on the development of kidneys in children. In 1998, Lifshitz and associates reported that SWL impaired bilateral renal growth in pediatric patients.[52] However, other pediatric series have shown no changes in blood pressure, predicted renal growth, mean body height, glomerular filtration rate, or split renal function after SWL treatment.[53–55] Most recently, Reisiger et al. compared SWL-treated kidneys with nontreated, contralateral kidneys for expected and actual kidney size and growth rate, but found no statistically significant differences.[56]

Although most clinical reports indicate that SWL in children is not associated with inevitable risk of adverse effects, shock wave treatment should always be applied with caution and with minimal dose and energy level in the pediatric population. At a high energy level and large number of shocks, lithotripsy has been shown to cause renal damage in animal models and may even result in transient damage of tubular function in children.[20,57–59] Furthermore, it has been demonstrated, in a porcine model, that small kidneys are more susceptible to SW-induced injury than their adult counterparts.[60]

24.2.3 Extrarenal Effects

24.2.3.1 Cardiovascular System

The main concern regarding SWL-associated adverse effects on the cardiovascular system is the induction of arrhythmic activity. Initially, it was considered that shock waves are capable of producing cardiac arrhythmia as they traverse through the body. Therefore, synchronizing the shock wave release rate with electrocardiogram was recommended to prevent extrasystolic cardiac arrhythmias.[61] With this mode of operation, SWL only rarely induces arrhythmic events[9,61–65]; however, the patient heart rate determines the shock wave release rate and, therefore, the duration of the procedure.

Ungated SWL procedures do not incorporate cardiac synchronization, allowing a higher number of shocks to be delivered per minute. Although ungated SWL was reported to be occasionally associated with cardiac arrhythmias, the procedure has been demonstrated to be safe and effective in the adult population.[66–70]

Myocardial injury produced by SWL and its potential connection with arrhythmic activity have been investigated by correlating measurements of creatinine kinase with isoenzymes, plasma troponin I, and serial ECGs.[71–73] The results indicated that lithotripsy is unlikely to cause damage to the heart and that SWL-induced arrhythmias do not appear to be associated with myocardial injury.

24.2.3.2 Lung

Several animal studies have demonstrated that direct exposure of lung tissue to high-energy shock waves can cause severe damage, such as hemorrhages, alveolar rupture, severe emphysema, congestion, edema, inflammation, loss of normal structure, and epithelial desquamation.[74,75] This is likely caused by the strong wave reflection and resultant stresses generated at the lung tissue–air interface due to their large differences in acoustic impedance.[75] Because of the anatomical separation between lung and kidneys, pulmonary injury during SWL is rarely observed clinically in adult patients.[69] However, great care should be taken to prevent pulmonary injury from SWL in children.[76,77]

24.2.3.3 Liver

Liver injury following SWL is extremely rare in clinical practice and has only been reported sporadically during the past decade. Examples of SWL-induced injury in liver include subcapsular hematoma, formation of amebic abscess, peritoneal liquid collection in perisplenic and paracolonic spaces, and bilateral pleural effusions.[78,79] Meyer et al. have suggested that known liver lesions, such as hemangioma in or near the shock path to the right kidney, should be a contraindication of SWL procedure.[78]

24.2.3.4 Pancreas

Several studies have evaluated the acute damage of the pancreas following SWL for upper urinary tract (UUT) calculi, but the results are controversial. A slight increase in blood amylase and lipase,[80] small pancreatic hematomas,[81] and acute pancreatitis[82] have been observed post-SWL. In contrast, other studies evaluating the changes in serum markers following SWL for kidney stones failed to detect any increase in serum amylase and lipase.[83] More recently, serum values of c-peptide, insulin, and glucagons, known to be reliable markers for determining acute pancreatic injury, were shown not to increase significantly over time after SWL.[84] Furthermore, no significant differences were found between the serum values of the group treated by SWL for proximal ureteric or kidney stones and the control group,[84] leading the authors to conclude that SWL for UUT calculi may not cause pancreatic trauma and the subsequent development of DM.[84] The discrepancies between these studies may be caused in part by the large variety of lithotripters used, each with differing focal zone characteristics and shock wave dosages. Because of the potential and occasional incidence of pancreatic injury caused by SWL, applying the minimal necessary shock wave dose and energy for treatment of patients with UTT stones is a logical recommendation.

24.2.3.5 Bowels

In a recent review, 62 of 3,423 (1.81%) patients experienced a documented gastrointestinal (GI) injury complication following SWL.[85] Reported complications from case studies in which shock waves traversed the peritoneal cavity include: small bowel and colon perforation, ureterocolic fistula formation, GI anastomosis dehiscence, cecal ulcers, colon erythema, bleeding per rectum, pancreatitis, peripancreatic hematoma and abscess formation, liver and spleen subcapsular hematomas, and ileus.[85] The results from these studies suggest that a higher dose of shock waves during SWL may pose injury risks to the GI system.

24.2.3.6 Ureter

To date, few studies have been performed to investigate SWL-induced bioeffects on the ureter. It was reported that shock wave exposure did not alter ureteral epithelial cells, although histological evidence indicated changes to the muscular layer in an animal model.[86] Interstitial and intracellular edemas were found by light microscopy. Marked chromatin and mitochondrial changes were observed at the subcellular level, and the adventitial layer was notably edematous initially. However, these changes returned to normal within 5 days after SWL treatment.[86] Clinically, no morphological abnormality of the ureter was detected by magnetic resonance imaging (MRI) in patients who underwent SWL for lower ureteral stones.[87]

In several case reports, though, ureteral rupture with retroperitoneal urinoma has been reported.[88] Ureteral complications of this nature, though rare, further emphasize the importance of adequate pre-and postoperative evaluation, as well as the precise identification of the cause of the persistent pain after SWL.[87] Well-controlled clinical studies need to be performed to more precisely determine the effect of SWL on morphology and function of the ureter.

24.2.3.7 Testes and Ovaries

Experimental and clinical studies have demonstrated fairly conclusively that SWL does not cause severe adverse changes in testicular and ovarian function.[89–91] Consequently, male and female fertility are not affected by SWL.[92,93]

24.2.3.8 Pregnancy

Although there have been reports of using extracorporeal shock wave lithotripsy (ESWL) during pregnancy, either knowingly or inadvertently,[94,95] pregnancy is still considered a contraindication of SWL because of the potential disruptive impact on the fetus.[96] Results from animal studies support the clinical observation of spontaneous miscarriages secondary to SWL.[89]

24.3 Other Therapeutic Applications of Shock Waves

24.3.1 Clinical Shock Wave Therapy for Bone and Tissue Healing

In addition to its widespread use in the treatment of kidney and ureteral stones, high-energy shock waves have been exploited for the treatment of musculoskeletal disorders and soft tissue healing. The application in these areas is generally referred to as shock wave therapy (SWT) or extracorporeal shock wave therapy (ESWT). Although the effect and indications for SWT are not completely clear, the number of orthopedic cases treated in Germany by SWT is similar to those of SWL for urolithiasis.[97] To date, SWT has been employed to facilitate the healing of delayed unions and nonunion fractures and for the treatment of calcifying tendonitis of rotator cuff, lateral epicondylitis, plantar fasciitis, and chronic ulcers of lower extremities. Furthermore, shock waves have been demonstrated to induce angiogenic and antibacterial effects. While the mechanisms associated with these therapies are still largely unknown, the range of applications for shock wave therapy outside of urology continues to expand.

24.3.1.1 Shock Wave Therapy for Healing of Chronic Ulcers

The adaptation of SWT for soft tissue healing has been investigated during the past decade. A dose-dependent effect of shock waves on the healing of partial-thickness wounds in a porcine model was observed by Haupt et al.[98] It was noted that high-energy treatments (100 shocks at 18 kV) induced inhibition of reepithelialization, while low-energy treatments (10 shocks at 14 kV) stimulated healing. In another study, 100 shocks at a very low energy density (0.037 mJ/mm^2) have been successfully employed to treat lower extremity ulcerations. A decrease in ulcer size with concomitant reduction in pain was noted after 4–6 treatment sessions.[99]

24.3.1.2 Shock Wave Therapy for Orthopedic Disorders

The applications of SWT for soft-tissue conditions, primarily in the management of lateral epicondylitis, plantar fasciitis, and other forms of tendonitis, have been investigated extensively. Significant relief in pain with concomitant radiographic improvement has been observed for calcific tendonitis of the shoulder and rotator cuff injury when low and high dose shock waves were delivered compared to the control group.[100,101] ESWT has also been used for the treatment of lateral epicondylitis (tennis elbow). In several randomized clinical trials, significant pain reduction was reported in the treatment group compared to the control.[102,103] In 2000, SWT was approved by the Food and Drug Administration (FDA) for treatment of plantar fasciitis in the USA. Studies have shown that the delivery of low energy shock waves correlates with reduced pain and increased mobility.[104,105]

While numerous studies have reported positive treatment outcomes in SWT of orthopedic disorders, several randomized double-blind studies have shown no statistical differences between treatment and sham groups, although improvement over the control group is often observed.[106–109] Thomson et al. performed a comprehensive review of the randomized clinical trials employing shock waves for alleviation of plantar fasciitis, concluding that, despite a statistically significant reduction in heel pain, SWT produced a small effect size and that the two trials yielding the greatest support for SWT were also of lower experimental quality.[110]

24.3.1.3 Shock Wave Therapy for Fracture Healing

Similar to its effects on urinary calculi, shock waves are believed to cause microfractures in bones, which, in turn, may stimulate neovascularization, osteoblast formation, and subsequent healing.[111–113] A dose-dependent relationship was observed in which higher energy shock waves, as opposed to a higher number of impulses, produced greater gross changes to the bone structure.[114] Based on these observations, it was postulated that controlled shock wave delivery could produce controlled microfractures and fracture hematoma, which in turn could stimulate bone growth via an osteogenetic response.[115] Several studies have demonstrated improved radiologic healing and better mechanical stability with morphologic indications of enhanced fracture healing in animal models following low energy shock wave treatment.[111,116,117]

The clinical application of SWT for fracture healing in Europe, particularly in Germany, has increased rapidly in popularity over the past decade. The ability to stimulate healing in cases of pseudarthrosis through a noninvasive modality appeals to clinicians seeking a nonsurgical intervention. Three phases of healing have been suggested following shock wave treatment: (1) shock-wave-induced callus formation at soft-tissue intersection, (2) subsequent fragment connection, and (3) cortical reorientation.[118] The use of shock waves was found to be effective in stimulating osteogenetic effects in a series of studies.[118–121] In particular, it has been observed that SWT was most successful in hypertrophic nonunions as opposed to atrophic nonunions.[121]

For treatment of pseudarthrosis and other forms of fracture healing, some have questioned the true effectiveness of shock wave treatment.[122,123] In a review of clinical studies, Biedermann conceded that, while the data has shown some promise, inconsistencies in experimental models suggest a lack of concrete evidence to support the use of SWT.[97] Others have questioned the impact of natural healing in clinical studies, believing that stabilization of fractures, as is common for shock-wave-induced fracture healing, may play a large role in the treatment.[97] Furthermore, the high level of variability in fractures and the impact of follow-up timelines may also obscure the interpretation of the experimental results. While the use of SWT for orthopedic indications and bone healing has increased in Europe, there have been relatively few investigations aimed at determining the primary mechanisms in shock-wave-induced fracture healing and osteogenesis.

24.3.1.4 Mechanisms of Shock-Wave-Induced Healing

In contrast to the significant number of clinical investigations on SWT for soft-tissue disorders and bone healing, relatively few studies have been carried out regarding the mechanisms of shock-wave-induced healing. Early studies suggested that the impact of shock waves on bone might disrupt calcium deposits while stimulating neovascularization, thus potentially inducing neural effects as well. Ohtori et al. observed nearly complete degeneration of nerve fibers in shock wave-exposed rat skin, followed by reinnervation of the epidermis 2 weeks after the treatment.[124] Direct damage to nerve fibers may be a primary effect of analgesic shock wave therapy.[124] The fact that SWT enhances both bone and tendon regeneration suggests that shock waves may induce cell signaling responsible for the growth and maturation of mesenchymal progenitors from bone marrow.[125] Wang et al. hypothesized that shock wave therapy promotes the growth and differentiation of bone marrow mesenchymal cells via the induction of osteogenic growth factors.[126] In a series of experiments using rat models, they found a correlation between SWT and the induction of transforming growth factor-beta (TGF-β1) and core binding factor alpha1 (CBFA1), as well as the activation of angiogenic transcription factors (HIF-1α[alpha]) and VEGF-A expression.[125–127] These findings suggest that shock wave therapy may affect healing through multiple mechanisms. Differentiation of mesenchymal stromal cells into osteoprogenitors could produce bone matrices for new bone growth, while angiogenic activity may also be stimulated by shock waves through the formation of reactive oxygen species.[126,127]

24.3.1.5 Treatment of Peyronie's Disease

Over the previous decade, shock wave therapy has been applied to the treatment and management of Peyronie's disease (PD). In PD, fibrous plaque formation results in an abnormal upward curvature of the penis, producing erectile pain and dysfunction. In early clinical studies employing the Storz Minilith SL1, approximately half of the patients experienced improved angulation (straightening) in the penis after 3,000 shocks at energy density of 0.11–0.17 mJ/mm,[2] with over half of those treated experiencing pain relief.[128,129] Minimal bruising was reported following the shock wave treatment, and no other significant side effects were reported.[129] Similar to other shock wave therapy procedures, the underlying mechanism for alleviation of PD curvature and pain is largely unclear. Possible effects speculated include the stimulation of an inflammatory reaction that stimulates plaque lysis, improved vascularity, and induction of contralateral scarring, which may provide a compensatory straightening effect.[130] However, subsequent investigations into the efficacy of shock wave treatment for PD have demonstrated that the procedure may only provide pain relief without significant straightening or functional improvement. In a prospective study by Hauck et al., the absence of serious side effects from shock wave treatment was confirmed; however, they also concluded that ESWT does not significantly affect penile curvature or sexual function, although some cases of notable improvement (about 30%) after treatment did occur. Pain alleviation, though, was reported by 76% of patients. In a metaanalysis of 17 clinical trials, Hauck et al. concluded that the efficacy of ESWT for PD is questionable, with inconsistent criteria for patient recruitment and posttreatment comparisons.[131] Recent studies in rat models have provided further evidence that shock waves do not significantly affect plaque volume or penile structure.[132] Therefore, despite anecdotal evidence that shock wave treatment may alleviate symptoms of PD, ESWT is not recommended as a standard therapy for Peyronie's disease.[133]

24.3.2 Shock-Wave-Mediated Gene and Drug Delivery

In addition to wound healing, other cellular level bioeffects of shock waves have been investigated for potential therapeutic applications. Cavitation is a well-known mechanism associated with shock waves, oftentimes associated with cell lysis.[134] However, it has also been observed that some cells not permanently damaged by cavitation bubbles could survive and uptake macromolecules that are normally incapable of passing through the cell membrane. This phenomenon was assumed to include a rapid opening and resealing of the plasma membrane.[135–137] This effect on cell membrane permeability has been termed sonoporation and was first demonstrated in the mid 1980s through the use of 20 kHz ultrasound to introduce fluorescein-labeled dextran molecules first into ameboid mold cells, then HeLa cells and fibroblasts.[136,137] Sonoporation has been the subject of intensive investigation for the past 2 decades as a possible means of gene and drug delivery. Specifically, it has the potential to be employed as a means of targeted gene therapy through nonviral means or for increased localized delivery of anticancer drugs.

The implementation of lithotripter shock waves for sonoporation research began in the mid 1990s. In one in vitro study, the accumulation of fluorescein-labeled dextran in L1210 cells was monitored after exposure to 1,000 shocks in an experimental lithotripter. These large macromolecules that are generally impermeable across cell membranes were observed in the cytoplasm of survival cells after shock wave treatment.[138] Also, red blood cells were loaded with fluorescent dextran by shock wave treatment for illustrating the uptake of molecules of relatively high molecule weight into erythrocytes.[139] When static excess pressure was applied during shock wave exposure to reduce the size and number of cavitation bubbles, membrane permeability effects were significantly diminished. This study provided strong evidence that shock-wave-induced sonoporation is feasible and strongly correlated with cavitation activities. Furthermore, Lauer et al. demonstrated plasmid DNA delivery using shock wave exposures in a variety of in vitro cell lines, including HepG2, CV-1 monkey kidney cells, HeLa cells, and L1210 mouse lymphocytic leukemia cells.[140] In these studies, while the ability to facilitate macromolecule transport into target cells showed much promise, shock wave exposures also induced high levels of cell lysis.

Most attempts at harnessing shock wave bioeffects for gene and drug delivery have been focused on cancer treatment applications, particularly tumor therapy. Due to the highly focused nature of lithotripter shock waves, sonoporation could be used for improving highly selective treatment of tumors with large toxic molecules. The concept of combined shock wave therapy and gene or drug delivery to tumors was demonstrated in a B16 murine melanoma model. Reporter gene expression was significantly improved in melanoma tumors exposed to 24.4 MPa shock wave therapy.[141] Progressing beyond reporter gene expression, 500 shocks of 7.4 MPa peak negative pressure were delivered to B16 and renal cancer cell (RENCA) carcinoma tumors following injections of air bubbles with recombinant interleukin-12 (rIL-12) protein or DNA plasmids coding for interleukin-12 (pIL-12). In these studies, both IL-12 treatments combined with shock waves produced significant reductions in tumor growth and increases in survival.[142] Similarly, shock waves were demonstrated to significantly increase the transfer, and subsequent action of, ribosome inactivating proteins gelonin and saporin in both L1210 and HeLa cells.[143] Overall, tumor cell killing was greatly enhanced by shock wave exposure. Furthermore, in a murine SSK2 fibrosarcoma tumor model, 500 shocks were administered to subcutaneous tumors after injections of gelonin and saporin. Significant remission of tumors was observed in 40% of mice when localized shock wave treatment was administered subsequent to systemic injection of toxins; however, regression was not observed in mice receiving only shock wave therapy or injections of gelonin and saporin.

While others have observed natural tumor cell killing capabilities with lithotripter shock waves alone, the combination of shock-wave-induced sonoporation with the administration of anticancer therapeutic agents may hold promise in a clinical setting. Zhong et al. have investigated methods of controlling permeabilization and cell death during shock wave exposure for improved sonoporation and delivery efficiency.[144] Using a Dornier XL-1 lithotripter with a modified reflector, a preceding weak shock wave of −0.96 to −1.91 MPa in tensile pressure was delivered prior to the primary lithotripter pulse (>60 MPa in peak positive pressure). This preceding wave induces the formation of inertial microbubbles, which are collapsed in situ by the ensuing lithotripter pulse, leading to intensified cavitation activities in the focal region. At low treatment exposures (less than 100 shocks), this strategy was found to produce higher membrane permeabilization efficiency in a T-cell hybridoma line. At higher exposures (>100 shocks), significant cell death was observed. This study emphasized the importance of microbubble dynamics in shock-wave-mediated gene or drug delivery, illustrating that shock wave–bubble interaction can be tailored for different biomedical applications.

More recent examinations have shed some light on the specific bubble–cell interactions that may occur to enable membrane permeabilization from shock waves or sinusoidal ultrasound exposures. Using low frequency (24 kHz) ultrasound, Schlicher et al. sought to determine whether sonoporation occurred through active transport via endocytosis, passive transport through nanometer-sized pores, or molecular influx via actively repairable wounds in the cell membrane.[145] Their work in DU145 prostate cells suggests that micronscale wounds form in the plasma membrane and reseal on the order of seconds by patching these pores with intracellular vesicles through a process that requires the influx of Ca^{2+}, a conclusion that is in agreement with observations by patch-clamp technique.[146] Due to the high level of cell lysis that generally occurs during sonoporation, particularly from shock waves, it was suggested that strategies to promote this repair mechanism may improve the overall efficacy with higher cell viability. Using high speed imaging of oscillating microbubbles in bovine endothelial cell cultures, others have proposed that shear stress from bubble oscillation may lead to the pore formation responsible for enhanced molecular uptake.[147] Moreover, Ohl et al. demonstrated that while shock waves from inertial bubble collapse may not be the primary cause for sonoporation, radial jet flow from bubble implosion close to cell surfaces can generate shear stresses sufficient for tearing in the cell membrane.[148] The effects of shear stresses associated with acoustic microstreaming and jet formation have been investigated previously within the context of ultrasound bioeffects, and the results are in agreement with these observations.[149–151]

The feasibility of directing focused lithotripter shock waves at tumor sites for combined therapy and drug delivery for enhanced destruction of tumor tissue has been demonstrated in several murine models. However, sinusoidal ultrasound exposures have been shown to produce more efficient gene delivery for therapeutic applications; in particular, shock wave exposures resulted in significantly reduced cell viability.[152] Thus, most efforts to harness shock-wave-induced sonoporation have been focused on tumor therapy, in which maintaining a high level of cell viability is not a primary concern. Investigations have shown that control of inertial cavitation and microbubble size can greatly influence sonoporation efficiency. Similar to other ultrasound studies, the incorporation of cavitation nucleation agents can significantly increase effects on membrane permeability.[153] Shock-wave-induced sonoporation has also been explored for treatment of thrombolysis[154,155] and disruption of the blood brain barrier.[156]

24.3.2.1 Other Bioeffects of Shock Waves

Besides stone fragmentation, soft-tissue and bone healing, and drug delivery, other bioeffects produced by high-energy shock waves have been observed. It is clear from the previously described applications that shock waves have a multitude of unexplored interactions with biological tissues, inducing significant changes through both physical and chemical processes. High-energy shock waves were found to induce a bactericidal effect on suspensions of *Staphylococcus aureus*.[157] This antibacterial effect was found to increase with energy and the number of impulses delivered, offering potential applicability to sterilization procedures. In fact, Nigri et al. have used laser-induced shock waves to enhance, in vitro, sterilization of infected vascular prosthetic grafts. Importantly, they note that the shock waves had little to no effect on their own; instead, they can interact synergistically with the standard antibiotic therapy for improved efficacy.[158] In line with results from Wang et al. concerning the effect of shock waves on promoting the production of osteoprogenitors, others have investigated angiogenic effects of SWT for applications in cardiology.[126] Nishida et al. employed low energy shock waves to ischemic myocardium, observing complete recovery of left ventricular ejection fraction and myocardial blood flow.[159] Furthermore, Nurzynska et al. observed in vitro that shock waves have a positive influence on the proliferation and differentiation of cardiomyocytes, smooth muscle, and endothelial cell precursors.[160] These investigations provide encouraging preliminary evidence that shock waves can promote angiogenesis as a potential therapy for ischemic heart disease. Finally, others have employed shock waves both in vitro and in vivo to manipulate stem cell differentiation. High-energy shock waves have been used as a pretreatment on cord blood CD34+ cells to improve progenitor cell expansion, presenting shock wave therapy as a potential utility for genetic applications.[161]

24.4 Conclusions

The range of biological effects produced by high-energy shock waves continues to expand from the well-established treatment of urolithiasis by SWL to new applications in musculoskeletal disorders, wound healing, and macromolecule delivery. In SWL, the most common side effects are hematuria, hematoma, and temporary functional deterioration of the kidney, all of which typically resolve over a short period of time. These short-term side effects are often related to energy level, dose, and pulse repetition rate of the shock waves, as well as patient history. For chronic adverse effects, such as diabetes mellitus and hypertension, the causal relationship with shock wave treatment and associated mechanisms are still under investigation. When SWL is administered at high-energy level with high pulse repetition rate, significant tissue injury with scar formation has been demonstrated, leading to renal function loss. Therefore, high-energy shock waves should be used judiciously (i.e., using energy level and pulse repetition rate as low as possible to fragment the kidney stones), especially for elderly and pediatric patients who are at increased risk for shock-wave-induced chronic injuries. Regarding extra-renal bioeffects, except for some anecdotal evidence, damage from SWL to other organs adjacent to the kidney is rare.

Beyond SWL, high-energy shock waves have been explored and employed extensively in Europe to facilitate the healing of soft tissue and bone fractures, as well as to alleviate other musculoskeletal disorders, such as epicondylitis. However, despite its growing use, debate continues over the effectiveness and efficacy of shock wave treatment for many of these indications. Similarly, investigation on the use of shock wave therapy for Peyronie's disease has been controversial, leading to the general recommendation that shock wave should not be considered as a standard therapy for Peyronie's disease.

Moreover, shock waves at low dose (i.e., a few hundred pulses) have been demonstrated to induce a transient cell membrane permeabilization, opening up a new avenue for potential applications in targeted drug and gene delivery. In particular, the promise of shock-wave- or ultrasound-mediated tumor therapy is intriguing, enabling noninvasive and site-specific combinations of different treatment modalities to enhance the overall efficacy while reducing systemic toxicity.

In summary, investigation into the multitude of bioeffects produced by high-energy shock waves continues to expand with current and potential applications in different clinical fields. Further mechanistic investigations on the cause of acute and chronic biological effects produced by high-energy shock waves are needed to improve the technology, treatment strategy, and overall patient outcome in SWL and ESWT, as well as to explore new applications in targeted drug and gene delivery, antibacterial, and angiogenic treatment.

References

1. Karlsen SJ, Smevik B, Hovig T. Acute morphological changes in canine kidneys after exposure to extracorporeal shock waves. A light and electron microscopic study. *Urol Res.* 1991;19:105-115.
2. Recker F, Hofmann W, Bex A, Tscholl R. Quantitative determination of urinary marker proteins: a model to detect intrarenal bioeffects after extracorporeal lithotripsy. *J Urol.* 1992;148:1000-1006.
3. Delius M, Jordan M, Eizenhoefer H, et al. Biological effects of shock waves: kidney haemorrhage by shock waves in dogs–administration rate dependence. *Ultrasound Med Biol.* 1988;14:689-694.
4. Evan AP, Willis LR, Connors B, Reed G, McAteer JA, Lingeman JE. Shock wave lithotripsy-induced renal injury. *Am J Kidney Dis.* 1991;17:445-450.
5. Evan AP, McAteer JA. Q-effects of shock-wave lithotripsy. In: Coe FL, Preminger GM, eds. *Kidney Stones: Medical and Surgical Management.* Philadelphia: Lippincott-Raven; 1996.
6. Chaussy C, Schüller J, Schmiedt E, Brandl H, Jocham D, Liedl B. Extracorporeal shock-wave lithotripsy (ESWL) for treatment of urolithiasis. *Urology.* 1984;23:59-66.
7. Coptcoat MJ, Webb DR, Kellett MJ, et al. The complications of extracorporeal shockwave lithotripsy: management and prevention. *Br J Urol.* 1986;58:578-580.
8. Knapp PM, Kulb TB, Lingeman JE, et al. Extracorporeal shock wave lithotripsy-induced perirenal hematomas. *J Urol.* 1988;139:700-703.
9. Roth RA, Beckmann CF. Complications of extracorporeal shock-wave lithotripsy and percutaneous nephrolithotomy. *Urol Clin North Am.* 1988;15:155-166.
10. Tillotson CL, Deluca SA. Complications of extracorporeal shock wave lithotripsy. *Am Fam Physician.* 1988;38:161-163.
11. Kaude JV, Williams CM, Millner MR, Scott KN, Finlayson B. Renal morphology and function immediately after extracorporeal shock-wave lithotripsy. *AJR Am J Roentgenol.* 1985;145:305-313.
12. Rubin JI, Arger PH, Pollack HM, et al. Kidney changes after extracorporeal shock wave lithotripsy: CT evaluation. *Radiology.* 1987;162:21-24.
13. Baumgartner BR, Dickey KW, Ambrose SS, Walton KN, Nelson RC, Bernardino ME. Kidney changes after extracorporeal shock wave lithotripsy: appearance on MR imaging. *Radiology.* 1987;163:531-534.

14. Skolarikos A, Alivizatos G, de la Rosette J. Extracorporeal shock wave lithotripsy 25 years later: complications and their prevention. *Eur Urol.* 2006;50:981-990. discussion 990.

15. Dhar NB, Thornton J, Karafa MT, Streem SB. A multivariate analysis of risk factors associated with subcapsular hematoma formation following electromagnetic shock wave lithotripsy. *J Urol.* 2004;172:2271-2274.

16. Krishnamurthi V, Streem SB. Long-term radiographic and functional outcome of extracorporeal shock wave lithotripsy induced perirenal hematomas. *J Urol.* 1995;154:1673-1675.

17. Hill DE, McDougal WS, Stephens H, Fogo A, Koch MO. Physiologic and pathologic alterations associated with ultrasonically generated shock waves. *J Urol.* 1990;144:1531-1534.

18. Jaeger P, Constantinidis C. Canine kidneys: changes in blood and urine chemistry after exposure to extracorporeal shock waves. In: Lingeman JE, Newman DM, eds. *Shock Wave Lithotripsy 2: Urinary and Biliary Lithotripsy.* Plenum Press: New York; 1989:7-10.

19. Grantham JR, Millner MR, Kaude JV, Finlayson B, Hunter PT 2nd, Newman RC. Renal stone disease treated with extracorporeal shock wave lithotripsy: short-term observations in 100 patients. *Radiology.* 1986;158:203-206.

20. Cimentepe E, Eroglu M, Oztürk U, et al. Rapid communication: renal apoptosis after shockwave application in rabbit model. *J Endourol.* 2006;20:1091-1095.

21. Yaman O, Sarica K, Ozer G, et al. Protective effect of verapamil on renal tissue during shockwave application in rabbit model. *J Endourol.* 1996;10:329-333.

22. Strohmaier WL, Koch J, Balk N, Wilbert DM, Bichler KH. Limitation of shock-wave-induced renal tubular dysfunction by nifedipine. *Eur Urol.* 1994;25:99-104.

23. Zhong P, Zhou Y, Zhu S. Dynamics of bubble oscillation in constrained media and mechanisms of vessel rupture in SWL. *Ultrasound Med Biol.* 2001;27:119-134.

24. Freund JB, Colonius T, Evan AP. A cumulative shear mechanism for tissue damage initiation in shock-wave lithotripsy. *Ultrasound Med Biol.* 2007;33:1495-1503.

25. Howard D, Sturtevant B. In vitro study of the mechanical effects of shock-wave lithotripsy. *Ultrasound Med Biol.* 1997;23:1107-1122.

26. Biri H, Oztürk HS, Büyükkoçak S, et al. Antioxidant defense potential of rabbit renal tissues after ESWL: protective effects of antioxidant vitamins. *Nephron.* 1998;79:181-185.

27. Ozguner F, Armagan A, Koyu A, Caliskan S, Koylu H. A novel antioxidant agent caffeic acid phenethyl ester prevents shock wave-induced renal tubular oxidative stress. *Urol Res.* 2005;33: 239-243.

28. Li B, Zhou W, Li P. Protective effects of nifedipine and allopurinol on high energy shock wave induced acute changes of renal function. *J Urol.* 1995;153:596-598.

29. Munver R, Delvecchio FC, Kuo RL, Brown SA, Zhong P, Preminger GM. In vivo assessment of free radical activity during shock wave lithotripsy using a microdialysis system: the renoprotective action of allopurinol. *J Urol.* 2002;167:327-334.

30. Russell JD, Churchill DN. Calcium antagonists and acute renal failure. *Am J Med.* 1989;87:306-315.

31. Schrier RW, Arnold PE, Van Putten VJ, Burke TJ. Cellular calcium in ischemic acute renal failure: role of calcium entry blockers. *Kidney Int.* 1987;32:313-321.

32. Finn WF. Prevention of ischemic injury in renal transplantation. *Kidney Int.* 1990;37:171-182.

33. Newman R, Hackett R, Senior D, et al. Pathologic effects of ESWL on canine renal tissue. *Urology.* 1987;29:194-200.

34. Morris JS, Husmann DA, Wilson WT, Preminger GM. Temporal effects of shock wave lithotripsy. *J Urol.* 1991;145:881-883.

35. Evan AP, Willis LR, Lingeman JE, McAteer JA. Renal trauma and the risk of long-term complications in shock wave lithotripsy. *Nephron.* 1998;78:1-8.

36. Lechevallier E, Siles S, Ortega JC, Coulange C. Comparison by SPECT of renal scars after extracorporeal shock wave lithotripsy and percutaneous nephrolithotomy. *J Endourol.* 1993;7:465-467.

37. Montgomery BS, Cole RS, Palfrey EL, Shuttleworth KE. Does extracorporeal shockwave lithotripsy cause hypertension? *Br J Urol.* 1989;64:567-571.

38. Janetschek G, Frauscher F, Knapp R, Höfle G, Peschel R, Bartsch G. New onset hypertension after extracorporeal shock wave lithotripsy: age related incidence and prediction by intrarenal resistive index. *J Urol.* 1997;158:346-351.

39. Knapp R, Frauscher F, Helweg G, et al. Age-related changes in resistive index following extracorporeal shock wave lithotripsy. *J Urol.* 1995;154:955-958.

40. Krambeck AE, Gettman MT, Rohlinger AL, Lohse CM, Patterson DE, Segura JW. Diabetes mellitus and hypertension associated with shock wave lithotripsy of renal and proximal ureteral stones at 19 years of followup. *J Urol.* 2006;175:1742-1747.

41. Knapp R, Frauscher F, Helweg G, et al. Blood pressure changes after extracorporeal shock wave nephrolithotripsy: prediction by intrarenal resistive index. *Eur Radiol.* 1996;6:665-669.

42. Bataille P, Cardon G, Bouzernidj M, et al. Renal and hypertensive complications of extracorporeal shock wave lithotripsy: who is at risk? *Urol Int.* 1999;62:195-200.

43. Jewett MA, Bombardier C, Logan AG, et al. A randomized controlled trial to assess the incidence of new onset hypertension in patients after shock wave lithotripsy for asymptomatic renal calculi. *J Urol.* 1998;160:1241-1243.

44. Sato Y, Tanda H, Kato S, et al. Shock wave lithotripsy for renal stones is not associated with hypertension and diabetes mellitus. *Urology.* 2008;71:586-591. discussion 591–582.

45. Tiselius HG. Commentary. *Eur Urol.* 2006;50:612.

46. Whitfield HN. Commentary. *Eur Urol.* 2006;51:281.

47. Lieske JC, de la Vega LS, Gettman MT, et al. Diabetes mellitus and the risk of urinary tract stones: a population-based case-control study. *Am J Kidney Dis.* 2006;48:897-904.

48. Krambeck AE, Gettman MT. Editorial comment. *Urology.* 2008; 71:591.

49. Mandel N, Mandel I, Fryjoff K, Rejniak T, Mandel G. Conversion of calcium oxalate to calcium phosphate with recurrent stone episodes. *J Urol.* 2003;169:2026-2029.

50. Parks JH, Worcester EM, Coe FL, Evan AP, Lingeman JE. Clinical implications of abundant calcium phosphate in routinely analyzed kidney stones. *Kidney Int.* 2004;66:777-785.

51. Newman DM, Coury T, Lingeman JE, et al. Extracorporeal shock wave lithotripsy experience in children. *J Urol.* 1986;136:238-240.

52. Lifshitz DA, Lingeman JE, Zafar FS, Hollensbe DW, Nyhuis AW, Evan AP. Alterations in predicted growth rates of pediatric kidneys treated with extracorporeal shockwave lithotripsy. *J Endourol.* 1998;12:469-475.

53. Goel MC, Baserge NS, Babu RV, Sinha S, Kapoor R. Pediatric kidney: functional outcome after extracorporeal shock wave lithotripsy. *J Urol.* 1996;155:2044-2046.

54. Thomas R, Frentz JM, Harmon E, Frentz GD. Effect of extracorporeal shock wave lithotripsy on renal function and body height in pediatric patients. *J Urol.* 1992;148:1064-1066.

55. Frick J, Sarica K, Kohle R, Kunit G. Long-term follow-up after extracorporeal shock wave lithotripsy in children. *Eur Urol.* 1991;19:225-229.

56. Reisiger K, Vardi I, Yan Y, et al. Pediatric nephrolithiasis: does treatment affect renal growth? *Urology.* 2007;69:1190-1194.

57. Willis LR, Evan AP, Connors BA, Blomgren P, Fineberg NS, Lingeman JE. Relationship between kidney size, renal injury, and renal impairment induced by shock wave lithotripsy. *J Am Soc Nephrol.* 1999;10:1753-1762.

58. Shao Y, Connors BA, Evan AP, Willis LR, Lifshitz DA, Lingeman JE. Morphological changes induced in the pig kidney by extracorporeal

shock wave lithotripsy: nephron injury. *Anat Rec A Discov Mol Cell Evol Biol.* 2003;275:979-989.

59. Villányi KK, Székely JG, Farkas LM, Jávor E, Pusztai C. Short-term changes in renal function after extracorporeal shock wave lithotripsy in children. *J Urol.* 2001;166:222-224.

60. Blomgren PM, Connors BA, Lingeman JE, Willis LR, Evan AP. Quantitation of shock wave lithotripsy-induced lesion in small and large pig kidneys. *Anat Rec.* 1997;249:341-348.

61. Chaussy CHSE, Jocham D, Fuchs G, Brendel W. Clinical experience with extracorporeal shock wave lithotripsy (ESWL). In: Chaussy C, ed. *Extracorporeal Shock Wave Lithotripsy: Technical Concept, Experimental Research, and Clinical Application.* New York: Karger: Basel; 1986.

62. Chaussy C, Brendel W, Schmiedt E. Extracorporeally induced destruction of kidney stones by shock waves. *Lancet.* 1980;2:1265-1268.

63. Vandeursen H, Tjandramaga B, Verbesselt R, Smet G, Baert L. Anaesthesia-free extracorporeal shock wave lithotripsy in patients with renal calculi. *Br J Urol.* 1991;68:18-24.

64. Delius M, Hoffmann E, Steinbeck G, Conzen P. Biological effects of shock waves: induction of arrhythmia in piglet hearts. *Ultrasound Med Biol.* 1994;20:279-285.

65. Ector H, Janssens L, Baert L, De Geest H. Extracorporeal shock wave lithotripsy and cardiac arrhythmias. *Pacing Clin Electrophysiol.* 1989;12:1910-1917.

66. Cass AS. The use of ungating with the Medstone lithotriptor. *J Urol.* 1996;156:896-898.

67. Greenstein A, Kaver I, Lechtman V, Braf Z. Cardiac arrhythmias during nonsynchronized extracorporeal shock wave lithotripsy. *J Urol.* 1995;154:1321-1322.

68. Lingeman JE, Newman DM, Siegel YI, Eichhorn T, Parr K. Shock wave lithotripsy with the Dornier MFL 5000 lithotriptor using an external fixed rate signal. *J Urol.* 1995;154:951-954.

69. Rodrigues Netto N Jr, Longo JA, Ikonomidis JA, Rodrigues Netto M. Extracorporeal shock wave lithotripsy in children. *J Urol.* 2002;167:2164-2166.

70. Winters JC, Macaluso JN Jr. Ungated Medstone outpatient lithotripsy. *J Urol.* 1995;153:593-595.

71. Parr KL, Lingeman JE, Jordan M, Coury TA. Creatinine kinase concentrations and electrocardiographic changes in extracorporeal shock-wave lithotripsy. *Urology.* 1988;32:21-23.

72. Greenstein A, Sofer M, Lidawi G, Matzkin H. Does shock wave lithotripsy of renal stones cause cardiac muscle injury? A troponin I-based study. *Urology.* 2003;61:902-905.

73. Eaton MP, Erturk EN. Serum troponin levels are not increased in patients with ventricular arrhythmias during shock wave lithotripsy. *J Urol.* 2003;170:2195-2197.

74. Chaussy C. *Extracorporeal Shock Wave Lithotripsy: New Aspects in the Treatment of Kidney Stone Disease.* Basel; New York: Karger; 1982.

75. Eroglu M, Cimentepe E, Demirag F, Unsal E, Unsal A. The effects of shock waves on lung tissue in acute period: an in vivo study. *Urol Res.* 2007;35:155-160.

76. Malhotra V, Gomillion MC, Artusio JF Jr. Hemoptysis in a child during extracorporeal shock wave lithotripsy. *Anesth Analg.* 1989;69:526-528.

77. Malhotra V, Rosen RJ, Slepian RL. Life-threatening hypoxemia after lithotripsy in an adult due to shock-wave-induced pulmonary contusion. *Anesthesiology.* 1991;75:529-531.

78. Meyer JJ, Cass AS. Subcapsular hematoma of the liver after renal extracorporeal shock wave lithotripsy. *J Urol.* 1995;154:516-517.

79. Bogdanovic J, Mirkovic M, Idjuski S, Popov M, Marusic G, Stojkov J. Liver injury related to extracorporeal shock wave lithotripsy in a quadriplegic patient. *BJU Int.* 1999;83:718-719.

80. Kirkali Z, Kirkali G, Tanci S, Tahiri Y. The effect of extracorporeal shock wave lithotripsy on pancreatic enzymes. *Int Urol Nephrol.* 1994;26:405-408.

81. Hung SY, Chen HM, Jan YY, Chen MF. Common bile duct and pancreatic injury after extracorporeal shock wave lithotripsy for renal stone. *Hepatogastroenterology.* 2000;47:1162-1163.

82. Hassan I, Zietlow SP. Acute pancreatitis after extracorporeal shock wave lithotripsy for a renal calculus. *Urology.* 2002;60:1111.

83. Apostolov I, Minkov N, Koycheva M, et al. Acute changes of serum markers for tissue damage after ESWL of kidney stones. *Int Urol Nephrol.* 1991;23:215-220.

84. Wendt-Nordahl G, Krombach P, Hannak D, et al. Prospective evaluation of acute endocrine pancreatic injury as collateral damage of shock-wave lithotripsy for upper urinary tract stones. *BJU Int.* 2007;100:1339-1343.

85. Maker V, Layke J. Gastrointestinal injury secondary to extracorporeal shock wave lithotripsy: a review of the literature since its inception. *J Am Coll Surg.* 2004;198:128-135.

86. Kirkali Z, Esen AA, Hayran M, et al. The effect of extracorporeal electromagnetic shock waves on the morphology and contractility of rabbit ureter. *J Urol.* 1995;154:1939-1943.

87. Kirkali Z, Diren B. Periureteric effects of electromagnetic shock waves. *Int Urol Nephrol.* 1993;25:147-151.

88. Turgut M, Can C, Yenilmez A, Akcar N. Perforation of the upper ureter: a rare complication of extracorporeal shock wave litho-tripsy. *Urol Res.* 2007;35:215-218.

89. Basar MM, Samli MM, Erbil M, Ozergin O, Basar R, Atan A. Early effects of extracorporeal shock-wave lithotripsy exposure on testicular sperm morphology. *Scand J Urol Nephrol.* 2004;38: 38-41.

90. Hellstrom WJ, Kaack MB, Harrison RM, Neal DE Jr, Thomas R. Absence of long-term gonadotoxicity in primates receiving extracorporeal shock wave application. *J Endourol.* 1993;7:17-21.

91. Recker F, Jaeger P, Knönagel H, Uhlschmid G, Diener P. Does extracorporeal shock wave lithotripsy injure the female reproductive tract? *Helv Chir Acta.* 1990;57:471-475.

92. Andreessen R, Fedel M, Sudhoff F, Friedrichs R, Loening SA. Quality of semen after extracorporeal shock wave lithotripsy for lower urethral stones. *J Urol.* 1996;155:1281-1283.

93. Vieweg J, Weber HM, Miller K, Hautmann R. Female fertility following extracorporeal shock wave lithotripsy of distal ureteral calculi. *J Urol.* 1992;148:1007-1010.

94. Frankenschmidt A, Sommerkamp H. Shock wave lithotripsy during pregnancy: a successful clinical experiment. *J Urol.* 1998;159: 501-502.

95. Asgari MA, Safarinejad MR, Hosseini SY, Dadkhah F. Extracorporeal shock wave lithotripsy of renal calculi during early pregnancy. *BJU Int.* 1999;84:615-617.

96. Ohmori K, Matsuda T, Horii Y, Yoshida O. Effects of shock waves on the mouse fetus. *J Urol.* 1994;151:255-258.

97. Biedermann R, Martin A, Handle G, Auckenthaler T, Bach C, Krismer M. Extracorporeal shock waves in the treatment of non-unions. *J Trauma.* 2003;54:936-942.

98. Haupt G, Chvapil M. Effect of shock waves on the healing of partial-thickness wounds in piglets. *J Surg Res.* 1990;49:45-48.

99. Saggini R, Figus A, Troccola A, Cocco V, Saggini A, Scuderi N. Extracorporeal shock wave therapy for management of chronic ulcers in the lower extremities. *Ultrasound Med Biol.* 2008;34(8): 1261-71.

100. Loew M, Daecke W, Kusnierczak D, Rahmanzadeh M, Ewerbeck V. Shock-wave therapy is effective for chronic calcifying tendinitis of the shoulder. *J Bone Joint Surg Br.* 1999;81:863-867.

101. Gerdesmeyer L, Wagenpfeil S, Haake M, et al. Extracorporeal shock wave therapy for the treatment of chronic calcifying tendonitis of the rotator cuff: a randomized controlled trial. *JAMA.* 2003;290:2573-2580.

102. Rompe JD, Hope C, Küllmer K, Heine J, Bürger R. Analgesic effect of extracorporeal shock-wave therapy on chronic tennis elbow. *J Bone Joint Surg Br.* 1996;78:233-237.

103. Pettrone FA, McCall BR. Extracorporeal shock wave therapy without local anesthesia for chronic lateral epicondylitis. *J Bone Joint Surg Am*. 2005;87:1297-1304.

104. Rompe JD, Hopf C, Nafe B, Burger R. Low-energy extracorporeal shock wave therapy for painful heel: a prospective controlled single-blind study. *Arch Orthop Trauma Surg*. 1996;115:75-79.

105. Ogden JA, Alvarez R, Levitt R, Cross GL, Marlow M. Shock wave therapy for chronic proximal plantar fasciitis. *Clin Orthop Relat Res*. 2001;387:47-59.

106. Schmitt J, Haake M, Tosch A, Hildebrand R, Deike B, Griss P. Low-energy extracorporeal shock-wave treatment (ESWT) for tendinitis of the supraspinatus. A prospective, randomised study. *J Bone Joint Surg Br*. 2001;83:873-876.

107. Speed CA, Richards C, Nichols D, et al. Extracorporeal shock-wave therapy for tendonitis of the rotator cuff. A double-blind, randomised, controlled trial. *J Bone Joint Surg Br*. 2002;84:509-512.

108. Speed CA, Nichols D, Richards C, et al. Extracorporeal shock wave therapy for lateral epicondylitis – a double blind randomised controlled trial. *J Orthop Res*. 2002;20:895-898.

109. Haake M, König IR, Decker T, et al. Extracorporeal Shock Wave Therapy Clinical Trial Group. Extracorporeal shock wave therapy in the treatment of lateral epicondylitis: a randomized multicenter trial. *J Bone Joint Surg Am*. 2002;84-A:1982-1991.

110. Thomson CE, Crawford F, Murray GD. The effectiveness of extra corporeal shock wave therapy for plantar heel pain: a systematic review and meta-analysis. *BMC Musculoskelet Disord*. 2005; 6:19.

111. Delius M, Draenert K, Al Diek Y, Draenert Y. Biological effects of shock waves: in vivo effect of high energy pulses on rabbit bone. *Ultrasound Med Biol*. 1995;21:1219-1225.

112. May TC, Krause WR, Preslar AJ, Smith MJ, Beaudoin AJ, Cardea JA. Use of high-energy shock waves for bone cement removal. *J Arthroplasty*. 1990;5:19-27.

113. Weber U, Nietert M, Jacob E. Possibilities and limits of ultrasound manipulation-removal of bone cements. *Aktuelle Probl Chir Orthop*. 1987;31:347-349.

114. Kaulesar Sukul DM, Johannes EJ, Pierik EG, van Eijck GJ, Kristelijn MJ. The effect of high energy shock waves focused on cortical bone: an in vitro study. *J Surg Res*. 1993;54:46-51.

115. McKibbin B. The biology of fracture healing in long bones. *J Bone Joint Surg Br*. 1978;60-B:150-162.

116. Haupt G, Haupt A, Ekkernkamp A, Gerety B, Chvapil M. Influence of shock waves on fracture healing. *Urology*. 1992;39:529-532.

117. Johannes EJ, Kaulesar Sukul DM, Matura E. High-energy shock waves for the treatment of nonunions: an experiment on dogs. *J Surg Res*. 1994;57:246-252.

118. Schleberger R, Senge T. Non-invasive treatment of long-bone pseudarthrosis by shock waves (ESWL). *Arch Orthop Trauma Surg*. 1992;111:224-227.

119. Valchanou VD, Michailov P. High energy shock waves in the treatment of delayed and nonunion of fractures. *Int Orthop*. 1991;15:181-184.

120. Rompe JD, Rosendahl T, Schollner C, Theis C. High-energy extracorporeal shock wave treatment of nonunions. *Clin Orthop Relat Res*. 2001;387:102-111.

121. Wang CJ, Chen HS, Chen CE, Yang KD. Treatment of nonunions of long bone fractures with shock waves. *Clin Orthop Relat Res*. 2001;387:95-101.

122. Augat P, Claes L, Suger G. In vivo effect of shock-waves on the healing of fractured bone. *Clin Biomech (Bristol, Avon)*. 1995;10: 374-378.

123. Forriol F, Solchaga L, Moreno JL, Canadell J. The effect of shockwaves on mature and healing cortical bone. *Int Orthop*. 1994;18: 325-329.

124. Ohtori S, Inoue G, Mannoji C, et al. Shock wave application to rat skin induces degeneration and reinnervation of sensory nerve fibres. *Neurosci Lett*. 2001;315:57-60.

125. Wang FS, Wang CJ, Sheen-Chen SM, Kuo YR, Chen RF, Yang KD. Superoxide mediates shock wave induction of ERK-dependent osteogenic transcription factor (CBFA1) and mesenchymal cell differentiation toward osteoprogenitors. *J Biol Chem*. 2002;277: 10931-10937.

126. Wang FS, Yang KD, Chen RF, Wang CJ, Sheen-Chen SM. Extracorporeal shock wave promotes growth and differentiation of bone-marrow stromal cells towards osteoprogenitors associated with induction of TGF-beta1. *J Bone Joint Surg Br*. 2002;84:457-461.

127. Wang FS, Wang CJ, Chen YJ, et al. Ras induction of superoxide activates ERK-dependent angiogenic transcription factor HIF-1alpha and VEGF-A expression in shock wave-stimulated osteoblasts. *J Biol Chem*. 2004;279:10331-10337.

128. Hamm R, McLarty E, Ashdown J, Natale S, Dickinson A. Peyronie's disease-the Plymouth experience of extracorporeal shockwave treatment. *BJU Int*. 2001;87:849-852.

129. Husain J, Lynn NN, Jones DK, Collins GN, O'Reilly PH. Extracorporeal shock wave therapy in the management of Peyronie's disease: initial experience. *BJU Int*. 2000;86:466-468.

130. Levine LA. Review of current nonsurgical management of Peyronie's disease. *Int J Impot Res*. 2003;15(Suppl 5):S113-120.

131. Hauck EW, Mueller UO, Bschleipfer T, Schmelz HU, Diemer T, Weidner W. Extracorporeal shock wave therapy for Peyronie's disease: exploratory meta-analysis of clinical trials. *J Urol*. 2004;171: 740-745.

132. Müller A, Akin-Olugbade Y, Deveci S, et al. The impact of shock wave therapy at varied energy and dose levels on functional and structural changes in erectile tissue. *Eur Urol*. 2008;53:635-642.

133. Hauck EW, Diemer T, Schmelz HU, Weidner W. A critical analysis of nonsurgical treatment of Peyronie's disease. *Eur Urol*. 2006;49:987-997.

134. Miller MW, Miller DL, Brayman AA. A review of in vitro bioeffects of inertial ultrasonic cavitation from a mechanistic perspective. *Ultrasound Med Biol*. 1996;22:1131-1154.

135. Bao S, Thrall BD, Miller DL. Transfection of a reporter plasmid into cultured cells by sonoporation in vitro. *Ultrasound Med Biol*. 1997;23:953-959.

136. Fechheimer M, Boylan JF, Parker S, Sisken JE, Patel GL, Zimmer SG. Transfection of mammalian cells with plasmid DNA by scrape loading and sonication loading. *Proc Natl Acad Sci USA*. 1987;84:8463-8467.

137. Fechheimer M, Denny C, Murphy RF, Taylor DL. Measurement of cytoplasmic pH in Dictyostelium discoideum by using a new method for introducing macromolecules into living cells. *Eur J Cell Biol*. 1986;40:242-247.

138. Gambihler S, Delius M, Brendel W. Biological effects of shock waves: cell disruption, viability, and proliferation of L1210 cells exposed to shock waves in vitro. *Ultrasound Med Biol*. 1990;16:587-594.

139. Miller DL, Williams AR, Morris JE, Chrisler WB. Sonoporation of erythrocytes by lithotripter shockwaves in vitro. *Ultrasonics*. 1998;36:947-952.

140. Lauer U, Bürgelt E, Squire Z, et al. Shock wave permeabilization as a new gene transfer method. *Gene Ther*. 1997;4:710-715.

141. Bao S, Thrall BD, Gies RA, Miller DL. In vivo transfection of melanoma cells by lithotripter shock waves. *Cancer Res*. 1998;58: 219-221.

142. Song J, Tata D, Li L, Taylor J, Bao S, Miller DL. Combined shockwave and immunogene therapy of mouse melanoma and renal carcinoma tumors. *Ultrasound Med Biol*. 2002;28:957-964.

143. Delius M, Adams G. Shock wave permeabilization with ribosome inactivating proteins: a new approach to tumor therapy. *Cancer Res*. 1999;59:5227-5232.

144. Zhong P, Lin H, Xi X, Zhu S, Bhogte ES. Shock wave-inertial microbubble interaction: methodology, physical characterization, and bioeffect study. *J Acoust Soc Am*. 1999;105:1997-2009.

145. Schlicher RK, Radhakrishna H, Tolentino TP, Apkarian RP, Zarnitsyn V, Prausnitz MR. Mechanism of intracellular delivery by acoustic cavitation. *Ultrasound Med Biol.* 2006;32:915-924.

146. Deng CX, Sieling F, Pan H, Cui J. Ultrasound-induced cell membrane porosity. *Ultrasound Med Biol.* 2004;30:519-526.

147. van Wamel A, Kooiman K, Harteveld M, et al. Vibrating microbubbles poking individual cells: drug transfer into cells via sonoporation. *J Control Release.* 2006;112:149-155.

148. Ohl CD, Arora M, Ikink R, et al. Sonoporation from jetting cavitation bubbles. *Biophys J.* 2006;91:4285-4295.

149. Brujan EA. The role of cavitation microjets in the therapeutic applications of ultrasound. *Ultrasound Med Biol.* 2004;30:381-387.

150. Brujan EA, Ikeda T, Matsumoto Y. Jet formation and shock wave emission during collapse of ultrasound-induced cavitation bubbles and their role in the therapeutic applications of high-intensity focused ultrasound. *Phys Med Biol.* 2005;50:4797-4809.

151. Wu J. Theoretical study on shear stress generated by microstreaming surrounding contrast agents attached to living cells. *Ultrasound Med Biol.* 2002;28:125-129.

152. Huber PE, Jenne J, Debus J, Wannenmacher MF, Pfisterer P. A comparison of shock wave and sinusoidal-focused ultrasound-induced localized transfection of HeLa cells. *Ultrasound Med Biol.* 1999;25:1451-1457.

153. Miller DL, Song J. Lithotripter shock waves with cavitation nucleation agents produce tumor growth reduction and gene transfer in vivo. *Ultrasound Med Biol.* 2002;28:1343-1348.

154. Katoh M, Haage P, Pfeffer JG, Wildberger JE, Günther RW, Tacke J. Noninvasive extracorporeal thrombolysis using electrical discharge-induced shock waves: in vitro experiments. *Invest Radiol.* 2004;39:244-248.

155. Belcaro G, Nicolaides AN, Cesarone MR, et al. Shock waves (SW) noninvasive extracorporeal thrombolysis treatment (NISWT). *Angiology.* 1999;50:707-713.

156. Kato K, Fujimura M, Nakagawa A, et al. Pressure-dependent effect of shock waves on rat brain: induction of neuronal apoptosis mediated by a caspase-dependent pathway. *J Neurosurg.* 2007;106:667-676.

157. Gerdesmeyer L, von Eiff C, Horn C, et al. Antibacterial effects of extracorporeal shock waves. *Ultrasound Med Biol.* 2005;31:115-119.

158. Nigri GR, Tsai S, Kossodo S, et al. Laser-induced shock waves enhance sterilization of infected vascular prosthetic grafts. *Lasers Surg Med.* 2001;29:448-454.

159. Nishida T, Shimokawa H, Oi K, et al. Extracorporeal cardiac shock wave therapy markedly ameliorates ischemia-induced myocardial dysfunction in pigs in vivo. *Circulation.* 2004;110:3055-3061.

160. Nurzynska D, Di Meglio F, Castaldo C, et al. Shock waves activate in vitro cultured progenitors and precursors of cardiac cell lineages from the human heart. *Ultrasound Med Biol.* 2008;34:334-342.

161. Berger M, Frairia R, Piacibello W, et al. Feasibility of cord blood stem cell manipulation with high-energy shock waves: an in vitro and in vivo study. *Exp Hematol.* 2005;33:1371-1387.

Jorge Gutierrez-Aceves, Oscar Negrete-Pulido,
and Marnes Molina-Torres

Abstract Introduced in the 1980s, shock wave lithotripsy (SWL) is still considered a primary treatment option. Actually,minimally invasive endourological procedures may have a similar or even major role as therapeutic options. Most of the stones requiere fragmentation and the urologist has several options of intracorporeal lithotripsy technologies. The ideal lithotripter should be usable in a variety of settings, multifunctional, with adjustable energy output, effective for all stone compositions, reusable, safe, and inexpensive. To decide which is the best alternative of the nonlaser options, it appears that the election needs to be individualized to the patient population, clinical scenario and to the physician practice.

25.1 Introduction

The introduction of shock wave lithotripsy (SWL) in the 1980s represented a great evolution in the management of urinary stones. Today, it is still considered as a primary treatment option in many clinical instances. Nevertheless, due to the outstanding technological evolution of the endoscopic instruments, as well as the development of different energy sources for intracorporeal lithotripsy, minimally invasive endourological procedures performed in a retrograde manner or through a percutaneous access have today a similar or even major role as therapeutic options to treat stones located in the urinary tract.

According to the American Urological Association (AUA) Guidelines published in 2007, ureteroscopy, as well as SWL, is considered a first-line treatment option for calculi located in the distal or even proximal ureter.[1]

Percutaneous nephrolithotripsy (PCNL) is the most effective treatment alternative for renal stones greater than 2 cm or other selected cases including lower pole stones larger than 1 cm, hard stones, stones in morbid obesity or in anatomical abnormalities, reconstructed urinary tracts, or even large proximal ureteral stones.[2,3] Intracorporeal lithotripsy—either transurethral or suprapubic through percutaneous approach— has replaced the open cystolithotomy as the first treatment choice for bladder stones.[4]

Small stones may be removed intact; nevertheless, most of the stones larger than 5 mm require fragmentation and extraction of the resultant fragments. At the present time, there is a large variety of intracorporeal lithotripsy technologies; electrohydraulic, ultrasound, ballistic or pneumatic, and various laser systems. The ideal lithotripter should be usable in a variety of settings, multifunctional, with adjustable energy output, effective for all stone compositions, reusable, safe, and inexpensive.[5]

Laser systems have become in the first choice among stone fragmentation devices in many centers; nevertheless, in the present era cost may represent an important issue to decide which lithotripsy alternative to use. Here, we review the clinical data of different lithotripsy technologies other than laser.

25.2 Electrohydraulic Lithotripsy

Electrohydraulic lithotripsy (EHL), first described by Yutkin in the 1950s, was the first intracorporeal lithotripsy modality available for clinical use.[6] Today, this is the less expensive alternative available, and even when it has proved to be highly effective, it is probably the least demanded, mainly due to the lowest safety profile.

Basically, the mechanism of fragmentation is through the effect of an electrical discharge produced in a liquid medium. This electrical discharge vaporizes the water surrounding the probe, creating a bubble of cavitation that rapidly expands and collapses. The result of this phenomenon is the generation of a shock wave that hits the calculi, producing fragmentation.[7]

O. Negrete-Pulido and M. Molina-Torres
Instituto de Endourología, Centro Medico Puerta de Hierro and Nuevo Hospital Civil, Zapopan, Jalisco, México

P.N. Rao et al. (eds.), *Urinary Tract Stone Disease*,
DOI 10.1007/978-1-84800-362-0_25, © Springer-Verlag London Limited 2011

The first device developed, the URAT-1, was used clinically to treat bladder stones with efficacy and relative safety.[8] Today, in the bladder, the fragmentation rate index is more than 80% with low complication rates.[9]

Indications in the treatment of ureteral stones began back in the 1970s. The initial experience reported high incidence of complications due to the use of the probe without the aid of endoscopic control: extravasations and ureteral perforations, inconsistent fragmentation, and ureteral strictures.[10,11] In contrast, later experiences with intraureteral EHL under endoscopic control demonstrated it to be an effective and safe method of stone fragmentation. Reduction in the diameter of EHL fibers from 9 to 1.9 Fr, controlled energy output, and the use of saline for irrigation add additional safety to intracorporeal EHL lithotripsy. A number of authors have reported success rates from 84% to >90%,[12,13] although the reported rate of complications varies from 6% to 17.6%, most frequently related to mucosal erosion, submucosal inflammation, hemorrhage, and ureteral perforation.[14–17]

From the intracorporeal devices, only EHL and laser systems are alternatives to be used in the treatment of intrarenal stones through flexible instruments. Elashry et al.[18] reported their experience with the use of 1.9 Fr fiber in the treatment of 32 ureteral and renal stones with an overall stone-free success rate of 98% and 87%, respectively, in a subgroup of patients with stones in the lower pole; they did not observed any complications related with the use of electrohydraulic energy.

In PCNL, Clayman reported a lower efficacy of EHL in comparison to other mechanical lithotripters as ultrasound or pneumatic lithotripsy; nevertheless, EHL may play an important role in the fragmentation and removal of stones located in nonaccessible calices using flexible endoscopes during PCN surgery.[19]

25.2.1 Surgical Tips on EHL

Because EHL has the narrowest margin of safety of all forms of intracorporeal lithotripsy, careful attention to the technique must be observed in order to reduce the potential risk of complications and damage to the instruments. The following recommendations may help to improve results and reduce risks:

- Be sure that the insulation layers of the probe are intact.
- The tip of the probe must be positioned at least 5 mm ahead of the endoscope in order to protect the lens.
- The probe must be positioned 1 mm from the stone to assure maximal effect of the shock wave.
- Maintain an adequate irrigation flow to keep the ureter distended and avoid accidental shooting to the urothelium.
- Use 1.9 Fr probes to improve the irrigation flow through the endoscope.

- Be sure that the tip of the probe is visible away from the urothelium.
- Do not activate the probe direct on the security guide wire.
- Start with low power and increase the energy as needed.
- Check periodically the insulation of the probe tip.
- Be aware to use EHL in patients with external pacemaker.

EHL is the less expensive intracorporeal lithotripter unit; depending on the place, the cost is around US $15,000 for the generator. The disposable probes have a cost of US $200 – their lifespan varies in a range of 20 to 60 s. The last generation of electrohydraulic devices, AEH-4 from Gyrus ACMI, has an integrated automatic circuit that prolongs the lifespan of the small probes.

25.3 Ultrasonic Lithotripsy

Ultrasonic lithotripsy, as well as EHL, has been slowly replaced by pneumatic or laser lithotripsy. Nevertheless, this technology maintains unique characteristics of fine fragmentation and simultaneous aspiration of stone particles, making this device still an interesting option for treating stones, especially in the kidney. In addition, this technology has the potential to be combined with pneumatic lithotripsy, increasing the spectrum of indications.

Ultrasonic waves are those acoustic frequencies that are beyond the range of audibility of the human ear. They are mechanical waves covering a frequency range of $20,000–10 \times 10$ cycles/s (Hz). Ultrasonic waves may be generated in a mechanical, thermal, electrostatic, or piezoelectric manner. Ultrasonic lithotripters use piezoelectric waves to generate energy. Current transmitted from a foot pedal to a piezoceramic crystal within a handpiece results in vibrational energy, which is transmitted along a solid or hollow probe, producing a drilling effect at the tip of the probe that results in fragmentation of the stone.[6,7]

In 1953, Mulvaney[20] described the first attempt to destroy urinary calculi with ultrasonic waves. The first clinical application started in 1970s; and in 1984 Hautmann[21] reported interesting results in the treatment of 412 patients with bladder stones. Same as with other lithotripters, initial experience was obtained with bladder stones. Since the 1970s, several series have reported efficacy as high as 99% in stone fragmentation with an adequate safety margin[4,22–24] either via transurethral or percutaneous suprapubic.

Since the 1980s, several reports proved the benefits of ultrasonic lithotripsy in ureter, with success rates between 69% and 100%.[7] While this modality of lithotripsy can be used in ureter in association with rigid ureteroscopy, the large probe size and rigid nature of the probe may limits its utility. Using a solid 2.5 Fr probe, Chaussy reported complete stone fragmentation in 96.6% of patients,[25] and Fuchs obtained successful fragmentation in 91%, 94%, and 98% for stones located in the proximal, middle, and distal ureter, respectively.[26] More recently, Gur,[27] using an 8 Fr ureteroscope in combination with a 4.5 Fr hollow probe, found 88% success without complications. Some other authors have suggested that ultrasonic lithotripsy is the method of election in ureter in selected cases like incrusted catheters or large steinstrasse due to the smooth and fine stone fragmentation.[28,29]

Ultrasonic lithotripsy is most commonly utilized to treat large stone burdens during PCNL. The advantages of this modality, particularly for treating large stones, include proven safety, minimal effect on tissue, and the possibility to aspirate stone material through hollow probes during fragmentation. The advantage of this device in PCNL has been reported since its early introduction in the 1970s.[30]

Recently, a new ultrasound dual probe ultrasonic lithotripter, CyberWand (Gyrus/ACMI), (Fig. 25.1) has been introduced. This device incorporates coaxial high frequency and low frequency ultrasonic probes, which provide a synergistic mechanism to improve stone fragmentation, maintaining at the same time the suction capability. The CyberWand consists of an ultrasonic hand piece and two concentric probes: a 27-mm outer diameter inner probe and a 3.75-mm outer diameter outer probe. The inner probe is fixed to the hand piece and it vibrates at 21,000 Hz. The outer probe is free to move in a reciprocate fashion. It is pushed outward by a sliding piston driven by the vibration energy of the inner probe, and it is returned to its starting position by resistance from a coil spring. The outer probe is 1 mm shorter than the inner probe and its movement never passes the tip of the inner probe. Calculi fragmentation occurs from the conventional high frequency ultrasonic effect of the inner probe and also from the ballistic action of the low frequency outer probe.[31]

Kim, et al.[31] showed in an in vitro study using artificial stone models that CyberWand has a better penetration capability and stone fragmentation compared to a standard combined ultrasound and pneumatic energy device. These results were not reproduced by Ferrandino et al.[32] who reported, also in an in vitro study, that a conventional combined ultrasound and pneumatic unit produce better results in terms of penetration, fragmentation, and extraction of stones than the CyberWand both in soft and in hard stone models. Miller et al.,[33] in an ongoing randomized clinical trial, compared the efficacy of CyberWand versus a standard ultrasound lithotripter. In 38 PCNL, they did not find statistically significant differences between both units in the analyzed parameters – mainly the time to clearance and the stone clearance rate. It is clear that the final results of this and others prospective and comparative studies are required to establish the efficacy and potential benefits of this device.

25.3.1 Surgical Tips on Ultrasonic Lithotripsy

- Because of the rigidity of the probes, endoscopes with straight and wide working channels are obligated.
- Saline or nonelectrolyte solution is useful for irrigation.
- The surgical probe must be in direct contact with the periphery of the calculi, it is suggested to use short energy discharges to produce small stone particles that can be easily evacuated in a simultaneous fashion.
- In large stone burden, a valid alternative is to fragment the calculi in a controlled manner to allow the removal of larger stone particles.
- Continuous irrigation is obligated when activating the generator, in order to avoid overheating of the probe.
- Avoid long energy discharge to reduce overheating of the probe; do not activate the probe if irrigation has been interrupted.
- Maintaining continuous irrigation improves suction of stone particles.
- The hand piece and the probes are reusable; nevertheless, both pieces must be periodically evaluated and replaced.

Conventional ultrasound technology costs range from US$15,000 to US$20,000; the disposable probes cost US$250 and may be reused in most parts of the world. The new dual probe generator CyberWand has an approximated cost of US$30,000 and the cost of the probes varies from US$250 to US$350.

25.4 Ballistic/Pneumatic Lithotripsy (Lithoclast)

The Swiss Lithoclast uses a direct contact solid rigid probe using a principle similar to a pneumatic jackhammer. In this system, clean pressure air acts as an energy source to propel a projectile contained in a hand piece against a metal rod in contact with the stone at a pressure of 3 atm and a frequency of 12 Hz. Repeated impacts of the probe tip against the stone

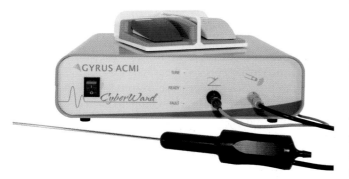

Fig. 25.1 The CyberWand ultrasonic lithotripter with probe (Courtesy of Gyrus ACMI, Inc., Southborough, Massachusetts)

results in a mechanical stone breakage. The device uses solid probes available in sizes ranging from 0.8 to 3.0 mm; they do not allow simultaneous evacuation of the stone particles; they do need to be used through a rigid endoscope.[6,7]

Studies of tissue effects of Lithoclast in animals have demonstrated the safety of the device. After probe firing, focal areas of hemorrhage were visible, but no perforation of the bladder or ureteral or mucosa injuries were observed, nor other long-term damage related to the use of the device.[34,35]

The Lithoclast is universally effective in kidney, ureter, and bladder stones, including very hard stones. Reported fragmentation rates range from 84% to 97% and stone-free rates in ureter is 70% to 95%, depending on the location of the stone within the ureter, with no complication related to the device.[36–41] Treating large stone burdens in kidney or bladder, most of the series report fragmentation rates greater than 95%.[42,43]

Successful lithotripsy with Lithoclast is facilitated with fixation of the stone against the urothelium in order to allow the jackhammer action of the probe. This fixation of the stone is relatively easy to achieve with stones in the kidney or in the bladder. Nevertheless, in the ureter, particularly in stones located in the proximal segment or when the ureter is dilated above the stone, retrograde migration of the stone is a potential problem. Trapping the calculi inside a Segura basket or similar tools, like the stone cone, prevents the proximal migration of the stone when using pneumatic lithotripsy in ureter.[44]

Trying to avoid the migration problem, EMS Company developed the Swiss Lithoclast System 2, which works on the principle of simultaneous fragmentation and suction, using variable air pressure and frequency (2–12 Hz). The foot pedal controls the frequency and the hand piece controls the suction mechanism, helping in stabilizing the stone, thereby preventing migration. Some authors have reported similar results when comparing this system with Ho-Laser in the treatment of ureteral stones.[45]

25.4.1 Surgical Tips on Pneumatic Lithotripsy

- Hold the stone against the urothelium to avoid continuous movement of calculi during lithotripsy in kidney or in the bladder.
- The probe must be in direct contact with the surface of the stone.
- Initiate the fragmentation on the periphery of the calculi and keep control on the resultant fragments.
- As the stone fragments are getting separated from the big stone mass, remove them with forceps.
- Avoid uncontrolled migration of large fragments to different calices.

- When the stone is in the ureter, trap it before activating the foot pedal.
- As the stone gets smaller inside the basket or similar tool, remove it without forcing against the ureteral wall.

The conventional Swiss Lithoclast system has a favorable cost, comparable with other intracorporeal lithotripters; the cost of the generator ranges from US$15,000 to US$20,000 and the reusable probes range from US$400 to US$600.

25.5 Combined Pneumatic and Ultrasound Lithotripsy

The combination between the efficacy in fragmentation of pneumatic lithotripsy with the aspiration and clearing capability of the ultrasound energy bring an important advance in intracorporeal lithotripsy. The Lithoclast Master (EMS, Bern, Switzerland), commercialized as Lithoclast Ultra (Boston Scientific, Natick, MA), represents an all-in-one or combo product that allows the possibility to use pure pneumatic lithotripsy with or without suction (Lithovac), pure ultrasound energy, or the combination of both energies with a better efficacy and versatility in fragmentation.

Pneumatic probes are available in different diameters (0.8, 1.0, 1.6, and 2.0 mm); the 1.0 mm probe may be inserted into a hollow 3.3 or 3.8 mm ultrasound probe. The tip of the pneumatic probe is positioned at the same distance of the ultrasound probe, to allow the contact with the calculi surface with both energies. The generator can be used either in separate pneumatic or ultrasound activation mode or in combined activation mode. The unit allows adjustments of the pulse frequency up to 12 Hz, number of pulses, and the pneumatic pressure level of the Lithoclast. The ultrasound power can be set from 10% to 100% with a frequency of 24–26 kHz.[7]

Due to the rigidity and size of the probe, the combination pneumatic/ultrasound lithotripter can be used only in the management of renal stones; nevertheless, it appears to be the most efficient device currently available for PCNL. In vitro studies demonstrated a significantly faster time to fragment phantom stones with the combined pneumatic/ultrasound unit (7.41 min) versus the ultrasound (12.87 min) or the pneumatic lithotripter (23.76 min) used individually.[46] Clinical studies have proved the fragmentation and clearance efficacy of the device, with stone-free rates after PCNL from 76% to 89.7%.[47,48] Pietrow et al. compared in a clinical study the combination mode versus the pure pneumatic mode and showed a faster fragmentation and clearance of stone fragments with the pneumatic/ultrasound lithotripter.[49] In another clinical study, Lehman et al. found a significant improvement of fragmentation using the combination mode in hard stones; they did not observed any difference between the combination and the pure ultrasound energy in soft stones.[50]

25.5.1 Surgical Tips on Combined Pneumatic/Ultrasound Lithotripsy

- Recommended star setting is 50% of ultrasound power and 100% of pneumatic power at 4 Hz. This may increase the probe lifespan.
- If stone is not efficiently fragmented, increase the ultrasound power step-wise by 10% to a maximum of 100% and the pneumatic power to a maximum of 12 Hz until adequate fragmentation occurs.
- When the power is increased, the fragmentation improves. Nevertheless, when the ultrasound power reaches 100% and the pneumatic energy reaches 12 Hz, the penetration power on the stone is mainly produced by the pneumatic energy; this may produce a noncontrolled number and size of stone fragments.[51]

The combined pneumatic and ultrasound Lithoclast system has a cost ranging from US$39,000 to US$45,000. The reusable probes have an approximate cost of US$500.

25.6 Electrokinetic Lithotripsy

At the end of 1990s, a new alternative of ballistic lithotripsy was developed. The principle of the electrokinetic lithotripsy (EKL) device is the same of a jackhammer as in Lithoclast; the only difference is that in EKL, instead of a projectile road, a magnetic core is accelerated electromagnetically. An electromagnetic field produced inside the hand piece allows vibration at 15–30 Hz; this drilling movement is transmitted to the distal tip of the probe and produces the jackhammer effect on the calculi.

In vitro studies have proved that the efficacy of EKL is equally effective as pneumatic lithotripsy.[52] Several clinical studies have evaluated the efficacy of this method. Keeley et al.[53] reported excellent results, in terms of ureteral stone fragmentation, of 99.3% with high security margins; nevertheless, they also reported only an 80% stone-free rate, due to the frequent retrograde migration of large stone fragments into the kidney. Comparative studies in the management of ureteral stones have also proved that success rates do not differ between EKL and pneumatic lithotripsy, but the requirements of stone baskets to trap the stone before fragmentation have been more necessary with EKL, due to a major propulsion of the electromagnetic energy.[53,54] More recently, De Sio et al., in a randomized study comparing EKL versus pneumatic lithotripsy, also demonstrated similar efficacy,

with stone-free rates of 94.7% and 89.4%, respectively, and excellent safety margins.[55]

Despite these results and despite that EKL is a low-cost attractive lithotripsy option, overall, the popularity of the technology is still poor.

25.7 Contact Ballistic Lithotripsy (LMA)

The LMA StoneBreaker™ (LMA Urology, Gland, Switzerland) is a portable, nonelectric, contact ballistic intracorporeal lithotripter. The device requires no extraneous electric or pneumatic connections; it is powered by a cartridge of high-pressure CO_2 gas, which delivers a pressure of 2.9 MPa at the tip of the probe.

Once the cartridge has been perforated by the built-in screw system, the gas passes through a preadjusted pressure regulator–reducer to fill an intermediate chamber. A spring-loaded hammer is activated when the trigger is depressed; the compressed gas expands and in doing so transmits energy to the hammer; this impacts a guided projectile, which in turn transmits energy directly to the probe. Expended gas leaves the chamber through a specially designed exhaust port and exhaust line. A spring pushes the hammer back to its starting position; when the trigger snaps back, the intermediate chamber is again filled with gas and the device is now ready for the next cycle and further use. One full cartridge allows delivery of at least 80 shocks.

Animal studies were conducted by Rané et al.[56] to evaluate the safety of the StoneBreaker in a model of acute ureteral perforation; there was no evidence of perforation even at artificially high-pressure settings of up to 5.0 MP. They compared the fragmentation efficiency with the Swiss Lithoclast; the number of "hits" required to break stones at different size. For large stone phantoms (mean 7.4 g), the Lithoclast required a mean of 307 firings versus 77 for the StoneBreaker ($P < 0.001$); for medium stones (mean 3.2 g), the respective values were 221 and 46 ($P < 0.001$); and for small stones (mean 0.50 g), 72 and 26 ($P < 0.01$).

Initial clinical experience reported by Rané et al.[56] in a small cohort of patients, demonstrates a high effectiveness and safety, with fragmentation rates reaching 100% for renal, ureteral, and bladder stones, requiring an average of 10 hits per centimeter of stone and no side effects related with lithotripsy. Nearly et al. found a fragmentation success of 100% in patients with ureteral stones without complications related to the lithotripsy; the number of shocks needed on average to fragment the stone was eight, and the incidence of stone retropulsion was 6.36%.[57]

This new pneumatic lithotripsy appeared to be an interesting option; it is portable, safe, and a cost-effective alternative. The only disposable item in this unit is the CO_2 cartridge,

Table 25.1 Comparison of lithotripsy procedures

Intracorporeal lithotripsy	Effectiveness (Stone-Free rates) (%)	Utility in Hard stones	Safety	Flexible probes	Versatility	Stone localization studied	Cost
Electrohydraulic	87–98	+	+	Yes	+	Kidney, ureter, bladder (KUB)	+
Ultrasound	88–98	+	++	No	+	KUB	++
CyberWand	56.25[a]	++	++	No	+	Kidney	++
Ballistic							
Pneumatic	86.5–94	+++	++	No	++	KUB	++
Electrokinetic	80–94.7	+++	+	No	++	Ureter	[b]
Stonebreaker	77–100	+++	++	No	+++	Kidney and ureter	+
Combination							
Ultrasonic/pneumatic	76–89.7	+++	+++	No	+++	Kidney	+++

[a]Preliminary report
[b]Ignored

which needs to be replaced after every 40–50 shocks. The cost of the device ranges from US$10,000 to US$15,000 and the cost of the cartridges is between US$5 and US$10, which, therefore, does not add significantly to the cost of the procedure. At the present time, proper and larger comparative studies are needed to evaluate the potential benefits of this technology.

25.8 Conclusions

A significant evolution over the last decade in technology for intracorporeal lithotripsy with a number and variety of devices currently available allow the urologist to deal with most stone situations (Table 25.1). Especially for difficult scenarios and complex cases, it would be desirable to have access to more than one technology. From the nonlaser alternatives to fragment a stone using intracorporeal lithotripsy, it seems that for dealing with kidney stones the best alternative is the combination of pneumatic and ultrasound energy—this device means an advance in terms of fragmentation and stone clearance. Pure ultrasound lithotripsy is still a commonly used lithotripter with rigid scopes during PCNL. The pneumatic Lithoclast technology is a safe and relatively inexpensive, cost-effective technology efficient for the whole urinary tract; for most urologists it is probably the best choice. The new LMA ballistic lithotripter seems to be an attractive, effective, and safe option to fragment stones in the kidney and ureter, but experience with this technology is still limited.

To decide which is the best alternative of the nonlaser options, it appears that the election needs to be individualized to the patient population and to the physician practice.

References

1. Preminger G, Tiselius H, Assimos D. 2007 Guidelines for the Management of Ureteral Calculi. *J Urol*. 2007;178:2418-2434.
2. Wen Ch, Nakada S. Treatment Selection and Outcomes: Renal Calculi. *Urol Clin N Am*. 2007;34:409-419.
3. Preminger G, Assimos D, Lingeman J, et al. Chapter 1: AUA Guideline on management of staghorn calculi: diagnosis and treatment recommendations. *J Urol*. 2005;173:1991-2000.
4. Papatsoris A, Varkarakis, Dellis A. Bladder lithiasis: from open surgery to lithotripsy. *Urol Res*. 2006;34:163-167.
5. Buchholz N. Intracorporeal lithotripters: selecting the optimum machine. *BJU Int*. 2002;89:157-161.
6. Zheg W, Denstedt J. Intracorporeal lithotripsy Update on technology. *Urol Clin N Am*. 2000;272:301-13.
7. Knudsen B, Denstedt J. Intracorporeal Lithotriptors. In: Smith A, Badlani G, Bagley D, et al., eds. *Textbook of Endourology*. 2nd ed. Hamilton.London: BC Decker Inc; 2006:27-36.
8. Bergman B, Nygaard E, Osterman G, et al. Vesical calculi Experience of electrohydraulic lithotripsy with URAT I. *Scand J Urol Nephrol*. 1982;16:217.
9. Razvi H, Song T, Denstedt J. Management of vesical calculi: comparison of lithotripsy devices. *J Endourol*. 1996;10:559.
10. Raney A, Handler J. Electrohydraulic nephrolithotripsy. *Urology*. 1975;6:439.
11. Reuter H, Kern E. Electronic lithotripsy of ureteral calculi. *J Urol*. 1973;110:181.
12. Yang S, Hong J. Electrohydraulic lithotripsy of upper ureteral calculi with semirigid ureteroscope. *J Endourol*. 1996;10:27-30.
13. Vorreuther R, Engelking R. Adjustable electrohydraulic lithotripsy for minimally invasive ureteroscopic stone treatment. *Urologe A*. 1992;31:76-80.
14. Vorreuther R, Engelking RVorreuther R, Corleis R, Klotz T, et al. Impact of shock wave pattern and cavitation bubble size on tissue damage during ureteroscopic electrohydraulic lithotripsy. *J Urol*. 1995;153:849-853.
15. Wu T, Hsu T, Li A, et al. Morphological change in the urothelium after electrohydraulic versus pulsed dye laser lithotripsy. *Br J Urol*. 1994;74:685-689.
16. Green D, Lytton B. Electrohydraulic lithotripsy in the ureter. *Urol Clin North Am*. 1988;15:361.

17. Hofbauer J, Hobarth K, Marberger M. Electrohydraulic versus pneumatic disintegration in the treatmet of ureteral stones: A randomized prospective trial. *J Urol.* 1995;153:623-625.
18. Elashry O, DiMeglio RB, Nakada SY, et al. Intracorporeal electrohydraulic lithotripsy of ureteral and renal calculi using small caliber (1.9F) electrohydraulic lithotripsy probes. *J Urol.* 1996;156:1581.
19. Clayman R. Techniques in percutaneous removal of renal calculi. Mechanical extraction and electrohydraulic lithotripsy. *Urology.* 1984;23:11.
20. Mulvaney W. Attempted disintegration of calculi by ultrasonic vibrations. *J Urol.* 1953;70:704.
21. Hautmann RTBRPGFLW. Ultrasonic litholapaxy of bladder stones - 10 years of experience with more than 400 cases. In: Ryall R, Brockis JG, Marshall V, eds. *Urinary Stones.* New York: Churchill Livingstone; 1984:120-4.
22. Fahiq S, Wallace D. Ultrasonic lithotriptor for urethral and bladder stones. *Br J Urol.* 1978;50:255.
23. Cetin S, Ozgur S, Yazicioglu A, et al. Ultrasonic lithotripsy of bladder stones. *Int Urol Nephrol.* 1988;20:361.
24. Razvi H, Song T, Denstedt J. Management of vesical calculi: comparison of lithotripsy devices. *J Endourol.* 1996;10:559.
25. Chaussy C, Fuchs G, Kahn R, et al. Transurethral ultrasonic ureterolithotripsy using a solid-wire probe. *Urology.* 1987;29:531.
26. Fuchs G. Ultrasonic lithotripsy in the ureter. *Urol Clin North Am.* 1988;15:347.
27. Gur U, Lifshitz D, Lask D, Livne P. Ureteral Ultrasonic Lithotripsy Revisited: A Neglected Tool? *J Endourol.* 2004;18(2):137-40.
28. Weinerth J, Flatt J, Carson C. Lessons learned in patients with large Steinstrasse. *J Urol.* 1989;142:1425-1427.
29. Grocela J, Dretler S. Intracorporeal lithotripsy: Instrumentation and development. *Urol Clin North Am.* 1997;24:13-23.
30. Kurth K, Hohenfellner R, Altwein J. Ultrasound litholapaxy of a staghorn calculus. *J Urol.* 1977;117:242.
31. Kim S, Matlaga B, Tinmouth W, Kuo R, et al. In Vitro Assessment of a Novel Dual Probe Ultrasonic Intracorporeal Lithotriptor. *J Urol.* 2007;177:1363-1365.
32. Ferrandino M, Simmons WN, Pierre S, Quin J, et al. Comparision of comminution and stone clearance between intracorporeal lithotripters. *J Urol.* 2008;179(4, Supplement):589.
33. Miller N, Humphreys M, Nakada S, Sterrett S, et al. Randomized controled trial comparing a dual probe ultrasonic lithotrite to a single probe lithotrite for percutaneous nephrolithotomy. *J Urol.* 2008; 179(4, Suppl):500.
34. Piergiovanni M, Desgrandchamps F, Cochand-Priollet B, et al. Ureteral and bladder lesions after ballistic, ultrasonic, electrohydraulic, or laser lithotripsy. *J Endourol.* 1994;8:293.
35. Denstedt J, Razvi H, Rowe E, et al. Investigation of the tissue effects of a new device for intracorporeal lithotripsy—the Swiss Lithoclast. *J Urol.* 1995;153:535.
36. Hofbauer J, Hobarth K, Marberger M. Lithoclast: new and inexpensive mode of intracorporeal lithotripsy. *J Endourol.* 1992;6:429.
37. Denstedt JD, Eberwein PM, Singh RR. The Swiss Lithoclast: a new device for intracorporeal lithotripsy. *J Urol.* 1992;148:1088.
38. Aghamir et al. Traetment of Ureteral Calculi with Ballistic Lithotripsy. *J Endourol.* 2003;10:887.
39. Sözen S, Küpeli B, Tunc L, et al. Management of ureteral stones with pneumatic lithotripsy: Report of 500 patients. *J Endourol.* 2003;17:721-724.
40. Yinghao S, Linhui W, Songxi Q, et al. Treatment of urinary calculi with ureteroscopy and Swiss lithoclast pneumatic lithotripter: report of 150 cases. *J Endourol.* 2000;14:281.
41. Sözen S, Küpeli B, Tunc L, et al. Management of ureteral stones with pneumatic lithotripsy: Report of 500 patients. *J Endourol.* 2003;17:721-724.
42. Denstedt J. Use of Swiss Lithoclast for percutaneous nephrolithotripsy. *J Endourol.* 1993;7:477.
43. Wollin TA, Singal RK, Whelan T, et al. Percutaneous suprapubic cystolithotripsy for treatment of large bladder calculi. *J Endourol.* 1999;13:739.
44. Gonen M, Cenker A, Istanbulluoglu O, Ozkardes H. Efficacy of Dretler stone cone in the treatment of ureteral stones with pneumatic lithotripsy. *Urol Int.* 2006;77:159-162.
45. Manohar T, Ganpule A, Desai M, et al. Comparative Evaluation of Swiss LithoClast 2® versus Holmium:YAG Laser Lithotripsy for Impacted Upper-Ureteral Stones. *J Endourol.* 2008;22:3.
46. Auge BK, Lallas CD, Pietrow PK, et al. In vitro comparison of standard ultrasound and pneumatic lithotrites with a new combination intracorporeal lithotripsy device. *Urology.* 2002;60:28.
47. Hormann R, Webe J, Heidenreich A, Varga Z, Olbert P. Experimental studies and first clinical experience with a new lithoclast and ultrasound combination for lithotripsy. *Eur Urol.* 2002;42:376-381.
48. Hormann R, Olbert P, Weber J, Wille S, Varga Z. Clinical experience with a new ultrasonic and LithoClast combination for percutaneous litholapaxy. *BJU Int.* 2002;90(1):16-19.
49. Pietrow PK, Auge BK, Zhong P, Preminger GM. Clinical efficacy of a combination pneumatic and ultrasonic lithotrite. *J Urol.* 2003;169:1247.
50. Lehman DS, Hruby GW, Phillips C, et al. Prospective randomized comparison of a combined ultrasonic and pneumatic lithotrite with a standard ultrasonic lithotrite for percutaneous nephrolithotomy. *J Endourol.* 2008;22(2):285-289.
51. Kuo R, Paterson R, Siqueira T, et al. In Vitro Assessment of Lithoclast Ultra Intracorporeal Lithotripter. *J Endourol.* 2004;18:2.
52. Vorreuther R, Klotz T, Heidenreich A, Nayal W, Engelmann U. Pneumatic vs electrokinetic lithotripsy in treatment of ureteral stones. *J Endourol.* 1998;12(3):233-6.
53. Keeley F, Pillai M, Smith G, Christofos M, Tolley DA. Electrokinetic lithotripsy: safety, efficacy and limitations of a new form of ballistic lithotripsy. *BJU Int.* 1999;84:261-263.
54. Menezes P, Kumar P, Timoney A. A randomized trial comparing lithoclast with an electrokinetic lithotripter in the management of ureteric stones. *BJU Int.* 2000;85:22-25.
55. De Sio M, Autorino R, Damiano R, Oliva A, et al. Comparing Two Different Ballistic Intracorporeal Lithotripters in the Management of Ureteral Stones. *Urol Int.* 2004;72(suppl 1):52-54.
56. Rané A, Kommu S, Kandaswamy, Rao P, Aron M, et al. Initial clinical evaluation of a new pneumatic intracorporeal lithotripter. *BJU Int.* 2007;100:629-631.
57. Nerli R, Koura A, Prabha V, Kamat G, et al. Use of LMA Stonebreaker as an Intracorporeal Lithotrite in the Management of Ureteral Calculi. *J Endourol.* 2008;22(4):621-643.

Laser Lithotripsy Physics

26

Andrew J. Marks, Jinze Qiu, Thomas E. Milner,
Kin Foong Chan, and Joel M.H. Teichman

Abstract The physics of laser lithotripsy are reviewed. The principal mechanisms by which lasers fragment urinary calculi are photomechanical or photothermal. Photomechanical effects are produced in lasers with short pulse durations, typically <1 μs. Such lasers include pulsed dye, Q-switched alexandrite, and FREDDY lasers. Photothermal effects are produced in lasers with long pulse durations, typically >10 μs. Such lasers include Ho:YAG and Er:YAG. Different fragmentation is seen with photomechanical and photothermal lasers. Photomechanical lasers tend to be more efficient whereas photothermal lasers are slower but produce smaller fragments and fragment all compositions. The physics of optical fibers used for Ho:YAG lithotripsy is reviewed.

26.1 Introduction

A laser is a relatively pure form of optical energy; i.e., light. The word "laser" is an acronym for light amplification by stimulated emission of radiation. A basic laser consists of a gain medium in a resonant optical cavity. The gain medium is an excitable material, gas, solid, or liquid, capable of releasing photons when its electrons are excited, "stimulated," or "pumped" by an external energy source. This external energy source can be electric current, chemical energy, or another light source. Since the gain medium is usually a homogeneous substance, electrons are stimulated to jump to uniform, higher energy orbitals and release photons with identical energy when they return to their more stable, lower energy orbitals. This process results in the emission of light at a single wavelength. Thus, lasers are fundamentally different than ordinary light from a household lightbulb or the sun's rays.

Amplification is usually achieved by placing the gain medium in a resonant cavity, the simplest of which is a box with two reflective surfaces on opposite ends. Imagine that the reflective surfaces act as mirrors on opposite sides and that there is no possible escape for the photons. Stimulated light emission is thus reflected back and forth in the resonator through the gain medium providing further excitation and emission, with each stimulated photon having the opportunity to collide into a nonstimulated atom, in a binomial expansion, until it reaches a certain balance and the signal saturates. Furthermore, the opposite position of the mirrors produces radiation that is directional and in-phase. The end result is the production of highly uniform, collimated light of a single wavelength of in-phase photons (Fig. 26.1).

In practice, the mirrors on the opposite ends of the gain medium consist of one total reflector and one partial reflector. The total reflector is ideally a 100% reflective mirror, while the partial reflector allows a portion of the light in the resonator to escape and is the output end of the laser cavity where the laser beam is emitted. This arrangement allows for continuous emission of laser energy and is appropriately referred to as a continuous wave laser. Alternatively, the light can be released in a pulsed fashion by various mechanisms. One example is a Q-switched laser, which uses a Venetian blind or shutter mechanism to intermittently release light. Another example is a mode-locked or phase-locked laser, which takes advantage of constructive and destructive interference in the resonant cavity to produce extremely short laser light pulses. The pulse duration has important implications for the mechanics of lithotripsy.

The first lithotripsy lasers produced used a synthetic ruby crystal as a gain medium and a flashlamp as an energy "pump".[2] Subsequently, multiple gain media with different pumping mechanisms have been devised to deliver laser energy of

J.M.H. Teichman (✉)
Department of Urologic Sciences, St. Paul's Hosiptal,
University of British Columbia, Vancouver, BC, Canada
e-mail: jteichman@providencehealth.bc.ca

P.N. Rao et al. (eds.), *Urinary Tract Stone Disease*,
DOI 10.1007/978-1-84800-362-0_26, © Springer-Verlag London Limited 2011

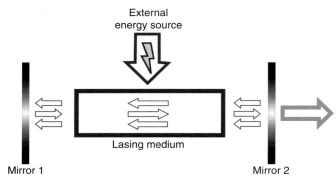

Fig. 26.1 A standard laser consists of a lasing medium, energized by an external energy source such as a flashlamp. Light oscillates between the mirrors, increasing in energy with each passage. Mirror 2 is partly transparent, and the laser beam emerges as a high-quality, collimated beam of laser energy[1] (Reprinted with permission from Teichman)

different wavelengths at different energy settings. Lasers used in medical applications differ from industrial lasers in that their construction requires them to be mobile, to be readily serviced, and to withstand the rigors of clinical use.

Gas lasers are among the oldest laser types for medical applications. These lasers use a gas such as carbon dioxide as the gain medium.[3] CO_2 lasers produce laser light with a wavelength of 10,600 nm. They are the highest power continuous wave lasers that are currently available and also quite efficient. CO_2 laser light is highly absorbed by water and thus has a narrow depth of penetration. As a result, CO_2 lasers have been useful in treating penile and vulvar lesions such as superficial squamous cell carcinoma and ablative skin resurfacing, but are yet to benefit stone fragmentation because fiber optic delivery of 10.6-µm wavelengths necessary for intracorporeal lithotripsy either suffers losses in the fiber or limitations of hollow waveguides in an aqueous environment.[4-6]

Dye lasers use an organic dye such as coumarin as the gain medium and are usually flashlamp pumped.[7] These lasers are both tunable (meaning the emitted wavelength can

be changed) and also produce short pulse durations with resultant high peak pressures. The coumarin dye laser has a wavelength of 504 nm, which is well absorbed by hemoglobin. Any excess or stray energy at 504 nm that "pass points" the stone and strikes the ureter is absorbed by hemoglobin and dissipated through blood flow, acting as an "energy sink," providing a high margin of safety during lithotripsy.[8] While they are safe, efficient lithotriptors, they tend to produce large fragments, and are poorly capable of fragmenting hard stones such as cystine, brushite, or calcium oxalate monohydrate stones.[8,9]

Solid-state lasers use a solid gain medium. The solid gain medium is often composed of a crystalline host material doped with ions, which can be excited to the desired energy levels. These lasers commonly produce high output power in the near infrared spectrum. A common laser crystal is yttrium aluminum garnet (YAG). Lasers using YAG doped with neodymium, holmium, erbium, and thulium have been produced and studied for application in urology. Of these, the long pulse (pulse duration 250–350 µs) holmium:YAG (Ho:YAG) laser has become the dominant laser currently used for lithotripsy due to its versatility and safety profile. Another solid-state laser lithotriptor is the FREDDY (frequency-doubled double-pulse Nd:YAG) laser. This laser uses a KTP crystal in the resonator of a Nd:YAG laser to produce and emit laser light at both 1,064 and 532 nm simultaneously. The relative absorptions of hemoglobin, melanin, and water of radiation from various laser types are shown in Fig. 26.2.

26.2 Laser Tissue Interaction

When laser energy strikes tissue, there are three possible interactions: photochemical, photothermal, and photomechanical interactions.[11] Photochemical interactions occur when laser light facilitates or catalyzes chemical reactions in tissues.

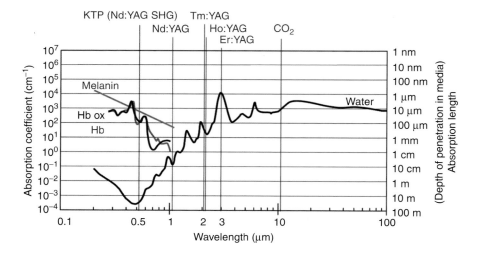

Fig. 26.2 Absorption spectrum of water, melanin, hemoglobin, and oxy-hemoglobin at various laser wavelengths (Reprinted with permission from Teichmann.[10] Copyright Springer-Verlag 2007)

This process is usually achieved by administering a photosensitive dye, which accumulates in a desired tissue. This process, known as photodynamic therapy, takes advantage of a particular dye's ability to produce singlet oxygen when stimulated by light of a certain wavelength, which can then rapidly react with any nearby biomolecules. Photosensitizers to stones have rarely been attempted for laser lithotripsy, and success has been limited. Photochemical laser mechanisms are not used for lithotripsy currently.

Photothermal interaction occurs when direct irradiation of tissues or materials by the laser light leads to vaporization and even ablation or fragmentation of tissues. Photothermal lithotripsy can occur either by direct absorption of photons by the stone crystalline structure and disruption of the lattice, or by water within the lattice rapidly heating and producing fast vapor flow that in turn disrupts the lattice ("explosive vaporization" as occurs when one microwaves popcorn). Photothermal interaction is the dominant mechanism when long pulse laser (approximately 2–500 μs per pulse) is applied.[12] For example, the free-running Ho:YAG and Er:YAG lasers fragment stones by photothermal mechanism. Efficient fragmentation or ablation through photothermal interaction is often associated with thermal confinement, where the laser energy is delivered within a pulse duration, usually <10 ms, shorter than the time it takes for heat to diffuse away from the immediate irradiated zone, causing adequate thermal buildup within the tissue for rapid vaporization.[13]

Photomechanical laser ablation occurs when the production of transient stress waves occurs from the deposition of laser energy on a tissue, material, or its surroundings, which then leads to cell death or ablation in tissues, and lithotripsy in stones. The pulsed dye and FREDDY lasers are examples of photomechanical lasers.[13–15] During laser lithotripsy using short pulse lasers (typically less than 10 μs), transient stress waves can be caused by three distinct mechanisms: thermoelastic expansion, recoil due to ejection of ablated material, and by expansion of materials undergoing phase change.[13,14] Thermoelastic expansion waves are generated when a tissue or material expands due to transient heating by laser energy. This expansion produces a pressure wave, which travels in all directions, but is reflected at the surface of the material producing a negative pressure wave traveling inward from the surface. If the negative pressure wave is strong enough, mechanical disruption may occur, a process known as spallation. Spallation occurs when a material undergoes rapid heating or cooling. An example of spallation is taking a hot ceramic plate from a dishwasher and running it under cold water. This rapid temperature cooling may produce irregular fragmentation. Secondly, when tissue ablation causes material to be ejected, conservation of momentum causes a recoil pressure wave, which may produce stress fracture deep to the actual surface of ablation.[16] Lastly, and most importantly in lithotripsy using short pulse lasers (<1 μs),

laser-induced phase changes produce significant transient pressure waves that can fragment urinary calculi.[13] One example of such a phase change is the production of plasma. Plasma is considered a fourth state of matter. It is produced by the vaporization of ions that exist in a cloud of shared, free electons. Due to plasma's instability, rapid plasma expansion and contraction produce pressure waves capable of inducing stress fractures in the matrix of a stone. Plasma occurs with extremely short pulse durations, typically <500 ns, such as achieved with Q-switched lasers.[13] Lasers that fragment stone via plasma mechanisms produce extremely high peak pressures at the tip of the optical fiber by virtue of the ultrashort pulse duration. Another example of phase change–induced pressure waves is the formation of cavitation bubbles, and cavitation occurs typically for lasers with pulse durations between 500 ns and 1 μs (although may continue to occur for pulse durations up to 10 μs). A cavitation bubble is caused by the rapid spherical expansion of laser-induced water vapor at the laser fiber tip.[13] The spherical bubble then rapidly collapses in the noncompressible surrounding water several hundred milliseconds later. When collapse occurs, it releases the energy stored from its generation in an instant, creating very strong pressure waves, which strain the crystal matrix of stones leading to fragmentation[13,15] Fragmentation due to plasma formation tends to produce larger fragments compared to laser-induced cavitation bubbles.[13] Cavitation bubbles produce a characteristic pressure transient pattern. An initial pressure transient is caused by cavitation bubble expansion, followed by bubble collapse after the end of the pulse duration. After bubble collapse, there is a higher pressure transient caused by the release of bubble energy, leading to fragmentation. The amplitude (force) of the pressure transient is related to the maximal bubble radius (raised to the power of three).[13] Thus, photomechanical laser lithotripsy is characterized by initial pressure transient (bubble expansion), termination of the laser pulse, bubble collapse, a second pressure transient, and subsequent lithotripsy.[13,14] The time course differs from photothermal lithotripsy so that photomechanical (cavitation-induced) lithotripsy produces an expanding spherical vapor bubble that after collapse produces mechanical energy that transmits to the stone and causes lithotripsy; photothermal lithotripsy produces direct irradiation of the stone and lithotripsy.[13,14] In general, efficient fragmentation or ablation through photomechanical interaction is often associated with stress confinement, where the laser energy was delivered within a pulse duration, usually <1 μs, shorter than the time it takes for mechanical stress to propagate away from the immediate irradiated zone, causing a rapid buildup of pressure and heat within the tissue and often generating a shock wave that causes physical dissociation of the target tissue or crystalline structure.

The distribution of laser energy in tissues is important in determining the applications of a particular laser. The choice of laser wavelength depends on the optical properties of the target tissue.[11] If the tissue causes a large amount of photon scattering, less radiation is absorbed per unit tissue volume and the optical penetration is diminished. If there is minimal scattering, the only limit to penetration of laser irradiation is laser absorption by the material. If a tissue absorbs a particular wavelength well and has a low scatter, the spatial confinement will be high (high fluence). In other words, the depth of penetration is small. Conversely, a poorly absorbing material with high scatter will lead to a deep depth of penetration or low fluence.[11] The width of the laser beam also affects the confinement of laser energy. A wide beam deposits energy over a large surface area, producing a lower fluence at the same depth within the tissue than that of a narrow laser beam of the same power level.[16,17] Finally, tissue pigmentation can affect laser distribution in tissues. Pigments preferentially absorb some wavelengths and can confine laser energy to their locations.[17] (Fig. 26.2).

26.3 Physics of Laser Lithotripsy

The ideal laser lithotrite produces predictable lithotripsy of all stone compositions, is simple to operate, efficient, and has a wide safety margin for surrounding tissues so there is maximal stone fragmentation with minimal collateral damage. As a general rule, photomechanical lasers have high safety margins for lithotripsy with efficient fragmentation; photothermal lasers have acceptable (but lower) safety margins with less efficient fragmentation.[14] However, photothermal lasers produce smaller fragments and fragment all stone compositions compared to photomechanical lasers.[18]

Pulsed dye lasers were among the first lasers to be used clinically in lithotripsy.[8,9,13] As mentioned previously, pulsed dye lasers (coumarin green) operate at 504 nm, a wavelength highly absorbed by hemoglobin (Fig. 26.2). They fragment stones by a photomechanical mechanism.[11,14,15] A key component to the effective photomechanical lithotripsy of pulsed dye lasers is the short (<1 μs) pulse duration. Cavitation bubble collapse is important in dye laser lithotripsy. One advantage of this mechanism is that it obviates the need to have the laser in direct contact with the stone since the laser-induced shock wave from cavitation bubble collapse propagates in all directions from the fiber tip and can thus be placed anywhere close to the stone to cause fragmentation. In fact, placing the fiber directly on the stone limits cavitation bubble expansion, thereby limiting the amplitude of the resultant shock wave and inhibits lithotripsy.[15] Another advantage of this system is the inherent safety of these lasers. Dye laser light at 504 nm is well absorbed by hemoglobin, which acts as a laser and heat sink and protects local tissues from thermal injury (Fig. 26.2). However, these lasers are limited by several factors. They tend to produce large, heterogeneous fragments.[18] Also, fragment

ejection and transient pressure waves can cause significant retropulsion of the stone, making lithotripsy more time-consuming and potentially more difficult.[16] Finally, fragmentation results with hard stones such as brushite, calcium oxalate monohydrate, and cystine are disappointing.[19]

With ultrashort laser pulse duration (<500 ns), high peak pressures are produced by the temporal confinement of laser energy. This temporal confinement is especially important in the production of plasma as a lithotripsy mechanism, which requires large amounts of energy.[20,21] Q-switched alexandrite and Nd:YAG lasers have been attempted for lithotripsy but a practical limitation is that the high peak power causes fiber tip destruction and shards of optical fiber can be created within the ureter.[22-24]

The FREDDY laser fragments stones by a similar photomechanical mechanism. By incorporating a KTP crystal in the resonator of a Nd:YAG laser, the FREDDY laser produces laser wavelengths of 532 and 1,064 nm, with pulse durations of 0.3–1.5 μs. At these pulse durations, the light at 532 nm wavelength induces plasma formation, which is further enhanced by the light at 1,064 nm, leading to high-energy pressure transients.[25-27] This laser design is cost effective, and has a high safety margin.[28,29] Although also effective for lithotripsy, the FREDDY laser is less effective in fragmenting hard calculi.[30,31]

The Ho:YAG laser fragments stones using a photothermal mechanism.[32] Most Ho:YAG lasers generate light of a wavelength of 2.12 μm, and operate at a pulse duration of 250–350 μs, significantly longer than pulse dye lasers. This long pulse duration precludes any significant stress confinement, so vapor bubble expansion and collapse are irregular in shape (i.e., not spherical) so that bubble collapse occurs at multiple loci at different times with no significant pressure transients created.[33] Time-resolved imaging studies and transient pressure wave studies of Ho:YAG lasers failed to show a significant photomechanical effect.[15,32,33] The pressure transients from Ho:YAG are typically between 8 and 20 bars, significantly lower than the pressure transients produced by photomechanical lasers (>300 bars).[13,15,32]

In a series of experiments, Vassar et al. demonstrated the photothermal mechanism of the Ho:YAG laser.[32] Each of the experiments showed evidence either of direct energy absorption by the stone, or paucity of pressure transients. When hydrated and dehydrated stones were irradiated in air or water, the dehydrated stones in air showed the more fragmentation. This finding indicates lack of photomechanical effect due to the lack of aqueous medium for plasma and cavitation bubble–induced pressure transients. It also shows that water literally impedes lithotripsy as it absorbs (and dissipates) energy from direct absorption by the stone. High-speed imaging also shows the dynamics of Ho:YAG laser lithotripsy: An initial period of up to 60 μs is required to vaporize the water between the fiber tip and the stone surface, after which the energy is more efficiently coupled through vapor to the stone—called the "Moses effect" (as if Moses parted the water on flight from Egypt).[14,15,32] Again, this phenomenon shows how water absorbs and dissipates long pulse Ho:YAG energy compared to photomechanical lithotripsy where water is required to produce a cavitation bubble. During Ho:YAG lithotripsy, fragment ejection begins 60 µs into a 250 µs pulse, while the laser continues to emit. This time course whereby lithotripsy occurs during the pulse (rather than after the pulse) is consistent with direct energy absorption as opposed to cavitation bubble collapse dynamics. Another finding is that the Ho:YAG laser produces more lithotripsy when oriented at 90° to the stone surface (normal incidence), indicating that direct irradiation is relevant, and energy density is critical to reach criterion threshold for ablation; when the laser fiber tip is placed in contact with the stone surface but oriented parallel to the stone surface (90° laser incidence) a large vapor bubble forms, but no ablation occurs.[34] In contrast to photomechanical lasers, the angle of orientation between the fiber tip and stone makes little difference in fragmentation. Indeed, other studies show that incident angle is correlated to Ho:YAG lithotripsy efficiency.[35-38] Further evidence of photothermal mechanism included the production of thermal breakdown products during lithotripsy with the Ho:YAG laser and enhanced

lithotripsy when stones were irradiated at room temperature versus cold.[32]

The impact of pulse duration is integral to mechanism. In an important experiment, Jansen et al. fired a holmium:YAG laser through an optical fiber in still water (no stone) varying the pulse duration and used high-speed images to document the vapor bubble dynamics for each pulse duration.[33] At 500 ns pulse duration (using a Q-switch), large spherical cavitation bubbles were created, which collapsed to a single locus, releasing significant ripples (pressure transients) in the water. As the laser pulse duration was expanded, the vapor bubble became less spherical, and the collapse events occurred at multiple loci, producing less ripples in water. As the pulse duration was lengthened to 260 µs, the bubble became pear shaped and collapsed asymmetrically with no ripples seen. Thus, the long pulse Ho:YAG laser used currently does not create any significant photomechanical effect (Fig. 26.3).[16,33]

Ho:YAG lasers do exhibit some limitations. The generation of small, powderized fragments means less efficient lithotripsy and longer procedure times.[39] This inefficiency can be overcome by simply increasing the energy or frequency settings, but the higher efficiency comes at the cost of more

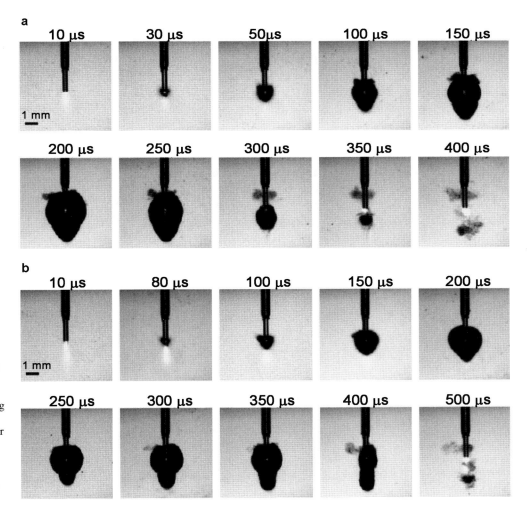

Fig. 26.3 Compilation of bubble expansion and collapse at room temperature for two pulse durations: (**a**) short pulse, (**b**) long pulse. Fiber diameter 365 µm, energy 800 mJ. Elapsed time after initiation of pulse shown above each image (Reprinted with permission from Kang.[16] Copyright 2006 Wiley-Liss, Inc., a subsidiary of Wiley)

retropulsion, higher risk of collateral tissue damage, and tip degradation with energy settings >1.0 J.[40] Retropulsion is an occasional issue with Ho:YAG lithotripsy at normal energy settings, but is less compared to other intracorporeal lithotripsy devices such as electrohydraulic lithotripsy, pulsed dye lasers, or pneumatic devices. With holmium:YAG, stone retropulsion occurs from vapor bubble expansion and the momentum imparted by debris ejection.[16]

Lee et al. showed that fragments always eject at a right angle from the stone surface, regardless of the incident angle.[16] A large diameter fiber creates a wide, shallow crater, allowing for greater x-axis vectors of plume ejection and increased retropulsion. In contrast, a small fiber creates narrow, deep craters, with more y-axis vectors ejecting less x-axis vectors debris, so retropulsion is minimized (Fig. 26.4). Another strategy to minimize retropulsion is to prolong the pulse duration. Since the recoil pressure is proportional to the radiant power (energy per pulse duration), shorter pulse durations with high-energy density produce higher retropulsion. Experimentally, extended long pulse duration holmium:YAG lasers achieve less retropulsion per pulse, and less retropulsion per unit of stone ablation.[16,42] Some commercially available holmium:YAG lasers offer a "normal" pulse duration and an "extended" pulse duration.

One way to overcome some of the limitations of current photothermal lithotripsy is to use lasers with wavelengths more efficiently absorbed by renal calculi. Experiments with free electron lasers showed that lithotripsy is more efficient at wavelengths between 2.9 and 3.1 μm as compared to 2.1 μm (Ho:YAG wavelength).[17] The Erbium:YAG laser has a wavelength of 2.9–2.94 μm, making it a potentially more efficient lithotriptor than the Ho:YAG laser. Similar to the Ho:YAG laser, experiments have shown the Er:YAG laser operates with a paucity of photomechanical effects, has similar vapor bubble characteristics, and ablates multiple stone types with symmetric ablation craters.[43,44] Er:YAG and Ho:YAG lasers were compared experimentally at similar energy levels. Er:YAG lasers produced more lithotripsy than Ho:YAG lasers, but with marginally larger fragments at 50 mJ. However, when Ho:YAG lasers were ramped up to 500 J, the amount of lithotripsy was similar to

the Er:YAG laser at 50 J. Although there was some difference at the same energy output, similar amounts of lithotripsy can be achieved by simply increasing the Ho:YAG power and frequency settings. But high-energy output may cause fiber tip damage and irregular beam output.[45] Erbium and Holmium lasers were also compared in vitro.[46] Both were controlled for focal length, energy density, and beam width and profile. Pulse energies varied between 0.2 and 1 J for each. For a single laser pulse, crater volumes were five times greater for all stone types with Er:YAG lasers than Ho:YAG lasers.[46] Clinical use of erbium lasers is limited most importantly by the lack of clinically useful laser fibers.[46] The relatively inexpensive and reusable low OH silica fibers used with holmium lasers do not transmit laser light from an erbium laser adequately. This is due to energy absorption at the input end of the laser, which can lead to thermal degradation and damage to the fiber and laser. Fluoride fibers are another option for laser fiber material, and do transmit Er:YAG irradiation successfully, but tend to be brittle, and have a hygroscopic structure. Single crystal sapphire fibers present another option, but their cost is prohibitive, they only transmit energy adequately up to 200 mJ if a diameter of 425 μm is chosen, and they risk damage at their output ends due to high peak power levels. Fibers still being considered include compound fibers of germanium oxide with silica tips and hollow wave guides. While compound fibers are still under investigation, hollow wave guide fibers have been tested experimentally. Some initial studies showed good flexibility and strength, with energy transmission sufficient to fragment calculi. However, problems remain, including the generation of hot spots and irregular ablation craters.[47,48]

26.4 Optical Fibers

Basic fiber design consists of an inner circular core surrounded by two to three layers of cladding and a surrounding jacket. Both glasses and polymers can be used as core

Fig. 26.4 Diagram of ejection of ablated stone particles from a wide versus narrow laser fiber. Note the total vector in the Y direction greater for the wider crater. (**a**) Wide and shallow crater. (**b**) Narrow and deep crater (Reprinted with permission from Lee et al.[41] Copyright Elsevier 2003)

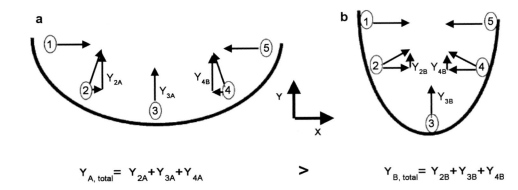

materials. Among the glasses, silica (amorphous silicon dioxide SiO2) is the dominant material.[49] The first lasers used clinically in urology used silica fibers. These are ideal laser fibers as they transmit laser energy well with minimal attenuation, are relatively inexpensive, and are small and flexible enough to be used in endoscopic instruments. Ho:YAG lasers use low OH silica fibers since the hydroxyl groups absorb light readily at 2,100 nm, thus reducing transmission of light and potentially causing fiber damage.[10] A high OH concentration is better for UV transmission. Cladding types can also differ. Cladding constructed of fluorine-doped silica has better laser light confinement and a smaller bending radius than fluoroacrylate cladding, which can generate light leakage and damage with lasers of 2 μm wavelength.[50] Most fibers also have a third layer of cladding, called a buffer layer. The buffer often consists of ethylene tetrafluoroethylene (ETFE, Tefzel), which protects the fiber from external mechanical damage.

The laser–fiber interface is usually composed of a protective connector that holds the proximal end of the laser fiber in the proper orientation to receive energy from the laser itself. The subminiature version A connector (SMA) is the industry standard connector, allowing different lasers to accept multiple laser fiber sizes and brands. It consists of a central reinforced housing surrounded by a connector shell. The housing is often a polymer material and the shell is usually composed of steel. The end of the laser fiber exiting the shell is shrinkwrapped in a plastic coating to guard against mechanical damage. With regular use, there will be some misalignment of the laser and the proximal fiber end, which can result in higher order rays, attenuation, or fiber breakdown. At the input end, stray laser light can be absorbed by the steel shell, which can then vaporize. The condensation of the vapor coats the outer surface of the laser, disrupting its optics and leading to failure (Fig. 26.5). Manufacturers use various mechanisms and engineering to couple the laser to the proximal fiber connector. There are advantages and disadvantages to each design, and a more detailed explanation may be found in Nazif et al.[50]

Urologists may confuse the collimated laser emission generated from ideal lasers as the output from laser fibers. The fiber designs used currently lead to noncollimated output. The collimated laser beam is focused through a lens so that a convergent beam is delivered from the lens to the proximal fiber tip, and the beam launches as a divergent beam down the fiber.[50] If the energy is not launched with a "bull's-eye," strike down the center of the fiber, off-axis rays are increased and proximal fiber failure risk is increased.[51] In order to conduct laser light without having excessive losses or thermal damage, most of the light must be reflected within the fiber to the very distal tip, where it is discharged. This principle, referred to as total internal reflection, is utilized in laser fiber technology. Photons bounce off the cladding and reflect back down the core fiber, where they bounce off the opposite wall cladding, like billiard balls bouncing off the side of a pool table. When light strikes a surface, a portion of it is reflected and a portion may be refracted, depending on the refractive index of both the environment and the material. The refractive index of a material describes how quickly it allows light to pass through it. When light coming from a denser environment strikes a less dense substance, the angle to the normal at which it refracts, or bends, is larger than the incident angle of incoming light. As the incident angle to normal becomes wider, the refracted light in the less dense substance will eventually travel at a 90° angle to the normal, or parallel to the surface of the substance. In other words, light will not penetrate into the less dense substance. At this angle of incident light, there is total internal reflection, and laser light is not absorbed by the cladding at all and reflects entirely inside the core fiber. In contrast, if laser approaches the cladding at a more normal incidence, the light refracts and may not reflect. As an example, a pebble can be skipped along the surface of water with a wide incident angle, whereas dropping the pebble at the water surface (narrow incident angle) causes the pebble to fall into the water. The implications for fiber transmission are significant: A laser that launches light with too divergent a beam risks refraction into

Fig. 26.5 Typical SMA connector. Connector interfaces between laser and laser fiber. Heat-shrink wrap overlaps laser fiber as it enters connector, providing stiffness and decreased mechanical stress at junction. Polymer adhesive envelops laser fiber inside connector. (Reprinted with permission from Nazif.[5] Review Copyright Mary Ann Liebert 2004)

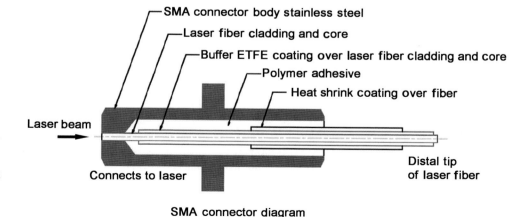

SMA connector body stainless steel
Laser fiber cladding and core
Buffer ETFE coating over laser fiber cladding and core
Polymer adhesive
Heat shrink coating over fiber
Laser beam
Connects to laser
Distal tip of laser fiber
SMA connector diagram

the cladding, whereas a laser that launches light with a narrowly divergent beam has less risk of refraction into the cladding. The limit of beam divergence a fiber can safely transmit is characterized by the numerical aperture (NA). NA provides a description of what maximum acceptance angle of laser light will provide total internal reflection for a certain fiber. The NA of Ho:YAG lasers ranges from 0.2 to 0.22. An NA of 0.21 corresponds to a maximum acceptance angle of 12°. Despite total internal reflection, some light will partially penetrate the cladding. These penetrating light waves, known as evanescent waves, can damage cladding if they are strong enough. They are accentuated by bending of the fiber.

Bending of the laser fiber can also affect the reflection of light. The high number of bends, or amount of bending, produces a greater number of internal reflections. If the reflected angles produced are smaller than the critical angle, some energy will transmit through the cladding. This is especially damaging in the case of near infrared lasers such as Ho:YAG as their wavelengths are well absorbed by plastics. This problem is occasionally encountered during retrograde ureteronephroscopy for lower pole renal calculi, where the flexible ureteroscope is maximally deflected to orient the fiber to the lower pole stone. Laser energy refracts into the cladding at the site of maximal deflection and causes fiber and ureteroscope destruction, and possible patient injury.[45,,52]

The positioning of the fiber during laser lithotripsy is also an important factor to consider. Since an important difference between short pulse and long pulse lasers for lithotripsy is that with short pulse duration lasers (<1 μs) where photomechanical lithotripsy occurs, a separation distance of 1 mm between the fiber tip and the stone surface yields maximal fragmentation due to the importance of maximal bubble expansion and collapse-induced pressure transients.[13,15] In contrast, long pulse Ho:YAG and Er:YAG laser (250–350 μs) achieve maximal lithotripsy efficiency in contact mode as the energy is absorbed efficiently by water.[14,17,32,33] To minimize the amount of Ho:YAG or Er:YAG lost to vaporize a water channel ("Moses effect"), the laser fiber should be placed in contact with the stone surface.

26.5 Conclusions

An understanding of the physics of laser design and function will allow the urologist to make informed decisions regarding the clinical application of laser technology in their practice. Central to the clinical application of lasers in urology is basic knowledge of the interaction of lasers with biological tissues and their environments. The physics of laser lithotripsy is one of the most studied applications of lasers in urology and its understanding is important clinically, and also relevant in the advent of new and better laser technology. Lastly, the optical delivery of laser energy is an important component of laser technology with implications for the types of lasers that can be used, how they can be used, and for urological instruments and equipment. In this chapter, we have summarized key points regarding laser physics, which should prove useful to the urologist as it applies to stone disease. As investigators gain further insight into the physics of lasers in urology, further advancements will make lasers in urology safer and more efficient.

References

1. Teichman JMH. Lasers. In: Smith AD, Badlani GH, Bagley DH, et al., eds. *Smith's Textbook of Endourology*. Hamilton, Ontario: BC Decker; 2007:37-40.
2. Maiman TH. Stimulated optical radiation in ruby. *Nature*. 1960;187:493-494.
3. Patel CK, Mc Farlane RA, Faust WL. Selective excitation through vibrational energy transfer and optical maser action in N2–CO2. *Physiol Rev*. 1964;13:617-619.
4. Rosemberg SK. Carbon dioxide laser treatment of external genital lesions. *Urology*. 1985;25:555-558.
5. Rosemberg SK. Lasers and squamous cell carcinoma of external genitalia. *Urology*. 1986;27:430-433.
6. Greenbaum SS, Glogau R, Stegman SJ, et al. Carbon dioxide laser treatment of erythroplasia of Queyrat. *J Dermatol Surg Oncol*. 1989;15:747-750.
7. Sorokin PP, Lankard JR. Stimulated emission observed from an organic dye, chloroaluminium phthalocyanine. *IBM J Res Dev*. 1966;10:162.
8. Dretler SP, Watson G, Parrish JA, Murray S. Pulsed dye laser fragmentation of ureteral calculi: initial clinical experience. *J Urol*. 1987;137:386-389.
9. Bhatta KM, Nishioka NS. Effect of pulse duration on microsecond-domain laser lithotripsy. *Lasers Surg Med*. 1989;9:454-457.
10. Teichmann HO, Herrmann TR, Bach T. Technical aspects of lasers in urology. *World J Urol*. 2007;25:221-225. Epub (2007) May 30.
11. Jacques SL. Laser-tissue interactions. Photochemical, photothermal, and photomechanical. *Surg Clin North Am*. 1992 Jun;72(3):531-558.
12. Berlien H-P, Muller G. *Applied Laser Medicine*. Germany: Springer; 2003.
13. Rink K, Delacrétaz G, Salathé RP. Fragmentation process of current laser lithotriptors. *Lasers Surg Med*. 1995;16:134-146.
14. Chan KF, Pfefer TJ, Teichman JMH, Welch AJ. A perspective on laser lithotripsy: the fragmentation processes. *J Endourol*. 2001;15:257-273.
15. Zhong P, Tong HL, Cocks FH, Pearle MS, Preminger GM. Transient cavitation and acoustic emission produced by different laser lithotripters. *J Endourol*. 1998;12:371-378.
16. Kang HW, Lee H, Teichman JM, Oh J, Kim J, Welch AJ. Dependence of calculus retropulsion on pulse duration during Ho: YAG laser lithotripsy. *Lasers Surg Med*. 2006;38:762-772.
17. Chan KF, Hammer DX, Choi B, et al. Free electron laser lithotripsy: threshold radiant exposures. *J Endourol*. 2000;14:161-167.
18. Teichman JM, Vassar GJ, Bishoff JT, Bellman GC. Holmium: YAG lithotripsy yields smaller fragments than lithoclast, pulsed dye laser or electrohydraulic lithotripsy. *J Urol*. 1998;159(1): 17-23.
19. Dretler SP. An evaluation of ureteral laser lithotripsy: 225 consecutive patients. *J Urol*. 1990;143:267-272.
20. Fradin D, Bass M. Electron avalanche breakdown induced by ruby laser light. *Appl Phys Lett*. 1973;22(5):206-208.

21. Doukas AG, Zweig AD, Frisoli JK, Birngruber R, Deutsch TF. Non-invasive determination of shock wave pressure generated by optical breakdown. *App Phy B*. 1991;53:237-245.

22. Denstedt JD, Chun SS, Miller MD, Eberwein PM. Intracorporeal lithotripsy with the Alexandrite laser. *Lasers Surg Med*. 1997;20: 433-436.

23. Tschepe J, Gundlach P, Leege N, Hopf J, Müller G, Scherer H. The endoscopic laser lithotripsy of salivary gland calculi and the problem of fiber wear. *Opt Fibers Med VII SPIE*. 1992;1649:254-263.

24. Pearle MS, Sech SM, Cobb CG, et al. Safety and efficacy of the Alexandrite laser for the treatment of renal and ureteral calculi. *Urol*. 1998;51:33-38.

25. Helfmann J. Untersuchung der physikalischen Phanomene bei der Zertrummerung von Korperkonkrementen durch laserinduzierte Plasmen. In: *Advances in Laser Medicine*. Landsberg, Zurich: ecomed; 1992.

26. Helfmann J, Muller G. Laser lithotripsy: process overview. *Med Laser Appl*. 2001;16:30-37.

27. Tischer CF, Koort H, Bazo A, Rasch R, Thiede C. Clinical experiences with a new frequency-doubled double-pulse Nd:YAG Laser (FREDDY) for the treatment of urolithiasis. In: *Proceedings of SPIE*, San Jose, California vol 4609; 2002.

28. Schafhauser W, Zorcher W, et al. *Erste klinische Erfahrungen mit neuem frequenzverdoppeltem Doppelpuls Neodym:YAG Laser in der Therapie der Urolithiasis. Poster presentation at the DGU*. Germany: Hamburg; 2000.

29. Stark L, Carl P, Zauner R. A new technique for Laser-Lithotripsy: FREDDY, the partially frequency-doubled double-Pulse Nd:YAG Laser. Poster presentation at: The 1st International Consultation on Stone Disease, 2001; Paris

30. Dubosq F, Pasqui F, Girard F, et al. Endoscopic lithotripsy and the FREDDY laser: initial experience. *J Endourol*. 2006;20:296-299.

31. Stark L, Car P. First clinical experiences of laser lithotripsy using the partially frequency-doubled double-pulse neodymium:YAG laser ("FREDDY") (abstract). *J Urol*. 2001;165:362A.

32. Vassar GJ, Chan KF, Teichman JM, et al. Holmium: YAG lithotripsy: photothermal mechanism. *J Endourol*. 1999;13:181-190.

33. Jansen ED, Asshauer T, Frenz M, Motamedi M, Delacretaz G, Welch AJ. Effect of pulse duration on bubble formation and laser-induced pressure waves during Holmium laser ablation. *LasersSurg Med*. 1996;18:278-293.

34. Schmidlin FR, Beghuin D, Delacretaz GP, et al. Laser lithotripsy with the Ho:YAG laser: fragmentation process revealed by time-resolved imaging. In: SPIE, San Jose, California 3245.123S, 1998.

35. Chan KF, Vassar GJ, Pfefer TJ, et al. Holmium:YAG laser lithotripsy: a dominant photothermal ablative mechanism with chemical decomposition of urinary calculi. *Lasers Surg Med*. 1999;25:22-37.

36. Freiha GS, Glickman RD, Teichman JM. Holmium:YAG laser-induced damage to guidewires: experimental study. *J Endourol*. 1997;11:331-336.

37. Teichman JM, Rogenes VJ, McIver BJ, Harris JM. Holmium:yttrium-aluminum-garnet laser cystolithotripsy of large bladder calculi. *Urology*. 1997;50:44-48.

38. Teichman JM, Rao RD, Glickman RD, Harris JM. Holmium:YAG percutaneous nephrolithotomy: the laser incident angle matters. *J Urol*. 1998;159:690-694.

39. Teichman JM, Rao RD, Rogenes VJ, Harris JM. Ureteroscopic management of ureteral calculi: electrohydraulic versus holmium:YAG lithotripsy. *J Urol*. 1997;158:1357-1361.

40. Spore SS, Teichman JM, Corbin NS, Champion PC, Williamson EA, Glickman RD. Holmium: YAG lithotripsy: optimal power settings. *J Endourol*. 1999;13:559-566.

41. Lee H, Ryan RT, Teichman JM, et al. Stone retropulsion during holmium:YAG lithotripsy. *J Urol*. 2003 Mar;169(3):881-885.

42. Finley DS, Petersen J, Abdelshehid C, et al. Effect of holmium:YAG laser pulse width on lithotripsy retropulsion in vitro. *J Endourol*. 2005;19:1041-1044.

43. Chan KF, Lee H, Teichman JMH, Kamerer A, McGuV HS, Welch AJ. Erbium:YAG laser lithotripsy. *J Urol*. 2002;168:436-441.

44. Lee H, Kang HW, Teichman JM, Oh J, Welch AJ. Urinary calculus fragmentation during Ho: YAG and Er:YAG lithotripsy. *Lasers Surg Med*. 2006;38:39-51.

45. Lee H, Ryan RT, Teichman JM, et al. Effect of lithotripsy on holmium:YAG optical beam profile. *J Endourol*. 2003;17:63-67.

46. Teichman JM, Chan KF, Cecconi PP, et al. Erbium: YAG versus holmium:YAG lithotripsy. *J Urol*. 2001;165:876-879.

47. Iwai K, Shi Y, Matsuura Y, Miyagi M. Rugged hollow fiber for the infrared and its use in laser lithotripsy. In: Proceedings of SPIE, vol 4916; 2002:115–119

48. Teichman JMH, Kang W, Glickman RD, Welch AJ. *Update on Erbium:YAG Lithotripsy. AIP Conference Proceedings 2007, Vol 900*. London: IOP Institute of Physics Publishing Ltd.; *Indianapolis, Indiana* 2007:216-227.

49. Gambling WA. The rise and rise of optical fibers. *IEEE J Sel Top Quant Electron*. 2000;6(6)):1084.

50. Nazif OA, Teichman JMH, Glickman RD, Welch AJ. Review of laser fibers: a practical guide for urologists. *J Endourol*. 2004;18: 818-829.

51. Marks AJ, Mues AC, Knudsen BE, Teichman JMH. Holmium: yttrium-aluminum-garnet lithotripsy proximal fiber failures from laser and fiber mismatch. *Urology*. 2008;71:1049-1051.

52. Knudsen BE, Glickman RD, Stallman KJ, et al. Performance and safety of holmium: YAG laser optical fibers. *J Endourol*. 2005;19: 1092-1097.

Alternative Laser Energy Sources: Clinical Implications

27

Andreas J. Gross and Thorsten Bach

Abstract The ongoing technical development over the last years made the laser one of the most important tools in endourology and daily urological practice. Today several laser types have been introduced for soft tissue surgery and stone treatment. To understand the differences between these lasers available for clinical use, one has to be aware of the possible variables the urologist has to deal with. In this chapter, we will review the differences of the introduced laser systems. These laser systems, in combination with modern fiber technology, shifted ureterorenoscopy from a diagnostic tool to a real therapeutic option in the treatment of patients with urolithiasis. However, one has to be aware of the differences to choose the right laser for the desired treatment.

27.1 Introduction

The ongoing technical development over the last years has made the laser one of the most important tools in endourology and daily urological practice.

To date, several laser types have been introduced for soft tissue surgery and stone treatment. To understand the differences between the lasers available for clinical use, one has to be aware of the possible variables with which the urologist has to deal. First of all the optical properties of the targeted tissue/stone are of major importance. Depending on the type of treatment one likes to perform, the parameters of the laser in use are critical for the surgical outcome: The laser wavelength defines absorption of the laser energy at the target tissue and may also cause possible side effects (light–tissue interaction). The other parameters to consider are the mode of operation (continuous wave versus pulsed), and last, but not least, the power output of the laser device.

In this chapter, we will review the differences of the introduced laser systems and their clinical impact.

27.2 Technical Requirements for Laser Use in Endourology

Endourology has to deal with calculi fragmentation within the bladder, the ureter, or the renal pelvis. The ongoing technical development in endourology in terms of semirigid and flexible endoscopy opened a demand for surgical tools to be compatible with these instruments. In stone fragmentation, two main tasks have to be fulfilled. First of all, the energy (laser) source should have the potential to fragment the calculi efficiently, but keep the risk for collateral damage as low as possible. Further, the delivery system (laser fiber) should carry the energy to the desired point within the collecting system without compromising the function of the instrument. Mechanical strain to fibers and to the instrument should be as low as possible. The fiber diameter should be small to maintain the cross section of the working channel for irrigation. By fulfilling these criteria, in most cases, modern endourological treatment has made open stone surgery redundant.

27.3 Light–Tissue Interaction

The most fundamental differentiation between lasers for surgical application is in their laser wavelength, which determines the absorption process of light in tissue. With regard to

A.J. Gross (✉)
Department of Urology, Asklepios Hospital Barmbek, Hamburg, Germany
e-mail: an.gross@asklepios.com

P.N. Rao et al. (eds.), *Urinary Tract Stone Disease*,
DOI 10.1007/978-1-84800-362-0_27, © Springer-Verlag London Limited 2011

this process, laser radiation simply is directed light of a narrow bandwidth, which is synonymous with a single color.

Absorption is the most important but not the only process of light–tissue interaction. When the laser beam encounters an object, a percentage of the laser beam is reflected at the boundary layer. The reflected radiation not only is lost for the surgical purpose but also may constitute a risk to surrounding tissue as it may cause heat where an increase in temperature is not desired. The process of reflection is not very dependent on wavelength and therefore is very similar between different lasers.

From an optical point of view, endourological targets are not homogenous and they will scatter an intruding laser beam. Scattering takes some of the beam out of its intended direction, and in most surgical applications, this portion is lost for the intended purpose. The degree of scattering depends on the size of the particles that the laser beam encounters and on the wavelength of the laser. Shorter wavelengths are scattered to a much higher degree than longer wavelengths.

Absorption is the most important light–tissue interaction process. On entering into an absorbing medium, the intensity of the laser beam decreases exponentially (Lambert-Beer's law). Absorbed laser radiation is converted into heat and causes an increase in temperature. Depending on the amount of heat involved, this will result in coagulation or even vaporization of tissue. The exponential behavior and the immediate onset of the absorption process on entering of the laser beam into the absorbing medium implies more generated heat next to the surface than further below. Hemoglobin and the water molecule are widely used as chromophores (absorber) for surgical lasers. The absorption length at familiar laser wavelengths in these body chromophores are shown in Fig. 27.1 and may help to understand the tissue effect of these laser systems.

27.4 Laser Emission Mode

The interaction between laser energy and the addressed target is not only determined by the laser wavelength, but also by the laser emission mode. Two ways of energy discharge are possible: The laser energy can be emitted either in a pulsed mode or in a continuous wave mode. Comparing two lasers of the same average power, the pulsed laser presents the higher peak (or maximum) power than the continuous wave laser. The pulse duration among pulsed lasers may differ. The shorter the pulses are, the higher the pulse peak power will be.

The criterion whether the duration of a laser emission on a target has a pulsed or continuous wave character is determined by the rate by which the laser energy is absorbed by the target compared to the heat flow out of the target area. In a continuous wave process, absorption of laser energy and dissipation of heat reach equilibrium.

A pulsed process is characterized by a buildup of heat in the target before dissipation takes it away. Depending on the amount of accumulated heat in the target during the pulse, a localized steam pressure may be generated or plasma formation takes place. An example is the absorption of a holmium laser pulse by a stone. The generated heat creates a localized steam pressure inside the stone that breaks the stone apart. Overall, the stone does not experience a significant increase of temperature.

Continuous wave lasers – for example, the GreenLight laser or the continuous wave Thulium:YAG laser (RevoLix) – are predominantly used in soft tissue surgery. It is important to keep in mind that the GreenLight laser technically is a QCW laser. This means quasicontinuous wave. With frequencies of around 1,000 Hz, the difference between quasicontinuous wave and real continuous wave within the target tissue seems negligible.

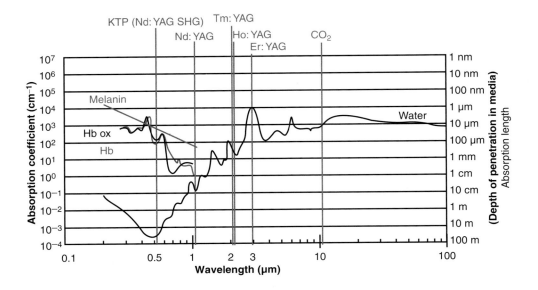

Fig. 27.1 Absorption spectrum of melanin, hemoglobin, and water in comparison to selected laser wavelengths. *Hb* hemoglobin, *ox* oxiginated

Continuous wave emission of the laser energy leads to cleaner cuts and therefore to more precise cutting performance[1] than laser systems with pulsed energy emission. However, in stone fragmentation, the continuous energy emission has some pitfalls.

The irradiation of calculi by a continuous wave laser results in an increase of temperature of the bulk until any water is driven out of the stone. The surface may start to melt, and the stone may disintegrate.

Although this way of stone destruction is possible in multiple stone compositions, the surrounding of the stone is heated excessively, which leads to an increased risk of collateral damage.[2]

Contrary pulsed energy emission generates only a small increase in temperature of the stone although localized high-energy density can be achieved.

In a stable power setting, the amount of released energy increases with decreasing pulse time.

Stone defragmentation is achieved by two different physical mechanisms. Either photothermal (Ho:YAG laser) or photomechanical (both discussed later in this chapter). By pulsed energy emission, efficient stone fragmentation may be achieved in all stone compositions. On the other hand, in soft tissue surgery, the pulsed mode leads to an uneven ruptured surface with a cotton-wool appearance.

In conclusion, one has to keep in mind that the physical laser parameters (wavelength, emission mode, power) determine the treatment outcome. Knowledge and understanding of these factors is essential to achieve the best result for the patient.

While pulsed mode laser systems have significant advantages in stone defragmentation, continuous wave laser systems seem to be superior for soft tissue surgery. Combined systems may be a way out of this dilemma.[3]

27.5 Fibers

To obtain an optimal combination of a laser energy device and an endoscopic instrument, be it flexible or semirigid, the laser fiber is of tremendous importance.

Usually laser fibers do have an inner circular optical core and up to three outer concentric layers. In general, the core of a laser fiber transmits the laser radiation. The next layer confines the radiation inside the core by total reflection. The outer layers provide mechanical stability and ruggedness.[4] Laser fibers made from low OH (low water content) silica with an optical cladding of fluorine-doped silica are the best choice in most endourological applications. These fibers allow a smaller bend radius. Alternative fibers with fluoroacrylate cladding are more rigid and laser radiation may leak through these fibers, which may cause serious damage to the working channel and the integrity of the scope.[5,6]

27.6 Individual Lasers for Stone Treatment

Several laser types for stone treatment are available. Laser systems differ in terms of wavelength, compatible fiber diameter, and pulse duration, which leads to different mechanisms of stone fragmentation.[7,8] Introduced laser systems may be divided into photoacoustic lasers and photothermal lasers. The different systems are reviewed in the following:

27.6.1 Photoacoustic Lasers

In photoacoustic lasers, the energy is delivered in water or stone and creates a vapor bubble.[9] With the collapse of the vapor bubble, a pressure effect occurs at the calculus and leads to fragmentation. To achieve maximum fragmentation efficacy, the fiber should be positioned with a little distance to the stone surface to allow best bubble expansion. Due to the circumferential spread of the photoacoustic effect, the fiber can be used sideways of the stone to achieve similar fragmentation effects. Lasers in the blue-green portion of the spectrum like the "FREDDY" laser (frequency-doubled double Nd:YAG laser, 532 nm) or the pulsed dye laser (504 nm) belong to this group. These laser devices emit laser energy at a wavelength where the energy is absorbed by stones of the right color and by hemoglobin. Due to the absorption in hemoglobin these lasers have a high safety margin,[10,11] since energy that accidentally hits the mucosa is absorbed and carried away by the blood flow. Hemoglobin acts as a "heat sink" for the laser energy.[12] Another laser in the category is the alexandrite laser (755 nm). However, photoacoustic lasers have deficiencies in the fragmentation of cystine as well as calcium oxalate monohydrate calculi.[13,14]

27.6.1.1 Pulsed Dye Laser

The pulsed dye was one of the first laser systems used in the treatment of urinary calculi. It has an emission wavelength of 504 nm. The short pulse duration of approximately 1 μs allows effective stone fragmentation. Since the energy is not absorbed in water, the risk of thermal damage to the urothelium during stone workup is diminished and thereby reduces the need for optimal visualization.[15] Calcium oxalate monohydrate and cystine as well as brushite stones cannot be treated efficiently with this laser since the optical absorption of the laser energy is reduced in these types of stones,[16] which pushed this laser out of the endourological routine.[17]

27.6.1.2 FREDDY Laser (Frequency-Doubled Double Pulse Nd:YAG)

The FREDDY laser has been designed for the fragmentation of urinary calculi. It was created by placing a potassium titanyl phosphate (KTP) crystal into the resonator of a Nd:YAG laser. Therefore, it creates pulses with two wavelengths of 1,064 and 532 nm. Other than the pulsed dye laser, this laser does not generate a steam but a plasma bubble on the stone due to absorption of the 532 nm laser pulse. The plasma on the surface of the stone absorbs the 1,064-nm laser radiation and heats up the plasma bubble further. This leads to its rapid expansion subsequently and then induces the collapse. From that point, the mechanism of action is comparable to that of the pulsed dye laser. The collapse of the plasma bubble generates a mechanical shock wave, which causes fragmentation. Regular pulse durations are within 0.3 and 1.5 μs.[18] Compared to the Ho:YAG laser, the risk of collateral damage during laser lithotripsy is lower with the use of the FREDDY laser. Santa-Cruz et al. showed that it would take about two pulses with a Ho:YAG laser to perforate an ureter, while 2,000 pulses of the FREDDY laser failed to do so.[19] Clinical results are good with the FREDDY laser. In ureteral stone treatment, stone-free rates of up to 95% are reported, whereas one study reports a combined stone-free rate of 87% for the whole collecting system.[20] However, comparable to the pulsed dye laser, the FREDDY laser cannot break up cystine stones, since its wavelengths are not absorbed by cystine.[21,22]

27.6.2 Photothermal Lasers

Photothermal lasers, like the Ho:YAG or the Erbium:YAG lasers, work in the mid-infrared range of the electromagnetic spectrum. At this wavelength, the laser energy is absorbed by water. Laser types causing photothermal effects do have relatively long pulse duration of approximately 300 μs. Therefore, energy deposit in water is slow[23] and the vapor bubble is pear shaped in the Ho:YAG laser and torpedo shaped in the Erbium:YAG laser. This leads to reduced cavitations and insignificant acoustic pressure waves.[24] Other than in photoacoustic lasers, the fiber in these types of lasers should be positioned with contact to the stone surface.[25] Compared to photoacoustic lasers, the generated fragments are smaller in photothermal stone fragmentation.[26] In contrast to photoacoustic lasers, photothermal lasers have a lower safety margin and can perforate the ureter or coagulate the ureter.[19] All types of calculi can be fragmented with these laser types.[27]

27.6.2.1 Holmium:Yttrium:Aluminum:Garnet (Ho:YAG) Laser

The Ho:YAG laser generates laser energy at a wavelength of 2.1 μm and at a pulse duration of 150–1,000 μs. Due to the wavelength, holmium laser energy is efficiently absorbed by water, leading to a high safety profile in an aqueous surrounding like the urinary tract.[28] It is currently the most widespread intracorporeal laser lithotripter. With the energy release, the irrigant surrounding the fiber tip is vaporized and a steam bubble is created.[29] The energy of the Ho:YAG laser is then transmitted through this "vapor-window" to the stone[30] (Moses effect). If this laser radiation is delivered to urinary calculi, some of the energy penetrates the stone and is absorbed by water inside the stone. This causes fragmentation by building up of pressure inside the stone.[4] Furthermore, the implosion of the vapor bubble causes a shock wave, which is transmitted to the stone and causes additional fragmentation. Decreasing the laser pulse duration at a given energy will lead to more effective stone fragmentation since the peak pulse power will increase. This characteristic is used in calculi fragmentation in combination with flexible silica fibers.[31] The Holmium:YAG laser is capable of fragmenting all types of stone composition. Other than photoacoustic lasers, the Ho:YAG laser can also cause fragmentation of cystine stones efficiently. Hereby, the percentage of stones treated by ureterorenoscopy have inclined and the need for percutaneous procedures in this group of patients has declined.[32]

Fragmentation efficacy is largely influenced by laser settings like the applied energy, pulse duration and frequency, as well as the fiber diameter. According to Kuo et al., optimal laser setting for small caliber fibers should be below 1.0 J and at 5–10 Hz.[33] These findings are supported by other workgroups.[34,35]

Another important point concerning Ho:YAG lithotripsy is the possibility to use small caliber fibers, with an optical core as small as 200 μm. This allows performing laser lithotripsy also in combination with flexible ureterorenoscopes. So access to virtually every point within the collecting system can be achieved. However, the stiffness of the laser fiber still leads to diminished deflection capacity of the flexible ureterorenoscope.[36–38]

Efficacy of stone treatment using the Holmium:YAG laser has been shown in a wide variety of clinical studies. In the treatment of urinary calculi, stone-free rates around 95% are published.[39,40]

Potential limitations are the risk of collateral soft tissue damage, which makes excellent visualization mandatory, and long-lasting surgery, especially in larger renal stones.[41,42]

27.6.2.2 Erbium:YAG laser

The Erbium:YAG laser has the potential to become a valuable substitute to the Ho:YAG laser. While already in use in dentistry and ophthalmology, the employment in urology is still experimental.[43] The potential of the Erbium:YAG laser to be valuable for stone treatment is based on the physics of energy absorption in urinary calculi. Maximum energy absorption seems to be at a wavelength of 2.9 μm. Theoretically, this makes the Erbium:YAG laser, with its wavelength of 2.9–2.94 μm, the optimal laser energy source for stone fragmentation. The pulse duration is 275 μs short.[44]

As described previously, the mechanism of stone fragmentation is photothermal and thereby comparable to that of the Holmium:YAG laser. However, as shown in vitro by Teichman et al., stone fragmentation with the Erbium:YAG seems to be up to five times more efficient than stone fragmentation with the Ho:YAG laser.[45] The problem with the Erbium:YAG laser to date is the lack of fibers that allow using this promising laser device in endourology. Therefore, the Erbium:YAG today is still excluded from clinical use in urology.

27.7 Conclusions

In summary, various laser systems are introduced on the market. Today, the Ho:YAG laser represents the widest spread and most efficacious laser lithotripter in endourology. In combination with small caliber ureterorenoscopes, of semirigid as well as flexible nature, virtually every point within the collecting system can be reached and treated endoscopically. Modern laser and fiber technology shifted ureterorenoscopy from a diagnostic tool to a real therapeutic option in the treatment of patients with urolithiasis.[46,47]

Acknowledgement The authors thank Dr. H.O. Teichmann (Lisa laser products, Katlenburg, Germany) for his support and advice.

References

1. Bach T, Herrmann TR, Cellarius C, Gross AJ. Bladder neck incision using a 70 Watt continuous wave laser (RevoLix) World. *J Urol.* 2007;25:263-267.
2. Mulvaney WP, Beck CP. The laser beam in urology. *J Urol.* 1968;99:112-115.
3. Bach T, Herrman TR, Gross AJ. The RevoLix duo - a new workhorse in urology. *J Endourol.* 2008;22:159. Abstract 102.
4. Teichmann HO, Herrmann TR, Bach T. Technical aspects of lasers in urology. *World J Urol.* 2007;25:221-225.
5. Nazif OA, Teichman JM, Glickmann RD, Welch AJ. Review of laser fibers: a practical guide for urologists. *J Endourol.* 2004;18:818-829.
6. Sung JC, Springhart WP, Marquet CG, et al. Location and etiology of flexible and semirigid ureteroscope damage. *Urology.* 2005;66:958-963.
7. Grocela J, Dretler SP. Intracorporal lithotripsy: instrumentation and development. *Urol Clin North Am.* 1997;24:13-23.
8. Watson GM. A survey of the action of lasers on stones. In: Steiner R, ed. *Laser lithotripsy: clinical use and technical aspects.* Berlin: Springer Verlag; 1988:15-24.
9. Rink K, Delacretaz G, Salanthe RP. Fragmentation process of current laser lithotripters. *Lasers Surg Med.* 1995;16:134-146.
10. Nishioka NS, Kelsey PB, Kibbi A, et al. Laser lithotripsy: animal studies of safety and efficacy. *Lasers Surg Med.* 1988;8:357-362.
11. Dretler SP. An evaluation of ureteral laser lithotripsy: 225 consecutive patients. *J Urol.* 1990;143:267-272.
12. Teichman JM. Lasers. In: Smith AD, Badlani GH, Bagley DH, Clayman RV, Docimo SG, Jordan GH, Kavoussi LR, Lee BR, Lingemann JE, Premiinger GM, Segura JW, eds. *Smith´s Textbook of Endourology.* 2nd ed. London: BC Decker Inc Hamilton; 2006:37-40.
13. Bhatta KM, Prien EL Jr, Dretler SP. Cystine calculi – rough and smooth: a new clinical distinction. *J Urol.* 1989;142:937-940.
14. Densted JD, Chun SS, Miller MD, Eberwein PM. Intracorporal lithotripsy with the Alexandrite laser. *Laser Surg Med.* 1997;20:433-436.
15. Zhong P, Tong HL, Cocks FH, et al. Transient cavitation and acoustic emission produced by different laser lithotripters. *J Endourol.* 1998;12:371-378.
16. Rink K, Delacretaz G, Salanthe RP. Fragmentation process of current laser lithotripters. *Laser Surg Med.* 1995;16:134-146.
17. Marks AJ, Teichman JM. Lasers in clinical urology: state of the art and new horizons. *World J Urol.* 2007;25:227-233.
18. Helfmann J, Muller G. Laser lithotripsy: process overview. *Med Las Appl.* 2001;16:30-37.
19. Santa-Cruz RW, Leveillee RJ, Krongrad A. Ex vivo comparison of four lithotripters commonly used in the ureter: What does it take to perforate ? *J Endourol.* 1998;12:417-422.
20. Schafhauser W, Radlmaier M, Schrott KM, Kuehn R. Erste klinische Erfahrungen mit neuem frequenzverdoppeltem Doppelpuls Neodymium:YAG Laser in der Therapie der Urolithiasis. *Urologe A Suppl.* 2000;39(1):39. Abstract P3.17.
21. Dubosq F, Pasqui F, Girard F, et al. Endoscopic lithotripsy and the FREDDY laser: initial experience. *J Endourol.* 2006;20:296-299.
22. Stark L, Carl P. First clinical experiences of laser lithotripsy using the partially frequency-doubled double pulse neodymium:YAG laser (FREDDY). *J Urol.* 2001;165(suppl):362A.
23. Jansen ED, Asshauer T, Frenz M, et al. Effect of pulse duration on bubble formation and laser-induced pressure waves during holmium laser ablation. *Lasers Surg Med.* 1996;18:278-293.
24. Chan KF, Lee H, Teichman JM, et al. Erbium:YAG lithotripsy mechanism. *J Urol.* 2002;168:436-441.
25. Freiha GS, Glickmann RD, Teichman JM. Holmium:YAG laser induced damage to guidewires: an experimental study. *J Endourol.* 1997;11:331-336.
26. Teichman JM, Vassar GJ, Bishoff JT, Bellmann GC. Holmium:YAG laser-induced lithotripsy yields smaller fragments than lithoclast, pulsed-dye or electrohydraulic lithotripsy. *J Urol.* 1998;159:17-23.
27. Sofer M, Watterson JD, Wollin TA, et al. Holmium:YAG laser lithotripsy for upper urinary tract calculi In 598 patients. *J Urol.* 2002;167:31-34.
28. Jansen ED, van Leeuwen TG, Motamedi M, Borst C, Welch AJ. Temperature dependence of the absorption coefficient of water

for midinfrared laser radiation. *Laser Surg Med.* 1994;14: 258-268.

29. Vassar GJ, Chan KF, Teichman JM, et al. Holmium:YAG lithotripsy: Photothermal mechanism. *J Endourol.* 1999;13:181-189.

30. Vassar GJ, Teichman JM, Glickman RD. Holmium:YAG lithotripsy efficiency varies with energy density. *J Urol.* 1998;160:471-476.

31. Teichman JM. Laser lithotripsy. *Curr Opin Urol.* 2002;12(4): 302-309.

32. Kourambas J, Munver R, Preminger GM. Ureteroscopic management of recurrent renal cystine calculi. *J Endourol.* 2000;14:489-492.

33. Kuo RL, Asian P, Zhong P, Preminger GM. Impact of holmium laser settings and fiber diameter on stone fragmentation and endoscope deflection. *J Endourol.* 1998;12:523-527.

34. Spore SS, Teichman JM, Corbin NS, Champion PC, Williamson EA, Glickman RD. Holmium:YAG lithotripsy: optimal power settings. *J Endourol.* 1999;13:559-566.

35. Pierre S, Preminger GM. Holmium laser for stone management. *World J Urol.* 2007;25:235-239.

36. Bach T, Geavlete B, Herrmann TRW, Gross AJ. Working tools in flexible ureterorenoscopy – influence on flow and deflection: What does matter? *J Endourol.* 2008 Aug;22(8):1639-1643.

37. Delvecchio FM, Preminger GM. Endoscopic management of urologic disease with the holium laser. *Curr Opin Urol.* 2000;10:233-237.

38. Wu CF, Shee JJ, Lin CL, Chen CS. Comparison between extracorporal shock wave lithotripsy and semi-rigid ureterorenoscopy with holmium:YAG laser lithotripsy for treating large proximal ureteral stones. *J Urol.* 2004;172:1899-1902.

39. Teichman JM, Rao RD, Rogenes VJ, Harris JM. Ureteroscopic management of ureteral calculi: electrohydraulic versus holmium:YAG lithotripsy. *J Urol.* 1997;158:1357-1361.

40. Razvi HA, Denstedt JD, Chun SS, Sales JL. Intracorporal lithotripsy with the holmium:YAG laser. *J Urol.* 1996;156:912-914.

41. Pearle MS, Lingemann JE, Leiveilee R, et al. Prospective randomized trail comparing shock wave lithotripsy and ureteroscopy for lower pole caliceal calculi 1 cm or less. *J Urol.* 2005;173: 2005-2009.

42. Finley DS, Petersen J, Abdelshehid C, Ahlering M, Chou D, Borin J, Eichel L, McDougall E, Clayman RV. Effect of holmium: YAG laser pulse width on lithotripsy retropulsion in vitro. *J Endourol.* 2005 Oct;19(8):1041-1044.

43. Visuri SR, Walsh JT, Wigdor HA. Erbium laser ablation of dentin hard tissue: effect of water cooling. *Laser Surg Med.* 1996;18:294-300.

44. Chan KF, Hammer DX, Choi B, et al. Free electron laser lithotripsy: threshold radiant exposures. *J Endourol.* 2000;14:161-167.

45. Teichman JM, Chan KF, Cecconi PP, et al. Erbium:YAG versus Ho:YAG. *J Urol.* 2001;165:876-879.

46. Grasso M, Bagley D. Small diameter, actively deflectable, flexible ureteropyeloscopy. *J Urol.* 1998;160:1648-1654.

47. Bagley DH. Ureteroscopic surgery: changing times and perspectives. *Urol Clin North Am.* 2004;31:1-4. vii.

Imaging for Stones

Alison J. Bradley and P. Nagaraja Rao

Abstract Imaging for stones covers the techniques available and evaluates the optimal techniques for the diagnosis of stone disease. This is mainly by multidetector computed tomography (MDCT), but the roles of intravenous urography (IVU), ultrasound (US), magnetic resonance imaging (MRI), fluoroscopic studies, and isotope renography are also discussed. Thin-section MDCT allows three-dimensional (3D) postprocessing with multiplanar reconstruction, thus providing an accurate assessment of stone burden and distribution. CT urography is explained, and its role in determining pelvicalyceal anatomy and for planning therapy is discussed. The section on evaluation of the results of therapy is divided into imaging for postoperative complications, and assessment for residual stones. The final section covers evaluation of function by isotope renography. An extensive review of the literature has been undertaken to bring an up-to-date and evidence-based slant to imaging, which is pivotal to stone management.

28.1 Introduction

Accurate confirmation of the presence of stone disease, and evaluation of the total stone burden, is crucial to optimal stone management, and is achieved by good quality imaging. Urinary tract stones can be visualized by many imaging modalities, from plain films to magnetic resonance scans. Plain abdominal radiographs still have an important role in the assessment and follow-up of stone disease. Ultrasound offers a quick and easy option with the advantage of avoiding radiation, albeit at the expense of diagnostic accuracy. Computed tomography (CT) has increasingly become the mainstay of evaluation of stone disease in both acute and elective situations. Function can be assessed crudely by post-contrast imaging techniques, and accurately by nuclear medicine techniques. An understanding of the physics of the various imaging techniques, together with their applications, is a useful tool for all involved in stone management.

28.2 Techniques

28.2.1 Abdominal Radiograph

This is a plain film exposure of the abdomen and pelvis, performed to look for opaque urinary tract stones. It should include both kidneys, ureters, and the bladder area, and is commonly requested as a "KUB" for this reason. The lower margin of the symphysis pubis should be visible on a good quality radiograph, as should be vertical collimation lines from a lead diaphragm, which reduces radiation scatter. Low kilovoltage techniques (60–70 kVp) optimize the contrast between stones and soft tissues; larger patients often require higher doses (70–80 kVp) to avoid under-exposure.

Conventional radiographs are produced by direct exposure onto a silver-containing screen film, resulting in a hard copy. Computed radiographic (CR) technology was developed in the 1980s, and its use is now widespread.[1] The CR plate is a reusable imaging medium that can be used many thousands of times; it is read and fed into a picture archiving and communication system (PACS). Digital radiography (DR) is a newer development whereby exposure is made directly onto the digital plate, which links directly into PACS. Although more costly, DR is becoming an attractive alternative. In many hospitals, both systems are in use and operate symbiotically.[1]

A.J. Bradley (✉)
Department of Radiology, University Hospital of South Manchester, Manchester, Lancashire, UK
e-mail: alison.bradley@uhsm.nhs.uk

P.N. Rao et al. (eds.), *Urinary Tract Stone Disease*,
DOI 10.1007/978-1-84800-362-0_28, © Springer-Verlag London Limited 2011

Unlike conventional radiography, both CR and DR offer a wide dynamic range (the range of exposure over which a diagnostic quality image will be produced) leading to a lower repeat rate. The radiation dose to the patient is usually less on CR and DR than on conventional radiography.[2] Studies have demonstrated that soft copy reporting is at least as accurate for stone detection as is conventional hard copy.[3,4]

Linear tomography allows selection of a 1 cm thick slice at a predetermined level within the patient. The level of the kidneys from the tabletop is usually 8–11 cm depending upon patient thickness. Structures above and below this level are blurred out, thus increasing detail within this slice.[5,6]

28.2.2 Intravenous Urography

Intravenous injection of iodinated contrast medium is excreted by the kidneys, and a series of films taken over the following 30 min constitutes the intravenous urography (IVU). Documented severe allergy to iodinated contrast medium is an absolute contraindication; pregnancy and renal impairment are relative contraindications. Patients with renal impairment are at an increased risk of developing contrast medium–induced nephrotoxicity, and the risk is greater with concomitant diabetes. Good hydration is the only factor that has been demonstrated to help prevent nephrotoxicity.[7,8] Bowel preparation does not improve the quality of the study, and is unpleasant for the patient.[9]

A control or preliminary view must be obtained to evaluate for the presence of stones. Following contrast medium injection, a series of radiographs is taken and abdominal compression applied if there is no obstruction or abdominal mass such as an aortic aneurysm. Compression of the ureters at the pelvic brim results in improved distension of the collecting systems. Protocols vary widely in their recommended film sequence[10]; the four film IVU is often adequate in our experience.[11] Linear tomography with a 20° arc is helpful when contrast opacification is poor, or there is considerable bowel gas overlying the kidney.[12] Supplementary views, such as oblique views of the renal areas, or a prone abdominal view (to improve ureteric distension) can be used as required.

28.2.3 Ultrasound

Ultrasound (US) waves in the 2–6 MHz range are employed in abdominal ultrasound, using a sector or curvilinear probe. The probe acts as both a transmitter and receiver of US waves, and calculation of the time interval between the two is used to calculate depth and build up an image. The kidney has good intrinsic contrast, with the parenchyma of low echogenicity compared with the echogenic renal sinus or "central echo complex" (due to the renal sinus fat) (Fig. 28.1). Unlike other imaging modalities, US is very operator dependant. Large patients are not ultrasound friendly due to the increased sound penetration required, and the increased scatter (noise) produced. Harmonic imaging has been developed to circumvent this problem. The second harmonic is an echo seen at twice the transmitted frequency, and has the effect of greatly reducing image noise. US has the advantage of

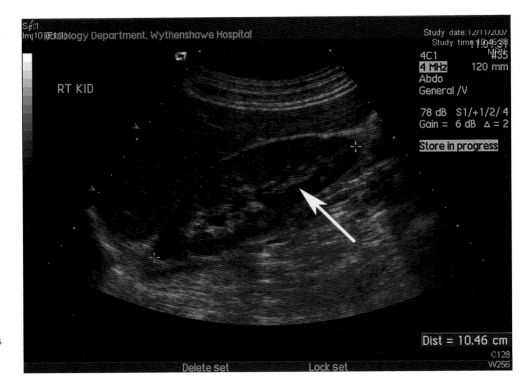

Fig. 28.1 Normal ultrasound of the right kidney. Note the echogenic renal sinus fat (*white arrow*). The collecting system is just seen in the center of the renal sinus

assessing the urinary tract in real time. Fluid ingestion prior to the study to fill the urinary bladder is routinely employed, although it probably is not required in the assessment of renal colic.[13]

The Doppler effect is a frequency change from the transmitted wave when it hits a moving target. The magnitude of the frequency shift can be used to calculate the velocity of the moving object, in this case blood. Color Doppler US can be useful in distinguishing between collecting system and blood vessel; it is particularly useful in the pelvis where the distal ureter crosses the iliac vessels. Arterial waveform within the kidney can be used to measure the resistive index (RI), which is a ratio of the diastolic to systolic flow within the kidney. Resistive indices of <0.7 are normal, and >0.7 are abnormal (obstruction reduces diastolic flow, hence increasing resistive index).[14]

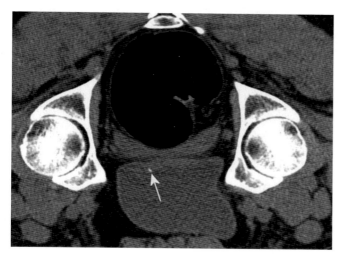

Fig. 28.2 Non-enhanced CT taken in the prone position. There is a small stone at the left VUJ (*white arrow*)

28.2.4 Computed Tomography

In recent years, computed tomography (CT) has evolved from single-detector row scanners into multidetector row scanners (MDCT), which are capable of covering large volumes of the body during a single breath-hold. Nonenhanced MDCT is performed to assess calculous disease; this is a quick and easy technique that requires no preparation for the patient.[15] In patients with acute flank pain, this can be performed in the prone position to distinguish between vesico-urethral junction (VUJ) calculi and bladder calculi, because free bladder calculi will fall anteriorly (being heavier than urine), and VUJ calculi will remain posteriorly at the VUJ[16] (Fig. 28.2).

When acquired in a helical scanner, the CT data set can be post processed to obtain different section thicknesses, depending upon the acquisition parameters. A full discussion of these is beyond the scope of this text, but it is sufficient to say that thinner sections require more radiation dose, with concomitant increased risks of cancer induction.[17–21]

The two-dimensional (2D) resolution will depend upon the number of picture elements (pixels) in the matrix; when reconstructed in 3D, these acquire volume and are thus termed voxels. When images are reconstructed at section thicknesses of 1 mm or less, the voxels have isotropic properties, in that they can be equally well resolved in any plane. The axial reconstruction data can be used to create non-axial two-dimensional images by means of multiplanar reformation (MPR). Multiplanar images can be thickened into slabs with projectional techniques such as maximum intensity projection (MIP) and volume rendering (VR).[22] MIP images are particularly useful in displaying the collecting system in CT urography.[23] These techniques are illustrated in Fig. 28.3a, b.

Fig. 28.3 Coronal reconstructions of a CT Urogram. (**a**) Maximum intensity projection (MIP), (**b**) volume rendered (VR). A small parenchymal calcification in the left upper pole is only appreciated on the VR images (*red arrows*)

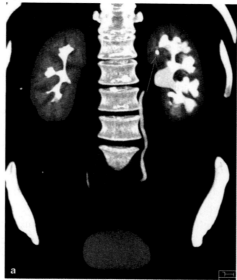
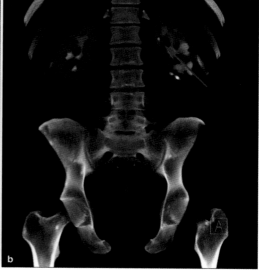

Table 28.1 CT urography technique using a split contrast bolus

- Scanner: Siemans Somatom 16 detector CT scanner
- Non-contrast acquisition
  - Settings: 100 effective mAs, 120 KVp, pitch 0.75, rotation time 0.5 s, beam width 24 mm (16 × 1.5 mm)
  - 75 mL of intravenous contrast agent
  - Administered by hand immediately after the initial acquisition
- Post-contrast acquisition
  - Performed 13 min following initial acquisition
  - Further 75 mL of contrast administered by an automated pump (3 mL/s)
  - Second acquisition performed 110 s following initiation of pump injection
  - Settings: 200 reference effective mAs, 120 KVp, pitch 0.75, rotation time 0.5 s, beam width (16 × 0.75 mm) 12 mm
- Siemens CARE Dose 4D automatic exposure control utilized

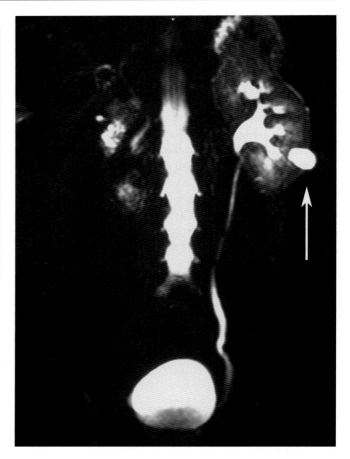

Fig. 28.4 T2W thick slab MR urogram, in a patient with a solitary left kidney. There is a small simple cyst within the left kidney (*white arrow*). Note that all fluid within the acquired volume is displayed; CSF, small intestine, and bile within the biliary tree

Different phases of contrast enhancement of the urinary tract can be obtained depending upon the timing of the bolus of contrast administration. A 30-s delay from the start of a dynamic injection will produce a cortico-medullary phase, where the cortex but not the medulla is enhanced. Imaging at 120 s produces a nephrographic phase, when there is uniform enhancement of normal renal parenchyma; and imaging after 10 min produces excretory phase images.

CT urography (CTU) is a term that causes some confusion, because it has been applied to various phases of imaging, including nonenhanced. However, CT urography should be reserved for post-contrast imaging that includes the excretory phase. The full technique includes pre-contrast, nephrographic, and excretory phase imaging.[24–26] The nephrographic and excretory acquisitions can be combined by employing a split contrast bolus technique as is suggested in Table 28.1.[19,24,27] The acquisition time for excretory phase imaging can be shortened by the addition of a small dose of furosemide (typically 10 mg). This can be given 3–5 min before the first contrast injection, allowing the delayed acquisition to be obtained at 5–10 min, instead of 13–15 min.[28–30] Furosemide has been shown to be more effective in improving distension (of the distal ureters in particular) than other methods such as compression and saline infusion.[29–32]

28.2.5 Magnetic Resonance Imaging

The urinary tract can be imaged either by static or dynamic techniques. The static technique uses heavily T2-weighted (T2W) spin echo sequences that will show urine as high signal intensity. Breath-hold T2W magnetic resonance urograms (MRUs) can be obtained as either thick (@ 8 cm) or thin (@ 3 mm) sections, using half Fourier techniques.[33] The thick slabs are usually displayed as MIP (maximum intensity projections) in a similar fashion to CT urograms. All fluid within the slice will be seen as bright in T2W MRU (Fig. 28.4). T2W techniques are excellent for evaluation of the dilated collecting system and bladder, but give no functional information.[34]

Dynamic or excretory MRU is the technique that is analogous to CTU and IVU; gadolinium-based contrast medium is injected intravenously in low doses in the region of 0.05 mmol/kg together with 5 mg of furosemide.[33] Gadolinium shortens the T1 relaxation time of urine, allowing it to appear bright on T1W sequences (Fig. 28.5). The diuretic improves flow and results in dilution and uniform distribution of contrast agent throughout the urine. Three-dimensional fat-suppressed gradient echo techniques are used to cover the urinary tract during a single breath hold. Dynamic MRU requires normal or near-normal renal function; the use of gadolinium in patients with significant renal impairment is now not advisable due to the association with Nephrogenic Systemic Sclerosis, a progressive and fatal condition that is without effective treatment.[35]

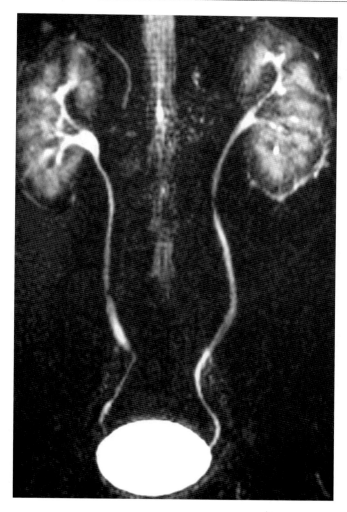

Fig. 28.5 Normal dynamic MR urogram, following injection of intravenous gadolinium chelate

28.2.6 Fluoroscopic Studies

Antegrade and retrograde studies during low-dose pulsed fluoroscopy with intra-luminal injection of iodinated contrast medium produce real time images of the urinary tract. Such studies are antegrade if injected via a nephrostomy tube, and retrograde if performed via a ureteric catheter.

28.2.7 Isotope Renography

Technetium-99 m mercaptoacetyltriglycine (MAG_3) is the isotope of choice for dynamic renography; it has twice the renal clearance rate of diethylene triamine penta-acetic acid (DTPA) and is an easier isotope to use than iodine-131. Furthermore, MAG_3 can be used to assess glomerular filtration rate based upon clearance from plasma samples.[36] Following injection, a time-activity curve is generated from regions of interest placed

around both kidneys and the bladder, over 15–30 min. The relative uptake of isotope by each kidney is calculated between the 2nd and 3rd min post injection.[36] Time to peak activity should normally occur by 5 min, and most isotope will have been excreted by 20 min in undilated collecting systems. Drainage from dilated collecting systems is more difficult to assess, so diuresis with IV furosemide may help. When furosemide is given 15 min before the start of the study, the kidneys are maximally stressed by a high flow rate of urine (F-15 MAG_3 renography) (Fig. 28.6). The rate of washout can be determined by calculating the T1/2, which is the time taken for the renal activity to decrease to half of the peak value.[37]

28.3 Establish Diagnosis of Stone Disease

28.3.1 Abdominal Film

The KUB remains the first radiological investigation that patients suspected of having stone disease will have. Approximately 90% of calculi are radio-opaque, although their visibility will also depend upon other factors, such as bowel gas overlying the urinary tract. The reviewer needs to be aware of different patterns of abdominal calcification (for example, gall stones or calcified mesenteric nodes) that may mimic a renal calculus.[38] A posterior oblique view of the affected side may help to distinguish between renal and other causes of calcification (Fig. 28.7a, b).

Roughly 90% of urinary calculi are radio-opaque due to the calcium content. Cysteine stones are poorly opaque, and uric acid stones are lucent. The incidence and radio-opacity of different types of stone are given in Table 28.2.[39] Plain radiographs are 60–70% sensitive and 70–80% specific in the detection of stone disease in renal colic when compared to CT or stone retrieval[40,41]; without colic, accuracy is less, but still better than the scout view on a CT scan.[42]

Different stone compositions may be recognized by the patterns of calcification they typically produce, for example calcium oxalate monohydrate tends to be smooth and densely opaque, whereas triple phosphate stones are commonly staghorn calculi (Fig. 28.8a, b)

28.3.2 Intravenous Urogram

Despite reports of its demise, due to the increasing role of multidetector CT (MDCT), the intravenous urogram (IVU) continues to be important in stone evaluation.[43–45] The topography of the pelvicalyceal system is readily appreciated, and the low mean radiation dose of 2.4 mSv for a standard four film series is much less than the mean dose of

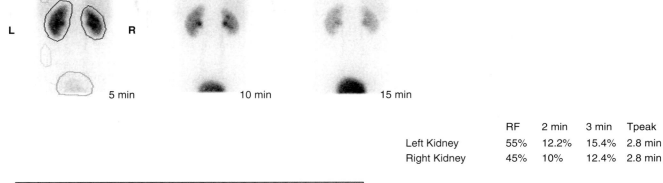

	RF	2 min	3 min	Tpeak
Left Kidney	55%	12.2%	15.4%	2.8 min
Right Kidney	45%	10%	12.4%	2.8 min

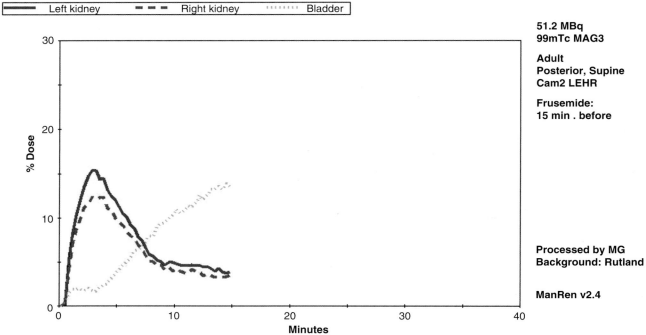

**51.2 MBq
99mTc MAG3**

**Adult
Posterior, Supine
Cam2 LEHR**

**Frusemide:
15 min . before**

**Processed by MG
Background: Rutland**

ManRen v2.4

Fig. 28.6 Normal diuresis renogram. Furosemide has been administered 15 min before the study

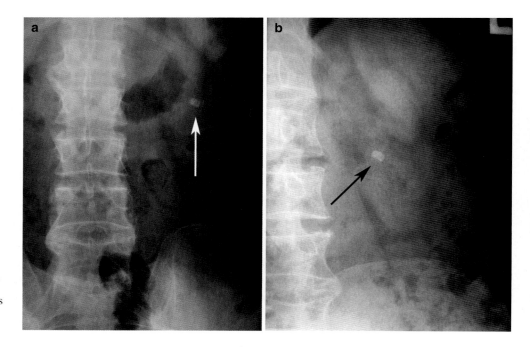

Fig. 28.7 (**a**) Antero-posterior, (**b**) left posterior oblique views of the left kidney. This confirms the calcification (*arrows*) to lie within the kidney

Table 28.2 Stone composition, frequency, and radio-opacity on plain films

Composition	Frequency (%)	Density
Calcium oxalate + phosphate	30–45	Opaque
Calcium oxalate	20–30	Densely opaque
Calcium phosphate	5–10	Opaque
Triple phosphate (struvite)	15–20	Variably opaque
Uric acid	5–10	Lucent
Cysteine	1–2	Poorly opaque

13 mSv for a CT urogram in our center.[18] In younger patients, the increased risk of fatal cancer induction from a CTU continues to make an IVU an attractive option. Nonenhanced CT carries a lower radiation dose, and this is discussed later in Sect. 28.2.4.

The diagnosis of obstruction by calculus is usually readily apparent on the initial film of the IVU series, when there is no contrast excretion or a dense nephrogram on the affected side (Fig. 28.9). It may take several hours to establish the site of obstruction, which is a disadvantage of the technique.[46] Conversely, a non-obstructing ureteric calculus may be overlooked when there is no delay in contrast excretion (Fig. 28.10a, b). Careful evaluation of a possible standing column of contrast within the ureter, and any subtle changes in caliber should be sought in symptomatic patients.[12] To this end, a post micturition view is often helpful (Fig. 28.11).

Prior to 1995, the IVU was considered to be the gold standard of imaging in renal colic patients,[47] but things changed when Smith et al. published the results of a study evaluating the findings at non-enhanced CT and IVU in 20 patients with acute flank pain. Of the 12 patients found to have obstruction on both modalities, 5 had a ureteric stone that was demonstrated on both non-enhanced CT scans and IVU radiographs, 6 had a stone that was depicted on non-enhanced CT scans only, and in 1 patient, a stone could not be detected by either modality.

They concluded that "non-enhanced CT was more effective than IVU in precisely identifying ureteric stones and is equally effective as IVU in the determination of the presence or absence of ureteric obstruction."[15] This paved the way for the gradual replacement of the IVU by non-enhanced CT in the evaluation of renal colic.[48] The appearances of a partly obstructing stone on both IVU and CT are shown in Fig. 28.12a–c.

28.3.3 Ultrasound

Ultrasound (US) has the advantages of being quick to perform, readily available, and avoids ionizing radiation. It is useful in the follow-up of stones that are nonopaque on KUB.[49] However, its accuracy is modest at best. Stones within the pelvicalyceal system can be reliably identified if they are greater than 5 mm in size, as smaller stones do not usually cast an acoustic shadow (Fig. 28.13a, b). Stones are more readily appreciated in the presence of hydronephrosis (Fig. 28.14). Fowler et al. compared US with nonenhanced CT, finding that 73% of undetected stones were 3 mm or less in size[50]; however, most stones of less than 3 mm are clinically insignificant. Sensitivity and specificity for stone detection were 24% and 90%, respectively. Only 39% of patients with multiple calculi were identified as such.[50] Ulusan et al. had slightly better results with sensitivity of 55% for stone detection in the right kidney and 36 % in the left.[51]

The twinkling artifact on color or power Doppler (seen as a comet tail appearance of rapidly changing color behind the stone) is seen in relation to 83–96% of stones in vivo, and can help to characterize them as stones.[52,53] This phenomenon has improved the accuracy of detection of intrarenal stones.

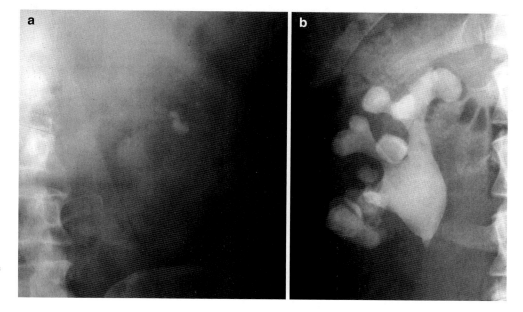

Fig. 28.8 (**a**) Three densely opaque stones are seen within the left kidney, (**b**) right staghorn stone

Fig. 28.9 IVU with delayed
excretion on the left, producing a
dense nephrogram

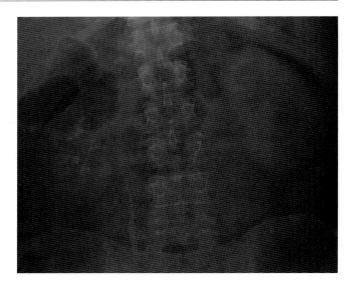

Fig. 28.10 (**a**) Control view,
(**b**) post-contrast view from an
IVU series. There is a left-sided
pelvic calcification that is
subsequently seen to lie in the
distal left ureter (*white arrows*)

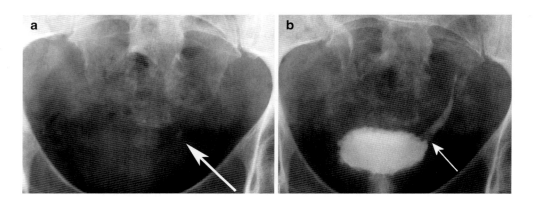

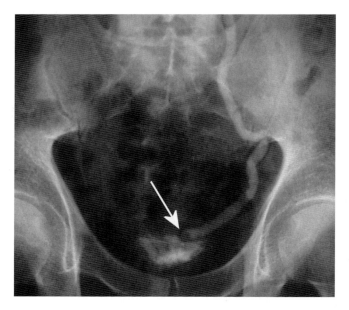

Fig. 28.11 Post micturition view from an IVU series. There is a small
left VUJ stone with a standing column of contrast in the left ureter

In the setting of renal colic, ultrasound performs better. In
a study by Sheafor et al.,[54] CT depicted 22 of 23 ureteric calculi (sensitivity, 96%), and US depicted 14 of 23 ureteric calculi (sensitivity, 61%). But when modalities were compared
for the detection of any clinically relevant abnormality (e.g.,
unilateral hydronephrosis and/or other stones in patients with
an obstructing stone), sensitivities of US and CT increased to
92% and 100%, respectively. Rosen et al.[55] prospectively evaluated the use of bedside US in renal colic patients, to detect
hydronephrosis and predict the likelihood of urolithiasis, and
found that the positive predictive value (PPV) and negative
predictive value (NPV) were 86% and 75%, respectively.

Patlas et al. evaluated 62 consecutive patients with flank
pain who were examined with both CT and US.[56] Forty-three
of the 62 patients were confirmed as having ureteric calculi
based on stone recovery or urological interventions. US
showed 93% sensitivity and 95% specificity in the diagnosis
of ureteric stones; CT showed 91% and 95%, respectively.
These results would be difficult to reproduce, but do endorse
the use of ultrasound as a first-line test in renal colic patients.

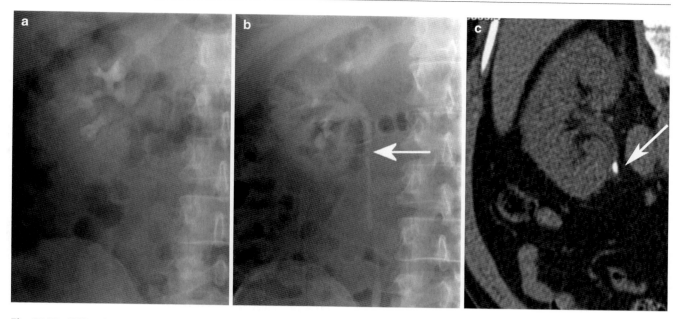

Fig. 28.12 IVU series (**a**, **b**). (**c**) A coronal reconstruction of non-enhanced CT from the same patient. There is low-grade obstruction of the right ureter on the IVU. The stone (*white arrows*) is much less easily appreciated than on the corresponding CT image

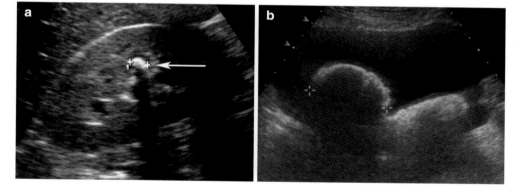

Fig. 28.13 (**a**) Ultrasound of the right kidney. An echogenic stone (*white arrow*) is casting a convincing acoustic shadow behind it. (**b**) Ultrasound of the bladder. There is a large stone seen between the two cursors. It measured 5 cm

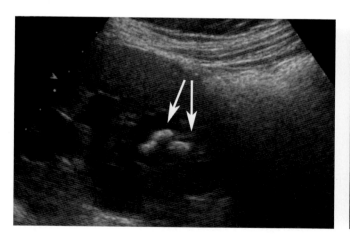

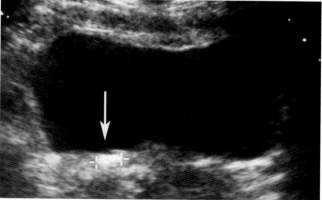

Fig. 28.14 Ultrasound of a moderately hydronephrotic left kidney. Three calculi are present within the lower pole (*white arrows*)

Fig. 28.15 Ultrasound of a non-obstructing right VUJ stone, seen through the bladder (*white arrow*)

Stones in the mid ureter are very difficult to detect, but stones in the upper ureter may be seen. VUJ stones can be assessed if the full bladder is used as a window (Fig. 28.15).

28.3.4 Computed Tomography

Since the initial paper by Smith et al. in 1995,[15] there have been multiple studies confirming the value of nonenhanced CT in the setting of acute loin pain.[46,57–60] Dalrymple et al.[58] studied 417 patients with acute flank pain who underwent nonenhanced helical CT, finding that helical CT diagnosed ureteric stone disease with 95% sensitivity, 98% specificity, and 97% accuracy, which is superior to any other imaging technique. Additionally, CT will diagnose other causes of flank pain, for example appendicitis, diverticulitis, or cholecystitis as the commoner non-renal causes.[61] This has led to widespread adoption of nonenhanced MDCT in patients with acute flank pain,[57] with the added advantage that virtually all stones, including uric acid, are opaque on CT.[62] The exception to this is protease inhibitor crystals, which are lucent on CT as well as plain films. Indinavir sulfate is the most widely used protease inhibitor in human immunodeficiency virus (HIV) therapy, with crystallization and stone formation occurring in as many as 20% of patients taking the medication.[63,64]

Sometimes a ureteric stone is not seen, or a calcification is considered to be indeterminate but suspicious, in which case secondary signs of obstruction are important for diagnosis. Ureteric dilatation has a sensitivity of 90% and a specificity of 93%, and perinephric stranding had a sensitivity 82% and specificity of 93%, respectively[65] (Fig. 28.16a, b). Collecting system dilatation and renal enlargement are also useful secondary signs.[65] Absence of the white pyramid and reduced attenuation of the renal parenchyma on the obstructed side (by approximately 5 Hounsfield units)

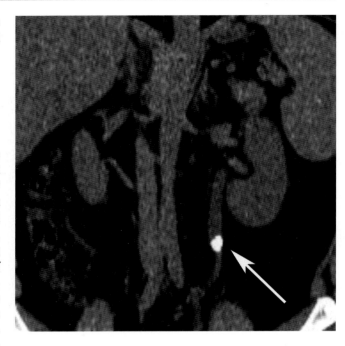

Fig. 28.17 Coronal reconstruction of a non-enhanced CT scan. There are two stones in the mid ureter, with a change in caliber back to normal below them (*white arrow*)

have subsequently been described as additional secondary signs.[66,67]

Distinguishing between a ureteric stone and a phlebolith in a pelvic vein can be difficult. The soft tissue rim sign has been described as a circumferential rim due to edema of the obstructed ureteric wall at the site of stone impaction and found to have a sensitivity of 77% and a specificity of 92% for distinguishing a stone from a phlebolith[68] The presence or absence of a tissue rim sign does not correlate with the degree of urinary obstruction present.[69] Conversely, phleboliths can have a comet tail sign, which is an important indicator that a suspicious calcification represents a phlebolith. The tail sign has a sensitivity of 65% and a specificity of 100% in

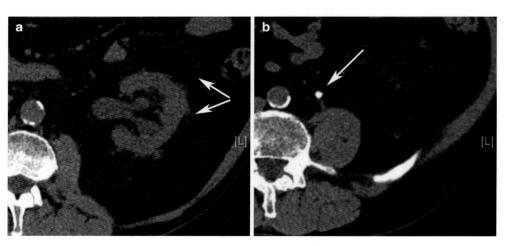

Fig. 28.16 Non-enhanced CT demonstrating the secondary signs of ureteric obstruction. (**a**) Note the mild hydronephrosis and perinephric stranding (*white arrows*). (**b**) A few sections more distally, a stone is seen in the upper left ureter (*white arrow*)

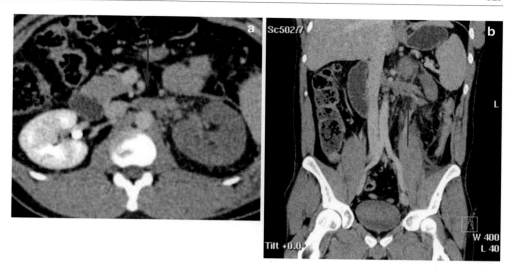

Fig. 28.18 (**a**) Axial section, (**b**) coronal reconstruction from a parenchymal phase renal CT. The patient presented with severe left loin pain and had a negative non-enhanced CT. There is no enhancement of the left kidney, and thrombus within the left renal vein (*red arrows*)

differentiating phleboliths from ureteric calculi.[70] Scrolling through a stack of images in cine mode allows the viewer to follow the course of the ureter, and coronal or curved multiplanar reconstruction (MPR) can demonstrate the relationship of a calcification to the ipsilateral ureter (Fig. 28.17).[66] In comparison with the IVU, which is easily interpreted by both radiologists and urologists, there is a small but real learning curve with the non-enhanced MDCT.[71]

The disadvantage of the technique is that it provides no functional information about the degree of obstruction present. There have been some studies evaluating the usefulness of secondary signs in predicting the severity of obstruction,[72] but they correlate poorly with MAG 3 renography and thus do not permit evaluation of the functional status of obstructed kidneys.[73,74] Another pitfall is the possibility of missing other serious causes of acute flank pain, which would be readily appreciated on post-contrast scans; for example, relatively rare conditions such as renal vein thrombosis (Fig. 28.18a, b). In a large study of 708 patients evaluating the utility of additional post-contrast imaging in patients with unexplained renal colic, 67 (9.4%) had abnormalities only seen on the post-contrast scans. The authors concluded that IV contrast is rarely helpful.[75]

Initial reports of nonenhanced CT for renal colic documented a radiation dose three times greater than that of an IVU,[17] but subsequent studies have evaluated low-dose techniques using 50–70 mAs. This has not resulted in a reduction in accuracy of stone detection with an effective radiation dose of 1.5 mSv.[76,77] Ultra-low-dose techniques producing effective doses of less than 1 mSv have been described but have yet to be fully evaluated.[78]

CT urography is rarely required in establishing the diagnosis of stone disease; occasionally, it is valuable in kidneys with abnormal anatomy due to previous surgery or parenchymal

scarring, as it can distinguish between calcifications within the parenchyma and the collecting system. This is discussed further in Sects. 28.5 and 28.6.

28.3.5 Magnetic Resonance Imaging

Although magnetic resonance imaging (MRI) offers superior contrast resolution to CT, spatial resolution is less. However, the main drawback of MRU in the assessment of urolithiasis is that stones show signal void, and thus appear black, making them much more difficult to resolve (Fig. 28.19). Additionally, not all low-signal-intensity filling defects are due to calculi, because blood clots and tumors can have similar appearances, although neoplasms will show enhancement following gadolinium-based contrast agents.[33]

The use of MRU is usually restricted to children and pregnant women, where avoidance of radiation is desirable, or patients with documented allergy to iodinated contrast media.[79] Static MRU is particularly useful in the evaluation of loin pain in pregnant patients, where it can distinguish effectively between hydronephrosis of pregnancy (HOP) and other causes of obstruction. In HOP, smooth tapering of the ureter between the gravid uterus and iliac vessels is seen, usually on the right. In other causes, such as obstruction by stone, the site of caliber change will be elsewhere (Fig. 28.20a, b).[80]

Static MRU does have the advantages of demonstrating the anatomy of the urinary tract, and in a study by Jung et al.,[81] it was superior to IVU in the detection of ureteric calculi in symptomatic patients. MRU detected 64 of 72 stones, compared with 49 of 72 stones at IVU. High-grade obstruction with non excretion of contrast was the major cause of IVU failure. Regan et al.[82] compared a combination of static MRU

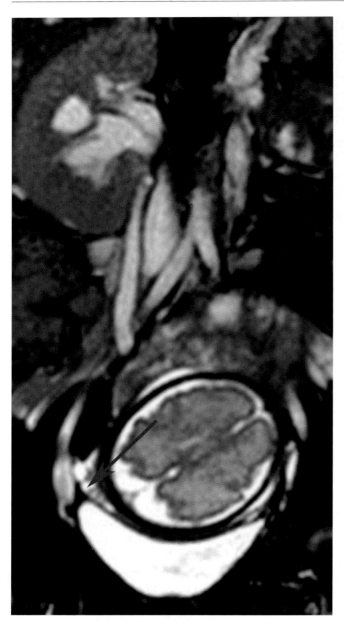

Fig. 28.19 Coronal thin-section T2W section from an MR urogram in a pregnant patient with right loin pain. There is a small stone (*red arrow*) in the distal right ureter

28.3.6 Fluoroscopic Studies

With the increasing use of CT, antegrade and retrograde studies do not have a role in establishing the diagnosis of stone disease. They are useful in pre- and posttherapeutic assessment, and this is discussed in Sects. 28.7 and 28.8.

28.3.7 Isotope Renography

The isotope renogram does not have a role in the diagnosis of stone disease as it does not resolve stones; its role in aiding management decisions is discussed in Sects. 28.6 and 28.8.

28.4 Assess Stone Burden and Distribution

Densely opaque stones can be readily assessed on KUB or IVU, but these will give a two-dimensional view of a three-dimensional structure, which can lead to errors of overestimation or underestimation of stone size.[85] Additionally, there is a small but real magnification effect, causing some overestimation of stone size, when compared to retrieved stone size.[85] Ultrasound can evaluate in 3D, but smaller stones will be missed, and it is difficult to reproduce planes of imaging in sequential examinations.[50,86] Stones within the renal pelvis, particularly the extra-renal pelvis, can be very difficult to locate at US. MR has little role because stones appear black, and thus can be easily overlooked.[33]

As discussed in Sects. 28.2 and 28.3, CT has the advantages of all stones (with the exception of protease inhibitor crystals and matrix stones) being opaque, and measurable in three dimensions.[22,87,88] A recent meta-analysis of the literature revealed that CT has better diagnostic performance than IVU in the evaluation of urolithiasis.[48] Different window settings (for example bone windows) and the use of MIP images can improve the conspicuity of stones (Fig. 28.21a, b).[89] Coronal reformations allow equally accurate and more rapid detection of urinary stones compared with axial images alone, but are best used in conjunction with axial data sets for the most accurate evaluation of stone burden.[90,91] The coronal reformations will give a longitudinal measurement of the stone size; depending upon the thickness of the reconstructed sections, there will be overestimation of the stone size of the order of 1 mm on thin slices.[92] Another study by Dundee et al.[93] found that CT underestimated stone size (as measured in its greatest

and KUB with nonenhanced MDCT in patients with renal colic, finding that the MRU/KUB combination detected only 72% of stones seen at CT. MRU was more sensitive in the detection of secondary findings of acute ureteric obstruction such as peri-renal fluid and ureteric dilatation. If dynamic MRU is used, then sensitivity and specificity of 96% and 100%, respectively, are achievable.[83] The same group (Sudah et al.) reported accuracy for stone detection by dynamic MRU that was similar to that of nonenhanced CT, but noted that patients would prefer to have a CT if a repeat test was required.[84]

Fig. 28.20 (**a**) Coronal, (**b**) sagittal reconstructions from a parenchymal phase renal CT demonstrating a partial staghorn stone in the left kidney (*red arrows*). The reconstructions were used to plan access via the upper pole collecting system

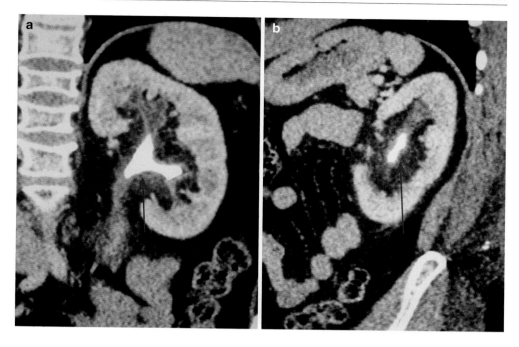

Fig. 28.21 Coronal reconstruction of a non-enhanced CT scan, (**a**) viewed on bone window settings, (**b**) viewed on soft tissue window settings. The stone (*white arrows*) is more conspicuous on the bone windows. Note that it appears larger on the soft tissue settings

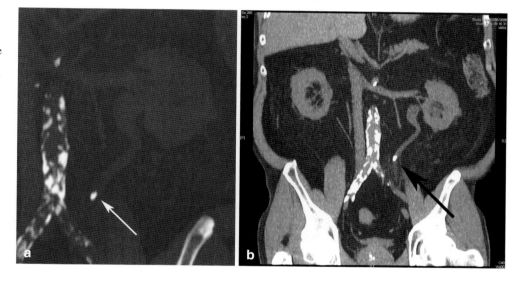

dimension) by 12% in comparison to KUB, but this was a small study of 24 patients. Section widths of >3 mm will also lead to a reduction in the number of renal and ureteric calculi detected.[94] So, on thin-section MDCT of 3 mm or less, measurement of stones is reasonably accurate so long as measurements are made. Kampa et al.[95] evaluated 421 responses from UK radiologists and urologists about how they evaluated stone size. Forty percent of radiologists and 60% of urologists guesstimated size on IVU or KUB. On CT or US, where electronic measurement is possible, 10–15% still guesstimated.[95] It is thus important to state in the imaging report how the stone(s) have been measured, as

size can affect management particularly of lower pole calculi, as discussed in Sect. 28.6.[96]

28.5 Determine Anatomy

The anatomy of the pelvicalyceal system can only be assessed on post-contrast studies; usually IVU or CT urography. If the patient has a nephrostomy tube in situ, then antegrade fluoroscopy can also be used (Fig. 28.22a, b). There has been some debate in the literature whether IVU

Fig. 28.22 Same patient as Fig. 28.20. (**a**) Control, (**b**) post-contrast views from an antegrade study. A percutaneous nephrostomy tube was placed into the left upper pole. The stone (*black arrows*) is poorly opaque, and difficult to appreciate on the post-contrast view

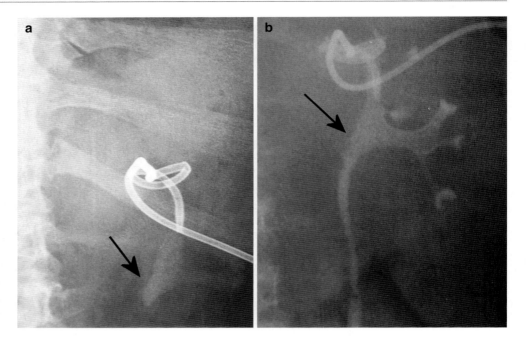

Fig. 28.23 (**a**) Control, (**b**) post-contrast view of the right kidney from an IVU series. On the initial view, the cluster of calcifications resembles gallstones, but are confirmed to lie within a large calyceal diverticulum in the right upper pole following contrast

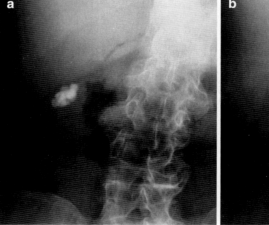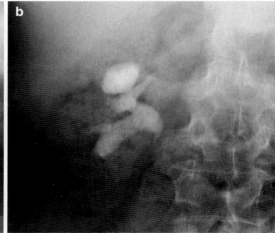

should be replaced by CT, or whether it still has a role in preoperative imaging.[45,97] As has been discussed in Sect. 28.2.4, CT urography has a much higher radiation dose than does IVU, but also the advantage of multiplanar reconstruction and 3D imaging, which gives superior anatomical resolution. Many stone formers will have to undergo repeated examinations and therapy over their lifetimes, so reduction of the radiation burden is desirable. The choice of imaging modality will be decided upon local resources, the level of anatomical detail required, and consideration of the risks of cancer induction.

Post-contrast imaging is important to confirm the location of calculi within the collecting system, and at which site(s). An IVU will suffice in most cases of straightforward anatomy,

and will readily appreciate abnormalities such as calyceal diverticulae (Fig. 28.23a, b). CT is playing an increasing role,[98] especially in abnormal renal anatomy such as a horseshoe or transplant kidney (Fig. 28.24a–c), or abnormal patient anatomy; for example, spina bifida.[99]

CT is usually performed with the patient supine and PCNL with the patient prone. Is there any difference in pelvicalyceal anatomy between the two positions? Sengupta et al.[100] evaluated CT scans in 14 patients, performed both supine and prone, and found that the position of the patient had a small effect on the orientation of the kidneys, with the mean angle changing from 56.6°, when supine, to 61.6°, when prone. However, no significant change in calyceal orientation or the relative projection of the anterior and

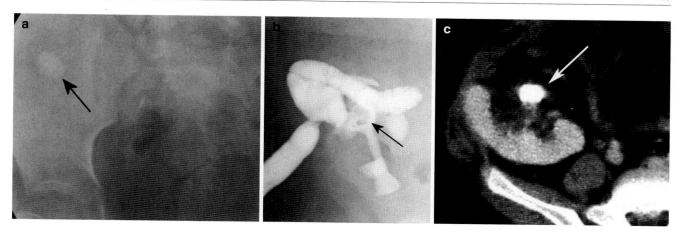

Fig. 28.24 (**a**) Plain radiograph, (**b**) loopogram, and (**c**) CT scan from a young patient with a transplanted kidney draining into an ileal loop. There is a stone in the renal pelvis (*arrows*). The loopgram and CT scan were performed to plan access prior to PCNL

posterior calices occurred as a result. There is thus no need to carry out preoperative imaging in the prone position.

The lower pole collecting system morphology is considered to be a factor in determining success of extracorporeal shock wave lithotripsy (ESWL); infundibulopelvic angles of less than 90°, infundibular width of less than 4 mm and infundibular length greater than 3 cm can be associated with poorer clearance rates. The lower pole ratio is calculated as a ratio of infundibular length: infundibular width as measured on preoperative intravenous urograms, with ratios less than 3.5 associated with poorer clearance by ESWL.[101,102]

28.6 Plan Therapy

Stone size and number form the basis of management pathways in patients with urolithiasis, so accurate evaluation of this is important. Knowledge of composition is also helpful.

28.6.1 Acute Management

The rate of spontaneous passage of ureteric stones does vary with stone size and location as determined by CT. Coll et al.[103] evaluated 172 cases of confirmed ureterolithiasis. For stones 2–4 mm, the rate was 76%; for stones 5–7 mm, 60%; for stones 7–9 mm, 48%; and for stones larger than 9 mm, 25%. The measurements were made in the axial plane. Spontaneous passage rate as a function of stone location was 48% for stones in the proximal ureter, 60% for mid ureteric stones, 75% for distal stones, and 79% for

VUJ stones.[103] This data correlates well with that previously published by the American Association of Urologists.[104] Conservative management is usually employed for stones 5 mm or less in size, and for slightly larger stones in the distal ureter. Stones larger than 7 mm and causing obstruction usually require intervention, particularly in the presence of sepsis, either by retrograde JJ stent or percutaneous nephrostomy insertion, depending upon local expertise.[105] MAG3 renography is the most accurate imaging technique for establishing whether obstruction is present or not, and is often used following non-contrast CT scan to evaluate the need for intervention. High-grade obstruction (Fig. 28.25) will require urgent decompression by PCN, whereas management of low-grade obstruction can be planned electively.

For stones that fail to pass spontaneously, the management options are ESWL or ureteroscopic retrieval.[102] A recent study by Pearle et al.[106] compared ureteroscopy (32 patients) and ESWL (32 patients) for distal ureteric stones, and found both were associated with high success and low complication rates. However, lithotripsy required significantly less operating time; was more often performed on an outpatient basis; and showed a trend toward less flank pain and dysuria, fewer complications, and quicker convalescence.[106]

28.6.2 Elective Management

Size, composition, and location of intrarenal stones will determine whether lithotripsy, percutaneous, or ureteroscopic extraction is more appropriate.

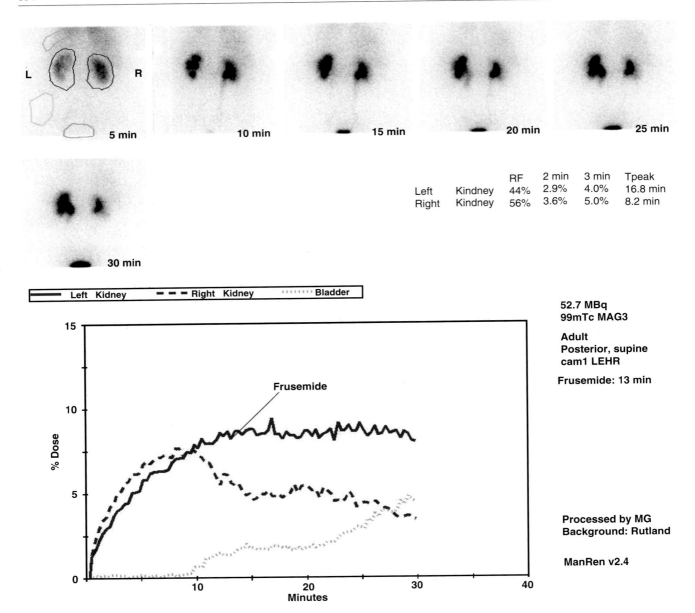

		RF	2 min	3 min	Tpeak
Left	Kindney	44%	2.9%	4.0%	16.8 min
Right	Kindney	56%	3.6%	5.0%	8.2 min

52.7 MBq
99mTc MAG3

Adult
Posterior, supine
cam1 LEHR

Frusemide: 13 min

Processed by MG
Background: Rutland

ManRen v2.4

Fig. 28.25 MAG3 renogram in a patient with a known left upper ureteric stone. There is reasonable uptake on the left but no elimination, despite furosemide

28.6.2.1 Stone Location

Non-enhanced CT is usually adequate prior to ESWL or straightforward PCNL, especially when 3D post processing is used[98,107,108] (Fig. 28.26). Three-dimensional reconstructions are particularly useful for complex calculi such as staghorns,[88] and simple trigonometric measurements can be performed to facilitate track planning for PCNL.[108] Although not routinely required, CT urography provides excellent understanding of collecting system anatomy, and confirms whether a stone is within the collecting system or the parenchyma/medullary pyramid (Fig. 28.27a, b).[109]

Anatomical location is important when considering ESWL therapy. Factors predicting a good response to ESWL include upper or mid pole calyceal stones, size less than 2 cm, and normal urinary tract anatomy; these features can allow stone-free rates of up to 90%.[110] Renal pelvic and PUJ stones clear better than do calyceal stones.[111]

Clearance of lower pole stones by ESWL is poor, varying from 37% to59%.[102,112]

28.6.2.2 Stone Size/Burden

Lower pole stones smaller than 1 cm in diameter can be managed with observation, shock wave lithotripsy, or ureteroscopy; those 1–2 cm in diameter are best managed with PCNL,

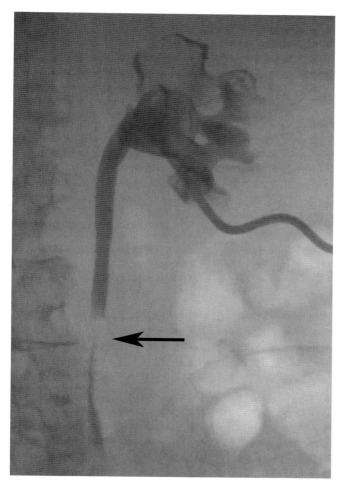

Fig. 28.26 Antegrade nephrostogram. There is a lucent stone in the mid left ureter (*black arrow*). Note further partial staghorn stone in the left upper pole collecting system

although ureteroscopy is an option in selected patients. Lower pole stones greater than 2 cm are best managed by PCNL. Upper or interpolar calyceal stones up to 2 cm can be treated with ESWL; stones larger than this will require percutaneous extraction.[102] Wang et al. evaluated factors that were associated with a poor outcome from ESWL and demonstrated that a stone number >2, stone size >12 mm, stone burden of more than 700 mL, and a maximal stone density of more than 900 HU ($P = 0.0430$) were statistically significant predictors of failure.[113]

28.6.2.3 Stone Composition

Most calcium-containing stones will fragment easily, but cystine and oxalate stones are relatively resistant to ESWL. Struvite staghorn–infected stones pose a real risk to the kidney, and need to be treated relatively urgently, usually by percutaneous extraction.[114,115] Determination of stone composition by radiographic means would be a useful tool in aiding management decisions. Plain radiographs alone will correctly predict stone composition in less than 40% of cases.[116] CT, however, can be used to predict composition for some types of stone. Matrix calculi are rare, but will be predominantly of soft tissue attenuation,[117] as will protease inhibitor crystals.[63] In a study by Nakada et al., 99 patients with predominantly (greater than 50%) calcium oxalate or uric acid composition had the attenuation value measured on nonenhanced CT scan. Values were compared with stone analysis; 82 calculi predominantly composed of calcium oxalate had a mean Hounsfield measurement of 652 (±490 HU), and 17 calculi predominantly composed of uric acid had a mean of 344 (±152 HU), which was a significant difference ($P = 0.017$, unpaired t test).[118] More recently, dual energy CT has been used in an anthropomorphic phantom model to accurately discriminate uric acid stones from other stone types.[119] Identification of uric acid calculi can allow pharmacological rather than surgical treatment.[120] CT has also been used to successfully characterize in vitro cystine

Fig. 28.27 CT urogram in a patient with known medullary sponge kidney. (**a**) Unenhanced CT shows multiple bilateral small calcifications. (**b**) Following contrast, some of these are seen to lie within dilated tubules within the medullary pyramids (*white arrow*)

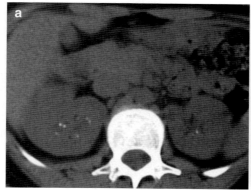
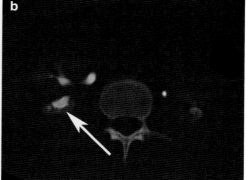

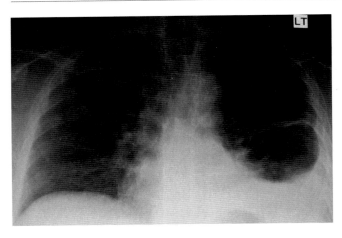

Fig. 28.28 Same patient as Figs. 28.20 and 28.22. Following PCNL via the upper pole, the patient developed a left pleural effusion due to accumulation of saline in the pleural space

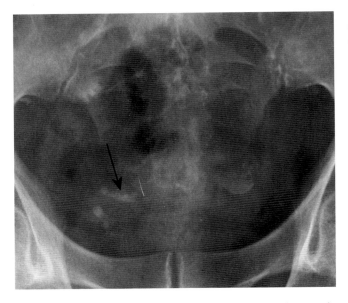

Fig. 28.29 Following ESWL, this patient has developed steinstrasse in the distal right ureter (*black arrow*). Calcifications below this in the right hemi-pelvis represent phleboliths

stones as rough or smooth, which is useful because rough cystine stones are more susceptible to ESWL.[121]

28.7 Evaluate Results of Therapy

28.7.1 Postoperative Complications

At PCNL, retained stone fragments can occasionally pass into the ureter, and if not recognized at the time of operation, can cause obstruction. This becomes apparent when the post procedural nephrostomy tube is clamped, causing pain, and is

an indication for an antegrade study or nephrostogram (Fig. 28.26). If appreciated at the time of surgery, a JJ stent can be placed antegradely. Poor nephrostomy drainage should also prompt an antegrade study, to confirm that the tube is still within the collecting system; if it is not, then an ultrasound is required to check for a urinoma or hydronephrosis.[102]

A chest radiograph is mandatory for all supra-12 rib punctures, as there is a possibility of irrigant fluid/saline accumulating in the pleural space (Fig. 28.28).

Postoperative bleeding is either early and venous, which usually responds to tamponade of the track, or delayed (>7 days) and arterial. This can be secondary to an arteriovenous fistula or pseudo aneurysm, and complicates less than 1% of PCNL procedures.[122]

CT scan in the arterial phase may show the cause of bleeding, but early angiography is indicated with a view to embolization of an arterial abnormality.[123]

Following ESWL, fragments may drop into the ureter and cause obstruction. This gives the characteristic appearance of steinstrasse on KUB (Fig. 28.29).

28.7.2 Assess for Residual Stones

The goal of therapy is to render the patient stone free, and the role of post therapeutic imaging is to detect residual stones as accurately as possible. Fluoroscopy at the time of surgery is not sufficiently reliable to detect these, and a KUB is required postoperatively. Ultrasound is not an effective method of assessment.[124,125] However, CT does assess for residual stones very effectively. Park et al.[126] prospectively compared the sensitivity of antegrade pyelography, plain film radiography, and non-enhanced CT for detecting residual stones after PCNL in

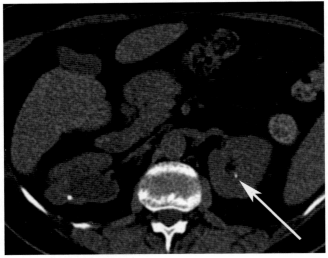

Fig. 28.30 Non-enhanced CT showing a small linear calcification within the left kidney, thought to represent a Randall's plaque (*white arrow*)

53 patients. Stone-free rates were 73.6% for antegrade pyelography, 62.3% for KUB, and 20.8% for CT. Some of the fragments detected at CT were considered to be clinically insignificant; however, this illustrates the greater sensitivity of CT. Other studies have found similar results.[125,127] Pearle et al.[127] compared non-enhanced CT with "second look" flexible nephroscopy following PCNL, and found CT to have a sensitivity of 100% and specificity of 62% for detection of residual stones. The specificity is lower because CT cannot always distinguish between Randall's plaques and stones within the collecting system (Fig. 28.30). It is not always practical to perform CT after every procedure, but after difficult procedures, or when residual calculus is shown to be present on a KUB, then it is advisable to plan further potential therapy. Small residual fragments can be treated by ESWL.[102]

28.8 Evaluate Function

The function of a kidney can be impaired by the effects of stone disease such as obstruction, which can be at calyceal, infundibular, pelvic, or ureteric level, and thus affect part or all of the kidney. Superimposed infection will hasten the loss of nephrons. Postoperative assessment of function is not routinely required in patients following ureteroscopic retrieval of stone(s),[128] but should be done after surgery for complex stones. Such patients will have had preoperative MAG3 renography to evaluate function and the presence of obstruction; postoperative renography will document improvement in drainage or function once obstruction has been relieved, and act as a baseline against further studies. Changes in function (either increase or decrease) can occur up to 6 months following surgery, a factor that needs to be considered in the timing of the postoperative renogram.[129] Recently, a study by Moskovitz et al. evaluating single-photon emission CT (SPECT) measurement of Tc-dimercaptosuccinic acid (DMSA) uptake by the kidneys in 88 patients has found that although the total functional volume of the treated kidney was slightly decreased following PCNL, neither total percent uptake nor percent of injected dose was reduced significantly.[130] This suggests that the surgery itself is not damaging the kidney, and a marked reduction in function following surgery should prompt further imaging to look for possible obstruction.

Various studies in the early 1990s evaluated the effect of ESWL upon kidney function.[130–133] Elgazzar et al.[131] demonstrated transient changes in relative uptake function, glomerular filtration rate, and time-activity curves, but these returned to baseline after a week. Gupta et al.[132] found that a small number of patients (3/42) had a reduction in relative function of greater than 5% at 3 months post treatment, and concluded that "newer generation lithotriptors may limit renal damage while permitting satisfactory treatment of renal

calculi." Today, evaluation of function is not routinely necessary following ESWL unless the stone burden is large or the kidney is known to be scarred or functioning poorly.

28.9 Conclusions

Advances in imaging techniques, particularly in the development of multidetector CT protocols, have revolutionized imaging for stones in the last decade. The high contrast between stones and soft tissues allows for easy recognition. Sub-millimeter isotropic voxels provide excellent detail, with the capability of reconstruction in any plane. Post-contrast imaging, where required, evaluates the anatomy and function of the urinary tract.

References

1. Cowen AR, Davies AG, Kengyelics SM. Advances in computed radiography systems and their physical imaging characteristics. *Clin Radiol.* 2007;62:1132–1141.
2. Slovis TL. The pictures are great but is the radiation dose greater than required? *Am J Roentgenol.* 2002;179:39–41.
3. Cervi PM, Bighi S, Merlo L, Lupi L, Vita G. Digital radiography versus conventional radiography during excretory urography: our experience. *Ann Radiol (Paris).* 1990;33:321–328.
4. Kim AY, Cho KS, Song KS, Kim JH, Kim JG, Ha HK. Urinary calculi on computed radiography: comparison of observer performance with hard-copy versus soft-copy images on different viewer systems. *AJR Am J Roentgenol.* 2001;177:331–335.
5. Goldwasser B, Cohan RH, Dunnick NR, Andriani RT, Carson CC III, Weinerth JL. Role of linear tomography in evaluation of patients with nephrolithiasis. *Urology.* 1989;33:253–256.
6. Schwartz G, Lipschitz S, Becker JA. Detection of renal calculi: the value of tomography. *AJR Am J Roentgenol.* 1984;143:143–145.
7. Thomsen HS. Current evidence on prevention and management of contrast-induced nephropathy. *Eur Radiol.* 2007;17(suppl 6): F33-F37.
8. Thomsen HS. European Society of Urogenital Radiology guidelines on contrast media application. *Curr Opin Urol.* 2007;17:70–76.
9. Bradley AJ, Taylor PM. Does bowel preparation improve the quality of intravenous urography? *Br J Radiol.* 1996;69:906–909.
10. Zagoria RJ, Donati DL, Chen MY, Gelfand DW, Ott DJ, Dyer RB. Cost-effective filming sequence for intravenous urography. *South Med J.* 1994;87:899–901.
11. Bradley AJ, Rajashanker B, Atkinson SL, Kennedy JN, Purcell RS. Accuracy of reporting of intravenous urograms: a comparison of radiographers with radiology specialist registrars. *Clin Radiol.* 2005;60:807–811.
12. Dyer RB, Chen MY, Zagoria RJ. Intravenous urography: technique and interpretation. *Radiographics.* 2001;21:799–821.
13. Ozden E, Gogus C, Turkolmez K, Yagci C. Is fluid ingestion really necessary during ultrasonography for detecting ureteral stones? A prospective randomized study. *J Ultrasound Med.* 2005;24:1651–1657.
14. Akcar N, Ozkan IR, Adapinar B, Kaya T. Doppler sonography in the diagnosis of urinary tract obstruction by stone. *J Clin Ultrasound.* 2004;32:286–293.

15. Smith RC, Rosenfield AT, Choe KA, et al. Acute flank pain: comparison of non-contrast-enhanced CT and intravenous urography. *Radiology*. 1995;194:789–794.

16. Levine J, Neitlich J, Smith RC. The value of prone scanning to distinguish ureterovesical junction stones from ureteral stones that have passed into the bladder: leave no stone unturned. *AJR Am J Roentgenol*. 1999;172:977–981.

17. Denton ER, Mackenzie A, Greenwell T, Popert R, Rankin SC. Unenhanced helical CT for renal colic–is the radiation dose justifiable? *Clin Radiol*. 1999;54:444–447.

18. Williams LR, Smith A, Hufton A, Bradley AJ. Comparison of effective radiation doses of conventional and two-phase CT Urography. *Eur Radiol*. 2008;18:C–402.

19. Chow LC, Kwan SW, Olcott EW, Sommer G. Split-bolus MDCT urography with synchronous nephrographic and excretory phase enhancement. *AJR Am J Roentgenol*. 2007;189:314–322.

20. Dalrymple NC, Prasad SR, El-Merhi FM, Chintapalli KN. Price of isotropy in multidetector CT. *Radiographics*. 2007;27:49–62.

21. McCollough CH, Bruesewitz MR, Kofler JM Jr. CT dose reduction and dose management tools: overview of available options. *Radiographics*. 2006;26:503–512.

22. Dalrymple NC, Prasad SR, Freckleton MW, Chintapalli KN. Informatics in radiology (infoRAD): introduction to the language of three-dimensional imaging with multidetector CT. *Radiographics*. 2005;25:1409–1428.

23. Kawashima A, Vrtiska TJ, LeRoy AJ, Hartman RP, McCollough CH, King BF Jr. CT urography. *Radiographics*. 2004;24(suppl 1): S35–S54.

24. Nolte-Ernsting C, Cowan N. Understanding multislice CT urography techniques: many roads lead to Rome. *Eur Radiol*. 2006;16:2670–2686.

25. Noroozian M, Cohan RH, Caoili EM, Cowan NC, Ellis JH. Multislice CT urography: state of the art. *Br J Radiol*. 2004;77(Spec No 1):S74–S86.

26. Van Der Molen AJ, Cowan NC, Mueller-Lisse UG, Nolte-Ernsting CC, Takahashi S, Cohan RH. CT urography: definition, indications and techniques. A guideline for clinical practice. *Eur Radiol*. 2008;18:4–17.

27. Van Der Molen AJ, Cowan NC, Mueller-Lisse UG, Nolte-Ernsting CC, Takahashi S, Cohan RH. CT urography: definition, indications and techniques. A guideline for clinical practice. *Eur Radiol*. 2008;18:4–17.

28. Morcos SK. Computed tomography urography technique, indications and limitations. *Curr Opin Urol*. 2007;17:56–64.

29. Nolte-Ernsting CC, Wildberger JE, Borchers H, Schmitz-Rode T, Gunther RW. Multi-slice CT urography after diuretic injection: initial results. *Rofo*. 2001;173:176–180.

30. Silverman SG, Akbar SA, Mortele KJ, Tuncali K, Bhagwat JG, Seifter JL. Multi-detector row CT urography of normal urinary collecting system: furosemide versus saline as adjunct to contrast medium. *Radiology*. 2006;240:749–755.

31. Caoili EM, Inampudi P, Cohan RH, Ellis JH. Optimization of multi-detector row CT urography: effect of compression, saline administration, and prolongation of acquisition delay. *Radiology*. 2005;235:116–123.

32. Roy C, Jeantroux J, Irani FG, Sauer B, Lang H, Saussine C. Accuracy of intermediate dose of furosemide injection to improve multidetector row CT urography. *Eur J Radiol*. 2007;17:1262–1266.

33. Leyendecker JR, Barnes CE, Zagoria RJ. MR urography: techniques and clinical applications. *Radiographics*. 2008;28:23–46.

34. Nolte-Ernsting CC, Adam GB, Gunther RW. MR urography: examination techniques and clinical applications. *Eur Radiol*. 2001;11:355–372.

35. Thomsen HS. ESUR guideline: gadolinium-based contrast media and nephrogenic systemic fibrosis. *Eur Radiol*. 2007;17: 2692–2696.

36. Taylor A. Radionuclide renography: a personal approach. *Semin Nucl Med*. 1999;29:102–127.

37. Taylor A Jr, Nally JV. Clinical applications of renal scintigraphy. *AJR Am J Roentgenol*. 1995;164:31–41.

38. Dyer RB, Chen MY, Zagoria RJ. Abnormal calcifications in the urinary tract. *Radiographics*. 1998;18:1405–1424.

39. Dyer RB, Zagoria RJ. Radiological patterns of mineralization as predictor of urinary stone etiology, associated pathology, and therapeutic outcome. *J Stone Dis*. 1992;4:272–282.

40. Eray O, Cubuk MS, Oktay C, Yilmaz S, Cete Y, Ersoy FF. The efficacy of urinalysis, plain films, and spiral CT in ED patients with suspected renal colic. *Am J Emerg Med*. 2003;21:152–154.

41. Levine JA, Neitlich J, Verga M, Dalrymple N, Smith RC. Ureteral calculi in patients with flank pain: correlation of plain radiography with unenhanced helical CT. *Radiology*. 1997;204:27–31.

42. Jackman SV, Potter SR, Regan F, Jarrett TW. Plain abdominal x-ray versus computerized tomography screening: sensitivity for stone localization after nonenhanced spiral computerized tomography. *J Urol*. 2000;164:308–310.

43. Amis ES Jr. Epitaph for the urogram. *Radiology*. 1999;213:639–640.

44. Becker JA, Pollack HM, McClennan BL. Urography survives. *Radiology*. 2001;218:299–300.

45. Gallagher HJ, Tolley DA. 2000 AD: still a role for the intravenous urogram in stone management? *Curr Opin Urol*. 2000;10:551–555.

46. Pfister SA, Deckart A, Laschke S, et al. Unenhanced helical computed tomography vs intravenous urography in patients with acute flank pain: accuracy and economic impact in a randomized prospective trial. *Eur Radiol*. 2003;13:2513–2520.

47. Mutazindwa T, Husseini T. Imaging in acute renal colic: the intravenous urogram remains the gold standard. *Eur J Radiol*. 1996;23:238–240.

48. Shine S. Urinary calculus: IVU vs. CT renal stone? A critically appraised topic. *Abdom Imaging*. 2008;33:41–43.

49. Pollack HM, Arger PH, Goldberg BB, Mulholland SG. Ultrasonic detection of nonopaque renal calculi. *Radiology*. 1978;127:233–237.

50. Fowler KA, Locken JA, Duchesne JH, Williamson MR. US for detecting renal calculi with nonenhanced CT as a reference standard. *Radiology*. 2002;222:109–113.

51. Ulusan S, Koc Z, Tokmak N. Accuracy of sonography for detecting renal stone: comparison with CT. *J Clin Ultrasound*. 2007;35:256–261.

52. Aytac SK, Ozcan H. Effect of color Doppler system on the twinkling sign associated with urinary tract calculi. *J Clin Ultrasound*. 1999;27:433–439.

53. Lee JY, Kim SH, Cho JY, Han D. Color and power Doppler twinkling artifacts from urinary stones: clinical observations and phantom studies. *AJR Am J Roentgenol*. 2001;176:1441–1445.

54. Sheafor DH, Hertzberg BS, Freed KS, et al. Nonenhanced helical CT and US in the emergency evaluation of patients with renal colic: prospective comparison. *Radiology*. 2000;217:792–797.

55. Rosen CL, Brown DF, Sagarin MJ, Chang Y, McCabe CJ, Wolfe RE. Ultrasonography by emergency physicians in patients with suspected ureteral colic. *J Emerg Med*. 1998;16:865–870.

56. Patlas M, Farkas A, Fisher D, Zaghal I, Hadas-Halpern I. Ultrasound vs CT for the detection of ureteric stones in patients with renal colic. *Br J Radiol*. 2001;74:901–904.

57. Chen MY, Zagoria RJ, Saunders HS, Dyer RB. Trends in the use of unenhanced helical CT for acute urinary colic. *AJR Am J Roentgenol*. 1999;173:1447–1450.

58. Dalrymple NC, Verga M, Anderson KR, et al. The value of unenhanced helical computerized tomography in the management of acute flank pain. *J Urol*. 1998;159:735–740.

59. Vieweg J, Teh C, Freed K, et al. Unenhanced helical computerized tomography for the evaluation of patients with acute flank pain. *J Urol*. 1998;160:679–684.

60. Chowdhury FU, Kotwal S, Raghunathan G, Wah TM, Joyce A, Irving HC. Unenhanced multidetector CT (CT KUB) in the initial imaging of suspected acute renal colic: evaluating a new service. *Clin Radiol.* 2007;62:970–977.

61. Rucker CM, Menias CO, Bhalla S. Mimics of renal colic: alternative diagnoses at unenhanced helical CT. *Radiographics.* 2004;24(suppl 1):S11-S28.

62. Dean TE, Harrison NW, Bishop NL. CT scanning in the diagnosis and management of radiolucent urinary calculi. *Br J Urol.* 1988;62:405–408.

63. Schwartz BF, Schenkman N, Armenakas NA, Stoller ML. Imaging characteristics of indinavir calculi. *J Urol.* 1999;161:1085–1087.

64. Gentle DL, Stoller ML, Jarrett TW, Ward JF, Geib KS, Wood AF. Protease inhibitor-induced urolithiasis. *Urology.* 1997;50: 508–511.

65. Smith RC, Verga M, Dalrymple N, McCarthy S, Rosenfield AT. Acute ureteral obstruction: value of secondary signs of helical unenhanced CT. *AJR Am J Roentgenol.* 1996;167:1109–1113.

66. Dalrymple NC, Casford B, Raiken DP, Elsass KD, Pagan RA. Pearls and pitfalls in the diagnosis of ureterolithiasis with unenhanced helical CT. *Radiographics.* 2000;20:439–447.

67. Goldman SM, Faintuch S, Ajzen SA, et al. Diagnostic value of attenuation measurements of the kidney on unenhanced helical CT of obstructive ureterolithiasis. *AJR Am J Roentgenol.* 2004;182: 1251–1254.

68. Heneghan JP, Dalrymple NC, Verga M, Rosenfield AT, Smith RC. Soft-tissue "rim" sign in the diagnosis of ureteral calculi with use of unenhanced helical CT. *Radiology.* 1997;202:709–711.

69. Kawashima A, Sandler CM, Boridy IC, Takahashi N, Benson GS, Goldman SM. Unenhanced helical CT of ureterolithiasis: value of the tissue rim sign. *AJR Am J Roentgenol.* 1997;168:997–1000.

70. Boridy IC, Nikolaidis P, Kawashima A, Goldman SM, Sandler CM. Ureterolithiasis: value of the tail sign in differentiating phleboliths from ureteral calculi at nonenhanced helical CT. *Radiology.* 1999;211:619–621.

71. Rosser CJ, Zagoria R, Dixon R, et al. Is there a learning curve in diagnosing urolithiasis with noncontrast helical computed tomography? *Can Assoc Radiol J.* 2000;51:177–181.

72. Boridy IC, Kawashima A, Goldman SM, Sandler CM. Acute ureterolithiasis: nonenhanced helical CT findings of perinephric edema for prediction of degree of ureteral obstruction. *Radiology.* 1999;213:663–667.

73. Lorberboym M, Kapustin Z, Elias S, Nikolov G, Katz R. The role of renal scintigraphy and unenhanced helical computerized tomography in patients with ureterolithiasis. *Eur J Nucl Med.* 2000;27:441–446.

74. Sfakianakis GN, Cohen DJ, Braunstein RH, et al. MAG3-F0 scintigraphy in decision making for emergency intervention in renal colic after helical CT positive for a urolith. *J Nucl Med.* 2000;41:1813–1822.

75. Miller FH, Kraemer E, Dalal K, Keppke A, Huo E, Hoff FL. Unexplained renal colic: what is the utility of IV contrast? *Clin Imaging.* 2005;29:331–336.

76. Meagher T, Sukumar VP, Collingwood J, et al. Low dose computed tomography in suspected acute renal colic. *Clin Radiol.* 2001;56:873–876.

77. Mulkens TH, Daineffe S, De WR, et al. Urinary stone disease: comparison of standard-dose and low-dose with 4D MDCT tube current modulation. *AJR Am J Roentgenol.* 2007;188:553–562.

78. Kluner C, Hein PA, Gralla O, et al. Does ultra-low-dose CT with a radiation dose equivalent to that of KUB suffice to detect renal and ureteral calculi? *J Comput Assist Tomogr.* 2006;30:44–50.

79. Kawashima A, Glockner JF, King BF Jr. CT urography and MR urography. *Radiol Clin N Am.* 2003;41:945–961.

80. Spencer JA, Chahal R, Kelly A, Taylor K, Eardley I, Lloyd SN. Evaluation of painful hydronephrosis in pregnancy: magnetic resonance urographic patterns in physiological dilatation versus calculous obstruction. *J Urol.* 2004;171:256–260.

81. Jung P, Brauers A, Nolte-Ernsting CA, Jakse G, Gunther RW. Magnetic resonance urography enhanced by gadolinium and diuretics: a comparison with conventional urography in diagnosing the cause of ureteric obstruction. *BJU Int.* 2000;86:960–965.

82. Regan F, Petronis J, Bohlman M, Rodriguez R, Moore R. Perirenal MR high signal–a new and sensitive indicator of acute ureteric obstruction. *Clin Radiol.* 1997;52:445–450.

83. Sudah M, Vanninen R, Partanen K, Heino A, Vainio P, la Opas M. MR urography in evaluation of acute flank pain: T2-weighted sequences and gadolinium-enhanced three-dimensional FLASH compared with urography. Fast low-angle shot. *AJR Am J Roentgenol.* 2001;176:105–112.

84. Sudah M, Vanninen RL, Partanen K, et al. Patients with acute flank pain: comparison of MR urography with unenhanced helical CT. *Radiology.* 2002;223:98–105.

85. Otnes B, Sandnes H. Comparison of radiological measurement and actual size of ureteral calculi. *Scand J Urol Nephrol.* 1978;12:155–156.

86. Sandhu C, Anson KM, Patel U. Urinary tract stonesLPart I: role of radiological imaging in diagnosis and treatment planning. *Clin Radiol.* 2003;58:415–421.

87. Foley WD. Renal MDCT. *Eur J Radiol.* 2003;45(suppl 1):S73–S78.

88. Hubert J, Blum A, Cormier L, Claudon M, Regent D, Mangin P. Three-dimensional CT-scan reconstruction of renal calculi. A new tool for mapping-out staghorn calculi and follow-up of radiolucent stones. *Eur Urol.* 1997;31:297–301.

89. Van Beers BE, Dechambre S, Hulcelle P, Materne R, Jamart J. Value of multislice helical CT scans and maximum-intensity-projection images to improve detection of ureteral stones at abdominal radiography. *AJR Am J Roentgenol.* 2001;177:1117–1121.

90. Lin WC, Uppot RN, Li CS, Hahn PF, Sahani DV. Value of automated coronal reformations from 64-section multidetector row computerized tomography in the diagnosis of urinary stone disease. *J Urol.* 2007;178:907–911.

91. Memarsadeghi M, Schaefer-Prokop C, Prokop M, et al. Unenhanced MDCT in patients with suspected urinary stone disease: do coronal reformations improve diagnostic performance? *AJR Am J Roentgenol.* 2007;189:W60-W64.

92. Narepalem N, Sundaram CP, Boridy IC, Yan Y, Heiken JP, Clayman RV. Comparison of helical computerized tomography and plain radiography for estimating urinary stone size. *J Urol.* 2002;167:1235–1238.

93. Dundee P, Bouchier-Hayes D, Haxhimolla H, Dowling R, Costello A. Renal tract calculi: comparison of stone size on plain radiography and noncontrast spiral CT scan. *J Endourol.* 2006;20: 1005–1009.

94. Memarsadeghi M, Heinz-Peer G, Helbich TH, et al. Unenhanced multi-detector row CT in patients suspected of having urinary stone disease: effect of section width on diagnosis. *Radiology.* 2005;235:530–536.

95. Kampa RJ, Ghani KR, Wahed S, Patel U, Anson KM. Size matters: a survey of how urinary-tract stones are measured in the UK. *J Endourol.* 2005;19:856–860.

96. Raman JD, Pearle MS. Management options for lower pole renal calculi. *Curr Opin Urol.* 2008;18:214–219.

97. Fielding JR, Steele G, Fox LA, Heller H, Loughlin KR. Spiral computerized tomography in the evaluation of acute flank pain: a replacement for excretory urography. *J Urol.* 1997;157:2071–2073.

98. Greenstein A, Beri A, Sofer M, Matzkin H. Is intravenous urography a prerequisite for renal shockwave lithotripsy? *J Endourol.* 2003;17:835–839.

99. Ghani KR, Rintoul M, Patel U, Anson K. Three-dimensional planning of percutaneous renal stone surgery in a horseshoe kidney

using 16-slice CT and volume-rendered movies. *J Endourol.* 2005;19:461–463.

100. Sengupta S, Donnellan S, Vincent JM, Webb DR. CT analysis of caliceal anatomy in the supine and prone positions. *J Endourol.* 2000;14:555–557.

101. Fong YK, Peh SO, Ho SH, Ng FC, Quek PL, Ng KK. Lower pole ratio: a new and accurate predictor of lower pole stone clearance after shockwave lithotripsy? *Int J Urol.* 2004;11:700–703.

102. Sandhu C, Anson KM, Patel U. Urinary tract stones–Part II: current status of treatment. *Clin Radiol.* 2003;58:422–433.

103. Coll DM, Varanelli MJ, Smith RC. Relationship of spontaneous passage of ureteral calculi to stone size and location as revealed by unenhanced helical CT. *AJR Am J Roentgenol.* 2002;178:101–103.

104. Segura JW, Preminger GM, Assimos DG, et al. Ureteral Stones Clinical Guidelines Panel summary report on the management of ureteral calculi The American Urological Association. *J Urol.* 1997;158:1915–1921.

105. Pearle MS, Pierce HL, Miller GL, et al. Optimal method of urgent decompression of the collecting system for obstruction and infection due to ureteral calculi. *J Urol.* 1998;160:1260–1264.

106. Pearle MS, Nadler R, Bercowsky E, et al. Prospective randomized trial comparing shock wave lithotripsy and ureteroscopy for management of distal ureteral calculi. *J Urol.* 2001;166:1255–1260.

107. Ng CS, Herts BR, Streem SB. Percutaneous access to upper pole renal stones: role of prone 3-dimensional computerized tomography in inspiratory and expiratory phases. *J Urol.* 2005;173:124–126.

108. Bilen CY, Kocak B, Kitirci G, Danaci M, Sarikaya S. Simple trigonometry on computed tomography helps in planning renal access. *Urology.* 2007;70:242–245.

109. Park S, Pearle MS. Imaging for percutaneous renal access and management of renal calculi. *Urol Clin N Am.* 2006;33:353–364.

110. Rassweiler JJ, Renner C, Chaussy C, Thuroff S. Treatment of renal stones by extracorporeal shockwave lithotripsy: an update. *Eur Urol.* 2001;39:187–199.

111. Weld KJ, Montiglio C, Morris MS, Bush AC, Cespedes RD. Shock wave lithotripsy success for renal stones based on patient and stone computed tomography characteristics. *Urology.* 2007;70:1043–1046.

112. Albala DM, Assimos DG, Clayman RV, et al. Lower pole I: a prospective randomized trial of extracorporeal shock wave lithotripsy and percutaneous nephrostolithotomy for lower pole nephrolithiasis-initial results. *J Urol.* 2001;166:2072–2080.

113. Wang LJ, Wong YC, Chuang CK, et al. Predictions of outcomes of renal stones after extracorporeal shock wave lithotripsy from stone characteristics determined by unenhanced helical computed tomography: a multivariate analysis. *Eur Radiol.* 2005;15:2238–2243.

114. Segura JW. Staghorn calculi. *Urol Clin N Am.* 1997;24:71–80.

115. Gettman MT, Segura JW. Struvite stones: diagnosis and current treatment concepts. *J Endourol.* 1999;13:653–658.

116. Ramakumar S, Patterson DE, Leroy AJ, et al. Prediction of stone composition from plain radiographs: a prospective study. *J Endourol.* 1999;13:397–401.

117. Bani-Hani AH, Segura JW, Leroy AJ. Urinary matrix calculi: our experience at a single institution. *J Urol.* 2005;173:120–123.

118. Nakada SY, Hoff DG, Attai S, Heisey D, Blankenbaker D, Pozniak M. Determination of stone composition by noncontrast spiral computed tomography in the clinical setting. *Urology.* 2000;55:816–819.

119. Primak AN, Fletcher JG, Vrtiska TJ, et al. Noninvasive differentiation of uric acid versus non-uric acid kidney stones using dual-energy CT. *Acad Radiol.* 2007;14:1441–1447.

120. Preminger GM. Pharmacologic treatment of uric acid calculi. *Urol Clin N Am.* 1987;14:335–338.

121. Kim SC, Hatt EK, Lingeman JE, Nadler RB, McAteer JA, Williams JC Jr. Cystine: helical computerized tomography characterization of rough and smooth calculi in vitro. *J Urol.* 2005;174:1468–1470.

122. Kessaris DN, Bellman GC, Pardalidis NP, Smith AG. Management of hemorrhage after percutaneous renal surgery. *J Urol.* 1995;153:604–608.

123. Gremmo E, Ballanger P, Dore B. Aubert J (Hemorrhagic complications during percutaneous nephrolithotomy. Retrospective studies of 772 cases). *Prog Urol.* 1999;9:460–463.

124. Lehtoranta K, Mankinen P, Taari K, Rannikko S, Lehtonen T, Salo J. Residual stones after percutaneous nephrolithotomy; sensitivities of different imaging methods in renal stone detection. *Ann Chir Gynaecol.* 1995;84:43–49.

125. Osman Y, El-Tabey N, Refai H, et al. Detection of residual stones after percutaneous nephrolithotomy: role of nonenhanced spiral computerized tomography. *J Urol.* 2008;179:198–200.

126. Park J, Hong B, Park T, Park HK. Effectiveness of noncontrast computed tomography in evaluation of residual stones after percutaneous nephrolithotomy. *J Endourol.* 2007;21:684–687.

127. Pearle MS, Watamull LM, Mullican MA. Sensitivity of noncontrast helical computerized tomography and plain film radiography compared to flexible nephroscopy for detecting residual fragments after percutaneous nephrostolithotomy. *J Urol.* 1999;162:23–26.

128. Bugg CE Jr, El-Galley R, Kenney PJ, Burns JR. Follow-up functional radiographic studies are not mandatory for all patients after ureteroscopy. *Urology.* 2002;59:662–667.

129. Chen KK, Chen MT, Yeh SH, Chang LS. Radionuclide renal function study in various surgical treatments of upper urinary stones. *Zhonghua Yi Xue Za Zhi (Taipei).* 1992;49:319–327.

130. Moskovitz B, Halachmi S, Sopov V, et al. Effect of percutaneous nephrolithotripsy on renal function: assessment with quantitative SPECT of (99 m)Tc-DMSA renal scintigraphy. *J Endourol.* 2006;20:102–106.

131. Elgazzar AH, Mahmoud AH, el Sayed M, et al. Evaluation of renal functional changes after extracorporeal piezoelectric lithotripsy (EPL) by radionuclide studies. *Nucl Med Commun.* 1990;11:579–583.

132. Gupta M, Bolton DM, Irby P III, et al. The effect of newer generation lithotripsy upon renal function assessed by nuclear scintigraphy. *J Urol.* 1995;154:947–950.

133. Michaels EK, Pavel DG, Orellana P, Montes A, Olea E. Use of radionuclide renal imaging for clinical followup after extracorporeal shock wave lithotripsy of renal stones. *J Urol.* 1992;148:1015–1021.

Gernot Schubert

Abstract The main urinary stone components as well as drug-induced stones are presented. The morphology of stones is described. The frequency of stone components as main component, the frequencies of occurrence of stone components, and the frequency of different combinations of components (stone types) are given. The importance and the forms of texture types and the core-shell relations are represented. The purposes and problems of stone analysis are discussed. The methods of stone analysis polarization microscopy, X-ray diffraction, and infrared spectroscopy are described, while the benefits and disadvantages of these methods are evaluated. The results of ring trials show that the X-ray diffraction method is the best method with regard to correctness. A combination of two or three methods including X-ray diffraction is recommendable.

29.1 Introduction

Urinary stones are solid biogenous formations of the urinary system. Mainly they have a crystalline structure; the size is more than 1 mm. About 95% of stones are crystalline components and 5% are organic components, as different kinds of proteins or the so-called matrix.[1]

29.2 Stone Components

29.2.1 Urinary Stone Components

There are different groups of urinary stone components (Table 29.1) with reference to mineralogical and chemical composition[2]:

- Inorganic crystalline substances: calcium oxalates, calcium phosphates, and magnesium-ammonium phosphates
- Organic crystalline substances: uric acid and several purine derivates and urates
- L-cystine
- Crystalline drug–induced stones

G. Schubert
Institute of Laboratory Diagnostics, Vivantes Klinikum im Friedrichshain, Berlin, Germany
e-mail: gernot.schubert@vivantes.de

- Organic noncrystalline substances: protein, matrix stones, blood coagulum
- Artifacts, falsifications

Some examples of crystalline drug–induced stones include: indinavir monohydrate, atanazavir sulfate, ceftriaxone (as calcium ceftriaxonate), N4-acetylsulfadiazine, N4-acetylsulfamethoxazole, amoxicillin trihydrate, and triamterene.[3,4]

Quartz, calcite, gypsum, and seedcorns are found as artifacts or falsifications among others.

29.2.2 Frequency of Stone Components

The abundance of the main groups of stone components is very different. Table 29.2 shows the frequencies of stone components as main component and the frequencies of occurrence of the different stone components.[1,2]

The most frequent components are the calcium oxalates whewellite and weddellite as calcium oxalate monohydrate and dihydrate. The occurrence frequency of whewellite is 78%; that of weddellite is 43%. A calcium oxalate trihydrate was described in the literature,[5] but the occurrence was not confirmed by other authors. Also the occurrence of a second form of calcium oxalate monohydrate has been observed.[6]

- Apatite (or carbonate apatite) is a very frequent stone component with a 33% occurrence rate.

Table 29.1 Urinary stone components

Mineral name	Chemical name	Chemical formula
Calcium oxalates		
Whewellite	Calcium oxalate monohydrate	$CaC_2O_4 \times H_2O$
Weddellite	Calcium oxalate dihydrate	$CaC_2O_4 \times 2\,H_2O$
Calcium phosphates		
Apatite	Calcium phosphate	$Ca_{10}(PO_4,CO_3)_6(OH,CO_3)$
Brushite	Calcium hydrogen phosphate dihydrate	$CaHPO_4 \times 2\,H_2O$
Whitlockite	Tricalciumphosphate	$Ca_3(PO)_4$
	Octa calcium phosphate	$Ca_8H_2(PO_4) \times 5\,H_2O$
Magnesium-Ammonium-Phosphates		
Struvite	Magnesium-ammonium-phosphate hexahydrate	$MgNH_4PO_4 \times 6\,H_2O$
Newberyite	Magnesiumhydrogen-phosphate trihydrate	$MgHPO_4 \times 3\,H_2O$
Purine derivates		
Uricite	Uric acid	$C_5H_4N_4O_3$
	Uric acid monohydrate	$C_5H_4N_4O_3 \times H_2O$
	Uric acid dihydrate	$C_5H_4N_4O_3 \times 2\,H_2O$
	Ammonium hydrogen urate	$NH_4C_5H_3N_4O_3$
	Natriumhydrogenurate monohydrate	$NaC_5H_3N_4O_3 \times H_2O$
	Kaliumhydrogenurate	$KC_5H_3N_4O_3 \times H_2O$
	Xanthine	$C_5H_4N_4O_2$
	2,8-Dihydroxyadenine	$C_5H_4N_5O_2$
L-cystine		$C_6H_{12}N_2O_4S_2$
Other substances		
	Organic substances	
	Drug-induced stones	
	Artifacts, falsifications	

Table 29.2 Frequency of urinary stone components (%)

Stone component	Main component ($n = 72.383$)	Frequency of occurrence ($n = 111,196$)
Whewellite	59.5	77.5
Weddellite	13.5	42.8
Apatite	9.7	32.5
Uric acid	7.5	10.0
Struvite	3.3	5.9
Uric acid dihydrate	2.0	5.5
Brushite	0.6	1.1
Ammoniumurate	0.4	0.9
Cystine	0.3	0.3
Octacalciumphosphate	0.02	0.2
Whitlockite	0.03	0.1
Na-, K-urate	0.03	0.03
Uric acid monohydrate	<0.01	<0.01
Newberyite	<0.01	<0.01
Calcite, aragonite	<0.01	<0.01
Drug stones	<0.01	<0.01
Organic stones	0.7	0.7
Artifacts, falsifications	2.3	2.3
Total	100.0	

- Brushite does not appear frequently (1–2% occurrence rate), but the frequency of brushite has increased in the last years.
- The other calcium phosphates such as whitlockite and octacalcium phosphate are very rare.
- The most typical infection stone component is struvite with a frequency of 6%.
- Struvite often forms big staghorn stones with apatite.
- Newberyite is a very rare transformation product of struvite.
- Uric acid is a frequent stone constituent with a frequency of 10% as well as uric acid dihydrate at a 6% occurrence rate.
- Uric acid monohydrate is very rare, and recently described by the author for the first time.[7]
- The very rare occurrence of a second form of uric acid[8] could be confirmed by the author.[9]
- Ammonium urate has a frequency of 1%.
- The other urates and purine derivates, such as xanthine and dihydroxyadenine, are absolutely rare.
- L-cystine is not that frequent with 0.3%, but it is important because of the high recurrence rate without metaphylaxis.

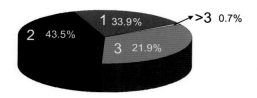

Fig. 29.1 Number of components in urinary stones ($n = 70{,}131$)

Only seven urinary stone components have a frequency of occurrence of greater than 1%. The other stone minerals, about 15, range from rare up to very, very rare. Noteworthy is the percentage of artifacts with a 2.3% frequency rate.

The majority of 44% of all stones ($n = 70{,}131$) consists of two minerals[1]; 34% are monominerals; 22% consist of three minerals; and only 0.7% consist of four, five, or six components.

The fact that mixtures of stone components play such an enormous role is important for stone analysis and for the classification of the stone patient in a metaphylactic group (Fig. 29.1).[10]

The author examined the frequency of different combinations of listed components in a more detailed analysis,[10] finding a considerable diversity resulting in 145 different combinations of stone components (stone types). However, the vast majority of these combinations have to be considered as rare stone types. Only 25 stone types (Table 29.3) show a frequency over 0.1%; they represent 99% of all urinary stones. Out of these, 12 types have a frequency of 0.1–1%, whereas the remaining 13 stone types are found more frequently; that is, more than 1%. The three stone types, whewellite and whewellite-weddellite and whewellite-weddellite-apatite, account for 70% of all calculi already on their own.

29.2.3 Morphology and Structure of Stone Components

29.2.3.1 Morphology

There is a very broad variety in appearance, color, and consistency of the different urinary stones. The composition and the localization of stone forming influence the appearance of urinary stones.

Whewellite stones usually have a dark-brown or black color. The lighter the color, the higher the content of organic material. The surface is often mulberry-like or morningstar-like (Fig. 29.2a). The stones are very hard.

Weddellite stones mostly have a loose structure and a gray-yellow color (Fig. 29.2b). Especially noteworthy are crystals of tetragonal-dipyramidal morphology. The crystals are sharp and in various orientations with the edges on the outer surface. The author mostly found the compact whewellite as the

Table 29.3 Frequency of stone types >0.1% ($n = 72{,}383$)

Stone type	%
Whewellite	28
Whewellite-weddellite	24.6
Whewellite-weddellite-apatite	17.8
Whewellite-apatite	4.8
Struvite-apatite	4.6
Uric acid-uric acid dihydrate	4.1
Artifacts, falsifications	2.5
Uric acid	2.1
Whewellite-uric acid	1.9
Weddellite-apatite	1.3
Whewellite-uric acid-uric acid dihydrate	1.3
Apatite	1.1
Whewellite-struvite-apatite	1.1
Weddellite	0.8
Organic substances	0.7
Struvite-apatite-ammoniumurate	0.4
Brushite-apatite	0.3
Whewellite-weddellite-uric acid	0.3
Cystine	0.3
Uric acid dihydrate	0.2
Whewellite-weddellite-struvite-apatite	0.2
Whewellite-weddellite-uric acid-uric acid dihydrate	0.2
Uric acid-ammoniumurate	0.1
Brushite	0.1
Brushite-apatite-whewellite	0.1
Total (frequency > 0.1%)	98.6

core and the weddellite crystals on the surface of mixed stones of whewellite-weddellite (Fig. 29.2c).

Apatite stones (Fig. 29.2d) have a white or gray color. The surface is mostly smooth, and the consistency ranges from solid to loose. Brushite stones (Fig. 29.2e) are usually very hard. The color differs between white and gray. They often have a cauliflower-like surface.

Struvite often forms with apatite mixed stones in the form of big staghorn stones (Fig. 29.2f). The color is mostly white to light gray. In most cases, they have a loose consistency.

The color of stones of uric acid and uric acid dihydrate (Fig. 29.2g) varies from light yellow via red-yellow to red-brown. The higher the content of uric acid hydrate, the more intensive the color in mixed stones. Their surfaces are mostly very smooth.

The rarely found uric acid monohydrate (Fig. 29.2h) and the urate stones mostly have a white to gray color and a loose consistency.

Stones of cystine (Fig. 29.2i) have a typical yellow color and a wax-like surface. The consistency is very solid.

The so-called matrix stones consist of pure protein or protein with struvite-apatite. The matrix stones have a very soft consistency in their native state, but become solid after drying.

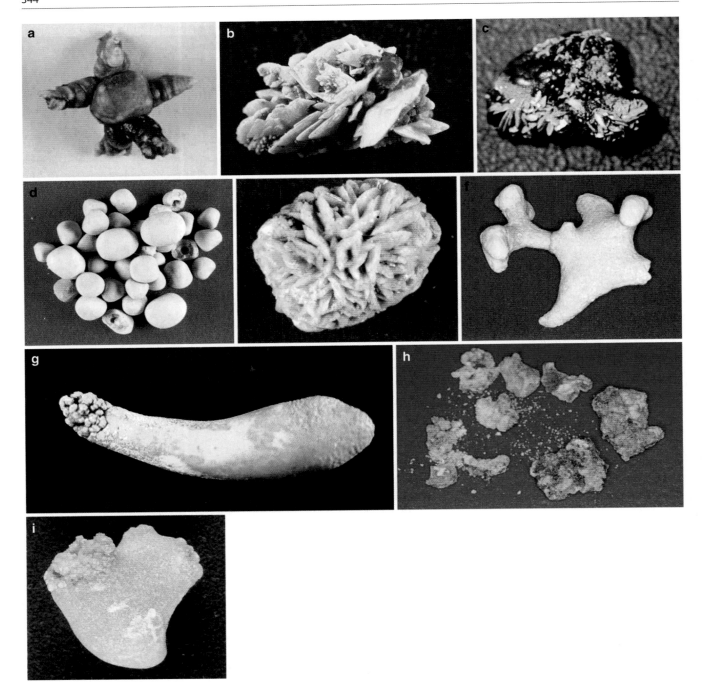

Fig. 29.2 Morphology of urinary stone. (**a**) Whewellite. (**b**) Weddellite. (**c**) Weddellite crystals on whewellite core. (**d**) Apatite. (**e**) Brushite. (**f**) Struvite-apatite. (**g**) Uric acid. (**h**) Uric acid monohydrate. (**i**) L-cystine

29.2.3.2 Texture

The term *texture* describes the shape and the morphological appearance of grains or crystals, and the relative arrangement of crystals to each other and relative to the geometry of stones.

The calcium oxalate stones show a large variety of morphological and structural forms of appearance due to the existence of the two hydrate levels (whewellite and weddellite) and the transformation phenomenon of weddellite into whewellite.[11,12]

The author has reduced the various forms of texture appearance of calcium oxalate calculi to four basic texture types:

- *Type 1*: concentrically laminated whewellite texture with differing degrees of fibrous-radial arrangement of whewellite crystals. This is the so-called annual ring texture (Fig. 29.3a).

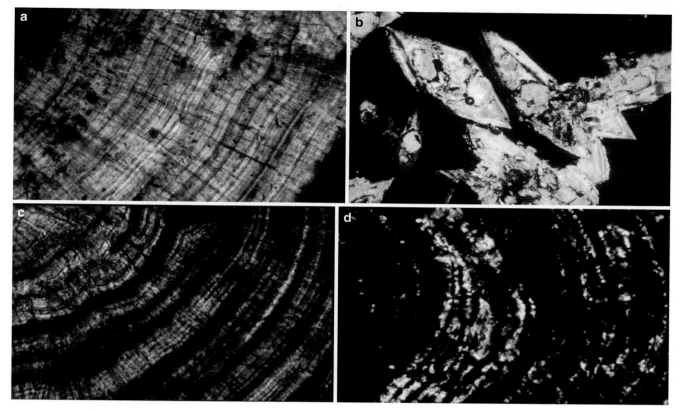

Fig. 29.3 Polarization microphotographs of texture types (thin sections). (**a**) Calcium oxalate type 1 – concentrically laminated texture with fibrous-radial arrangement of whewellite crystals. (**b**) Calcium oxalate type 4 – irregular texture of idiomorphic weddellite crystals.

(**c**) Uric acid type 2 – concentrically laminated texture with radial arrangement of uric acid crystals. (**d**) Struvite-apatite texture type 2 with concentrically laminated texture with a pearl necklace-like arrangement of struvite crystals

- *Type 2*: fine to very fine-grained irregular whewellite texture.
- *Type 3*: mosaic texture of irregularly oriented whewellite single crystals, often containing morphological weddellite residues.
- *Type 4*: irregular texture of idiomorphic weddellite crystals (Fig. 29.3b).

The occurrence of these texture types is not random, but is determined by certain pathogenetic factors such as hypercalciuria.[13] Also, the other urinary stones show different texture types. The uric acid/uric acid dihydrate stones have:

1. A fine-grained irregular texture
2. A concentrically laminated texture, sometimes with a radial arrangement of uric acid crystals (Fig. 29.3c)

The struvite-apatite stones show three texture types:

1. Irregular mosaic texture of struvite crystals with apatite as basic matter
2. Concentric laminated texture with a pearl necklace-like arrangement of struvite crystals in apatite basic matter (Fig. 29.3d)
3. Fibrous-radial arrangement of mostly very big struvite crystals

29.2.3.3 Core–Shell Relations

The different components in mixed stones can be homogenously distributed over the total stone or the different components are arranged separately in core and different shells (Fig. 29.4). Approximately 25% of all stones show qualitative differences

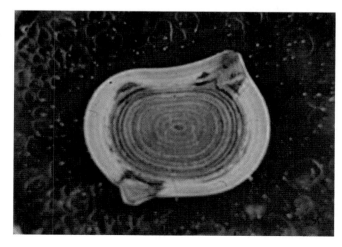

Fig. 29.4 Urinary stone with core of uric acid and shell of whewellite (grind)

of the composition of central and peripheral stone parts. With respect to metapylaxis, the differences between core and shell appear to be most important for the following stone types: calcium oxalate-uric acid, calcium oxalate-struvite, and uric acid-struvite. These types represent up to 5% of all calculi.[10,14]

29.3 Purposes and Problems of Stone Analysis

The purpose of stone analysis is the extensive qualitative differentiation of all stone components, especially of the different hydrate forms, the urates and purine derivates, and of the several calcium phosphates. Furthermore, another purpose is the semiquantitative determination of all components in mixtures.

The analysis of demanding stone phases, such as rare purine derivates, drug-induced stones, and artifacts in some cases, presents a certain problem. The consideration of inhomogeneities (core-shell, disintegrates in stones) and problems of cost efficiency are important, too.

The stone analysis is of importance to the therapy and metaphylaxis of residual and recurrent stones.

- Composition and structure refer to the choice of therapy methods:

    - Litholysis in case of uric acid and struvite
    - The choice of ureteroscopy or percutaneous nephrolithotomy as alternative methods for shockwave-resistant stones such as whewellite, brushite, and cystine[15]

- The exact stone analysis is the basic requirement for an effective metaphylaxis.

The correct determination of the stone type is essential for the classification of the stone patient in the matching metaphylactic group. The main component in mixed stones is not decisive for the classification of patients in the metaphylactic group in every case. A content of 30% struvite in a mixed stone with apatite would be a reason for the classification of a patient in the infection stone group and not in the calcium stone group, for example.

29.4 Methods of Stone Analysis

29.4.1 Overall View of Methods of Stone Analysis

A large number of methods in the past were used for the determination of the composition of urinary stones. Table 29.4 shows an overall view of the several methods

Table 29.4 Methods of urinary stone analysis and their evidence

Methods of analysis	Possible information on		
	Chemical composition	Mineralogical composition	Texture
Chemical analysis	x	(x)	
Thermal analysis	(x)	(x)	
Electron diffraction		x	
Scanning electron microscopy		(x)	x
Electron microprobe	x	(x)	
Laser microprobe	x	(x)	
X-ray microradiography		(x)	
Polarization microscopy		x	x
Infrared spectroscopy		x	
X-ray diffraction		x	

x – full information (x) – limited information

used for stone analysis and their validity. Only some methods can give the exact stone composition as per the stone components in Table 29.1. Some methods can only give a content of atoms and molecules (chemical methods, for example). Only the methods like polarization microscopy and scanning electron microscopy deliver findings to the texture of urinary stones.

In the last years, three methods turned out to be the best methods of stone analysis: X-ray diffraction, infrared spectroscopy, and polarization microscopy. These methods meet the demands for stone analysis (see previous section).

The principles, benefits, and disadvantages of polarization microscopy, X-ray diffraction, and infrared spectroscopy are described in the following sections.

29.4.2 Polarization Microscopy

Polarization microscopy is based on the interaction of polarized light with the crystals of stones. The internal morphology, color, the refraction of light, and birefringence of crystals or crystal aggregates are parameters for the identification of stone minerals.[16,17] The principal pattern of the polarization investigation is shown in Fig. 29.5. Some micrographs of grain preparations are depicted in Fig. 29.6a–f.

The benefits of polarization microscopy are:

- Cost efficiency
- Quick examinations and analyses of very small samples are possible

    - This method is really the final analysis for simple stones as whewellite or weddellite.
    - Very small contents of components in the stones are detectable.

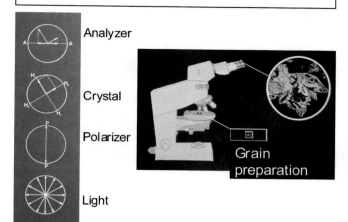

Fig. 29.5 Principal pattern of polarization investigation

The disadvantages are:

- High subjective experience is necessary.
- Differentiation of components is difficult in some cases in the groups of uric acid and purine derivates and calcium phosphates.
- The quantitative analysis in mixtures is difficult in some cases.

29.4.3 Infrared Spectroscopy

The infrared spectroscopy is based on the interaction of infrared-light and the molecules in the stone components.[4,18,19] The light stimulates atomic vibrations, and the consequence is energy absorption. The energy absorption results in absorption bands in the infrared spectrum (Fig. 29.7).

A new technique in the infrared spectroscopy is the method of *Attenuated Total Reflection* – the diamond ATR method (Fig. 29.8). The advantages of this technique are the easy preparation and the application for soft samples. The infrared spectra of some stone components are shown in Fig. 29.9a, b, d–f.

The benefits of the infrared spectroscopy are:

- Moderate costs.
- Quick examination using Fourier transformation infrared-technique.
- Examinations of small samples are possible.
- The preparation is easy using ATR-technique.

- Semiautomatic evaluations are possible, applying search-match functions.
- Noncrystalline substances (as proteins or fat) are detectable.

The disadvantages are:

- Time-consuming preparation applying the usual tablets technique with potassium bromide.
- Differentiation and qualitative analyses are in some cases difficult; for example, in the case of uric acid, purines, and calcium phosphates.
- The detection of small contents of components is in some cases difficult; for example, whewellite in weddellite or reverse, or urates and uric acid dihydrate in uric acid and others.

29.4.4 X-ray Diffraction

X-ray diffraction is based on the diffraction of X-rays on crystal lattice.[20,21] Subject to certain conditions, there are diffraction maxima corresponding to the Bragg-equation (Fig. 29.10).

Figure 29.11 shows X-ray equipment, used by our laboratory, with the X-ray tube, the sample changer, and the detector. The measurement of up to 12 samples is programmable. An autoquan program allows the exact and easy quantitative analysis of the stone components.

Figure 29.12a–f show the X-ray diffractograms of some stone components. The benefits of this method are:

- Easy preparation.
- Automatic measurement (using a sample changer).
- Semiautomatic evaluation of the X-ray diffractogram (search-match program).
- Quantitative analyses (applying the autoquan system).
- Exact differentiation of all crystalline components is possible.

The disadvantages are:

- High costs of X-ray equipment.
- Noncrystalline substances are not detectable.
- Time per measurement is up to 30 min (the time per measurement using X-ray diffraction can be reduced considerably by means of up-to-date equipment).

29.5 Evaluation of Analysis Methods

The previously described methods – X-ray diffraction, polarization microscopy, and infrared spectroscopy – all have their benefits and their disadvantages. All benefits of

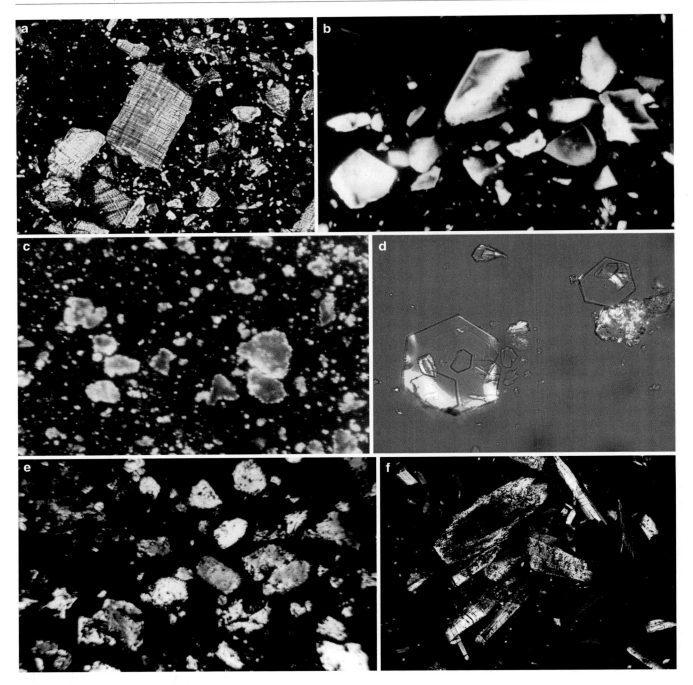

Fig. 29.6 Polarization microphotographs of grain preparations. (**a**) Whewellite. (**b**) Weddellite. (**c**) Uric acid. (**d**) L-cystine. (**e**) Struvite. (**f**) Brushite

the applied methods can be used to the best advantage with a combination of two or three of the mentioned methods.

Very beneficial is the combination of all three methods. Figure 29.13 shows a flow chart of such a combined analysis. The analysis starts with the polarization microscopic

investigation of a grain preparation of the stone. A final result can be expected for simple monomineralic stones (whewellite or weddellite for example).

The following investigation by X-ray diffraction is necessary for the stone groups uric acid (and urates) and the phosphates and for polymineralic stones. After that, we obtain a

Fig. 29.7 Principal pattern of infrared spectroscopy

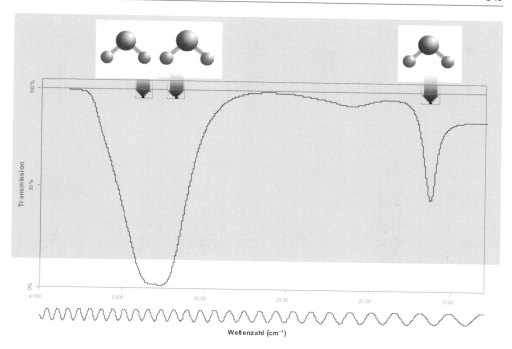

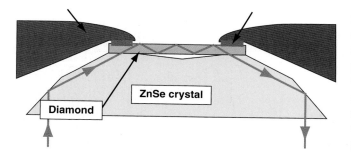

Fig. 29.8 The principle of ATR Technique

qualitatively and quantitatively exact result of the stone composition. For organic stones (protein, fat, gallstones) and drug-induced stones, the use of the infrared spectroscopy using the ATR-technique is very helpful.

The German Society of Clinical Chemistry and Laboratory Medicine (DGKL) periodically organizes a survey for urinary calculi analyses for quality control in stone analysis. The result of the survey for urinary stone analysis in the year 2008 is helpful for the evaluation of the different methods. One sample consisted of 60% apatite, 20% whewellite, and 20% uric acid. This is a relatively rare mixture; however, the material came from a native urinary stone. The qualitative correctness for the participants using X-ray diffraction was 100% for apatite, whewellite, and uric acid. There were no false analyses. Referring to the

infrared spectroscopy, 93% of the participants detected apatite correctly, but only 61% detected whewellite correctly and 57% detected uric acid correctly. Thirty-eight percent of participants gave false analyses with struvite, weddellite, uric acid dihydrate, and protein. The participants using chemical methods could only give simplified analyses results with 100% of all participants for calcium oxalate and calcium phosphate, but only 33% for uric acid.

29.6 Conclusions

Unfortunately, many urologists make no use of stone analysis due to cost reasons, ignorance, or convenience. The results of the ring trials reveal that the quality of stone analysis has room for improvement, despite the use of exact methods such as infrared spectroscopy. A professional and accurate stone analysis in special stone analysis centers is absolutely necessary.

The results of the evaluation of stone analyses for recurrent stone formation show significant differences in the stone composition in 35% of all patients, and at stone formation in different sides of the urinary tract in 30% of all patients.[22] For that reason, one stone analysis for each stone episode per patient is required for an effective therapy and metaphylaxis.

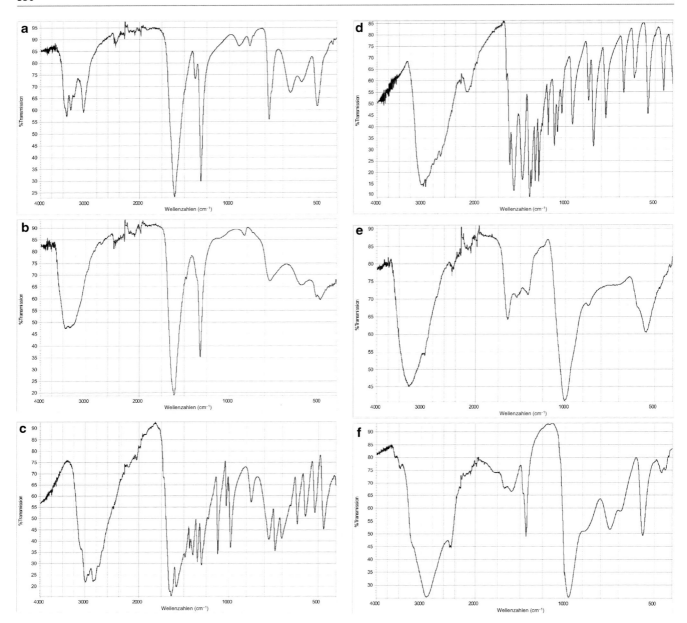

Fig. 29.9 Infared spectra of some stone components. (**a**) Whewellite. (**b**) Weddellite. (**c**) Uric acid. (**d**) L-cystine. (**e**) Apatite. (**f**) Struvite

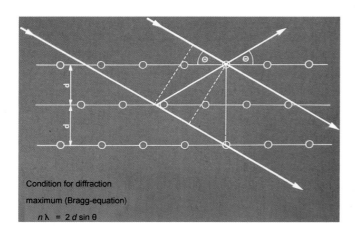

Condition for diffraction

maximum (Bragg-equation)

$n\lambda = 2d\sin\theta$

Fig. 29.10 Diffraction of X-rays on the crystal lattice

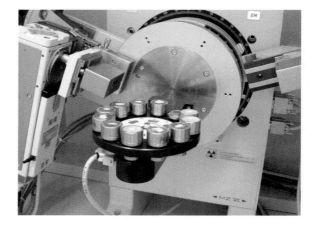

Fig. 29.11 X-ray diffraction equipment

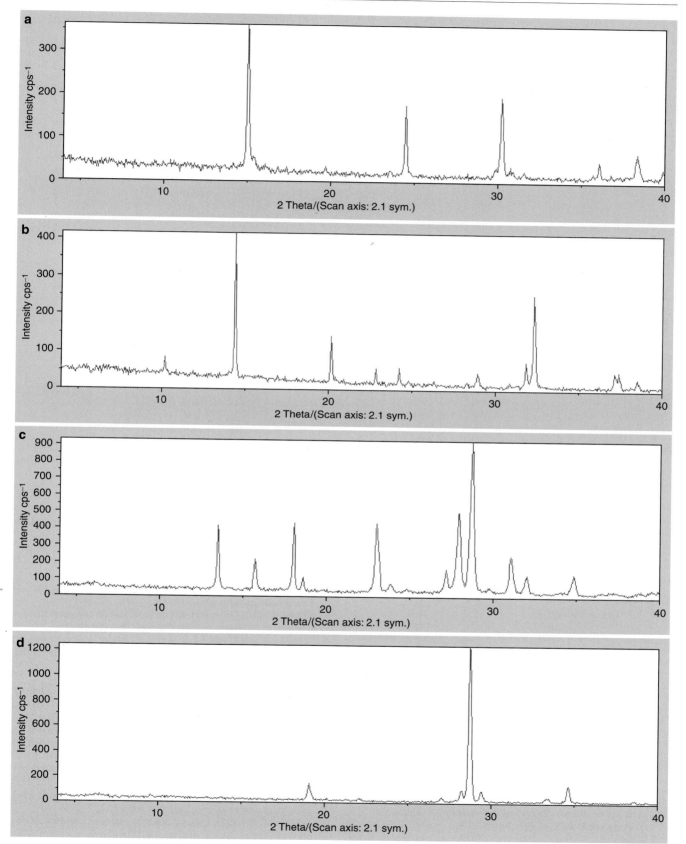

Fig. 29.12 X-ray diffractograms of some stone components. (**a**) Whewellite. (**b**) Weddellite. (**c**) Uric acid. (**d**) L-cystine. (**e**) Struvite. (**f**) Brushite

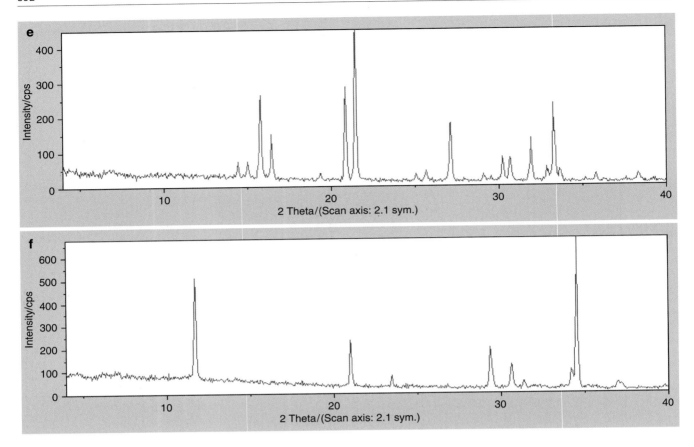

Fig. 29.12 (continued)

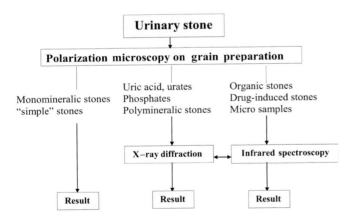

Fig. 29.13 Flow pattern of urinary stone analysis

References

1. Schubert G. Stone analysis. *Urol Res*. 2006;34:146–150.
2. Schubert G. Stone composition in Germany – evaluation of 110, 000 stone analysis. *Urol Res*. 2005;33:138.
3. Schubert G. Incidence and analysis of drug-induced urinary stones. In: Rodgers AL, Hibbert BE, Hess B, Khan SR, Preminger GM, eds. IXth Intern. Symp. *Urolithiasis*, publ. University Cape Town, South Africa 2000:416–418.
4. Dao NQ, Daudon M. *Infrared and Raman Spectra of Calculi*. Paris: Elsevier; 1997.
5. Heijnen W, Jellinghaus W, Klee WE. Calcium oxalate trihydrate in urinary calculi:. *Urol Res*. 1985;13:281–283.
6. Schubert G, Ziemer B. A new calcium oxalate monohydrate produced by thermal dehydration of Weddellite. *Cryst Res Technol*. 1981;16:1025–1031.
7. Schubert G, Reck G, Jancke H, et al. Uric acid monohydrate – a new urinary calculus phase. *Urol Res*. 2005;33:238.
8. Shirley R, Sutor DJ. Anhydrous uric acid: nature and occurrence of a new form in urinary calculi. *Science*. 1968;159:544.
9. Schubert G. Stone analysis of very rare urinary stone components. In: Tiselius HG, ed. *Renal Stones - Aspects on Their Formation, Removal and Prevention*. Stockholm VIth Europ. Symp. *Urolithiasis* 1995:134–135.
10. Schubert G. 70.000 Urinary stone analyses - analytical and metaphylactic aspects. In: Pak CYC, Resnick MI, Preminger GM, eds. *Urolithiasis 1996*. Dallas: Millet the Printer; 1996:452–453.
11. Schubert G, Brien G, Lenk S, Koch R. Texture examinations on grain preparations of calcium oxalate calculi and their relations to pathogentic parameters. *Urol Res*. 1982;11:111–115.
12. Schubert G, Brien G. Crystallographic investigations of urinary calcium oxalate calculi. *Intern Urol Nephrol*. 1981;13:249–260.
13. Schubert G, Strohmaier WL. Clinical significance of texture types in calcium oxalate stones. *Urol Res*. 2004;32:157.
14. Schubert G, Brien G, Bick C. Separate examinations on core and shell of Urinary calculi. *Urol Int*. 1983;38:65–69.
15. Strohmaier WL, Schubert G, Rosenkranz T, Weigl A. Comparison of extracorporeal shock wave lithotripsy and ureteroscopy in the treatment of ureteral stones: a prospective study. *Eur Urol*. 1999;36:376–379.

16. Prien EL. Crystallographic analysis of urinary calculi: a 23 year survey study. *J Urol*. 1963;89:917.

17. Prien EL, Prien EL Jr. Composition and structure of urinary stones. *Am J Med*. 1968;45:654.

18. Beischer DE. Analysis of renal calculi by infrared spectroscopy. *J Urol*. 1955;73:653.

19. Hesse A, Sanders G. *Atlas of Infrared Spectra for the Analysis of Urinary Concrements*. Stuttgart: Thieme; 1988.

20. Debye P, Scherrer P. Interferenzen an regellos orientierten Teilchen im Röntgenlicht. *Phys Zschr*. 1917;17:291.

21. Seifert HH, Gebhardt MAH. Quantitative röntgenographische Harnsteinanalyse mittels Guinier-Diffraktometer. *Fortschr Urol Nephrol*. 1979;14:275.

22. Schubert G. Change of the stone composition at recurrent stone formation and in different sides of urinary tract. *Urol Res*. 2008; 36:164.

Risk Indices

30

Norbert Laube and Lisa Kleinen

Abstract Risk indices combine biological and physico-chemical knowledge with epidemiological data and calculate a single number from an array of measured or observed quantities. This single number can be used to classify the health status of the examined person with respect to the investigated disease on a standardized scale.

This chapter discusses the issue of risk indices in urolithiasis research and treatment. On the example of the most frequent stone type, calcium oxalate, several approaches with different complexity are introduced. On the example of a set of urinalyses of stone formers and controls, discriminative power and predictive value of the presented risk indices are determined using receiver operating characteristics for each index. The advantages and disadvantages of risk indices in urolithiasis treatment and clinical routine are discussed.

Abbreviations

AP(CaOx)	Ion-activity product index for calcium oxalate
AUC	Area under curve
BRI	BONN-Risk-Index
CA	Citric acid
CaOx	Calcium oxalate
ESWL	Extracorporeal shock wave lithotripsy
M	Mean value
MD	Median value
NH_4Ox	Ammonium oxalate
NSF	Non stone former (healthy subject)
OA	Oxalic acid
PV+	Positive predictive value
PV−	Negative predictive value
ROC	Receiver operating characteristic
RSS	Relative supersaturation
SD	Standard deviation
SE	Sensitivity
SF	Calcium oxalate stone former
SP	Specificity
UA	Uric acid

(X)	Titrated amount of substance X
[X]	Concentration of substance X
{X}	24-h excretion of substance X

N. Laube (✉)
Medizinisches Zentrum Bonn Friedensplatz, Academic Teaching
Center of the University of Bonn, Bonn, Germany
e-mail: n.laube@deutsches-harnsteinzentrum.de

30.1 Introduction

Risk Indices are indicators that facilitate the choice of an appropriate therapy for the individual patient based on laboratory data and epidemiological observations. While their usefulness is discussed with some controversy,[1–7] they are widely used in all medical disciplines. Prominent non-urological examples are, for example, the Goldman risk index for determination of the risk of perioperative cardiac complications for patients older than 40 years of age about to be operated on looking at nine variables,[8] and the Multinational Association for Supportive Care in Cancer (MASCC) risk index, which can be used to identify low-risk patients for serious complications of febrile neutropenia,[9] and several others.[10–12]

In general, risk indices combine biological and physico-chemical knowledge with epidemiological data to calculate a single number from an array of measured or observed quantities. This single number then classifies the health status of the examined person with respect to the investigated disease on a standardized scale. It can be translated into an individual risk for the person to contract the disease. This way, a risk

P.N. Rao et al. (eds.), *Urinary Tract Stone Disease*,
DOI 10.1007/978-1-84800-362-0_30, © Springer-Verlag London Limited 2011

index transforms an otherwise unmanageable amount of data into decision-making information.

Risk indices can be used to characterize a patient's base line risk and to monitor the success of the prescribed treatment scheme. Generally, under therapy a decreasing risk index confirms the choice of treatment strategy, while an unchanged or even increasing risk index requires an adjustment in therapeutic measures.

To be of any practical relevance, a risk index should meet (at least) two demands: It should be relatively easy to determine within the daily clinical or practice routine at reasonable costs, and – even more important – it needs to distinguish accurately between persons at high risk and persons at low risk to develop symptoms. This leads to the main issue of risk index development: the right choice of measured or observed quantities and their correct interdependence. Most risk indices include values for commonly known or assumed so-called risk factors, quantities that (potentially) promote or inhibit the development of symptoms. In case of urolithiasis, risk factors definitely include all lithogenic components (e.g., concentrations of calcium ions [Ca^{2+}] and oxalic acid [OA]), lack of inhibitory urinary components (e.g., hypocitraturia), and – with different relevance – parameters like gender or age or various underlying or associated diseases (e.g., osteoporosis or renal tubular acidosis). To calculate the risk index, the interrelation between the different risk factors has to be known or at least plausibly estimated in order to deduce the mathematical function that weighs the impact of the measured values correctly.

Frequently, different biological, chemical, and physical processes within the body are related to a certain disease pattern. Depending on the number of identified or assumed causative factors, usually several, often quite different risk indices for the same disease pattern exist. This is also the situation for the multi-factorial disease pattern "urolithiasis",[13] as can be seen in the next section in which a selection of risk indices for the most common stone type in urolithiasis, the calcium oxalate,[14] is presented.

30.2 Risk Indices for Calcium Oxalate Formation

From the first attempt to determine the risk of calcium oxalate stone formation by measuring one of the main promotoric factors, the urinary calcium concentration,[15–17] to the latest methods, sophisticatedly combining several measurands,[18,19] iterative computation of urinary supersaturation based on thermodynamic models,[20–22] or inducing crystallization processes in vitro in native urine samples,[23] risk indices have been continuously developed and refined[24,25] during the past decades: a trend that reached its preliminary peak in the 1970s and 1980s.

With the innovation of the extracorporeal shockwave lithotripsy (ESWL) in the late 1970s,[26] the urologists' interest in the causes of stone formation and metaphylactic stone treatment began to dwindle. The ESWL was considered a "comfortable" tool (for patient as well as urologist) making the need for primary prevention and metaphylaxis of stone formation obsolete, although the propensity for stone recurrence remains unaltered by removal of stones with ESWL.[27] At the same time, the increased interest on research topics in the field of tumor diseases of the urinary tract also eclipsed stone research.

Nowadays, provoked by the globally increasing prevalence and incidence of urolithiasis[28–31] with growing number of patients and considerably increasing treatment costs, urolithiasis research, and with it risk index development, is currently experiencing a comeback. Stone metaphylaxis, individually matched to the patient's needs, becomes more important as no or insufficient stone treatment results in negative effects on the etiopathology.[25,32,33] This and the patients' expectations[34] bring biochemical risk evaluation and risk indices back into focus as they are essential for the development of an efficient metaphylaxis program on an individual level.

As already mentioned in the introduction, the right choice of measured or observed quantities and the correct analysis of their interdependence are required in order to develop a meaningful risk index. After decades of investigation into the causes of urolithiasis, a multitude of different risk factors have become available.[35–38] Certainly, all of them are more or less relevant for treatment of stone diseases, but only a few are relevant for the determination of the patient's health status concerning stone formation, hence the risk index development.

Since the driving force of crystal formation from urine is urinary supersaturation and since a risk index for urinary stone formation always predicts the probability of a physico-chemical process to occur, most risk indices consider at least one lithogenic urinary component. In order to better predict true urine supersaturation and ion-activity products with respect to the investigated stone type, the major promotoric and inhibitoric urinary constituents – as known from, for example, crystallization experiments – are combined into the mathematical expression of a risk index.

Also, numerous intrinsic and extrinsic epidemiologic risk factors (with different impacts) have been identified as playing a role in the etiology of stone disease and thus could be considered for inclusion in a risk index. For example, gender, age, anatomical abnormalities of the urinary tract, underlying or associated diseases (e.g., gout, osteoporosis, hypertension, hyperparathyroidism, renal tubular acidosis, diabetes, recurrent urinary infections), or disease patterns (e.g., metabolic syndrome), as well as climate, occupation, and lifestyle (including dietary habits, physical inactivity, stress) are, inter alia, made responsible for the occurrence of urolithiasis [e.g.,[39–43]]. In particular, changes in lifestyle factors during the past decades are considered causative for the dramatic increase of the occurrence of urolithiasis.[44] These factors are certainly relevant for therapeutic recommendations, as many of them should be adjusted for general health improvement quite independently of the stone disease.

However, compared to a laboratory (biochemical) analysis of a urine sample, data of these epidemiological risk factors are gathered with more effort and are difficult to comprise mathematically as their contributions to a particular patient usually cannot be quantified. In contrast to the biochemical data that always refer to the particular individual delivering the urine sample with a

potential supersaturation, most of the epidemiological factors are connected to the individual only by statistics, often with weak significance to the particular case.

For this reason, from the multitude of urolithiasis risk indices currently available[13,24,45] only those based on biochemical analysis are presented here. A selection of risk indices developed since 1976 for the evaluation of the individual risk of stone formation for the most common stone type in urolithiasis, the calcium oxalate, is given in Table 30.1.[46-65] Their main underlying concepts will be exemplarily discussed in the following subsections.

Table 30.1 Examples of risk indices of calcium oxalate stone formation with different underlying approaches and methods to estimate urinary (relative) supersaturation, urinary ion-activity products. They distinguish between urines of calcium oxalate stone formers and urines of normal subjects. Some of them provide the patient's gender. Some indices have been repeatedly refined

Index	Abbreviation	Special features	Reference
Activity product ratio	APR		Pak and Holt (1976)[46]
Formation product ratio	FPR		Pak and Holt (1976)[46]
Supersaturation inhibition index	SII	Combination of calculated urine saturation and measured inhibitor activity	Robertson et al. (1976)[47]
Approximation equation	$\log \Pi/\Pi_n$	Computational approach	Achilles et al. (1976)[48]
Probability index	P_{SF}		Robertson et al. (1978)[49]
Relative supersaturation	RSS	Computational approach (EQUIL)	Finlayson (1978)[50]
Inhibitor activity		Induction of crystal formation in gel system	Bothor et al. (1982)[51]
Activity product index	AP(CaOx)	EQUIL-based non-iterative estimate of the CaOx activity product with reduced number of input variables	Tiselius (1982)[18]
Discrimination index		Induction of crystal formation in urine	Sarig et al. (1982)[52]
Risk quotients			Berg et al. (1983)[53]
Supersaturation		Computational approach	Achilles and Ulshöfer (1984)[54]
Calcium oxalate crystallization risk	CaOx-CR	Induction of crystal formation in urine	Tiselius et al. (1985)[55]
Oxalate tolerance value		Induction of crystal formation in urine	Briellmann et al. (1985)[56]
Crystal growth rate	V_{kr}	Induction of crystal formation in gel system	Achilles and Ulshöfer (1985)[57,58]
Saturation degree			Marangella et al. (1985)[59]
Relative Supersaturation	RSS	Computational approach (EQUIL2)	Werness et al. (1985)[22]
Discriminant score			Parks and Coe (1986)[60]
Standardized activity product index	AP(CaOx)$_s$		Tiselius (1989)[19]
			Tiselius and Sandvall (1990)[61]
Saturation coefficient			Robert et al. (1994)[62]
Crystallization risk index	CRI		Daudon et al. (1996)[63]
Evaluation of a urine's capacity to crystallize calcium salts		Color reaction of urine on a micro-structured reactive substrate after 24-h incubation	Grases et al. (1997)[64]
Saturated solution model		Computational approach (SEQUIL)	Ashby and Gyory (1997)[1]
BONN-Risk-Index	BRI	Induction of crystal formation in urine	Laube et al. (2000)[23]
Metastable limit		Induction of crystal formation in urine; 96 well-plate assay	Kavanagh et al. (2000)[65]
Turbitidy rate index		Induction of crystal formation in urine; 96 well-plate assay	Kavanagh et al. (2000)[65]
Risk factor model			Robertson (2003)[24]

30.2.1 Single Quantities

Historically, the first indicators to classify risk of stone formation were based on the determination of one risk factor, preferably that known or assumed as most influential on etiopathology of urolithiasis. If the analytical value of this particular factor is used to classify the patient's status in the sense of "hyper-," "normo-," or "hypo-," this factor can be considered as an index.[16,17]

In the case of calcium oxalate lithiasis, the concentrations or excretions of calcium, oxalate, citrate and pH are examined. This diagnostic procedure follows the major recommendations of the European and German guidelines on urolithiasis in order to evaluate specific abnormalities in urine composition.[66,67] For example, mild hypercalciuria starts at Ca-excretions exceeding 5 mmol/d. In general practice, values exceeding this limit call for dietary measures,[66] while in terms of risk indices, this value could be translated into an indicator of increased crystallization risk caused by abnormally high calcium excretions. Values exceeding 8 mmol Ca-excretion per day require medication[66] and can be translated into an indicator of very high risk for calcium stone formation.

Similar classifications can be done to transform other important biochemical risk factors (e.g., hyperoxaluria, hypocitraturia, and low urinary pH-levels) into risk indices. Although they are not considered classic risk indices, on closer inspection, they are definitely used as such, detecting lithogenic diseases and defining the first measures for treatment.

These parameters, however, are in most cases recorded without further mathematically correlation, neglecting the possibility of, for example, inhibitory effects when only looking at promotoric quantities.

30.2.2 Simple Ratios

If a history of stone formation exists and the concentration and excretion values of the lithogenic, promotoric, and inhibitoric urine parameters plot without pathological findings within their respective normal range, their single values alone cannot be used for the evaluation of the person's stone formation risk. For this idiopathic stone formation, consideration of single quantities relative to one another can improve the diagnostic information.

In these cases, urinary concentrations or excretions of several lithogenic and other promotoric and inhibitoric substances and, where appropriate, of further urinary characteristics, such as 24-h volume and urinary pH, are taken. They are suitable as input variables for the calculation of multiparameter ratios or other mathematical correlations. As these approaches account for the antagonistic processes involved

in urinary stone formation, they promise better distinction between stone formers (SF) or persons prone to form stone, respectively, and normal subjects and successfully treated former stone patients.

Based on urinalysis parameters, simple quotients with promotoric variables in the numerator and inhibitoric ones in the denominator are calculated. Examples are the concentration-based ratios: [Ca]/[CA], ([Ca] × [OA])/[CA] and ([Ca] × [OA])/([CA] × [Mg]), or, focusing on urinary excretions, the {Ca}/{CA} and ({Ca} × {OA})/{CA} ratios. A variety of further indices exists.[53,60,68,69]

Since most stone formers are idiopathic and since absence of a single quantity reflects that stone formation is mainly caused by a complex imbalance between all promoting and inhibiting urinary factors,[70,71] at least one of these ratios should be chosen as a tool for exploratory risk evaluation.

30.2.3 Iterative Model Calculations

Another type of risk indices is based on computer simulations of commonly accepted thermodynamic equilibrium models of complex chemical interactions in urine, taking into account the most important urinary components. The simulations iteratively calculate from an initial chemical analysis of several urinary components (e.g., $[H_3O^+]$, $[Na^+]$, $[K^+]$, $[Ca^{2+}]$, $[Mg^{2+}]$, $[NH_4^+]$, $[SO_4^{2-}]$, $[PO_4^{3-}]$, [CA], [OA]) the ion activities and the concentrations of potentially formed coexisting complexes, and finally the relative supersaturations for all potentially precipitating salts. Computer programs providing these features include EQUIL,[20,22] JESS[72,73]). Among these, EQUIL is the most often used program in urolithiasis research to estimate the relative urinary supersaturation (RSS).

To date, the RSS risk index – based on the supersaturation calculated from urinalysis with EQUIL – is one of the most sophisticated risk indices that bases on a biochemical analysis. RSS is computed from the concentrations of at least 12 independent primary cations and anions commonly found in urine. Based on this data set and a set of thermodynamic stability constants of complexes that may form in urine from these ions, a set of nonlinear simultaneous equations can be developed. Taking the conservation of mass into account, the nonlinear equation system rapidly converges to self-consistency by iterative approximation, in order to obtain the equilibrium concentrations of potentially occurring complexes. The less-soluble stone-salt complexes are of particular interest. From these complex concentrations, the urinary supersaturation of important mineral components in kidney stones (e.g., calcium oxalate) can be computed. Since its first release, the computer program has experienced several improvements.[20–22,50,74]

Although this classic thermodynamic approach promises the best results for estimation of urinary supersaturation by including a number of urinary components (23 at the most enhanced program version, EQUIL93[20]), it seems that this variety of input variables in fact hinders more widespread use of the EQUIL tool.

30.2.4 Complex Combined Parameters

A prominent example of a more complex risk index for calcium oxalate is the widely used AP(CaOx) index, which estimates the urinary ion-activity product with respect to calcium oxalate from urinalysis data. With the AP(CaOx), Tiselius developed an analytical, non-iterative approach to approximate the more laboriously obtained ion-activity product.[18] Starting with an average urine composition, the relative contribution of selected urine components to the ion-activity product was determined. Under systematic variation of each of the urine components, the ion-activity product was calculated based on the principles of Robertson[75] and Finlayson,[74] the latter supplying the EQUIL program for use. The most influencing parameters were combined to a quotient according to the results obtained from the previous calculations.

AP(CaOx) is computed from Eq. (30.1)[13]:

$$AP(CaOx) = 1.9 \times \frac{\{Ca\}^{0.84} \times \{OA\}}{\{CA\}^{0.22} \times \{Mg\}^{0.12} \times V^{1.03}} \quad (30.1)$$

with $\{Ca\}$, $\{OA\}$, $\{CA\}$, $\{Mg\}$, and V as the urinary 24-h excretions of calcium, oxalic acid, citric acid, magnesium, and the 24-h urine volume, respectively. The different exponents in Eq. (30.1) reflect the different influences of each of the quantities on the ion-activity product of calcium oxalate and thus calcium oxalate formation. The exponents as well as the factor were continuously adjusted to improve the approximation to the updated calculations of ion-activity products.

Out of all risk indices, the AP(CaOx) index found its way into many national guidelines on urolithiasis.[66,67] The great success of the AP(CaOx) index in comparison to RSS can be ascribed to its convenient application due to the manageable number of laboratory parameters and the implicit use of background information considering the important role of urinary supersaturation in stone-forming processes provided by EQUIL. The use of excretion values as commonly accepted by the clinicians for evaluation of the patient's metabolic state instead of the concentration values intuitively increases the willingness for AP(CaOx) application.

30.2.5 In Vitro Crystallization Experiments with Native Urine

Initially, the development of novel risk indices was mainly characterized by the preferential consideration of an increasing number of risk factors. These approaches reached considerable mathematical complexity. Some of them give an acceptable differentiation between stone formers and healthy subjects.[76] However, these risk indices are conceptually unable to include all of the important physico-chemical factors of stone formation that influence – either as promoters or as inhibitors – processes such as heterogeneous nucleation, aggregation, and agglomeration. Especially the macromolecular urinary constituents belonging to the groups of glycosaminoglycans, glycoproteins, and polypeptides are not accounted for in any of the common or aforementioned risk indices. Although a number of these molecules were identified (e.g., heparin, chondroitin, hyaluronic acid, bikunin, prothrombin-1-fragment, fibronectin, osteopontin, uromodulin) and their respective effect on crystallogenesis has been extensively investigated,[37,77–81] their role in urolithiasis remains enigmatic, as their cumulative effect on each of the processes of crystal and stone formation depends not only on their individual concentrations but also on their chemical environment itself. Furthermore, most of these macromolecular urinary constituents are either not yet routinely accessible or analysis would be too laborious or too costly.

In vitro crystallization tests investigating initial steps of stone formation in native or processed urine samples implicitly consider the influence of all urinary components contained in the sample. Risk indices based on these methods are therefore bound to score well with respect to accuracy and discriminatory power.

Various methods for urine preparation and induction of crystal formation were developed to investigate the propensity of urine specimens for urolithiasis.[23,56,65,82–86] These approaches in general trigger lithiasis-related processes with different techniques (e.g., evaporation, dialysis, addition of oxalate-solution, or seeding). In principle, they allow for the investigation of the influence of any substance on nucleation, growth, agglomeration, and aggregation of insoluble urinary salts.[84,87,88] Based on experiment-derived measures, possibly in combination with one or a few quantities from urinalysis, a risk index predicting individual risk of stone formation can be developed.

As an example for a crystallization experiment–based risk index, the BONN-Risk-Index (BRI) is chosen. In brief, it was shown that in whole native urine, the ratio of the initial urinary ionized calcium concentration $[Ca^{2+}]$ to the amount of oxalate anions (Ox^{2-}) necessary to be titrated to a 200 ml aliquot to that urine to induce the precipitation of calcium oxalate salts can be used as a diagnostic marker to monitor a person's risk to form calcium oxalate stones. This quotient was termed the BONN-Risk-Index. The easy-to-determine index effectively distinguishes between urines of stone formers and controls.[89,90]

The advantage of risk indices determined from experimental crystallization models in native urine is their potential consideration of both kinetic and thermodynamic influences on the urine's "crystallization risk." The interaction of all urinary constituents in their native chemical environment, as presented by the patient, is considered.

The major disadvantage of this principle approach is the fact that it alone fails to answer the question as to why the patient is assigned with an increased risk. When no comprehensive urinalysis is performed, the chemical causes of stone formation may remain unspecific. In these cases, at least the apparent biochemical risk factors related to, for example, hypercalciuria or hypocitraturia have to be evaluated separately in order to establish a specific therapy. Once the individual cause for urolithiasis is found and a specific therapy is established, its efficacy is best controlled by use of crystallization experiment–based risk indices as therapy-related effects that are beyond (routine) analytical accessibility are considered.

Risk indices based on a crystallization experiment are often assumed to be more suitable for clinical research rather than for clinical routine application, because they sometimes require a relatively laborious preparative work prior to measurement and expertise in result interpretation. Therefore, their popularity only slowly increases, as can be observed for the BRI.[91–94]

Table 30.2 Statistical key figures of the underlying data sets used for calculation of the presented risk indices

	Unit	NSF			SF		
		M	MD	SD	M	MD	SD
[pH]	–	6.24	6.29	0.43	6.32	6.45	0.49
[Na]	mmol/L	69.56	54.94	32.50	58.46	56.63	24.56
[K]	mmol/L	29.49	26.00	12.08	*24.04	23.77	7.89
[Ca]	mmol/L	1.66	1.50	0.91	**2.37	2.14	1.25
[Ca²⁺]	mmol/L	0.32	0.28	0.21	**0.75	0.72	0.36
[Mg]	mmol/L	2.17	1.99	1.14	*1.73	1.61	0.70
[NH₄]	mmol/L	14.51	14.17	6.64	*12.77	10.96	7.66
[Cl]	mmol/L	68.05	56.00	28.21	62.87	59.95	26.95
[PO₄]	mmol/L	12.82	11.09	5.98	11.83	10.97	4.65
[UA]	mmol/L	1.56	1.31	0.74	1.37	1.25	0.56
[OA]	mmol/L	0.15	0.13	0.11	**0.22	0.14	0.25
[CA]	mmol/L	1.48	1.22	1.14	**0.86	0.70	0.63

Uric acid, Oxalic acid, Citric acid, BONN-Risk-Index [1/L]. * and ** difference statistically significant versus H, if $p \leq 0.05$ and if $p \leq 0.005$, respectively. Non-parametric two-sided test (Mann-Whitney-U) for independent (i.e., H versus P). Mean values (M, geometric mean for BRI, otherwise arithmetic mean), median values (MD), and standard deviations (SD) of molar concentrations of important urinary constituents determined from 24-h urines of healthy volunteers (NSF, n = 90), untreated recurrent calcium oxalate stone formers (SF, n = 100) at start of their metabolic workup. Ca²⁺ was analyzed using a calcium-selective electrode.

30.3 Application to a Selected Data Set

In order to illustrate the different qualities of exemplary risk indices of calcium oxalate stone formation, non-infected 24-h urines of 90 healthy volunteers (NSF) and of 100 untreated recurrent calcium oxalate stone formers (SF) at start of their metabolic workup were collected and assayed for calcium, phosphate, oxalate, citrate, and other electrolytes. Based on these analyses, three quotients of concentrations of selected urinary constituents, as described in Sect. 30.2.2, as well as the risk indices RSS and AP(CaOx) were calculated. Furthermore, from all urines, the BONN-Risk-Index (BRI) was determined according to the standardized method described in Sect. 30.2.5.[23] All subjects were under free diets at the time of urine collection, and none of the patients was undergoing pharmacologic treatment with respect to stone disease.

The statistical key characteristics (mean, median, SD) of the determined urinary parameters (concentrations, related renal excretions, volume, and pH) are depicted in Tables 30.2 and 30.3. These summaries indicate that mean urinary concentrations and mean 24-h excretions of some urinary parameters differ significantly, as expected, between controls and stone formers, in particular for total calcium, free calcium, oxalic acid and citric acid.

As risk indices should be the key tools in the process of therapeutic decision making, their ability to distinguish

Table 30.3 Mean values (M), median values (MD), and standard deviations (SD) of renal 24-h excretions determined from the same set of urinalyses that was taken as basis of Table 30.1

	Unit	NSF			SF		
		M	MD	SD	M	MD	SD
{V}	mL/d	2802	2695	1320	2503	2463	823
{Na}	mmol/d	172.10	142.68	74.66	139.94	138.14	53.68
{K}	mmol/d	43.29	45.55	38.94	ᵇ57.91	57.27	20.20
{Ca}	mmol/d	4.21	3.66	2.32	ᵇ5.75	5.63	2.64
{Ca²⁺}	mmol/d	0.93	0.81	0.68	ᵇ1.83	1.77	0.99
{Mg}	mmol/d	5.32	5.11	2.15	ᵇ4.23	4.11	1.81
{NH₄}	mmol/d	36.79	34.47	18.28	ᵃ29.13	25.77	14.19
{Cl}	mmol/d	169.77	146.45	69.26	148.84	147.39	58.48
{PO₄}	mmol/d	30.87	29.49	10.11	27.15	27.87	7.28
{UA}	mmol/d	3.76	3.53	1.27	ᵃ3.18	3.11	0.93
{OA}	mmol/d	0.33	0.33	0.11	0.50	0.36	0.59
{CA}	mmol/d	3.54	3.16	1.86	ᵇ2.14	1.99	1.56

Abbreviations and symbols see Table 30.1

between the patients' alternative states of health should be reliable and accurate. Both given the applicability and usefulness of a risk index determines its practical value.

The diagnostic accuracy, the most fundamental property of any laboratory test and especially a risk index as a classification device, can be measured as pairs of diagnostic sensitivity (true positive rate) and diagnostic specificity (true negative rate). For each defined decision threshold, dividing the examined subjects into the two subgroups, the test or risk index displays a certain diagnostic sensitivity and specificity – the high value of one usually trading off the high value of the other quantity. Only the entire spectrum of sensitivity/specificity pairs provides a complete picture of the test's accuracy[95] and its discriminative power. Receiver operating characteristics (ROC) graphs plot all of the sensitivity/specificity pairs resulting from continuous variation of the decision thresholds and demonstrate the test's ability to correctly classify subjects into clinically relevant subgroups.[95,96] The actually chosen decision threshold refers to the so-called operating point of the ROC graph indicating the sensitivity and specificity of the test performed with this threshold.

For the selected risk indices examined in this section, the diagnostic sensitivity and specificity were calculated for decision thresholds varying over the entire range of observed results. Next, ROC graphs were drawn by plotting the true positive rate (or sensitivity) against the false positive rate (1-specificity). Often, the diagnostic accuracy of a test determined by ROC is quantified by a single number – mostly the area under curve (AUC). The values for AUC range by definition between 0.5 (in average true positive rate equals false positive rate with no discriminatory power of the test) and 1.0 (only true positives, no false positives with perfect separation of the test values of the two groups). The implied conclusion that ROC plots with higher AUCs always exhibit higher discriminatory powers of the corresponding tests is only conditionally valid.[95] Nevertheless, the area under the ROC curve (AUC) was determined for the ROC plot of each selected risk index and is discussed in Sect. 30.3.6.

30.3.1 Evaluation of Single Quantities as Risk Indices

For the previously described samples, ROC curves of the important urinary parameters of calcium oxalate lithiasis, Ca^{2+}, total Ca, Mg, citric acid, and oxalic acid, are plotted for their concentrations (Fig. 30.1) and their related excretions (Fig. 30.2). All other investigated urinary single parameters, such as the concentrations and 24-h excretions of K, Na, or uric acid, are indicated by poor discriminatory power (AUC < 0.6) and are therefore not shown. Surprisingly, the often discussed urinary 24-h volume is also of poor discriminatory power as the negligibly small AUC of 0.57 indicates; for orientation, this parameter was also included in Fig. 30.1 as well as later in Fig. 30.3 as one of the input parameters for calculation of AP(CaOx).

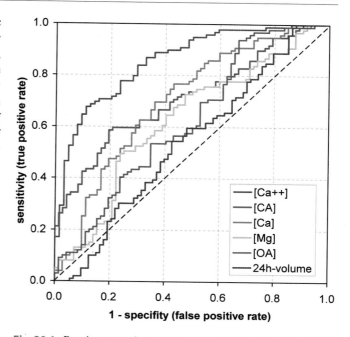

Fig. 30.1 Receiver operating curves (ROC) comparing discriminatory power of the indicated urinary concentrations. The parameter "urinary concentration of free Ca^{2+}-ions" shows by far the highest discriminatory power. Citric acid, total calcium, and magnesium show similar curves, whereas oxalic acid and 24-h urine volume are of no discriminatory value. The legend gives the indices in order of increasing "area under the curve" (AUC)

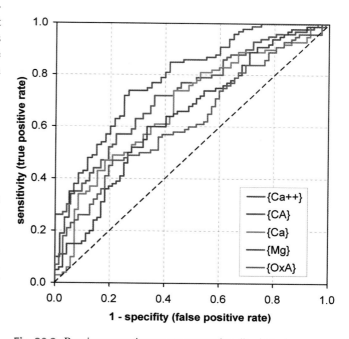

Fig. 30.2 Receiver operating curves comparing discriminatory power of the indicated urinary 24-h excretions. The parameter "24-h excretion of free Ca^{2+}-ions" shows by far the highest discriminatory power. The legend gives the indices in order of increasing "area under the curve" (AUC)

ROC graphs for urinalyses of the subjects included in this study show a high discriminative power of the free calcium ions, in particular their concentration. Within this data frame, the single value of free calcium concentration ($[Ca^{2+}]$) proved to be an acceptable risk index and can be used to discriminate between CaOx-SF and NSF. Total calcium and citric acid as single quantities used as risk indices show only moderate discriminatory power, whereas magnesium and oxalic acid and, in particular, the 24-h volume cannot distinguish accurately between SF and NSF.

The good performance of free calcium concentration as a risk index for discrimination between CaOx-SF and NSF is possibly due to the limited groups of subjects, consisting only of CaOx-SF and NSF. Once an adequately large group of other calcium stone formers (e.g., of brushite or of carbonate-apatite) is admitted to the study, the single quantity "calcium concentration" no longer discriminates between CaOx-SF and NSF. As therapies for CaOx-SF and calcium-phosphate-SF may differ significantly, a risk index based solely on urinary free calcium concentration has no value in the decision-making process. In practice, the occurrence of calcium-containing stones not composed of CaOx has a probability of less than 10%. Under this consideration, the concentration of free calcium can be expected to continue to discriminate between CaOx-SF and controls.

30.3.2 Evaluation of Simple Ratios as Risk Indices

Diagnostic sensitivity and specificity were determined for the quotients [Ca]/[CA], [Ca][OA]/[CA], and ([Ca][OA])/([CA][Mg]) calculated from the data set. The corresponding ROC graphs are shown in Fig. 30.4. While the first two quotients show similar discriminatory power, inclusion of the magnesium concentration in the latter quotient enhances its discriminator power as the increase of area under curve from 0.87 and 0.86, respectively, to 0.9 indicates. However, [Mg] as single quantity showed only negligible discriminatory power. Compared to the single quantities, at a comparable sensitivity the specificity of the test is higher, resulting in a lower false positive rate as can be seen in the respective ROC graphs.

30.3.3 Evaluation of Iterative Model Calculations as Risk Indices

The relative supersaturation (RSS) for calcium oxalate was determined from the urinalyses of the respective subjects groups using a program based on EQUIL. Sensitivity and specificity were obtained from the results. The respective ROC graph is shown in Fig. 30.5 together with ROC graphs of the later on discussed risk indices AP(CaOx) and BRI. Although an area under curve from nearly 0.8 indicates

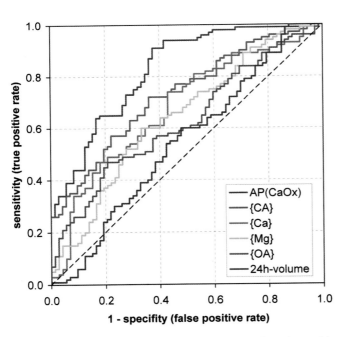

Fig. 30.3 Receiver operating curves illustrating the effect of a combination of five single parameters to a meaningful risk index. The AP(CaOx)-Index is calculated from Eq. (30.1) and shows, compared to each of the input parameters, the highest differentiation potential between urines from stone formers and controls

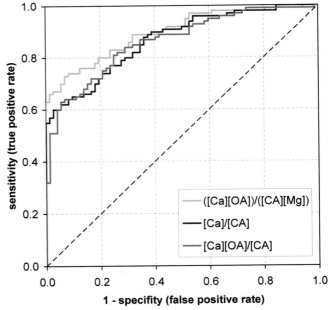

Fig. 30.4 Receiver operating curves comparing discriminatory power of the concentration-based risk indices ([Ca]/[OA]/([CA][Mg]), [Ca]/[CA] and [Ca]/[OA]/[CA]). The legend gives the indices in order of increasing "area under the curve" (AUC)

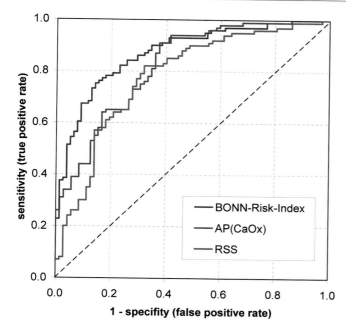

Fig. 30.5 Receiver operating curves comparing discriminatory power of the risk indices BRI, AP(CaOx), and RSS. The legend gives the indices in order of increasing "area under the curve" (AUC)

30.3.5 Evaluation of In Vitro Crystallization Experiments with Native Urine

As an example of a crystallization experiment–based risk index for calcium oxalate lithiasis, the recently developed, easily accessible BONN-Risk index (BRI) was chosen. From each of the collected urines, the BRI was determined as described in Sect. 30.2.5. Diagnostic sensitivity and specificity were determined for the BRI and are plotted against each other in the ROC graph of Fig. 30.5 together with the ROC graphs of AP(CaOx) and RSS.

30.3.6 Discriminatory and Predictive Power of Selected Risk Indices

In this section, the ability of selected risk indices to discriminate between just two alternatives, calcium oxalate stone former (SF) or non-calcium oxalate stone formers (NSF), is examined. As with all empirical data, in both groups, some subjects are diagnosed falsely. In the group of subjects declared as SF, NSF can be found (false positives), and in the group of NSF, SF can be found (false negatives). The number of false diagnoses in each group depends on the decision criterion set for the index.

In order to compare the discriminatory power of the examined risk indices, for each risk index, the value resulting in the same false positive rate and false negative rate was chosen as an example threshold (cutoff value) for decision making. As false negative rate equals 1-sensitivity and false positive rate equals 1-specificity, the corresponding operating point for each ROC graph then lies on the intersection between the ROC plot and the diagonal line with sensitivity = specificity. Actually, the appropriate decision criterion for a particular risk index depends strongly on the benefits ascribed to the correct outcomes and the costs ascribed to the incorrect ones.[96] For example, if a therapy based on the risk index' classification provides only general advice (e.g., solely influencing dietary habits and physical activity with positive side effects to the general health status), a threshold value resulting in a higher false positive rate is clearly acceptable. If a treatment scheme provokes severe side effects (e.g., due to heavy medication), a lower false positive rate would be preferable.

In Table 30.4, the area under curve, decision threshold or cutoff value, true positive and false positive rates, as well as positive and negative predictive values are given for each of the investigated risk indices at the example thresholds in order of decreasing sensitivity. All six risk indices – the three simple quotients as well as AP(CaOx), RSS, and BRI – have sensitivities higher than 0.7 and false positive rates lower than 0.3 for the corresponding example threshold. The area

acceptable discriminatory power, only low sensitivity at high specificity of the test is found within this subject groups. Especially for the detection of SF, a high sensitivity – hence a high true positive rate – would be preferable. Sensitivity above 0.9 is achieved at costs of low specificity below 0.4. For comparison, the quotient $([Ca][OA])/([CA][Mg])$ displays a specificity of 0.6 at the same sensitivity of 0.9 (Fig. 30.4).

30.3.4 Evaluation of Complex Combined Parameters as Risk Indices

AP(CaOx) for each urine analysis was calculated according to Eq. (30.1). Diagnostic sensitivity and specificity were determined for this risk index and are plotted against each other in the ROC graph of Fig. 30.3, together with the respective ROC graphs of the input parameters {Ca}, {Mg}, {CA}, {OA} and 24-h volume. While the single quantities show only low-to-moderate potential to distinguish between SF and NSF, the combination of these parameters in the AP(CaOx) leads to a risk index whose discriminatory power exceeds that of each of the included risk factors alone; a good example for how risk indices increase knowledge superior to single consideration of risk factors. In Fig. 30.5, AP(CaOx) is shown in comparison to RSS and BRI. Their differences will be discussed in Sect. 30.3.6.

Table 30.4 Key numbers derived from ROC-analysis of various biochemical risk factors and risk indices of calcium oxalate stone formation analyzed and calculated from urine samples summarized in Tables 30.2 and 30.3

Risk factor/risk index	Unit	AUC	Cutoff value	SE	1 – SP	PV+	PV–
([Ca][OA])/([Mg][CA])	dim. less	0.90	0.15	0.80	0.20	0.851	0.026
BRI	1/L	0.87	1.43	0.79	0.21	0.833	0.025
[Ca^{2+}]	mmol/l	0.86	0.45	0.77	0.23	0.835	0.027
[Ca][OA]/[CA]	mmol/l	0.86	0.27	0.76	0.24	0.817	0.026
[Ca]/[CA]	dim. less	0.87	1.94	0.76	0.24	0.817	0.026
{Ca^{2+}}	mmol/d	0.79	1.15	0.73	0.27	0.820	0.027
AP(CaOx)	(mmol/d)$^{1.5}$/ml$^{1.03}$	0.82	0.67	0.72	0.28	0.783	0.025
RSS	dim. less	0.78	3.35	0.72	0.28	0.783	0.025
[Ca]	mmol/l	0.70	1.88	0.66	0.34	0.722	0.023
{CA}	mmol/d	0.73	2.49	0.65	0.35	0.685	0.021
[CA]	mmol/l	0.71	0.92	0.63	0.38	0.722	0.023
[NH$_4$]	mmol/l	0.62	12.13	0.62	0.38	0.476	0.011
{NH4}	mmol/d	0.63	29.13	0.61	0.39	0.476	0.011
{Ca}	mmol/d	0.68	5.01	0.61	0.39	0.685	0.021
[Mg]	mmol/l	0.63	1.74	0.61	0.39	0.476	0.011
{Mg}	mmol/d	0.64	4.74	0.60	0.40	0.476	0.011
{OA}	mmol/d	0.63	0.34	0.57	0.43	0.648	0.019
[OA]	mmol/l	0.62	0.13	0.57	0.43	0.644	0.019
24-h volume	ml/d	0.54	2550	0.55	0.45	0.523	0.014

Area under the ROC curve, Sensitivity (i.e., true positive rate) at cutoff value (decision threshold), 1 – Specificity (i.e., false positive rate) at cutoff value, Positive predictive value at decision threshold for the examined study sample, Negative predictive value at decision threshold for the examined study sample.

under curve of the respective ROC graphs exceeds 0.75 for these indices. With the exception of [Ca^{2+}] and {Ca^{2+}}, all single quantities show less discriminatory power and a lower sensitivity. Concentration and excretion of free calcium rank between the more sophisticated risk indices for the examined subject groups, within the limits discussed in Sect. 30.3.1. The laboriously calculated RSS and the simplified estimate of the ion-activity product, AP(CaOx), show comparable sensitivity, accuracy, and discriminatory power, confirming the good approximation of complex physico-chemical processes by a thoroughly developed formula.

However, the performance of a diagnostic test cannot be evaluated by area under curve or any other single number derived from the ROC plot since a particular discriminatory pattern can only be recognized from the curvature of the whole plot.[95] In Fig. 30.5, the ROC graphs of three different risk indices, each reflecting different methods of determination, are compared directly with each other: the AP(CaOx), the EQUIL-based relative supersaturation (RSS), and the BONN-Risk-Index (BRI). Among all ROC graphs of the risk indices presented in this section, the ROC graph of BRI shows the most typical convex curvature. The ROC plot for BRI passes closer to the upper left corner of the diagram than those for AP(CaOx) and RSS, allowing choice of an operating point with higher sensitivity and specificity and thus indicating higher discriminatory power for BRI. The slope of a tangent to a differentiable function fitted to the BRI-ROC data decreases continuously with an increasing false positive rate. The decision threshold can be shifted up to values corresponding to the sensitivity and specificity of an operation point with a tangent slope of one, gaining more true positives than false positives with each increment. Shifting the decision threshold to values with higher sensitivity, the false positive rate increases more than the true positive rate (slope of a tangent <1). Up to a certain limit, in case of urolithiasis, the gain of even a few more true positives at the cost of an increased number of false positives can be accepted as severe side effects in stone therapy are uncommon.

In practice, the ideal operating point and hence the decision threshold to be chosen cannot be evaluated by these mathematical or statistical considerations. Here, the cost of misclassifications and the epidemiological prevalence are usually taken into account to determine the slope of a straight line drawn as a tangent to the ROC graph as described by Zweig et al.[95] For ROC graphs with a continuously decreasing slope of the fitted function, as with one for the BRI, one distinct operating point can be easily defined for each slope calculated on the basis of any selected evaluation criterion.

In this chapter, sensitivity and specificity are used to evaluate the risk indices, especially their discriminatory power. Both properties are inherent to the test and can be seen as a measure of performance independent from the prevalence of the examined symptom.

The predictive power of a test can be described in terms of predictive value, either the fraction of all correct positive results (PV+) or all correct negative results (PV−). Both quantities are strongly correlated to prevalence within the examined group and evaluate the test's predictive performance within this particular subject group. They are given in Table 30.4 for each of the examined risk indices for the previously specified cutoff values. As the prevalence of calcium oxalate stone formers in the study sample (= 1.11) is not representative for prevalence of urolithiasis in the target population (e.g., 0.05 in Germany or 0.13 in USA[97]), the positive predictive values for each risk index given in Table 30.4 are most likely too high. All data shown in Table 30.4 will change not only with cutoff value but also with increasing total number of subjects and changing ratios between number of SF and NSF, respectively.

30.4 Benefits and Limits

Urinary calculi are the symptom and the manifestation of a (mostly) complex disease pattern altering urinary composition toward a thermodynamically instable solution with supersaturation exceeding the metastable limit.[28,98,99] Quite frequently, initial causes cannot be identified and remain unknown.

A suitable and advisedly used risk index can be an effective tool for classifying an otherwise almost unmanageable amount of analysis data, facilitating diagnoses, improving prevention, therapy monitoring, and sometimes providing even a first indicator of the potentially underlying diseases. The main benefit of risk index application is the evaluation of the impact of medication and of adjunct dietary recommendations in the course of treatment. In case of a non-sufficient therapeutic outcome, the measures can then be individually fine-tuned step by step to best meet the patient's requirements. Especially, the crystallization experiment–based indices consider all individual, otherwise probably not detected, urinary properties influencing stone formation. In addition to the already mentioned macromolecular fraction, even urinary compositions altered by, for example, metabolites of drugs are included in the result.

Despite the advantages, mostly urologists at clinics specializing in urolithiasis treatment are regularly using risk indices of different complexities for patient characterization

and follow-up examination. In particular, the urologists in private practice often forgo the advantages of a powerful tool. Amount of efforts and (sometimes extra) costs associated with the determination of the input parameter of a risk index are often overrated but quite frequently cited as reasons for a lack of risk index acceptance. Also, occasional "negative experiences" with a certain index may explain the cautious application of risk indices in general. Certainly, the user of a particular risk index must be aware of the index-individual restrictions – for example, the correct input parameters (e.g., concentrations, excretions, units) and the pitfalls that may occur during urine collection and analysis (e.g., the use of spot urine instead of 24-h urine, or wrong urine-storage during collection). It is often overlooked that the considerable day-to-day variation of the urinary parameters requires repeated (24-h) urine collections and risk index determination for sufficient risk evaluation,[66,100,101] especially at the beginning of a therapy, not only to characterize the patient's baseline crystal formation risk, but also to obtain a meaningful set of urinalyses for evaluation of biochemical risk factors. When deciding on the crystallization risk from spot urines, the fraction should be carefully chosen in order to evaluate that moment most characteristic for the stone formation risk while within-day variation of urinary composition.[102] Furthermore, urine collection must be performed at a moment that does reflect the person's normal life conditions. In case of the patient suffering from stone load during urine collection, alteration of the concentration of the lithogenic parameters toward "false-low" analysis values should be taken into consideration when interpreting urinalysis data.[103,104] Also, in case of risk indices including urinary pH as input parameter, the exclusion of a urinary tract infection is recommended.

Risk indices without therapy concepts are of limited value, as they are only indicators and do not provide a specific conclusion. Nevertheless, with the correct diagnosis and a valuable treatment scheme, an appropriate risk index determined by following the respective instructions yields a gain in information that justifies the effort – especially when the results are carefully interpreted by a physician familiar with the limits of the model concerned.

30.5 Conclusions

Quantification of risk has already gained importance in many disciplines, including medicine where for almost every disorder at least one risk index exists. In urolithiasis research, several risk indices assessing the probability of stone formation are available. Due to the advances in diagnosis and urinalysis, new risk factors can be identified and risk factors of minor impact may consequently be disposed. Thus, existing risk indices can be optimized and improved.

As complex indices are actually only rarely used in daily routine, newly developed risk indices should not only provide a high discriminatory power but should also use preferably easy-to-access parameters and an easy-to-calculate algorithm.

There are efforts to develop risk indices including only general patient data such as age, sex, urine volume, smoking, alcohol intake, family history, stone number, and history of gouty arthritis for the so-called Stone Recurrence Predictive Score (SRPS),[105] or age at onset of the disease, gender, urinary pH and specific gravity, serum calcium and uric acid, stone burden, side and location, treatment modality and recurrence history as combined in an approach of Unal et al.[106] Because these risk indices require few or even no laboratory data, they offer – at least for the two above cited studies – a convenient method for prognosis of stone recurrence. However, the applications of risk indices like the SRSP, which forgo any kind of information about urine composition, are limited to preliminary investigations whether more cost-intensive analyses are recommended. They offer no hints about the physico-chemical causes of urolithiasis and cannot be used for monitoring of individual treatment success.

Another new approach in assessing the risk of urolithiasis is the use of artificial neuronal networks (ANN).[107,108] Since ANNs can recognize patterns in highly complex data sets, they are supposed to be more accurate in multivariate analysis than classical statistical analysis and are increasingly used in medical decision processes. Dussol et al. used ANNs to define the best risk factors among 19 medical and laboratory parameters. ANNs pointed out calcium oxalate supersaturation and 24-h urinary urea concentration as the most discriminant variables and allowed for the compilation of a two-dimensional map including these parameters for risk-determination of calcium oxalate stone formation.

All these examples show, with increasing detailed knowledge in the processes governing stone formation and with successive progress in the analytical methods, risk formulas will be developed exceeding the predictive power of the present approaches.

Acknowledgments The authors gratefully acknowledge the editorial help of Mrs. Sabine Dentler.

References

1. Ashby R, Gyory AZ. A thermodynamic equilibrium model for calcium salt urolithiasis: clinical application. *Exp Nephrol.* 1997;5:246–252.
2. Kavanagh JP. A critical appraisal of the hypothesis that urine is a saturated equilibrium with respect to stone-forming calcium salts. *BJU Int.* 2001;87:589–597.
3. Laube N, Pullmann M. The use of risk indices - do they predict recurrence? Yes, they (at least some) do. *Urol Res.* 2006;34:118–121.
4. Rathore SS, Weinfurt KP, Foody JM, et al. Performance of the Thrombolysis in Myocardial Infarction (TIMI) ST-elevation myocardial infarction risk score in a national cohort of elderly patients. *Am Heart J.* 2005;150:402–410.
5. Roger VL. To score or not to score? *Am Heart J.* 2005;150:371–372.
6. Sutton RAL. The use of risk indices: do they predict recurrence? *Urol Res.* 2006;34:122–125.
7. van Loo IHM, van Keulen PHJ, Kluytmans JAJW. Recent developments in the prevention of surgical site infections: preoperative screening and postoperative surveillance. *Expert Rev Anti-Infect Ther.* 2003;1:261–266.
8. Goldman L, Caldera DL, Nussbaum SR, et al. Multifactorial index of cardiac risk in noncardiac surgical procedures. *N Engl J Med.* 1977;297:845–850.
9. Klastersky J, Paesmans M, Rubenstein EB, et al. The Multinational Association for Supportive Care in Cancer risk index: A multinational scoring system for identifying low-risk febrile neutropenic cancer patients. *J Clin Oncol.* 2000;18:3038–3051.
10. Avolio AW, Siciliano M, Barbarino R, et al. Donor risk index and organ patient index as predictors of graft survival after liver transplantation. *Transplant Proc.* 2008;40:1899–1902.
11. Cereda E, Zagami A, Vanotti A, et al. Geriatric Nutritional Risk Index and overall-cause mortality prediction in institutionalised elderly: a 3-year survival analysis. *Clin Nutr.* 2008;27:717–723.
12. Feringa HH, Bax JJ, Hoeks S, et al. A prognostic risk index for long-term mortality in patients with peripheral arterial disease. *Arch Intern Med.* 2007;167:2482–2489.
13. Tiselius HG. Risk formulas in calcium oxalate urolithiasis. *World J Urol.* 1997;15:176–185.
14. Schubert G. Stone analysis. *Urol Res.* 2006;34:146–150.
15. Flocks RH. Studies on nature of urinary calcium; its role in calcium urolithiasis. *J Urol.* 1959;64:633–637.
16. Nordin BE. The estimation of "free" calcium in the urine and its relevance to calculus formation. *Br J Urol.* 1959;31:404–413.
17. Nordin BEC, Tribedi K. Ionized calcium in normal and stone-forming urine. *Lancet.* 1962;279:409–410.
18. Tiselius HG. An improved method for the routine biochemical evaluation of patients ith recurrent calcium oxalate stone disease. *Clin Chim Acta.* 1982;122:409–418.
19. Tiselius HG. Standardized estimate of the ion activity product of calcium oxalate in urine from renal stone formers. *Eur Urol.* 1989;16:48–50.
20. Brown CM, Ackermann DK, Purich DL. EQUIL93: a tool for experimental and clinical urolithiasis. *Urol Res.* 1994;22:119–126.
21. Finlayson B, Miller GH. Urine ion equilibria – a numerical approach demonstrated by application to antistone therapy. *Invest Urol.* 1969;6:428–440.
22. Werness PG, Brown CM, Smith LH, et al. EQUIL 2: a basic computer program for the calculation of urinary supersaturation. *J Urol.* 1985;134:1242–1244.
23. Laube N, Schneider A, Hesse A. A new approach to calculate the risk of calcium oxalate crystallization from unprepared native urines. *Urol Res.* 2000;28:274–280.
24. Robertson WG. A risk factor model of stone formation. *Front Biosci.* 2003;8:1330–1338.
25. Tiselius HG. Factors influencing the course of calcium oxalate stone disease. *Eur Urol.* 1999;36:363–370.
26. Chaussy C, Eisenberger F, Forssmann B. Extracorporeal shockwave lithotripsy (ESWL): a chronology. *J Endourol.* 2007;21:1249–1253.
27. Fine JK, Pak CYC, Preminger GM. Effect of medical management and residual fragments on recurrent stone formation following shock wave lithotripsy. *J Urol.* 1995;153:27–33.

28. Curhan GC. Epidemiology of stone disease. *Urol Clin North Am.* 2007;34:287–293.
29. Hesse A, Brändle E, Wilbert D, et al. Study on the prevalence and incidence of urolithiasis in Germany comparing the years 1979 vs. 2000. *Eur Urol.* 2003;44:709–713.
30. Ramello A, Vitale C, Marangella M. Epidemiology of nephrolithiasis. *J Nephrol.* 2000;13(Suppl 3):S45–S50.
31. Stamatelou KK, Francis ME, Jones CA, et al. Time trends in reported prevalence of kidney stones in the United States: 1976–1994. *Kidney Int.* 2003;63:1817–1823.
32. Strohmaier WL. Course of calcium stone disease without treatment. What can we expect? *Eur Urol.* 2000;37:339–344.
33. Worcester EM, Coe FL. Nephrolithiasis. *Prim Care.* 2008;35: 369–391. vii.
34. Tiselius HG. Patients' attitudes on how to deal with the risk of future stone recurrences. *Urol Res.* 2006;34:255–260.
35. Nakagawa Y, Kaiser ET, Coe FL. Isolation and characterization of calcium oxalate crystal growth inhibitors from human urine. *Biochem Bioph Res Co.* 1978;84:1038–1044.
36. Pak CY. Medical stone management: 35 years of advances. *J Urol.* 2008;180:813–819.
37. Ryall RL. Macromolecules and urolithiasis: parallels and paradoxes. *Nephron Physiol.* 2004;98:37–42.
38. Ryall RL, Harnett RM, Marshall VR. The effect of urine, pyrophosphate, citrate, magnesium and glycosaminoglycans on the growth and aggregation of calcium oxalate crystals in vitro. *Clin Chim Acta.* 1981;112:349–356.
39. Daudon M, Junggers P. Diabetes and nephrolithiasis. *Curr Diab Rep.* 2007;7:443–448.
40. Ekeruo WO, Tan YH, Young MD, et al. Metabolic risk factors and the impact of medical therapy on the management of nephrolithiasis in obese patients. *J Urol.* 2004;172(1):159–163.
41. Lewandowski S, Rodgers AL. Idiopathic calcium oxalate urolithiasis: risk factors and conservative treatment. *Clin Chim Acta.* 2004;345:17–34.
42. Obligado SH, Goldfarb DS. The association of nephrolithiasis with hypertension and obesity: a review. *Am J Hypertens.* 2008;21: 257–264.
43. Sakhaee K. Nephrolithiasis as a systemic disorder. *Curr Opin Nephrol Hypertens.* 2008;17:304–309.
44. López M, Hoppe B (2008) History, epidemiology and regional diversities of urolithiasis. Pediatr Nephrol (Epub ahead of print)
45. Hussain F, Billimoria FR, Singh PP. Predictive value of some biochemical indices in stone formers. *Int J Urol Nephrol.* 1990;22: 25–31.
46. Pak CYC, Holt K. Nucleation and growth of brushite and calcium oxalate in urine of stone formers. *Metabolism.* 1976;25:665–673.
47. Robertson WG, Peacock M, Marshall R, et al. Saturation inhibition index as a measure of the risk of calcium oxalate stone formation in the urinary tract. *N Eng J Med.* 1976;294:249–252.
48. Achilles W, Cumme GA, Scheffel M. Investigation of complex chemical equilibria in urinary systems with respect to calcium oxalate formation. In: Fleisch H, Smith LH, Robertson WG, Vahlensieck W, eds. *Urolithiasis research.* New York/London: Plenum; 1976:229–232.
49. Robertson WG, Peacock M, Heyburn PJ, et al. Risk factors in calcium stone disease of the urinary tract. *Brit J Urol.* 1978;50: 449–454.
50. Finlayson B. Physicochemical aspects of urolithiasis. *Kidney Int.* 1978;13:344–360.
51. Bothor C, Berg W, Börner RH, et al. Gelmodell zur Messung von Kristallisationsinhibitoraktivitäten. *Zschr Urol Nephrol.* 1982;75:689–698.
52. Sarig S, Garti N, Azoury R, et al. A method for discrimination between calcium oxalate kidney stone formers and normals. *J Urol.* 1982;128:645–649.

53. Berg W, Mäurer F, Brundig P, et al. Possibilities of computing urine parameters as a means of classification of normals and patients suffering from calcium oxalate lithiasis. *Eur Urol.* 1983;9:353–358.
54. Achilles W, Ulshöfer B (1984) Calculation of complex chemical equilibria in urine; estimate of stone formation risks and derivation of prophylactic measures. In: Proceedings of the 5th international symposium on urolithiasis and related clinical research, abstracts; Urol Res 12:96
55. Tiselius HG. Measurement of the risk of calcium oxalate crystallization in urine. *Urol Res.* 1985;13:297–300.
56. Briellmann T, Hering F, Seiler H, et al. The oxalate-tolerance-value: a whole urine method to discriminate between calcium oxalate stone formers and others. *Urol Res.* 1985;13:291–295.
57. Achilles W, Ulshöfer B. A computer program for the calculation of activity products and solubilities of stone forming constituents in urine. In: Schwille PO, Smith LH, Robertson WG, Vahlensieck W, eds. *Urolithiasis and related clinical research.* New York/London: Plenum; 1985:770–780.
58. Achilles W, Ulshöfer B. Die GKV-Messung relativer Kristallwachtumsgeschwindigkeit von Kalziumoxalat in 24-Stunden Sammelurinen von Normalpersonen und Steinträgern mit rezidivierender Kalzium Urolithiasis. In: Gasser G, Vahlensieck W, eds. *Pathogenese und Klinik der Harnsteine XI, Fortschritte Urologie und Nephrologie,* vol. 23. Darmstadt: Steinkopff; 1985:261–266.
59. Marangella M, Daniele PG, Ronzani M, et al. Urine saturation with calcium salts in normal subjects and idiopathic calcium stoneformers estimated by an improved computer model system. *Urol Res.* 1985;13:189–193.
60. Parks JH, Coe FL. A urinary calcium-citrate index for the evaluation of nephrolithiasis. *Kidney Int.* 1986;30:85–90.
61. Tiselius HG, Sandvall K. How are urine composition and stone disease affected by therapeutic measures at an outpatient stone clinic? *Eur Urol.* 1990;17(206):212.
62. Robert M, Boularan AM, Colette C, et al. Urinary calcium oxalate supersaturation in 'stone formers' and normal subjects: an application of the EQUIL2 program. *Br J Urol.* 1994;73:358–361.
63. Daudon M, Labrunie M, Ivaldi A, et al. A new crystallisation risk index (CRI) for calcium oxalate (CaOx) stone formers. In: Pak CYC, Resnick MI, Preminger GM, eds. *Urolithiasis.* Dallas: Millet the Printer; 1996:357–358.
64. Grases F, García-Ferragut L, Costa-Bauzá A, et al. Simple test to evaluate the risk of urinary calcium stone formation. *Clin Chim Acta.* 1997;263:43–55.
65. Kavanagh J, Jones L, Rao N. Calcium oxalate crystallization kinetics studied by oxalate-induced turbidity in fresh human urine and artificial urine. *Clin Sci.* 2000;98:151–158.
66. Straub M, Strohmaier WL, Berg W, et al. Diagnosis and metaphylaxis of stone disease. Consensus concept of the national working committee on stone disease for the upcoming German urolithiasis guideline. *World J Urol.* 2005;23:309–323.
67. Tiselius HG, Alken P, Buck C, et al. *Guidelines on urolithiasis.* Arnhem: European Association of Urology (EAU); 2008.
68. King JS Jr, O'Connor FJ Jr, Smith MJ, et al. The urinary calciummagnesium ratio in calcigerous stone formers. *Invest Urol.* 1968;6:60–65.
69. Tiselius HG. Different estimates of the risk of calcium oxalate crystallization in urine. *Eur Urol.* 1983;9:231–234.
70. Batinić D, Milosević D, Blau N, et al. Value of the urinary stone promoters/inhibitors ratios in the estimation of the risk of urolithiasis. *J Chem Inf Comput Sci.* 2000;40:607–610.
71. Laube N, Allie-Hamdulay S, Rodgers A, et al. Calcium oxalate stone formation risk - a case of disturbed relative concentrations of urinary components. *Clin Chem Lab Med.* 2008;46:1134–1139.
72. May PM, Murray K. JESS, a joint expert specification system – I. *Talanta.* 1991;38:1409–1417.

73. May PM, Murray K. JESS, a joint expert specification system – II. The thermodynamic database. *Talanta*. 1991;38:1419–1426.

74. Finlayson B. Calcium stones: some physical and clinical aspects. In: David DS, ed. *Calcium metabolism in renal failure and nephrolithiasis*. New York/Chichester: Wiley; 1977:337–382.

75. Robertson WG. Measurement of ionized calcium in biological fluids. *Clin Chim Acta*. 1969;24:149–157.

76. Roca P, Conte A, Riera T, et al. Can a relationship reflect the risk of calcium oxalate urolithiasis? *Int Urol Nephrol*. 1990;22:215–222.

77. Khan SR, Kok DJ. Modulators of urinary stone formation. *Front Biosci*. 2004;9:1450–1482. Comment in: J Urol 2005 Feb;173(2):478.

78. Kumar V, Lieske JC. Protein regulation of intrarenal crystallization. *Curr Opin Nephrol Hypertens*. 2006;15:374–380.

79. Rodgers AL, Jappie D. Studies on the role of urinary macromolecules in urolithiasis: review of methodologies and a proposal for a standard reference crystallization system. *Scan Microsc*. 1996;10:535–545.

80. Ryall RL, Chauvet MC, Grover PK. Intracrystalline proteins and urolithiasis: a comparison of the protein content and ultrastructure of urinary calcium oxalate monohydrate and dehydrate crystals. *BJU Int*. 2005;96:654–663.

81. Sheng X, Jung T, Wesson JA, et al. Adhesion at calcium oxalate crystal surfaces and the effect of urinary constituents. *Proc Natl Acad Sci USA*. 2004;102:267–272.

82. Achilles W. In vitro crystallization systems for the study of urinary stone formation. *World J Urol*. 1997;15:244–251.

83. Baumann JM, Ackermann D, Brown CM, et al. Problems related to the measurement of crystallization in whole urine. *Urol Res*. 1989;17:143–151.

84. Guerra A, Meschi T, Allegri F, et al. Concentrated urine and diluted urine: the effects of citrate and magnesium on the crystallization of calcium oxalate induced in vitro by an oxalate load. *Urol Res*. 2006;34(6):359–364.

85. Hess B, Ryall RL, Kavanagh JP, et al. Methods for measuring crystallization in urolithiasis research: why, how and when? *Eur Urol*. 2001;40:220–230.

86. Kavanagh JP. Methods for the study of calcium oxalate crystallisation and their application to urolithiasis research. *Scan Microsc*. 1992;6:685–704. discussion 704–5.

87. Cerini C, Geider S, Dussol B, et al. Nucleation of calcium oxalate crystals by albumin: involvement in the prevention of stone formation. *Kidney Int*. 1999;55:1776–1786.

88. Guerra A, Meschi T, Schianchi T, et al. Crystalline aggregation in vitro: interaction between urinary macromolecules and the micromolecular environment. *Acta Biomed*. 2002;73:11–26.

89. Kavanagh J, Laube N. Why does the Bonn risk index discriminate between calcium oxalate stone formers and healthy controls? *J Urol*. 2006;175:766–770.

90. Laube N, Hergarten S, Hoppe B, et al. Determination of the calcium oxalate crystallization risk from urine samples - the BONN-Risk-Index in comparison to other risk formulas. *J Urol*. 2004;172:355–359.

91. Ahmed B, Sultan S, Hussain I, et al. Urinary crystallization index: A risk marker for calcium oxalate lithiasis. *J Ped Urol*. 2008;4:S26.

92. Lewandowski S, Rodgers AL, Laube N, et al. Oxalate and its handling in a low stone risk vs a stone-prone population group. *World J Urol*. 2005;23:330–333.

93. Porowski T, Zoch-Zwierz W, Konstantynowicz J, et al. A new approach to the diagnosis of children's urolithiasis based on the Bonn risk index. *Pediatr Nephrol*. 2008;23:1123–1128.

94. Porowski T, Zoch-Zwierz W, Wasilewska A, et al. Normative data on the Bonn risk index for calcium oxalate crystallization in healthy children. *Pediatr Nephrol*. 2007;22:514–520.

95. Zweig HG, Campbell G. Receiver-operating characteristic (ROC) plots: a fundamental evaluation tool in clinical medicine (erratum in Clin Chem 1993;39:1589). *Clin Chem*. 1993;39:561–577.

96. Swets JA. Measuring the accuracy of diagnostic systems. *Science*. 1988;240:1285–1293.

97. Bartoletti R, Cai T, Mondaini N, et al. Epidemiology and risk factors in urolithiasis. *Urol Int*. 2007;79(Suppl 1):3–7.

98. Miller NL, Evan AP, Lingeman JE. Pathogenesis of renal calculi. *Urol Clin North Am*. 2007;34:295–313.

99. Rao PN. Debate: The key to stone formation is. *Urol Res*. 2006;34:79–80.

100. Hess B, Hasler-Strub U, Ackermann D, et al. Metabolic evaluation of patients with recurrent idiopathic calcium nephrolithiasis. *Nephrol Dial Transplant*. 1997;12:1362–1368.

101. Parks JH, Goldfisher E, Asplin JR, et al. A single 24-hour urine collection is inadequate for the medical evaluation of nephrolithiasis. *J Urol*. 2002;167:1607–1612.

102. Ogawa Y, Yonou H, Hokama S, et al. Urinary saturation and risk factors for calcium oxalate stone disease based on spot and 24-hour urine specimens. *Front Biosci*. 2003;8:a167–a176.

103. Laube N, Pullmann M, Hergarten S, et al. Influence of urinary stones on the composition of a 24-hour urine sample. *Clin Chem*. 2003;49:281–285.

104. Pullmann N, Hergarten S, Laube N. The influence of a variable differential function on the stone growth-related urinary depletion effect. *Clin Chem*. 2004;50:1675–1678.

105. Lee YH, Huang WC, Lu CM, Tsai JY, Huang JK. Stone recurrence predictive score (SRPS) for patients with calcium oxalate stones. *J Urol*. 2003;170:404–407.

106. Unal D, Yeni E, Verit A, Karatas OF. Prognostic factors effecting on recurrence of urinary stone disease: a multivariate analysis of everyday patient parameters. *Int Urol Nephrol*. 2005;37:447–452.

107. Dussol B, Verdier JM, LeGoff JM, et al. Artificial neuronal networks for assessing the risk of urinary calcium stone among men. *Urol Res*. 2006;34:17–25.

108. Dussol B, Verdier JM, LeGoff JM, et al. Artificial neural networks for assessing the risk factors for urinary calcium stones according to gender and family history of stone. *Scand J Urol Nephrol*. 2007;41:414–418.

Blood and Urinary Tests in Stone Formers

31

Michelle Jo Semins and Brian R. Matlaga

Abstract Kidney stone disease is highly prevalent, has a rising incidence, and a high recurrence rate. Stone events greatly impact quality of life of patients and pose a great financial burden on society. Over several decades, the surgical treatment of stone disease has advanced significantly. While surgical technique has evolved, evidence demonstrates medical therapy decreases stone recurrence rates and prevention should not be overshadowed by surgical advances. A thorough metabolic evaluation of stone formers helps guide therapy for prevention. Herein we review the specific blood and urine tests that can be done in stone formers to identify specific treatable metabolic abnormalities.

31.1 Introduction

Kidney stone disease is a common malady, estimated to affect approximately 10% of the US population: The lifetime prevalence among males is 13%, and among females is 7%.[1-3] However, recent evidence suggests that the prevalence of stone disease is increasing among women such that the gender distribution is moving closer to parity.[4] Alarmingly, the incidence of upper urinary tract stone disease is increasing; between 1980 and 1994, there was a 37% increase in the prevalence of this disorder.[2] It should also be noted that kidney stones are a recurrent phenomenon; the lifetime recurrence rate has been reported to be greater than 50%.[5,6]

The surgical treatment of patients suffering from symptomatic kidney stones has undergone great advances over the previous 2 decades. Whereas kidney and ureteral stones were once commonly treated with open surgical lithotomy, such procedures are now rarely performed. In the present era, almost all urinary calculi are treated either in a minimally invasive endoscopic fashion with ureteroscopy or percutaneous nephrolithotomy, or in a completely noninvasive fashion with shock wave lithotripsy (SWL).[7] Perhaps as a consequence of the great advancements in the surgical treatment of stone-forming patients, some attention has shifted away from efforts to prevent the actual formation of a kidney stone.

In fact, though, medical therapy has been demonstrated to significantly decrease stone recurrence rates; given the high recurrence rates associated with stone disease, such preventive efforts are cost-effective as well.[8]

Kidney stone pathogenesis is often a multi-factorial process. However, in the majority of stone formers, a thorough metabolic evaluation will identify factors that can be modified in order to reduce the risk for recurrent stone formation.[1,3,5,9-11] Herein, we will review the laboratory studies that comprise a metabolic evaluation.

31.2 Blood Tests

All stone formers, including first-time uncomplicated stone formers, should undergo blood screening tests as part of their general diagnostic evaluation (Table 31.1). Blood testing should include serum electrolyte, calcium, and uric acid measurements. Patients should also undergo an assessment of renal function with the measurement of serum creatinine. Such tests are associated with a low cost, and are useful in the screening for certain metabolic abnormalities that may predispose to recurrent stone formation.

Hypercalcemic states, such as primary hyperparathyroidism, may be diagnosed by serum studies. If serum calcium is elevated, an intact serum parathyroid hormone level should be obtained, as well as serum phosphorous, to determine whether the patient has primary hyperparathyroidism. In patients with primary hyperparathyroidism, the intact

B.R. Matlaga (✉)
James Buchanan Brady Urological Institute,
The Johns Hopkins Hospital, Baltimore, MD, USA
e-mail: bmatlaga@jhmi.edu

P.N. Rao et al. (eds.), *Urinary Tract Stone Disease*,
DOI 10.1007/978-1-84800-362-0_31, © Springer-Verlag London Limited 2011

Table 31.1 Blood tests

All stone formers
Sodium
Potassium
Chloride
Carbon dioxide
Blood urea nitrogen
Creatinine
Calcium
Uric acid
Special circumstances
If calcium elevated:
Intact serum parathyroid hormone level
Phosphorous
If albumin abnormal:
Ionized calcium
If primary hyperoxaluria suspected:
Oxalate level
If sarcoidosis suspected:
Angiotensin-converting enzyme (ACE)
Calcitriol

parathyroid hormone level is usually elevated and phosphorous depressed. If serum albumin is abnormal, ionized calcium may be measured as well, which can increase the likelihood of detecting the disease. In some cases, though, hypercalcemia due to hyperparathyroidism may be intermittent; as a result, it is sometimes necessary to repeatedly measure serum calcium levels over time. Alternatively, the administration of a short course of thiazide-type diuretic can "unmask" occult cases as the patients will often become hypercalcemic on such therapy.

Renal tubular acidosis, a spectrum of clinical syndromes of metabolic acidosis that result from defects in renal tubular hydrogen ion secretion and urinary acidification, may also be suggested by serum studies. Distal renal tubular acidosis, which is generally associated with calcium phosphate stone formation, may be suggested by hypokalemia and low carbon dioxide levels.

Patients suffering from gouty diathesis may form renal calculi composed of uric acid. Such patients often manifest their disorder of uric acid metabolism with the symptoms of gouty arthritis. In general, uric acid levels in such patients are elevated; hyperuricemia can be diagnosed on the basis of serum testing.

Other blood tests are less commonly performed, although there are certain situations that may make their measurement appropriate. Patients suffering from primary hyperoxaluria will reveal elevated serum oxalate levels. Hypervitaminosis D can have a causative role for urinary calculi, and may be diagnosed by evaluating serum vitamin D levels. Measurement of serum angiotensin-converting enzyme (ACE) may provide supportive evidence of sarcoidosis, a disease associated with hypercalcemia and urinary calculi. The mechanism of hypercalcemia in sarcoidosis may be related to elevated circulating levels of calcitriol, which induces gastrointestinal absorption of calcium as well as bone resorption; in such patients one would expect blood tests to demonstrate elevated serum calcitriol.

31.3 Urine Tests

All patients should undergo a simple urinalysis, a modest study that can be very informative (Table 31.2). The specific gravity of urine can reveal the general state of hydration of a patient, an important parameter in the evaluation of stone formers. Urine pH can be revealing. A persistently elevated urinary pH (greater than 7.0) can be associated with distal renal tubular acidosis or the presence of urease-producing bacteria. The latter may be particularly likely with the

Table 31.2 Urinary tests

All stone formers
Simple urinalysis:
Specific gravity, urine pH, nitrites, leukocyte esterase, and bacteria
Urine sediment:
Crystals (hexagonal, rectangular "coffin-lid," tetrahedral "envelope")
Urine culture
More extensive evaluation
Two 24-h urine collection
Stone risk factors:
Volume, calcium
Oxalate: If primary hyperoxaluria suspected → glyoxalate and glycerate
Citrate, urinary pH, uric acid
Urinary supersaturation: calcium oxalate, calcium phosphate, uric acid
Dietary risk factors:
Sodium, potassium, magnesium, phosphorous, sulfate, urea nitrogen
Marker for completeness of collection:
Creatinine
Normalized values:
Calcium per kilogram
Calcium per gram of creatinine
Loading studies (rarely indicated):
Fasting, calcium loading, and calcium restriction metabolic studies
Ammonium chloride loading test
Purine loading test
One 24-h urine collection 4–6 weeks post-intervention

concomitant presence of nitrites, leukocyte esterase, and bacteria. If the pH is persistently low (less than 5.5), the patient may be at risk for the formation of uric acid calculi.

The urine sediment should be analyzed with a microscopic examination. In some cases, crystals identified by microscopy can predict the composition of stones formed by the patient. The presence of hexagonal crystals is pathognomonic for cystinuria.[5] Rectangular "coffin-lid" crystals are commonly encountered in patients with struvite calculi. Calcium oxalate stone formers may demonstrate tetrahedral "envelope" crystals.

In addition to the previously described evaluations, a urine culture should also be obtained. Should urine culture demonstrate the presence of a urea-splitting organism, such as *Proteus*, *Pseudomonas*, or *Klebsiella*, a struvite calculus may be present. In addition, patients with a positive urine culture should be treated with appropriate antibiotic therapy prior to any surgical procedure for the removal of a stone. The surgical treatment of a stone in the presence of active, untreated infection confers on the patient a great risk for infection-related complications.

There are certain patients who should undergo a more extensive evaluation than the aforementioned urinalysis (Table 31.3). Recurrent stone formers are one group that will likely benefit from a more extensive evaluation. Recurrence of stone formation suggests that either persistent or severe metabolic abnormalities may be present. However, select first-time stone formers should also undergo a more extensive evaluation. Such patients include those who have a solitary kidney or renal insufficiency, where further stone events could have a profound impact on the patient's health. Another group is those patients harboring residual stones, especially when the burden is large or high volume. Other patients who may be at higher risk for a subsequent stone event, such as those with intestinal disease or chronic diarrhea, those with pathologic skeletal fractures or osteoporosis, and those with gout, should

also be considered for a more extensive metabolic evaluation. Similarly, patients with stones composed of cystine, uric acid, or struvite may be at greater risk of recurrence and may benefit from an extensive evaluation. All children should undergo a complete investigation as the pediatric stone former has an increased risk of an underlying metabolic disturbance.[12,13]

For those patients undergoing a comprehensive metabolic evaluation, the cornerstone of such a study is the 24-h urine collection test. There is some controversy as to whether a single 24-h urine collection is sufficient for diagnosing metabolic abnormalities, or if two 24-h urine collections are required. Pak and associates have suggested that a single 24-h urine collection is adequate for the diagnosis of metabolic disturbances that may predispose to stone formation.[14] In their study of this matter, they found that the reproducibility of stone risk factors was adequate in repeated samples. However, Parks and associates reported that, in a comparison of two separate 24-h urine collections, there were significant disparities from one collection to the other.[15] In fact, within nearly 70% of the comparisons, the differences were great enough that clinical care may have been altered. As no clear consensus exists, it may be most prudent to proceed with two 24-h urine collections so as to maximize the utility of the investigation. When the results of the 24-h urine collections mandate an intervention, a post-intervention urine collection should be obtained 4–6 weeks following to ensure that the desired effect has occurred.

In general, minimal preparation is required prior to performing 24-h urine collections. The urine collections should be performed on an outpatient basis; if occurring after a urologic intervention, generally at least 1 month should elapse between intervention and collection to ensure that the patient has returned to their normal lifestyle and diet.[9] A urinary tract infection should be eradicated prior to the collection, to prevent bacterial citrate degradation (causing a pseudohypocitraturia) as well as bacteria-induced elevated urine pH. Some have suggested that patients cease consuming items such as antacids, diuretics, thiazides, H2 blockers, allopurinol, vitamin C/D, calcium, and magnesium supplements as they may interfere with the results of the collection.[1,9] However, such instructions may be problematic as some patients' health status may be dependent on these medications. If there is a strong suspicion that a medication is inducing a specific abnormality, a more focused collection may be performed.

Table 31.3 Indications for more extensive evaluation

Recurrent stone formers
Select first-time stone formers
Solitary kidney
Renal insufficiency
Patients harboring residual stones
Patients at high risk for recurrence
Intestinal disease
Chronic diarrhea
Pathologic skeletal fractures
Osteoporosis
Gout
Cystine stones
Uric acid stones
Struvite
All children

31.4 Stone Risk Factors

31.4.1 Volume

The finding of a low urine volume is one of the most common abnormalities detected on a 24-h urine metabolic evaluation. Although a low urine volume may strictly be defined as a volume less than 1 L/day, one may consider that for stone formers a volume less than 2 L/day is inadequate.[16] Although this abnormality is generally a consequence of a low dietary fluid intake, a low urine volume may also be encountered in patients who have large volume fluid losses by other mechanisms, such as chronic diarrheal states. A low urine volume may be associated with hypocitraturia, another factor that can increase the risk of stone formation.

31.4.2 Calcium

Elevated levels of calcium excretion, defined as greater than 200 mg in women and 250 mg in men over a 24-h period, in a patient with normal serum calcium, may be considered idiopathic hypercalciuria. Alternative methods to quantify calcium excretion would be indexing to creatinine, in which case less than 140 mg/g creatinine is considered to be normal, or indexing to body weight, in which case less than 4 mg/kg for either sex would be considered to be normal. Patients with idiopathic hypercalciuria excrete more calcium in their urine than is considered to be normal. In some cases, idiopathic hypercalciuria may be due to an absorptive phenomenon. The patients absorb and excrete an elevated fraction of dietary calcium. In other cases, idiopathic hypercalciuria may be due to reduced renal tubular calcium reabsorption. Resorptive hypercalciuria is a manifestation of hyperparathyroidism, and causes increased urinary calcium through a process of increased intestinal absorption of calcium, increased resorption of bone, and increased renal synthesis of $1,25(OH)_2$ vitamin D.

Rarely, urine calcium may be elevated as a consequence of other, less common medical conditions.[9] Certain malignancies may alter calcium balance and lead to hypercalciuria, such as multiple myeloma, lymphoma, leukemia, and other metastatic disease processes. Sarcoidosis, Paget's disease, hyperthyroidism, vitamin D intoxication, and milk-alkali syndrome, too, can give rise to increased urinary calcium levels.

31.4.3 Oxalate

Urinary oxalate excretion should be less than 40 mg/day; values greater than this amount are abnormal. In the majority of cases, the etiology of hyperoxaluria is idiopathic, and the central treatment point is dietary modification. Enteric hyperoxaluria should be suspected in patients with hyperoxaluria and small bowel pathology. Enteric hyperoxaluria may be associated with other physiologic disorders, such as low urine volume, low urine citrate, and low urine magnesium, which may also promote stone formation. When urinary oxalate is above 100 mg/day, a diagnosis of primary hyperoxaluria

should be in the patient's differential diagnosis. If primary hyperoxaluria is suspected, the urine should also be tested for glyoxalate and glycerate.[17]

31.4.4 Citrate

Urine citrate excretion should be greater than 450 mg/day in men and greater than 550 mg/day in women. Citrate inhibits stone formation by forming soluble complexes with calcium, which inhibit crystal nucleation and growth.[3,18] Hypocitraturia is present in more than 30% of stone patients; in up to 10% of cases, it is an isolated finding, whereas in 50% of cases it is one of multiple abnormalities present.[19] The etiology of hypocitraturia is variable. Most commonly, though, hypocitraturia is a result of idiopathic conditions, although other states, such as distal renal tubular acidosis, chronic diarrhea, urinary tract infection, and thiazide medication, can also induce hypocitraturia.

31.4.5 Urinary pH

The 24-h urine pH may affect stone formation, serving as an inhibiter in some cases, and a promoter in others. In general, urine pH should be between 5.8 and 6.2. Uric acid calculi can form when the urine pH is below the pKa of uric acid, which is 5.75. Urinary pH may be increased via pharmacologic intervention with alkali therapy, such as potassium citrate to reduce this likelihood. The crystallization process of cystine, too, is pH dependent; the pKa of cystine is 8.3. If urine pH can be increased beyond this value with alkali therapy, the likelihood of cystine stone formation will be reduced.

There are some situations, though, where an increased urinary pH may promote, rather than inhibit, stone formation. Calcium phosphate stones form in a pH-dependent manner. Distal renal tubular acidosis, a condition associated with calcium phosphate stones, should also be suspected when urinary pH is above 6.5. The presence of urea-splitting bacterial infection will raise urine pH above 8, and should be suspected if such pH measurements are present.

31.4.6 Uric Acid

Urinary uric acid greater than 800 mg/day in men and 750 mg/day in women is abnormally elevated. Hyperuricosuria is encountered in up to 35% of metabolic evaluations, although it is often one of multiple abnormalities detected.

Interestingly, of patients found to be hyperuricosuric, up to 20% of these patients will suffer from calcium oxalate calculi.[9] The etiology of hyperuricosuria calcium oxalate nephrolithiasis has not been explicitly defined, although it may be due to either a heterogeneous nucleation process or a consumption of inhibitors, or a combination thereof.

Certain medical conditions are associated with hyperuricosuria, including gouty diathesis and Lesch–Nyhan syndrome. Some patients suffering from malignancy, particularly those with increased cell death, which can elaborate large amounts of purine such as tumor lysis syndrome or myeloproliferative disorders, may develop hyperuricosuria. A diet rich in animal protein will also increase the uric acid load excreted by the kidney.

31.4.7 Urinary Supersaturation

Urinary supersaturation is a measure of the potential of urine to form and enlarge a crystal complex that will ultimately become a stone. Supersaturation calculations for stone-forming salts – such as calcium oxalate, calcium phosphate, and uric acid – are reliable predictors of stone formation. The supersaturation value for each salt depends on the concentration of dissolved salt relative to its solubility, and is calculated using the total concentration of urinary sodium, potassium, calcium, magnesium, ammonia, phosphate, sulfate, oxalate, citrate, uric acid, pyrophosphate, carbon dioxide, chloride, and pH.

31.5 Dietary Risk Factors

31.5.1 Sodium

Urinary sodium excretion should be less than 150 mg/day. Increased levels of urinary sodium will increase urinary calcium excretion, and may also blunt the hypocalciuric effects of thiazide medications. For every 100 mmol increase in dietary sodium, urinary calcium excretion will increase by 25 mg.[3] Sodium also reduces citrate excretion and increases cystine excretion.[16]

31.5.2 Potassium

Urine potassium levels should be monitored in stone formers; ideally, urine potassium excretion should be between 20 and 100 mmol/day. A hypokalemic state, which can promote hypocitraturia, may be reflected in urinary potassium levels. Certain conditions associated with low urinary potassium levels include bowel diseases with chronic diarrhea, diuretic

usage, or laxative abuse. Importantly, urine potassium levels may also be markers of medical therapy. One would expect that following potassium citrate prescription, the patient's urine potassium would increase at a level corresponding to the dosage of medication; absence of an increase may be a marker of noncompliance. Patients prescribed thiazide-type medications for hypercalciuria, without supplemental potassium, may exhibit a decline in urinary potassium levels, reflecting a relative hypokalemia.

31.5.3 Magnesium

Urine magnesium excretion should be between 30 and 120 mg/day. Magnesium is a divalent cation, which can complex with oxalate and reduce its urinary station. Calcium oxalate stone formation may thereby be inhibited. Supplemental magnesium therapy may also increase urinary citrate excretion by decreasing its tubular reabsorption. Urine magnesium may be low in conditions associated with poor nutritional status, laxative abuse, and certain malabsorption syndromes. Up to approximately 7% of patients, undergoing metabolic evaluation will demonstrate low magnesium levels and it is generally not an isolated finding, most commonly associated with low urine citrate and low urine volume.[10]

31.5.4 Creatinine

Urinary creatinine is a marker that will confirm the accuracy and comparability of the urine collection. When comparing specimens collected on different days, the creatinine should be examined first, to insure the consistency of urine collection. Urine creatinine should be between 20–27 mg/kg in males and 14–21 mg/kg in females.

31.5.5 Other

Increased consumption of protein can be associated with subsequent stone formation. Urinary analytes, such as phosphorus, sulfate, and urea, can be indicative of the amount of animal protein consumed.

31.5.6 Loading Studies

There are a number of loading-type studies that at one point were quite commonly utilized, although in modern times are much rarely indicated. Fasting, calcium loading, and calcium restriction metabolic studies of hypercalciuric patients were previously done to differentiate absorptive versus renal hypercalciuria. However, as the treatment of these disorders is similar, and given the cumbersome nature of the test protocols, they are seldom performed.[1,3,9] At one time the ammonium chloride loading test was used to diagnose complete and incomplete renal tubular acidosis. Presently, though, renal tubular acidosis is generally diagnosed without this test. Latent hyperuricosuria can be diagnosed via a purine loading test; presently, though, such a test is not commonly utilized.[20]

31.6 Conclusions

Nephrolithiasis is a highly prevalent and increasingly common disease; as such, it has great social and economic impact on our society. Medical therapy for prevention has been shown to be effective to decrease recurrence rate. Yet, diagnostic evaluations that would lead to medical therapy are not commonly performed. Although such evaluations do hold certain subtleties, in general their interpretation is straightforward. As reviewed herein, metabolic studies are designed to capture certain information that will enhance our understanding of the stone former's pathophysiology so that targeted medical therapy may be administered.

References

1. Levy FL, Adams-Huet B, Pak CYC. Ambulatory evaluation of nephrolithiasis: an update of a 1980 protocol. *Am J Med.* 1995;98:50.
2. Stamatelou KK, Francis ME, Jones CA, et al. Time trends in reported prevalence of kidney stones in the United States: 1976–1994. *Kidney Int.* 2003;63:1817.
3. Heilberg IP, Schor N. Renal stone disease: causes, evaluation, and medical treatment. *Arq Bras Endocrinol Metab.* 2006;50:823.
4. Scales CD, Curtis LH, Norris RD, et al. Changing gender prevalence of stone disease. *J Urol.* 2007;177:979.
5. Prezioso D, Di Martino M, Galasso R, et al. Laboratory assessment. *Urol Int.* 2007;79:20.
6. Odvina CV, Pak CYC. Medical evaluation of stone disease. In: Stoller ML, Men MV, eds. *Current Clinical Urology. Urinary Stone Disease: A Practical Guide to Medical and Surgical Management*, vol. 1. Totowa: Humana; 2007.
7. Pearle MS, Calhoun EA, Curha GC, et al. Urologic diseases in America project: urolithiasis. *J Urol.* 2005;173:848.
8. Lotan Y, Cadeddu JA, Pearle MS. International comparison of cost effectiveness of medical management strategies for nephrolithiasis. *Urol Res.* 2005;33:223.
9. Begun FP, Foley WD, Peterson A, et al. Patient evaluation laboratory and imaging studies. In: Resnick M, ed. *The Urologic Clinics of North America, Urolithiasis*, vol. 24. Philadelphia: W.B. Saunders; 1997:97–116.
10. Preminger GM. Medical evaluation and treatment of nephrolithiasis. *Semin Urol.* 1994;12:51.
11. Pak CYC, Britton F, Peterson R, et al. Ambulatory evaluation of nephrolithiasis. Classification, clinical presentation and diagnostic criteria. *Am J Med.* 1980;69:19.
12. DeFoor W, Asplin J, Jackson E, et al. Urinary metabolic evaluations in normal and stone forming children. *J Urol.* 2006;176:1793.
13. DeFoor W, Minevich E, Jackson E, et al. Urinary metabolic evaluations in solitary and recurrent stone forming children. *J Urol.* 2008;179:2369.
14. Pak CYC, Peterson R, Poindexter JR. Adequacy of a single stone risk analysis in the medical evaluation of urolithiasis. *J Urol.* 2001;165:378.
15. Parks JH, Goldfisher E, Asplin JR, et al. A single 24-hour urine collection is inadequate for the medical evaluation of nephrolithiasis. *J Urol.* 2002;167:1607.
16. Porena M, Guiggi P, Micheli C. Prevention of stone disease. *Urol Int.* 2007;79:37.
17. Leumann E, Hoppe B. The primary hyperoxalurias. *J Am Soc Nephrol.* 2001;12:1986.
18. Seltzer MA, Low RK, McDonald M, et al. Dietary manipulation with lemonade to treat hypocitraturic calcium nephrolithiasis. *J Urol.* 1996;156:907.
19. Coe FL, Kavlach AG. Hypercalciuria and hyperuricosuria in patients with calcium nephrolithiasis. *N Engl J Med.* 1974; 291:1344.
20. Hesse A, Vahlensieck W. Loading tests for diagnosis of metabolic anomalies in urinary stone formers. *Int Urol Nephrol.* 1986;18:45.

Crystallization and Other Studies

Dirk J. Kok

Abstract Crystallization is a prerequisite for forming a urinary stone. Whether abnormalities in the process or location of crystallization are the cause of stone formation is less clear. A kidney that performs its task to conserve water will form supersaturated fluid, urine. This occurs in each person. The supersaturation provides the driving force for crystal formation. After sufficient time crystals will form. From there on things are less obvious. If crystals are found in urine, were they formed in the bottle after collection, in the bladder after collection, in the pyelum, or in the nephrons? Is stone formation related to crystal formation per se, to massive crystal formation, or to crystal formation in the wrong place? What is a normal or wrong place – the nephron, the renal tissue, the pelvic space, free in fluid, or fixed to a surface? For all these questions, answering them involves assessing how crystallization proceeds under the specific conditions that exist at a specific site. The aim of this chapter is to describe these conditions, to review literature data in the light of what they tell us about the likelihood and regulation of crystallization at these sites, and to give leads for promising further studies on crystallization in the field of urinary stone formation.

32.1 Crystallization: From Solution to Solid

Ultimately, crystals and stones form because somewhere fluid became supersaturated with respect to the stone mineral and it was energetically favorable to form a solid. In the long term, thermodynamics ensure that in any solution where the concentration of a compound exceeds the maximum that can remain in solution – its solubility – the supersaturation results in the formation of a solid. On a short timescale, however, the first step of crystallization, nucleation, will only start when an energy barrier is taken. Thus, some degree of supersaturation, metastability, can be tolerated for some time before nucleation starts: nucleation lag-time. For the supersaturation range found in urine this lag-time varies from seconds to minutes. Urine travels through a nephron in a comparable time frame with variations related to the nephron length and the water load. Thus, variations in nucleation lag-time and variations in

transit time may well dictate whether or not crystals form inside a nephron. It thus becomes of interest to determine where in the nephron supersaturation first occurs, what happens to that supersaturation after that point, and what the residence time is for distinct nephron compartments. Crystals will only form inside the nephron when the residence time exceeds the nucleation lag-time.[1] On the other hand, for events that take place in the renal interstitium or at a fixed position – for instance, attached to cells – this time limit will be less relevant. In addition to all this, the urine is also not constant in composition. During the nephron passage as well as over time, concentrations of relevant compounds go up and down and this influences the crystallization processes. Again, for crystallization taking place at a fixed site or closed compartment in the kidney these changes may be different.

With these points in mind, I will review what literature data teaches us about:

- Intratubular crystallization in different nephron segments.
- Crystallization in the renal interstitium.
- Crystallization beyond the nephron.

This is always done from the viewpoint: Does it contribute to crystal formation and to stone formation?

D.J. Kok (✉)
Department of Pediatric Urology, Erasmus Medical Center,
Rotterdam, The Netherlands
e-mail: d.kok@erasmusmc.nl

P.N. Rao et al. (eds.), *Urinary Tract Stone Disease*,
DOI 10.1007/978-1-84800-362-0_32, © Springer-Verlag London Limited 2011

32.2 Crystallization in the Nephron

32.2.1 Experimental Studies Related to Crystallization in the Nephron

Whether and how often crystals are formed inside the nephron is a subject of debate. Two approaches have been used to investigate this question.

First, an in vitro approach with crystallization studies that employ conditions that mirror the fluid composition at the different nephron segments and the transit times of the fluid through those segments.[1–4] This approach leads to the conclusion that in the proximal tubule calcium salt precipitation will only occur at levels of oxalate that are very high for that segment and that correspond to serum values of well over 10 μmol per ml. Such values are encountered regularly in extreme cases of hyperoxaluria but also possibly after ingestion of an acute oxalate load.[5] Cells in a proximal tubule should usually not encounter crystals. This concurs with the finding from cell-culture studies that proximal tubule cells, LLC-PK1, bind calcium oxalate crystals and are damaged by them; two reactions that do not ensure safe passage of crystals.[6,7] A massive load of oxalate from the glomerular filtrate causes large-scale proximal tubule deposition of calcium oxalate crystals in in vivo models.[8]

One segment downstream, in the loop of Henle, the situation is completely different. In the loop of Henle, the concentrating process takes a large step. As a by-product of the loop's action, the intratubular pH increases up to 7.4. This causes a strong drive to precipitate calcium phosphates. In in vitro experiments, this occurs in an amorphous form and as hydroxyapatite.[1,3,4] Also other compounds of which the solubility is pH sensitive may precipitate like the human immunodeficiency virus (HIV) medication indinavir that is known to have indinavir stone formation as a side effect.[9,10] This drive will exist in each loop that is just doing its work efficiently, also in someone who does not form stones. Although it is never sure that such in vitro experiments truly mimic what happens in the real nephron, they do pose the advantage that the conditions employed can be manipulated easily. Doing so, it becomes clear that the drive to form calcium phosphate crystals in the loop of Henle increases when the local calcium concentration increases. This would happen when the glomerular filtered load of calcium increases due to chronic hypercalcemia; for example, in hyperparathyroidism, or during transient slight hypercalcemia; for example, after a systemic acid load like a high protein meal. The drive also increases when the citrate concentration decreases, another effect of a high animal protein meal. Such changes will speed up the nucleation processes in the loops where they already occur under the "normal" conditions.

They also will induce nucleation earlier in the descending limb of the longest loops, but also in shorter loops that are less efficient in concentrating fluid and where the rise in pH is smaller. Since there are four to five times as many short loops as long loops, the total drive to form crystals for the whole kidney increases exponentially.[11] This could explain the massive crystalluria that is encountered in patients with hyperparathyroidism.

Beyond the loop of Henle, in the distal tubule and collecting ducts, the conditions become favorable for the formation of calcium oxalates. Formation of calcium oxalates may occur for instance at high oxalate conditions that exist chronically in primary hyperoxaluria and transiently after consumption of high oxalate content food, like a load of dark chocolate.[5] In addition, the formation of calcium oxalate may be enhanced by what is called heterogeneous nucleation. The fluid that enters the distal tubule may contain calcium phosphate nuclei that were formed in the loop of Henle. As the pH drops from above 7 at the tip of the loop of Henle to a low 6 value in the distal tubule, these nuclei start to dissolve. In vitro the presence of these dissolving calcium phosphate nuclei was found to decrease the energy barrier for nucleation of calcium oxalate and to induce calcium oxalate formation at supersaturation levels that do not support homogeneous nucleation.[1,12,13] Thus, factors that regulate calcium phosphate formation and dissolution may also direct the formation of calcium oxalate crystals and should be considered as risk factors for forming calcium oxalate stones. However, this relation is not one on one. In animal models, calcium oxalate can precipitate without involvement of calcium phosphate.[14] The results from crystallization experiments correspond to those from crystal-cell interaction studies. Whereas the crystallization studies implicate that the presence of crystals in the lumen of distal tubules and collecting ducts may be a normal event, cells with an origin from these segments, Madin Darby Canine Kidney (MDCK), are well prepared to such a presence. When these cells are fully functional, they resist binding of calcium crystals[6] and seem unharmed by their presence. When such cells are not fully functional, they bind calcium salt crystals and are further damaged by such crystals.

An interesting feature of crystallization in the nephron is that many of the proteins that are present in urine and that are known to have strong effects on all parts of the crystallization process[15] first enter the fluid there. This has several consequences. When studies are performed to investigate how tubule cells react to the presence of crystals, by producing a specific protein like osteopontin (OPN) for example, it must be remembered that the crystals that can be expected at those sites most likely will be small and at best a few minutes in existence. For calcium oxalate, for instance, this raises the possibility that part of the material is still in the calcium oxalate trihydrate form.[13] For studies on the effect of these proteins on the crystallization process, the experiments should employ the conditions (concentrations and experimental time) that exist inside the nephron. In general, this will mean that the protein concentration will be much lower than its value for the final urine.

32.2.2 In Vivo Data on Crystallization in the Nephron

The second test of whether crystals are formed inside the nephrons is to look directly at these nephrons. This has been done using tissue from animal experiments, with the advantage of possible manipulation of the renal conditions, and with human material, both postmortem studies and biopsies obtained during surgery.

Intratubular crystals are found in rat models of severe hyperoxaluria, in all nephron segments up to the proximal tubule as free crystals, attached to the tubule cells, and blocking the tubule by sheer size.[8,16,17] That calcium oxalate crystals can form under severe hyperoxaluric conditions in the proximal tubule already fits with the crystallization experiments described previously. When the same animals that have a urine calcium concentration of 1–2 mM, which would be considered low in humans, receive a moderate oxaluric diet, the urine is still supersaturated with respect to calciumoxalate but no intratubular crystals are found.[18] Translating this to the human situation, where calcium concentration of the urine usually is 1.5–2 times higher, the formation of calcium oxalate crystals inside the distal parts of the nephron thus is a likely event at high urine oxalate concentrations, a possible event at moderately elevated oxalate concentrations, and an unlikely event with normal calcium and oxalate concentrations – although the urine is still supersaturated with respect to calcium oxalate under those conditions. In so-called idiopathic stone formers, the formation of calcium phosphate in the tubules is expected to predominate. Increases in the filtered load and decreases in the reabsorption of calcium, in response to a dietary load for instance, will further increase the drive to form calcium phosphates more than it will increase the drive to form calcium oxalates. This concurs with the findings in hypercalciuric rat models.[19] An interesting aspect here is the possible role of other urine compounds on the calcium phosphate – calcium oxalate crystallization sequence. Osteopontin (OPN) and Tamm Horsfall protein (THP) are two urine proteins that in various in vitro crystallization studies proved to affect calcium oxalate and calcium phosphate crystallization in various manners.[15,20–22] Genetic removal of these crystallization inhibitors in mice results in the formation of interstitial

calcium phosphate deposits in 10% of the OPN mice, 14.3% of the THP mice, and 39.3% of the OPN/THP mice, while the wild type mice did not show such deposits.[23] The increased propensity to produce calcium phosphate made the OPN/THP mice vulnerable to increases in oxalate consumption. A hyperoxaluric diet that did not induce calcium oxalate crystallization in wild-type mice caused widespread intratubular calcium oxalate crystallization and stone formation in the double-null mice. The urine from all three mutant mice strains in addition showed a significant loss in the ability to inhibit adhesion of calcium oxalate to renal cell cultures in vitro.

Data obtained from studies on human renal materials confirm the above.

Under acute and chronic hyperoxaluria, calcium oxalate crystals are found both intratubular and interstitial and up to the proximal tubule.[24] The studies of large series of postmortem obtained kidneys reveal that intratubular crystals are found in kidneys of both stone formers and non-stone formers.[25] Despite the fact that the staining techniques used may result in remarkable loss of crystals from the tissue, a later study with whole kidneys showed intratubular crystals in 32–500 kidney specimens.[26] The lower limit of detection was 0.2 μm. More recent studies that investigated renal biopsies show that intratubular crystals are present under conditions of abnormal urine composition.[27] In four intestinal bypass patients who formed stones, intratubular crystals were present as aggregates blocking the collecting ducts and as crystalline overlays of tubule cells. The latter sites also show presence of hyaluronan,[27] which indicates that cell damage repair and possibly adherence of crystals to that hyaluronan[28] may have taken place. The crystal material was calcium oxalates plus calcium apatite. However, in contrast to the studies on cadaver kidneys, no intratubular crystals were found under the normo-oxaluric conditions in four non-stone formers and in "idiopathic" stone formers.[27] An explanation for this seeming discrepancy is that intratubular crystals are passed out of the nephron during normal transit as long as they are allowed to move freely. Large structures like the aggregates that form in the intestinal bypass patients thus get stuck while the smaller particles are not hindered by their size but maybe only by adherence to (damaged) tubule cells. In an animal model where transient hyperoxaluria was induced in rats by injection, intratubular crystals were seen immediately after the injection but were washed out within 1 h.[29] When a period of prolonged dietary-induced hyperoxaluria was followed by a low-oxalate diet, all free intratubular crystals were washed out within 1 day while attached crystals were removed by other means (see next section). In light of this data, it is well possible that the period of fasting (usually 12 h) in combination with sufficient hydration that is standardly applied before surgery is a good method to remove intratubular crystals. Next to reduction of the supersaturation, a beneficial effect of increased hydration that is shown to effectively reduce stone formation[30] could thus be washing out crystals from the tubules.

32.2.3 Data from Crystallization Experiments Related to Intratubular Events

There have been numerous studies where the effect of urine and urine compounds on different aspects from the crystallization process – supersaturation, nucleation, crystal growth, and crystal aggregation – have been studied. Results related to supersaturation and nucleation may help to understand where crystals are formed in the urinary tract. Data on crystal growth and crystal aggregation bear relevance to crystal–cell interactions and to the possibility that crystals are retained by their sheer size. From the latter two, aggregation may be the more relevant one. As said before, when particles are found in renal tissue they tend to be in the aggregate form,[31] and this role of aggregates is found not only with calcium salt crystals but also with cystine crystals.[27] Furthermore, microscopic examination of a urinary stone reveals that it consists of multiple microcrystallites that have, together with organic material, combined into one large structure.[32] From theoretical models it was concluded that crystals that are formed inside the tubules cannot grow fast enough to become "too large" during normal kidney transit times of urine.[1,2,33] However, through aggregation of the small individual crystals the size may approach the limit of what can be passed within normal transit times. The most likely nephron segment for aggregation to play a role will be the collecting ducts where crystals from multiple nephrons meet. Thus, the data from crystallization studies should be related to the conditions that exist in collecting ducts.

Many investigators have investigated how individual urine compounds and complete urine affect crystal aggregation. Urine studies have shown that urine from a non-stone former very efficiently inhibits calcium oxalate crystal agglomeration.[34,35] This ability is diminished or even lost in calcium oxalate stone formers and the extent of this loss is even directly related to the stone frequency.[35] Which part of the urine composition is responsible for this agglomeration inhibition has partly been answered. High molecular weight (MW) molecules with multiple calcium binding sites in cooperation with small molecules, especially like citrate, appear to be responsible.[36] The decrease in agglomeration inhibition in stone formers can partly be attributed to a decrease of citrate content of their urine.[34,37] However, changes in the action of the high MW compounds also play

a role that still has not been revealed completely. A molecule or a molecular aggregate that contains multiple sites with affinity for calcium ions is very efficient in binding to the surface of a calcium oxalate crystal where calcium ions are available. Thus, they can both strongly influence nucleation and crystal agglomeration.[22,36,38] In this process, they will bind preferentially to that crystal face that provides the best structural match of available calcium ions for its binding sites.[22] However, when these structures become large enough to bridge from one crystal surface to another they may reverse their action to stimulation of agglomeration. Compounds like THP may cross this fine line due to changed urine composition, low pH, low citrate, high calcium, high ionic strength, and due to intrinsic changes.[39] Exactly how crystal aggregation is regulated in the kidney is still not completely known and further research into this matter will be useful.

The question is how this type of research could benefit the actual stone former. One way is to use the effect of urine on agglomeration as a marker for the hard end point to allow early assessment of the efficacy of a specific treatment. The marker inhibition of crystal agglomeration correlates well with the positive effect of citrate therapy[37,40] and with the negative effect of animal protein consumption.[37]

Another question is how you could manipulate the ability of urine to inhibit crystal agglomeration. As mentioned before, one way is by increasing the urine citrate content. The approach to increase high MW agglomeration inhibitors in the urine is more of a challenge. Most will not pass the glomerular filtration step. It has, however, proven possible to supply animals with polyanions that can have an agglomeration inhibitory effect.[41] This promising approach awaits further assessment of its effects on the crystallization process in the urine and the translation to patients.

Data from crystallization experiments also help to understand crystal–cell interactions. Crystals present in the urine contain organic molecules both on their surface, for instance THP, and inside the crystal matrix. The latter, termed crystal matrix protein, contains among others OPN and prothrombin fragment 1 (PTF1). When crystals are produced freshly in vitro in urine, there also appears to be specificity of proteins toward crystal types.[42] OPN was found in COD but not in calcium oxalate monohydrate (COM) crystals, while PTF1 was found in calcium oxalate dihydrate (COD), at a lesser degree than OPN, but also in COM. Since OPN has been shown to have affinity for COM,[20] an explanation may be that OPN is so effective in preventing COM nucleation that instead COD is formed. What role preferential formation of COD over COM might play for stone formation is as of yet unclear.

A next question that can be investigated in crystallization studies is what characteristics determine the effect of a compound on crystallization. For OPN, the aspartic and

glutamic acid residues and phosphate groups appear to determine the affinity of OPN for the COM crystal {100} surface.[20,22] When the structure of PTF1 was modified in vitro by removing sialic acid residues and glycolic moieties,[43] PTF1 became less effective in inhibiting crystal aggregation and promoting COM nucleation. The changes did not (glycosylic moieties) or only slightly (sialic acid) reduce the capacity to inhibit crystal growth. Furthermore, when trying to distinguish stone formers from non-stone forming persons on the basis of urine chemistry, a set of proteins including PTF1 showed the best result.[44] These findings subscribe the results from studies with urine where the inhibition of crystal aggregation was related to its citrate content,[34,37,40] but through a cooperation of citrate with high MW compounds,[45] while inhibition of crystal growth appeared to be a feature that can be exerted by many urine compounds. An explanation for this may be that inhibition of crystal growth is something that can be accomplished by any compound that contains groups with an affinity for calcium ions. Such groups include carboxylic acid, phosphate, and sulfate, and can be assisted by nearby hydroxyl and amino groups.[38] Small compounds may bind with equal affinity to available calcium ions at any crystal surface. Although they may concentrate on growth sites where most calcium ions will be available, they will also bind to other surfaces. In contrast, larger compounds with multiple calcium binding sites will show a preference for crystal sites where calcium ions are available for binding by more than one of those calcium binding groups. This means that there not only should be more calcium ions available, but also spaced in a way that fits the calcium binding groups of the inhibitor. These compounds will show a preference for the fastest growing faces and growth sites. Because of this selective adsorption to the sites where crystal growth is regulated, this automatically means that they will retard crystal growth at much lower concentrations. OPN, for instance, has been shown to possess this selective behavior.[21] The peculiar COM crystal shapes found in crystalluria may be a direct consequence of such face-specific adsorption. When the concentration of such compounds is increased to even higher levels, COM will no longer form and COD, with different surface characteristics, is formed.[38] Similar actions have been described for urine proteins like urinary trefoil factor I.[46] However, in urine there occurs an overload of compounds that can inhibit COM crystal growth from small compounds like citrate magnesium and phytate to many of the proteins that are normally present.[15,45,47] In urine, the proteins present inhibit the growth of calcium oxalate at the lowest concentrations and are probably the compounds responsible for most of the crystal growth inhibition by urine. However, when all proteins are removed, the inhibition of COM crystal growth does not decrease

significantly. The role of the proteins is replaced by smaller compounds that were not removed by the filtration process.[45]

The importance of proteins inside the crystals may reside in the fact that they can be degraded in vitro by proteinase activity and that they decrease the solidity of the particle.[48] The inclusion of these proteins may be more than random and provide the organism with the means to locate and remove calcium oxalate crystals when they appear at unwanted places. The proteins involved are all formed at the level of the loop of Henle and beyond. This mechanism may thus not protect the kidney against crystals that are formed and retained in the proximal tubule.

32.3 Crystallization in the Interstitium

In the hyperoxaluric animal models, as well as in the human samples of hyperoxaluria,[18] calcium oxalate crystals are also found in the interstitium. These interstitial crystals appear to start as intratubular crystals that attach to the tubular cells and are subsequently overgrown by tubular epithelium. In the animal models, when the hyperoxaluric diet was stopped and followed by a diet that induces slight hyperoxaluria, the intratubular crystals were washed out, but the interstitial crystals remained present or even grew in size. When this approach is continued, the animals eventually form stones. When a follow-up diet that gives a low urine oxalate concentration was provided, not only were the intratubular crystals washed out within 2 days but also all interstitial crystals disappeared.[18] This data raises some interesting questions that relate to the crystallization aspects involved. First, although there is no free exchange between tubular fluid and interstitial fluid, the composition of the latter apparently does respond to the composition of the intratubular fluid. Second, the conditions in the interstitium are such that they do not allow nucleation of calcium oxalate, otherwise all kidneys would be one large stone, and only allow further growth of existing crystals when the urine supersaturation is also increased. Thus, the interstitial situation will be metastable with respect to calcium oxalate/calcium phosphate and/or nucleation and the growth of existing crystals is hindered by the location or the presence of organic material on the crystal surface. These latter effects are not complete since the crystals do grow when the oxalate concentration is increased. A second important aspect is the mechanism for removal of calcium oxalate crystals from the interstitium. The interstitial crystals attract macrophages and/or macrophage precursor cells that fuse into multinuclear giant cells. The latter take up the crystals in specialized vesicles that can be acidified and show proteolytic activity. In animal models, this macrophage system can remove interstitial crystals when the hyperoxaluric pressure is gone.[17,18,24]

This raises the question: What attracts these macrophages to the crystals? To answer this question, you must first establish how the crystals in a stone, in renal tissue, and in crystalluria actually look like.

Macroscopically, most stones show a pattern of alternating layers of mineral and organic matrix. The outer mineral layers consist of multiple crystals present in an ordered fashion. In the center of the stone, the crystals are present as random agglomerates. Microscopically, what at first sight appear to be individual crystals in a stone actually themselves are aggregates of tiny crystallites, from several nanometers to micrometer size[49] covered and segregated by protein. This structure is revealed when the crystal material from a stone is dissolved and the remaining so-called crystal ghosts are studied.[49,50] Several proteins have been identified in these organic layers including OPN (uropontin) and osteocalcin. A similar microcrystalline buildup with intracrystalline protein has been demonstrated for crystals produced in urine.[48,51] The proteins are accessible to proteolytic activity and this feature facilitates the degradation of crystals by cultured renal cells.[52] The organic material present in these urine-derived crystals, termed crystal matrix protein, has been characterized and contains, among others, OPN and PTF1, while several proteins like THP that are also found in stones are found attached to the outside of the larger crystal structures.[42]

A second calcium salt found in the interstitium is calcium phosphate and is present as the well-known Randall's plaques. Here the etiology may be different. The plaques occur outside the tubular lumen and preferentially in the region where the bends in long loops of Henle and the latter parts of collecting ducts are present. This crystal material is found in stone formers as well as in non-stone formers, although more often in the first group. Their presence increases continuously with age, in contrast to stone formation that has a peak incidence during the active life period. Apparently, the formation of these plaques is a long-term event that has something to do with the normal kidney function, but under special circumstances can lead to or increase the risk of stone formation. To study the crystallization involved in the formation of these plaques you need to perform experiments that involve fluid compositions and variations thereof as they exist in the interstitium of the papillary tip, possibly are performed in a confined volume,[53] allow for decreasing calcium and phosphate concentrations locally due to consumption in the crystallization process when exchange of ions is not free, and examine heterogeneous nucleation and the influence of surfaces that can act as a nucleator or otherwise an inhibitor of growth.

32.4 Stone Attached to the Papillary Surface

Finally, in all the previous scenarios the total size of the crystal deposit will still be small. To reach the size of the stones that actually cause the colic pain, the main reason why you would want to remove the stone, crystallization processes of other dimensions must take place. The time frame moves from minutes, hours, and days to days, months, and years. The amount of material involved increases greatly. Variations in fluid flow and composition have a different meaning for material that resides fixed to the papillary epithelium or in a dead end of the pelvic collection area. Furthermore, from the buildup of stones, alternating layers of crystals and organic material, it may well be concluded that the crystal material of a growing stone is not, or not fully, exposed to the urine fluid. If so, the crystallization processes that increase the size of a stone may take place in confined spaced. It has been suggested that this may be some gel-like environment and several techniques have been devised to study crystallization under such conditions.[47,53] For crystallization in a gel, smaller compounds may play a larger role as they can more freely move through the space. Phytate, for instance, strongly retards the formation of stones in the stone farm technique.[47] If this type of research leads to understanding of how a stone actually grows and to ways of interfering with that growth, this might allow patients to keep stones at a size that do not cause symptoms.

32.5 Conclusions

This chapter has described the information that crystallization studies have produced with respect to understanding urinary stone formation. Many questions remain unanswered. Further crystallization studies are needed to answer these questions. When performing such experiments, it is important to apply test conditions that resemble the natural conditions; which conditions those are will depend on the specific aspect of urinary stone formation that you would want to explore. In Fig. 32.1 showing a nephron in a papilla, seven sites are described plus the specific aspects of crystallization that may occur there and may be relevant to stone formation. Examples for experimental conditions that resemble those sites can be found, for instance, in a review by Kok.[1]

Acknowledgments DJ Kok Jr. is gracefully thanked for producing the figure on crystallization in a nephron.

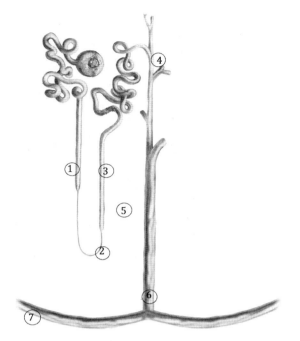

Fig. 32.1 (1) Possible sites of crystallization in the kidney. Crystallization in the proximal tubule. Under normal situations, the solution composition in the proximal tubule should not allow crystal nucleation to occur during the transit time of the fluid. A likely characteristic of the abnormal situation thus will be rapid nucleation driven by extreme SS. Examples are animal and human cases of hyperoxalaemia. **(2)** Crystallization in the long loop of Henle. The conditions in the loop of Henle are clearly distinct from the rest of the kidney. In the longest loops, the concentration of lithogenic compounds approaches (oxalate) or may supersede (calcium) the final concentrations in the urine. Furthermore, the pH is always high. The normal situation here may well be inevitable nucleation, especially of pH sensitive minerals like calcium phosphates and indinavir.[9,10] The question here will be how the kidney can handle such crystal formation. **(3)** Crystallization in the distal tubule. **(4)** Crystal–cell interaction in the distal tubule and beyond. In the distal tubule, the presence of (remnants of) crystals originating from the loop of Henle may be a normal situation. Cells are prepared as they show anti-adherence capability. Heterogeneous nucleation may occur here. **(5)** Interstitial crystal handling. The presence of crystalline calcium phosphate around the loop of Henle is relatively common (75% of stone formers and up to 43% of non-stone formers)[25,27] and does not seem to evoke a cellular response. In contrast, interstitial presence of calcium oxalate crystals induces strong cellular reactions.[24] Calcium oxalate crystals that enter the interstitium are readily surrounded by giant multinuclear macrophages and dissolved over time. These cells and/or their precursors must somehow sense the presence of the crystals. Proteins attached to or present inside the crystals may be important for this recognition and the consequent removal process.[18] **(6)** Crystal aggregation in the collecting ducts. A special feature of the collecting ducts/ducts of Bellini is the fact that multiple nephrons shed their content into one such tubule. Crystalline particles emerging from different nephrons have an increased chance of meeting each other and forming larger structures inside these still confined structures. The study of aggregation will be most relevant under these conditions. **(7)** Stone attached to the papillary surface. Crystal material that is attached to the outside of a papilla, for instance starting from a Randall's plaque where the cell surface was eroded or from a precipitate blocking the duct of Bellini, may grow as it is continuously exposed to the urine. The characteristic stone buildup may be governed by these conditions (Illustration courtesy of DJ Kok Jr.)

References

1. Kok DJ. Free and fixed particle mechanism, a review. *Scan Electron Microsc.* 1996;10:471-486.
2. Kok DJ, Khan SR. Calcium oxalate nephrolithiasis, a free or fixed particle disease. *Kidney Int.* 1994;46:847-854.
3. Luptak I, Bek-Jensen H, Fornander AM, Hoigaard I, Nilsson MA, Tiselius HG. Crystallization of calcium oxalate and calcium phosphate at supersaturation levels corresponding to those in different parts of the nephron. *Scan Microsc.* 1994;8:47-54.
4. Asplin J, Mandel NS, Coe Fl. Evidence for calcium phosphate supersaturation in the loop of Henle. *Am J Physiol.* 1996;270: F604-F613.
5. Balcke P, Zazgornik J, Sunder-Plasmann G, et al. Transient hyperoxaluria after ingestion of chocolate as a risk factor for calcium oxalate calculi. *Nephron.* 1989;51:32-34.
6. Verkoelen CF, van der Boom BG, Kok DJ, et al. Cell type-specific acquired protection from crystal adherence by renal tubule cells in culture. *Kidney Int.* 1999;55:1426-1433.
7. Verkoelen CF, Van Der Boom BG, Kok DJ, Schroder FH, Romijn JC. Attachment sites for particles in the urinary tract. *J Am Soc Nephrol.* 1999;10:S430-S435.
8. Khan SR. Animal models of kidney stone formation: an analysis. *World J Urol.* 1997;15:236-243.
9. Dieleman JP, Salahuddin S, Hsu YS, et al. Indinavir crystallisation under loop of Henle conditions: experimental evidence. *J Acq Immun Def Synd.* 2001;28:9-13.
10. Salahuddin S, Hsu YS, Buchholz NP, Dieleman JP, Gyssens IC, Kok DJ. Is indinavir crystalluria an indicator for indinavir stone formation? *AIDS.* 2001;15:1079-1080.
11. Kok DJ, Schell-Feith. Risk factors for crystallisation in the nephron: the role of renal development. *J Am Soc Nephrol.* 1999;10: S364-S370.
12. Tang R, Nancollas GH, Giocondi JL, Hoyer JR, Orme CA. Dual roles of brushite crystals in calcium oxalate crystallisation provide physicochemical mechanisms underlying renal stone formation. *Kidney Int.* 2006;70:71-78.
13. Guan X, Wang L, Dosen A, et al. An understanding of renal stone development in a mixed oxalate-phosphate system. *Langmuir.* 2008;24(14):7058-7060.
14. Khan SR, Glenton PA. Calcium oxalate crystal deposition in kidneys of hypercalciuric mice with disrupted type IIa sodium-phosphate cotransporter. *Am J Physiol Renal Physiol.* 2008;294: F1109-F1115.
15. Khan SR, Kok DJ. Modulators of urinary stone formation. *Front Bioscience.* 2004;1:1450-1482.
16. de Bruijn WC, Boevé ER, van Run PRWA, et al. Etiology of experimental calcium oxalate monohydrate nephrolithiasis in rats I. Can this be a model of human stone formation? *Scanning Microsc.* 1995;9:103-114.
17. De Water R, Boevé ER, van Miert PPMC, et al. Pathological and immunocytochemical changes in chronic calcium oxalate nephrolithiasis in the rat. *Scanning Microsc.* 1996;10(2):577-590.
18. De Water R, Noordermeer C, Houtsmuller AB, et al. Role of macrophages in nephrolithiasis in rats: an analysis of the renal interstitium. *Am J Kidney Dis.* 2000;36:615-625.
19. Bushinsky DA, Frick KK, Nehrke K. Genetic hypercalciuric stone-forming rats. *Curr Opin Nephrol Hypertens.* 2006;15:403-418.
20. Grohe B, O'Young J, Ionescu DA, et al. Control of calcium oxalate crystal growth by face-specific adsorption of an osteopontin phosphopeptide. *J Am Chem Soc.* 2007;129:14946-14951.
21. Taller A, Grohe B, Rogers KA, Goldberg HA, Hunter GK. Specific adsorption of osteopontin and synthetic polypeptides to calcium oxalate monohydrate crystals. *Biophys J.* 2007;93:1768-1777.

22. Wang L, Guan X, Tang R, Hoyer JR, Wierzbicki A, De Yoreo JJ, Nancollas GH. Phosphorylation of osteopontin is required for inhibition of calcium oxalate crystallization. J Phys Chem B. 9 Jul 2008 [Epub ahead of print].

23. Mo L, Liaw L, Evan AP, Sommer AJ, Lieske JC, Wu XR. Renal calcinosis and stone formation in mice lacking osteopontin, Tamm-Horsfall protein, or both. Am J Physiol Renal Physiol. 2007;293: F1935-F1943.

24. De Water R, Noordermeer C, van der Kwast TH, et al. Calcium oxalate nephrolithiasis: effect of renal crystal deposition on the cellular composition of the renal interstitium. Am J Kidney Dis. 1999;33:761-771.

25. Randall A. Papillary pathology as a precursor of primary renal calculus. J Urol. 1940;44:580-589.

26. Bennington JL, Haber SL, Smith JV, Warner NE. Crystals of calcium oxalate in the human kidney. Studies by means of electron microprobe and X-ray diffraction. J Clin Pathol. 1964;41:8-14.

27. Evan AP, Coe FL, Gillen D, Lingeman JE, Bledsoe S, Worcester EM. Renal intratubular crystals and hyaluronan staining occur in stone formers with bypass surgery but not with idiopathic calcium oxalate stones. Anat Rec (Hoboken). 2008;291:325-334.

28. Verkoelen CF. Crystal retention in renal stone disease: a crucial role for the glycosaminoglycan hyaluronan? J Am Soc Nephrol. 2006;17:1673-1687.

29. Khan SR, Finlayson B, Hackett RL. Histologic study of the early events in oxalate induced intranephronic calculosis. Invest Urol. 1979;17:199-202.

30. Borghi L, Schianchi T, Meschi T, et al. Comparison of two diets for the prevention of recurrent stones in idiopathic hypercalciuria. N Engl J Med. 2002;346:77-84.

31. Khan SR, Hacket RL. Retention of calcium oxalate crystals in renal tubules. Scanning Microsc. 1991;5:707-712.

32. Sandersius S, Rez P. Morphology of crystals in calcium oxalate monohydrate kidney stones. Urol Res. 2007;35:287-293.

33. Finlayson B, Reid F. The expectation of free and fixed particles in urinary stone disease. Invest Urol. 1978;15:442-448.

34. Kok DJ, Papapoulos SE, Bijvoet OLM. Excessive crystal agglomeration with low citrate excretion in recurrent stone formers. Lancet. 1986 May 10;1(8489):1056-1058.

35. Kok DJ, Papapoulos SE, Bijvoet OLM. Crystal agglomeration is a major element in calcium oxalate urinary stone formation. Kidney Int. 1990;37:51-56.

36. Kok DJ, Papapoulos SE, Bijvoet OLM. Modulation of calcium oxalate monohydrate growth kinetics in vitro. Kidney Int. 1988;34:346-350.

37. Kok DJ, Iestra J, Doorenbos JC, Papapoulos SE. The effects of chronic dietary loads with salt and animal protein on the calcium oxalate crystallization kinetics in urines of healthy men. J Clin Endocrin Metab. 1990;71:861-867.

38. Kok DJ. Inhibitors of calcium oxalate crystallization. In: Khan SR, ed. Calcium oxalate in biological systems, chapter 2. Boca Raton, FL: CRC press; 1995:23-36.

39. Hess B, Jordi S, Zipperle L, Ettinger E, Giovanoli R. Citrate determines calcium oxalate crystallization kinetics and crystal morphology-studies in the presence of Tamm-Horsfall protein of a healthy subject and a severely recurrent calcium stone former. Nephrol Dial Transplant. 2000;15:366-374.

40. Erwin DT, Kok DJ, Alam J, et al. Predicting recurrent renal stone formation and therapy using crystal agglomeration inhibition. Am J Kidney Dis. 1994;24:893-900.

41. Kleinman JG, Alatalo LJ, Beshensky AM, Wesson JA. Acidic polyanion poly(acrylic acid) prevents calcium oxalate crystal deposition. Kidney Int. 18 Jun 2008.

42. Ryall RL, Chauvet MC, Grover PK. Intracrystalline proteins and urolithiasis: a comparison of the protein content and ultrastructure of urinary calcium oxalate monohydrate and dihydrate crystals. BJU Int. 2005;96:654-663.

43. Webber D, Rodgers AL, Sturrock ED. Glycosylation of prothrombin fragment 1 governs calcium oxalate crystal nucleation and aggregation, but not crystal growth. Urol Res. 2007;35:277-285.

44. Bergsland KJ, Kelly JK, Coe BJ, Coe FL. Urine protein markers distinguish stone-forming from non-stone-forming relatives of calcium stone formers. Am J Physiol Renal Physiol. 2006;291:F530-F536.

45. Fuselier HA, Moore K, Lindberg J, et al. Urinary Tamm-Horsfall protein increased after potassium citrate therapy in calcium stone formers. Urology. 1995;45:942-946.

46. Thongboonkerd V, Chutipongtanate S, Semangoen T, Malasit P. Urinary trefoil factor 1 is a novel potent inhibitor of calcium oxalate crystal growth and aggregation. J Urol. 2008;179:1615-1619.

47. Saw NK, Chow K, Rao PN, Kavanagh JP. Effects of inositol hexaphosphate (phytate) on calcium binding, calcium oxalate crystallisation and in vitro stone growth. J Urol. 2007;177:2366-2370.

48. Fleming DE, Van Riessen A, Chauvet MC, et al. Intracrystalline proteins and urolithiasis: a synchrotron X-ray diffraction study of calcium oxalate monohydrate. J Bone Miner Res. 2003;18:1282-1291.

49. De Bruijn WC, de Water R, van Run PRWA, et al. Ultrastructural osteopontin localization in papillary stones induced in rats. Eur Urol. 1997;32:360-367.

50. McKee MD, Nanci A, Khan SR. Ultrastructural immunodetection of osteopontin and osteocalcin as major matrix components of renal calculi. J Bone Miner Res. 1995;10:1913-1929.

51. Ryall RL, Fleming DE, Doyle IR, Evans NA, Dean CJ, Marshall VR. Intracrystalline proteins and the hidden ultrastructure of calcium oxalate urinary crystals: implications for kidney stone formation. J Struct Biol. 2001;134:5-14.

52. Grover PK, Thurgood LA, Fleming DE, van Bronswijk W, Wang T, Ryall RL. Intracrystalline urinary proteins facilitate degradation and dissolution of calcium oxalate crystals in cultured renal cells. Am J Physiol Renal Physiol. 2008;294:F355-F361.

53. Achilles W, Freitag R, Kiss B, Riedmiller H. Quantification of crystal growth of calcium oxalate in gel and its modification by urinary constituents in a new flow model of crystallisation. J Urol. 1995;154:1552-1556.

Experimental Models for Investigation of Stone Disease

33

Kemal Sarica

Abstract The incidence of stone disease has been rising in recent years and calcium-containing stones (calcium oxalate) are the most prevalent stone types of all. In an attempt to mimic the stone formation process in humans and to understand the mechanisms involved, a number of theoretical, chemical, and animal models have been developed.

In these experimental models, formation of calcium oxalate deposits in the kidney can be demonstrated in a short period of time by enabling the physicians to study the processes involved in stone maturation, as well as for examining the role of inhibitors and promoters of crystal growth. Although rabbits and dogs have also been used, rats are the most commonly used animals for the study of nephrolithiasis.

An accurate and reliable animal model may allow us to develop newer treatment algorithms and medications that may help to better understand the pathogenesis of stone formation and direct improved methods of stone prevention.

There are many similarities between experimental nephrolithiasis-induced rat model and human kidney stone formation where oxalate metabolism is considered to be almost identical between rats and humans. The accumulated data so far have clearly shown that rat models of nephrolithiasis may help us to evaluate the various phases of stone formation including nucleation, aggregation, and retention of crystals.

Last but not least, although the pathogenesis of stone formation can be studied in animal models, the limitations of these models should always be kept in mind.

33.1 Introduction

The incidence of stone disease has been rising in recent years and calcium-containing stones(calcium oxalate) are the most prevalent stone types detected in cases suffering from this disease.[1,2] In an attempt to mimic the stone formation in humans and to understand well the mechanisms involved in this extraordinary complex process, a number of theoretical, chemical, and animal models have been developed.[3–7] Such models helped the physician not only to demonstrate the formation of urinary stones in animal kidneys, but also at the same time they enabled an understanding of the different aspects of urinary stone disease as well as the possible underlying mechanisms involved. Moreover, development of the

newer treatment algorithms and medications that may help to better understand the pathogenesis of stone formation and search for improved methods of stone prevention were among the goals to be achieved by using these models. There is no doubt that such experimental models gave a great chance to the physicians in providing a significant contribution to the study of renal stones. Since a vast majority of urinary stones contain calcium oxalate (CaOx) crystals, CaOx urolithiasis has been studied in greater detail.[8–11]

On the other hand, among the different animal models used, the rat is the most frequently used animal in the majority of these studies. As spontaneous calcium oxalate urolithiasis is very rare in these animals, the experimental induction of hyperoxaluria has been found to be of paramount importance to promote CaOx urolithiasis in rats, where the animals are generally made hyperoxaluric either by administration of excess oxalate, exposure to the toxin ethylene glycol, or various nutritional manipulations. All of the experimental models did show renal injury associated with crystal deposition.[2,3,12–16]

K. Sarica (✉)
Department of Urology, University of Yeditepe, Medical School, Istanbul, Turkey
e-mail: ksarica@yeditepe.edu.tr

P.N. Rao et al. (eds.), *Urinary Tract Stone Disease*,
DOI 10.1007/978-1-84800-362-0_33, © Springer-Verlag London Limited 2011

Studies have clearly demonstrated that in such models, calcium oxalate deposit formation in animal kidneys can be demonstrated in a short period of time, with the macroscopic presence of renal and ureteral stones. Therefore, experimental animal models are ideal to study both the processes involved in stone maturation and the role of inhibitors and promoters of crystal growth.[1–3,17–20]

33.2 Induction of Hyperoxaluria

To evaluate and understand the complex nature of calcium oxalate stone disease in humans, excess urinary excretion of urinary stone forming risk factors (with or without manipulation of urinary pH and/or deficient excretion of crystallization inhibitors) has been the principal mechanism used to induce experimentally crystallization in the urine and formation of stones in the kidneys. With this aim, induction of hyperoxaluria has been well accomplished in different animal models by either addition of oxalate or an oxalate precursor (such as ethylene glycol, glycolate, and hydroxyproline) to the diet, or by intraperitoneally injecting them into the animal used. Additionally, hyperoxaluria has also been induced by other dietary manipulations including pyridoxine-deficient diets, low phosphate diets, and high protein diets. In these experimental models, ethylene glycol (EG) has generally been used either by itself or in combination with ammonium chloride (NH4Cl, by generating acidic urine pH) or vitamin D3 in an attempt to form calcium oxalate crystals in urine and calcium oxalate deposits in the kidneys of rats. However, EG, NH4Cl, and vitamin D3 each has been found to be nephrotoxic, and at high doses these agents may further worsen the general condition of the rats.[1–4,6,9,18,20] Use of these compounds has also been found to be advantageous not only for economical reasons, but also for their practical administration via drinking water where CaOx crystal deposition is observed in a short period of time.

Although EG-induced hyperoxaluria in animal models is the most common way of experimental stone formation, this method has been criticized for the nephrotoxic nature of EG and some of its metabolites as well as the subsequent formation of metabolic acidosis. Last but not least, both oxalate (Ox) and CaOx crystals have also been found to be injurious to renal epithelial cells, making it difficult enough to distinguish the effects of EG and its metabolites from those induced by Ox and CaOx crystals.

33.3 Calcium Oxalate Stone Formation

Urinary stones form following a complex sequence of events for which the oversaturation of the urine with calculogenic risk factors, urinary levels of crystallization inhibitors, and various urinary promoters of crystal aggregation and growth play certain roles in this specific process. Related with this subject again, nucleation, crystal growth, aggregation, and retention of the concrements within the urinary system are the main steps in the pathogenesis of urinary stones. This complex sequence of events, however, may be controlled by a variety of modulators, which may ultimately promote, inhibit, or modify them. In the final phase of urinary stone formation, retained crystals within the urinary system will evolve into urinary stones – a process that has not yet been experimentally examined in detail.[21–24]

In the early process of urinary stone formation, contact of the urinary crystals with renal epithelial cells and an eventual retention phase have been proposed as critical events where cell injury has also been proposed as one of the important factors involved in the development of small crystals into mature stones. In the present experimental models of urinary stone formation, calcium oxalate crystal deposition has often been associated with severe kidney dysfunction and renal damage.

Studies have clearly demonstrated that deposition of calcium oxalate crystals in wide areas of the kidneys is a common finding noted shortly after hyperoxaluria induction, and this condition has been accepted as indicating an abnormal physiological condition. Taking this fact into account, to investigate cell injury originating from mild hyperoxaluria and crystaluria along with the attachment of the crystals to renal epithelial cells, more physiological conditions should be searched to mimic the events occurring in the human body. It is necessary to establish a suitable model for calcium oxalate crystaluria with minimal or no renal damage.

Lastly, crystal–cell interaction has also been studied in in vitro models using calcium oxalate crystals and many kinds of kidney cells, which have been grown in cell culture models. Crystal–cell interaction during calcium oxalate stone formation has been well evaluated in animal models with appropriate conditions for hyperoxaluria and calcium oxalate crystaluria without concomitant renal damage.[25–28]

33.3.1 Crystal Formation in the Kidney

Much information about how and where the crystals of CaOx are formed in the kidneys has been provided by in vivo studies using mainly the rat models. Documented cases of spontaneous urinary stone formation in rats are rare. Although, renal calcium phosphate and/or ammonium magnesium phosphate stones have been reported, there are no reports of spontaneously formed oxalate stones in the rat upper urinary tract. Rarely, oxalate stones have been found in the bladder. Of 100 male Sprague–Dawley rats in a toxicity study, only 2 rats were found to have oxalate calculi and these were associated with calcium carbonate and calcium or ammonium phosphate.[2,3,6,9]

Provided that there is no spontaneous production of urinary stones by normal rats (especially the calcium oxalate type), induction of hyperoxaluria seems to be the initial and essential step. This condition could be accepted as similar to humans because the presence of hyperoxaluria is regarded as the critical factor of idiopathic CaOx urolithiasis in humans too.

Induction of acute hyperoxaluria or moderate- to high-grade chronic hyperoxaluria in male Sprague–Dawley rats (a condition somewhat similar to primary hyperoxaluria in humans) results in urinary CaOx supersaturation and subsequent deposition of the formed crystals in the proximal segments of the renal tubules. On the other hand, however, a low-grade chronic hyperoxaluria (a condition probably similar to most hyperoxaluric stone formers) results in a deposition of crystals in the papillary segments of the renal tubules.

Crystals are seen in the kidneys up to 7 days after the challenge. They are initially seen in the tubular lumen and later by day 7 in the interstitium. Calcium oxalate crystals deposit first in the papillary collecting ducts. Crystal deposition in the kidneys is preceded by calcium oxalate crystalluria and starts with the retention of aggregated calcium oxalate crystals in the renal tubules. Retained crystals move from the tubules to the interstitium, and in the process, become anchored to the tubular basement membrane. Crystal aggregates present in the superficial peripheral collecting ducts of the renal papillae ulcerate through to the papillary surface and grow into the stones. In addition, it has been shown that interstitial crystals surrounded by cells are generally involved in the inflammatory processes.[5,6,10]

33.3.2 Animal Models of Stone Formation

In an attempt to work the pathophysiologic pathways of CaOx stone formation occurring in the human body in an experimental basis, several animal models have been developed and used. As the models are used to imitate the complex events taking place in the human body, physicians aimed to benefit from these models to a considerable extent by dividing the whole process into separate segments in an attempt to simplify it and reproduce the events whenever needed. An additional aim was to validate the hypotheses by evaluating the effect and consequences of certain therapeutic modalities in these models.[2–4,6,29–33]

Taking the fairly complex nature of urinary stone formation into account, (which involves urinary oversaturation with stone-forming salts, the presence and certain effects of various urinary inhibitors and promoters of crystal aggregation and growth) various animal models ranging from rats to dogs have been used, including diet-induced urolithiasis, drug-induced urolithiasis, and genetically altered animals that form stones to evaluate the process of calculous formation in detail. In addition to the nearly identical oxalate metabolism of the

rat to that in humans, experimental calcium oxalate urolithiasis in the rat has also been found to be similar to calcium oxalate stone disease in humans.[2–4,10,13,14,33–35]

However, although there is a sufficient knowledge about the phases of stone formation in humans, it is clear that adequate information about human and model animal kidney anatomy, and to some extent urinary chemistry, is necessary. Studies have demonstrated that there are basic anatomical differences between kidneys of humans and those of animals such as dogs, rabbits, and rats. With this aim in addition to study the renal ultrastructure and physiology, rats have been extensively used in the development of models of many renal diseases. Basically, the kidneys of these animals are much smaller, are unipapillate, and have fewer urinary tubules, a simpler pelvis, and a smaller urinary space. However, the medulla-to-cortex volume ratio is very similar, being 1:2 in the rat, the dog, and the human, and 1:16 in the rabbit. In the light of these differences, especially with respect to the size of the animal model kidney, one may appreciate that model kidneys with relatively smaller renal structures (especially the renal pelvis) will produce only a small miniature imitation of the human stone.[2–4,6,8,17,35]

Last, but not least, to set up and evaluate the complex phases of urolithiasis in different animal models, authors have stated that the desired model should form calculi in a reproducible manner and stone-forming agents should not be toxic to the normal urinary tissues. With this aim, as the most easily available and commonly used laboratory animal, rats have been used in a number of experimental models to study calcium oxalate urolithiasis.[6,9,12–15,36,37]

33.3.3 Evaluation of Stone Formation in Different Models

As mentioned earlier, to evaluate and discuss the different steps of the complex stone formation process, a number of models have been developed and used as reported in the literature. Although the data obtained from the use of these models did produce valuable data to a certain extent, regarding the very complex nature of the urinary stone formation, it is clear that there is no unique model that will provide adequate information about all aspects of the pathogenesis of urinary calculi. Some of these models provide limited information regarding only one aspect of the whole process. Related with this subject, while crystal nucleation and growth parts of stone formation have been well studied by using various types of crystallizers, tissue-culture studies are currently being used to outline the possible interaction between oxalate and/or calcium oxalate crystals and renal tubular epithelial cells. On the other hand, theoretical computational models could provide limited information concerning the crystallization potential of urine itself.[38–44]

In addition to the information obtained in the pathogenesis of calcium oxalate stone formation, some experimental animal models did provide additional data regarding the anatomical and physiological role of kidneys as well as the renal tubules in this specific complex process. Although rats are the most commonly used animal type to study the different phases of stone formation, rabbits and dogs have also been used for this aim. As calcium oxalate (CaOx) stones constitute the most commonly diagnosed and treated type (75–80%), formation of these stones has been subjected to the majority of these experimental models.

Evaluation of the experimental models used in the literature did clearly show that *diet-induced urolithiasis* was commonly used, mainly in rat models, to both induce and evaluate stone formation.[2,6,45–48] Much of the information in the pathogenesis of uric acid calculi has been derived from these models. Induction of severe hyperuricemia as well as severe hyperuricosuria were produced in male Wistar rats by feeding dietary supplements of oxonic acid and uric acid. Long-term renal histological alterations in this animal model (drug-induced hyperuricemia) have been found to be similar to the changes noted in human gouty nephropathy. Authors have claimed that this type of model may provide an opportunity to investigate certain factors influencing the renal alterations during sustained hyperuricemia.[49]

Another example of this type of model was "a high protein diet model" using casein in rats. Following the institution of increased dietary protein in these animals (a substantial acid load), significantly decreased urinary pH and urinary citrate have been well noted, which at the same time resulted in increased urinary calcium and calcium phosphate saturation. Researchers noted that, despite the lack of evident stone formation, this model might provide valuable information regarding the mechanisms of protein-induced nephrolithiasis due to the higher consumption of animal protein.[50,51] Last, but not least, a pyridoxine-deficient rat model with the addition of 3% glycolic acid has been found to induce hyperoxaluria in Wistar rats. Researchers have used these models to evaluate the effects of dietary modifications on stone formation, among which vitamin E and selenium have been commonly tested.[52]

In *drug-induced animal models,* CaOx calculi formation has been evaluated following the induction of hyperoxaluria by classical application of ethylene glycol (EG) in rats. While hyperoxaluria formation alone after EG administration alone does not result in stone formation, as a potent nephrotoxic agent causing renal tubular injury, gentamicin application was also found to be essential to induce renal crystals. These models support the concept that renal cellular damage must be associated with an underlying metabolic defect, in this case hyperoxaluria, to induce nephrolithiasis.[2,6,53,54]

More recently, hydroxyproline (HP) has been used to induce hyperoxaluria and subsequently to investigate possible stone formation. Gross morphological and microscopic histopathological analyses did reveal CaOx crystal deposition, and renal tubular injury were noted on the renal papillae. This model successfully mimics the most common type of metabolic abnormality as well as the most common type of stone seen in humans.[1,55,56]

As a promising animal model of urolithiasis, "genetic hypercalciuric stone-forming animals," primarily rats and mice, have been genetically inbred for more than 54 generations in an attempt to serve as a model for the most common metabolic abnormality: hypercalciuria. Metabolic abnormalities noted in these animals were similar to patients with idiopathic hypercalciuria. Genetic hypercalciuric rats have been found to absorb excessive amounts of intestinal calcium, fail to adequately reabsorb filtered calcium, and their bone resorption is uniquely sensitive to 1,25(OH)2D3. All of these characteristics are apparently due to an increase in the number of receptors for vitamin D. Studies have demonstrated that these rats spontaneously form calcium phosphate stones in the absence of dietary related hyperoxaluria. Both hypercalciuric rats and humans appear to be predisposed to initially form calcium phosphate stones and not the commonly observed calcium oxalate stones. Thus, these findings suggest that rats and humans appear to be protected against calcium oxalate stone formation unless a nucleation site, such as the more easily formed calcium phosphate crystal, is present.[12,14,15]

As an inhibitory urinary protein in CaOx crystal formation, Tamm-Horsfall protein (THP) has been investigated using a THP knockout mouse model for the spontaneous formation of calcium crystals in the kidney. Experimentally induced renal crystal formation was achieved by administering ethylene glycol and vitamin D3 that increase calcium absorption. In this model, inactivation of the THP gene in mouse embryonic stem cells caused the spontaneous formation of calcium crystals in adult kidneys. As the most common type of risk factors for human renal stones, diet-related hypercalciuria and hyperoxaluria did apparently increase the frequency and the severity of renal calcium crystal formation in THP-deficient mice. These results in turn provide the first in vivo evidence that THP is a critical urinary defense factor against calcium oxalate crystal formation. Thus, deficiency of THP could play an important role in calcium oxalate stone formation.[57]

Although it is not as common as hypercalciuria and/or hyperoxaluria, cystinuria has been well studied by using the Newfoundland dog model as the most widely used model. Hexagonal microcrystals indicative for cystine calculi were found in the urine of all homozygous animals. However, renal and/or bladder calculi were reported in all homozygous males and about 23% of homozygous females. This gender prevalence is also noted in dogs and wolves.[58]

Finally, the role of the enteric bacteria *Oxalobacter formigenes*, which colonizes in the colon and regulates oxalate homoeostasis, primarily by preventing enteric oxalate absorption, has been evaluated in some animal models. It has been clearly postulated that the loss of this bacterium from intestinal flora is associated with an increased risk of hyperoxaluria and calcium oxalate urolithiasis. In such models, noncolonized Sprague–Dawley rats were colonized with live bacteria or treated with oxalate-degrading enzymes derived from *O. formigenes* to determine the response to a high oxalate load and they were found to excrete lower levels of oxalate, without crystalluria, and that of calcium oxalate crystals in the nephrons, as observed in control rats. In the light of the published data, *O. formigenes* has been found to be important for maintaining oxalate homeostasis, absence of which has been shown to increase the risk of hyperoxaluria and recurrent kidney stone disease. Data derived from these models demonstrated that the replacement therapy might be an efficient procedure to prevent hyperoxaluria and related complications.[59–62]

33.4 CaOx Nephrolithiasis

Induction of acute or chronic hyperoxaluria by using a variety of agents such as sodium oxalate, ammonium oxalate, hydroxy-L-proline, ethylene glycol, and glycolic acid in different animal models was the main step for the formation of CaOx stones in animals (mainly in rats).

Although these agents are generally applied orally in food or water or by gavage, intraperitoneal injection has also been used to induce hyperoxaluria. Lastly, such agents have often been used in association with vitamin D or a magnesium-deficient diet and, sometimes, with a pH-reducing protocol of ammonium chloride administration.[1,3,7,18,20,30,45,46,63]

Studies have clearly demonstrated that following the induction of acute hyperoxaluria by way of intraperitoneal sodium oxalate injection increased urinary excretion of oxalate; and accumulation of CaOx crystals in lumina of the renal proximal tubules could easily be demonstrated as well. Crystals were later seen in collecting ducts of the cortex and papilla. The amount of the injected hyperoxaluric agent affected the duration of urinary excretion of excess oxalate and the size, number, and location of crystals within the kidneys. The largest amount of oxalate was excreted within the first 6 h of the challenge. Depending on the dose of the injected agent, crystals either were restricted to the tubular lumens with lower doses and disappeared within a few days or they were initially located in tubular lumina and later seen in the interstitium with higher doses of the agent. On the other hand, while some crystals and crystal aggregates remained small and did not adhere to the renal epithelium being subsequently flushed out with the urine, relatively larger crystals did move slowly and they were attached to the

renal epithelium being too large to move with the urine migrated to the interstitium. Lastly, histologic evaluation after hyperoxaluria induction has clearly demonstrated that the main sites of crystal retention were the renal papillary tips and the corticomedullary junction.[2,3,6]

Another way of hyperoxaluria induction was oral chronic administration of ethylene glycol (EG) as a 0.75% aqueous solution in drinking water to male Sprague–Dawley rats. While excretion of oxalate was found to increase significantly, excretion of calcium, magnesium, and citrate decreased, leading to an increased urinary CaOx supersaturation accordingly. During chronic hyperoxaluria induced by the administration of 0.75% EG alone or with 2% ammonium chloride (AC), persistent crystalluria was present in all rats by day 3 and nephrolithiasis by day 7. It has also been observed that it took rats approximately 12 days of chronic administration of EG alone to show persistent crystalluria and about 3 weeks to start depositing crystals in their kidneys. In addition to the induction of hyperoxaluria, a magnesium-deficient diet has accelerated and exaggerated crystalluria and nephrolithiasis in male rats receiving 1% EG in drinking water. The crystals were located in both the cortex and the medulla. Administration of magnesium oxide to male rats receiving a 1% aqueous solution of EG significantly reduced their urinary oxalate excretion and stopped their CaOx nephrolithiasis.[2,3]

Another important observation derived from these studies was the size and distribution of these crystals during the chronic hyperoxaluric phase, and it has been noted that the crystals were initially formed randomly in the renal medulla. In later stages of hyperoxaluric phase, however, the collecting ducts at the renal papillary tip and papillary base were the preferred sites of crystal deposition. After 4–6 weeks, crystals were also seen between the tubular epithelial cells as well as inside the epithelial cells and the interstitium. After only 1 week of EG+AC treatment or 8 weeks of EG alone, the kidneys of some rats had nephroliths or stones attached to their renal papillary surfaces. These stones contained both CaOx mono – and dihydrate crystals and calcified the entire papillary tip. Examination of the papillary stones by light microscopy and scanning and transmission electron microscopy revealed that they originated in the lumina of collecting ducts near the renal papillary surface.[2,6]

In addition to evident hyperoxaluria and subsequent crystal formation in animal models, acute or chronic induction of hyperoxaluria did also cause the increased urinary excretion of some certain enzymes.[2,6,64,65] As a lysosomal enzyme, urinary levels of N-acetyl-3-glucosaminidase increased in mild chronic hyperoxaluria without crystal deposition in the kidneys. On the other hand, by causing tubular damage, deposition of CaOx crystals has been found to be associated with increased urinary excretion of the membrane marker enzymes such as alkaline phosphatase, leucine aminopeptidase, and gamma-glutamyl transpeptidase. Severe damage has been shown in membranes of the tubules containing the crystals.[2,3,6]

With respect to the gender difference of the animals used as a model, all studies described were carried out in male rats. EG solutions of low concentration that induce CaOx nephrolithiasis in male rats were not found to produce similar results in females. Male rats have been found to be more prone to crystal formation and deposition than female ones.

In conclusion, studies in rats with EG-induced hyperoxaluria have shown that CaOx nephrolithiasis can be induced experimentally and is associated with enzymuria. The renal papillary tip and calyces were the preferential sites for crystal deposition in chronic hyperoxaluria. Chances for crystal deposition elsewhere in the kidneys, including the renal cortex, increased with increasing levels of urinary oxalate and duration of the hyperoxaluric state. Magnesium deficiency was found to exacerbate nephrolithiasis. Experimentally produced crystals and stones did contain an organic matrix of carbohydrates, lipids, and proteins. On the other hand, studies have demonstrated that the female rats are more prone to CaP nephrolithiasis than male rats. Increased urinary excretion of calcium and phosphate and decreased excretion of magnesium promote CaP nephrolithiasis. Both testosterone and estrogen appeared to play a significant role in the pathogenesis.[2,66–68]

33.4.1 Comparison Between Rat and Human Nephrolithiasis

Detailed evaluation as well as comparison of the stones formed in models of rat kidneys revealed the following findings: In addition to the ultrastructural characteristics, despite the small size of the calculi formed, the nature and the composition of stone crystals and matrix have been found to be identical in both human and rat kidney stones. Moreover, formation of the calculi has been found to be initiated by crystal deposition in collecting ducts of the renal papilla and the subsequent stones have been found to be located on the papillary surfaces. These findings again have been reported as similar in humans and mildly hyperoxaluric rats. Concerning the underlying factors in stone formation in both humans and rats, chronic mild hyperoxaluria was found to be the main factor initiating these specific events. Taking the fact that not all the rats with similar urinary oxalate and CaOx supersaturation do produce CaOx nephroliths, it has been stated that factors other than supersaturation might be involved in kidney stone formation where experimental nephrolithiasis in rats has also been found to be associated

with a reduction in the urinary excretion of citrate. Unlike these findings, although a majority of idiopathic stone formers are hypercalciuric, experimentally induced stone formation in rats has been found to be associated with lower than normal urinary excretion of calcium.[2,6,69]

Last, but not least, renal crystal deposition in experimentally induced rats was in all conditions associated with cell injury. Cell damage can be detected during crystal formation, and it has been reported that the damage may occur either prior to or subsequent to crystal deposition.

However, enzymuria in the absence of nephrolithiasis indicated the possibility of impairment prior to crystallization and suggested that challenge to the renal epithelial cell could be an initiating event. The development of stones on Randall's plaques, enzymuria of proximal tubular origin, and functional or structural tubular abnormalities and/or tubular damage demonstrated in different studies implicate renal injury in human nephrolithiasis. The interaction between crystals and organic material appears critical in the attachment and growth of urinary stones. All crystals, whether experimentally induced in rats or spontaneously formed in humans, were found to contain organic material occluded within and on their surfaces.[70–73]

33.5 Conclusions

In the light of the findings presented in this chapter, it is clear that valuable data on the pathogenesis of kidney stone formation can be derived from the animal models, among which the rat is the most contributive one. Similarity of the oxalate metabolism in humans and rats may allow us to propose several strategies for experimental modeling of stones in rats. With respect to the complex nature of stone formation and the unanswered questions in the etiopathogenesis, by evaluating the sequence of events in animal models of nephrolithiasis, valuable data could be derived regarding the initial events; the site of early response to hyperoxaluric challenge; the nucleation, aggregation, and retention of crystals; and the involvement of macromolecules during these processes in the kidneys. Two key processes of stone formation, namely, stone nucleation and nidus formation in the study of nephrolithiasis and stone growth in the study of foreign-body encrustation have been well studied in animal models allowing us to compare them with the human stone formation.

In summary, animal models could provide reliable and valuable data to understand the pathogenetic steps of human nephrolithiasis. Given the similarities in pathophysiology, perhaps the treatment strategies used in animal urolithiasis models can be extrapolated to human stone disease.

Acknowledgment It is my pleasure to thank Saeed Khan for his highly contributive original experimental publications in forming animal designs for urolithiasis research and enabling us to benefit from them to an extraordinary extent.

References

1. Khan SR, Glenton PA, Byer KJ. Modeling of hyperoxaluric calcium oxalate nephrolithiasis: experimental induction of hyperoxaluria by hydroxy-L-proline. *Kidney Int.* 2006;70(5):914-923.
2. Khan SR. Animal models of kidney stone formation: an analysis. *World J Urol.* 1997;15(4):236-243. Review.
3. Khan SR. Experimental calcium oxalate nephrolithiasis and the formation of human urinary stones. *Scanning Microsc.* 1995; 9(1):89-100; discussion 100-101. Review.
4. Kumar S, Sigmon D, Miller T, Carpenter B, Khan S, Malhotra R, Scheid C, Menon M. A new model of nephrolithiasis involving tubular dysfunction/injury. *J Urol.* 1991;146(5):1384-1389.
5. Itatani H, Itoh H, Yoshioka T, Namiki M, Koide T, Okuyama A, Sonoda T. Renal metabolic changes relating to calculogenesis in an experimental model of calcium containing renal stone formation in rabbits. *Invest Urol.* 1981;19(2):119-122.
6. Khan SR, Hackett RL. Calcium oxalate urolithiasis in the rat: is it a model for human stone disease? A review of recent literature. *Scan Electron Microsc.* 1985;(Pt 2):759-774. Review.
7. Wolkowski-Tyl R, Chin TY, Popp JA, Heck HD. Chemically induced urolithiasis in weanling rats. *Am J Pathol.* 1982;107(3): 419-421.
8. Marnie R. Robinson, Regina D. Norris, Roger L. Sur, Glenn M. Preminger: Urolithiasis: Not Just a 2-Legged Animal Disease. *J Urol.* 2008;179:46-52.
9. Yamaguchi S, Wiessner JH, Hasegawa AT, Hung LY, Mandel GS, Mandel NS. Study of a rat model for calcium oxalate crystal formation without severe renal damage in selected conditions. *Int J Urol.* 2005;12:290-298.
10. de Bruijn WC, Boevé ER, van Run PR, van Miert PP, de Water R, Romijn JC, Verkoelen CF, Cao LC, Schröder FH. Etiology of calcium oxalate nephrolithiasis in rats. I. Can this be a model for human stone formation? *Scanning Microsc.* 1995;9(1):103-114.
11. Robertson WG. Kidney models of calcium oxalate stone formation. *Nephron Physiol.* 2004;98(2):21-30.
12. Bushinsky DA, Frick KK, Nehrke K. Genetic hypercalciuric stone-forming rats. *Curr Opin Nephrol Hypertens.* 2006;15(4):403-418.
13. Worcester EM, Chuang M, Laven B, Orvieto M, Coe FL, Evan AP, Gerber GS. A new animal model of hyperoxaluria and nephrolithiasis in rats with small bowel resection. *Urol Res.* 2005;33(5): 380-382. Review.
14. Bushinsky DA. Bench to bedside: lessons from the genetic hypercalciuric stone-forming rat. *Am J Kidney Dis.* 2000;36(3):LXI-LXIV.
15. Bushinsky DA. Genetic hypercalciuric stone forming rats. *Semin Nephrol.* 1996;16(5):448-457. Review.
16. Yasui T, Fujita K, Sasaki S, Sato M, Sugimoto M, Hirota S, Kitamura Y, Nomura S, Kohri K. Expression of bone matrix proteins in urolithiasis model rats. *Urol Res.* 1999;27(4):255-261.
17. Bouropoulos N, Bouropoulos C, Klepetsanis PG, Melekos M, Barbalias G, Koutsoukos PG. A model system for the investigation of urinary stone formation. *Br J Urol.* 1996;78(2):169-175.
18. Sarica K, Bakir K, Yağci F, Topçu O, Akbay C, Sayin N, Korkmaz C. Limitation of shockwave-induced enhanced crystal deposition in traumatized tissue by verapamil in rabbit model. *J Endourol.* 1999;13(5):343-349.
19. Burgess NA, Reynolds TM, Williams N, Pathy A, Smith S. Evaluation of four animal models of intrarenal calcium deposition and assessment of the influence of dietary supplementation with essential fatty acids on calcification. *Urol Res.* 1995;23(4):239-242.
20. Sarica K, Soygür T, Yaman Ö, Özer G, Sayin N, Akbay C, Küpeli S, Yaman LS. Stone recurrence after shock wave lithotripsy: Evaluation of possible enhanced crystal deposition in traumatized tissue in rabbit model. *J Endourol.* 1996;10(6):513-517.
21. Itatani H, Yoshioka T, Namiki M, Koide T, Takemoto M, Sonoda T. Experimental model of calcium-containing renal stone formation in a rabbit. *Invest Urol.* 1979;17(3):234-240.
22. Kohjimoto Y, Ebisuno S, Tamura M, Ohkawa T. Adhesion and endocytosis of calcium oxalate crystals on renal tubular cells. *Scanning Microsc.* 1996;10(2):459-468; discussion 468-470.
23. Khan SR. Calcium oxalate crystal interaction with renal tubular epithelium, mechanism of crystal adhesion and its impact on stone development. *Urol Res.* 1995;23(2):71-79. Review.
24. Khan SR. Role of renal epithelial cells in the initiation of calcium oxalate stones. *Nephron Exp Nephrol.* 2004;98(2):55-60. Review.
25. Verkoelen CF. Crystal retention in renal stone disease: a crucial role for the glycosaminoglycan hyaluronan? *J Am Soc Nephrol.* 2006;17(6):1673-1687. Review.
26. Verkoelen CF, van der Boom BG, Schröder FH, Romijn JC. Cell cultures and nephrolithiasis. *World J Urol.* 1997;15(4):229-235. Review.
27. Hackett RL, Shevock PN, Khan SR. Alterations in MDCK and LLC-PK1 cells exposed to oxalate and calcium oxalate monohydrate crystals. *Scanning Microsc.* 1995;9(2):587-596.
28. Verkoelen CF, Schepers MS, van Ballegooijen ES, Bangma CH. Effects of luminal oxalate or calcium oxalate on renal tubular cells in culture. *Urol Res.* 2005;33(5):321-328.
29. Schepers MS, Duim RA, Asselman M, Romijn JC, Schröder FH, Verkoelen CF. Internalization of calcium oxalate crystals by renal tubular cells: a nephron segment-specific process? *Kidney Int.* 2003;64(2):493-500.
30. Sarica K, Erbagci A, Yağci F, Bakir K, Erturhan S, Uçak R. Limitation of apoptotic changes in renal tubular cell injury induced by hyperoxaluria. *Urol Res.* 2004;32(4):271-277.
31. Sarica K, Yağci F, Bakir K, Erturhan S, Uçak R. Renal Tubular injury induced by hyperoxaluria: Evaluation of apoptotic changes. *Urol Res.* 2001;29(1):34-37.
32. Karalezli G, Göğüş O, Bedük Y, Kököuslu C, Sarica K, Köksal O. Histopathologic effects of ESWL on rabbit kidney. *Urol Res.* 1993;21:67-70.
33. Mandel NS, Henderson JD Jr, Hung LY, Wille DF, Wiessner JH. A porcine model of calcium oxalate kidney stone disease. *J Urol.* 2004;171(3):1301-1303.
34. Paterson RF, Lingeman JE, Evan AP, Connors BA, Williams JC Jr, McAteer JA. Percutaneous stone implantation in the pig kidney: a new animal model for lithotripsy research. *J Endourol.* 2002;16(8): 543-547.
35. Webb DR, Fitzpatrick JM. A canine model for the investigation of human calculus disease. *Eur Urol.* 1985;11(6):406-409.
36. Meimaridou E, Lobos E, Hothersall JS. Renal oxidative vulnerability due to changes in mitochondrial-glutathione and energy homeostasis in a rat model of calcium oxalate urolithiasis. *Am J Physiol Renal Physiol.* 2006;291(4):F731-F740.
37. Sarica K, Türkölmez K, Koşar A, Alçığır G, Özdiler E, Göğüş O. Evaluation of basal membrane antibody (immunoglobulin G) formation after high energy shockwave application in rats. *J Endourol.* 1998;12(6):505-508.
38. Kavanagh JP. In vitro calcium oxalate crystallisation methods. *Urol Res.* 2006;34(2):139-145.
39. Achilles W. In vitro crystallisation systems for the study of urinary stone formation. *World J Urol.* 1997;15(4):244-251.
40. Achilles W, Jöckel U, Schaper A, Burk M, Riedmiller H. In vitro formation of "urinary stones": generation of spherulites of calcium phosphate in gel and overgrowth with calcium oxalate using a new

flow model of crystallization. *Scanning Microsc.* 1995;9(2):577-585; discussion 585-586.

41. Grases F, Costa-Bauzá A, March JG. Artificial simulation of the early stages of renal stone formation. *Br J Urol.* 1994;74(3):298-301.

42. Achilles W, Jöckel U, Schaper A, Burk M, Ulshöfer B, Riedmiller H. Formation of spherulites of calcium phosphate and crystallization of calcium oxalate in gel in a new experimental model of urinary stone formation. *Investig Urol (Berl).* 1994;5:218-221.

43. Achilles W. Crystallization in gel matrices: a new experimental model of calcium stone formation. *Contrib Nephrol.* 1987;58:59-64.

44. Nancollas GH, Singh RP. In vitro system for calcium stone formation: the constant composition model. *Contrib Nephrol.* 1987;58:49-58.

45. Mourad B, Fadwa N, Mounir T, Abdelhamid E, Mohamed Fadhel N, Rachid S. Influence of hypercalcic and/or hyperoxalic diet on calcium oxalate renal stone formation in rats. *Scand J Urol Nephrol.* 2006;40(3):187-191.

46. Morozumi M, Ogawa Y. Impact of dietary calcium and oxalate ratio on urinary stone formation in rats. *Mol Urol.* 2000;4(4):313-320.

47. de Water R, Boevé ER, van Miert PP, Vermaire CP, van Run PR, Cao LC, de Bruijn WC, Schröder FH. Pathological and immunocytochemical changes in chronic calcium oxalate nephrolithiasis in the rat. *Scanning Microsc.* 1996;10(2):577-587; discussion 587-590.

48. Mourad B, Fadwa N, Mounir T, Abdelhamid E, Mohamed Fadhel N, Rachid S. Influence of hypercalcic and/or hyperoxalic diet on calcium oxalate renal stone formation in rats. *Scand J Urol Nephrol.* 2006;40(3):187-191.

49. Sakly R, Bardaoui M, Neffati F, Moussa A, Zakhama A, Najjar MF, Hammami M. Effect of hyperprotidic diet associated or not with hypercalcic diet on calcium oxalate stone formation in rat. *Ann Nutr Metab.* 2005;49(2):132-138.

50. Bluestone R, Waisman J, Klinenberg JR. Chronic experimental hyperuricemic nephropathy. *Lab Invest.* 1975;33(3):273-279.

51. Amanzadeh J, Gitomer WL, Zerwekh JE, Preisig PA, Moe OW, Pak CY, Levi M. Effect of high protein diet on stone-forming propensity and bone loss in rats. *Kidney Int.* 2003;64(6):2142-2149.

52. Creedon A, Cashman KD. The effect of high salt and high protein intake on calcium metabolism, bone composition and bone resorption in the rat. *Br J Nutr.* 2000;84(1):49-56.

53. McAfee JG, Thomas FD, Roskopf M, Ritter K, Lyons B, Lilien OM, Schoonmaker JE. Changes in renal uptake of Tc-99m methylene diphosphonate (MDP) in stone-forming rats. *Invest Radiol.* 1984;19(6):543-548.

54. Jones WT, Waterhouse RL, Resnick MI. The evaluation of urinary protein patterns in a stone-forming animal model using two-dimensional polyacrylamide gel electrophoresis. *J Urol.* 1991;145(4):868-874.

55. Hackett RL, Shevock PN, Khan SR. Cell injury associated calcium oxalate crystalluria. *J Urol.* 1990;144(6):1535.

56. Knight J, Jiang J, Assimos DG, Holmes RP. Hydroxyproline ingestion and urinary oxalate and glycolate excretion. *Kidney Int.* 2006;70(11):1929-1934.

57. Ogawa Y, Hossain RZ, Ogawa T, Yamakawa K, Yonou H, Oshiro Y, Hokama S, Morozumi M, Uchida A, Sugaya K. Vitamin B6 deficiency augments endogenous oxalogenesis after intravenous L-hydroxyproline loading in rats. *Urol Res.* 2007;35(1):15-21.

58. Mo L, Huang HY, Zhu XH, Shapiro E, Hasty DL, Wu XR. Tamm-Horsfall protein is a critical renal defense factor protecting against calcium oxalate crystal formation. *Kidney Int.* 2004;66(3):1159-1166.

59. Peters T, Thaete C, Wolf S, Popp A, Sedlmeier R, Grosse J, Nehls MC, Russ A, Schlueter V. A mouse model for cystinuria type I. *Hum Mol Genet.* 2003;12(17):2109-2120.

60. Sidhu H, Allison MJ, Chow JM, Clark A, Peck AB. Rapid reversal of hyperoxaluria in a rat model after probiotic administration of Oxalobacter formigenes. *J Urol.* 2001;166(4):1487-1490.

61. Sidhu H, Schmidt ME, Cornelius JG, Thamilselvan S, Khan SR, Hesse A, Peck AB. Direct correlation between hyperoxaluria/oxalate stone disease and the absence of the gastrointestinal tract-dwelling bacterium Oxalobacter formigenes: possible prevention by gut recolonization or enzyme replacement therapy. *J Am Soc Nephrol.* 1999;10 Suppl 14:S334-S340.

62. Milliner D. Treatment of the primary hyperoxalurias: a new chapter. *Kidney Int.* 2006;70(7):1198-2000.

63. Oliver J, MacDowell M, Whang R, Welt LG. The renal lesions of electrolyte imbalance. IV. The intranephronic calculosis of experimental magnesium depletion. *J Exp Med.* 1966;124:263-265.

64. Liu J, Cao Z, Zhang Z, Zhou S, Ye Z. A comparative study on several models of experimental renal calcium oxalate stones formation in rats. *J Huazhong Univ Sci Technolog Med Sci.* 2007;27(1):83-87.

65. Khan SR, Hackett RL. Hyperoxaluria, enzymuria and nephrolithiasis. *Contrib Nephrol.* 1993;101:190-193. No abstract available.

66. Khan SR, Shevock PN, Hackett RL. Acute hyperoxaluria, renal injury and calcium oxalate urolithiasis. *J Urol.* 1992;147(1):226.

67. Khan SR, Glenton PA. Deposition of calcium phosphate and calcium oxalate crystals in the kidneys. *J Urol.* 1995;153:811-817.

68. Lee YH, Huang WC, Chiang H, Chen MT, Huang JK, Chang LS. Determinant role of testosterone in the pathogenesis of urolithiasis in rats. *J Urol.* 1992;147:1134-1138.

69. Lyon ES, Borden TA, Vermeulen CW. Experimental oxalate nephrolithiasis produced with ethylene glycol. *Invest Urol.* 1966;4:143-151.

70. Khan SR. Pathogenesis of oxalate urolithiasis: lessons from experimental studies with rats. *Am J Kidney Dis.* 1991;17(4):398-401.

71. Jaeger P, Portman L, Ginalski J-M, Jacqeut A-F, Temler E, Burkhardt P. Tubulopathy in nephrolithiasis: consequence rather than cause. *Kidney Int.* 1986;29:563-575.

72. Baggio B, Gambaro G, Ossi E, Favaro S, Borsatti A. Increased urinary excretion of renal enzymes in idiopathic calcium oxalate nephrolithiasis. *J Urol.* 1983;129:1161-1165.

73. Randall A. The etiology of primary renal calculus. *Int Abstr Surg.* 1940;71:20-24.

Clinical Trials in Stone Disease

34

Loris Borghi, Umberto Maggiore, Antonio Nouvenne, and Tiziana Meschi

Abstract Randomized controlled trials (RCTs) are considered the most reliable form of scientific evidence in medicine because they eliminate bias and spurious causality. Correctly performing RCTs require some well-defined rules. In kidney stone disease a relatively small number of clinical trials have been performed. In this chapter, the main principles to plan and implement nephrolithiasis clinical trials are focused. The best way to select study population, to randomize, to perform study design, and to assess adherence and outcomes is discussed. Finally, practical examples and a brief literature review should be useful for the reader to work out a critical point of view about this field.

34.1 Introduction

In spite of the important morbidity linked to the high prevalence of kidney stones in the general population, a relatively small number of clinical trials have been performed so far in the treatment of this disorder. In this chapter, we will address some of the problems most commonly encountered in the planning and implementation of clinical trials dealing with kidney stone treatment. Our focus will be on the pharmacological and dietary treatments aimed at reducing the risk of kidney stone formation, viewed from the perspective of the methodological issues involved in the clinical trials.

The clinical trial is the most reliable tool at our disposal for assessing the efficacy of a treatment. Some authors believe that efficacy should be distinguished from effectiveness in an intervention. The former refers to what the intervention accomplishes in an ideal setting, the latter to what it accomplishes in actual practice, taking into account the incomplete adherence of the participants to the protocol. We do not agree with this distinction. In fact, the quality of the scientific evidence provided by a clinical trial depends on the specificity of the setting in which the intervention is tested, namely its indications, characteristics, and degree of compliance achieved.[1]

The clinical trial is a prospective study performed on human beings to compare the effect of intervention(s) against a control.[2] At baseline, the control group must be sufficiently similar in all relevant aspects to the intervention group, allowing to reasonably attribute the differences in outcome to the effect of the intervention. Randomization, a method resembling the tossing of a coin, is the preferred way of assigning participants to the control group or to the intervention group. The main advantage of randomization is that it tends, in the long run, to balance evenly all prognostic factors, including those that are unmeasured and/or unknown. It is crucial that randomization be performed only after the patient has already been enrolled in the study. This ensures that the investigator has no knowledge of how treatments will be assigned before deciding whether or not the patient is eligible for the study.

A special type of clinical trial is the crossover study, which allows each participant to act as his (or her) own control. The assumption underlying this study design is that the effects of the first intervention do not carry over to the second treatment period. However, in the clinical setting of kidney stone treatment, such an assumption is untenable when the primary end point regards "stone recurrence rate," whereas it might be appropriate when the effect regards the urinary stone risk factors.

In a clinical trial, the outcome should be assessed in a consistent and unbiased manner in all patients. Whenever feasible, blinding of the treatment to the investigator and to the participant would fulfill this requirement. Another important advantage of blinding is that it minimizes the risk of concomitant or compensatory treatments being prescribed differently in the groups under comparison. While widely

L. Borghi (✉)
Department of Clinical Sciences, University of Parma, Parma, Italy
e-mail: loris.borghi@unipr.it

P.N. Rao et al. (eds.), *Urinary Tract Stone Disease*,
DOI 10.1007/978-1-84800-362-0_34, © Springer-Verlag London Limited 2011

391

used for testing the effectiveness of drugs, blinding is, obviously, of virtually impossible implementation for assessing the effectiveness of dietary interventions.

34.2 Choice of Study Population

Before starting the trial, it is essential to specify the category of patients to be investigated, and the strategy to be used for patient recruitment.[3]

The category of patients under investigation is defined by the inclusion and exclusion criteria. These criteria are usually chosen in such a way as to select the patients who would most likely benefit from the treatment being studied. For instance, a dietary treatment would be less efficacious in case of hereditary or well-defined acquired diseases such as cystinuria, primary hyperoxaluria, medullary sponge kidney, primary hyperparathyroidism, infections, and anatomical alterations of the urinary tract. Therefore, these conditions should be listed among the exclusion criteria. Whether or not the results of the study can then be extended to these categories, it is merely a matter of clinical judgment.

The practical strategy of patient enrolment is also important. For instance, enrolment implemented only in tertiary centers rather than by the general practitioners tends to select the most severe cases of kidney stone recurrence and the most motivated patients who are more likely to comply with the assigned treatment. As a matter of fact, we know only one double-blind RCT made in a general practice setting that, despite a catchment area of 17,000 inhabitants, was able to include 50 subjects only, who were followed up for an average of 40 months.[4]

The study population should be as homogeneous as possible. First of all, a precise characterization of stone phenotype is mandatory (i.e., calcium nephrolithiasis, uric acid, cysteine, struvite, etc.). This purpose might be difficult to implement due to inadequate availability of stone composition analysis. In calcium nephrolithiasis, stone composition analysis should allow to distinguish between calcium oxalate (CaOx), calcium phosphate, and mixed stones with various percentages because these stones differ in natural history, severity, recurrence rate, and response to treatment. On this account, several published studies are not easily comparable. According to current criteria, CaOx urolithiasis is defined by a stone CaOx (monohydrate and dihydrate) content exceeding 79%.[5–7] Accordingly, the study populations should be homogeneous as to the metabolic alterations, such as hypercalciuria, hyperoxaluria, hyperuricosuria, and hypocitraturia. Because these abnormalities are known to increase the risk of nephrolithiasis, several studies selected patients on the basis of the type of metabolic alterations.[5,7–12] An exception to this rule is the case in which a treatment might be equally effective on two or more stone types: for example, potassium citrate on calcium and uric stones.

Many other aspects, such as severity of disease, surgery, number of stones, etc. are to be taken also into consideration and will be discussed later in Sect. 34.4.

34.3 Sample Size Estimates and Assumptions

Each clinical trial must enroll a sufficient number of participants to achieve an adequate statistical power. The power is the probability that the trial will detect a true difference between treatments as statistically significant. The power depends on the magnitude of the difference between treatments, the variability of the response, and the statistical analysis being used, namely, the level of statistical significance and the type of the statistical test.[13] Commonly, a sample size is chosen such as to achieve a power ranging from 80% to 95%. When only a single statistical primary hypothesis is planned, a two-sided alpha of 5% is regarded as the level of statistical significance. The complement of the power is the probability of a false-negative finding. For instance, a sample size that achieves an 80% power runs a 20% risk of finding a falsely negative result.

The chapter authors feel that a clinical trial on kidney stone recurrence should last at least 3 years, but a duration of 5 years would appear safer. Most experts share this opinion since almost every prophylactic treatment shows its significant effect on stone episode recurrence after 2 years, on average. In fact, perhaps due to the "stone clinic effect" and to other still unknown factors, the most effective prophylactic treatments described in literature (i.e., potassium citrate, thiazide, allopurinol, water, and diet) are able to induce a rapid (weeks or months) decrease of urinary stone risk factors, while the greater reduction of recurrence rate occurs later (>2 years).[5–9,14–17]

To calculate the power, the investigator must specify beforehand the presumed difference in response between the intervention and control group, that is, the effect of the intervention. The effect of the intervention is usually inferred from previously published studies. Often, however, previous references regarding the effects of the treatment are lacking and only the prognostic information regarding patients under the standard treatment (i.e., the control group) is available. When this is the case, a minimum difference that can be regarded as clinically meaningful may be postulated. For instance, data from several studies – both retrospective and prospective[9,14,18,19] – show that, at 5 years, patients with urolithiasis not receiving any specific therapeutic intervention run a 20% risk of stone recurrence after the first episode, and of almost 40% after two episodes, with the mean interval periods decreasing along with the increase in the frequency of recurrences.[18] One might calculate the power of detecting a treatment effect that halves this 5-year risk of recurrence. Figure 34.1 (upper leftmost panel) reports the total number of patients required for planning a trial in which participants are assigned to either the treatment or control group (with a 1:1 probability). Calculations are based on the estimated risk of recurrence in the control group, the effect of treatment halving this risk, and refer to the use of the Mantel–Cox (Log-rank) statistical test with a two-sided significant level of 5%. These computations make use of the recurrence probabilities at 5 years.

Remember that, in all likelihood, some patients will withdraw from the study during a 5-year follow-up period. This is a very common problem in all clinical trials, including those regarding kidney stone recurrence. Therefore, before calculating sample size requirements, it is important to estimate how many patients will withdraw from the study. Figure 34.1 reports how sample size changes with different rates of patient withdrawals.

Note that these computations assume that the participants not withdrawing from the study will be followed up for the entire duration planned for the study. Therefore, if, for example, the study duration is planned over 5 years, the clinical trial will not close until the last patient enrolled in the study has completed the 5-year study period. On the contrary, if the plan foresees to stop the trial at a preset calendar date, then by that time some of the participants might not have completed the entire planned study period. In this instance, the duration of accrual and the accrual rate must be taken into account in the sample size computations.

Sometimes, rather than verifying whether a treatment effect differs from the standard (control) treatment, we might wish to assess whether this treatment is equivalent or, more simply, noninferior. The hypothesis of equivalence is defined by setting the maximum difference between treatments that we would accept to conclude that the two treatments are equivalent. Usually, study results are presented as a $(1-\alpha[alpha])\%$ confidence interval for the difference between the two treatments.[20] The equivalence is declared whenever the upper and lower bounds of the confidence intervals lie within the prespecified equivalence limits. Non-inferiority trials use the same approach except that they only look at the lower side of the confidence interval. Equivalence and non-inferiority trials are often planned whenever the standard (control) treatment is either costly or causes an excessive burden for the patients, thus making an equally efficacious yet simpler alternative preferable.

In Sect. 34.8, we will discuss the use of outcome measures that can be considered surrogates of kidney stone formation such as urinary stone risk factors.

The Appendix reports simple formula that can be used for sample size computation, thus avoiding the need for specific computer programs.

Table 34.1 lists all published interventional RCTs on nephrolithiasis and reports data that might be the basis for the assumption needed for sample size computation when planning a clinical trial on kidney stone disease.[21–32]

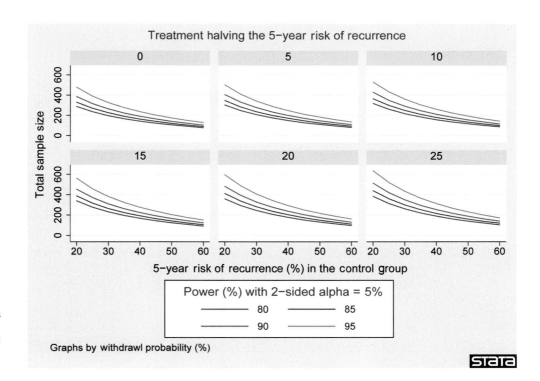

Fig. 34.1 Total number of patients required for planning a trial in which participants are assigned to either the treatment or control group (with a 1:1 probability)

Table 34.1 Data needed for sample size computation based on all published interventional RCT

End point	Study population	Intervention	Central tendency	Variability	Reference
Urinary calcium excretion	CaOx stone formers with hypercalciuria Males and females	Low-salt diet	Ca 271 mg	SD 86	Nouvenne[47]
			Ox 28 mg	SD 8	
			Na 68 mmol	SD 43	
			Cl 74 mmol	SD 62	
			Uric Acid 539 mg	SD 153	
			P 801 mg	SD 237	
Urinary oxalate excretion	CaOx stone formers with hyperoxaluria Males and females	Probiotics (Oxadrop)	52.6 mg	IQR 44.6–68	Goldfarb[12]
Urinary stone risk factors	Healthy subjects in bed rest on metabolic diet Males and females	KMgCitrate	Ca 222 mg	SD 71	Zerwekh[21]
			K 82 mEq	SD 11	
			Mg 165 mg	SD 45	
			Cit 976 mg	SD 330	
			pH 6.56	SD 0.41	
			RSR CaOx 3.37	SD 1.50	
			RSR brush 1.82	SD.01	
			Undissociated Uric acid 70 mg	SD 91	
Urinary stone risk factors	Healthy subjects and CaOx stone formers on metabolic diet Males and females	Orange juice	Cit 1,000 mg	Range 450–1,400	Odvina[22]
			NAE 17.3	SD 20.8	
			Mg 108 mg	SD 28	
			K 85 mEq	SD 21	
			Amm 23 mEq	SD 8	
			Ox 35 mg	SD 6	
			RS CaOx 3.71	SD 1.58	
			RS brush 0.82	SD 0.56	
Stone recurrence	Recurrent CaOx stone formers Males and females	Thiazide diuretics (Hydrochlorothiazide)	32% at 3 years	-	Fernandez-Rodriguez[48]
Oxalate excretion, absorption, endogenous synthesis	Healthy subjects and CaOx stone formers on metabolic diet Males and females	Ascorbic acid	Ox ur 51.2 mg	SD 12.5	Massey[23]
			Ox absorption% 10.5	SD 3.2	
			Ox endogenous 49 mg	SD 12	
Urinary calcium, oxalate, Tiselius Risk Index (TRI)	Healthy subjects on metabolic diet Males	Ca carbonate	Ox 11.7 mg	SD 4.5	Domrongkitchaiporn[24]
			Cit 159 mg	SD 109	
			Ca 207 mg	SD 104	
			TRI 0.57	SD 0.22	
Urinary stone risk factors	Healthy subjects on metabolic diet Males and females	Low Ca diet	Ca 148 mg	SD 55	Heller[25]
			Ox 25 mg	SD 7	
			Vol 1,814 ml	SD 626	
			pH 6.25	SD 0.31	
			RS CaOx 4.3	SD 2.2	
			Cit 849 mg	SD 299	

(continued)

Table 34.1 (continued)

End point	Study population	Intervention	Central tendency	Variability	Reference
Urinary stone risk factors	Healthy subjects Males	Cranberry juice	Ca 121 mg	SD 44	McHarg[26]
			Ox 9.9 mg	SD 1.8	
			Cit 714 mg	SD 129	
			Vol 1,805 ml	SD 176.53	
			Metastable limit 0.007	SD 0.45	
			RS CaOx 1.46	SD 9.16	
			RS uric a 0.96	SD 7.48	
			RS brushite 0.68	SD 7.48	
Stone recurrence	Recurrent idiopathic hypercalciuric CaOx stone formers Males	Normal-Ca, low-salt, low-protein diet	20% at 5 years	-	Borghi[9]
Stone recurrence	CaOx stone formers post-lithotripsy Males and females	KCitrate	0% at 1 year	-	Soygur[27]
Stone recurrence	Recurrent CaOx stone formers Males and females	KMgCitrate	12.9% at 3 years	-	Ettinger[15]
Stone recurrence	Calcium stone formers (first episode) Males and females	Water	12.1% at 5 years	-	Borghi[14]
Stone recurrence	Recurrent CaOx stone formers Males and females	NaKCitrate	69% at 3 years	-	Hofbauer[28]
Stone recurrence and stone rate	Recurrent hypocitraturic CaOx and CaOx-CaP stone formers Males and females	KCitrate	27.8% at 3 years Stone rate 0.1	- SD 0,2	Barcelo[8]
Stone recurrence and stone rate	Recurrent hypercalciuric CaOx and CaOx-CaP stone formers Males and females	Diet, fluid, indapamide, and allopurinol	12.5% at 3 years Stone rate 0.04	- SD 0,11	Borghi[5]
Stone recurrence	CaOx stone formers (first episode) Males and females	Low animal protein, high fiber, normal calcium diet	Stone recurrence 7,1/100 person/years	-	Hiatt[49]
Stone recurrence and stone rate	Recurrent hypercalciuric CaOx and CaOx-CaP stone formers Males and females	Thiazide diuretics (Trichlormethiazide)	8.3% at 2 years Stone rate 0.13	- SD 0,33	Ohkawa[7]
Stone recurrence and stone rate	Recurrent calcium stone formers Males	Thiazide diuretics (Trichlormethiazide) and Allopurinol	51% at 4,6 years Stone rate 0.20	- -	Kohri[16]
Stone recurrence and stone rate	Recurrent CaOx stone formers Males and females	Thiazide diuretics (Chlortalidone)	13% at 3 years Stone rate 0.05	- -	Ettinger[6]

(continued)

Table 34.1 (continued)

End point	Study population	Intervention	Central tendency	Variability	Reference
Stone recurrence and stone rate	Recurrent normocalciuric and hyperuricosuric CaOx stone formers Males and females	Allopurinol	31% at 3 years Stone rate 0.12	- -	Ettinger[11]
Stone recurrence and stone rate	Recurrent CaOx stone formers Males and females	Thiazide diuretics (Chlortalidone)	23% at 2.4 years Stone rate 0.06	- -	Ettinger[10]
Stone recurrence	Recurrent CaOx stone formers Males and females	Allopurinol	22% at 1 year 25% at 5 years	-	Smith[50]
Stone rate	Recurrent calcium stone formers Males and females	Ortophosphate	0.20	-	Robertson[17]
Stone recurrence	Recurrent calcium stone formers Males and females	Thiazide diuretics (Hydrochlorothiazide)	22% at 3 years	95% CI	Laerum[4]
Stone recurrence	Recurrent calcium stone formers Males and females	Water	5,3% at 2 years	-	Ulman[29]
Stone area doubled and stone recurrence (new stones)	Struvite stone formers with infection with urea-splitting organism Males and females	Acetohydro xamic acid	0% at 1.3 years 0% at 1.3 years	- -	Williams[19]
Stone recurrence Urinary calcium	Recurrent calcium stone formers Males and females	Thiazide diuretics (Hydrochlorothiazide)	24% at 1 year Ca 153 mg	- SD 110	Scholz[30]
Stone recurrence and rate (stone number/patient/year)	Recurrent stone formers Males and females	Thiazide diuretic (Bendroflumethiazide)	15% at 1,5 years Stone rate 0.09	- -	Brocks[31]
Stone recurrence and urinary calcium	Recurrent CaOx stone formers on Low Ca diet Males and females	Low Ca diet	30% at 3 years Ca 183 mg	- SD 43	Ettinger[32]

TRI tiselius risk index, *SD* standard deviation, *IQR* inter quantile range, *RS* relative supersaturation, *CaOx* calcium oxalate, *NAE* net acid excretion; *Stone Recurrence*% of patients recurrent during intervention, *Stone Rate* stone number/patient/year, *CI* confidential interval

34.4 Baseline Assessment

Before starting the intervention, all relevant baseline characteristics should be measured in all study participants. Reporting the baseline characteristics of the randomized groups allows us to evaluate their comparability (i.e., the success of the randomization process), and how the findings from the present study compare with those from other studies.

Identifying imbalances does not invalidate the study results, but it makes their interpretation more complicated. Usually, multiple regression or stratification techniques are used to adjust the study results when baseline imbalances are present. It is worth noting that the statistical tests comparing randomized groups at baseline (as reported in several research articles) are meaningless, since randomization makes the "null hypothesis" true by definition.

Most of the kidney stone patients are repeatedly evaluated before enrolment in a clinical trial by physical examination and laboratory data. It is crucial that the definition of "baseline" be uniform for the entire study population, and that the baseline characteristics reflect clinical conditions at the time of randomization as closely as possible.

Table 34.2 shows the ideal baseline setting for performing correctly an RCT for evaluating the effect of an intervention on stone rate recurrence. This approach can be applied both in tertiary centers and in general practice, because it is simple and the major items are easily obtained through an accurate medical history. As described previously, the

Table 34.2 Baseline characteristics to collect for each stone former enrolled in an interventional RCT, to assess the effects of both pharmacological and non-pharmacological treatments in the prevention of stone recurrences

Mandatory baseline information	
Age	
Gender	
Body weight	Concomitant relevant diseases
Height	Concomitant pharmacological treatments
Blood pressure	Dietary habit (essential for trials on dietary treatment)
Family history of stones	
Stone composition	Serum creatinine
Total stones formed	Serum calcium
	Serum uric acid
Age at first stone	Standard urine analysis
Recurrence rate (stone number/patient/year)	Urine culture analysis (essential for trials on struvite stones)
Number of retained stones	
Number of urological procedures to remove stones	
Very useful baseline information	
Serum sodium	
Serum chloride	24-h urine pH
Serum potassium	24-h urine calcium
Serum magnesium	24-h urine oxalate
	24-h urine uric acid
	24-h urine citrate
	24-h urine ammonium (for trials on struvite stones)
Serum phosphorus	Cystine screening or 24-h cystine (for trials on cystine stones)
Serum PTH	
Serum bicarbonate	
24-h urine volume	
24-h urine creatinine	
Ancillary baseline information	
24-h urine urea	24-h urine magnesium
24-h urine sodium	24-h urine sulfate
24-h urine chloride	Relative saturation for: CaOx
24-h urine potassium	- CaP
24-h urine phosphorus	- Uric acid

characterization of stone composition is crucial. By contrast, measurement of urinary stone risk factors is not mandatory if the primary end point is clearly fixed as "stone recurrence." In this setting, knowledge of urinary composition is helpful to support the findings regarding the primary end point, but not essential to evaluate the efficacy of the intervention.

34.5 Intervention and Concomitant Medications

Table 34.3 shows the main published RCT with "recurrence" as primary end point, classified by stone composition.

As usual, pharmacological or dietary interventions are conceivable if based on a well-defined scientific background. Considering literature, it is useful to note that, nowadays, as far as nephrolithiasis is concerned, it is not ethically acceptable to perform any intervention without prescribing an adequate increase in fluid intake, either in the control or active groups. This safeguard apart, no other ethical constraints distinguish nephrolithiasis from other medical conditions.

Concomitant medications are a crucial point: Any drugs not provided for in the study protocol that are likely to exert a positive or negative effect on the natural history of the nephrolithiasis should be avoided. Regular supplements with calcium, vitamin C, vitamin D, and biphosphonates therapy are acceptable only if they are equally balanced in the group being compared, or if they are the object of a subgroup analysis planned beforehand.

34.6 Random Allocation

Randomization is a critical issue since it removes the investigator's bias in assigning treatments and produces, in the long run, groups that are comparable for prognostic factors. Several methods for randomly allocating participants are currently in use. They share the prerequisite that neither the participant nor the investigator should know what the assignment will be before inclusion of the participants in the study.

Among the special methods of randomization that may be applicable in trials on kidney stone disease, we will mention the stratified randomization, the blocked randomization, and the adaptive randomization methods. Stratified randomization is a process that is performed separately for each stratum. It is especially useful when subgroup analyses are planned in the study protocol and in case of multicenter trials where each stratum is represented by a single center. Blocked randomization is meant to prevent imbalance in the number of patients assigned to each group. The blocks are short sequence blocks at the end of which the number of treatment assignments is evenly distributed (for instance, ABBA AB ABABBBAA). Adaptive randomization procedures change the allocation probabilities as the study progresses.[33] It may be employed to correct imbalance of baseline characteristics for those clinical trials enrolling only a limited number of patients.

Despite the importance of randomization, often published RCT on nephrolithiasis do not provide details about the methods used to randomize study participants.

Table 34.3 Randomized controlled trials with "recurrence" as primary endpoint

Reference	Study population	No. of patients who completed the study	Type of intervention	Mean duration of treatment	Recurrence%	p
Calcium stones						
Fernandez-Rodriguez[48]	Recurrent calcium stone formers Males and females	150	Hydrochlorothiazide 50 mg + KCl 20 mEq/die (I) vs. Hydrochlorothiazide 50 mg (II) vs. No therapy (III)	3 years	30% (I) vs. 32% (II) vs. 56% (III)	*p* <0.05
Borghi[9]	Recurrent idiopathic hypercalciuric CaOx stone formers Males	103	Normal-calcium, low-protein, low-salt diet vs. Traditional low calcium diet	5 years	20% vs. 38%	*p*=0.04
Soygur[27]	CaOx stone formers post-lithotripsy both stone free and with residual fragments Males and females	60	KCitrate 60 mEq vs. no treatment	1 years	0% vs. 28.5% (Stone free) 12.5% vs. 44.5% (residual fragments)	*p*<0.05 *p*<0.05
Ettinger[15]	Recurrent CaOx stone formers Males and females	41	K-Mg-Citrate (42-21-63 mEq) vs. Placebo	3 years	12.9% vs. 63.6%	Not done
Borghi[14]	Stone formers (first episode) Males and females	199	Water intake to achieve urine volume >2 L vs. no treatment	5 years	12.1% vs. 27%	*p*=0.008
Hiatt[49]	CaOx stone formers (first episode) Males and females	99	Low animal protein, high fiber, normal calcium diet + Hydropinic therapy vs. Normal calcium diet + Hydropinic therapy	4,5 years	32% vs. 5%	*p* = 0.006
Hofbauer[28]	Recurrent CaOx stone formers Males and females	22	Na-K-Citrate tid to obtain pH 7–7.2 vs. General prophylactic instructions	3 years	69% vs. 73%	*p*=0.65
Barcelo[8]	Recurrent hypocitraturic CaOx and CaP stone formers Males and females	38	K Citrate 20 mEq tid vs. Placebo	3 years	27.8% vs. 80%	Not done
Borghi[5]	Recurrent, stone free at baseline, hypercalciuric CaOx and CaOx-CaP stone formers	64	Diet and fluid (I) vs. Diet and fluid + Indapamide 2.5 mg (II) vs. Diet and fluid + Allopurinol 300 mg (III)	3 years	42.8% (I) vs. 15.8% (II) vs. 12.5% (III)	*p*=0.02 (II and III vs. I)
Ohkawa[7]	Recurrent hypercalciuric CaOx and CaOx-CaP stone formers Males and females	175	Trichlormethiazide 4 mg vs. no therapy	2 years	8.3% vs. 14.1%	0.05<*p*>0.1

Author	N	Population	Intervention	Duration	Outcome	p-value
Ettinger[6]	124	Recurrent CaOx stone formers Males and females	Placebo vs. Milk of magnesia 325 mg bid (group A) vs. Milk of Magnesia 650 mg bid (group B) vs. Chlorthalidone 25 mg (group C) vs. Chlorthalidone 50 mg (group D)	3 years	45% (Plac) vs. 27% (A) vs. 33% (B) vs. 16% (C) vs. 13% (D)	$p<0.05$ (group D vs. others)
Ettinger[11]	60	Recurrent normocalciuric and hyperuricosuric CaOx stone formers Males and females	Allopurinol 100 mg tid vs. Placebo	3 years	31% vs. 58%	$p<0.001$
Laerum[4]	48	Recurrent calcium stone formers in general practice Males and females	Hydrochlorothiazide 25 mg vs. placebo	3 years	22% vs. 48%	$p=0.05$
Ulman[29]	51	Recurrent calcium stone formers Males and females	Idropinic therapy (I) vs. Idropinic Therapy + Hydrochlorothiazide 50 mg (II) vs. Phosphorous 750 mg bid (III)	2 years	5.3% (I) vs. 26% (II) [% (III) n.d.]	$p<0.05$
Scholz[30]	48	Recurrent calcium stone formers Males and females	Hydrochlorothiazide 25 mg bid vs. Placebo	1 year	24% vs. 23%	$p=$ns (values not shown)
Brocks[31]	62	Recurrent calcium stone formers Males and females	Bendroflumethiazide 2.5 tid vs. Placebo	1.5 years	15% vs. 17%	Not done
Smith[50]	92	Recurrent CaOx stone formers Males and females	Allopurinol 100 mg vs. Placebo	1 years	22% vs. 48%	Not done
Ettinger[32]	71	Recurrent CaOx stone formers on Low Ca diet (600 mg)	K Acid Phosphate (1,4 g of P) (I) vs. Placebo (II) vs. Low Ca diet alone (III)	3 years	50% (I) vs. 30% (II) vs. 53% (III)	Not done

Struvite stones

Author	N	Population	Intervention	Duration	Outcome	p-value
Williams[19]	33	Struvite stone formers with infection with urea-splitting organism. Males and females	Acetohydroxamic acid 15 mg/Kg/day vs. Placebo	1.3 years	0% vs. 37%	$p<0.01$

Uric acid stones

No RCTs available

Cystine stones

No RCTs available

34.7 Participant Adherence and Compliance: Monitoring Response Variables

Many potential adherence problems can be prevented or minimized before enrolling the participants. Once a participant is enrolled, taking measures to motivate and monitor the participants' adherence is of fundamental importance.

After being enrolled in a trial, some patients may withdraw from the study because they are unwilling or unable to return for the follow-up visits. Other patients, assigned to the control group, might follow the intervention regimen or vice versa ("crossover"). Others apparently adhering to the assigned treatment do not, in fact, comply with the treatment prescriptions.

By "lost to follow-up" we mean the irremediable loss of contact with the patient, hence there is no way of assessing his/her outcome. By "withdrawal from treatment" we mean the patient who continues to report for the scheduled visits, but is not complying with the treatment assignment. Some authors refer to the latter category as "dropouts." By "withdrawal from the study" we mean the patient who is unwilling to continue the scheduled visits but can still be contacted (say, by a telephone call). The worst scenario is, of course, that of the "lost to follow-up." Investigators should make every effort to avoid having even a single patient "lost to follow-up." As we will show in Sect. 34.9.1, it is possible to retrieve information on withdrawals without invalidating the study results; but it is safer not to have to resort to this means of retrieval but, rather, to encourage, through the implementation of appropriate strategies, the patients' adherence and compliance.

Due to the natural history and characteristics of the disease, it is very hard to minimize withdrawals in kidney stone trials; in fact, nephrolithiasis usually affects "healthy" subjects who adhere strictly to their doctors' advice and treatments at the time of an acute episode of renal colic but soon lose interest and compliance. Accordingly, the number of withdrawals in published RCTs on nephrolithiasis is considerable, particularly for those with a long-term follow-up. This pitfall notwithstanding, monitoring adherence is a precise target for the study personnel and it is possible to enact a number of strategies to deal with the withdrawal phenomenon and to minimize the loss of compliance. For instance, it could be helpful to arrange scheduled visits (i.e., every 3 months), make frequent phone contacts, and provide illustrative material for patients to take home. It is also useful to inform the general practitioner; moreover, a periodic 24-h urine collection could interest the patient enabling him/her to see the practical results of his/her efforts. Also performing a simple study intervention, agreeable to the patient, decreases withdrawals. In case of dietary intervention, it is important to have an assessment carried out by a dietician: this encourages the patient to adhere to the protocol and reduces the loss of compliance. Additionally, at the beginning of the study before randomization, a patient follow-up period, without intervention, may be conducted with the aim of assessing the compliance and the baseline characteristics (a "run-in" period).[6,9,11]

Finally, it is helpful to provide, as far as it is possible, some "facilities," such as a dedicated outpatients' department, some free exams, and avoiding waiting lists.

34.8 Outcome Assessment and Surrogate Endpoints

Studies confirm that, when available, noncontrast helical computed tomography scanning (spiral CT) has superior sensitivity and specificity in the detection of stones.[34] In RCTs on nephrolithiasis, the primary outcome should be "recurrence." It is important to specify the method employed to diagnose the relapses. The most simple case is when at the first episode there is a single stone that is then ejected; in this situation, a new acute colic episode or the appearance of new asymptomatic stone detected by imaging techniques easily permit diagnosis. If, on the other hand, the first episode presents as a case of multiple or residual stones, then the colic is not synonymous with recurrence, which can be diagnosed only if the retained stones are increased in number or size. However, due to interobserver variability, such diagnosis is often not easily available. In either case, the radiologist should be blind to treatment assignment.

In conclusion, the ideal setting is that where the patient is stone-free after the first episode, and, in case of residual stones, a good CT imaging, possibly with a urographic phase, may be useful.

When examinations are planned at yearly intervals, the use of renal ultrasound with/without abdominal flat plate might be adequate for asymptomatic patients. If renal stones are detected, CT imaging is also performed.

The achievement of the "ideal" end point, namely recurrence, requires a long-term follow-up period; lacking which, one might evaluate the surrogate end points[21] – commonly the urinary stone risk factors. This is an acceptable method based on the knowledge that the imbalance of urinary stone risk factors exposes patients to a greater recurrence rate. Studies, either prospective or retrospective, have shown that urinary stone risk factors, particularly low volume and high calcium, are associated with a shorter relapse interval.[35]

However, besides being a surrogate end point, urinary indexes also present the disadvantage of being multiple, thus needing multiple comparisons implying an increase above the nominal value of the chances of incurring in the type I error rate (i.e., false-positive findings). When dealing with multiple end points, the classical solutions are: (1) to select a single urinary index beforehand as primary end point, which is appropriate whenever the treatment is specifically aimed at correcting its abnormal values; (2) to "cut down" the alpha level used to declare statistical significance according to the number of tests performed; this procedure, however, substantially increases sample size requirements; (3) to use multivariate tests for simultaneously comparing several urinary indexes, but this approach usually requires a number of rigid statistical assumptions; and (4) to create a composite end point; that is, to declare the effect of intervention in each individual when at least one of a prespecified list of results is reached, an approach that can, however, cause substantial interpretation problems.[36–39]

34.9 Issues in Data Analysis

34.9.1 The Intention-to-Treat Principle

Randomizing the participants between the treatment groups is the fundamental step adopted for preserving the study from biases. Even randomization, however, would not allow achieving this goal fully unless two other requirements are met:

1. Outcome is to be assessed in even and unbiased ways in every patient. As outlined before, to accomplish this requirement one has to "blind" (i.e., mask) whenever possible treatment assignments to both patients and clinical staff including those assessing the outcome.
2. Safeguards have to be taken to prevent missing data from randomized patients becoming an important source of bias in the comparison of the treatment groups.[40]

To accomplish the latter goal, the investigator has to implement steps aimed at evaluating all randomized patients at the scheduled visits. All the randomized participants must be included in the final analyses. Even more importantly, they have to be analyzed according to the treatment they were originally allocated to, regardless whether they had not received all the treatment, or had received the wrong treatment (out of mistake or outside drug prescription), or had withdrawn from treatment because of adverse effects. In an intent-to-treat study, treatment interruption ("dropouts") should never lead to withdrawal from the study. Any analysis that involves post hoc exclusions of information (such as "per protocol" analysis, in which patients are analyzed according to the treatment actually administered), can substantially alter the comparability between the study groups, which is the very primary goal of the randomization process. Patients should not be withdrawn from treatment because of lack of "success" or compliance failure, unless safety considerations dictate patients be administered alternative

treatments. Even in such instances, the patients' follow-up should continue as scheduled. Thus, irrespective of the causes of withdrawal from the treatment, every patient should continue to be followed-up and to undergo all scheduled outcome evaluations until the study is completed, or withdrawal becomes unavoidable because of the patient's death. This approach also requires the patients never be labeled as "dropouts." Of course, the patient is free to withdraw his/her consent to participate in the trial at any time, because of changes or adversity in their everyday life or whatever other reason. Their request should always be complied with without prejudice. Obviously, patients will be welcomed back into the trial whenever they wish to be reinserted under their original follow-up schedule, and analyzed within their originally randomized treatment allocation.

34.9.2 Subgroup Analyses

An analysis technique commonly employed is to divide the study population into subgroups, such as to allow the comparison between control and intervention within each subgroup. The aim is to identify the categories of patients most likely to benefit from the treatment. Great caution must be exercised in performing such analyses because they lead to multiple testing, which implies an increase in the type I error rate (i.e., the probability of false-positive findings), and a loss of power leading to false-negative findings.[41]

The weakest type of subgroup analyses are the "post hoc" analyses – the analyses suggested by the data themselves. Subgroup analyses should, on the other hand, be based on sound prior knowledge. Ideally, they should be planned before starting the trial by explicitly stating this purpose in the study protocol.

An example of subgroup analyses that seems appropriate in trials on kidney stones concerns those regarding the gender, the degree of severity of the disease, and the type of kidney stones when the study population is heterogeneous in this regard. For example, in our RCT on the effect of normal-calcium, low-salt, low-protein diet in hypercalciuric recurrent men, based on the assumption that the diet cannot be effective upon stones already in formation, we performed a subgroup analysis by selecting men at high risk, namely those with a history of five or more episodes of colic in the year before randomization and/or ten or more stones formed. This permitted us to assess that dietary treatment was poorly effective in the more severely affected patients.[9] Furthermore, in RCTs testing the prophylactic effect of allopurinol on stone recurrences, the subgroup analysis showed a greater reduction of relapse rate in the hyperuricosuric than in non-hyperuricosuric patients.[11,16]

Subgroup analyses are usually performed by computing the confidence intervals of the intervention effects in each subgroup separately.[41] The formal statistical test is the "test of interaction," which is the test for the difference between the effects observed in each subgroup. This test, however, lacks statistical power.

34.9.3 Longitudinal Data Analysis

When examining the effect of a treatment on urinary indexes, we have to deal with the baseline measures and their change over the follow-up. Statistical comparisons in this setting can be made in several ways. In the absence of baseline imbalance, the simple comparison of urinary indexes at the end of the trial (posttreatment) is usually adequate. If, however, there is a data imbalance at baseline, the commonest approach is to adjust posttreatment differences for baseline difference using a regression technique known as ANCOVA (ANalysis of COVAriance). Alternatively, a "change" variable can be created (posttreatment minus pretreatment value). The latter approach, however, does not eradicate the spurious statistical correlation between baseline and posttreatment values: If, for instance, a patient has by chance a high value at baseline, this abnormality will subsequently tend to disappear by virtue of the statistical phenomenon known as "regression to the mean."

When examining a long series of measurements over the course of the follow-up, regression methods for repeated measurements should be used.[42]

34.9.4 Interim Analysis

Sometimes an interim analysis of the treatment effects may become necessary to decide whether the difference between the two arms is large enough as to permit the earlier termination of the study. This may happen whenever the study findings have an urgent public impact, whenever new evidence emerges to suggest that one of the treatments under evaluation is potentially hazardous or ineffective or the study design was wrong, and/or precious economic or human resources are being wasted. Issues of this kind rarely emerge, however, in RCTs on kidney stone disease. Anyway, if interim analyses are planned, they imply that the alpha level used to declare statistical significance must be corrected in order to maintain the type I error probability. At each interim analysis, the level of significance is chosen in such a way as to be the more stringent (more conservative); the lower is the number of patients and length of follow-up cumulated up to the time of the interim analysis. For the subsequent statistical tests, the original alpha level (say 0.05) is to be cut down by the amount of "significance" spent for performing the previous interim statistical tests.[43]

34.10 Peculiar Types of Study Design

34.10.1 Within-Subject Study: The Crossover Design

The crossover design, by eliminating the error (the "noise") due to between-patient variability, requires fewer subjects to be recruited compared to the parallel group design, with a considerable saving of resources.

Subjects are given all the treatments in sequence. As outlined previously, the assumption underlying this study design is that the effects of the first intervention do not carry over to the second treatment period. To provide a safe ground to this assumption, it is necessary to perform an adequate "washout period." Moreover, if all subjects receive the two treatments in the same order, observed differences between treatments would be confounded with any other changes that occur naturally over time. The two treatment, two-period crossover trial overcomes this difficulty by having half of the subjects receive treatment A followed by treatment B, while the other half receive B followed by A. Any temporal trend that might favor B over A in one group will favor A over B in the other group and cancel out of the treatment comparison.[44]

In nephrolithiasis intervention trials, if the primary end point is "stone rate," crossover protocol is not applicable. On the other hand, this kind of study design lends itself more profitably for assessing the effect of pharmacological or dietary interventions on urinary stone risk factors. Several kidney stone RCTs have chosen this approach to assess the changes in urinary stone risk factors associated with the intervention.[22–26]

34.10.2 Additivity and Synergism: The Factorial Study

Sometimes the question might arise on whether two different treatments exert additive or synergic effect on the risk of kidney stones. This issue is best examined by planning a "factorial study," whereby each treatment arm represents one of all the possible combinations of the treatments being tested.[45] Imagine, for instance, a factorial study in which calcium stone formers are randomized to thiazide diuretic or KCitrate with the outcome measure being the stone rate recurrence. The 2×2 design would imply four treatment groups namely, Diuretic and KCitrate ("withDiuretic–withCitrate"), Diuretic and Placebo ("withDiuretic–withoutKCitrate"), Placebo and KCitrate ("withoutDiuretic–withKCitrate"), and Placebo and Placebo ("withoutDiuretic–withoutKCitrate"). *Additivity* occurs whenever the joint effect of the two treatments results from the sum of their separate effects. On the other hand, s*ynergism* occurs when the joint effect of two treatments is greater than would be expected from the sum of their separate effect. The formal statistical hypothesis of synergism is the test for an *interaction* between the effects (i.e., departure from an additive model). In our hypothetical example, *additivity* occurs whenever the higher the number of treatments the higher is the efficacy. In other words, the "withDiuretic/withKCitrate" combination (two treatments) is more efficacious than either "withDiuretic–withoutKcitrate" or "withoutDiuretic–withKCitrate" (one treatment), and all these are in turn more efficacious than "withoutDiuretic–withoutKCitrate" (zero treatments). On the other hand, *synergism* occurs when the efficacy of Thiazide Diuretic used in combination with KCitrate (which is measured as the difference between "withDiuretic–withKCitrate" and "withoutDiuretic–withKCitrate") is superior to the efficacy of Thiazide Diuretic used without KCitrate (which is measured as the difference between "withDiuretic–withoutKCitrate" and "withoutDiuretic–withoutKCitrate"). In other words, the use of KCitrate modifies (potentiates) the effect of thiazide diuretic.

34.10.3 The Dose-Response Study

Sometimes the trial, whether based on parallel groups or crossover comparison, aims at assessing what is the most efficacious dose of the intervention to administer to the patients. Accordingly, patients are allocated to the placebo arms or to groups corresponding to each one of distinct levels of the dose of the drug or the intake of a nutrient or element. This is a powerful design, in that it not only reinforces the evidence about the efficacy of the treatment being tested, but also provides information about the minimal efficacious intervention. The latter issue is particularly important when the treatment is poorly tolerated by the patients, thus causing problems of compliance. As an example, such design would be useful to investigate the effect of different levels of NaCl intake on kidney stone recurrence in calcium stone formers.

34.11 Conclusions

The general rules recommended for the correct implementation of the RCTs[2] apply also to kidney stones, namely,: a study population of adequate size and adequate length of follow-up, accurate definition of the therapeutic intervention and clinical setting, randomization for treatment allocation, outcome assessed in a like manner, minimal missing information, and intention-to-treat principle as a guide for data analysis. However, in many published studies these rules often have not been complied with; certainly not out of carelessness, but because of the difficulties inherent in the natural history of kidney stone disease, a disorder that affects otherwise "healthy" subjects who become hardly interested in prophylaxis once the acute pain of the colic has became a remote memory.

In spite of the relatively high prevalence of the disorder, it is striking to notice the lack of large trials recorded in the medical literature, especially with regard to the general practice setting. This neglect can be partially attributed to the lack of interest by the pharmaceutical industry. Due to the paucity of effective drugs available in the pharmaceutics market, nephrolithiasis can be rated almost as a drug "orphan" disease. For these reasons, effort should be made by institutional researchers to fill this gap.

Appendix

Sample Size Formulas

All the formulas include the following quantities: $Z_{\beta(beta)}$, which reflects the power of the study, and $Z_{\alpha(alpha)/2}$, which reflects the level of significance of the statistical test. $Z_{\beta(beta)}$ is chosen according to the following table:

Power (%)	$Z_{\beta(beta)}$
80	0.842
85	1.036
90	1.282
95	1.645

Usually, $Z_{\alpha(alpha)/2} = 1.960$ (it means that the two-sided alpha level is 5%)

In the formulas that follow, "2N" is the total sample (half that number being allocated to each treatment arm).

Continuous Measurement (e.g., Urinary Indexes)

In the following formulas, δ(delta) is the hypothesized difference (or the clinically relevant difference) between means of the intervention and control group; σ(sigma) is the standard deviation of each group (based on results obtained from earlier trials). The formulas assume a large sample (say, well above 30) and the outcome measure being normally distributed.

Parallel Group Design

When the comparison is performed between the mean of the urinary index taken at the end of the study period (e.g., two sample *t*-test), the formula is the following:

$$2N = \frac{4 \times (Z_{\alpha/2} + Z_\beta)^2 \times \sigma^2}{\delta^2}$$

On the other hand, in a longitudinal study in which each subject has *n* measurements of the same urinary index, and the outcome is the average response of these *n* measurements, the formula is the following:

$$2N = \frac{4 \times (Z_{\alpha/2} + Z_\beta)^2 \times \sigma^2}{\delta^2} \times \frac{\{1 + (n-1) \times \rho\}}{n}$$

Where ρ(rho) is the correlation between measurements within each subject.

Crossover Study

$$N = \frac{(Z_{\alpha/2} + Z_\beta)^2 \times \sigma_d^2}{\delta_d^2}$$

Where δ_d(delta$_d$) is the difference on the same patient between the two treatments (PRE e POST) and σ_d(sigma$_d$) is the standard deviation of this difference. The latter quantity can be obtained from the following formula:

$$\sigma_d^2 = 2 \times \sigma^2 \times (1 - \rho)$$

where ρ(rho) is the correlation between the PRE and POST measurements.

Time to Failure (i.e., Recurrence Rate)

In the following formula, λ_I(lambda$_I$) is the hazard rate of recurrence in the intervention group and λ_C(lambda$_C$) the hazard rate of recurrence in the control group.

$$2N = \frac{2 \times (Z_{\alpha/2} + Z_\beta)^2 \times [\varphi(\lambda_C) + \varphi(\lambda_I)]}{(\lambda_I - \lambda_C)^2}$$

Where:

$$\varphi(\lambda) = \frac{\lambda^2}{1 - e^{\lambda T}}$$

where $\phi(\lambda_C)$ [phi(lambda$_C$)] and $\phi(\lambda_I)$ [phi(lambda$_I$)] are obtained by replacing λ(lambda) in $\phi(\lambda_C)$ [phi(lambda$_C$)] with λ_C(lambda$_C$) or λ_I(lambda$_I$), respectively; T is the follow-up period.

Consider, however, the instance in which the investigator has access only to data on the recurrence risk in the control group, such as probabilities of recurrence-free survival, hazard ratio, or median time until recurrence. The latter parameters can be derived from the hazard rate, and easily converted into one another provided that a couple of assumptions are met, namely that survival probability follows a mono-exponential model (i.e., survival probability changes as a fixed proportion per unit time because the rate of recurrence is constant over the follow-up) and the proportional hazard assumption (i.e., the relative reduction in the stone recurrence due to treatment is constant over the entire study period). Below we show how to perform the conversions.

If λ(lambda) = hazard rate of recurrence (incidence rate of recurrence), M = median time until recurrence, R_t = recurrence at time t, S_t = probability of being free of recurrence at time t, HR = relative Hazard (Hazard Ratio), then:

$$M = -\text{Log}_e(0.5) / \lambda(\text{lambda})$$

$$S_t = 1 - R_t$$

$$R_t = 1 - S_t$$

$$\Lambda(\text{lambda}) = -\text{Log}_e(1 - R_t) / t$$

$$HR = \lambda(\text{lambda})^{\text{intervention}} \div \lambda(\text{lambda})^{\text{control}}$$

$$HR = M^{\text{control}} \div M^{\text{intervention}}$$

$$HR = \text{Log}_e(1 - R_t^{\text{intervention}}) \div \text{Log}_e(1 - R_t^{\text{control}})$$

$$R_t = 1 - exp(-\lambda(\text{lambda}) * t)$$

$$R_t^{\text{intervention}} = 1 - (1 - R_t^{\text{control}})^{RR}$$

For instance, a 25% and 50% 5-year risk of stone recurrence (i.e., 0.25 and 0.50 risk of recurrence) corresponds to a 1−0.25 = 0.75 (i.e., 75%), and 1−0.5 = 0.5 (i.e., 50%) probability of recurrence-free survival. The incidence rate of recurrence is −Log(0.75)÷5 = 0.058 (i.e., 5.8 recurrences per 100 person-years follow-up) and −Log(0.50)÷5 = 0.139 (i.e., 13.9 recurrences per 100 person-years follow-up), respectively. The median time until recurrence is −Log(0.5) ÷ 0.058 = 12 years, and −Log(0.5) ÷ 0.139 = 5 years, respectively. The Hazard Ratio (HR) is Log(0.75) ÷ Log(0.50) = 0.42.[13,46]

References

1. Miettinen OS (2001) The modern scientific physician: 5. the useful property of an intervention. Can Med Assoc J 165:1059–1060

2. Altman DG, Schulz KF, Moher D, for the CONSORT Group et al (2001) The revised CONSORT statement for reporting randomized trials: explanation and elaboration. Ann Intern Med 134:663–694

3. Gross CP, Mallory R, Heiat A et al (2002) Reporting the recruitment process in clinical trials: who are these patients and how did they get there? Ann Intern Med 137:10–16

4. Laerum E, Larsen S (1984) Thiazide prophylaxis of urolithiasis. A double-blind study in general practice. Acta Med Scand 215:383–389

5. Borghi L, Meschi T, Guerra A et al (1993) Randomized prospective study of a nonthiazide diuretic, indapamide, in preventing calcium stone recurrences. J Cardiovasc Pharmacol 22:S78–S86

6. Ettinger B, Citron JT, Livermore B et al (1988) Chlorthalidone reduces calcium oxalate calculous recurrence but magnesium hydroxide does not. J Urol 139:679–684

7. Ohkawa M, Tokunaga S, Nakashima T et al (1992) Thiazide treatment for calcium urolithiasis in patients with idiopathic hypercalciuria. Br J Urol 69:571–576

8. Barcelo P, Wuhl O, Servitge E et al (1993) Randomized double-blind study of potassium citrate in idiopathic hypocitraturic calcium nephrolithiasis. J Urol 150:1761–1764

9. Borghi L, Schianchi T, Meschi T et al (2002) Comparison of two diets for the prevention of recurrent stones in idiopathic hypercalciuria. N Engl J Med 346:77–84

10. Ettinger B, Citron JT, Tang A et al (1985) Prophylaxis of calcium oxalate stones: clinical trials of Allopurinol, magnesium hydroxide and chlorthalidone. In: Schwille PO et al (eds) Urolithiasis and Related Clinical Research. Plenum Press, New York, pp 549–552

11. Ettinger B, Tang A, Citron JT et al (1986) Randomized trial of allopurinol in the prevention of calcium oxalate calculi. N Engl J Med 315:1386–1389

12. Goldfarb DS, Modersitzki F, Asplin JR (2007) A randomized, controlled trial of lactic acid bacteria for idiopathic hyperoxaluria. Clin J Am Soc Nephrol 2:745–749

13. Lachin JM (1981) Introduction to sample size determination and power analysis for clinical trials. Control Clin Trials 2:93–113

14. Borghi L, Meschi T, Amato F et al (1996) Urinary volume, water and recurrences in idiopathic calcium nephrolithiasis: a 5-year randomized prospective study. J Urol 155:839–843

15. Ettinger B, Pak CY, Citron JT et al (1997) Potassium-magnesium citrate is an effective prophylaxis against recurrent calcium oxalate nephrolithiasis. J Urol 158:2069–2073

16. Kohri K, Kodama M, Katayama Y et al (1990) Allopurinol and thiazide effects on new urinary stone formed after discontinued therapy in patients with urinary stones. Urology 36:309–314

17. Robertson WG, Peacock M, Selby PL et al (1985) A multicentre trial to evaluate three treatments for recurrent idiopathic calcium stone disease – a preliminary report. In: Schwille PO et al (eds) Urolithiasis and Related Clinical Research. Plenum Press, New York/London, pp 545–548

18. Parks JH, Coe FL (1994) An increasing number of calcium oxalate stone events worsens treatment outcome. Kidney Int 45:1722–1730

19. Williams JJ, Rodman JS, Peterson CM (1984) A randomized double-blind study of acetohydroxamic acid in struvite nephrolithiasis. N Engl J Med 311:760–764

20. Piaggio G, Elbourne DR, Altman DG, for the CONSORT group et al (2006) Reporting of non-inferiority randomized trials. An extension of the CONSORT statement. JAMA 295:1152–1160

21. Zerwekh JE, Odvina CV, Wuermser LA et al (2007) Reduction of renal stone risk by potassium-magnesium citrate during 5 weeks of bed rest. J Urol 177:2179–2184

22. Odvina CV (2006) Comparative value of orange juice versus lemonade in reducing stone-forming risk. Clin J Am Soc Nephrol 1:1269–1274

23. Massey LK, Liebman M, Kynast-Gales SA (2005) Ascorbate increases human oxaluria and kidney stone risk. J Nutr 135:1673–1677

24. Domrongkitchaiporn S, Sopassathit W, Stitchantrakul W et al (2004) Schedule of taking calcium supplement and the risk of nephrolithiasis. Kidney Int 65:1835–1841

25. Heller HJ, Doerner MF, Brinkley LJ, Adams-Huet B, Pak CY (2003) Effect of dietary calcium on stone forming propensity. J Urol 169(2):470–474

26. McHarg T, Rodgers A, Charlton K (2003) Influence of cranberry juice on the urinary risk factors for calcium oxalate kidney stone formation. BJU Int 92:765–768

27. Soygür T, Akbay A, Küpeli S (2002) Effect of potassium citrate therapy on stone recurrence and residual fragments after shockwave lithotripsy in lower caliceal calcium oxalate urolithiasis: a randomized controlled trial. J Endourol 16:149–152

28. Hofbauer J, Höbarth K, Szabo N et al (1994) Alkali citrate prophylaxis in idiopathic recurrent calcium oxalate urolithiasis – a prospective randomized study. Br J Urol 73:362–365

29. Ulmann A, Sayegh F, Clavel J et al (1984) Fréquence des récidives lithiasiques après une cure de diurèse simple ou associée à un traitement par un diurétique ou le phosphore. Presse Méd 13:1257–1260

30. Scholz D, Schwille PO, Sigel A (1982) Double-blind study with thiazide in recurrent calcium lithiasis. J Urol 128:903–907

31. Brocks P, Dahl C, Wolf H et al (1981) Do thiazides prevent recurrent idiopathic renal calcium stones? Lancet 18:124–125

32. Ettinger B (1976) Recurrent nephrolithiasis: natural history and effect of phosphate therapy. A double-blind controlled study. Am J Med 61:200–206

33. Scott NW, McPherson GC, Ramsay CR et al (2002) The method of minimization for allocation to clinical trials: a review. Control Clin Trials 23:662–674

34. Richmond J (2007) Radiological diagnosis of Kidney stones. Nephrology 12:S34–S36

35. Strauss AL, Coe FL, Deutsch L et al (1982) Factors that predict relapse of calcium nephrolithiasis during treatment: a prospective study. Am J Med 72:17–24

36. Freemantle N, Calvert M, Wood J et al (2003) Composite outcomes in randomized trials. Greater precision with greater uncertainty? JAMA 289:2554–2559

37. Hochberg Y (1988) A sharper Bonferroni procedure for multiple tests of significance. Biometrika 75:800–802

38. Holm S (1979) A simple sequentially rejective multiple test procedure. Scand J Stat 6:65–70

39. O'Brien PC, Shampo MA (1988) Statistical considerations for performing multiple tests in a single experiment. 5. Comparing two therapies with respect to several endpoints. Mayo Clin Proc 63:1140–1143

40. Lachin JM (2000) Statistical considerations in the intent-to-treat principle. Control Clin Trials 21:167–189

41. Lagakos SW (2006) The challenge of subgroup analyses – reporting without distorting. N Engl J Med 354:16

42. Everitt BS (1995) The analysis of repeated measures: a practical review with examples. Statistician 44:113–135

43. DeMets DL, Lan KKG (1994) Interim analysis: the alpha spending function approach. Stat Med 13:1341–1352

44. Hills M, Armitage P (1979) The two-period cross-over clinical trial. Br J Clin Pharmacol 8:7–20

45. Fleiss JL (1986) Factorial experiments. In: The Design and Analysis of Clinical Experiments. Wiley, New York

46. Giggle PJ, Liang K, Zeger SL (1994) Sample Size Calculations in: Analysis of Longitudinal Data. Oxford Science Publications, Oxford

47. Nouvenne A, Meschi T, Prati B et al (2010) Effects of a low-salt diet on idiopathic hypercalciuria in calcium-oxalate stone formers: a 3-mo randomized controlled trial. Am J Clin Nutr 91:565–570

48. Fernandez-Rodriguez A, Arrabal-Martin M, Garcia-ruiz MJ et al (2006) Role of thiazides in prophylaxis of relapsing calcium stones. Actas Urol Esp 30:305–309

49. Hiatt RA, Ettinger B, Caan B et al (1996) Randomized controlled trial of a low animal protein, high fiber diet in the prevention of recurrent calcium oxalate kidney stones. Am J Epidemiol 144:25–33

50. Smith MJV (1977). Placebo versus Allopurinol for renal calculi. J Urol 117:690–692

Epidemiology of Pediatric Urolithiasis

35

José Manuel Reis-Santos and Alberto Trinchieri

Abstract The current epidemiology of urolithiasis in children has been described in numerous surveys conducted in various countries showing different patterns of the disease. A pattern of relatively rare calcium-based upper tract stones is prevalent in children from industrialized countries. Endemic bladder stones, composed of uric acid and calcium oxalate in the presence of sterile urine, are typical of children living in developing countries, especially in rural areas. However, the incidence of endemic bladder stones is gradually decreasing, as poverty and infantile malnutrition disappear and affluence spreads to all social classes.

Other patterns of urolithiasis can also be observed in relation to genetic and socioeconomic or climatic factors. Cystinuria and hyperoxaluria account for up to 5–15% of pediatric stones.

Infection stones, mainly composed of struvite and carbonate apatite, are associated with chronic infection and often related to poor health conditions. In particular, boys are prone to infected stones, although this type of calculi is decreasing in Western countries. Upper urinary stones composed of calcium oxalate mixed with calcium phosphate and uric acid are becoming frequent in tropical regions where the risk of stone formation is compounded by low urine volume.

Prematurity, neurological problems, ketogenic diet, and reconstructed or augmented bladders are increased risk factors for stones in babies.

35.1 Introduction

Urolithiasis can occur in children even in neonatal life. It has been characterized by a pattern of either relatively rare calcium-based upper tract stones in children of industrialized countries or endemic bladder stones in young ones in developing countries – especially in rural areas. In the course of the twentieth century, there has been a gradual decrease in the incidence of endemic bladder stones, as poverty and infantile malnutrition have gradually disappeared and affluence has spread to all social classes.

At the present time, upper urinary tract stones are prevalent in children living in economically developed countries, whereas bladder stones, composed of uric acid and calcium oxalate in the presence of sterile urine, are still present in developing countries, although upper urinary tract stones are becoming more frequent also in these geographical areas.

J.M. Reis-Santos (✉)
Faculdade De Engenharia, Universidade Católica Portuguesa,
Rio de Mouro, Portugal
e-mail: j.reissantos@gmail.com

35.2 Western Countries

During the first years of life, the incidence of urolithiasis varies greatly according to where we are born with all extrinsic risk factors and other intrinsic risks carried individually.[1] This variance occurs not only in the way it presents itself but also in its frequency, being very rare in industrialized countries, but constituting a serious threat to public health in undeveloped areas. Stone type and composition also change from industrialized countries to developing ones and also the associated metabolic alterations.[2] Worldwide, girls have a slightly decreased risk for renal stone disease compared to boys, but there was no clear gender preference in either Western Europe or the USA; and the age distribution shows that for half of the children suffering from calculi, diagnosis was made before they reached school age.

Studies analyzing race and childhood stones found that in the USA, 80% of children with stone disease are Caucasian.[1] In Germany, Borgmann and Nagel found that Turkish children who were born in West Berlin suffer from urolithiasis 2–2.5 times as often as German children of the same age groups.[3] Stone localization is moving toward the upper

P.N. Rao et al. (eds.), *Urinary Tract Stone Disease*,
DOI 10.1007/978-1-84800-362-0_35, © Springer-Verlag London Limited 2011

urinary tract. In the past, people had mainly urinary bladder stones, and in these cases, the majority of patients were male. Today, stones containing oxalate are being found more often. In children, a high proportion of mixed concrements in stone analysis is more common now. The rate of recurrence for children also varies, but is very high and figures between 15% and 25% are frequently found. These figures will be even higher if we have children with cystine stones or urinary infections not controlled by antibiotics.[1]

In industrialized countries today, renal and ureteric stones are the most common, whereas in developing countries, vesical stones are most frequently found, as was the case in nineteenth century Europe.[4] In societies of abundance, lithiasis usually occurs in the upper urinary tract in patients with malformations and/or urinary infection often associated with metabolic disorders such as hypercalciuria, hyperoxaluria, or inborn errors of metabolism such as cystine and other dibasic amino acids. It is not uncommon to find hypercalciuria associated with urinary infection, thus altering the composition of the stone, as we have already stressed. In cases of urinary infection, struvite stones, caused by the urease-splitting organisms *Proteus* and *Klebsiella*, are expected, but may have additional components, such as oxalate, due to a different metabolic environment.[5–9]

Stones of different composition can be found when there are additional risks such as prematurity, dehydration, use of furosemide in the neonatal period, or in human immunodeficiency virus (HIV) patients taking Indinavir.[10–13] Other drugs can be involved. A prospective study shows the possibility that use of ceftriaxone may also be associated with stone formation in children.[14] Also sulfadiazine-associated stone has been described in HIV-positive adult patients but rarely in children. Catalano-Pons et al.[15] report two pediatric cases and review 45 adult cases. The first child had a hyper-immunoglobulin M (IgM) syndrome and was treated with sulfadiazine for cerebral toxoplasmosis, the other had toxoplasmosis retinitis. Both developed multiple bilateral stones with acute renal failure. Normalization of renal function and reduction of calculi size were rapidly achieved after discontinuation of sulfadiazine, encouragement of hyper-hydration, and alkalinization.

Whenever there is a situation of hyperparathyroidism, renal tubular acidosis, hypervitaminosis D, sarcoidosis, immobilization, etc., stones are often found related to hypercalciuria. Stones are also present as a result of malabsorption syndromes.[1,4]

Stones have been associated with use of the ketogenic diet in children with refractory seizure disorders. Clinical characteristics of 18 children presenting with stones (8 uric acid stones, 6 mixed calcium/uric acid stones, 1 calcium oxalate/phosphate stone, 3 stones not evaluated) were compared with characteristics of non-stone-forming children initiating the ketogenic diet at Johns Hopkins, by Furth et al.[16] Since July 1996, 112 children initiating the ketogenic diet have been followed. Prospectively, children initiating the ketogenic diet revealed that almost 40% had elevated fasting urine calcium/

creatinine ratios at baseline; increasing to 75% after 6 months on the diet. Hypercalciuria, acid urine, and low urinary citrate excretion are found if the diet is maintained; these added to a low fluid intake increased the risk for both uric acid and calcium stone formation.

Kielb et al.[17] stressed the risk of nephrolithiasis with this ketogenic diet and reported it as being as high as 10%. They also found hypercalciuria, elevated urinary uric acid and hypocitruria and serum acidosis. Fluids and bicitrate are recommended as a prophylactic measure.

The most recent accident caused by addition of melamine to milk for children, retailed in China, stresses the importance of extrinsic factors on the etiopathogeny of stones. On the 13th September, 2008, the Chinese health minister confirmed the death of 1 child and the appearance of stones in the urinary tracts of 452 other children all under 1 year of age and fed with a milk formula containing one of the triazines isomers. These figures increased dramatically weeks later, and older children were also involved.

The triazine structure is a heterocyclic ring, analogous to the six-membered benzene ring but with three carbons replaced by nitrogen. The three isomers of triazine are distinguished from each other by the positions of their nitrogen atoms. The best-known 1,3,5-triazine derivative is melamine.

Melamine is a thermosensitive polymer used in industry for making plastics, fertilizers, and resins. In 2007, this substance was responsible for the death of numerous domestic dogs and cats in the USA. It was incorporated into dry pet food with the same idea of appearing to increase the protein content when being tested. This additive thickens watered down milk and, when tested, the milk appears to have normal protein content. The appearance of renal stones in Chinese babies is a valid epidemiological experimental model showing the importance of food additives that can alter urine composition, cause renal lesions or crystalluria, all of which are responsible for the formation of renal stones. Very quickly it was understood that the number of child deaths in China had increased, that about 50,000 children were drinking formula containing melamine and that all products containing milk with this additive (biscuits, sweets, chocolate milk, etc.) were being retailed in Chinese supermarkets throughout Europe. Therefore, we can assume that this will be an influential agent on the stone population in general, although on a smaller scale than in China.

General speaking, in children, the results from different case series show that the frequency of different stone composition is between 45% and 65% for calcium oxalate, 14–30% to calcium phosphate, 13% to struvite, 4% for acid uric, and 4% for mixed miscellaneous.[9,18]

The various epidemiological studies available show differences between the USA and Europe. In the USA, lithiasis accompanies the metabolic alterations responsible for hypercalciuria whereas in Europe, urinary infection is by far the most frequent risk factor, often associated with malformation of the urinary tract. In Europe, studies show that urinary infection occurs in 30–90% of children with lithiasis whereas in the USA, it only affects around 20%.

A recent study in *England* (1987–2004) compares data from this period with data from a previous study done 30 years ago and concludes that: there has been a shift in the epidemiology of pediatric renal stone disease in the UK over the past 30 years.[19] Underlying metabolic causes are now the most common but can be masked by coexisting urinary tract infection. From 121 patients, a metabolic abnormality was found in 44% of the children, 30% were classified as infective, and 26% idiopathic. Bilateral stones on presentation occurred in 26% of the metabolic group compared to 12% in the infective/idiopathic group. Coexisting urinary tract infection was common (49%) in the metabolic group.

In 1975 from England and Ireland, Ghazali[20] gave us the results of 152 children with urinary stones followed between 1972 and 1973 and stated, "There was a marked male preponderance particularly evident in early life. In 124 children the urine was infected on admission, in 87, particularly the younger children, this was with the *Proteus* species. Awareness of the relationship between *Proteus* urinary infection and matrix calculi is stressed."

In another more recent study, van't Hoff[21] analyzes etiological factors in pediatric urolithiasis and concludes that children, particularly boys, are prone to infective stones, although this type of calculi is decreasing in Western countries. Cystinuria and hyperoxaluria each account for 5–15% of pediatric stones. Prematurity, neurological problems, ketogenic diet, and reconstructed or augmented bladders are increased risk factors for stones.

In *Italy*, Trinchieri et al.[22] give us some useful information about children in a group of 2,086 consecutive patients who visited the stone clinic in Milan over a period of 15 years. In all of the group, calcium stones accounted for 61% of cases; infection, uric acid/calcium oxalate, and cystine stones accounted for 24%, 8%, 5%, and 2%, respectively. Nephrolithiasis was more prevalent in males (male-to-female ratio 1:0.76), while infected stones were more frequent in females (male-to-female ratio 1:1.6). The peak age incidence of renal calcium stones occurred in the third to fifth decades, although about 3.4% reported onset of disease in the first and second decades of life. The onset of cystine stones was always in the first and second decades. Recurrence was around 50%. Cystine and uric acid groups had the highest recurrence rate. A metabolic defect could be found in 54% of the patients with idiopathic calcium stones. The prevalence rate of hypercalciuria was 33%. In struvite stone patients, the incidence of persistent infection was 46% (*Proteus* 18%). In this group, an underlying disease of the urinary tract was diagnosed in 18.8%, whereas a positive metabolic alteration was demonstrated in 8.5%, a urinary risk factor for metabolic

stone disease in 42%, and a previous episode of metabolic stone disease in 33%.

Another study was done by La Manna et al.[23] on Italian children with symptoms of recurrent abdominal pain, dysuria, and hematuria, occurring alone or in combination. Hematuria was the presenting symptom in 41% of patients and was the only urinary finding in more than one-third. Clinical data from 196 children aged 0.9–15.9 years were studied. Renal ultrasound examination revealed hyperechogenic spots in renal calyces (<3 mm in diameter) assumed as "calyceal microlithiasis." There was a history of urolithiasis in 70.4% of patients in at least one first- or second-degree relative. Hypercalciuria was present in about one-third and hyperuricuria in one-fifth of the patients. Of 29 patients who were followed for at least 2 years, 9 developed calculi 4–7 mm in diameter. For the authors, "calyceal microlithiasis" possibly represents the first step in stone formation and possibly Randal's Plaques.

Results from a *Spanish* study – including 130 children suffering from urinary stones, aged between 4 and 6 years, and a male-to-female ratio of 2.5:1 – show the reality of another country.[24] There were 108 cases of reno-ureteric lithiasis and 23 vesico-urethral lithiasis. In 69 cases, pyelocalyceal lithiasis predominated. Bilateral stones were found in 30% of the children, and in 19%, a staghorn calculi was present. Study of these cases failed to indicate whether obstruction of the upper urinary tract (14%) or infection (27%) was the cause or the effect of the lithiasis. In this study, eight cases of cystinuria (6%), one of glycinuria, one of hyperoxaluria, and seven of hypercalciuria were identified. It is the author's belief that, at least in Spain, lithiasis in children would appear to be essentially idiopathic. However, 40% of these cases of lithiasis were secondary to obstruction of the urinary tract and/or urinary infection. All types of entero-uroplasty were lithogenic (six cases) and 32% of the children had a *Proteus* infection, in contrast with a recent study in adult males with enteric bladders substitutions showing stone incidence in only 1%.[25]

Fourteen children were treated medically and 125 surgically: 70% are stone free and 7% have a residual lithiasis. The low recurrence rate achieved according to the conclusions is due to a complete surgical removal of the stone.

The incidence of nephrourolithiasis among children in *Denmark* was studied during the period 1994–2003. Thirty-two cases were admitted, diagnosed, and treated in two Danish pediatric departments.[26] All patients underwent radiological examination and metabolic evaluation. Kidney stone analysis was performed in 14 of the 32 cases (44%). In 21 children (66%), there were one or more predisposing factors to stone formation, the most common being urinary tract malformation, found in 40% of the cases, of which 42% presented with hypercalciuria.

When looking at data from countries like *Germany*, we must take into account that modern Germany includes what used to be two separate countries with different development and economic characteristics as well as the fact that many patients are children of immigrant parents, as can be seen from the following study by Borgmann and Nagel.[3] One hundred eighty-one of 2,606 patients hospitalized due to urolithiasis during a 12-year period were younger than 15 years (6.9%). They found the incidence of urolithiasis in children to be 1–5%, which, at least in Central Europe, corresponds approximately with that in adults. The risk factors involved were: malformation of urinary tract in 35.9%, infection in 80.7%, and metabolic disorders in only 5.5% of patients. Stone analysis showed a predominance of phosphate-containing calculi. Follow-up was done in 154 children over periods of 6 months to 11 years. "Recurrent stones" were seen in 32 patients; however, the exact comparison of pre- and postoperative X-ray films showed that in 17 cases the calculi had not been completely removed during surgery (11%). Consequently, the true recurrent stones were present only in 15 children (9.9%). Since the population of West Berlin includes a high percentage of Turkish people, they conclude from the data presented that even those Turkish children who were born in West Berlin suffer from urolithiasis 2–2.5 times as often as German children of the same age groups.

For additional information from autopsied patients, it is worthwhile to look at two studies from *Germany* and *the Ukraine*. Both these studies compare stone data from children with that from adults, and from countries not too far from each other but certainly with different realities.

In 27,133 autopsies done at Pathologisch-Anatomisches Institut Stralsund in the area of Rügen-Stralsund, the frequency of urolithiasis was 6%. Data show that obesity, hypertension, and diabetes mellitus may increase the tendency of cholelithiasis patients to develop additional urolithiasis. Urethral and urinary bladder calculi are more frequent among male patients. In the autopsy material, multiple calculi and bilateral cases occur more frequently. Some of the calculi may develop at a very advanced age.[27]

The other study that also uses data from autopsies and carried out in Central Europe shows that children in the first years of life can have lithiasis.[28] With this autopsy data, Kurennaia et al. show that urolithiasis is found in 3.6% of 100 cases, most frequently in men (62 cases) over 40 years of age. In two-thirds of patients, the length of the disease was under 8 years, rarer over 15 years. In most cases, renal involvement was bilateral (72 patients). More than 70% had two or three operations. A pathogenetic relationship was found between urolithiasis and malformations of urinary tract, urinary stasis neurogenic related, prostate hyperplasia, and metabolic disorders.

France follows the rest of Europe, although some changes are noted from one region to another. For detailed information on stone composition found in children, important for making an etiological diagnosis of the disease, we resume the results found by Daudon.[29] Detailed calculi analyzed from 727

children confirmed that calcium oxalate was the main component in 36.7% of cases, followed by calcium phosphate (31%), struvite (9.9%), and purines (7.7%). The most frequently observed crystalline form was carbapatite (26%), then whewellite (21%) and weddellite (15.7%). As regards the etiopathogenic aspect in adults, the relations between hypercalciuria and weddellite, and between hyperoxaluria and whewellite are also found in the child: In subjects with hypercalciuria, 82% of the calculi contained over 20% weddellite; and in subjects with hyperoxaluria, whewellite was the major constituent in 79% of cases (or 95% in the absence of associated hypercalciuria). In 27 calculi mainly composed of whewellite, the morphological analysis indicated primary hyperoxaluria. Urinary infection is associated with stones, but its lithogenic role cannot be confirmed without stone analysis. Also from France and confirming the importance of metabolic anomaly and infection, Naoumis[30] presents a study carried out on 33 stone children. Four out of 12 had hyperoxaluria, 6 hypercalciuria, and 2 cystinuria. In 14 children, stones were associated with infection. No metabolic defect or anatomic malformation could be found in seven of the children.

In *Portugal*, in a national survey conducted by Reis-Santos[31] in 1975 involving all the country, based on a sample of 43,033 persons, the standardized lifetime stone prevalence in children under 15 was 0.4% in females and 0.2% in males. Table 35.1 and Fig. 35.1 show the distribution of standardized

Table 35.1 Lifetime stone prevalence (%) in Portugal by gender and age group found in 43,033 individuals

Urolithiasis in Portugal lifetime prevalence (%)						
	Age					
Gender	<15	<30	<45	<60	<75	<90	<105
FEM	0.4	1.9	6.2	6.9	7.1	7.1	7.1
MALE	0.2	1.2	4.2	6.1	7	7.2	7.2

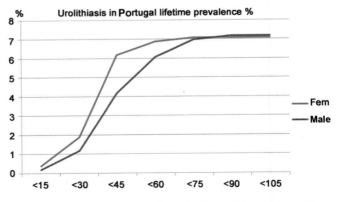

Fig. 35.1 Lifetime stone prevalence in Portugal by gender and age group

lifetime stone prevalence (%) by gender stratified by age group (15 years) in Portugal.

Results from the study population show a lifetime prevalence of urolithiasis in Portugal of 7.2% in the general population. When analyzed by gender, the global sample ($n = 43,032$) shows similar figures for male (7.217%) and female (7.096%).

Distribution of lifetime prevalence (%) stratified by age group (5 years) can be seen in Fig. 35.2. As regards the youth population, the initial peak up to school age and the beginning of a new high at 15 years should be noted.

In this survey, univariate analysis shows that stones were gender related only in two age groups, summarized in Table 35.2. The same survey gives some information about the recurrence rate expected in this group (Table 35.3).

Defining the true stone incidence rate as the rate of new stones formed in individuals with no previous history of stones, we have analyzed the incidence of stones in Portugal in the year prior to the survey. For the whole group, the incidence rate was $701/10^5$ persons per year. See results stratified by age group in Table 35.4.

Recently, the same author (Reis-Santos, J) studied the incidence of urolithiasis in children based on hospital admission, collecting Portuguese hospital data from 2002 to 2007. This chapter presents unpublished data and analyzes the data collected during the last 6 years (2002–2007) from all admissions in all the Portuguese hospitals connected to the National Health Service. There were 5,663,903 admissions to the 85 hospitals covering the country, 1,113,836 of which were individuals of 18 years of age or younger. Over the period in question, 279 children were admitted and treated with a diagnosis of lithiasis. Figures 35.3–35.6 present data relating to their age, distribution by gender, and year of admission.

Table 35.5 summarizes data related to 279 patients age 18 or under with urolithiasis, treated during hospital admission between 2002 and 2007 in Portugal. The study of these patients (age 18 or under) shows slight differences as regards gender, as well as variations in the incidence of admission for lithiasis over the years in question, with a marked increase in 2007. These variations may not only be due to the illness itself but also to changes in the health system policy. For example, the majority of patients treated by extracorporeal shock wave lithotripsy (ESWL) are now treated as outpatients – even children. It should be noted that because the group has been extended to 18 years, we are encountering more young women with lithiasis. Figures 35.5–35.9 summarize age separated by gender as well as incidence of lithiasis for each year in the group of children admitted. It can be said that the incidence values, at present time, calculated

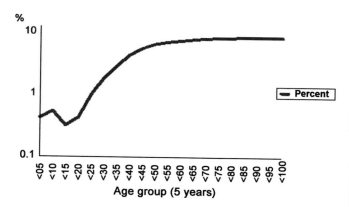

Fig. 35.2 Results of lifetime stone prevalence (%) in all the population stratified by age group (5-year intervals)

Table 35.3 One stone episode versus stone recurrence. Distribution by age group (15-year intervals)

Age group	One stone episode		Recurrent	
	FEM	MALE	FEM	MALE
	% ($n = 657$)	% ($n = 576$)	% ($n = 683$)	% ($n = 528$)
0–14	1.2	0.3	0.1	0.2
15–29	10.2	6.8	6.9	4
30–44	48.6	41.1	42.3	27.8
45–59	19.2	31.1	28.8	40.3
60–74	15.1	14.6	16.4	21.6
75–89	5.2	5.9	5.3	4.9
≥90	0.5	0.2	0.2	1.2

Table 35.4 Stone incidence per year, by age group, in Portugal

Age group ($n = 40,033$)	0–14	15–29	30–44	45–59	60–74	>75
Incidence rates (stones/10^5 persons-year)	35	407	917	1,086	835	1,119

Table 35.2 Summary of univariate analysis of ratio between gender and formation or non-formation of stones, taking into account the various age groups

Age (age group)	SIG *	Odds ratio	IC 95%	X^2 (mantel-Haenaszel)	P value
0–14	N	2.34	0.71, 8.49	2.34	0.126
15–29	Y	1.59	1.19, 2.11	11.00	0.0009
30–44	Y	1.21	1.07, 1.36	9.53	0.0020
45–59	N	0.90	0.78, 1.04	2.00	0.1577
60–74	N	0.93	0.77, 1.13	0.57	0.452
≥75	N	0.90	0.63, 1.27	0.41	0.521

*Significant at $P < 0.01$

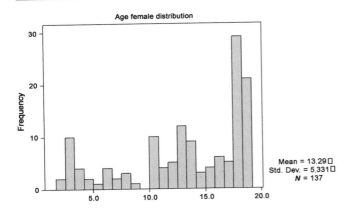

Fig. 35.3 Female distribution of lithiasis by age

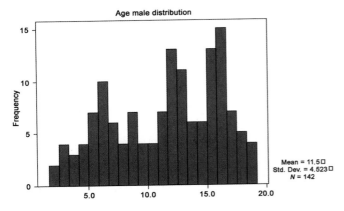

Fig. 35.4 Male distribution of lithiasis by age

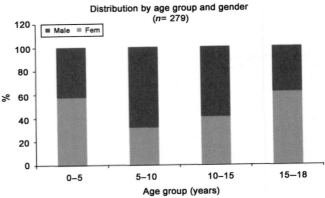

Fig. 35.5 Distribution of lithiasis by age group and gender

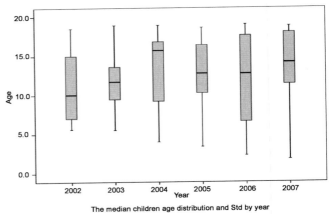

Fig. 35.6 Median child age distribution and Std by year of lithiasis

from hospital registers, are lower than those found, for example, in other European countries and the USA. However, it must be noted that these values may reflect several biases and may, for various reasons not related to the natural history of the illness, overestimate the sample values. Based on data taken from the 1975 survey, it can be added that in Portugal only 3.9% of individuals did not go to the doctor during their first stone episode. Out of the whole sample, regardless of age, 31.6% (*n* = 935) of those who were medically assisted were admitted to hospital but, if we only consider children, this figure is 100%. These data show the importance of the hospital in this type of pathology and also give credibility to all the information collected from there – information that relates to the majority of stone patients. The standardized values found for lifetime prevalence in the 1975 survey are within those found throughout Western Europe and show that, in Portugal, prevalence in women is increasing and now approximates the values for men, with the first stone episode occurring at the beginning of adulthood. Table 35.5 presents the results of stone incidence from the same survey.[31] In Portugal, composition of the first stone is now calcium oxalate and not struvite as it used to be in the past.[32,33]

A study recently carried out in *Iceland*,[34] a country with a high standard of living, shows some very interesting results. All children under 18 who, with a first episode of kidney stones, were seen at pediatric referral centers in Iceland during the years 1995–2000 were studied retrospectively. Clinical and imaging studies support the diagnosis of stones: 15 females and 11 males, median age 9.4 (range 0.2–14.9) years, experienced 34 episodes of kidney stones. The incidence was 5.6 and 6.3 per 100,000 children younger than 18 and 16 years of age, respectively. Microhematuria was present in 21 patients (80.8%), sterile pyuria in 17 (65%), and 2,8-dihydroxyadeninuria in 2. Six patients (23%) had urinary infection at the time of diagnosis and five (20%) had urinary tract anomalies. One-third of the patients gave a family history of kidney stones. Metabolic risk factors were identified in 22 of 23 patients (96%) who underwent evaluation. Hypercalciuria was present in 18 patients (78%), 9 patients (35%) spontaneously passed the stone, and 6 had recurrent stone episodes. In Iceland, kidney stone incidence in children is high compared with other Western populations, curiously affecting females more than males, underlying that metabolic risk factors were common. It should be emphasized that, until October 2008, Iceland had the highest standard of living in the world.

Table 35.5 Summary of data related to 279 patients aged 18 or younger with urolithiasis, treated during hospital admission between 2002 and 2007 in Portugal

Year	Total admissions	Children with stones Age ≤ 18	Total children admissions Age ≤ 18 years	Incidence/1,000/ children admissions/ year
2002	948,933	32	200,329	0.15973
2003	969,615	47	199,051	0.23612
2004	943,701	50	184,743	0.27064
2005	942,778	28	179,891	0.15565
2006	949,269	46	179,724	0.25594
2007	909,607	76	170,098	0.44680
	Total 5,663,903	Total 279	Total: 1,113,836	

In the *USA*, incidence of lithiasis in the pediatric community varies between 1 in 1,000 and 1 in 1,760 hospital admissions, depending on whether or not the child lives in the known "stone belt" region.[1] In the USA, as in other parts of the world, the prevalence of stones changes geographically. A study involving more than one million individuals carried out in the USA clearly shows a north-south and west-east gradient, with the highest prevalence occurring in southeastern areas.[1] Other risk factors are involved such as infection, metabolic alterations, diet, malformations, genetics, and others like anywhere else.[35]

In the early 1980s, O'Regan et al.[36] found pediatric urolithiasis accounting for 1:4,090 hospital admissions. Forty percent of patients had no identifiable predisposition to urolithiasis. Eight patients presented with hematuria in the absence of renal colic, suggesting that pediatric urolithiasis, although uncommon, is an important cause of painless hematuria.

VanDervoort et al.[37] in the Schneider Children's Hospital, New York, conducted a retrospective, single-site review to test the hypotheses that the incidence of urolithiasis in pediatric patients increased from 1994 to 2005, and that metabolic abnormalities were more common in patients with renal stones in the final 3 years of the study period. Medical files from two time periods were reviewed, 1994–1996 (period 1) and 2003–2005 (period 2). Clinical and laboratory data were recorded. The results show that the number of stone patients increased from 7 in period 1 to 61 in period 2. When expressed as cases per 100 new patients, the incidence increased 4.6 times ($p = 0.014$). Considering period 2, 28% of patients were younger than 10 years. While blood tests were generally normal, 76% of patients had at least one abnormality in the 24-h urine collection. Hypocitraturia, the most common metabolic abnormality, was registered in 52% of patients. Surgery and/or ESWL was needed in 12 children and recurrence found in 39%. The study confirmed a fivefold increased incidence of stones in children during the last decade. Hypocitraturia, follow by hypercalciuria, is the most common metabolic abnormality. A high recurrence rate, around 40%, was recorded.

Gearhart et al.[38] between June 1979 and June 1989, studied 54 children with urolithiasis at the Johns Hopkins Children's Center. Symptoms of flank or abdominal pain (58%) and gross hematuria (28%) were common. In 46 children (86%), stones were secondary to a preexisting condition, and in only 8 (14%), no apparent cause of stone formation could be found. Thirty-six patients (66%) had a solitary stone, most commonly found in the kidney. Urinary tract infections were present in 25 (47%) of the patients. Stones composed either of calcium oxalate or struvite were the most frequently recovered in these patients with infections. Thirty-nine percent spontaneously passed their stones whereas 43% required either surgery or ESWL. Twenty percent had recurrence, with follow-up periods ranging from 1 month to 10 years.

From University of Florida, Lim et al.[39] report the results of managing pediatric urolithiasis during a 10-year period. A retrospective review is presented of 100 patients up to age 18 years who were treated for urolithiasis between 1984 and 1994. The mean follow-up was 36 months. They found in 42 patients structural anomalies of the urinary tract requiring additional management. Metabolic abnormalities in 48 included hypercalciuria, and 76 of the 100 patients had identifiable predisposing factors. Procedures included ESWL in 42 cases, basket extraction with or without ureteroscopy in 20, percutaneous nephrostolithotomy in 11, litholapaxy in 12, and open surgery in 25 cases.

35.3 Non-Western Countries

The current epidemiology of urolithiasis in children from non-Western countries is described in numerous surveys conducted by various countries showing different patterns of the disease.

Endemic infantile bladder calculi composed of ammonium urate and calcium oxalate are still fairly widespread in huge rural areas, although their incidence is decreasing in proportion as social conditions gradually improve. This form

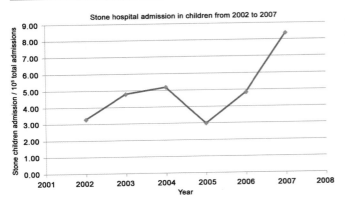

Fig. 35.7 Prevalence in children admitted for lithiasis

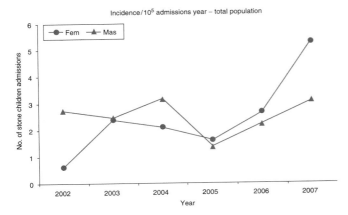

Fig. 35.8 Lithiasis incidence/10^5 admissions year of the total population

of urolithiasis is due to malnutrition in the very early years of life and, more particularly, to precocious weaning together with a cereal diet. Other patterns of urolithiasis can also be observed in relation to different socioeconomic and climatic factors. Infection stones mainly composed of struvite and carbonate apatite are associated with chronic infection and are often related to poor health conditions. Calcium oxalate and phosphate reno-ureteric stones similar to those observed in children of Western countries are a common pattern in highly industrialized areas of East Asia such as Japan or in white populations of Australia or South Africa.

Finally, upper urinary stones composed of calcium oxalate mixed with calcium phosphate and uric acid are becoming frequent in tropical regions where the risk of stone formation is compounded by low urine volume.

In some geographical regions, different patterns can be observed in the same geographical area during different periods of time due to concomitant variations in socioeconomic conditions.

According to UNICEF data, non-industrialized countries can be divided in some relatively homogeneous regions in terms of economic and health conditions: Sub-Saharan Africa, North Africa and Middle East; South Asia, East Asia and Pacific; Latin America and Caribbean; Central Eastern Europe and Commonwealth of Independent States (CEE & CIS).

South Asia and Sub-Saharan Africa have the highest levels of children suffering from poor nutrition (respectively 46% and 38%). Accordingly, the list of the least developed territories with per capita income of less than $438 (US dollars) includes most countries of Sub-Saharan Africa and South Asia together with a few countries of East Asia (Laos, Cambodia, Timor) and the Middle East (Yemen).

South Asia includes *India, Pakistan, Afghanistan, Nepal*, and other countries with a PNL per capita of 777 USD in the year 2006.

Although some areas of India are now rapidly developing, bladder stones in Indian children are still reported in high prevalence in the Hindu populations of slum areas in association with poor incomes and consumption of cereal-based diets with minimal or poor protein intake.[40,41]

Bladder stones account for a large proportion of surgical admissions also in Nepal with a striking prevalence of male subjects.[42]

Reports from Afghanistan[43] described prevalent endemic bladder stones in particular in males younger than 5 years of age. Stones consisted of calcium oxalate and uric acid, and their formation was related to poor nutrition mainly based on wheat bread with very low intakes of milk and dairy products, eggs, and meat.

Also in the least developed countries of other regions of East Asia and the Middle East, endemic childhood bladder stones with a high male-to-female ratio are frequent.

In the 1970s, bladder stone was a common disease of childhood in *Indonesia* with an estimated incidence of 8.3/100,000 population per year, a peak age of onset of 2–4 years, and a male/female ratio of 12:1.[44] Diarrhea was common in the majority of the patients who were from poor families with a diet low in protein and phosphate. The stones were primarily composed of ammonium acid urate and associated to high levels of urinary ammonia in sterile urine. This urinary pattern is consistent with excretion of a high acid load, due to both an acidogenic rice diet combined with a low level of phosphate intake and to chronic diarrhea.

In Laos,[45] bladder stone removal is still the commonest of all surgical procedures performed on children, who often present a history of frequent episodes of diarrhea associated with the introduction of white rice into their diet as early as the first week of life.

Bladder stones were the commonest stones in children in Sub-Saharan Africa, although in more recent years, there has been a progressive increase in the number of operations for upper tract stone, suggesting a change in the pattern of urolithiasis also in this region.

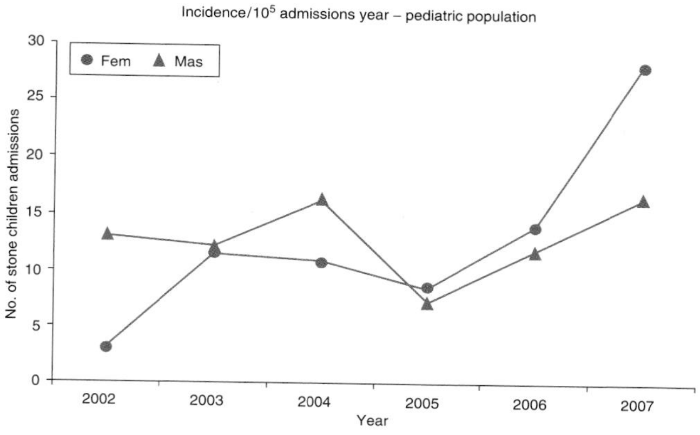

Incidence/10^5 admissions year – pediatric population

Fig. 35.9 Lithiasis incidence/10^5 admissions year of the pediatric population

In *Sudan*,[46,47] calcium oxalate stones were the most frequent (about 40% of all childhood stones), but ammonium urate stones typical for underdeveloped countries are still common (30%). Infectious stones (struvite and carbonate apatite) accounted for 5% of stones in children.

In the northern Sahelian belt of *Cameroon*,[48] pediatric endemic bladder stone disease is still present with mixed stones of ammonium urate, struvite, and whewellite. Infection associated with malnutrition seemed to be the most common cause of stone formation associated with a low level of socioeconomic development as a predisposing factor, especially in male rural dwellers.

A similar pattern of bladder stones with ammonium acid urate and calcium oxalate monohydrate as the major constituents was described in young children in *Niger*.[49]

On the contrary, in other countries of Central and Southern Africa, urinary calculi are generally reported as uncommon in black people and mainly related to infection and concomitant diseases of the lower urinary tract. In spite of widespread poverty, vesical lithiasis in infancy is rarer, probably because prolonged breast feeding is common practice (>50% children still breast feeding at 20–23 months).

Bladder stones in children were once endemic in North Africa and in a belt of countries from the Balkans through Asia, but this pattern has been recently changing.

Until the end of the twentieth century, in some areas of North Africa, stones in children were described as predominantly located in the bladder, more frequent in males, and composed of calcium oxalate, with ammonium as the main component of the nuclei.[50]

More recently, in *Algeria*, upper tract stones became predominant in children, especially in males.[51] Stone composition remained similar but ammonium urate was now less frequently found in the nucleus of the stone. The presence of struvite stones has not decreased over recent years, accounting for about 30% of all stones and being more frequently observed in women.

Also in *Tunisian* children, urinary stones are mainly composed of whewellite and located in the upper urinary tract in up to 75% of cases with a male-to-female ratio of 2:1.[52,53]

Endemic urolithiasis, defined by its nucleus composed of ammonium urate without struvite, represented 40% of cases, whereas the analysis of the stone suggested that urinary tract infection was involved in the nucleation or growth of a third of all calculi. Exclusive metabolic factors, including genetic diseases, such as primary hyperoxaluria or cystinuria, and hypercalciuria, were responsible for less than 25% of cases.

Pediatric urolithiasis is still endemic in the southeast of *Turkey*,[54] but stones are now localized mainly in the upper urinary tract, with metabolic disorders, anatomical defects, and infected stones as the most relevant etiological factors.

Also in *Iraq*,[55] primary endemic bladder calculi are now less frequent than in the past, but urolithiasis remains a serious problem. Upper tract stones, often multiple and bilateral, are frequent, whereas bladder stones account for only 10% of cases. Early onset of presentation, high male-to-female ratio, family history of stones, and consanguinity were common features. Metabolic disorders are considered the commonest causes (50–75%) of urinary stones, although they can be masked by associated urinary tract infections. Staghorn calculi associated with recurrent urinary tract infection still occurred in 15% of the cases.

In *Armenia*,[56] renal stones are more prevalent than bladder stones and male patients predominate. Calcium oxalate is the most frequent constituent in stone composition, but infectious calculi and endemic stones are still common, although progressively decreasing.

In *Iran*,[57] urolithiasis amounts to 1 case in 300 pediatric hospitalizations. The location of the stones is more frequent in the upper urinary tract, with calcium oxalate as the most frequent component followed by ammonium acid urate. Metabolic disorders, including cystinuria and xanthinuria (6%), as well as anatomic malformations were identified in about 25% of the cases. Staghorn calculi accounted for 11% of the total.

In the Arabian Peninsula, upper tract location of stones is prevalent in children and stones are more frequent in males. In *Kuwait*[58,59] the incidence of urolithiasis in the pediatric age group was estimated in only 6.9 per 100,000 population. Calcium oxalate was the main component of all stones but the proportion of urate stones was also relatively high (25%); whereas in *Yemen*[60] the nucleus and/or the main component of the stones was ammonium urate in about 75% of the cases. In Kuwaiti children, metabolic causes were found to be the major predisposing factors to stone formation (hypercalciuria, hyperoxaluria, cystinuria, and xanthinuria) and strong family aggregation of stone disease was reported. Also in *Saudi Arabia*,[61] hereditary disorders are common. Urinary tract infection and obstruction were demonstrated in less than 10% of the cases.

In *Jordan*,[62] most pediatric patients had upper tract stones, with males dominating the series and prevalence of calcium oxalate and uric acid stones. The causative factors or cofactors were infection, malformations, and urodynamic abnormalities, whereas metabolic disorders were rare.

In *Israel*,[63–65] urinary stone disease was frequently found in Oriental Jewish children, as well as in Arab children (0.29/1,000 and 0.26/1,000, respectively), but was rare in Jewish children of Ashkenazic European origin (0.04/1,000). In southern Israel, urolithiasis is predominant in Bedouin toddlers. Prevalence was greater for Bedouin than for Jewish children (1.02 versus 0.13 cases/1,000 inhabitants at risk respectively, $P < 0.01$). The more frequent stone location was the upper urinary tract (about 90%), with stones made of calcium salts in 80% and urinary tract infections associated in 24% of cases. A family history of stones is frequent, suggesting that hereditary factors could have a role in the higher incidence of the disease.

In particular, the higher incidence of childhood urolithiasis in Arab children in Israel has been related to a higher frequency of hypercalciuria (57%) (and to a lesser extent of hyperuricosuria).[66]

Cystinuria is especially common among Libyan Jews who suffer from non-type I associated with disease mutations in SLC7A9, with the high carrier rate resulting from a single missense mutation (V170M).[67]

A peculiar form of stone disease has been described in Aboriginal children living in tropical and desert regions of *Australia* who are at risk of developing urate stones in their upper urinary tract not associated with anatomic anomalies.[68,69]

This pattern of urolithiasis differs from the usual pattern of either endemic bladder stones in young children in developing countries or predominantly calcium-based stones in the upper tract of older children in affluent industrialized countries.

A report from the Goldfields region of Western Australia[70] described urate renal stones as a common finding in Aboriginal children. In a community, stone attack rate was nearly one in ten children presented per year. Stones present at a very young age (<5 years) with urinary tract infections and failure to thrive. These radiolucent calculi were only recognized with the availability of ultrasound diagnosis and often require surgical removal. Stone disease appears to resolve spontaneously after the weaning period, but in some cases results in ureteric obstruction and infection, which may lead to renal damage including renal scarring and hypertension.

Carbohydrate intolerance might be an etiological factor together with chronic diarrhea and intraluminal breakdown of sugars by enteric bacteria, resulting in a condition of chronic metabolic acidosis.[71]

In Australia, stone disease in Caucasian children presents at a later age (median 10.5 years) and most calculi are associated with an underlying urological or metabolic abnormality.[72]

In *Japan*,[73] the prevalence of urolithiasis in children is low and it has been associated with a low prevalence of hypercalciuria. An extensive screening for cystinuria was done demonstrating chemical cystinuria 920 to 1, cystine crystalluria 16,000 to 1, and homozygous cystinuria 18,000 to 1.[74]

35.4 Conclusions

The pattern of urolithiasis in children still varies according to the region of the world paralleling with the socioeconomic and health level of the particular population. In developing countries, presenting patterns are similar to those observed in other parts of the world, but the relative frequency of the various patterns remains different. However, features of urinary stone disease are tending to evolve in the same direction as in industrialized countries.

References

1. Santos-Vistoriano M, Brouchard BH, Cunningham RJ III. Renal stone disease in children. *Clin Pediatr*. 1998;37:583-600.
2. Tekin A, Tekgul N, Atsu N, Sahin A, Ozen H, Bakkaloglu M. A study of the etiology of idiopathic calcium urolithiasis in children: hipocitratúria is the most importante risk factor. *J Urol*. 2000;164:162-165.
3. Borgmann V, Nagel R. Urolithiasis in childhood. A study of 181 cases. *Urol Int*. 1982;37:198-204.
4. Gault MH, Chafe L. Relationship of frequency, age, sex, stone weight and composition in 15, 624 Stones: comparisons of results for 1980–1983 and 1995–1998. *J Urol*. 2000;164:302-307.
5. Cappuccio FP, Kalaitzidis R, Duneclift S, Eastwood JB. Unraveling the links between calcium excretion, salt intake, hypertension, kidney stones, and boné metabolism. *J Neprhol*. 2000;13:3.
6. Curhan GC, Willet WC, Rimm EB, Stampher MJ. A prospective study of dietary calcium and other nutrients and the risk of symptomatic kidney stones. *N Engl J Med*. 1993;328:833.
7. Curhan GC, Rimm EB, Willet WC, Stampfer MJ. Regional variation in nephrolithiasis incidence and prevalence among United States men. *J Urol*. 1994;151:838-841.
8. Curhan GC, Curhan SG. Diet and urinary stone disease. *Curr Opin Urol*. 1997;7:222.
9. Johnson CM, Wilson DM, O'Fallon WM, Malek RS, Kurland LT. Renal stone epidemiology: a 25-year study in Rochester, Minnesota. *Kid Int*. 1979;16:624-631.
10. Sowers MR, Jannausch M, Wood C, Pope SK, Lachance LL, Peterson B. Prevalence of renal stones in a population-based study with dietary calcium, oxalate, and medication exposures. *Am J Epidemiol*. 1998;147:914-920.
11. Reiter WJ, Schon-Pernerstorfer H, Dorfinger K, Hofbauer J, Marberger M. Frequency of urolithiasis in individuals seropositive for human immunodeficiency virus treated with indinavir is higher than previously assumed. *J Urol*. 1999;161:1082-1084.
12. Merck and Co. *Indavir sulfate (Crixivan) package insert*. West Point: Merck and Co; 1996.

13. Wu DS, Stoller ML. Indinavir urolithiasis. *Curr Opin Urol*. 2000; 10:557-561.

14. Mohkam M, Karimi A, Gharib A, et al. Ceftriaxone associated nephrolithiasis: a prospective study in 284 children. *Pediatr Nephrol*. 2007;22:690-694.

15. Catalano-Pons C, Bargy S, Schlecht D, et al. Sulfadiazine-induced nephrolithiasis in children. *Pediatr Nephrol*. 2004;19:928-931.

16. Furth SL, Casey JC, Pyzik PL, et al. Risk factors for urolithiasis in children on the ketogenic diet. *Pediatr Nephrol*. 2000;15:125-128.

17. Kielb S, Koo HP, Bloom DA, Farber GJ. Nephrolithiasis associated with the ketogenic acid. *J Urol*. 2000;164:464-466.

18. Stapleton FB, McKay CP, Noe HN. Urolithiasis in children: the role of hypercalciuria. *Pediatr Ann*. 1987;16:980.

19. Coward RJ, Peters CJ, Duffy PG, et al. Epidemiology of paediatric renal stone disease in the UK. *Arch Dis Child*. 2003;88:962-965 (Erratum in: Arch Dis Child. 2004;89:797.).

20. Ghazali S. Childhood urolithiasis in the United Kingdom and Eire. *Br J Urol*. 1975;47:739-743.

21. van't Hoff WG. Aetiological factors in paediatric urolithiasis. *Nephron Clin Pract*. 2004;98:c45-c48.

22. Trinchieri A, Rovera F, Nespoli R, Currò A. Clinical observations on 2086 patients with upper urinary tract stone. *Arch Ital Urol Androl*. 1996;68:251-262.

23. La Manna A, Polito C, Cioce F, et al. Calyceal microlithiasis in children: report on 196 cases. *Pediatr Nephrol*. 1998;12:214-217.

24. Gosalbez R, Garat JM, Piro C, Martin JA. Urinary lithiasis in the child. *J Urol (Paris)*. 1980;86:665-670.

25. Dhar NB, Hernadez Av, Reinhardt K, et al. Prevalence of nephrolithiasis in patients with ileal bladder substitutes. *J Urol*. 2008; 71:128-130.

26. Wason MP, Hansen A. Renal and urinary calculi in children. *Ugeskr Laeger*. 2005;167:3786-3789.

27. Grosse H. Frequency, localization and associated disorders in urinary calculi. Analysis of 1671 autopsies in Urolithiasis. *Z Urol Nephrol*. 1990;83:469-474.

28. Kurennaia SS, Uzun GV, Gerasimenko AI. The incidence of urolithiasis (based on autopsy data from the Donetsk Province Clinical Hospital). *Lik Sprava*. 1992;3:77-79 [Article in Russian].

29. Daudon M. Component analysis of urinary calculi in the etiologic diagnosis of urolithiasis in the child. *Arch Pediatr*. 2000;7:855-865.

30. Naoumis A, Dumas R, Belon C, Averous M. Urinary calculi in children. Etiologic survey. *Arch Fr Pédiatr*. 1989;46:347-349.

31. Reis-Santos JM. The epidemiology of stone disease in Portugal. In: Jungers P, Daudon M, eds. *Renal Stone Disease – Proceedings of the 7th European Symposium on Urolithiasis*. Paris: Elsevier; 1997:12-14.

32. Reis-Santos JM. Composition and frequency of stone minerals in the South of Portugal. In: Ryall R, Brockis JG, Marshall V, Finlayson B, eds. *Urinary Stone*. Melbourne/Edinburgh/London/New York: Churchill Livingstone; 1984:231-260.

33. Reis-Santos JM. Composition of urinary calculi in the south of Portugal. In: Ryall R, Bais R, Marshall VR, Rofe AM, Smith LH, Walker VR, eds. *Urolithiasis 2 – Proceedings of VII International Symposium on Urolitiasis*. Cairns (Australia)/New York: Plenum; 1994. Abstract G31.

34. Edvardsson V, Elidottir H, Indridason OS, Palsson R. High incidence of kidney stones in Icelandic children. *Pediatr Nephrol*. 2005;20:940-944.

35. Soucie J, Coatees R, McClellan W, et al. Relation between geographic variability in kidney stones prevalence and risk factors for stones. *Am J Epidemiol*. 1996;143:487-495.

36. O'Regan S, Homsy Y, Mongeau JG. Urolithiasis in children. *Can J Surg*. 1982;2:566-568.

37. Van Dervoort K, Wiesen J, Frank R, et al. Urolithiasis in pediatric patients: a single center study of incidence, clinical presentation and outcome. *J Urol*. 2007;177:2300-2305.

38. Gearhart JP, Herzberg GZ, Jeffs RD. Childhood urolithiasis: experiences and advances. *Pediatrics*. 1991;87:445-450.

39. Lim DJ, Walker RD 3rd, Ellsworth PI, et al. Treatment of pediatric urolithiasis between 1984 and 1994. *J Urol*. 1996;156:702-705.

40. Shah AM, Kalmunkar S, Punekar SV, Billimoria FR, Bapat SD, Deshmukh SS. Spectrum of pediatric urolithiasis in western India. *Indian J Pediatr*. 1991;58:543-549.

41. Hussain F, Billimoria FR, Singh PP. Urolithiasis in northeast Bombay: seasonal prevalence and chemical composition of stones. 1. *Int Urol Nephrol*. 1990;22:119-124.

42. Sharma N, Furber A, Lemaster J. Study on urinary bladder stone cases at Okhaldhunga Hospital, Nepal. 1988–1994. *Nepal Med Coll J*. 2004;6:49-52.

43. Srivastava RN, Hussainy MA, Goel RG, Rose GA. Bladder stone disease in children in Afghanistan. *Br J Urol*. 1986;58:374-377.

44. Thalut K, Rizal A, Brockis JG, Bowyer RC, Taylor TA, Wisniewski ZS. The endemic bladder stones of Indonesia: epidemiology and clinical features. *Br J Urol*. 1976;48:617-621.

45. Sayasone S, Odermatt P, Khammanivong K, et al. Bladder stones in childhood: a descriptive study in a rural setting in Saravan Province, Lao PDR. *Southeast Asian J Trop Med Public Health*. 2004; 35(Suppl 2):50-52.

46. Kambal A, Wahab SM, Khattab AH. The pattern of urolithiasis in the Sudan. *Br J Urol*. 1978;50:376-377.

47. Balla AA, Salah AM, Khattab AH, et al. Mineral composition of renal stones from the Sudan. *Urol Int*. 1998;61:154-156.

48. Angwafo FF 3rd, Daudon M, Wonkam A, Kuwong PM, Kropp KA. Pediatric urolithiasis in sub-saharan Africa: a comparative study in two regions of Cameroon. *Eur Urol*. 2000;37:106-111.

49. Vanwaeyenbergh J, Vergauwe D, Verbeeck RM. Infrared spectrometric analysis of endemic bladder stones in Niger. *Eur Urol*. 1995;27:154-159.

50. Harrache D, Mesri A, Addou A, Semmoud A, Lacour B, Daudon M. Urolithiasis in children in West Algeria. *Ann Urol*. 1997; 31:84-88.

51. Djelloul Z, Djelloul A, Bedjaoui A, et al. Urinary stones in Western Algeria: study of the composition of 1, 354 urinary stones in relation to their anatomical site and the age and gender of the patients. *Prog Urol*. 2006;16:328-335.

52. Kamoun A, Daudon M, Abdelmoula J, et al. Urolithiasis in Tunisian children: a study of 120 cases based on stone composition1. *Pediatr Nephrol*. 1999;13:920-925.

53. Alaya A, Bouri A, Najjar MF. Paediatric renal stone disease in Tunisia: a 12 years experience. *Arch Ital Urol Androl*. 2008; 80:50-55.

54. Ece A, Ozdemir E, Gürkan F, Dokucu AI, Akdeniz O. Characteristics of pediatric urolithiasis in south-east Anatolia. *Int J Urol*. 2000;7: 330-334.

55. Ali SH, Rifat UN. Etiological and clinical patterns of childhood urolithiasis in Iraq. *Pediatr Nephrol*. 2005;20:1453-1457.

56. Sarkissian A, Babloyan A, Arikyants N, Hesse A, Blau N, Leumann E. Pediatric urolithiasis in Armenia: a study of 198 patients observed from 1991 to 1999. *Pediatr Nephrol*. 2001;16:728-732.

57. Kheradpir MH, Bodaghi E. Childhood urolithiasis in Iran with special reference to staghorn calculi. *Urol Int*. 1990;45:99-103.

58. el-Reshaid K, Mughal H, Kapoor M. Epidemiological profile, mineral metabolic pattern and crystallographic analysis of urolithiasis in Kuwait. *Eur J Epidemiol*. 1997;13:229-234.

59. Al-Eisa AA, Al-Hunayyan A, Gupta R. Pediatric urolithiasis in Kuwait. *Int Urol Nephrol*. 2002;33:3-6.

60. Holman E, Khan AM, Flasko T, Toth C, Salah MA. Endoscopic management of pediatric urolithiasis in a developing country. *Urology*. 2004;63:159-162.

61. Abdurrahman MB, Elidrissy AT. Childhood renal disorders in Saudi Arabia. *Pediatr Nephrol*. 1988;2:368-372.

62. Dajani AM, Abu Khadra AL, Baghdadi FM. Urolithiasis in Jordanian children. A report of 52 cases. *Br J Urol*. 1988;61:482-486.

63. Sokol Y, Winter ST, Boxer J, Kana'aneh H. Urinary calcium excretion in schoolboys. Ethnic group differences. *Isr J Med Sci.* 1978;14:432-435.

64. Drachman R, Lotan D, Aladjem M, Boichis H, Hertz M. Urolithiasis in Isreali children. *Arch Fr Pédiatr.* 1981;38:117-120.

65. Freundlich E, Saab K, Bitterman W. Urinary calculi in children. *Urology.* 1982;20:503-505.

66. Landau D, Tovbin D, Shalev H. Pediatric urolithiasis in southern Israel: the role of uricosuria. *Pediatr Nephrol.* 2000;14:1105-1110.

67. Sidi R, Levy-Nissenbaum E, Kreiss I, Pras E. Clinical manifestations in Israeli cystinuria patients and molecular assessment of carrier rates in Libyan Jewish controls. *Isr Med Assoc J.* 2003; 5: 439-442.

68. Jones TW, Henderson TR. Urinary calculi in children in Western Australia: 1972–86. *Aust Paediatr J.* 1989;25:93-95.

69. Williams WM, Nicholas JJ, Nungurrayi PB, Napurrula CR. Paediatric urolithiasis in a remote Australian aboriginal community. *J Paediatr Child Health.* 1996;32:344-346.

70. Baldwin DN, Spencer JL, Jeffries-Stokes CA. Carbohydrate intolerance and kidney stones in children in the Goldfields. *J Paediatr Child Health.* 2003;39:381-385.

71. Carson PJ, Brewster DR. Unique pattern of urinary tract calculi in Australian Aboriginal children. *J Paediatr Child Health.* 2003;39:325-328.

72. Cheah WK, King PA, Tan HL. A review of pediatric cases of urinary tract calculi. *J Pediatr Surg.* 1994;29:701-705.

73. Kaneko K, Tsuchiya K, Kawamura R, et al. Low prevalence of hypercalciuria in Japanese children. *Nephron.* 2002;91:439-443.

74. Ito H, Murakami M, Miyauchi T, et al. The incidence of cystinuria in Japan. *J Urol.* 1983;129:1012-1014.

Metabolic Stone Disease in Children

Kemal Sarica and Mustafa Berber

Abstract When compared with the adult population, with an overall 1–2% incidence, urinary stone disease in children is relatively rare but often associated with metabolic abnormalities that can lead to recurrent stone episodes, emphasizing the necessity of full metabolic evaluation after the first stone episode. As a recurrent pathology, which may reveal functional as well and morphologic changes in the urinary tract, each child should be evaluated thoroughly on an individual basis.

The pathology is associated with considerable morbidity, with recurrence rates of 6.5–44%. Without close follow-up and medical management, stone recurrence rates have been reported to be as high as 50% within 5 or 6 years. In children, stone recurrence rates range widely from 3.6% to 67% and appears to be highest in children with metabolic abnormalities. The rate of stone recurrence in our previous report was 4% during a 5-year follow-up period.

Given the high risk of subsequent calculus formation, it could be argued that all children should undergo some form of evaluation to determine the cause of their kidney stone and to help plan proper management strategies. It is well-known that certain groups of children should undergo a full metabolic workup due to the high risk of recurrence. Through these efforts future stone formation and/or growth may be controlled in the pediatric population, limiting the morbidity of this disease.

36.1 Introduction

Pediatric urolithiasis is a relatively rare disease in developed countries, and in different series the prevalence values have been reported to be ranging from 2% to 2.7%.[1,2] Although recent studies have shown that the annual incidence is increasing in Western populations,[3,4] stone formation is uncommon in children younger than 2 years of age. In contrast to the marked predominance of male stone formers in adults, boys seem to be affected slightly higher by stone formation than girls.[5,6] While the majority of the calculi (up to 90%) are located in the upper urinary tract in developed countries,[7] lower urinary tract calculi are seen more frequently in developing ones. Calcium-containing calculi (calcium oxalate and calcium phosphate) constitute the most common stone type and nearly 75% of all stones are of this composition.[5,8] Several factors predispose children to urolithiasis, of which metabolic and genitourinary anomalies are particularly important. These factors are frequently combined with dietary, environmental, and infectious causes where underlying metabolic abnormalities may be present in approximately 50–75% of patients.[5,8] Due to the common presence of metabolic abnormalities, stone disease may recur in this specific population more often than adults. Therefore, children require a thorough anatomic and metabolic evaluation for a proper treatment plan to prevent further stone formation. Remarkable improvements in the understanding of both physicochemical principles and pathophysiology of stone formation have increased the need for a thorough metabolic evaluation, and medical treatment is crucial in the prevention of the recurrences in these patients.

36.2 Pathophysiology

Stone formation is a complex process beginning with crystallization and followed by crystal growth, aggregation, and adherence (Fig. 36.1), among which crystal formation has

K. Sarica (✉)
Department of Urology, Yeditepe University, Medical School, Istanbul, Turkey
e-mail: ksarica@yeditepe.edu.tr

P.N. Rao et al. (eds.), *Urinary Tract Stone Disease*,
DOI 10.1007/978-1-84800-362-0_36, © Springer-Verlag London Limited 2011

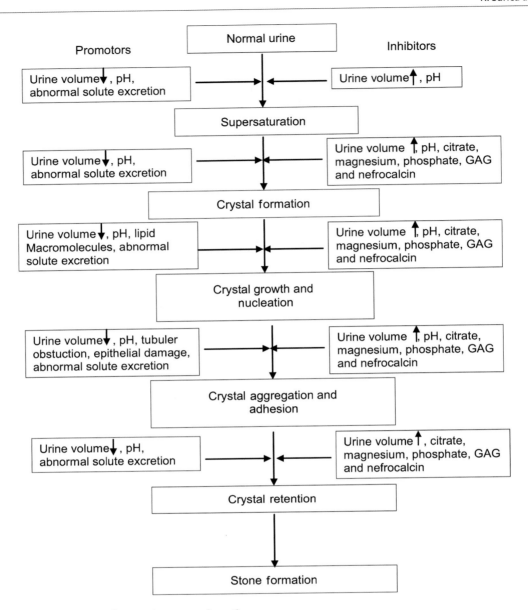

Fig. 36.1 The sequence of events leading to urinary stone formation

been defined as an important step for the initiation and growth of urinary stones.

These steps are promoted or inhibited by a number of chemical and environmental factors. Supersaturation is defined as the concentration of a solute that is higher than the solubility for that substance and necessary for the crystallization process. It depends on the total daily excretion of the substances and urine volume. Although the concentration of solutes is the principal determinant, ionic strength, pH, promoter and inhibitor factors also play important roles in stone formation. Although urine is often supersaturated with calcium oxalate, calcium phosphate, or sodium urate, concentrations of mineral solutes vary throughout the day. In a large series study, the relative risk for stone formation was found to be strongly correlated with urinary calcium concentration.[9]

In addition to the supersaturation of the urine, some promoting factors were also found to be necessary to trigger new stone formation. Of these factors, some urinary macromolecules, salt crystals and lipids, which may act as a nuclei or an aggregation factor for crystals, have been evaluated in different studies.[10-13] Another important factor for stone formation is pH of the urine, which may closely affect the solubility of urinary stone forming risk factors, resulting in an increased risk of crystal formation. While alkaline pH may ease the formation of calcium-containing stones, acidic urine lowers the solubility of uric acid and cystine crystals.[14] So urine pH may act either as a promoter or an inhibitor factor, making this parameter sometimes important as a therapeutic approach. Inhibitors are the substances that interfere well with the crystal surface, resulting in crystal growth limitation or formation of soluble complexes.[15–17] These natural inhibitors include citrate, magnesium, pyrophosphate, glycosaminoglicans, and nefrocalcin. To form a stone, crystals must reach a sufficient size to obstruct or adhere to a renal tubuli. After this step, these crystals may act as a nuclei and promote the stone formation. But these steps are very variable and in the majority of cases they do not form urinary stones. Children who form stones usually have underlying predisposing metabolic factors and/or anatomical abnormalities causing higher excretion of solutes, urinary obstruction, or urinary tract infection.[18]

36.3 Clinical Presentation

In adults, the typical features of nephrolithiasis are flank pain and/or hematuria being present in more than 90% of the cases. But in children, these typical symptoms are less common, and age is the key factor for signs and symptoms. While in adolescence, approximately 90% of affected children present with pain and hematuria, at school-age these symptoms may be present only in 70% of the cases. Under 5 years of age, however, these symptoms may be found only in 50% of patients.[5,19] Although infants with urinary calculi, usually present with colic pain, in younger children abdominal pain is more common than renal colic.

Hematuria (macroscopic or microscopic) was found in 14–90% of the cases in different age groups of children.[20–23] Sometimes hematuria may be present in children with hypercalciuria and hyperuricosuria without any urinary stone.[24–27] Urinary stones may be present with urinary infection or sterile pyuria, especially at preschool age children. Usually the diagnosis is made during investigation of a urinary tract infection or sterile pyuria with radio-sonographic findings.[5] Dysuria and urinary frequency are manifestations of bladder or urethral stones being rare in children.

In developed countries, approximately 90% of urinary stones found in upper urinary tract and bladder calculi commonly originate from the kidneys. Primary bladder stones were usually seen in developing countries and referred to as endemic bladder stones.[28,29] These stones were seen in younger children and related with dietary factors.[30,31] Especially a diet with whole grain cereals, oxalate rich vegetables with low calcium, animal protein, and phosphate increases the risk for developing such stones.[29,32] In Western countries, however, primary bladder stones are usually related to bladder malformations.

Calcium-containing stones are the most common types of nephrolithiasis, and of all the calculi evaluated 40–60% were calcium oxalate, 15–25% were calcium phosphate, 10–25% mixed stones, 17–30% magnesium ammonium phosphate (struvite), 10% cystine, and 2–10% were uric acid calculi in different series.[5,7,8,28,33–35]

36.4 Metabolic Factors

The majority of children with stone disease have at least one predisposing factor and these factors are identifiable in approximately 75% of the patients.[5,34–36] Tekin et al.,[23] evaluated the metabolic status of 78 cases with idiopathic calcium stone formation and demonstrated that hypocitruria and hyperoxaluria were 4.3- and 3-fold more common in stone formers than in normal controls, respectively. Due to the presence of underlying metabolic disorders, recurrence rates have been found to be higher (65%) than the normal population.[5] In a long-term follow-up study, Noe et al., investigated the recurrence rate in hypercalciuric patients and found that 33% of patients had at least one recurrence in 4–15 years and 40% of patients had multiple recurrences.[37] Patients who had abnormal urinary tract structure also had metabolic abnormalities and chronic infection being 39% and 29%, respectively.[37] Certain medical conditions have been shown to be associated with renal lithiasis in children. Calcium oxalate stones have been found to be quite common in malabsorptive states, resulting in enhanced uptake of oxalate and subsequent increased urinary oxalate excretion.[38] Children with cystic fibrosis had significantly elevated oxalate excretion compared to normal healthy children.[39] All these data show that there is a tendency for stone recurrence in children with these identifiable risk factors that should be investigated carefully.[40,41]

Metabolic risk factors for nephrolithiasis are as follows:

- Hypercalciuria
- Hyperoxaluria
- Cystinuria
- Hyperuricosuria
- Hypocitraturia

36.4.1 Hypercalciuria

Hypercalciuria was defined as excess urinary calcium excretion greater than 4 mg/kg/day measured in a 24-h urine collection or urinary calcium/creatinine ratio greater than 0.21 while taking a normal daily diet.[39–43] During the first 2 years of life, children tend to have higher calcium and lower creatinine excretion. Adolescents, however, may have slightly higher calcium excretion during rapid growth periods. Hypercalciuria is the most common cause of pediatric urolithiasis and can be found in 4% of the normal population.[44,45] It is not a single disease or entity but it is a condition that may be associated with genetic, endocrine, dietary, and renal disorders (Table 36.1). Children with hypercalciuria generally have normal blood calcium and, in most cases, no underlying pathology being described as idiopathic hypercalciuria.

Table 36.1 Factors associated with urolithiasis

Factors	Pathology	Conditions
Hypercalciuria	Genetic	Idiopathic
		Dent's disease
		Seyberth syndrome
		Williams syndrome
	Dietary	Dietary calcium excess
		Vitamin D excess
		Ketogenic diet
		Phosphate depletion
	Drugs	Corticosteroid
		Loop diuretics
	Endocrine diseases	Hyper-hypothyroidism
		Adrenocorticoid excess
		Hyperparathyroidism
	Bone metabolism	Immobilization
		Rickets
		Malignancies
		JRA
	Renal tubular	Renal tubular phosphate leak
	Dysfunction	Impaired renal tubular calcium absorption
		Type 1 (distal) renal tubular acidosis
		Bartter syndrome
	Other	Prematurity
		Metabolic acidosis
		Increased renal prostaglandin E2 production
Hyperoxaluria	Dietary excess or chronic malabsorption	Primary hyperoxaluria I and II
Cystinuria	Genetic	Cystinuria
Hyperuricosuria	Genetic	HPRT deficiency
	Dietary	Ketogenic diet
		High protein diet
	Drugs	Salicylates
		Phenylbutazone
		Sulfinpyrazone
	Other	Malignancies
		Tumor lysis syndrome
		Diabetes
		SIADH
Hypocitraturia	Tubular dysfunction	Distal RTA
		Hypokalemia
	Dietary	Ketogenic diet

HPRT hypoxanthine phosphoribosyltransferase, *RTA* renal tubular acidosis, *SIADH* syndrome of inappropriate secretion of antidiuretic hormone, *JRA* juvenile rheumatoid arthritis

Two different types of idiopathic hypercalciuria were described, the first type of which was related to excess gastrointestinal calcium absorption. The calcium–creatinine ratio is normal in fasting condition in these children. The second type is related to excess renal excretion, and dietary calcium restriction does not affect the urinary calcium levels.[46–48] Although the pathophysiology of idiopathic hypercalciuria is unclear, some patients with this pathology have an increased number of vitamin D receptors compared with controls.[49]

Some of these patients have familial penetrance, but the responsible gene has not been identified so far. The disease appears to be transmitted as an autosomal dominant trait with incomplete penetrance, as 40–65% of patients have a positive family history.[50–53] Hypercalciuria could be assessed in nearly half of the children with urinary stones and it is strongly associated with hematuria despite the absence of a stone. In a prospective study, Stapleton et al., found that 27% of children with unexplained hematuria had hypercalciuria, and when urinary calcium was reduced by treatment, hematuria resolved in the majority of the cases.[6] Hypercalciuria may also cause dysuria, urinary urgency, and perhaps recurrent urinary tract infections.[52–55] While in some studies 4–17% of patients did develop urinary stones,[51–53] in a prospective study, 8 of 65 patients with hypercalciuria and hematuria developed calculi in a 4-year follow-up period.[56] Garcia et al., revealed that 17% of patients developed urolithiasis where the mean period between hematuria and stone formation was 13.1 months without any predictive factor.[54]

Dent's disease is a rare X-linked recessive disorder related to a specific chloride channel (CLCN5), which is located on Xp11.22. This pathology affects proximal tubule, loop of Henle, and medullary thick ascending limb, and causes hypercalciuria, low molecular weight proteinuria, nephrolithiasis, and nephrocalcinosis.[57,58] The same chloride channel is associated with four different entities: Dent's disease, X-linked recessive hypophosphatemic rickets, and low molecular weight proteinuria with hypercalciuria and nephrocalcinosis.[59]

Other causes of hypercalciuria, such as use of corticosteroids and loop diuretics, distal renal tubuler acidosis, dietary excess calcium intake, hyperparathyroidism, immobilization, hypo- or hyperthyroidism, osteolytic metastases, idiopathic hypercalcemia of infancy, sarcoidosis, and hypervitaminosis D could be mentioned.

36.4.2 Hyperoxaluria

Hyperoxaluria is found in up to 20% of children with nephrolithiasis.[5,60] Oxalate is an end product of normal purine and aminoacid metabolism where endogenous oxalate is produced in the liver. Dietary oxalate is also important, and beets, turnips, strawberries, sweet potatoes, wheat bran, tea, cocoa, pepper, chocolate, spinach, dill, nuts, and citrus juices are defined as oxalate rich foods. Dietary oxalate normally combines with calcium in the intestine, and under normal conditions, 10% of the total oxalate excreted in urine comes from food, but in malabsorption syndromes fatty acids combine with calcium and leads to the excess oxalate absorption.[61,62] Renal oxalate excretion reflects endogenous and exogenous oxalate load.

Primary hyperoxaluria is a rare autosomal recessive disorder caused by deficiency of hepatic alanine glyoxylate transferase (AGT) (Type 1) or glyoxylatereductase/hydroxypy ruvate reductase (Type 2). This deficiency leads to a moderate to marked hyperoxaluria.[63,64] The gene of the enzyme of type 1 disease is located on chromosome band 2q37.3 and the type 2 enzyme is located on chromosome 9.[65] The enzyme deficiency also leads to hyperglyceric aciduria. Type 1 disease is more severe than type 2 disease and patients with type 2 disease usually do not have any symptoms until the second or third decade of life.[66] Due to moderate to marked hyperoxaluria, recurrent nephrolithiasis occurs during infancy in type 1 disease. Stone disease may progress to end-stage renal failure at early ages. When the glomerular filtration rate (GFR) decreased to 30 mL/min/m², blood oxalate level increases rapidly, resulting in calcium oxalate depositions in multiple organ systems (oxalosis). At this stage, aggressive dialysis is the primary treatment alternative.

Pyridoxine is the cofactor for AGT enzyme and, in cases with type 1 disease, pyridoxine should be a part of the treatment regimen. One-third of patients do respond to pyridoxine treatment.[67,68] Additionally, neutral phosphate administration, alkalinization of urine pH, and high fluid intake are beneficial measures to prevent urinary supersaturation with calcium oxalate and to reduce the stone-forming activity.[67] Diagnosis of hyperoxaluria requires a 24-h urine collection, and hyperoxaluria is defined if urine oxalate level exceeds 1.0–1.5 mmol/1.73 m²/24 h. Urine oxalate excretion is higher during infancy.[66]

Secondary hyperoxaluria may occur due to malabsorption states, ethylene glycol poisoning, renal tubular acidosis (RTA), pyridoxine deficiency, sarcoidosis, and ingestion of large amounts of vitamin C.[69]

36.4.3 Cystinuria

Cystinuria is an autosomal recessive disorder of renal tubular and intestinal reabsorptive transport of cystine and the dibasic amino acids (ornithine, arginine, and lysine).[70] Mutations of the SLC3A1 gene on chromosome arm 2p and the SLC7A9 gene of chromosome 19 are responsible for the disease.[71–73] Cystine stones account for only 6–8% of all urinary calculi in children in developed countries. Cystinosis has a wide range of incidence worldwide,[74] where the estimated incidence is 1/2,000 in England and 1/15,000 in the USA. A large amount of cystine is excreted in urine that cannot be absorbed by the tubules. Due to the low solubility, soluble cystine is limited to 1,000 µ(micro)mol/L (240 mg/L) in normal urine, and cystine crystals form in children with high excretion.[75] Cystine crystals have a characteristic flat hexagonal shape. These crystals can be seen in 25% of patients.[66] In suspected cases, a positive nitroprusside test indicates excess excretion of cystine, which needs to be confirmed by a 24-h urine collection.

Cystine stones are radiopaque stones, which generally begin to form during the first decade of life in these children. Therefore, a diagnosis of cystinuria often is delayed for several years. The majority of cases are asymptomatic until the second or third decade of life. Patients with homozygous forms of cystinuria have lifelong recurring stone formation.[76] First-line therapy consists of increased oral fluid intake and a low-salt diet. Alkaline pH increases the solubility of cystine, and alkalinization of the urine is an important part of treatment.[75] If stone formation cannot be controlled, D-penicillamine can be added to the therapy.

36.4.4 Hyperuricosuria

As a weak acid, uric acid is the end-product of purine metabolism. Its solubility is mainly dependent with urinary pH and decreases in acidic urine. Idiopathic uricosuria is often familial and asymptomatic where a defect in renal tubular reabsorption or increased secretion may cause the disease.[77–79] Although uric acid crystals may combine with calcium oxalate crystals and act as a nidus, this condition is uncommon in children. Uric acid stones are responsible for 3–4% of urinary calculi in pediatric patients. Hematuria is a common sign of idiopathic hyperuricosuria[77] and usually accompanies hypercalciuria.[5] These stones may also occur in children in case of a uric acid overproduction. Hereditary disorders associated with overproduction of uric acid include Lesch–Nyhan syndrome (hypoxanthine-guanine phosphoribosyl transferase deficiency), and Type I glycogen storage disease.[80] Increasing cell activity in lymphoproliferative or myeloproliferative disorders and tumor lysis syndrome may also raise the uric acid levels. Urolithiasis may present as early as the first year of life in patients with Lesch–Nyhan syndrome. Another inborn error of metabolism with hyperuricosuria is hypoxanthine-guanine phosphoribosyltransferase deficiency. The accumulation of phosphoribosyl pyrophosphate leads to the overproduction of uric acid.[18] Patients who have partial hypoxanthine-guanine phosphoribosyltransferase deficiency also may have gouty arthritis.[81]

During early months of life, uric acid excretion is relatively high and remains higher than adult values through infancy.[80] However, beginning with 2 years of age, the amount of uric acid excreted per deciliter of glomerular filtrate does not vary with age.[77] A normal value of less than 0.56 mg of uric acid per deciliter of glomerular filtrate may be used after 2 years of age.

Treatment of hyperuricosuria requires a high fluid intake along with the restriction of dietary purines. Alkalinization of urinary pH increases the solubility of uric acid. In addition to the classical clinical cases, allopurinol may also be recommended in an attempt to limit uric acid excretion in patients with Lesch–Nyhan syndrome or tumor lysis syndrome during chemotherapy.[81,82]

36.5 Diagnostic Evaluation

Evaluation of pediatric patients with stone disease include:

- Patient history (including diet)
- Family history of stone disease and genetic disorders
- Physical examination
- Detailed urine analysis (urinalysis, urine culture sensitivity tests)
- Blood biochemistry including calcium, renal profile
- Radio-sonographic imaging
- Twenty-four hours urine collection
- Stone analysis (if possible)

Evaluation of these children should begin with a detailed patient history including the history of prematurity. Patient's age at presentation, signs and symptoms of urinary and other systems may provide clues for an underlying systemic disease. Family history of hematuria, renal failure, urolithiasis, arthritis, and gouty disease is also important. Detailed dietary history including fluid intake, medications, dietary excesses and deficiencies should be obtained. The physical examination again includes growth evaluation, bone development, body deformities, and blood pressure. Urinalysis is performed for the presence of crystalluria, pyuria, or hematuria; and

urinary tract infection could be excluded with urine culture and sensitivity tests. Chemical analysis of stone is also important to focus on an appropriate metabolic workup. A 24-h urine collection will be helpful while the patient is healthy, under normal diet, and usual fluid intake, without any additional medication (Table 36.2). The presence and excretion rate of urinary stone forming risk factors (calcium, cystine, uric acid, sodium, oxalate, and citrate) should be measured. Ideally, the urine collection can be obtained at least 6 weeks after the passage of a stone. Abnormal values might be verified with a repeat collection when necessary. But determination of urinary supersaturation for calcium oxalate, calcium phosphate, and urate may be helpful if the urine volume is greater than 1 mL/kg/h.[83] The creatinine excretion rate may be used to verify an adequate urine collection where the majority of the children excrete 15–20 mg/kg/24 h.[18] Plasma levels of calcium, magnesium, phosphorus, creatinine, bicarbonate, and uric acid should be investigated. Lastly, intact parathyroid hormone (PTH) levels should be determined in children with hypercalciuria or hypophosphatemia.

If a 24-h urine collection cannot be obtained, random spot urine specimen measuring the solute to creatinine ratio can be used. But daily urine volume should be measured. The normal values of solute to creatinine ratio are given in Table 36.3.

Radiological imaging is an important part of the diagnostic evaluation of urolithiasis. Most of the calcium containing stones is radiopaque on plain films if the size is adequate. While struvite and cystine stones are less radiopaque than calcium stones,[5] uric acid and xanthine stones are radiolucent being diagnosed easily with ultrasonography and computed tomography (CT). Ultrasonography can diagnose all kind of stones with a false-negative rate of 30% where small papillary or calyceal stones along with ureteral calculi may

Table 36.2 Normal urinary values in school age children: 24-h urine collection[20]

Calcium	<4 mg/kg/day
Oxalate	<50 mg/1.73 mg^2/day
Cystine	<60 mg/1.73mg^2/day
Citrate	>400 mg/g creatinine
Uric acid	<0.56 mg/dL GFR
Volume	>20 mL/kg/day

Table 36.3 Normal urinary values in children[20]

	Age	mg/mg	mmol/mmol	mmol/mmol
Calcium/creatinine	0–6 months	<0.8	<2.24	
	6–12 months	<0.6	<1.68	
	2–18 years	<0.2	<0.56	
Oxalate/creatinine	<1 year	<0.3	<0.061	
	1–5 years	<0.15	<0.036	
	5–12 years	<0.1	<0.03	
	>12 years	<0.1	<0.013	
Cystine/creatinine	All ages	<0.02	<0.01	
Citrate/creatine	All ages	<0.51	*Male*	*Female*
	Infant		<1.9	<0.63
	Child		<0.27	<0.33
Magnesium	>2 years	0.12		
Uric acid	>3 years	<0.56 mg uric acid/dL of glomerular filtrate	<0.03 mmol uric acid/dL of glomerular filtrate	

GFR: (Urine uric acid × blood creatinine)/urine creatinine

be missed.[84,85] Additionally, ultrasonography can outline the presence of urinary obstruction or nephrocalcinosis. In a study evaluating the sensitivity for plain film, ultrasonography, and CT, these values were found to be 57%, 77%, and 100%, respectively.[86,87] CT has a high sensitivity and specificity (96–98%) and does not require any contrast.[20] Currently, for the prompt evaluation of acute renal colic, non contrast CT is the first imaging choice because of its high sensitivity for ureteral stones compared to other modalities.[88]

36.6 Treatment

36.6.1 Medical Treatment

Because of high recurrence rates of urolithiasis in children, a medical approach is an important part of the treatment regimen for urolithiasis (Table 36.4). For all kinds of stones, increased fluid intake is the main and essential part of the therapy. A high fluid intake prevents the supersaturation of the urine and reduces the concentration of the solutes. Again, the increased urinary flow helps to remove the crystals before they obstruct the renal tubulus. However, it is clear that maintenance of the daily urine output over 2 L for an adolescent is usually difficult for a long-term treatment period.

36.6.2 Hypercalciuria

High fluid intake and dietary sodium restriction are the initial steps for the management of hypercalciuria. Also excessive calcium intake should be restricted to that of the recommended daily allowance recommendations. Children should

avoid vitamin C and D supplementation and high protein intake. If the hypercalciuria cannot be well treated with dietary measures, thiazide diuretics may be added to the therapy. Thiazides mainly affect the renal tubulus by increasing the absorption of calcium. The effect of thiazide diuretics are increased when combined with salt restriction.[89,90] Common adverse effects of these drugs are hypokalemia and hyperlipidemia. Hypokalemia may cause decreased citrate excretion and potassium supplementation might be required if necessary. Citrate therapy is helpful in patients with hypocitrauria and hypercalciuria[91,92]. Lastly, amiloride may increase the distal tubular calcium reabsorption and may be useful with thiazide diuretics. Phosphate is another adjuvant therapy in cases with hypercalciuria.[6]

36.6.3 Hyperoxaluria

Initial therapy is similar to hypercalciuria with the recommendation of high fluid and low sodium intake. Additionally, avoidance of oxalate rich foods is essential. Citrate, magnesium, and phosphate supplements may also help to increase oxalate solubility. In case of an accompanying hypercalciuria, thiazides could be given. In primary hyperoxaluria Type 1, approximately 30% of patients respond to pyridoxine medication. Pyridoxine could be given at a dose of 25 mg/day initially and may be increased to 100 mg/day. Calcium intake should not be restricted, but excess calcium intake may be prohibited.

36.6.4 Uric Acid Lithiasis

A high urinary flow rate is essential for the management of hyperuricosuria. Limiting sodium intake may be useful by lowering the uric acid excretion. If these precautions fail, supplementation with citrate or bicarbonate will be indicated for alkalinization of the urine. In case of failure, allopurinol treatment may be necessary to decrease uric acid levels and that of excretion. Allopurinol decreases uric acid synthesis by inhibiting xanthine oxidase and is useful in disorders associated with excess uric acid production.

36.6.5 Cystinuria

For cystine stones, treatment aims to increase the urinary flow rate abundantly ($1.5 L/m^2$) and increase the urine pH above 7.5. Potassium citrate is the preferred choice for urinary alkalinization. The aim of the fluid therapy is keep the

Table 36.4 Selected medications used in the treatment of nephrolithiasis[20]

Chlorothiazide	<6 months: 10–40 mg/kg/day 1–2 doses 6–12 years: 10–20 mg/kg/day 2 doses >12 years: 500–2,000 mg/day in 1–2 doses
Hydrochlorothiazide	<6 months: 3.3 mg/kg/day 2 doses 6–12 years: 2–2.2 mg/kg/day 2 doses >12 years: 25–100 mg/day in 1–2 doses
Urinary alkalinization	Children: 2–3 mEq HCO3/kg/day 3–4 doses Adolescents: 30–60 mEq HCO_3 3–4 times daily
Alkalinizing agents	Potassium citrate: 2 mEq HCO_3/mL Sodium citrate/citric acid: 1 mEq HCO_3/mL Baking soda: 1 tsp = 42 mEq HCO_3 Sodium bicarbonate IV solution: 8.4%=1 mEq HCO_3/mL (given orally): 4.2%= 0.5 mEq HCO_3/mL

urinary cystine concentration less than 300 mg/dL. D-penicillamine and *a*-mercaptopropionyl glycine can be used as adjunctive therapies, if the first-line therapies fail.

36.7 Conclusions

The objective of stone management in children should be complete stone clearance, prevention of stone recurrence and regrowth, preservation of renal functions, control of UTI's, correction of anatomic abnormalities and correction of the underlying metabolic disorders. Long-term postoperative follow-up is mandatory; especially after using newer technical innovations for urinary calculus management during childhood. Regarding the management of stone forming children for metaphylaxis, there is a great choice of different treatment modalities, on which the clinicians have to decide about based on metabolic evaluation, stone analysis data, as well as the frequency of stone events.

Because of the multifactorial causes of stones in children (metabolic, anatomic and/or recurrent UTI), long-term follow-up treatment can only be successful when combined with appropriate prophylaxis to prevent recurrence. Numerous treatment regimens for preventing recurrent formation of calcium stones have been designed and published during recent decades. The patients can be treated conservatively by an increased fluid intake with or without dietary manipulations or by administering pharmacological agents. As a pharmacological agent, potassium citrate has been used with acceptable success rates.

However, it is really very troublesome to keep the child under a certain preventive measure for a long-period of time. Cooperative parents with children at older ages are the cases that may demonstrate acceptable successful outcomes following these measures.

References

1. Vahlensieck EW, Bach D, Hesse A. Incidence, prevalence and mortality of urolithiasis in the German Federal Republic. *Urol Res.* 1982;10:161–164.
2. Borghi L, Ferretti PP, Elia GF, et al. Epidemiological study of urinary tract Stones in a Northern Italian City. *Br J Urol.* 1990;65:231–235.
3. Tellaloğlu S, Ander H. Stones in children. *Turk J Pediatr.* 1984;26:51–60.
4. Edvardsson V, Elidottir H, Indridason O, Palsson R. High incidence of kidney stones in Icelandic children. *Pediatr Nephrol.* 2005;20:940–944.
5. Milliner DS, Murphy ME. Urolithiasis in pediatric patients. *Mayo Clin Proc.* 1993;68:241–245.
6. Stapleton FB, Roy S, Noe HN, Jerkins G. Hypercalciuria in children with hematuria. *N Engl J Med.* 1984;310:1345–1348.
7. Gearhart JP, Herzberg GZ, Jeffs RD. Childhood urolithiasis: experiences and advances. *Pediatrics.* 1991;87:445–450.
8. Stapleton FB, McKay CP, Noe HN. Urolithiasis inchildren: the role of hypercalciuria. *Pediatr Ann.* 1987;16:980–992.
9. Curhan GC, Willett WC, Speizer FE, et al. Twenty-four-hour urine chemistries of kidney stones among women and men. *Kidney Int.* 2001;59(6):2290–2298.
10. Khan SR, Glenton PA, Backov R, et al. Presence of lipids in urine, crystals and stones: implication for the formation of kidney stones. *Kidney Int.* 2002;62:2062–2072.
11. Pak CYC, Arnold LH. Heterogenous nucleation of calcium oxalate by seeds of monosodium urate. *Proc Soc Exp Biol Med.* 1975;149:930–932.
12. Fleisch H. Inhibitors and promoters of stone formation. *Kidney Int.* 1978;13:361–371.
13. Sarica K. Pediatric urolithiasis: etiology, specific pathogenesis and medical treatment. *Urol Res.* 2006;34:96–101.
14. Pak CYC. Potential etiologic role of brushite in the formation of calcium (renal) stones. *J Cryst Growth.* 1981;53:202–208.
15. Lingeman JE, Smith LH, Wood JR, et al. Basic considerations of urinary stone formation. In: Moster MB, ed. *Urinary calculi.* Philadelphia: Lea and Febiger; 1989:51–76.
16. Burdette DC, Thomas WC, Finlayson B. Urinary supersaturation with calcium oxalate before and during orthophosphate therapy. *J Urol.* 1976;115:418–422.
17. Pak CYC, Fuller C, Sakhaee K, et al. Long-term treatment of calcium nephrolithiasis with potassium citrate. *J Urol.* 1985;134:11–19.
18. Polinsky MS, Kaiser BA, Baluarte HJ. Urolithiasis in childhood. *Pediatr Clin North Am.* 1987;34:683–710.
19. Stapleton FB, Roy S, Noe HN. Hypercalciuria in children with hematuria. *N Engl J Med.* 1984;310:1345–1348.
20. Gillespie RS, Stapleton FB. Nephrolithiasis in children. *Pediatr Rev.* 2004;25(4):131–138.
21. Van Savage JG, Palanca LG, Andersen RD, et al. Treatment of distal ureteral stones in children: similarities to the American Urological Association guidelines in adults. *J Urol.* 2000;164:1089–1093.
22. Smith SL, Somers JM, Broderick N, Halliday K. The role of the plain radiograph and renal tract ultrasound in the management of children with renal tract calculi. *Clin Radiol.* 2000;55:708–710.
23. Tekin A, Tekgul S, Atsu N, et al. A study of the etiology of idiopathic calcium urolithiasis in children: hypocitruria is the most important factor. *J Urol.* 2000;164:162–165.
24. Nijman RJM, Ackaert K, Scholtmeijer RJ, et al. Long-term results of extracorporeal shock wave lithotripsy in children. *J Urol.* 1989;142:609–612.
25. Payne SR, Ford TF, Wickharnd EA. Endoscopic management of upper urinary stones. *Br J Surg.* 1985;72:822–825.
26. Smith LH. Stone activity. In: Roth RA, Finlayson B, eds. *Stones: Clinical Management of Urolithiasis.* Baltimore: Williams & Wilkins; 1983:183–185.
27. Vandeursen H, Devos P, Baert LUC. Electromagnetic extracorporeal shock wave lithotripsy in children. *J Urol.* 1991;145:1229–1232.
28. Sarkissian A, Baloyan A, Arikyants N, et al. Pediatric urolithiasis in Armenia: a study of 198 patients observed from 1991 to 1999. *Pediatr Nephrol.* 2001;16:728–732.
29. Milliner DS. Epidemiology of calcium oxalate urolithiasis in man. In: Kahn S, ed. *Calcium oxalate in Biological Systems.* Boca Raton: CRC Press; 1995:169–188.
30. Anderson DA. The nutritional significance of primary bladder stones. *Br J Urol.* 1962;34:160–163.
31. Ashworth M. Endemic bladder stones. *BMJ.* 1990;301:826–827.
32. Robertson WG. What is the aetiology of urinary calculi? *Pediatr Nephrol.* 1996;10:763.
33. Walther PC, Lamm D, Kaplan GW. Pediatric urolithiasis: a 10-year review. *Pediatrics.* 1980;65:1068–1072.

34. Lim DJ, Walker RD III, Ellsworth PI, et al. Treatment of pediatric urolithiasis between 1984 and 1994. *J Urol.* 1996;156: 702–705.

35. Choi H, Snyder HM, Duckett JW. Urolithiasis in childhood: current management. *J Pediatr Surg.* 1987;22:158–164.

36. Pietrow PK, Pope JC, Adams MC, et al. Clinical outcome of pediatric stone disease. *J Urol.* 2002;167:670–673.

37. Noe HN. Hypercalciuria and pediatric stone recurrences with and without structural abnormalities. *J Urol.* 2000;164: 1094–1096.

38. Faerber GJ. Pediatric urolithiasis. *Curr Opin Urol.* 2001;11: 385–389.

39. Turner MA, Goldwater D, David TJ. Oxalate and calcium excretion in cystic fibrosis. *Arch Dis Child.* 2000;83:244–247.

40. Sarica K. Medical aspect and minimal invasive treatment of urinary stones in children. *Arch Ital Urol Androl.* 2008;80(2):43–49. Review.

41. Erbagci A, Erbagci AB, Yilmaz M, et al. Pediatric urolithiasis – evaluation of risk factors in 95 children. *Scand J Urol Nephrol.* 2003;37(2):129–133.

42. DeSanto NG, DiLorico B, Capasso G, et al. Population based data on urinary excretion of calcium, oxalate, phosphate and uric acid in children from Cimitile. *Pediatr Nephrol.* 1992;6:149–157.

43. Hillman LS, Hoff N, Salmon S, et al. Mineral homeostasis in very premature infants: serial evaluation of serum 25 hydroxyvitamin D, serum minerals and bone mineralization. *J Pediatr.* 1985;106: 970–980.

44. Kruse K, Kracht U, Kruse U. Reference values for urinary calcium excretion and screening for hypercalciuria in children and adolescents. *Eur J Pediatr.* 1984;143:25–31.

45. Moore ES. Hypercalciuria in children. *Contrib Nephrol.* 1981;27: 20–32.

46. Stapleton FB, Noe HN, Jenkins GR, et al. Urinary excretion of calcium following an oral calcium loading test in healthy children. *Pediatrics.* 1982;69:594–597.

47. Hymes LC, Warshaw BL. Idiopathic hypercalciuria: renal and absorptive subtypes in children. *Am J Dis Child.* 1984;138: 176–180.

48. Pak CYC, Kaplan R, Bone H, et al. A single test for the diagnosis of absorptive, resorptive, and renal hypercalciuria. *N Engl J Med.* 1975;292:497–500.

49. Favus MJ, Karnauskas AJ, Parks JH, et al. Peripheral blood monocyte vitamin D receptor levels are elevated in patients with idiopathic hypercalciuria. *J Clin Endocrinol Metab.* 2004;89(10): 4937–4943.

50. Mehes K, Szelid Z. Autosomal dominant inheritance of hypercalciuria. *Eur J Pediatr.* 1980;133:239–242.

51. Coe FL, Parks JH, Moore ES. Familial idiopathic hypercalciuria. *N Engl J Med.* 1979;300:337–340.

52. Vachvanichsanong P, Malagon M, Moore ES. Urinary tract infection in children associated with idiopathic hypercalciuria. *Scand J Urol Nephrol.* 2001;35:112–116.

53. Stapleton FB. Idiopathic hypercalciuria: association with isolated hematuria and risk for urolithiasis in children. *Kidney Int.* 1990;37: 807–811.

54. Garcia CD, Miller LA, Stapleton FB. Natural history of hematuria associated with hypercalciuria in children. *Am J Dis Child.* 1991; 145:1204–1207.

55. Polito C, La Manna A, Cioce F, et al. Clinical presentation and natural course of idiopathic hypercalciuria in children. *Pediatr Nephrol.* 2000;15:211–214.

56. Stapleton FB. Idiopathic hypercalciuria. Association with isolated hematuria and risk for urolithiasis in children. The Southwest Pediatric Nephrology Study Group. *Kidney Int.* 1990;37: 807–811.

57. Devuyst O, Christie PT, Courtoy PJ, et al. Intra-renal and subcellular distribution of the human chloride channel, CLC-5, reveals a pathophysiological basis for Dent's disease. *Hum Mol Genet.* 1999;8:247–257.

58. Dent CE, Friedman M. Hypercalciuric rickets associated with renal tubular damage. *Arch Dis Child.* 1964;39:240–249.

59. Scheinman SJ. X-linked hypercalciuric nephrolithiasis: clinical syndromes and chloride channel mutations. *Kidney Int.* 1998; 53:3–17.

60. Neuhaus TJ, Belzer T, Blau N, et al. Urinary oxalate excretion in urolithiasis and nephrocalcinosis. *Arch Dis Child.* 2000;82(4): 322–326.

61. Hesse A, Schneeberger W, Engfeld S, et al. Intestinal hyperabsorption of oxalate in calcium oxalate stone formers: application of a new test with ($^{13}C_2$) oxalate. *J Am Soc Nephrol.* 1999;10: 329–333.

62. Monico CG, Ford GC, Persson XMT, et al. Potential mechanisms of marked hyperoxaluria not due to primary hyperoxaluria I or II. *Kidney Int.* 2002;62:392–400.

63. Danpure CJ. Primary hyperoxaluria. In: Schriver CR, Beaudet AL, Sly WS, et al., eds. *The metabolic and molecular bases of inherited disease.* 8th ed. New York: McGraw-Hill; 2001:3323–3367.

64. Giafi CF, Rumsby G. Primary hyperoxaluria type 2: enzymology. *J Nephrol.* 1998;11:29–31.

65. Cramer SD, Ferree PM, Lin K, et al. The gene encoding hydroxypyruvate reductase (GRHPR) is mutated in patients with primary hyperoxaluria type II. *Hum Mol Genet.* 1999;8: 2063–2069.

66. Thomas S, Stapleton FB. Pediatric urolithiasis: diagnosis and management. In: Gonzales E, Bauer SB, eds. *Pediatric Urology Practice.* Philadelphia: Lippincott-Raven; 1999: 607–621.

67. Milliner DS, Eickholt JT, Bergstralh E, et al. Primary hyperoxaluria: results of long-term treatment with orthophosphate and pyridoxine. *N Engl J Med.* 1994;331:1553–1558.

68. Toussaint C. Pyridoxine-responsive PHI: treatment. *J Nephrol.* 1998;11:49–50.

69. Stapleton FB. Childhood stones. *Endocrinol Metab Clin N Am.* 2002;31:1001–15.

70. Rosenberg LE, Durant JL, Holland JM. Intestinal absorption and renal extraction of cystine and cysteine in cystinuria. *N Engl J Med.* 1965;273:1239–1245.

71. Purroy J, Bisceglia L, Calonge MJ, et al. Genomic structure and organization of the human rBAT gene (SLC3A1). *Genomics.* 1996;37:249–252.

72. Chesney RW. Mutational analysis of patients with cystinuria detected by a genetic screening network: powerful tools in understanding the several forms of the disorder. *Kidney Int.* 1998;54:279–280.

73. Feliubadalo L, Font M, Purroy J, et al. Non-type I cystinuria caused by mutations in SLC7A9, encoding a subunit (bo, + AT) of rBAT. *Nat Genet.* 1999;23(1):52–57.

74. Rutchik SD, Resnick MI. Cystine calculi. Diagnosis and management. *Urol Clin N Am.* 1997;24:163–171.

75. Dent CE, Senor B. Studies on the treatment of cystinuria. *Br J Urol.* 1955;27:317–332.

76. Milliner DS. Urolithiasis. In: Avner ED, Harmon WE, Niaudet P, eds. *Pediatric nephrology.* Philadelphia: Lippincott Williams & Wilkins; 2004:1091–1101.

77. Stapleton FB. Hematuria associated with hypercalciuria and hyperuricosuria: a practical approach. *Pediatr Nephrol.* 1994;8: 756–761.

78. Baldree LA, Stapleton FD. Uric acid metabolism in children. *Pediatr Clin North Am.* 1990;2:391–418.

79. Benjamin D, Sperling O, Weinberger A. Familial hypouricemia due to isolated renal tubular defect. *Nephron.* 1977;18:220–225.

80. Stapleton FB. Renal clearance of uric acid in human neonates. *J Pediatr.* 1984;14:337–339.

81. Kelley WN. Gout and other disorders of purine metabolism. In: *Harrison's Principles of Internal Medicine.* 9th ed. New York: McGraw-Hill; 1980:483.

82. Lingeman JE, Smith LH, Wood JR, et al. Medical evaluation and treatment of the stone patient. In: Moster MB, ed. *Urinary calculi.* Philadelphia: Lea and Febiger; 1989:133.

83. Greene ML, Fujimoto WY, Seegmiller JE. Urinary xanthine stones: a rare complication of allopurinol therapy. *N Engl J Med.* 1969;280:426–427.

84. Diament MJ, Malekzadeh M. Ultrasound and the diagnosis of renal and ureteral calculi. *J Pediatr.* 1986;109:980–983.

85. Vrtiska TJ, Hattery RR, King BF, et al. Role of ultrasound in medical management of patients with renal stone disease. *Urol Radiol.* 1992;14:131–138.

86. Nimkin K, Lebowitz RL, Share JC, et al. Urolithiasis in a children's hospital: 1985–1990. *Urol Radiol.* 1992;14:139–143.

87. Mendelson RM, Arnold-Reed DE, Kuan M, et al. Renal colic: a prospective evaluation of non-enhanced spiral CT versus intravenous pyelography. *Aust Radiol.* 2003;47(1):22–28.

88. Smergel E, Greenberg SB, Crisci KL, et al. CT urograms in pediatric patients with ureteral calculi: do adult criteria work? *Pediatr Radiol.* 2001;31:720–723.

89. Stapleton FB, Kroovand RL. Stones in childhood. In: Coe FL, Favres MJ, Pak CYC, Parks JH, Preminger GM, eds. *Kidney Stones: Medical and Surgical Management.* Philadelphia: Lippencott-Raven; 1996:1065–1080.

90. Cohen TD, Ehreth J, King LR, Preminger GM. Pediatric urolithiasis: medical and surgical management. *Urology.* 1996;47(3):292–305.

91. Gillespie RS, Stapleton FB. Nephrolithiasis in children. *Pediatr Rev.* 2004;25(4):131–139.

92. Lande MB, Varade W, Erkan E, et al. Role of urinary supersaturation in the evaluation of children with urolithiasis. *Pediatr Nephrol.* 2005;20:491–494.

Ben Thomas and David Tolley

Abstract Since the introduction of minimally invasive techniques such as extracorporeal shock wave lithotripsy (ESWL), percutaneous nephrolithotomy (PCNL), and ureteroscopy (URS) in the early 1980s, the management of renal and ureteral stones in adults has changed dramatically. Introduction of these techniques in the management of stones in children has been slow. However, experience in the last decade or so has clearly demonstrated that these minimally invasive techniques are equally effective in the pediatric population.

37.1 Introduction

Up until the mid-1980s, surgery for urinary stones in both children and adults was almost exclusively by open techniques. The only real exception was cystolitholopaxy for small stones in the bladder. Progress with extracorporeal shock wave lithotripsy (ESWL), percutaneous nephrolithotomy (PCNL), and ureteroscopy in the adult population generated interest in their application within pediatric stone management. This evolution is elegantly highlighted in a paper from 1987 in which Choi, Snyder, and Duckett reviewed a series of 62 children treated for stone disease at the Children's Hospital of Philadelphia between 1972 and 1984, of which 43 required surgery. All stones were removed by an open surgical procedure except for three cystolitholopaxies. At the time, the authors concluded that even in those early days, 60% of the cases would have been suitable for the newer, less invasive methods. Such changes have meant that open surgery for stones has become almost obsolete.[1]

37.2 Extracorporeal Shock Wave Lithotripsy

Extracorporeal shockwave lithotripsy (ESWL) was first used to treat urinary lithiasis in adults in the early 1980s,[2] and it was not long before use of ESWL was described in children.[3]

The first commercially available lithotripter, the Dornier HM3, was only recommended by the manufacturers for treating patients greater than 135 cm in height. Further limitations of the original machine were the need for general anesthesia for the majority of treatments and that only stones visible with fluoroscopy could be treated. However, several authors reported the successful treatment of children less than 135 cm tall, by making modifications to the patient gantry, and adjusting the water level.[4,5]

The introduction of second-generation lithotripters, which did not require a water bath and included improved imaging with ultrasound, further facilitated the treatment of stone disease in children. Van Horn et al., compared their experience with a Dornier HM3 machine and the second-generation Siemens Lithostar® machine. Stone-free rates were comparable between the two machines (65% for HM3 and 71% for Lithostar). However, 67% of treatments on the HM3 were performed under general anesthesia (GA), whereas only 14% of children treated on the Lithostar required GA, with the rest receiving intravenous sedation.[6]

There is general agreement that the ureter in children, whilst smaller in diameter, is more efficient at transporting stone fragments than in adults. Early series suggested that larger stones could be cleared in children without excessive numbers of treatments or risk of complications, such as ureteric obstruction from steinstrasse. Thornhill et al., treated 22 children between 2 and 13 years of age, with stones ranging from 3 to 50 mm. A stone-free rate of 79% was achieved, with only two children (9%) encountering complications.[7] The authors surmise that a child's ureter is more capable of clearing fragments, a view also shared by Jayanathi et al.[8] This was formally assessed by Gofrit et al., who directly

D. Tolley (✉)
Department of Urology, Western General Hospital,
Scottish Lithotripter Centre, Edinburgh, UK
e-mail: datolley@tiscali.co.uk

P.N. Rao et al. (eds.), *Urinary Tract Stone Disease*,
DOI 10.1007/978-1-84800-362-0_37, © Springer-Verlag London Limited 2011

compared stone passage in children against a matched group of stones treated in adults.[9] The stone-free rate was higher (95% for children versus 79% for adults) and the stone-free state was achieved more rapidly in the children. None of the children developed steinstrasse, whereas this complication was seen in 5% of adults. There are two possible reasons for the better results in children: there is less attenuation of the shock wave as it is propagated more efficiently through the smaller body volume of the child, and the ureter is also more efficient at clearing stone fragments.

Elsobky compared 148 children treated on two second-generation lithotripters, the Dornier MFL 5000 spark-gap machine and the Toshiba Echolith piezoelectric machine.[10] Overall 51% of children were treated under general anesthesia, and all of these were aged less than 12. The stone-free rates between the two machines were similar (85% for MFL 500 and 87% for Echolith) but the retreatment rate on the piezoelectric machine was significantly higher (55% for MFL 5000 and 80% for Echolith). The only significant predictor of stone-free rate was the diameter of the stone, with those <10 mm having significantly better stone-free rates than those >10 mm in diameter.

Piezoelectric machines can generate the highest peak pressures, but their power is lower due to the small volumes of the focal zone (F2). Thus, these machines are perceived to be less painful. Hence, Marberger et al. demonstrated that it was possible to treat all but the youngest children (younger than 3 years) without anesthesia.[11] The indication for anesthesia was mainly due to issues of cooperation rather than because of pain. At 3 months, 96% of children were stone free, with a retreatment rate of 40%.

Longo and Netto treated 70 children between 3 and 14 years of age (mean 8) using a Siemens Lithostar or Lithostar Plus machine, and none required general anesthesia.[12] Intravenous sedation was utilized in 72.9% of cases, whilst 27.1% required no anesthesia. Overall success rate was 98.5% of patients rendered stone free, with a 29.4% retreatment rate. This series also demonstrated the intuitive observation that larger stones require more treatments.

In adults, treatment of larger and staghorn calculi is generally considered less effective due to the requirement for multiple treatments and higher complication rates. However, in children the improved efficiency of ESWL described previously has prompted some centers to treat larger and more complex stones with ESWL. Orsola et al., treated 15 children with staghorn calculi on a Siemens Lithostar-ULTRA machine.[13] After an average of two treatments, 73.3% were rendered stone free, and there were no cases of ureteric obstruction, but one case of fever. All treatments were performed without general anesthesia.

Lottmann et al., reported a series of 23 children treated with ESWL for complete or partial staghorn calculi.[14] All procedures were performed under a general anesthetic and achieved an overall stone-free rate of 82.6%. Further subdivision of the treatment groups by age found that in children 2 and under, the stone-free rate was 87.5% compared to 71.4% in children aged 6–11 years. The older children also required more treatment sessions. Only one case of ureteric obstruction was seen in an older child from a single obstructing fragment. Over a followup period ranging from 9 months to 9 years, no cases of hypertension were observed, and DMSA renography did not reveal any evidence of scarring. The poorest results were seen in those children with cystine stones, and thus the authors do not advocate ESWL for larger stones in this subgroup.

The largest single series of pediatric ESWL has been reported by Muslumanoglu et al.[15] They treated 408 calculi in 344 children, aged between 6 months and 14 years, in the same center. General anesthesia was used in 38.4% of cases, primarily for children under 3 years of age, whilst 40.1% were treated with intravenous sedation, and 21.5% required no anesthesia. The mean number of treatment sessions was 1.9 per stone and the stone-free rate was 79.9% at 3 months. Retreatment was required in 53.9% of cases. Stone size and location were the most significant factors for predicting outcome. All renal pelvis stones less than 1 cm, and stones in the proximal and mid-ureter were cleared. The least favorable results were seen in stones larger than 2 cm in any location, and stones in the calyces. Steinstrasse developed in 7.8% of children, all with initial stones larger than 1 cm; all were successfully treated with either in situ ESWL or managed conservatively. A similar overall stone-free rate was demonstrated in 78.3% of 225 unselected stones treated by Chamssuddin et al., and stone size predicted the need for multiple treatments.[16]

In our own center, 140 renal stones in children were treated with ESWL. The first 102 were treated with a Piezolith 2300 machine, and the remainder with a Compact Delta lithotripter. To enable treatment, 91% of children under 6 years of age required general anesthesia, compared with only 34% of those aged over 6 years. In agreement with other series, stone size was the most important determinant of the stone-free rate as well as predicting the need for multiple treatments and ancillary procedures. Overall, the stone-free rate for non-staghorn stones less than 20 mm was 84%, which dropped to 54% for non-staghorn stones larger than 20 mm. For partial or complete staghorn stones, the overall stone-free rate was 40%, with 45% of children requiring an ancillary procedure. There were six cases of steinstrasse after ESWL for complex stones, of which four required intervention (three ureteroscopy [URS] and one ESWL). Hence, for stones greater than 20 mm and staghorn stones, our practice is to perform PCNL in such cases, as our experience is that fewer treatment sessions are required and hence, fewer general anesthetic sessions.[17]

Since many children treated with ESWL are still growing, there has been concern about the effects of ESWL on the developing kidney. Early in vivo study suggested that, in rats,

ESWL led to decreased renal function and histological changes in the kidney.[18] Lifshitz et al., followed 29 children after ESWL for a mean of 9 years, and found that there was a trend towards reduced renal growth in the treated kidneys.[19] One case of hypertension was detected. However, the authors consider that the observed changes were due to abnormalities with the kidneys themselves, which led to the formation of calculi, rather than the ESWL. Subsequently, followup of 39 children treated with ESWL found no cases of hypertension or renal parenchymal scarring, as evidenced by DMSA scanning, after a range of 6 months to 8 years.[20]

Villanyi et al., examined the short-term effects of ESWL on the pediatric kidney.[21] In 16 children between the ages of 6 and 14, the authors measured a variety of enzymes and electrolytes in the urine up to 90 days after a session of shock wave treatment. Whilst there was no deterioration in renal function as evidenced by changes in electrolytes, excretion of various surrogate markers of renal damage, such as β(beta)2-microglobulin, rose transiently before returning to baseline levels by 7 days. This resulted in the recommendation that an interval of at least 15 days should be left between two successive ESWL treatments. However, as yet there is no significant evidence to suggest that ESWL in the prepubertal population has any significant long-term detrimental effects.

37.3 Percutaneous Nephrolithotomy

Following its original description in adults in 1976,[22] interest in pediatric PCNL led to the publication, in mid-1980s, of the first case-series utilizing the technique in children.[23,24] Inevitably, these early series were mainly performed on older children, as the instruments used were still relatively large, but they demonstrated the feasibility of the technique in the pediatric population. Boddy et al., described their first percutaneous procedures on ten children between 5 and 16 years of age.[4] In 6 children the stone was lifted out intact and no nephrostomy tube was left at the end of the procedure. Ultrasound was used to fragment the stones in the other four cases, two of which required a two-stage procedure during the same hospital admission. In these four cases, a 24 Fr nephrostomy tube was placed postoperatively. After one procedure, the stone-free rate was 80%, and stone-free status was achieved in 90% in one hospital admission. The only significant complication was intraoperative bleeding requiring termination of the case and a second look procedure was performed. However, a blood transfusion was not required.

The technique of PCNL is relatively standard and similar to the technique used in adults. The majority of authors perform an initial cystoscopy in order to place a retrograde ureteric catheter, which is subsequently utilized to opacify the renal pelvis and calyces with contrast when required.

Following cystoscopy the patient is then turned to the prone position for the remainder of the procedure. Radio-opaque contrast is then injected, via the ureteric catheter, to both opacify and distend the renal pelvis and calyces. This contrast can be mixed with methylene blue to allow simple identification of entry into the collecting system. A needle is then advanced under fluoroscopic guidance into the calyx of choice. Confirmation of entry into the collecting system is by aspiration of the blue-colored contrast mixture. An alternative method of obtaining needle access to the collecting system is with the aid of ultrasound. Both Desai et al., and Boormans et al., use this method as their standard access technique.[25,26] Ultrasound can also be particularly useful in situations where the anatomy of the lower urinary tract makes placement of a retrograde catheter difficult or impossible, such as ileal conduit or continent urinary diversion where urethral access no longer exists.

Having confirmed antegrade access to the required calyx, a guidewire is then passed through the needle and into the collecting system. The needle can then be removed and replaced by an access catheter to allow better manipulation of the wire. Ideally, the wire should be placed past the stone and down the ipsilateral ureter into the bladder to provide track stability. Once the wire is correctly positioned, the track can be dilated. This can be achieved using a series of graduated dilators, which may be metal (Alken dilators) or semirigid (Amplatz dilators), or alternatively dilation can be performed using a pressurized balloon dilator.

Most pediatric endourologists and radiologists seem to prefer either of the graduated dilator systems, although Khairy Salem et al., described the successful use of balloon dilation in 45% of their series of 20 PCNL in children between 4 and 15 years.[27] The aim of the study was to assess whether tubeless PCNL was feasible in children. However, they found no adverse outcomes from using balloon dilators compared to the metal dilators used in the other 55%. It has been suggested by Turna et al., that balloon dilation is associated with less hemorrhage than dilators.[28] In 193 patients, aged between 5 and 74, undergoing PCNL they retrospectively extrapolated risk factors for hemorrhage, and found significantly less bleeding where balloon dilation had been deployed. Although the series included patients as young as 5, there was no separate subgroup analysis of the pediatric patients.

Following dilation of the track, a sheath is placed to maintain the track and permit access by the nephroscope, which can then be inserted and withdrawn on multiple occasions if required. The size of the sheath depends on the size of the nephroscope being used and should be kept to a minimum depending on the equipment available. A wide variety of sheath sizes is available ranging from 12 up to 34 Fr, as well as differing lengths. Generally, the size of the sheath and nephroscope is tailored to the size of the patient and the stone, although the diameter of the access calyx may also influence the decision. Earlier series simply avoided treating the youngest patients percutaneously because only adult-sized instruments were available,[4,24] although there was no good evidence for this practice. However, as smaller instruments were developed, the use of such instruments on smaller children gained popularity. Although for most surgeons use of smaller instruments in younger patients was instinctive, Gunes et al., provided some basis for this practice.[29] In 25 PCNL operations, age range 27 months to 16 years, a 24 or 26 Fr nephroscope was utilized through a 24–30 Fr sheath. Complications were described in 40% (10/25) of cases, and as 71% of these complications occurred in children under 7 years of age, the authors concluded that adult equipment should not be used in the under 7s. Similarly, Desai et al., and Zeren et al., also found that one of the factors that significantly affected hemorrhage and transfusion rates was sheath size, but age of the patient was not a determining factor in Zeren's series.[26,30]

Others now routinely advocate use of smaller tracks and instruments in younger children,[31–33] whereas Boormans uses 18 Fg sheath in all pediatric patients up to 16.8 years.[25] However, in our own series of 43 PCNL, we routinely used a 24 Fr sheath and a 22 Fr nephroscope on all patients (range 1–15 years), without any increased complication rate in the younger children.[17] These findings were confirmed by Badawy who treated children as young as 3 with 26 Fr sheath and Khairy Salem who used a 24 Fr sheath in children as young as 4; neither series reported higher complications in the younger patients.[27,34]

Commonly only one track is needed or used in the majority of cases,[25,27,29,33,35] but in the treatment of larger and more complex calculi, more than one track may be required. Desai et al., and Ozden et al., report the use of multiple tracks in 60% and 40% respectively for the management of complex calculi.[26,32] Neither series reports any increased adverse effect on renal function compared to series where only one track is predominantly used.

For complex and staghorn calculi, use of supracostal punctures can give an extra dimension to improve access to the calyces and the upper ureter. The use of supracostal punctures has been well proven in adult practice; however, due to the slightly increased complication rate their use has been limited in children.[36] El-Nahas et al., have reviewed their series of 20 supracostal punctures and compared them with 40 similar subcostal punctures.[37] There were no significant differences in complication rates or hospital stay between the two groups, and the stone-free rates were equally comparable. Thus, if used judiciously in appropriate cases, supracostal puncture can be a useful adjunct to aid clearance of complex stones.

After inspection of the collecting system with the nephroscope, a variety of instruments can be used for removal and fragmentation of stones. Simple graspers and hybrid basket devices are available for lifting out small stones or stone fragments. If fragmentation is required, ultrasound[4,17,25,27,34] and ballistic lithotripsy[29,31] or a combination of both[30,32,35] are the most commonly deployed modalities. Devices are available that include active suction of fragments out of the collecting system, and one such device combines all three elements of ultrasound, ballistic lithotripsy, and suction. Although earlier series included electrohydraulic lithotripsy,[38,39] this is no longer used due to higher complication rates observed. Use of a flexible cystoscope down the sheath can improve access to all calyces, and this can be combined with the holmium laser for fragmentation and a basket to extract or manipulate the stone.

It is still usual to leave a nephrostomy tube draining the kidney after percutaneous surgery[17,25,26,29–35,38,39] in children, although in adult practice tubeless PCNL is gaining popularity. Following the early series of Boddy et al., where no nephrostomy was placed in 6/10 cases after a simple lift out procedure, without any reported adverse effects,[4] Khairy Salem et al., recently reported a study of tubeless PCNL.[27] In this nonrandomized trial, 20 PCNL were performed on children between 4 and 15 years, with a mean stone burden of 2.3 cm (range 2–5 cm). A nephrostomy tube was not placed, but a ureteric catheter was inserted for 24–48 h postoperatively. These cases were compared against ten similar cases where a nephrostomy was inserted. Postoperative complication rates were similar, with fever in 25% of tubeless cases versus 30% of nephrostomy cases. Perirenal hematoma was reported in 10% in both groups. Although the authors found that the mean postoperative pain scores were lower in the tubeless group compared to those with a nephrostomy (4.6 versus 5.5), the potential benefit of a tubeless procedure in children is less clear than in adults.

Overall success rates for PCNL, as gauged by stone-free rates, range from 58% to 96% after one treatment, rising to 81–100% after additional treatment, by second PCNL or ESWL.[4,17,25–27,29–35,38,39] Most pediatric urologists only consider cases that are truly stone free to be a success, since children have a longer future period in which to develop recurrence.

Given that PCNL in children is a relatively uncommon procedure, series are very heterogeneous and not always directly comparable due to the varied case mix. In some, stone burdens are measured as the maximal transverse diameter, whilst others describe the area of stone, calculated by measuring the "height" and the "width" of the stone and multiplying the two together. As a result, preoperative stone burdens are similarly very variable and difficult to compare.

In their series of complex calculi, Ozden et al., used multiple tracts in 40% of cases for larger or staghorn calculi.[32] After one PCNL, 73.6% of patients were stone free, and this rose to 86.8% after a second procedure – either PCNL or ESWL. Clearance rates were similar in cases with one tract and those with multiple tracts. However, the stone-free rate was influenced by the preoperative stone burden. Where the stone was less than 675 mm² the clearance rate was 97.4%, but this fell to 66.7% for stones larger than 675 mm².

Serious complications of PCNL are rare. Intraoperative bleeding can obscure vision and may necessitate cessation of the operation, placement of a nephrostomy tube, and a "second look" procedure at a later time. In some earlier series, troublesome bleeding resulted in conversion to an open operation in a very small number of cases.[30,34] However, with experience it is now widely held that this is unnecessary. In their pioneering series Boddy et al., encountered problematic bleeding in only 1 case, which was managed with a nephrostomy and "second look."[4] Reported transfusion rates after PCNL vary from 0%[4,17,27,38,39] to 23.9%.[30] In this latter series, most of the transfused cases occurred early in their experience and the authors observe that refinements of their operative technique reduced this complication. Further analysis of the transfused cases showed that the risk of transfusion was significantly correlated to operating time, sheath size, and stone burden, but the age of the patient was not an associated risk. Ozden et al., report a 17% transfusion rate in their recent series of "complex" stones.[32] Hemoglobin drop was significantly associated with the size and number of tracks used, whilst the transfusion rate was correlated with the initial stone burden. Desai et al., similarly showed that hemoglobin drop was significantly associated with the size and number of tracks, although the transfusion rate was not correlated.[26] These authors also observe that the hemoglobin decrease was greater during the earlier part of the learning curve.

Transient fever after PCNL is common and reported in up to 43% of cases[33]; in the vast majority of cases, it is associated with negative cultures and resolves without antimicrobial therapy. Septicemia and septic shock is fortunately much less common, although the rate of proven urinary tract infection has been reported in as many as 12% of cases.[29] Choong et al., reported that 23% of cases developed fevers higher than 38°C, which were treated with broad-spectrum intravenous antibiotics, but it is not clear whether any of these had positive cultures.[38]

Other complications are generally rare, and those described include renal pelvis perforation in 1/72,[35] 3/43,[17] and 3/25.[29] In two series, extravasation occurred in 5.6%[32] and 4%[29] of cases. Hydropneumothorax occurred in one case in each of the reports from Gunes et al., and Ozden et al.,[29,32] and one case of a pyeloo-colonic fistula was reported by Badawy et al.[34] The relatively infrequent use of upper pole punctures in the pediatric population explains the low occurrence of thoracic complications.

In the longer term, PCNL does not appear to have any significant deleterious effects on the kidney. Boddy et al., found none of their cases showed evidence of reduced renal growth or scarring, assessed by intravenous urography, during followup of 3 months to 5 years.[4] Dawaba et al.,

specifically examined the longer term effects of PCNL with followup ranging from 6 to 72 months.[35] Out of 72 PCNLs (age range 9 months–16 years), only 4 patients (5.6%) showed an immediate postoperative drop in glomerular filtration rate, 3 of which subsequently improved during followup, and the fourth remained static. Using DMSA renography, no evidence of renal scarring was demonstrated in any patient. Similarly, in their series of PCNL in patients under 5, Mahmud et al., found no decrease in renal function, no evidence of renal scarring, and no effect on blood pressure in any of the 30 children, over a median follow-up of 24.9 months.[31]

37.4 Ureteroscopy

The technique of ureteroscopy in children adheres to basic principles of upper tract endoscopy. Initial retrograde placement of a guidewire into the renal pelvis under fluoroscopic control, to act as a safety wire, is the essential first step. Differing methods of obtaining access to the bladder are described. The initial cystoscopy and wire placement can either be through a pediatric cystoscope[40–42] or directly through the ureteroscope.[17,43] A floppy-tip guidewire is used, and placed under fluoroscopy, ensuring that screening time is kept to a minimum. Guidewire diameters range from 0.018 to 0.035 in., with the choice of size largely determined by the preference of the surgeon. If difficulty in negotiating past the stone is encountered during the insertion of a standard PTFE (Teflon) coated guidewire, then softer hydrophilic coated wires, such as Sensor® or Terumo®, can prove very useful in passing the stone. However, once the upper tract is accessed, such a wire may be exchanged for a stiffer working wire, through an appropriate open-ended ureteric catheter. Having placed a wire to the renal pelvis, the ureteroscope can then be introduced, either over the wire[17] or alongside the wire.[40–42,44,45] The decision to dilate the ureteric orifice again largely rests with individual preference, since the risk of ureteric reflux is low and transient. Some authors report performing dilatation routinely,[8,41,43,44] whilst others will only dilate if it is not possible to pass the ureteroscope.[17,39,40,46,47] Van Savage describes the use of a second guidewire to negotiate the ureteric orifice if difficulty is encountered, and has not found the need to perform dilation.[42]

Just as there is variation in opinion regarding the need to dilate, the method of dilation is also variable. Balloon dilation is the favored option of some groups,[40,41,44,47] whilst others opt for a coaxial dilation technique.[8,17,39,43,46] Herndon et al., have challenged the need for any dilation and in their retrospective series of 34 ureteroscopies found that with routine use of a 4.5 or 6.5 Fr tapered semirigid ureteroscope, dilation was not required in any child.[45] Their reported complication rates are comparable to any other series.

A variety of different caliber ureteroscopes is available, depending on the manufacturer, and individual preference will usually dictate which instrument is utilized. Inevitably, older series tended to describe the use of larger ureteroscopes, with the more recently developed smaller scopes now being preferred. A balance exists between keeping the instrument small enough to access the ureter with the minimum of trauma, without making the working and irrigation channels so small that their usefulness is limited. As many series take several years to accrue, and given the fragility of these instruments, most authors report the use of a variety of ureteroscopes over the course of their experience. Currently, semirigid ureteroscopes of around 7 Fr (6.5–7.2 Fr) are the most commonly used.[17,39,43,46,47] Van Savage and latterly Heardon both report favorable results with the 4.5 Fr "needle scope," which allows utilization of either ballistic lithotripsy and or lasertripsy.[42,45]

Where flexible ureteroscopy is used, most authors favor an instrument between 6.9 and 7.5 Fr.[41,43,46,47] Similarly, the type of intracorporeal lithotripsy utilized tends to vary depending on the date of publication. Earlier series tend to describe use of electrohydraulic lithotripsy, lithoclast, and the pulsed dye laser,[40,48–50] whereas authors now tend to favor the holmium laser.[6,17,43,45–47]

The use of postoperative stents is variable. Absolute indications for stent insertion, such as ureteric trauma or perforation, are recognized by all. However, the routine use of ureteric drainage is more debated. Schuster advocates the use of a stent if the duration of the procedure is longer than 90 min.[41] In early series, when the techniques were still relatively new to pediatric practice, most authors were more cautious and would thus leave some form of ureteric drainage for all cases.[8,48–50] Temporary drainage of the ureter can also be achieved by either the placement of a straight ureteric catheter, which is brought out through the external urethral meatus and removed after 24–48 h, or by placement of a formal double pigtail ureteric stent. Initially, removal of such stents would necessitate a second general anesthetic, however, exteriorizing the string or "danglers" through the external urethral meatus will usually permit removal of the stent without the need for full anesthesia. Even in more contemporary reports many authors still advocate use of ureteric drainage in the majority of cases (85–91%).[43,46,47] However, as in adult practice, others have challenged this view. Herndon et al., (6/27) and Raza et al., (11/52) only used ureteric drainage in 21% of cases, and neither series reported a higher rate of complications than others who routinely drain the ureter.[17,45]

Overall, ureteroscopy for the treatment of ureteric stones in children has a high success rate. After one treatment, stone-free rates range between 72% and 100%.[6,8,17,39–50] Not all authors analyze the reasons for failure, but the type of intracorporeal lithotripsy used, position of the stone, and anatomical factors are all implicated as affecting outcome.

Stone sizes that are tackled by ureteroscopy range from 2 to 23 mm, but no authors report a correlation between stone size and success. Since the numbers in many series are small, it is difficult to draw meaningful conclusions regarding factors influencing stone-free rates. Al-Bussaidy et al., showed that the position of the stone affected the stone-free rate.[48] In their series of 50, overall stone-free rate after one treatment was 84%, which rose to 94% after a second treatment. When the position of the stone was analyzed, the overall stone-free rates were 78%, 100%, and 97%, for upper, mid, and lower ureteric stones, respectively. Influence of the type of lithotripsy on stone-free rate has been highlighted by both Bassiri and Raza. In Bassiri's series of 66 cases they achieved a stone-free rate of 88% after one treatment. In six out of the eight cases that failed, proximal migration of the stone whilst deploying the ballistic lithoclast was identified as the primary reason for failure.[40] Raza et al., also reported an effect of lithotripsy method on the stone-free rates. In 52 cases, the stone-free rates after one treatment were 72% where the pulsed-dye laser was used, 92% for electrohydraulic lithotripsy, and 100% for holmium laser.[17] The mean stone sizes were similar in all groups.

Other miscellaneous failures of ureteroscopy at the first attempt include failure to pass the ureteroscope despite dilation, either due to a tight or anatomically abnormal ureter, such as after a ureteric reimplantation. Perforation of the ureter with either a guidewire or the ureteroscope may occur, particularly at the site of an impacted stone, and should trigger abandonment of the procedure accompanied by drainage of the kidney by either retrograde placement of a stent or antegrade insertion of a percutaneous nephrostomy. Failure to render the patient stone free at the first sitting can be addressed by either a repeat attempt at retrograde ureteroscopy, which may be facilitated by prior placement of a ureteric stent at the primary procedure, or percutaneous access to allow antegrade ureteroscopy if the distal ureteric anatomy precludes retrograde instrumentation. ESWL is also a very useful adjunct procedure to aid stone clearance.

Complications of ureteroscopy are relatively uncommon, but the most serious are pyleonephritis and ureteric perforation. Complication rates are reported between 0% and 30%; however, detail of the description of complications is somewhat variable. Al-bussaidy reported the highest level of complications, but reported in the most detail, including children who had hematuria (10%), pain (4%), and pyrexia (12%). Bassiri reported hematuria in 17% of children, but only 1.5% experienced pain,[48] whilst Raza et al., describe pyrexia in 9% of cases.[17] Many other authors do not actually report on such complications. Pyelonephritis is reported in 0–4% of cases.[40,41,47] Perforation rates vary between 0% and 7%.[17,42,45,48] Causes of perforation may be easily apparent, such as impacted stone or secondary to use of a basket.[42,45] When analyzed by type of lithotripsy deployed, electrohydraulic lithotripsy (EHL) has the highest complication rate. Al-bussaidy reported two perforations in their series, which utilized EHL in the majority of cases.[48] Raza et al., similarly confirmed EHL to have the most complications.[17] Where EHL had been used, perforation occurred in one patient, and five children experienced fever, compared to one perforation and one ureteric stricture when the pulsed-dye laser was utilized and no complications in the holmium laser treated cases. Al-bussaidy also reported pyrexia in six patients in their mainly EHL-treated patients.[48] However, when holmium laser fragmentation is performed, complication rates are lowest.[17,43,46,47] No perforations related to use of the holmium laser itself have been reported.

Following the initial descriptions, there were concerns about potential damage to urethra, ureter, and the vesicoureteric junction (VUJ). In early series, dilatation of the ureteric meatus was commonly performed, particularly where larger (11.5 Fg) instruments were utilized. Due to the relatively infrequent occurrence of pediatric ureteroscopy, even large centers can take several years to accrue a meaningful sized series. Hence, a historical perspective is inbuilt, allowing comparison of older instrumentation and techniques with the more modern. Thomas et al., performed dilation of the ureteric orifice in all five children they ureteroscoped with an 11.5 Fr instrument,[51] but subsequently, when instruments of 8.5 Fr or smaller were used, only 3 of 11 children required dilation. However, even where dilation of the VUJ was performed the incidence of reflux is low, and where it does occur, is usually transient. In Thomas's series, a followup cystogram was performed in nine children (64%), and only one case of reflux was detected. Although this was grade III, the reflux resolved within 12 months.[51] Similar findings of transient reflux were reported by Schuster et al., who used voiding cystourethrography to examine for reflux in the first 11 children in their series. Of seven cases that had undergone balloon dilation to 15 Fg, two children were found to have grade I reflux, which resolved within 1 month. These authors still routinely dilate the ureteric meatus, as they believe it facilitates smooth passage of the ureteroscope.[41] However, they advocate that routine assessment for postoperative reflux is not necessary, and should only be reserved for children who are symptomatic, a view that is shared by others.[17,46]

Other authors have not routinely evaluated for reflux. Jayanathi et al., reported 11 successful ureteroscopies, with almost all cases undergoing balloon dilation of the VUJ. There was no incidence of infection in any child postoperatively, and thus, the authors postulate that even if reflux occurs, it is of no significance.[8]

Experience of flexible ureteroscopy for treating proximal ureteric and renal stones in children is very limited. Tanaka et al., describe their use of flexible ureteroscopy as initial treatment in 52 cases of children under 14 years of age (range 1.2–13.6) with a mean stone diameter of 8 mm (range 1–16).[47]

Over half of the cases required prior placement of a ureteric stent, of which 58% were felt necessary to dilate the ureter. The initial stone-free rate was 50%, which increased to 58% with extended followup. Additional procedures were required in 34.6% of cases, of which the majority were repeat ureteroscopy. The need for additional procedures increased with the size of the stone at presentation.

37.5 Conclusions

The full endourological armamentarium is now available for the treatment of stone disease in children. Due to the relative rarity of pediatric stone disease, and the heterogeneity of the presenting stones and treatment techniques, direct comparison of many studies is not possible. However, some simple underlying principles can be applied. Careful assessment of each stone, together with an assessment of the anatomy of the drainage system of the affected kidney, should enable an informed decision regarding treatment selection. Clearly, the key aim should be to obtain stone clearance with the minimum of treatment episodes and the minimum of complications.

ESWL remains the most appropriate first-line treatment method for many children with stones, but larger stones, staghorn calculi, and stones associated with abnormal anatomy will often necessitate use of other minimally invasive techniques.

When PCNL is undertaken, the smallest possible track and instruments should be used and the track should be dilated with coaxial dilators. Children will tolerate the placement of nephrostomy tube, and current evidence suggests that this should be routine.

Pediatric ureteroscopy, if required, should similarly be performed with the smallest available instruments and meticulous attention to technique. The holmium laser should be the intracorporeal lithotripsy method of choice, and placement of a ureteric stent is not routinely required, as the child's ureter is highly efficient at facilitating the passage of stone fragments. At the current time, there is very limited evidence to support the use of flexible ureteroscopy in the pediatric population.

References

1. Choi H, Snyder HM III, Duckett JW. Urolithiasis in childhood: current management. *J Pediatr Surg*. 1987;22:158–164.
2. Chaussy C, Brendel W, Schmiedt E. Extracorporeally induced destruction of kidney stones by shock waves. *Lancet*. 1980; 2:1265–1268.
3. Newman DM, Coury T, Lingeman JE, et al. Extracorporeal shock wave lithotripsy in children. *J Urol*. 1986;136:238–240.

4. Boddy SM, Kellett MJ, Fletcher MS, et al. Extracorporeal shock wave lithotripsy and percutaneous nephrolithotomy in children. *J Pediatr Surg.* 1987;22:223–227.

5. Kramolowsky EV, Willoughby BL, Loening SA. Extracorporeal shock wave lithotripsy in children. *J Urol.* 1987;137:939–941.

6. Van Horn AC, Hollander JB, Kass EJ. First and second generation lithotripsy in children: Results comparison and follow-up. *J Urol.* 1995;153:1969–1971.

7. Thornhill JA, Moran K, Mooney EE, et al. Extracorporeal shock-wave lithotripsy monotherapy for paediatric urinary tract calculi. *Br J Urol.* 1990;65:638–640.

8. Jayanathi VR, Arnold PM, Koff SA. Strategies for managing upper tract calculi in young children. *J Urol.* 1999;162:1234–1237.

9. Gofrit ON, Pode D, Meretyk S, et al. Is the paediatric ureter as efficient as the adult ureter in transporting fragments following extracorporeal shock wave lithotripsy for renal calculi larger than 10 mm. *J Urol.* 2001;166:1862–1864.

10. Elsobky E, Sheir KZ, Madbouly K, Mokhtar AA. Extracorporeal shock wave lithotripsy in children: experience using two second-generation lithotripters. *BJU Int.* 2000;86:851–856.

11. Marberger M, Turk C, Steinkogler I. Piezoelectric extracorporeal lithotripsy in children. *J Urol.* 1989;142:349–352.

12. Longo JA, Netto Jnr NR. Extracorporeal shockwave lithotripsy in children. *Urology.* 1995;46:550–552.

13. Orsola A, Diaz I, Caffaratti J, et al. Staghorn calculi in children: monotherapy extracorporeal shockwave lithotripsy. *J Urol.* 1999;162:1229–1233.

14. Lottmann HB, Traxer O, Archambaud F, Mercier-Paygeyral B. Monotherapy extracorporeal shockwave lithotripsy for the treatment of staghorn calculi in children. *J Urol.* 2001;165:2324–2327.

15. Muslumanoglu AY, Tefekli A, Sarilar O, et al. Extracorporeal shock wave lithotripsy as first line treatment alternative for urinary tract stones in children: a large scale retrospective analysis. *J Urol.* 2003;170:2405–2408.

16. Chamssuddin A, Khalili A, Roumani J. Monotherapy extracorporeal shockwave lithotripsy for the treatment of different size stones in children. *Eur Urol.* 2003;Suppl 2(No 1):11, number 35.

17. Raza A, Smith G, Moussa S, Tolley D. Ureteroscopy in the management of pediatric urinary tract calculi. *J Endourol.* 2005;19:151–158.

18. Claro Jde A, Denardi F, Ferreira U, et al. Effects of extracorporeal shockwave lithotripsy on renal growth and function: an animal model. *J Endourol.* 1994;8:191–194.

19. Lifshitz DA, Lingeman JE, Zafar FS, et al. Alterations in predicted growth rates of pediatric kidneys treated with extracorporeal shock-wave lithotripsy. *J Endourol.* 1998;12:469–475.

20. Traxer O, Lottmann H, Archambaud F, et al. Extracorporeal lithotripsy in children. Study of its efficacy and evaluation of renal parenchymal damage by DMSA-Tc 99m scintigraphy: a series of 39 children. *Arch Pediatr.* 1999;6:251–258.

21. Villanyi KK, Szekely JG, Farkas LM, et al. Short-term changes in renal function after extracorporeal shock wave lithotripsy in children. *J Urol.* 2001;166:222–224.

22. Fernstrom I, Johannson B. Percutaneous pyelolithotomy. A new extraction technique. *Scand J Urol Nephrol.* 1976;10:257–259.

23. Hulbert JC, Reddy PK, Gonzalez R, et al. Percutaneous Nephrostolithotomy: an alternative approach to the management of paediatric calculus disease. *Pediatrics.* 1985;76:610–612.

24. Woodside JR, Stevens GF, Stark GL, et al. Percutaneous stone removal in children. *J Urol.* 1985;134:1166–1167.

25. Boormans JL, Scheepe JR, Verkoelen CF, Verhagen PCMS. Percutaneous nephrolithotomy for treating renal calculi in children. *BJU Int.* 2005;95:631–634.

26. Desai MR, Kukreja RA, Patel SN, Bapat SD. Percutaneous nephrolithotomy for complex pediatric renal calculus disease. *J Endourol.* 2004;18:23–27.

27. Khairy Salem H, Morsi HA, Omran A, Daw MA. Tubeless percutaneous nephrolithotomy in children. *J Pediatr Urol.* 2007;3:235–238.

28. Turna B, Nazli O, Demiryoguran S, et al. Percutaneous nephrolithotomy: variables that influence hemorrhage. *Urology.* 2007;69:603–607.

29. Gunes A, Ugras MY, Yilmaz U, et al. Percutaneous nephrolithotomy for pediatric stone disease. *Scan J Urol Nephrol.* 2003;37:477–481.

30. Zeren S, Satar N, Bayazit Y, et al. Percutaneous nephrolithotomy in the management of pediatric renal calculi. *J Endourol.* 2002;16:75–78.

31. Mahmud M, Zaidi Z. Percutaneous nephrolithotomy in children before school age: experience of a Pakistani centre. *BJU Int.* 2004;94:1352–1354.

32. Ozden E, Sahin A, Tan B, et al. Percutaneous renal surgery in children with complex stones. *J Pediatr Urol.* 2008;4:295–298.

33. Samad L, Aquil S, Zaidi Z. Paediatric percutaneous nephrolithotomy: setting new frontiers. *BJU Int.* 2006;97:359–363.

34. Badawy H, Salama A, Eissa M, et al. Percutaneous management of renal calculi: experience with percutaneous nephrolithotomy in 60 children. *J Urol.* 1999;162:1710–1713.

35. Dawaba MS, Shokeir AA, Hafez AT, et al. Percutaneous nephrolithotomy in children: early and late anatomical and functional results. *J Urol.* 2004;172:1078–1081.

36. Munver R, Delvecchio FC, Newman GE, Preminger GM. Critical analysis of supracostal access for percutaneous renal surgery. *J Urol.* 2001;166:1242–1246.

37. El-Nahas AR, Shokeir AA, El-Kenawy MR, et al. Safety and efficacy of supracostal percutaneous nephrolithotomy in paediatric patients. *J Urol.* 2008;180:676–680.

38. Choong S, Whitfield H, Duffy P, et al. The management of paediatric urolithiasis. *BJU Int.* 2000;86:857–860.

39. Kurzrock EA, Huffman JL, Hardy BE, Fugelso P. Endoscopic treatment of pediatric urolithiasis. *J Pediatr Surg.* 1996;31:1413–1416.

40. Bassiri A, Ahnadnia H, Darabi MR, Yonessi M. Transureteral lithotripsy in pediatric practice. *J Endourol.* 2002;16:257–260.

41. Schuster TG, Russell KY, Bloom DA, et al. Ureteroscopy for the treatment of urolithiasis in children. *J Urol.* 2002;167:1813–1816.

42. Van Savage JG, Palanca LG, Andersen RD, et al. Treatment of distal ureteral stones in children: similarities to the American Urological Association guidelines in adults. *J Urol.* 2000;164:1089–1093.

43. Sofer M, Binyamini J, Ekstein PM, et al. Holmium laser ureteroscopic treatment of various pathologic features in pediatrics. *Urology.* 2007;69:566–569.

44. Dogan H, Tekgul S, Akdogan B, et al. Use of the holmium: YAG laser for ureterolithotripsy in children. *BJU Int.* 2004;94:131–133.

45. Herndon CEA, Viamonte L, Joseph DB. Ureteroscopy in children: is there a need for ureteral dilation and postoperative stenting? *J Pediatr Urol.* 2006;2:290–293.

46. Minevich E, Rousseau MB, Wacksman J, et al. Pediatric ureteroscopy: technique and preliminary results. *J Pediatr Surg.* 1997;32:571–574.

47. Tan AHH, Al-Omar M, Denstedt JD, Razvi H. Ureteroscopy in pediatric urolithiasis: an evolving first-line therapy. *Urology.* 2005;65:153–156.

48. Al Busaidy SS, Prem AR, Medhat M. Pediatric ureteroscopy for ureteric calculi: a 4-year experience. *Br J Urol.* 1997;80:797–801.

49. Minevich E, Defoor W, Reddy P, et al. Ureteroscopy is safe and effective in prepubertal children. *J Urol.* 2005;174:276–279.

50. Scarpa RM, De Lisa A, Porru D, et al. Ureterolithotripsy in children. *Urology.* 1995;46:859–862.

51. Tanaka ST, Makari JH, Pope JC IV, et al. Pediatric ureteroscopic management of intrarenal calculi. *J Urol.* 2008;180:2150–2154.

Indications for Surgical Removal, Including Asymptomatic Stones

38

J. Graham Young and Francis X. Keeley

Abstract The advent of minimally invasive methods of treating renal calculi has widened the indications for treatment beyond those stones causing significant pain, urinary tract infection, or obstruction. Despite the low morbidity of minimally invasive treatments, we must continue to balance risks and benefits of treatment versus conservative management in individual patients. For each patient there will be considerations relating to their age, occupation, comorbidity, stone history, and anatomy amongst many factors that will shape the most appropriate clinical treatment of their stone. We attempt to help rationalize these decisions and examine the knowledge we have in particular of the natural history of asymptomatic renal calculi, whose treatment remains most controversial.

38.1 Preoperative Evaluation

Before embarking on extracorporeal shock wave lithotripsy (SWL) or surgical treatment of calculi, a thorough preoperative evaluation of the patient must be performed. Patient occupation is relevant, as professions such as airline pilots may be required to be completely stone free before resuming duties. Women planning pregnancy may influence treatment of asymptomatic stones if they look likely to progress. A general medical history with attention to comorbidity and concomitant medication is clearly required, particularly with increasing use of anticoagulant medication such as warfarin, clopidogrel, and aspirin. Discussion should clearly take place with the patient to ensure understanding of the risks, benefits, and limitations of the various treatment modalities to ensure informed consent.

Body habitus should be noted and blood pressure checked, in particular before SWL to reduce risk of hematoma formation.[1] High quality imaging to evaluate stone burden, location, and variations in anatomy are necessary. Most commonly, this is now in the form of unenhanced computed tomography (CT), although plain X-ray, renography and contrast studies may give additional necessary information. Urine dipstick testing plus microscopy and culture is mandatory before treatment. Previous stone composition from the patient is also extremely important. Cystine, calcium oxalate monohydrate, and calcium hydrogen phosphate dihydrate (brushite) stones are all notoriously resistant to fragmentation with SWL. Such stones are likely to require invasive procedures with fragmentation with higher energy sources such as holmium laser. Furthermore, if such stones are of a borderline large size, preference may be given toward a percutaneous procedure rather than SWL.

Clinical suspicion of cystinuria presenting de novo may be raised in younger patients with multiple recurrent stones. Imaging features suggestive of cystine include low radio density, a ground-glass appearance with smooth edges, and the presence of multiple or bilateral stones. Cystine crystals should be present on urinalysis, a necessary screening instrument before treatment decision.

Many stones may also contain bacteria within a biofilm environment even when bacteriuria is only intermittently present. The fragmentation of stones may release bacterial endotoxins as well as viable bacteria that place the patient at risk for septic complications.[2] Therefore, patients who have clinical features of urine infection or struvite stones should receive appropriate antibiotics before surgery to reduce the risk of sepsis. They may benefit from fairly prolonged preoperative treatment, such as 1 week of a quinolone before percutaneous nephrolithotomy (PCNL).[3]

J.G. Young (✉)
Department of Minimally Invasive, Surgery and Stone Disease,
University Hospital of South Manchester, Manchester, UK
e-mail: grahamy31@yahoo.co.uk

P.N. Rao et al. (eds.), *Urinary Tract Stone Disease*,
DOI 10.1007/978-1-84800-362-0_38, © Springer-Verlag London Limited 2011

38.1.1 Indications for Treatment of Stones

When considering how we arrive at the current treatment consensus in our medical specialty, we should bear in mind historical factors. This is all the more so when the evidence base does not clearly point to a particular answer. Before the advent of endourological and minimally invasive methods of treating stones, the only options for treatment were conservative or open surgical methods. Due to the latter's significant morbidity, there was a natural reluctance in particular to treat incidental, or essentially asymptomatic calyceal calculi.

In the modern age, there remain clear indicators for surgical treatment whether a stone is large or small and independent of its location in the kidney or ureter. These consist of persistent pain, urinary tract infection, nonprogression of a ureteric calculus, and obstruction to urine drainage without spontaneous passage of a stone. However, with less invasive treatments, with lower morbidity and faster recovery, we can now rationally consider treatment of patients with mild symptoms. We can also consider treatment of asymptomatic calculi on the basis of possible reduction of risk of progression of their stone disease. Such calculi are increasingly found either in isolation or in the presence of symptomatic calculi, due to the increasing use of CT.[4]

38.1.2 Asymptomatic Stones and Treatment

There is conflicting evidence of the natural history of calyceal stones from a number of small-scale studies. Hübner et al., studied 63 patients for an average 7.4 years.[5] Of 80 stones studied, 38% remained unchanged, 16% passed spontaneously, and 40% required surgical intervention. During the 7.4 years of follow-up, 45% of the stones increased in size, 68% of the patients experienced symptoms suggestive of urinary tract infection, and 51% of the patients experienced pain. Eight of the patients developed staghorn calculi during follow-up. They concluded that conservatively treated calyceal stones are likely to increase in size, resulting in further pain or infection. Furthermore, the likelihood of spontaneous stone passage decreased over the long term, as did the risk of developing complications. Overall, it was felt that 83% of all calyceal stones required intervention within 5 years of diagnosis.

Glowacki[6] reviewed 107 patients with asymptomatic calyceal stones and found that the cumulative 5-year probability of a symptomatic event occurring was 48.5%, half of these events requiring active intervention. There was also an association between the development of symptoms and the number of previous stones, as well as the number of asymptomatic stones at presentation.

In a smaller, more recent study,[7] Inci et al., reported 24 patients who were followed up for an average of 4.4 years with CT scanning, ultrasound, as well as clinical evaluation. Progression in stone size was demonstrated in 9 of 27 renal units (33.3%) with 2 (11.1%) requiring intervention. There was no need for intervention during the first 2 years of follow-up. Three stones passed spontaneously without any symptoms. Pain developed in three patients during follow-up, and two of them passed a stone and responded to the analgesics without further treatment. Their conclusion was that observation was safe, provided that there was adequate supervision during follow-up. This study provides another example of the difficulty in comparing CT versus plain X-ray data, in that some stones seen on CT are not apparent on plain X-rays. This may provide a lead-time bias in that stones are smaller and therefore have a more benign natural history.

Further data is available indirectly from the study of so-called clinically insignificant residual fragments (CIRFs) – fragments of less than 4 mm following SWL in particular. The term remains controversial, as persisting fragments might be important risk factors for stone growth and recurrence. Osman et al.,[8] evaluated 173 patients who had been treated by SWL and discharged with CIRF. Mean follow-up was 4.9 years. Seventy-eight percent of the patients were recurrent stone formers with more than two stone episodes. In 78.6%, CIRF cleared spontaneously within a few weeks and did not recur within 5 years. However, residual stones led to stone recurrence and need of retreatment in 21.4%. There was no difference in stone growth between different locations in the kidney, with 23% of renal pelvis CIRF growing compared with 26.5% in lower pole calyces, and 27% and 26% respectively in middle and upper pole calyces. The authors concluded that whilst most CIRF pass spontaneously, one-fifth of the patients developed new stones at the side of residual fragments, thus it was clear that close follow-up is required. Given the data on stone-free rates following SWL as judged by CT scans, however, one might justifiably conclude that the stone recurrences in this study were, in fact, growth of fragments that never cleared but were too small to be seen on plain X-rays.

In one of the few prospective, randomized, controlled studies in urolithiasis, the results of conservative treatment versus SWL were compared for small, asymptomatic calyceal stones.[9] Two hundred twenty-eight patients with <15 mm total diameter asymptomatic calyceal stones were randomized to SWL or observation. In a mean 2.2 years of follow-up, there was no statistically significant difference in stone-free rates, noninvasive interventions, quality of life, renal function, or symptoms between the two groups, but ten patients in the observation group required invasive procedures, compared with none in the SWL group. There was also a trend towards higher stone-free rates in the treatment group, although this did not reach statistical significance. The main conclusion of this trial was unfortunately that longer follow-up was likely to be required to identify significant differences between the groups.

There is thus, no consensus on the safety of observation for asymptomatic renal calculi, but it seems likely that larger stones at least require very careful follow-up if not early intervention, whilst very small fragments present little hazard to the majority of patients. In a world of increasing scrutiny of health economics, it is not justified to spend resources in extended close follow-up of such patients. Many stones will clearly fall between these two scenarios and the clinical decision may best be guided by patient and physician preference.

38.1.3 Asymptomatic Stones: Staghorn Calculi

The presentation of patients with staghorn calculi may vary from no symptoms up to a devastating presentation with urosepsis or renal failure. Whilst a poorly defined term, it is generally agreed that these are calculi filling a major part of a renal collecting system, usually occupying the renal pelvis and one or more calyces. Most staghorn calculi consist of struvite.[10] As with small asymptomatic calyceal stones, it had been thought by some that they could be left untreated. However, Blandy and Singh[11] compared 60 patients having untreated staghorn stones with 125 staghorn stone patients who underwent operative removal. The 10-year mortality for untreated staghorn stone patients was 28% versus 7.2%, for patients having their stones removed by open surgery. Similar results were obtained by a great number of other authors including Koga,[12] Teichmann,[13] and Rous.[14] In separate studies, they examined more than 400 patients with follow-up in each of almost 8 years. Patients in nonsurgical groups suffered both higher renal failure and morbidity and mortality rates. The evidence became overwhelming for intervention, although it should be noted that none of the studies were randomized controlled trials.

The American Urological Association (AUA) Report on the Management of Staghorn Calculi, recommends percutaneous nephrolithotomy as the first-line treatment for staghorn calculi.[15] Open stone surgery is now rarely performed for reasons later discussed.

38.2 Treatment Options

Debate continues on the optimum treatment for different stone sizes and locations. Present options for treatment of renal and ureteric stones remain shock wave lithotripsy (SWL), percutaneous nephrolithotomy (PCNL), rigid and flexible ureterorenoscopy (URS), and laparoscopic stone surgery. Combinations of each may also be utilized, in particular the "sandwich technique" of alternating SWL with PCNL for the treatment of staghorn calculi. Open stone surgery (OSS) was demonstrated to have greater intraoperative and postoperative complication rates than percutaneous nephrolithotomy in a recent randomized prospective trial of 79 patients.[16] Major complications including bleeding requiring blood transfusion, and pleural, vascular, or ureteral injuries were reported in over 37% of patients with OSS. Similar stone-free rates and faster discharge and recovery were reported with PCNL. Given appropriate access to, and skills with the aforementioned techniques, OSS is rarely required for stone management. Furthermore, OSS has declined to the extent that operative experience of OSS is becoming increasingly rare and complications may therefore become more likely.

38.2.1 Extracorporeal Shock Wave Lithotripsy

In many centers, SWL has effectively become the first-line treatment for the great majority of renal and indeed ureteric stones. This is due to its very low morbidity, high acceptability to patients and physicians, and the fact that general anesthesia is usually not required with modern lithotriptors. In addition, there is increased access to lithotriptors due to capital cost reduction, in association with relatively generous payment under most health care systems.

In our algorithm of how to treat an individual stone, the first question is therefore "Are the stone and patient suitable for SWL?" Assuming the patient is suitable (for absolute and relative contraindications to SWL see Table 38.1), the three principles for successful SWL are: (1) ability to transmit the shock wave to the patient's stone, (2) the shock wave to act upon a breakable stone of a reasonable size, and (3) for the anatomy and physiology of the pelvicalyceal system, ureter, and indeed bladder to be such that fragments can spontaneously pass.

Table 38.1 Contraindications to SWL

Absolute	Relative
Pregnancy	Distal stones in young women
Uncontrolled coagulopathy	Aneurysms
Uncontrolled hypertension	Abnormal renal anatomy (ectopia, acute infundibulo-pelvic angles)
Distal obstruction	
	Ureteric anatomy (e.g., PUJ obstruction)
Untreated urinary tract infection	
	Cystine
	Mental abnormality/poor compliance
	Obesity
	Spinal abnormalities

For the majority of renal calculi and ureteric calculi not overlying the sacrum these criteria are indeed met.[17,18] Failures, however, may occur in the following circumstances.

38.2.1.1 Failure to Transmit Sufficient Energy to the Stone

The shock waves generated by different lithotripter machines clearly vary and this has been demonstrated to have significant effects on the success of SWL, in terms of fragmentation, stone-free rates, and retreatment rates.[19] The relatively large focal zone, overall power of the machine, and the efficiency of shock wave propagation using a full water bath rather than gel cushion appears to confer great advantage on the original Dornier HM-3 spark gap lithotripter. The ultrasound gel used for third-generation lithotriptors may be an overlooked factor in the lower success rates.[20]

In addition, failure to adequately transmit the shock wave to the target may be experienced in obese patients both by attenuation and inability to focus the shock wave. Power settings may need to be increased to uncomfortable levels to allow any chance of efficacy. Furthermore, those patients with morbid obesity may be simply too heavy for the SWL table.

Stones overlying bone may be in the acoustic shadow of the shock wave, or may make SWL painful and therefore poorly tolerated. Finally, stones that are non- or poorly radio-opaque cannot be adequately treated unless the lithotriptor has ultrasound capability and can be targeted effectively.

38.2.1.2 Large Stone Size

It is intuitive that SWL is not an appropriate treatment for particularly large stones, as the energy required to fragment the stone would require an unreasonably large number of treatments. Furthermore, the volume and size of fragments produced may well exceed the capacity of the ureter to pass them, resulting in steinstrasse. This risk is approximately 5% with renal stones smaller than 10 mm, 15% for 10–20 mm stones, and 25% for stones greater than 20 mm. For ureteric stones, steinstrasse rates were around 3% for stones less than 10 mm and 10% for stones 10–20 mm.[21] Whilst prophylactic stenting reduces the incidence of steinstrasse, it is clearly invasive and may reduce the spontaneous passage of fragments.[22] Since Grasso's 1995 review[23] of SWL failure in 121 patients, showing stones greater than 22 mm were associated with SWL failure, this has generally been the "cutoff" accepted by urologists for renal pelvis and upper/mid pole calyceal stones. Since the Lower Pole I randomized trial publication,[24] for lower pole stones the cutoff has generally been 10 mm, although not because of the risk of complications but rather because of the low reported success rate. One should still consider SWL to be a reasonable option for lower pole stones between 11 and 20 mm in size, but other options, especially PCNL, become more attractive.

38.2.1.3 Failure of Stone Fragmentation and Passage of Fragments

Grasso's paper also noted the association of SWL failure with stones composed of calcium oxalate monohydrate and brushite, where energy required to fragment the crystal structure is greater than can be produced and transmitted. The poor results of SWL on cystine stones are well established.[25]

Anatomy, particularly of the lower pole infundibulopelvic angle, infundibular length and width has been shown to be relevant to success; a smaller number of lower pole minor calyces, obtuse infundibulopelvic angles, short infundibular length and wide-necked infundibula being clearly favorable to the passage of fragments.[26–28] Once stone fragments have passed into the ureter, an unobstructed peristalsing ureter is needed to propel fragments into the bladder before eventual excretion. Clearly any condition affecting the ureter (e.g., pelviureteric junction obstruction or ureteric stricture) or the bladder (such as bladder outflow obstruction or neuropathic bladder) will have a negative impact on success.

The great variety of factors affecting the success of SWL for ureteric and renal stones has led several groups to develop nomograms to help predict the success of SWL. Kanao et al., have recently attempted to develop a predictive nomogram for stone-free status at 3 months following single session of SWL using stone size, location, and number.[29] Gomha et al., showed site, length, and width of the stone and the presence of a ureteral stent were the only significant predictors of success of SWL therapy for ureteric stones.[30] A similar group has also drawn up a further nomogram for renal stones.[31]

38.2.1.4 The Success Rates of SWL

The EAU/AUA Ureteral Stones Clinical Guidelines Panel analyzed all available studies, the vast majority of which were single-center case series. They found that following in-situ SWL monotherapy, median stone-free rates for stones less than 1 cm in diameter were 86% and 82% in the distal and proximal ureter, respectively.[32] One must keep in mind, however, that results of SWL for ureteric stones from randomized, prospective studies, as summarized by a recent Cochrane review, were between 51% and 100%.[33] Thus, reporting bias appears to play a major role in the SWL literature.

Success rates for renal calculi vary considerably, based on the definition of success. Traditionally, a plain abdominal X-ray was used to assess outcomes and many authors defined success to include residual fragments up to 4 mm in size, the so-called clinically insignificant residual fragments (CIRF) discussed previously. This is clearly not an adequate endpoint of "success", particularly for recurrent stone formers where fragments may act as nuclei for further stone growth. For example, the results of fixed and mobile lithotriptors audited from the south-west region of England showed stone-free rates were disappointingly low (16.7–26.7%); however, the results improved when fragments of <4 mm were included as "successful", giving an overall success rate of 45.9–66.7%.[34] Another clear example of the discrepancy between SWL outcomes as reported by single centers compared with randomized controlled trials (RCTs) is the Lower Pole Study Group publications. When plain X-rays were used to assess success, SWL had an overall stone-free rates of only around 37%, compared with 95% for percutaneous surgery.[24] Furthermore, when CT scans were used to assess outcomes for the treatment of small lower pole stones, the stone-free rate following SWL dropped further to 25%.

It is not absolutely known why the results of treatment of lower pole stones with SWL are poorer than those stones in middle and upper pole calyces. It is clearly suspected and there is strong circumstantial evidence that, just as with horseshoe kidneys, drainage from the lower pole is relatively impaired compared with other calyces. Interestingly, in support of the idea that gravity-dependent areas of the kidney lead to reduced expulsion of SWL fragments, there is some evidence that percussion, diuresis, and inversion (PDI) therapy may be beneficial in increasing clearance of lower pole fragments,[35] including randomized controlled studies.[36,37] Perhaps disappointingly it has not gained widespread use.

Elbahnasy et al., examined various anatomical factors relating to the lower pole and found that based on a pretreatment IVU, infundibulopelvic angle 90° or greater, infundibular length less than 3 cm and width greater than 5 mm all correlated with an improved stone-free rate after SWL.[38] In a prospective trial, Sampaio and associates found that 72% of patients became stone free after SWL when the infundibulopelvic angle was greater than 90°, but only 23% of patients were stone free when the angle was less than 90°.[39] There have been many other mainly retrospective studies investigating the influence of lower pole anatomy on stone clearance. Keeley et al.,[26] reported on 116 patients with lower pole stones between 11 and 20 mm who underwent SWL. An obtuse infundibulopelvic angle, lack of calyceal distortion, and a large infundibular diameter were all associated with a stone-free status, but the infundibulopelvic angle was the only factor to attain statistical significance in predicting stone-free status. The Lower Pole I Study failed to show an influence of lower pole anatomy on success rates.[24] In summary, many anatomical factors may play a role in the relatively poor clearance of stones from the lower pole. No consensus has been reached, however, in using these factors to predict outcomes.

38.2.2 Flexible and Rigid Ureterorenoscopy

Whilst originally developed for use in the ureter, the advent of fully deflectable ureterorenoscopes together with holmium laser fragmentation has increased their indications in stone treatment to include renal calculi, including many lower pole calculi. Relative contraindications to ureterorenoscopy (URS) include difficult ureteric access, abnormal ureteric anatomy, in particular strictures, or a convoluted ureter. Relative indications include obesity, as the ureteroscopic approach to the renal collecting system is not greatly affected by the presence of adipose tissue. Ureterorenoscopy may be the preferred treatment for morbidly obese patients when the stone burden is not excessively large.[40] Ureterorenoscopy is also the preferred treatment modality in anticoagulated patients, particularly those for whom anticoagulation cannot be safely temporarily discontinued. Grasso and Chalik reported that even when patients' coagulopathies were not fully corrected, stones could be successfully treated with no increase in complications from bleeding.[41]

Clearly, for the great majority of patients with ureteric stones of less than 5 mm spontaneous passage of stone is the expected natural history of acute ureteric colic.[42,43] For the minority of stones that require intervention, the remaining options comprise SWL or ureteroscopy. The recently updated AUA/EAU guidelines[32] from 2007 reviewed the published literature, which suggested that stone-free rates are somewhat superior with ureteroscopy for all sizes of stone and for all positions in the ureter apart from proximal ureteric stones under 10 mm. Ureteroscopy has a slight advantage over SWL at removing stones less than 10 mm in diameter; it eliminates stones in 93% of patients versus 86% with SWL. URS removes 87% of stones larger than 10 mm, whereas SWL removes 67%. The data on which these recommendations relied were generally, however, of poor quality, with many retrospective series included and few randomized clinical trials. They did, however, suggest the relative ascendancy of ureteroscopy in ureteric stone management, compared with the former guidelines published in 1997.[44]

A recent Cochrane review[33] included higher quality prospective multicenter studies. It concluded that stone-free rates were lower in patients treated with SWL than those treated with ureteroscopy. Furthermore, these rates were usually measured at a generous interval of up to 3 months. Thus, those patients treated unsuccessfully with SWL may have a long wait before receiving definitive treatment or passing stone fragments. Retreatment rates were also lower in the ureteroscopy group. The rate of complications and length of hospital stay were, however, higher in the ureteroscopy group. The great majority of complications were minor, such as hematuria. The specific and major complications of ureteroscopy essentially revolve around significant ureteric trauma, either manifesting as peri-operative ureteric avulsion, perforation, or late stricture formation.

Studies considered in this analysis did include techniques and equipment that might now be considered obsolete: ureteroscopes up to 11.5 Fr diameter and stone fragmentation with electrohydraulic, pneumatic, and ultrasound probes. More modern semirigid ureteroscopes, such as the Gyrus ACMI Bagley™, measure only 6.9 Fr. This reduced diameter significantly improves success rates and reduces perioperative ureteric trauma, likely leading to lower complication rates.[45]

For work in the upper ureter, these series commonly included only rigid ureteroscopy; by contrast, current practice is often to use a smaller diameter flexible ureteroscope. The now widespread use of the holmium/YAG laser enables safer fragmentation of stones compared with older electrohydraulic and pneumatic technologies. Furthermore, laser fragmentation frequently obviates the need for basket extraction. This further reduces the risk of operative damage to the ureter from a basket becoming trapped. The holmium/YAG laser's inherent properties, with penetration of only around 0.5 mm if misfired into the ureteric wall, reduce risk of ureteric perforation. Advances in ureteroscopic techniques continue, with the recent introduction of improved optical performance from ureteroscopes with inbuilt digital cameras at their distal end, the so-called "chip at the tip", and improved extraction baskets. Thus, ureteroscopy may continue to improve in both ease and safety in the future.

The main disadvantage of ureterorenoscopy compared with other modalities is clearly the frequent need for postoperative stenting, which many centers still practice as standard. The presence of a ureteric stent is clearly associated with a decreased quality of life, and lower urinary tract symptoms.[46] This increasing awareness amongst clinicians of how stents affect quality of life has led to a more critical approach when deciding whether post ureteroscopy stenting is obligatory in an individual patient.[47]

38.2.3 Percutaneous Nephrolithotomy

Percutaneous nephrolithotomy (PCNL), performed in the traditional manner, involves the puncture of an appropriate renal calyx and subsequent dilatation to introduce a 28–30 Fr working sheath, such as an Amplatz sheath, into the kidney. This allows fragmentation and removal of larger stones with instruments utilized via a nephroscope. Postoperatively a nephrostomy would be placed to produce tamponade of the potentially bleeding kidney as well as divert urine in case of obstructing small fragments of stone or blood clot. Clearly, the biggest risk with the procedure has been the initial puncture, which could inadvertently damage a major renal vessel, or even neighboring bowel or pleura.

Just as technology has changed ureterorenoscopes, in recent years many variations of PCNL have been described.

"Mini perc" or PCNL through a smaller sheath is an attempt to reduce the pain and morbidity of the renal puncture.[48–50] The term is, however, rather poorly defined and has been applied to a sheath from 11Ch up to 26Ch. It may be used in conjunction with "tubeless PCNL",[48] where no nephrostomy is placed postoperatively. This may be appropriate if there is deemed to be no significant bleeding, no residual stone load, an intact pelvicaliceal system, and no evidence of a residual ureteral stone.

PCNL is in general indicated for larger renal calculi, in harder to reach locations, such as calyceal diverticula, horseshoe kidneys, or in stones unlikely to fragment with the use of SWL, such as cystine or calcium oxalate monohydrate. SWL is generally contraindicated in cystine stones, and certainly can only be used on an extremely selective basis.[51] Recently, Rudnick et al.,[52] reported that ureterorenoscopy in six patients with cystine stones 1.5–3 cm achieved a stone-free rate of 83%. They suggested that flexible ureterorenoscopy (FURS) be considered an alternative to PCNL in cystinuric patients with stones 1.5–3 cm. The lower morbidity of FURS over PCNL makes it an attractive option for cystinuric patients likely to face repeated surgery during their lifetime.

As well as hard stones, PCNL is also preferred to SWL in treating soft matrix calculi that are associated with urea-splitting organisms and are mainly composed of gelatinous glycocalyx or biofilm matrix with interspersed struvite crystals.[53,54] Matrix stones are relatively radiolucent and are best managed with PCNL, usually with ultrasonic energy sources to disrupt their structure combined with suction evacuation.

Stones in calyceal diverticula may be difficult, if not impossible, to reach with the flexible ureterorenoscope. Historic treatment was with open stone surgery, but this has become very uncommon. In general, it is advantageous to obliterate the diverticulum at the same time as treating the stone, in order to prevent recurrence. This can be performed with ureterorenoscopy. Stone-free rates of up to 84% have been claimed for ureterorenoscopic approaches,[55] although there was clear anecdotal evidence that lower pole diverticula were difficult to locate, with five of seven such procedures abandoned. Successful ureteroscopy as a single modality is therefore somewhat limited to upper and middle calyceal diverticula with stones <1 cm. Successful treatment requires location at the narrow infundibulum and infundibulotomy performed with Nd:YAG laser or balloon dilatation before stones are treated and the diverticulum similarly obliterated.

Diverticula may also present an excessively narrow infundibulum to allow fragments to pass even after successful fragmentation with SWL. Obliteration of the diverticulum clearly cannot be achieved with SWL. However, in one of the largest studies, whilst stone-free rates for calyceal diverticular stones treated with SWL were disappointingly low at around 21%,[56] many more patients (61%) became asymptomatic following SWL. Results with PCNL were, however, significantly superior: 15 patients (83%) were stone free in the short term. PCNL is thus, the most widely used endourological option for calyceal diverticular stones.[57] In another non comparative study of 31 cases treated with PCNL, 1-year stone-free rates were 84%, and 88% of patients were asymptomatic at an average 2-year follow-up.[58] Furthermore, PCNL may allow for the obliterative management of the diverticulum itself.

PCNL is further indicated as the primary treatment modality when there is evidence of poor urinary drainage, such as may occur with ureteric stricture, pelviureteric junction obstruction, or horseshoe kidney. The results of PCNL for stones in horseshoe kidneys are generally superior to those of SWL. Stone-free rates after a single PCNL procedure have been quoted at 77%[59] compared with 66% for SWL for significantly smaller stones in the same study, and 81% in a separate study.[60]

Although many retrospective studies would seem to suggest that lower pole anatomy plays a significant role in predicting stone clearance (see previous discussion), the prospective, randomized Lower Pole I study[24] failed to demonstrate any difference in lower pole anatomical measurements between kidneys in which complete stone clearance did or did not occur. This study suggested simply that it was stone burden that played the overwhelming role in predicting SWL success or failure. This had previously been suggested in the meta-analysis by Lingeman,[61] showing stone-free rates of 74%, 56%, and 33% for stones 10 mm or smaller, 11–20 mm, and larger than 20 mm, respectively.

Indeed, with smaller stones <10 mm there is certainly little evidence that there is a significant difference between SWL and URS. Pearle et al.,[62] performed a multicenter prospective randomized study and found nonsignificant differences in stone-free rates at 3 months of 35% and 50% in SWL and URS, respectively. This was based on postoperative non contrast CT. This study was terminated early because of poor recruitment combined with an interim analysis that suggested that no difference was likely to be shown by completing the study. The small sample size, however, makes it more difficult to reach definitive conclusions.

Thus, SWL is the preferred initial approach for most patients with lower pole stones less than 1 cm in size, whereas PCNL is the primary therapy for stones greater than 2 cm. For patients with stones between 1 and 2 cm, there is still some controversy. PCNL, URS, and SWL are all acceptable. Considerations clearly include stone composition, as well as lower pole anatomy. Who would deny a patient with a 2 cm stone with a short, wide infundibulum and "shallow" lower pole the option of SWL? Unfortunately, with increasing use of non contrast CT, this anatomical information may not be clearly available for the individual

patient. In answer to this, CT reconstruction can be used to provide adequate information and, in fact, may prove to be more useful by showing a three-dimensional image.[63]

38.2.4 Laparoscopic Nephrolithotomy and Ureterolithotomy

When natural orifice or percutaneous surgery has failed or is considered inappropriate, a patient may be considered for a laparoscopic procedure in the same way that an open procedure might formerly have been the treatment of choice. Transperitoneal[64] and retroperitoneal approaches[65] to the kidney and ureter were both described early in the development of techniques. Furthermore, either approach can also be combined with URS.[64] Keeley et al.,[66] reported 14 patients undergoing transperitoneal laparoscopic ureterolithotomy. This represented only 1.1% of 1,240 stone patients treated during a 5-year period. The indications included stones that could not be accessed ureteroscopically or failed to fragment with other treatment modalities. Large (greater than 1.5 cm) proximal ureteric stones were also considered a relative indication. All patients in this series were rendered stone free after a single procedure. El-Moula et al.,[67] considered the procedure as a primary treatment for large impacted stones or as a salvage procedure after failed shock wave lithotripsy or ureteroscopy. Successful completion of the procedure occurred in 95% of cases.

The results of Keeley et al., (14 patients) and also El-Moula (74 patients over 4 years) indicate that even in tertiary centers, laparoscopic stone surgery is an uncommon procedure. Clinicians encountering patients in whom they are considering such surgery must clearly consider this in judging the optimum treatment for their patient, both in terms of which facility and which clinician performs this procedure.

38.3 Conclusions

For every stone and every patient, there is clearly a wide variety of considerations in choosing a treatment for their stone disease. Our own approach is generally first to consider if treatment is truly necessary – conservative treatment carrying few risks in many patients. Then, in consideration of stone size, location, symptoms, anatomy, stone composition, and patient factors, we consider which surgical treatments may be offered. It is only then and after full and open discussion with the patient of the merits and disadvantages of each choice that a treatment is selected. No algorithm can reproduce the exact decision-making process of treatment for stones, but Figs. 38.1–38.3 illustrates some general principles. Treatment preferences are indicated by thickness of arrows in the flow chart.

Fig. 38.1 Treatment algorithm
for ureteric stones

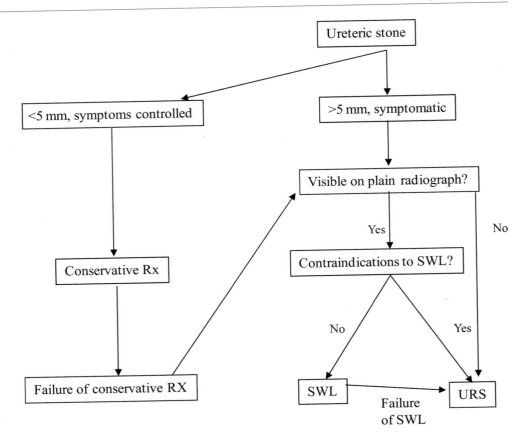

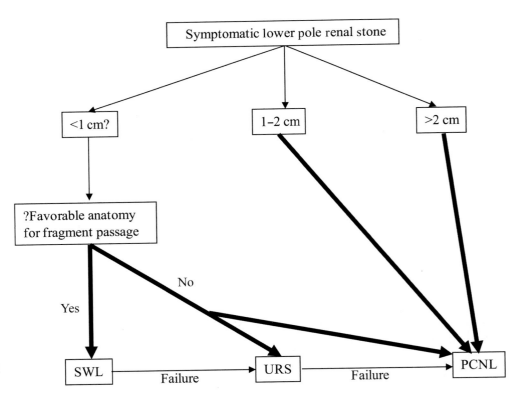

Fig. 38.2 Treatment algorithm
for symptomatic lower pole renal
stones

Fig. 38.3 Treatment algorithm for symptomatic non-lower pole renal stones

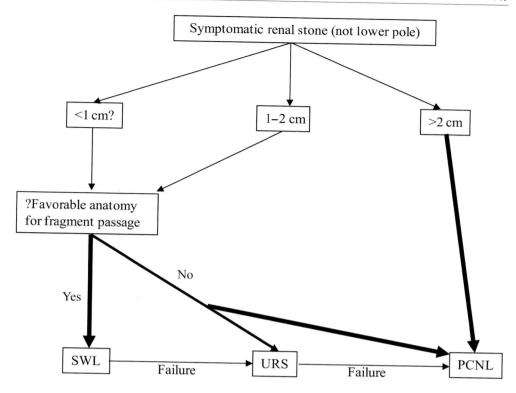

References

1. Knapp PM, Kulb TB, Lingeman JE, et al. Extracorporeal shock wave lithotripsy-induced perirenal hematomas. *J Urol*. 1988;139(4): 700-703.
2. Reid G, Jewett MA, Nickel JC, McLean RJ, Bruce AW. Effect of extracorporeal shock wave lithotripsy on bacterial viability. Relationship to the treatment of struvite stones. *Urol Res*. 1990;18(6):425-427.
3. Mariappan P, Smith G, Moussa SA, Tolley DA. One week of ciprofloxacin before percutaneous nephrolithotomy significantly reduces upper tract infection and urosepsis: a prospective controlled study. *BJU Int*. 2006;98(5):1075-1079.
4. Chen MY, Zagoria RJ, Saunders HS, Dyer RB. Trends in the use of unenhanced helical CT for acute urinary colic. *AJR Am J Roentgenol*. 1999;173(6):1447-1450.
5. Hübner W, Porpaczy P. Treatment of caliceal calculi. *Br J Urol*. 1990;66(1):9-11.
6. Glowacki LS, Beecroft ML, Cook RJ, Pahl D, Churchill DN. The natural history of asymptomatic urolithiasis. *J Urol*. 1992;147(2): 319-321.
7. Inci K, Sahin A, Islamoglu E, Eren MT, Bakkaloglu M, Ozen H. Prospective long-term follow up of patients with asymptomatic lower pole caliceal stones. *J Urol*. 2007;177(6):2189-2192.
8. Osman MM, Alfano Y, Kamp S, et al. 5-year-follow-up of patients with clinically insignificant residual fragments after extracorporeal shockwave lithotripsy. *Eur Urol*. 2005;47(6):860-864. Epub 19 Jan 2005.
9. Keeley FX Jr, Tilling K, Elves A, et al. Preliminary results of a randomized controlled trial of prophylactic shock wave lithotripsy for small asymptomatic renal calyceal stones. *BJU Int*. 2001;87(1):1-8.
10. Segura JW, Preminger GM, Assimos DG, et al. Nephrolithiasis clinical guidelines panel summary report on the management of staghorn calculi. *J Urol*. 1994;151:1648-1651.

11. Blandy J, Singh M. The case for a more aggressive approach to staghorn stones. *J Urol*. 1976;115:505-506.
12. Koga S, Arakai Y, Matsuoka MD, et al. Staghorn calculi: long-term results of management. *Br J Urol*. 1991;68:122-124.
13. Teichman JMH, Long RD, Hulbert JC. Long-term renal fate and prognosis after staghorn calculus management. *J Urol*. 1995;153:1403-1407.
14. Rous SN, Turner WR. Retrospective study of 95 patients with staghorn calculus disease. *J Urol*. 1977;118:902.
15. Preminger GM, Assimos DG, Lingeman JE, Nakada SY, Pearle MS, Wolf JS Jr. AUA Nephrolithiasis Guideline Panel. Chapter 1: AUA guideline on management of staghorn calculi: diagnosis and treatment recommendations. *J Urol*. 2005;173(6):1991-2000.
16. Al-Kohlany KM, Shokeir AA, Mosbah A, et al. Treatment of complete staghorn stones: a prospective randomized comparison of open surgery versus percutaneous nephrolithotomy. *J Urol*. 2005;173(2):469-473.
17. Lupu AN, Fuchs GJ, Chaussy CG. Treatment of ureteral calculi by extracorporeal shock-wave lithotripsy. UCLA experience. *Urology*. 1988;32(3):217-222.
18. Wickham JE. Treatment of urinary tract stones. *BMJ*. 1993;307(6916): 1414-1417.
19. Gerber R, Studer UE, Danuser H. Is newer always better? A comparative study of 3 lithotriptor generations. *J Urol*. 2005;173(6):2013-2016.
20. Jain A, Shah TK. Effect of air bubbles in the coupling medium on efficiency of extracorporeal shock wave lithotripsy. *Eur Urol*. 2007;51:1680-1687.
21. Soyupek S, Armağan A, Koşar A, et al. Risk factors for the formation of a steinstrasse after shock wave lithotripsy. *Urol Int*. 2005;74(4):323-325.
22. Lennon GM, Thornhill JA, Grainger R. Double pigtail ureteric stent versus percutaneous nephrostomy: effects on stone transit and ureteric motility. *Eur Urol*. 1997;31(1):24-29.
23. Grasso M, Loisides P, Beaghler M, Bagley D. The case for primary endoscopic management of upper urinary tract calculi: I. A critical review of 121 extracorporeal shock-wave lithotripsy failures. *Urology*. 1995;45(3):363-371.

24. Albala DM, Assimos DG, Clayman RV, et al. Lower pole I: a prospective randomized trial of extracorporeal shock wave lithotripsy and percutaneous nephrostolithotomy for lower pole nephrolithiasis-initial results. *J Urol.* 2001;166(6):2072-2080.

25. Cranidis AI, Karayannis AA, Delakas DS, Livadas CE, Anezinis PE. Cystine stones: the efficacy of percutaneous and shock wave lithotripsy. *Urol Int.* 1996;56(3):180-183.

26. Keeley FX Jr, Moussa SA, Smith G, Tolley DA. Clearance of lower-pole stones following shock wave lithotripsy: effect of the infundibulopelvic angle. *Eur Urol.* 1999;36(5):371-375.

27. Elbahnasy AM, Shalhav AL, Hoenig DM. Lower caliceal stone clearance after shock wave lithotripsy or ureteroscopy: the impact of lower pole radiographic anatomy. *J Urol.* 1998;159(3): 676-682.

28. Sumino Y, Mimata H, Tasaki Y, et al. Predictors of lower pole renal stone clearance after extracorporeal shock wave lithotripsy. *J Urol.* 2002;168(4 Pt 1):1344-1347.

29. Kanao K, Nakashima J, Nakagawa K, et al. Preoperative nomograms for predicting stone-free rate after extracorporeal shock wave lithotripsy. *J Urol.* 2006;176(4 Pt 1):1453-1456.

30. Gomha MA, Sheir KZ, Showky S. Can we improve the prediction of stone-free status after extracorporeal shock wave lithotripsy for ureteral stones? A neural network or a statistical model? *J Urol.* 2004;172(1):175-179.

31. Abdel-Khalek M, Sheir KZ, Mokhtar AA, et al. Prediction of success rate after extracorporeal shock-wave lithotripsy of renal stones – a multivariate analysis model. *Scand J Urol Nephrol.* 2004;38(2):161-167.

32. Preminger GM, Tiselius HG, Assimos DG, et al. EAU/AUA Nephrolithiasis Guideline Panel. 2007 guideline for the management of ureteral calculi. *J Urol.* 2007;178(6):2418-2434.

33. Nabi G, Downey P, Keeley F, Watson G, McClinton S. Extra-corporeal shock wave lithotripsy (ESWL) versus ureteroscopic management for ureteric calculi. *Cochrane Database Syst Rev.* 2007;24(1):CD006029.

34. Parkin J, Keeley FX Jr, Timoney AG. Re-auditing a regional lithotripsy service. *BJU Int.* 2002;89(7):653-657.

35. Brownlee N, Foster M, Griffith DP, Carlton CE Jr. Controlled inversion therapy: an adjunct to the elimination of gravity-dependent fragments following extracorporeal shock wave lithotripsy. *J Urol.* 1990;143(6):1096-1098.

36. Chiong E, Hwee ST, Kay LM, Liang S, Kamaraj R, Esuvaranathan K. Randomized controlled study of mechanical percussion, diuresis, and inversion therapy to assist passage of lower pole renal calculi after shock wave lithotripsy. *Urology.* 2005; 65(6):1070-1074.

37. Pace KT, Tariq N, Dyer SJ, Weir MJ, D'A Honey RJ. Mechanical percussion, inversion and diuresis for residual lower pole fragments after shock wave lithotripsy: a prospective, single blind, randomized controlled trial. *J Urol.* 2001;166(6):2065-2071.

38. Elbahnasy AM, Shalhav AL, Hoenig DM, et al. Lower caliceal stone clearance after shock wave lithotripsy or ureteroscopy: the impact of lower pole radiographic anatomy. *J Urol.* 1998; 159(3):676-682.

39. Sampaio FJ, D'Anunciação AL, Silva EC. Comparative follow-up of patients with acute and obtuse infundibulum-pelvic angle submitted to extracorporeal shockwave lithotripsy for lower caliceal stones: preliminary report and proposed study design. *J Endourol.* 1997;11(3):157-161.

40. Nguyen TA, Belis JA. Endoscopic management of urolithiasis in the morbidly obese patient. *J Endourol.* 1998;12(1):33-35.

41. Grasso M, Chalik Y. Principles and applications of laser lithotripsy: experience with the holmium laser lithotrite. *J Clin Laser Med Surg.* 1998;16(1):3-7.

42. Miller OF, Kane CJ. Time to stone passage for observed ureteral calculi: a guide for patient education. *J Urol.* 1999;162(3 Pt 1): 688-690.

43. Coll DM, Varanelli MJ, Smith RC. Relationship of spontaneous passage of ureteral calculi to stone size and location as revealed by unenhanced helical CT. *AJR Am J Roentgenol.* 2002;178(1): 101-103.

44. Segura JW, Preminger GM, Assimos DG, et al. Ureteral Stones Clinical Guidelines Panel summary report on the management of ureteral calculi. The American Urological Association. *J Urol.* 1997;158(5):1915-1921.

45. Harmon WJ, Sershon PD, Blute ML, Patterson DE, Segura JW. Ureteroscopy: current practice and long-term complications. *J Urol.* 1997;157(1):28-32.

46. Joshi HB, Newns N, Stainthorpe A, MacDonagh RP, Keeley FX Jr, Timoney AG. Ureteral stent symptom questionnaire: development and validation of a multidimensional quality of life measure. *J Urol.* 2003;169(3):1060-1064.

47. Nabi G, Cook J, McClinton S. Outcomes of stenting after uncomplicated ureteroscopy: systematic review and meta-analysis. *BMJ.* 2007;334:572. doi:10.1136/bmj.39119.595081.55.

48. Jackman SV, Hedican SP, Peters CA, Docimo SG. Percutaneous nephrolithotomy in infants and preschool age children: experience with a new technique. *Urology.* 1998;52(4):697-701.

49. Jackman SV, Docimo SG, Cadeddu JA, Bishoff JT, Kavoussi LR, Jarrett TW. The "mini-perc" technique: a less invasive alternative to percutaneous nephrolithotomy. *World J Urol.* 1998;16(6): 371-374.

50. Monga M, Oglevie S. Minipercutaneous nephrolithotomy. *J Endourol.* 2000;14(5):419-421.

51. Kachel TA, Vijan SR, Dretler SP. Endourological experience with cystine calculi and a treatment algorithm. *J Urol.* 1991;145(1):25-28.

52. Rudnick DM, Bennett PM, Dretler SP. Retrograde renoscopic fragmentation of moderate-size (1.5–3.0-cm) renal cystine stones. *J Endourol.* 1999;13(7):483-485.

53. Nickel JC, Emtage J, Costerton JW. Ultrastructural microbial ecology of infection-induced urinary stones. *J Urol.* 1985; 133(4):622-627.

54. Shah HN, Kharodawala S, Sodha HS, Khandkar AA, Hegde SS, Bansal MB. The management of renal matrix calculi: a single-centre experience over 5 years. *BJU Int.* 2009;103(6): 810-814.

55. Batter SJ, Dretler SP. Ureterorenoscopic approach to the symptomatic caliceal diverticulum. *J Urol.* 1997;158(3 Pt 1):709-713.

56. Turna B, Raza A, Moussa S, Smith G, Tolley DA. Management of calyceal diverticular stones with extracorporeal shock wave lithotripsy and percutaneous nephrolithotomy: long-term outcome. *BJU Int.* 2007;100(1):151-156.

57. Auge BK, Munver R, Kourambas J, Newman GE, Preminger GM. Endoscopic management of symptomatic caliceal diverticula: a retrospective comparison of percutaneous nephrolithotripsy and ureteroscopy. *J Endourol.* 2002;16(8):557-563.

58. Landry JL, Colombel M, Rouviere O, et al. Long term results of percutaneous treatment of caliceal diverticular calculi. *Eur Urol.* 2002;41(4):474-477.

59. Symons SJ, Ramachandran A, Kurien A, Baiysha R, Desai MR. Urolithiasis in the horseshoe kidney: a single-centre experience. *BJU Int.* 2008;102(11):1676-1680. Epub 8 Sep 2008.

60. Mosavi-Bahar SH, Amirzargar MA, Rahnavardi M, Moghaddam SM, Babbolhavaeji H, Amirhasani S. Percutaneous nephrolithotomy in patients with kidney malformations. *J Endourol.* 2007; 21(5):520-524.

61. Lingeman JE, Siegel YI, Steele B, Nyhuis AW, Woods JR. Management of lower pole nephrolithiasis: a critical analysis. *J Urol.* 1994;151(3):663-667.

62. Pearle MS, Lingeman JE, Leveillee R, et al. Prospective, randomized trial comparing shock wave lithotripsy and ureteroscopy for lower pole caliceal calculi 1 cm or less. *J Urol.* 2005;173(6):2005-2009.

63. El-Assmy A, Abo-Elghar ME, El-Nahas AR, Youssef RF, El-Diasty T, Sheir KZ. Anatomic predictors of formation of lower

caliceal calculi: is it the time for three-dimensional computed tomography urography? *J Endourol.* 2008;22(9):2175-2180.

64. Wuernschimmel E, Lipsky H. Laparoscopic treatment of an upper ureteral stone. *J Laparoendosc Surg.* 1993;3(3):301-307.

65. Gaur DD. Laparoscopic operative retroperitoneoscopy: use of a new device. *J Urol.* 1992;148(4):1137-1139.

66. Keeley FX, Gialas I, Pillai M, Chrisofos M, Tolley DA. Laparoscopic ureterolithotomy: the Edinburgh experience. *BJU Int.* 1999;84(7): 765-769.

67. El-Moula MG, Abdallah A, El-Anany F, et al. Laparoscopic ureterolithotomy: our experience with 74 cases. *Int J Urol.* 2008;15(7):593-597. Epub 8 May 2008.

Renal Stones

Tamer El-Husseiny, Athanasios Papatsoris, Junaid Masood, and Noor N.P. Buchholz

Abstract Renal stone disease is a significant and worldwide health problem, and extracorporeal shock-wave lithotripsy (SWL) has revolutionized the treatment for most patients with urolithiasis since its introduction in the early 1980s. In SWL, shock waves are generated by a source external to the patient's body and are then propagated into the body and focused on a kidney stone. Types of shock-wave generators are the electrohydraulic (spark gap) generator, the electromagnetic generator, and the piezoelectric generator. Imaging used during SWL includes fluoroscopy, ultrasonography, and combination of both fluoroscopy and ultrasonography. Initial SWL treatment required general or regional anesthesia, but the development of new-generation lithotripters has led to the reduction of shock wave–induced pain, thus minimizing the anesthetic requirement. Complications of SWL are mainly those related to stone fragments, infectious complications, and tissue damage through SWL. Contraindications to SWL treatment are pregnancy, blood clotting disorders, urinary tract infection, aortic and/or renal artery aneurysms, severe obesity, and certain malformations. Today, about 80% of all urinary stones and the majority of kidney stones can be successfully treated with SWL in a minimally invasive fashion. Most renal stones in adults can be treated in a day case setting.

39.1 Introduction

The concept of using shock waves to fragment stones was noted in the 1950s in Russia. However, it was during the investigation of pitting on supersonic aircraft that Dornier, a German aircraft corporation, rediscovered that shock waves originating from passing debris in the atmosphere can crack something that is hard. It was the ingenious application of a model developed with the hope of understanding such shock waves that extracorporeal shock-wave lithotripsy (SWL) emerged.[1]

Renal stone disease is a significant and worldwide health problem,[2,3] and extracorporeal shock-wave lithotripsy (SWL) has revolutionized the treatment for most patients with urolithiasis since its introduction in the early 1980s.[4,5]

The majority of urinary tract stones can be treated with SWL. Contraindications to SWL treatment in renal stone include pregnancy, uncontrolled blood clotting disorders, active urinary tract infection, aortic and/or renal artery aneurysms, severe obesity, and certain malformations precluding correct patient positioning. Relative contraindications are stone size, stone location in the lower pole calyx or within a calyx diverticulum, stone composition, pain tolerance, and the inability of a patient to remain still during treatment. A pacemaker is, however, not a contraindication.[6,7]

The HM-1 (Human Model-1) lithotripter underwent modifications in 1982 leading to the HM-2 and, finally, to the widespread application of the HM-3 in 1983. Since then, thousands of lithotripters have been put into use around the world, with millions of patients successfully treated.[1]

39.2 Physics of SWL

In SWL, shock waves are generated by a source external to the patient's body and then propagated into the body and focused on the kidney stone. The uniqueness of this device lies in its exploitation of shock-wave focusing. Relatively weak, non-intrusive waves are generated externally and transmitted through the body. The shock waves build up to sufficient strength only at the target, where they generate enough force to fragment a stone. Stones are broken by

T. El-Husseiny (✉)
Department of Urology, Barts and the London NHS Trust, London, UK
e-mail: d_tamer@hotmail.com

P.N. Rao et al. (eds.), *Urinary Tract Stone Disease*,
DOI 10.1007/978-1-84800-362-0_39, © Springer-Verlag London Limited 2011

different mechanisms, including both compressive and tensile forces.[8]

Currently, there are three different shock-wave generators in use worldwide:

1. The *electrohydraulic* (spark gap) generator produces a spherically expanding shock wave by an underwater spark discharge.[9]
2. The *electromagnetic* generators produce either plane or cylindrical shock waves. The plane waves are focused by an acoustic lens; the cylindrical waves are reflected by a parabolic reflector and transformed into a spherical wave.[8]
3. The *piezoelectric* lithotripter also produces plane shock waves with directly converging shock fronts.[8]

39.3 Imaging

Imaging for localization of a stone and focusing onto it is a crucial part of every SWL treatment. The better the imaging, the better the clinical outcome that can be expected. However, stones <5 mm will be difficult to locate with any of the methods available.

39.3.1 Fluoroscopy

The original Dornier HM3 lithotripter used two X-ray converters arranged at oblique angles to the patient and 90° from each other to localize the stone effectively at F2. To reduce the cost of lithotripters, an adjustable C-arm has been subsequently introduced on many devices.[8]

The primary *advantages* of fluoroscopy include its familiarity to most urologists, the ability to visualize radiopaque calculi throughout the urinary tract, the ability to use iodinated contrast agents to aid in stone localization, and the ability to display anatomic detail.[8]

The *disadvantages* include the exposure of the staff and patient to ionizing radiation, the high maintenance demands of the equipment, and the inability to visualize radiolucent calculi without the use of radiographic contrast agents.[8] During follow-up after SWL the appropriate use of hemi-KUB X-rays is a simple and effective way of significantly reducing the radiation exposure of such patients.[10,11]

39.3.2 Ultrasonography

Ultrasound has the advantage of real-time (continuous) imaging, absence of exposure to ionizing radiation, the ability to image radiolucent calculi, and much lower costs than fluoroscopic systems.[12]

There are a number of significant disadvantages of ultrasound imaging. Sonographic localization of a kidney stone requires a highly trained operator. It is almost impossible to view a kidney stone in areas such as the middle third of the ureter or when there is an indwelling ureteral catheter. Stones <5 mm may not be located, and once a stone is fragmented, it can be difficult to identify the remaining stone fragments.[8]

39.3.3 Combination of Ultrasonography and Fluoroscopy

As the demand for interdisciplinary lithotripters has increased, the lithotripsy industry has responded, in some cases, by combining ultrasonography and fluoroscopy for stone localization. There are clear advantages to these set-ups, but each system has a drawback that limits one of the functions of the system.[8]

39.4 Anesthesia

Initial SWL treatment required general or regional anesthesia, but the development of new-generation lithotripters has led to the reduction of shock wave–induced pain, thus minimizing the anesthetic requirement.[13,14]

Modern lithotripters generate less powerful but more accurate shock waves that produce less pain, and patients need not be anesthetized or sedated during the procedure.[13,14] Nevertheless, some form of analgesia may still be needed to avoid patient discomfort.[15]

The pathogenesis of SWL-related pain is not clear. It has been postulated that pain results from stimulation of nociceptive nerve endings in tissues along the shock-wave path; this is not considered a direct mechanical effect but rather is mediated by cavitation and generation and movements of gas bubbles in the body fluids or tissues.[16]

Several techniques have been used to reduce shock wave–induced pain: topical creams, infiltrating local anesthesia, nonsteroidal anti-inflammatory drugs (NSAIDs), intravenous sedation, and opioids. Topical anesthetic agents such as EMLA cream (lidocaine and prilocaine)[17] and infiltrating local anesthesia have been reported to decrease the need for opioid-based analgesia in patients undergoing SWL.[18,19]

Intravenous administration of opioids, such as fentanyl and its analogs, has been effective in controlling pain during SWL, either alone or combined with other forms of analgesia or sedation.[20–23] Despite their effectiveness, however, opioid analgesics may potentially cause severe adverse events, such as nausea and vomiting, over-sedation, significant respiratory depression, and oxygen desaturation,[24,25] which may limit their use, particularly in the outpatient setting of SWL.

39.5 Indications

The indication for SWL treatment of renal stones is dependent on the stone size.

For patients harboring non-staghorn stones <10 mm, SWL is usually the primary approach.[8]

For patients with stones between 10 and 20 mm, SWL can still be considered a first-line treatment unless factors of stone composition, location, or renal anatomy suggest that a more optimal outcome may be achieved with a more invasive treatment modality such as percutaneous nephrolithotomy (PCNL) or rigid/flexible ureteroscopy (URS).[8]

Patients with stones larger than 20 mm should primarily be treated by PCNL unless specific indications for ureteroscopy are present (e.g., bleeding diathesis, obesity). If SWL is used, a double-J stent may be needed to prevent steinstrasse (the obstruction of the ureter through the line up of stone fragments).[26] In patients harboring stones that are resistant to fragmentation (cystine, brushite, calcium oxalate monohydrate), SWL should be tried only when the stone burden is small. If there is no fragmentation after the initial two sessions, a different surgical approach should be chosen.[8]

The management of patients with staghorn stones by a combined approach of SWL and PCNL is called a *sandwich therapy*. Usually, an initial debulking PCNL is followed by further fragmentation of residual stones with SWL. The existing tract is then used for a second-look PCNL to remove remaining fragments. This approach requires, however, a readily available lithotripter and the infrastructure to plan consecutive surgery, which cannot be done in all health systems. It has therefore been replaced widely by multiple tract PCNLs with the use of flexible ureterorenoscopy (URS) and nephroscopy to evacuate residual fragments in the initial session.

SWL has a definite role in the treatment of residual fragments after more invasive treatments of renal stones, and of resulting steinstrasse.[8]

39.6 Contraindications

Pregnancy is an absolute contraindication to SWL because of the potential disruptive effects of the shock-wave energy on the fetus.[27]

SWL in anticoagulated patients may lead to severe subcapsular and intrarenal hematomas (Fig. 39.1) and persistent hematuria with renal colic through blood clots. Although SWL in patients with uncorrected coagulopathy can result in life-threatening hemorrhage, such patients can be safely treated once the bleeding diathesis has been corrected. However, if the patient's coagulopathy is the result of a pharmacologic therapy that cannot be safely discontinued, ureteroscopy with laser lithotripsy is the preferable approach.[28]

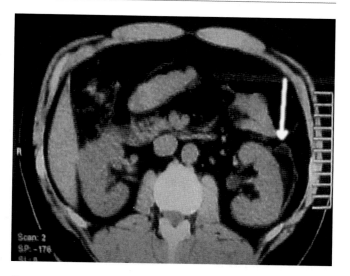

Fig. 39.1 Subcapsular hematoma following SWL

For patients on antiplatelets drugs such as aspirin, this treatment should be stopped prior to SWL for a period that depends on the dose they are receiving (i.e., 1 week for low dose aspirin [75 mg] and 2 weeks for full dose aspirin [325 mg]). In general, peri-SWL blood clotting adjustments follow the same principles as for small-to-moderate surgical procedures (i.e., heparinization, INR monitoring).

Urinary tract infections should be treated prior to SWL. It has been shown that bacteremia and fever are common after SWL, and urosepsis can result. However, although stones should be regarded as potentially infectious, general antibiotic prophylaxis for SWL has not been recommended.[29]

Patients with renal artery or aortic *aneurysms* are usually excluded from SWL treatment. It cannot be excluded that shock waves may go through the area of the aneurysm that could in theory lead to fragmentation and migration of atherosclerotic plaques or – worse – to a bursting of the thinned aneurysmatic wall.[30]

Patient size may exceed the manufacturer's specifications for the SWL treatment table – i.e., for weight (>135 Kg) and height (adults >200 cm, children <120 cm) – in which case another treatment option must be chosen such as flexible URS or PCNL with extra-long instruments.[31,32]

Malformations – i.e., spina bifida (Fig. 39.2) or contractures – may make it impossible to properly position the patient on the SWL table, thus making it impossible to properly couple the shock-wave generator and localize the stone.[33]

For the same reason, patients with pulmonary or cardiac *breathing difficulties* may not be able to lie flat enough to allow for effective coupling.

Patients who cannot tolerate low-grade *pain* may not be eligible for SWL without anesthesia. This may be a contraindication if the lithotripter has no operating theater setup; i.e., supply and removal of narcotic gases.

The same restrictions apply to patients who are *unable to lie still* through SWL treatment for whatever reason.

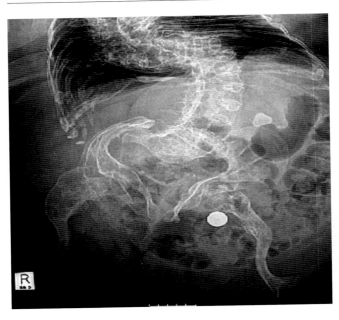

Fig. 39.2 Left renal stone in a patient with spina bifida

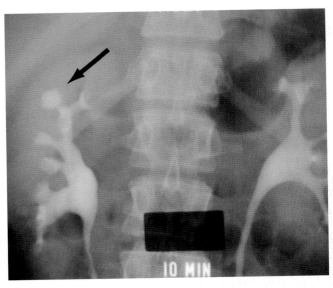

Fig. 39.4 Same patient with a right upper pole calyceal diverticulum stone (IVP)

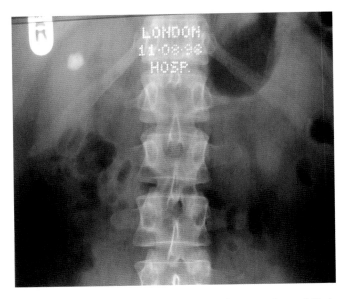

Fig. 39.3 Right upper pole calyceal diverticulum stone (control film)

Obstruction distal to the stone may hamper the proper passage of resulting fragments. This may be a (temporary) contraindication requiring treatment before SWL can be performed. Such obstructions include calyceal neck stenosis, renal calyx diverticulum (Figs. 39.3 and 39.4), ureteropelvic junction stenosis, ureter strictures, benign prostatic hyperplasia, and urethral as well as meatal strictures.[34]

Patients with known *very hard stones* such as cystine-, brushite-, and calcium monohydrate stone formers, in particular if they had previously failed SWL treatment, may be considered contraindicated and channeled toward other primary treatments such as URS and PCNL.[8]

39.7 Complications of SWL

Table 39.1 lists complications following SWL for urinary stones.

39.7.1 Immediate Complications

39.7.1.1 Complications Related to Stone Fragments

Incomplete fragmentation resulting in residual stone fragments, steinstrasse, and consecutive renal obstruction is one of the problems that urologists confront when SWL fails to completely fragment the stone treated.[35] These may result in renal colic, renal obstruction, upper urinary tract infection, pyonephrosis, and urosepsis.

Predisposing factors for incomplete stone fragmentation are stone composition, size, location, and number, as well as renal morphology and shock-wave rate and energy.[27,36] The larger the stone, the higher is the possibility of residual fragments of a significant size.

Also, the harder the stone the higher is the possibility of residual fragments of a significant size. The fragmentation rates of cystine and calcium oxalate monohydrate stones are notoriously low.[37]

If more than two residual fragments line up in the ureter and lead to renal obstruction, this is called *steinstrasse* (meaning "stone street" in German) (Fig. 39.5). Usually, a larger lead fragment gets stuck within the ureter, leading to a pile-up of other fragments proximally.

Table 39.1 Complications after SWL for urinary stones

Immediate	Delayed
Related to stone fragments	Chronic renal injury:
Infectious	• Function?
Tissue effects:	• Hypertension?
• Renal	Fertility?
• Extrarenal	

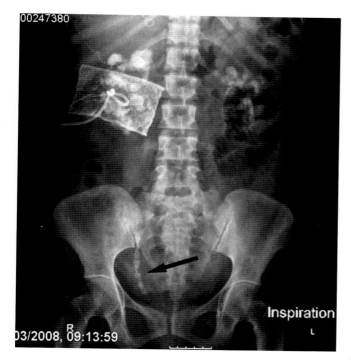

Fig. 39.5 Right-sided steinstrasse following right SWL in a patient after PCNL-debulking of complete staghorn stone on the right

The cause of steinstrasse is usually a large stone burden, and thus, in most cases, stones >2.5 cm in diameter are today considered unsuitable for SWL monotherapy. It was also found that using high energies during the initial treatment for renal stones can cause steinstrasse through the rapid breakup of the stone into large fragments. A confounding factor is the presence of any stenosis in the course of the ureter. If an initial debulking PCNL does not fragment enough stone, this also may lead to steinstrasse.[38–41]

Steinstrasse is most commonly located in the distal ureter (64%), followed by the proximal (29%) and mid-ureter (8%).[38,39]

Steinstrasse can be prevented by the following:

1. Thorough patient selection
2. Using low energies at the start of treatment, i.e., increasing the voltage gradually (a high initial voltage causes large fragments to pass directly into the ureter and obstruct it)

3. Excluding patients with suspected narrowing of the ureter, or treating any stricture endoscopically prior to SWL

A careful follow-up after SWL is essential to detect any steinstrasse and to avoid damaging the renal unit, especially in asymptomatic patients, as silent renal loss after SWL can occur.[42]

The conservative management of uncomplicated steinstrasse is effective in about half of patients.[38,43] Repeated ureteric SWL is successful in most remaining patients, with SWL used to disintegrate and to loosen the (leading) fragments. Placing a nephrostomy in patients with obstruction or infection can relieve obstruction and decrease the intrapelvic pressure, which re-establishes ureteric peristalsis and thus the passage of fragments. A nephrostomy may also lead to a decrease in ureteric edema around the fragments, which helps to dislodge them and allow them to pass without further treatment.[44]

Ureteroscopy can be used in nonfebrile patients, after the failure of SWL, and after placing a nephrostomy in cases where the steinstrasse did not clear under these measures.[45,46]

Placing a ureteric stent before SWL does not always prevent steinstrasse but can prevent their complications. Stenting before SWL can be considered in patients with large renal stones >2 cm, single kidney, and faint ureteric stones (especially those over the pelvic bones) to aid in stone location.[26,43]

39.7.2 Infectious Complications

The renal trauma and vascular disruption associated with SWL may allow bacteria in urine to enter the bloodstream. Moreover, when infected calculi are destroyed, bacteria are released from the stone into the urine and may be absorbed systemically. As a consequence, bacteriuria, bacteremia, clinical urinary tract infection (UTI), urosepsis, perinephric abscess formation, endocarditis, candidal and *Klebsiella* endophthalmitis, candidal septicemia, tuberculosis, and (rarely) death have all been reported after SWL.[47]

Careful post-SWL monitoring is important, and in an outpatient setting, patients must be made aware of possible infection and the need of re-attendance in case of symptoms. Clinical symptoms (pain, fever), erythrocyte sedimentation rate (ESR), white blood count (WBC), and urine and blood cultures are all helpful in detecting post-SWL bacteriuria and bacteremia.[48]

Yet, the role of routine prophylactic antibiotics is controversial. Preoperative antibiotics should routinely be given to patients with infection-related stones (staghorn and struvite calculi), positive urine cultures, or a history of recurrent UTIs and to those who undergo instrumentation at the time of SWL.[47,49–51]

39.7.3 Tissue Damage Through Shock Waves

39.7.3.1 Acute Renal Injury

The two most common renal side effects seen immediately after SWL are hemorrhage and edema within or around the kidney. Patients receiving more than 200 shocks show gross hematuria (which is the result of direct injury to the renal parenchyma), which generally resolves within 12 h.[31,52]

These changes are not specific to any particular lithotripter, and numerous reports have documented identical renal bioeffects induced by second- and third-generation lithotripters.[53–56] However, the size of a lesion induced by electromagnetic lithotripter is much larger as compared to electrohydraulic lithotripter.[57]

Likewise, the renal function can be acutely affected in some patients. The primary change appears to be a vasoconstrictive response resulting in a fall in renal blood flow and glomerular filtration rate.[8]

Risk factors that may predispose SWL patients to acute renal injury are age, obesity, coagulopathies, thrombocytopenia, diabetes mellitus, coronary heart disease, and preexisting hypertension.[8]

The harmful effects of SWL can be minimized by pretreating with low-energy shock waves and treating at the lowest power setting that fractures the stone. Using a more gentle approach, stone breakage can still be promoted by treating at slower rates, such as 1 Hz (60 shocks per minute).[8]

39.7.3.2 Extrarenal Injury

SWL induces acute injury in a variety of extrarenal tissues.[58,59] The unmodified HM3 has been associated with significant trauma to organs such as the *liver* and *skeletal muscle*, as detected by elevated levels of bilirubin, lactate dehydrogenase LDH, serum aspartate transaminase, and creatine phosphokinase within 24 h of treatment.[22,60,61]

Changes such as *gastric* and *duodenal erosion* have been identified and are thought to represent a common extrarenal complication of SWL therapy.[62]

The *lung parenchyma* can suffer injury if it is exposed directly to shock waves.[63] Several cases of clinically typical *acute pancreatitis*, associated with a marked rise in serum amylase and lipase levels, have been observed, and even in the absence of the symptoms of overt pancreatitis, increased amylase levels have been detected.[4,60]

Myocardial infarctions, cerebral vascular accidents, and *brachial plexus palsy* have been noted after SWL. In addition, clinical studies noted that shock waves could induce *cardiac*

arrhythmia, an observation that led to electrocardiographic synchronization with R-wave triggering on the Dornier HM3 device.[32]

39.7.4 Delayed Complications

39.7.4.1 Chronic Renal Injury

Although there still remains a paucity of information on the subject, four potential chronic renal changes that follow SWL have been discussed. They are an accelerated *rise in systemic blood pressure,* a *decrease in renal function,* an *increase in the rate of stone recurrence,* and the *induction of brushite stone disease.* All four effects appear to be linked to the observation that the acute injury does progress to scar formation at the site of previous stone fragmentation within the kidney.[8]

Although biochemical evidence of renal injury is apparent immediately after SWL, blood and urine markers such as renin, creatinine, N-Acetyl-b-D-glucosaminidase (NAG), b-galactosidase (BGAL), b-2-microglobulin (B2M), and proteinuria return to near-normal levels within a few days.[64–66]

Perhaps the most discussed and significant chronic change is a possible late rise in blood pressure. The incidence of newly diagnosed hypertension after lithotripsy was initially reported to be 8%. This does not, however, significantly differ from the incidence of new onset hypertension in the general population, which is approximately 6%.[67] Systolic hypertension per se has not been shown to rise after SWL, but diastolic hypertension has been found increased. This may be a dose-related phenomenon as an increasing number of shock waves correlate with more severe diastolic hypertension.[68] The question of whether or not SWL leads to significant hypertension has to date not been conclusively answered.

39.7.4.2 Fertility

Shock wave application was of concern in young patients because of the fear that it may adversely affect fertility. To date, there is sufficient evidence from experimental and clinical studies that SWL does not have severe permanent effects on testicular and ovarian functions. Consequently, male and female fertilities are not affected by SWL.[69,70]

39.8 Predictive Clinical Outcome Factors

Failure of stone disintegration results in unnecessary exposure of the renal parenchyma to shock waves and the requirement of an alternative additional treatment procedure, which increases medical costs. Hence, it is important to identify patients who will benefit from SWL.[71]

39.8.1 Stone Position

Lower pole stones have been consistently associated with lower stone-free rates following SWL when compared with upper and middle pole stones. Theories attempting to explain this finding include the tendency for stones to remain in dependent portions of the collecting system owing to gravity regardless of the degree of fragmentation.[72]

Various measurements of the lower pole dimensions were proposed to have an effect on the outcome of SWL, such as the lower pole infundibulopelvic angle, and the infundibular length and width.[73]

The lower pole of the kidney poses an anatomical challenge to stone fragments migrating into the renal pelvis. The lower infundibulopelvic angle has the greatest impact on fragment clearance (Fig. 39.6) followed by the infundibular length (Fig. 39.7). An angle of more than 70° and a length of less than 5 cm yield the best clinical results. Infundibular width (Fig. 39.7) appears to be associated with a more favorable outcome when >5 mm. These measurements can be easily

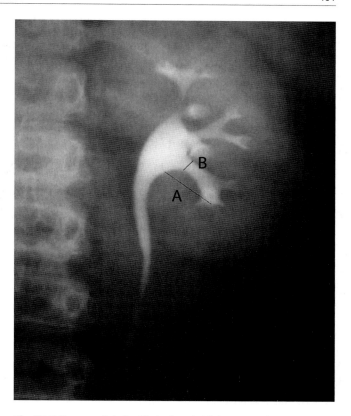

Fig. 39.7 Lower pole infundibular length (**A**) is measured as the distance from the most distal point at the bottom of the calyx harboring the stone to the midpoint of lower lip of renal pelvis. The infundibular width (**B**) is measured at the narrowest point of the lower pole infundibulum

measured off a standard IVP film and thus be used to select SWL as a treatment modality with a predictably favorable outcome in individual cases.[74]

39.8.2 Stone Burden

The first variable shown to consistently affect the success rate of SWL was stone burden. Accurate preoperative radiological assessment of stone burden is pivotal in predicting the outcome of SWL.[72]

It is controversial whether two-dimensional measurement of largest diameters is sufficient or whether a more-dimensional approach is warranted for proper treatment planning.[75]

Historically, plain KUB radiographs have been used for the initial evaluation; recently, computed tomography (CT) scanning has become the imaging study of choice for most clinicians owing to an improved measurement of stone size. If one wants to be more accurate, either CT coronal reconstructions may be obtained or both CT and X-KUB may be combined.[76]

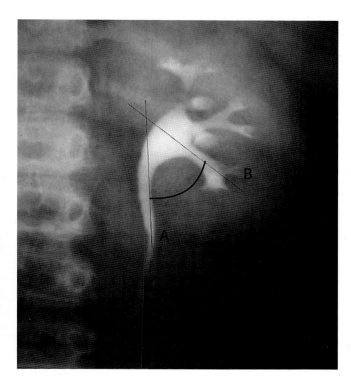

Fig. 39.6 The lower infundibulopelvic angle is the angle between the ureteropelvic axis (**A**) and the vertical axis of the lower infundibulum (**B**)

39.8.3 Stone Composition/Density

In contrast to failures resulting from a high stone burden resulting in difficulties in the clearance of fragments, failures related to stone composition result from a primary failure of stone fragmentation.[76]

Cystine, brushite, and calcium oxalate monohydrate stones have demonstrated a high degree of resistance to fragmentation by SWL owing to their high density, whereas less dense stones (calcium oxalate dihydrate, hydroxyapatite, and uric acid) are more susceptible to SWL.[77]

Preoperative determination of stone composition has been proposed using radiological findings such as smooth edges, a homogenous appearance, and a density greater than bone (compared with the twelfth rib) on plain KUB.[77,78]

The use of preoperative non-contrast CT attenuation values (HU) to predict stone composition and/or amenability to SWL has recently been proposed as a significant predictor of failure to fragment renal stones by SWL. An alternative treatment should be devised for patients with stone density >1,000 HU.[71,79–81]

To date, determining stone composition before treatment remains difficult and may not be sufficient to allow prediction of the response to SWL. Therefore, pre-SWL radiographic examinations should focus on those radiological stone characteristics that influence SWL outcome rather than on stone composition.[71]

39.8.4 Renal Abnormalities and SWL

The role of SWL in renal abnormalities is gradually being clarified. For stones in renal diverticula, it is generally agreed that stone clearance remains poor, and stone fragmentation is not always achieved.[82]

In other renal anomalies, the number of renal units (i.e., duplex kidney), the kidney shape (horseshoe, malrotated), and the kidney location (ectopic, crossed) are associated with difficult localization, incomplete clearance, and the presence of pelviureteric junction obstruction, which in itself may hamper stone clearance.[83]

Simple renal cysts and stones in polycystic kidneys are no contraindication for SWL treatment.[84]

39.8.5 Obesity and SWL

Obesity has become an epidemic, predisposing to a number of serious illnesses including stone disease.[85] For these patients, many issues have to be dealt with for successful SWL outcome.

The first problem is diagnosis. Symptoms and physical examination are often not helpful. Imaging studies pose another challenge: Weight restrictions might preclude the use of a KUB film; a stone might be missed because of poor penetration. Ultrasound cannot always identify a stone, and CT might be unavailable in morbidly obese patients or those with respiratory problems due to limitation of the equipment.

For SWL treatment, reinforced tables may be required in such patients, but the distance between F1–F2 focal points may remain insufficient. Abdominal straps to reduce the distance between shock-wave generator and stone, and high-power settings to treat a stone in the extended stone pathway may be helpful.[86]

Flexible ureteroscopy may be a better option in these patients, albeit slightly more invasive.

39.9 Improving the Success Rate of SWL

39.9.1 Shock-wave Rate

Lowering of the shock-wave frequency from usually 120–60 Hz has been reported to increase the fragmentation rates of renal stones.[87]

There is a minimal increase in the procedure time, but it favorably decreases the total number of shock waves to fragment a stone and, in consequence is associated with fewer complications and lower re-treatment rates.[88,89]

The exact mechanism responsible for a rate effect on the efficiency of SWL is still controversial: It may be related to decreased acoustic impedance mismatch, improved cavitation bubble production on the stone surface, or improved bubble dynamics due to water gas content surrounding the stone.[90]

Cavitation bubbles on the surface of the stone implode against the stone surface, and develop high-speed jets that erode the stone surface.[91] Firing a lithotripter at a high rate may cause the second shock to strike the bubbles formed from the first shock before they collapse, thus combining with each other to form a bubble cloud, which results in absorption or dissipation of energy from the second shock wave.[92]

39.9.2 Adjuvant Drug Therapy

Several studies have demonstrated the usefulness of pharmacological therapy in promoting spontaneous ureteral stone passage, thus reducing the time and pain associated with stone expulsion. Medical therapy helps by reducing spasm, edema, and infection.[93] Drugs used are calcium channel blockers, corticosteroids, nonsteroidal anti-inflammatory drugs (NSAIDs), and alpha-blockers.

Medical therapy following SWL to facilitate ureteral stone expulsion results in increased 1- and 2-month stone-free rates and in a lower percentage of those needing re-treatment. The efficacy of nifedipine for the upper-mid ureteral tract associated with ketoprofene makes expulsive medical therapy suitable for improving overall outcomes of SWL treatment for ureteral stones.[94]

In particular, alpha-adrenergic receptors have been detected in the human ureter with a predominance of alpha 1 D receptor subtypes in the lower ureter.[95] *Alpha 1 adrenergic inhibitors* reduce the frequency and intensity of peristalsis of the ureter, with an increase in the flow of urine.[96] They also reduce spasm by relaxing the smooth muscle of the ureter, and act on the C fibers blocking pain conduction.[97,98]

In cases with residual fragments after SWL, re-growth and persistence are common. Citrate therapy significantly improves the stone clearance rate in sterile and infection stone patients, and prevents residual fragment growth or re-aggregation in subjects in whom complete clearance was not achieved.[99]

39.9.3 Percussion, Diuresis, and Inversion (PDI) Therapy

Lower pole stones treated with SWL are less likely to clear than stones in other regions of the collecting system.[87] A combination of percussion (manual or mechanical), inversion (45–70°), and diuresis (500 ml water or 20 mg furosemide with or without 1–2 l of IV fluid) has been used to improve stone clearance after SWL for lower pole stones.[100–104]

39.10 Success Rates of SWL

Factors that significantly affect the success rate include the following:

39.10.1 Stone Size (Largest Diameter)

Stone size is a significant predictor of SWL outcome.[105–108] The success rate for stones <10 mm in diameter is about 90%. For 10–20 mm stones, the overall rate was 66%, while the rate for stones >20 mm was further reduced to 47%. Therefore, SWL is not recommend as primary therapy for stones >20 mm in diameter.[109]

39.10.2 Stone Site

The stone-free rate is significantly higher for pelvic and upper calyceal stones compared to lower calyceal ones. For upper and middle calyceal stones, stone-free rates are between 70–90%, compared to 50–70% for lower calyceal stones.[105,109–112]

39.10.3 Stone Number

Stone number is a significant predictor for success of SWL.[109] In patients with a small-to-medium stone burden, the number of stones is more important than the total stone burden.[105]

The success rate for single stones is 78.3% as compared to 62.8% for multiple ones.[109]

39.10.4 Obstruction

Kidneys obstructed prior to SWL treatment have a significantly lower stone-free rate compared with non-obstructed kidneys. This may be due to a weak peristalsis leading to poor clearance of the fragments.[36,109,113]

The success rate for patients with unobstructed renal units is 83% and 76% for obstructed units.[109]

39.10.5 Congenital Anomalies

The treatment of lithiasis in this entity is controversial due to problems derived from the anatomy of the kidney and its drainage when stones are treated with SWL.[114]

SWL is safe and reliable for treatment of urolithiasis in anomalous kidneys. It should be the primary therapy when the stones are <20 mm. The SWL outcome is comparable for normal and anomalous kidneys when the calculus size is considered. Neither the type of renal anomaly nor the type of lithotripter had any impact on the stone-free rate. The overall stone-free rate in malformed kidneys was 72.2%.[115]

Notably in this group, patients with ureteral duplication had the overall best stone-free rates.[116]

39.11 Special Considerations in SWL

39.11.1 SWL for Uric Acid Stones

Uric acid stones were once regarded as a relative contraindication for SWL with the Dornier HM3 lithotripter because of the difficulty in localizing the radiolucent stones with fluoroscopy.[117,118] However, with the help of intravenous contrast administration, SWL can be the first-line therapy for radiolucent stones[10,11] in particular for fragments entering the ureter. In this case, shock waves should focus 5 mm beyond the end of the column of contrast medium, except where a stone becomes clearly visible within the column.[10,11]

Today, the second generation of lithotripters is equipped with ultrasound guidance, which allows for more accurate and less invasive localization of radiolucent stones.[119] Sonographic localization of a kidney stone requires a highly trained operator. Also, it is almost impossible to view stones in areas such as the middle third of the ureter or when there is an indwelling ureteral catheter. Once a stone is fragmented, it is difficult to identify each individual stone piece. Unfortunately, these disadvantages tend to overshadow the advantages of ultrasound imaging.[8]

Treatment of uric acid stones with ultrasound-guided lithotripters is effective with concurrent application of alkali therapy. Most patients can be stone-free with a minimal risk of complications.[119]

39.11.2 SWL in Children

SWL is currently the first-line treatment for urinary lithiasis in the pediatric age group. The overall stone-free rates are excellent even with SWL monotherapy because children are able to clear stone fragments better than adults[120] due to a shorter and more elastic ureter.[121] Re-treatments with SWL can boost the stone-free rate to up to 100%.[122]

The new generation of lithotripters allows treatments without general anesthesia also in children. These machines have ultrasound real-time tracking systems, which reduce the irradiation needed.[122]

There is a 10–20% loss of shock-wave energy per 6 cm of the body tissue penetrated. Given the smaller body volume of children, shock waves are transmitted with little loss of energy.[123] As a result, a lower kilo-voltage can be used resulting in less pain and complications.[124]

39.11.3 SWL in Pregnancy

Although there have been reports of the inadvertent treatment of pregnant patients with SWL with no adverse sequelae to the fetus, pregnancy remains an absolute contraindication for this treatment modality[125,126] because of the potential disruptive effects of the shock-wave energy on the fetus as proven in numerous experimental studies.[70]

39.11.4 Pacemakers and Implantable Cardioverters/Defibrillators (ICD)

The following protocol has been developed and recommended for patients with pacemakers and implantable cardioverters/defibrillators (ICDs):[127]

- Patients should be monitored via telemetry.
- Equipment for pacemaker/defibrillator interrogation and programming must be readily available, with a resuscitation cart in the lithotripsy suite; a programmer plus a trained physician/nurse must be on site.
- SWL should be immediately terminated when significant arrhythmia develops, and the consulting cardiologist and/or pacemaker/ICD clinic should be notified.
- A decrease in the heart rate consistent with failure of pacing output or an unexplained tachycardia consistent with rate-response activation mandates device interrogation and reprogramming.
- SWL may be continued if premature atrial beats, premature ventricular beats, or controlled atrial fibrillation are the only observed arrhythmia.
- Should pacemaker output be suppressed, the device should be reprogrammed to nonsensing, fixed output mode for the duration of the procedure.
- A magnet may be considered to deactivate tachycardia therapies, especially where the distance between the ICD and F2 is <15 cm.
- Should any concern regarding device function arise, interrogation should be performed before discharge to ensure that there has been no change in programming or battery voltage.

39.12 Conclusions

Renal stone disease is a significant and worldwide health problem, and extracorporeal shock-wave lithotripsy (SWL) has revolutionized the treatment for most patients with urolithiasis since its introduction in the early 1980s. Today, about 80% of all urinary stones and the majority of kidney stones can be successfully treated with SWL in a minimally invasive fashion and most renal stones in adults can be treated in a day case setting.

References

1. Stoller ML. Urinary stone disease. *Smith's general Urology.* 16th edn. 2004;16:275-278.
2. Pak Y. Kidney stones. *Lancet.* 1998;351:1797-1801.
3. Soucie JM, Thun MJ, Coates RJ, et al. Demographic and geographic variability of kidney stones in the United States. *Kidney Int.* 1994;46:893-899.

4. Drach GW, Dretler S, Fair W, et al. Report of United States cooperative study of extracorporeal shock wave lithotripsy. *J Urol.* 1986;135:1127-1133.

5. Ehreth JT, Drach GW, Arnett ML, et al. Extracorporeal shock wave lithotripsy: multicenter study of kidney and upper ureter versus middle and lower ureter treatment. *J Urol.* 1994;152: 1379-1385.

6. Ignatoff JM, Nelson JB. Use of extracorporeal shock wave lithotripsy in a solitary kidney with renal artery aneurysm. *J Urol.* 1993;149:359-360.

7. Loughlin KR. Management of urologic problems during pregnancy. *Urology.* 1994;44:159-169.

8. Lingeman JE, Matalga BR, Evan AP. *Campbell-Walsh Urology.* 9th edn. Saunders, 2007; 44:1465–1485.

9. Cleveland RO, Bailey MR, Hartenbaum B, et al. Design and characterization of a research electrohydraulic lithotripter patterned after the Dornier HM3. *Rev Sci Instrum.* 2000;71:2514-2525.

10. Buchholz NP, van Rossum M. Shock wave lithotripsy treatment of radiolucent ureteric calculi with the help of contrast medium. *Eur Urol.* 2001;39:200-203.

11. Buchholz NP, Van Rossum M. The radiolucent ureteric calculus at the end of a contrast-medium column: where to focus the shock waves. *BJU Int.* 2001;88:325-328.

12. Preminger GM. Sonographic piezoelectric lithotripsy: more bang for your buck. In: Lingeman JE, Newman DM, eds. *Shock Wave Lithotripsy II: Urinary and Biliary Lithotripsy.* New York: Plenum Press; 1989:437-443.

13. Cass AS. Comparison of first generation (Dornier HM3) and second generation (Medstone STS) lithotripters: treatment results with 13, 864 renal and ureteral calculi. *J Urol.* 1995;153: 588-592.

14. Mobley TB, Myers DA, Grine WB, Jenkins JM, Jordan WR. Low energy lithotripsy with the Lithostar: treatment results with 19, 962 renal and ureteral calculi. *J Urol.* 1993;149:1419-1424.

15. Tauzin-Fin P, Delort-Laval S, Krol-Houdek MC, Maurette P, Bannwarth B. Effect of balanced analgesia with buprenorphine on pain response and general anaesthesia requirement during lithotripsy procedures. *Eur J Anaesthesiol.* 1998;15: 147-152.

16. Scheling G, Weber W, Mendl G, Braun H, Cullmann H. Patient controlled analgesia for shock wave lithotripsy: the effect of self-administered alfentanil on pain intensity and drug requirement. *J Urol.* 1996;155:43-47.

17. Bierkens AF, Maes RM, Hendrikx JM, Erdos AF, de Vries JD, Debruyne FM. The use of local anaesthesia in second generation shock wave lithotripsy: eutectic mixture of local anesthetics. *J Urol.* 1991;146:287-289.

18. Loening S, Kramolowsky EV, Willoughby B. Use of local anaesthesia for extracorporeal shock wave lithotripsy. *J Urol.* 1987;137: 626-628.

19. Rasmussen YH, Dahl C. Analgesic requirements for ESWL treatment. A double blind study. *Scand J Urol Nephrol.* 1994;28: 225-227.

20. Alhashemi JA, Kaki AM. Anesthesiologist-controlled versus patient-controlled propofol sedation for shockwave lithotripsy. *Can J Anaesth.* 2006;53:449-455.

21. Gesztesi Z, Rego MM, White PF. The comparative effectiveness of fentanyl and its newer analogs during extracorporeal shock wave lithotripsy under monitored anaesthesia care. *Anesth Analg.* 2000;90:567-570.

22. Parr KL, Lingeman JE, Jordan M, et al. Creatinine kinase concentrations and electrocardiographic changes in extracorporeal shock-wave lithotripsy. *Urology.* 1988;32:21-23.

23. Zommick J, Leveille R, Zabbo A, Colasanto L, Barrette D. Comparison of general anaesthesia and intravenous sedation-analgesia for SWL. *J Endourol.* 1996;10:489-491.

24. Beloeil H, Corsia G, Coriat P, Riou B. Remifentanil compared with sulfentanil during extra-corporeal shock wave lithotripsy with spontaneous ventilation: a double-blind, randomized study. *Br J Anaesth.* 2002;89:567-570.

25. Ozcan S, Yilmaz E, Buyukkocak U, Basar H, Apan A. Comparison of three analgesics for extracorporeal shock wave lithotripsy. *Scand J Urol Nephrol.* 2002;36:281-285.

26. Sulaiman MN, Buchholz NP, Clark PB. The role of ureteral stent placement in the revention of Steinstrasse. *J Endourol.* 1999;13(3): 151-155.

27. Madbouly K, Sheir KZ, Elsobky E, Eraky I, Kenawy M. Risk actors for the formation of steinstrasse after extracorporeal hock wave lithotripsy: a statistical model. *J Urol.* 2002;167: 12349-12442.

28. Streem SB, Yost A. Extracorporeal shock wave lithotripsy in patients with bleeding diatheses. *J Urol.* 1990;144:1347-1348.

29. Gasser TC, Frei R. Risk of bacteraemia during extracorporeal shock wave lithotripsy. *Br J Urol.* 1993;71(1):17-20.

30. De Graaf R, Veith FJ, Gargiulo NJ 3rd, Lipsitz EC, Ohki T, Kurvers HA. Endovascular abdominal aortic aneurysm repair to prevent rupture in a patient requiring lithotripsy. *J Vasc Surg.* 2003;38(6): 1426-1429.

31. Chaussey C, Schmiedt E, Jocham D, Schuller J, Brandl H, Liedl B. ESWL experience in 1,100 patients. Proceedings of the 2nd World Congress on Percutaneous Renal Surgery; 1984; Mainz (Abstract No. 50).

32. Chaussy C, Schmiedt E. Extracorporeal shock wave lithotripsy (ESWL) for kidney stones. An alternative to surgery? *Urol Radiol.* 1984;6:80-87.

33. Vaidyanathan S, Johnson H, Singh G, et al. Atrophy of kidney following extra corporeal shock wave lithotripsy of renal calculus in a paraplegic patient with marked spinal curvature. *Spinal Cord.* 2002;40(11):609-614.

34. Fuchs G, Miller K, Eisenberger F. Extracorporeal shockwave lithotripsy: one year experience with Dornier Lithotripter. *Eur Urol.* 1985;11:145-149.

35. Moody JA, Evans AP, Lingeman JE. Extracorporeal shockwave lithotripsy. In: Weiss RM, George NJR, ÓReilly PH, eds. *Comprehensive Urology.* London: Mosby International Limited; 2001: 623-636.

36. Abdel-Khalek M, Sheir KZ, Mokhtar AA, Eraky I, Kenawy Bazeed M. Prediction of success rate after extracorporeal hock-wave lithotripsy of renal stones – a multivariate analysis model. *Scand J Urol Nephrol.* 2004;38:161-167.

37. Zhong P, Preminger GM. Mechanisms of differing stone ragility in extracorporeal shock wave lithotripsy. *J Endourol.* 1994;8:263-268.

38. Kim SC, Oh CH, Moon YT, Kim KD. Treatment of steinstrasse with repeat extracorporeal shock wave lithotripsy: experience with piezoelectric lithotripter. *J Urol.* 1991;145:489-491.

39. Coptcoat MJ, Webb DR, Kellett MJ, Whitfield HN, Wickham JEA. The steinstrasse: a legacy of extracorporeal lithotripsy? *Eur Urol.* 1988;14:93-95.

40. Fedullo LM, Pollack HM, Banner MP, Amendola MA, Van Arsdalen KN. The development of steinstrassen after ESWL. Frequency, natural history and radiologic management. *AJR Am J Roentgenol.* 1988;151:1145-1147.

41. Roth RA, Beckmann CF. Complications of extracorporeal shock wave lithotripsy and percutaneous nephrolithotomy. *Urol Clin North Am.* 1988;15:155.

42. Hardy MR, McLeod DG. Silent renal obstruction with severe functional loss after extracorporeal shock wave lithotripsy: a report of 2 cases. *J Urol.* 1987;137:91-92.

43. Sayed MAB, El-Taher AM, Aboul-Ella HA, Shaker SE. Steinstrasse after extracorporeal shockwave lithotripsy: aetiology, prevention and management. *BJU Int.* 2001;88:675-678.

44. Dretler S. Management of ureteral calculi. Presented at the 5th World Congress on Endourology and ESWL; November 1–4, 1987: Cairo, Egypt, p 21.

45. Sigman M, Laudone V, Jenkins AD. Ureteral meatotomy as a treatment of steinstrasse following extracorporeal shock wave lithotripsy. J Endourol. 1988;2:41.

46. Riehle RA Jr, Naslund E. Patient management and results after ESWL. In: Riehle RA Jr, Newman RC eds. Principles of Extracorporeal Shock Wave Lithotripsy, Chapter 8. New York: Churchill Livingstone; 1987: 121–144.

47. Yilmaz E, Batislam E, Tuglu D, et al. C-reactive protein in early detection of bacteraemia and bacteriuria after extracorporeal shock wave lithotripsy. Eur Urol. 2003;43:270-274.

48. Dincel C, Ozdiler E, Ozenci H, Tazici N, Kosar A. Incidence of urinary tract infection in patients without bacteriuria undergoing SWL: comparison of stone types. J Endourol. 1998;12:1-3.

49. Pearle MS, Roehrbom CG. Antimicrobial prophylaxis prior to shock wave lithotripsy in patients with sterile urine before treatment: a meta-analysis and cost-effectiveness analysis. Urology. 1997;49:679-686.

50. Basar MM, Samli MM, Erbil M, Ozergin O, Basar R, Atan A. Early effects of extracorporeal shock-wave lithotripsy exposure on testicular sperm morphology. Scand J Urol Nephrol. 2004;38:38-41.

51. Bierkens AF, Hendrikx AJ, Ezz el Din KE, et al. The value of antibiotic prophylaxis during extracorporeal shock wave lithotripsy in the prevention of urinary tract infections in patients with urine proven sterile prior to treatment. Eur Urol. 1997;31:30-35.

52. Kaude JV, Williams CM, Millner MR, et al. Renal morphology and function immediately after extracorporeal shock-wave lithotripsy. AJR Am J Roentgenol. 1985;145:305-313.

53. Kohrmann KU, Rassweiler JJ, Manning M, et al. The clinical introduction of a third generation lithotriptor: Modulith SL 20. J Urol. 1995;153:1379-1383.

54. Piper NY, Dalrymple N, Bishoff JT. Incidence of renal hematoma formation after ESWL using the new Dornier Doli-S lithotripter. J Urol. 2001;165:377.

55. Thuroff S, Thorsten B, Chaussy C. Anatomy related shockwave power using Siemens Lithostar multiline. J Urol. 1988;159(suppl): 34.

56. Ueda S, Matsuko K, Yamashita T, et al. Perirenal hematomas caused by SWL with EDAP LT-01 lithotriptor. J Endourol. 1993;7:11-15.

57. Roessler W, Wieland WF, Steinbach P, et al. Side effects of high-energy shockwaves in the human kidney: first experience with model comparing two shockwave sources. J Endourol. 1996;10:507-511.

58. Evan AP, Willis LR, Connors B, et al. Shock wave lithotripsy–induced renal injury. Am J Kidney Dis. 1991;17:445-450.

59. Evan AP, Willis LR, Lingeman JE, et al. Renal trauma and the risk of long-term complications in shock wave lithotripsy. Nephron. 1998;78:1-8.

60. Lingeman JE, Newman D, Mertz JH, et al. Extracorporeal shock wave lithotripsy: the Methodist Hospital of Indiana experience. J Urol. 1986;135:1134-1137.

61. Ruiz Marcellan FJ, Ibarz Servio L. Evaluation of renal damage in extracorporeal lithotripsy by shock waves. Eur Urol. 1986; 12:73-75.

62. AlKarawi MA, Mohamed AR, El-Etaibi KE, et al. Extracorporeal shock-wave lithotripsy (ESWL)–induced erosions in upper gastro-intestinal tract. Prospective study in 40 patients. Urology. 1987;30:224-227.

63. Chaussy C, Fuchs GJ. Extracorporeal lithotripsy in the treatment of renal lithiasis. 5 years' experience [in French]. J Urol (Paris). 1986;92:339-343.

64. Recker F, Hofmann W, Bex A, Tscholl R. Quantitative determination of urinary marker proteins: a model to detect intrarenal bioeffects after extracorporeal lithotripsy. J Urol. 1992;148:1000-1006.

65. Perez-Blanco FJ, Arrabal Martin M, Ocete Martin C, et al. Urinary glycosaminoglycans after extracorporeal shock wave lithotripsy in patients with kidney lithiasis. Arch Esp Urol. 2001;54:875-883.

66. Neal DE Jr, Kaack MB, Harmon EP, et al. Renin production after experimental extracorporeal shock wave lithotripsy: a primate model. J Urol. 1991;146:548-550.

67. Jewett MA, Bombardier C, Logan AG, et al. A randomized controlled trial to assess the incidence of new onset hypertension in patients after shock wave lithotripsy for asymptomatic renal calculi. J Urol. 1998;160:1241-1243.

68. Yokoyama M, Shoji F, Yanagizawa R, et al. Blood pressure changes following extracorporeal shock-wave lithotripsy for urolithiasis. J Urol. 1992;147:553-557.

69. Vieweg J, Weber HM, Miller K, Hautmann R. Female fertility following extracorporeal shock wave lithotripsy of distal ureteral calculi. J Urol. 1992;148:1007-1010.

70. Ohmori K, Matsuda T, Horii Y, Yoshida O. Effects of shock waves on the mouse fetus. J Urol. 1994;151:255-258.

71. El-Nahas AR, El-Assmy AM, Mansour O, Sheir KZ. A prospective multivariate analysis of factors predicting stone disintegration by extracorporeal shock wave lithotripsy: the value of high-resolution noncontrast computed tomography. Eur Urol. 2007;51:1688-1694.

72. Kim FJ, Rice KR. Prediction of shockwave failure in patients with urinary tract stones. Curr Opin Urol. 2006;16:88-92.

73. Ghoneim IA, Ziada AM, El-Katib SE. Predictive factors of lower calyceal stone clearance after Extracorporeal Shockwave Lithotripsy (ESWL): a focus on the Infundibulopelvic anatomy. Eur Urol. 2005;48:296-302.

74. Skolarikos A, Alivizatos G, de la Rosette J. Extracorporeal shock wave lithotripsy 25 years later: complications and their prevention. Eur Urol. 2006;50:981-990.

75. Buchholz NP, Rhabar HM, Talati J. Is the measurement of stone surface area necessary for the shock wave treatment of non-staghorn calculi? J Endourol. 2002;16(4):215-220.

76. Pittomvils G, Vandeursen H, Wevers M, et al. The influence of internal stone structure upon the fracture behavior of urinary calculi. Ultrasound Med Biol. 1994;20:803-810.

77. Bon D, Dore B, Irani J, et al. Radiographic prognostic criteria for extracorporeal shock-wave lithotripsy: a study of 485 patients. Urology. 1996;48:556-561.

78. Mostafavi MR, Ernst RD, Saltzman B. Accurate determination of chemical composition of urinary calculi by spiral computerized tomography. J Urol. 1998;159:673-675.

79. Saw KC, McAteer JA, Fineberg NS, et al. Calcium stone fragility is predicted by helical CT attenuation values. J Endourol. 2000;14:465-468.

80. Saw KC, McAteer JA, Monga AG, et al. Helical CT of urinary calculi: effect of stone composition, stone size, and scan collimation. AJR Am J Roentgenol. 2000;175:329-332.

81. Albala DM, Assimos DG, Clayman RV, et al. Lower pole I: a prospective randomized trial of extracorporeal shock wave lithotripsy and percutaneous nephrostolithotomy for lower pole nephrolithiasis initial results. J Urol. 2001;166:2072.

82. Bilgasem S, Pace KT, Dyer S, Honey RJ. Erect and supine radiographs to assess effectiveness of SWL for stones in a calyceal diverticulum or dilated calyx. J Endourol. 2003;17:7-9.

83. Gross AJ, Herrmann TR. Management of stones in calyceal diverticulum. Curr Opin Urol. 2007;17:136-140.

84. Ng CS, Yost A, Streen SB. Nephrolithiasis associated with autosomal dominant polycystic kidney disease: contemporary urological management. J Urol. 2000;163(3):726-729.

85. World Health Organisation. *Obesity: Preventing and Managing the Global Epidemic.* Geneva: World Health Organisation; 1997.

86. Thomas R, Cass AS. Extracorporeal shock wave lithotripsy in morbidly obese patients. *J Urol.* 1993;150:30-32.

87. Kekre NS, Kumar S. Optimizing the fragmentation and clearance after shock wave lithotripsy. *Curr Opin Urol.* 2008;18: 205-209.

88. Kenneth TP, Daniela G, Melanie H. Shockwave lithotripsy at 60 or 120 shocks per minute: a randomized, double-blind trial. *J Urol.* 2005;174:595-599.

89. Derek W, Courtney L, Roland U, Manoj M. Impact of shockwave coupling of efficacy of extracorporeal shockwave lithotripsy. *J Endourol.* 2007;21:137-140.

90. Choi MJ, Coleman AJ, Saunders JE. The influence of fluid properties and pulse amplitude on bubble urodynamics in the field of shock wave lithotripter. *Phys Med Biol.* 1993;38:1561-1573.

91. Coleman AJ, Saunder JE. A survey of the acoustic output of commercial extracorporeal shockwave lithotriptors. *Ultrasound Med Biol.* 1989;15:213-217.

92. Allancien G, Munoz R, Borghi M, et al. Relationship between the frequency of piezoelectric shock waves and the quality of renal stone fragmentation. *Eur Urol.* 1989;16:41-44.

93. Porpiglia F, Destefanis P, Fiori C, Fontana D. Effectiveness of nifedipine and deflazocort in the management of distal ureteral stones. *Urology.* 2000;56:579-582.

94. Micali S, Grande M, Sighinolfi MC, De Stefani S, Bianchi G. Efficacy of expulsive therapy using nifedipine or tamsulosin, both associated with ketoprofene, after shock wave lithotripsy of ureteral stones. *Urol Res.* 2007;35(3):133-137.

95. Sigala S, Dellabella M, Milanese G, et al. Evidence for the presence of alpha 1 adrenoceptor subtypes in the human ureter. *Neurourol Urodyn.* 2005;24:142-158.

96. Dellabella M, Milanese G, Muzzonigro G. Efficacy of tamsulosin in the medical management of juxtavesical ureteral stones. *J Urol.* 2003;170:2202-2205.

97. Ishigooka M, Nakada T, Hashimoto T, et al. Spinal substance P immunoreactivity is enhanced by acute chemical stimulation of the rat prostate. *Urology.* 2002;59:139-144.

98. Kinnman E, Nygards EB, Hansson P. Peripheral alpha adrenoreceptors are involved in the development of capsaicin induced ongoing and stimulus evoked pain in humans. *Pain.* 1997; 69:79-85.

99. Cicerello E, Merlo F, Gambaro G, et al. Effect of alkaline citrate therapy on clearance of residual renal stone fragments after extracorporeal shock wave lithotripsy in sterile calcium and infection nephrolithiasis patients. *J Urol.* 1994;151(1):5-9.

100. Brownlee N, Foster M, Griffith DP, et al. Controlled inversion therapy: an adjunct to the elimination of gravity-dependent fragments following extracorporeal shock wave lithotripsy. *J Urol.* 1990;143:1096-1098.

101. Rodrigues Netto N Jr, Claro JF, Cortado PL, et al. Adjunct controlled inversion therapy following extracorporeal shockwave lithotripsy for lower pole caliceal stones. *J Urol.* 1991;146: 953-954.

102. Pace KT, Tariq N, Dyer SJ, et al. Mechanical percussion, inversion and diuresis for residual lower pole fragments after shockwave lithotripsy: a prospective single blind, randomized controlled trial. *J Urol.* 2001;166:2065-2071.

103. Honey JD, Luymes J, Weir MJ, et al. Mechanical percussion inversion can result in relocation of lower pole stone fragments after shock wave lithotripsy. *Urology.* 2000;55:204-206.

104. Chiong E, Hwee STP, Kay LM, et al. Randomized controlled study of mechanical percussion, diuresis and inversion therapy to assist passage of lower pole renal calculi after shock wave lithotripsy. *Urology.* 2005;65:1070-1074.

105. Ackermann DK, Fuhrimann R, Pfluger D, et al. Prognosis after extracorporeal shock wave lithotripsy of radiopaque renal calculi: a multivariate analysis. *Eur Urol.* 1994;25:105-109.

106. Cohen TD, Preminger GH. Management of calyceal calculi. *Urol Clin North Am.* 1997;24:81-86.

107. Lalak NJ, Moussa SA, Smith G, Tolley DA. The Dornier compact Delta lithotriptor: the first 500 renal calculi. *J Endourol.* 2002;16:3-7.

108. Sorensen CM, Chandhoke PS. Is lower pole calyceal anatomy predictive of extracorporeal shock wave lithotripsy success for primary lower pole kidney stones? *J Urol.* 2002;168:2377-2382.

109. Al Ansari A, As-Sadiq K, Al-Said S, et al. Prognostic factors of success of extracorporeal shock wave lithotripsy (ESWL) in the treatment of renal stones. *Int Urol Nephrol.* 2006;38:63-67.

110. Rassweiller J, Kohrmann KU, Alken P. ESWL, including imaging. *Curr Opin Urol.* 1992;2:291-299.

111. Tolon M, Miroglu C, Erol H, et al. A report on extracorporeal shock wave lithotripsy results on 1569 units in an outpatient clinic. *J Urol.* 1991;145:695-698.

112. Zanetti G, Montanari E, Mandressi A, et al. Long-term results of extracorporeal shock wave lithotripsy in renal stone treatment. *J Endourol.* 1991;5:61-64.

113. Poulakis V, Dahm P, Witzsch U, et al. Prediction of lower pole stone clearance after shock wave lithotripsy using an artificial renal network. *J Urol.* 2003;169:1250-1256.

114. Gómez Pascual JA, Soler Martínez J, García Galisteo E, et al. Extracorporeal shock-wave lithotripsy as treatment of lithiasis in horseshoe kidney. *Arch Esp Urol.* 2003;56(1):39-44.

115. Sheir KZ, Madbouly K, Elsobky E, Abdelkhalek M. Extracorporeal shock wave lithotripsy in anomalous kidneys: 11-year experience with two second-generation lithotripters. *Urology.* 2003;62(1): 10-15. discussion 15–6.

116. Küpeli B, Isen K, Biri H, et al. Extracorporeal shockwave lithotripsy in anomalous kidneys. *J Endourol.* 1999;13(5):349-352.

117. Chaussy CG, Schmiedt E. Shock wave treatment for stones in the upper urinary tract. *Urol Clin North Am.* 1983;10:743-746.

118. Royce PL, Fuchs GJ, Lupu AN, et al. The treatment of uric acid calculi with extracorporeal shock wave lithotripsy. *Br J Urol.* 1987;60:6-9.

119. Sun XZ, Zhang ZW. Shock wave lithotripsy for uric acid stones. *Asian J Surg.* 2006;29(1):36-39.

120. Gofrit ON, Pode D, Meretyk S, et al. Is the pediatric ureters as efficient as the adult ureter in transporting fragments following ESWL for renal calculi larger than 10 mm? *J Urol.* 2001;166:1862-1864.

121. Jayanthi VR, Arnold PM, Koff SA. Strategies for managing upper tract calculi in young children. *J Urol.* 1999;162:1234-1237.

122. D'Addessi A, Bongiovanni L, Sasso F, et al. Extracorporeal shock-wave lithotripsy in pediatrics. *J Endourol.* 2008;22(1):1-11.

123. Spirnak JP, Resnick MJ. Extracorporeal Shockwave Lithotripsy. In: Resnick MJ, Pak CYC, eds. *Urolithiasis: A Medical and Surgical References.* Philadelphia: WB Saunders; 1990:351-363.

124. Longo JA, Rodrigues Netto N Jr. Extracorporeal shockwave lithotripsy in children. *Urology.* 1995;46:550-552.

125. Chaussy C, Fuchs GJ. Current state and future developments of noninvasive treatment of human urinary stones with extracorporeal shock wave lithotripsy. *J Urol.* 1989;141(pt 2):782-789.

126. Frankenschmidt A, Sommerkamp H. Shock wave lithotripsy during pregnancy: a successful clinical experiment. *J Urol.* 1998;159: 501-502.

127. Platonv MA, Gillis AM, Kavanagh KM. Pacemakers, implantable cardioverter/defibrillators, and extracorporeal shockwave lithotripsy: evidence-based Guidelines for the modern era. *J Endourol.* 2008;22:243-247.

Extracorporeal Shock Wave Lithotripsy for Ureteral Stones

Jay D. Raman and Margaret S. Pearle

Abstract Shock wave lithotripsy has been utilized for the management of ureteral calculi since its introduction in the 1980s, although historically its use was limited to the treatment of proximal ureteral calculi. Currently, stones in all locations of the ureters can be treated successfully with SWL, albeit occasionally with the need for special positioning or use of ureteral catheters or intravenous contrast to facilitate localization. The feasibility and success of SWL for ureteral calculi are influenced by stone size, location, and composition, as well as on patient anatomy and comorbidities. Recent investigations have demonstrated that treatment parameters can be optimized and a variety of adjuvant measures can be utilized to enhance success rates and increase the safety of the procedure. Current guidelines endorse the use of SWL for the management of most patients with small-to-moderate-sized ureteral calculi.

40.1 Introduction

Since the initial report by Chaussy and colleagues almost 30 years ago, shock wave lithotripsy (SWL) has revolutionized the management of urolithiasis.[1] Presently, it remains the sole noninvasive surgical treatment modality for urinary tract calculi. The minimally invasive nature, relative lack of serious adverse sequelae, and, in some cases, avoidance of general anesthesia make SWL an attractive option for many patients. However, success with SWL is not universal, and stone fragmentation and passage depend on a variety of factors including patient characteristics, stone composition and location, renal anatomy, and choice of lithotriptor.

Since the introduction of SWL, proximal ureteral calculi have generally been considered amenable to successful SWL treatment. However, middle and lower ureteral calculi were initially excluded from SWL therapy owing to challenging patient positioning and difficult stone localization with first-generation lithotripters. With the introduction of newer generations of lithotripters with alternate shock wave (SW) sources, multifunctional tables, and improved imaging systems, indications expanded to include ureteral calculi in all locations. However, what is possible is not always appropriate. As such, it is advisable to carefully review clinical indications, outcomes, and complications when considering SWL for the management of ureteral calculi. This chapter highlights clinical considerations and new concepts with regard to SWL treatment of ureteral calculi.

40.2 Indications and Contraindications

40.2.1 Indications

The indications for surgical management of ureteral calculi include refractory pain, high grade or prolonged obstruction, concomitant infection, and failure or low likelihood of spontaneous stone passage.[2] In the setting of an obstructing stone with clinical signs of infection, definitive surgical management is deferred in lieu of adequate drainage of the obstructed, infected kidney. In this setting, either nephrostomy drainage or ureteral stent placement is acceptable drainage modality and should be instituted promptly.[3]

Although most ureteral stones will pass spontaneously, many do so with significant pain, morbidity, and potential loss of work. The introduction of medical expulsive therapy has resulted in an increased likelihood of spontaneous stone passage and reduced pain associated with passage. In a

J.D. Raman (✉)
Department of Surgery, Penn State Milton S. Hershey Medical Center,
Hershey, PA, USA
e-mail: jraman@hmc.psu.edu

P.N. Rao et al. (eds.), *Urinary Tract Stone Disease*,
DOI 10.1007/978-1-84800-362-0_40, © Springer-Verlag London Limited 2011

meta-analysis of nine randomized clinical trials (RCTs), Hollingsworth and associates found a risk ratio of 1.65 (95% CI 1.45–1.88, $p < 0.0001$) in favor of medical expulsive therapy.[4] Both alpha adrenergic receptor antagonists and calcium channel blockers showed efficacy in improving spontaneous passage rates, and some trials have additionally demonstrated reduced need for analgesics. Consequently, medical expulsive agents have changed the natural history of ureteral stones by increasing spontaneous passage rates and reducing the need for surgical intervention.

For patients with stones that fail or are unlikely to pass, or those with high grade or prolonged obstruction, the primary surgical modalities are shock wave lithotripsy (SWL) and ureteroscopy (URS). Additional, less commonly utilized treatment modalities include percutaneous antegrade ureteroscopy and ureterolithotomy (either open or laparoscopic), which are primarily used for large proximal or mid ureteral calculi or for SWL or URS failures, respectively.

40.2.2 Contraindications

Historically, contraindications to SWL have included pregnancy, middle or distal ureteral calculi in young girls or women of childbearing age, infected urine, irreversible coagulopathy or bleeding diathesis, implanted cardiac devices, and calcified vascular aneurysms (Table 40.1). Of these, pregnancy remains an absolute contraindication to SWL due to a theoretical risk to the fetus from shock waves[5]; although an anecdotal report of six women who were retrospectively found to be 1–4 weeks pregnant at the time of SWL found that all women bore healthy children without chromosomal abnormalities.[6] There is, however, continued debate regarding the potential deleterious effect of SWL on ovarian tissues when treating middle and distal ureteral calculi. In 1988, McCullough and colleagues exposed rat ovaries directly to shock waves and found no associated histologic changes.[7] Furthermore, in a retrospective study of human patients, Vieweg and colleagues reported no increased incidence of miscarriage or infertility in 84 women of childbearing age, among whom 6 women collectively gave birth to 7 healthy babies.[8] Although the experimental and limited clinical data suggests that the ovary is resistant to the effects of shock waves, absolute safety for SWL of middle/distal calculi cannot be assured.

Calcified vascular aneurysms, implantable cardiac devices, and bleeding diathesis have been historically believed to be contraindications to SWL. However, increasing evidence suggests that SWL can be safely performed in many of these clinical scenarios, particularly in patients with ureteral calculi.[2] Both Abber and colleagues and Vasavada and co-workers demonstrated in in vitro models that calcified vascular tissue is relatively resistant to the effects of shock waves.[9,10] Furthermore, clinical experience has shown that patients with asymptomatic ipsilateral calcified aneurysms with a diameter <2 cm for renal artery aneurysms and <5 cm for aortic aneurysms that are located >5 cm from the target stone can be safely treated with SWL.[11]

When treating patients with implantable cardiac devices, secondary backup equipment should be made available and the device should be tested both before and immediately after the procedure. Of note, shock waves can damage the piezoelectric crystals of abdominally implanted cardiac devices thus excluding patients with these specific devices from SWL therapy.[12]

Finally, SWL is an acceptable treatment modality in patients with a *reversible* coagulopathy due to hemophilia, von Willebrand's disease, or advanced liver disease, provided the coagulopathy is corrected both before and for 24–48 h following therapy.[13] Furthermore, close observation is warranted as treatment in these patients poses a higher risk of post-procedural bleeding. Patients in whom the coagulopathy cannot or should not be reversed can be managed by an alternative treatment modality, such as ureteroscopy.[14,15]

40.3 Factors Impacting Outcomes of SWL for Ureteral Calculi

Outcomes of SWL for ureteral calculi depend on a variety of intrinsic factors, including stone characteristics (size and composition), stone location, and ureteral anatomy, and are impacted by type of lithotripter, treatment-related variables (shock wave rate and energy), and use of adjuvant medical therapy (Table 40.2).

40.3.1 Intrinsic Factors

40.3.1.1 Stone Size

In general, success rates for SWL vary inversely with stone size. According to the 2007 Ureteral Stones Clinical Guidelines Panel, median stone-free rates for proximal,

Table 40.1 Contraindications for shock wave lithotripsy (SWL) of ureteral calculi

Absolute contraindications
Pregnancy
Uncorrectable coagulopathy
Active infection
Relative contraindications
Women of childbearing age
Implantable cardiac devices
Calcified vascular aneurysms
Reversible bleeding diathesis

Table 40.2 Factors impacting outcomes of SWL for ureteral calculi

Intrinsic factors

    Stone size

    Stone composition

    Stone location

    Presence of impaction or obstruction

Patient factors

    Body habitus

    Patient positioning

    Stone localization

Extrinsic factors

    Type of lithotriptor

    Treatment parameters

    Adjuvant medical therapies

middle, and distal ureteral calculi were higher for ≤10 mm stones than stones >10 mm (90% versus 68%, respectively, for proximal stones; 84% versus 76%, respectively, for middle ureteral stones; and 86% versus 74%, respectively, for distal stones).[16,17]

40.3.1.2 Composition

Stone composition plays a significant role in determining the clinical efficacy of SWL. Effective stone fragmentation by shock waves requires transmission through an acoustic interface between the stone and a fluid medium. By different mechanisms, matrix and cystine calculi provide poor acoustic interfaces. Shock waves are limited in their ability to penetrate through the amorphous structure of matrix stones, that are comprised of a gelatinous mixture of water, sugars, and protein.[18] On the other hand, cystine calculi are uniquely hard stones owing to the multiple disulfide bonds that collectively stabilize its crystalline structure. Consequently, cystine stones generally require more shockwaves with higher amplitude for fragmentation, thereby limiting the size of cystine stones that can be successfully managed by SWL.[19] However, Bhatta and colleagues recognized two morphologic subtypes of cystine stones, "rough" and "smooth," that differed in their response to SWL.[20] Using micro-computed tomography (CT) imaging, Kim and associates validated these two morphologic subtypes and showed differences in the internal structure of "rough" (stones with internal low attenuation areas) and "smooth" (stones with a homogeneous CT appearance) subtypes that corresponded in vitro to fragmentation efficiency with SWL.[21]

The precise stone composition for most patients undergoing SWL is not known in advance. In addition, the responsiveness of stones to SWL varies considerably even among patients with chemically similar calculi.[22] Attempts to predict the composition of stones preoperatively using computed tomography attenuation coefficients has met with limited success, largely because of overlapping values, particularly among calcium-containing stones.[23] However, CT attenuation coefficients may predict the likelihood of successful SWL fragmentation, without regard to precise stone composition. Sacco and associates retrospectively evaluated 112 patients undergoing SWL for ureteral calculi and found that SWL success correlated with stone size and Hounsfield units (HU).[24] In this study, no patients with ureteral calculi >6 mm in size and HU > 1,000 were rendered stone free by SWL monotherapy. Likewise, Pareek and colleagues reviewed 50 patients with upper urinary tract calculi including 30 with ureteral calculi.[25] Among the patients with ureteral calculi, those rendered stone free (70%, 21/30) had a mean HU of 505 compared with a mean HU of 889 in the nine patients with residual fragments. Collectively, these studies suggest that use of attenuation coefficients measured on unenhanced CT may predict the treatment outcome of SWL, thereby facilitating treatment selection.

40.3.1.3 Stone Location

Stone location factors prominently into SWL success rates for a variety of reasons. Even well-fragmented proximal ureteral stones have a longer distance to traverse and a greater chance of being retained before reaching the bladder than more distally located stones. In addition, location in the ureter impacts stone visibility on fluoroscopy and dictates the patient position required to facilitate or enable stone targeting. For example, middle ureteral stones are often obscured by the underlying pelvic bone, which additionally attenuates shock waves. As such, patients with middle ureteral calculi are optimally treated in the prone position in order to provide a shorter path to the anteriorly located stone and to avoid attenuation of the shock waves by the pelvic bone. As a result of these confounding factors, SWL stone-free rates differ with stone location in the ureter. According to the Ureteral Stones Clinical Guidelines Panel analysis, stones in the proximal, middle, and distal ureter were associated with stone-free rates of 83%, 73%, and 74%, respectively.

40.3.1.4 Impacted/Obstructing Ureteral Calculi

Experimental evidence suggests that shock waves do not fragment ureteral calculi as efficiently as renal calculi. Several investigators proposed that stone impaction and the lack of a sufficient stone-fluid interface account for this poorer fragmentation. Indeed, both Muller and colleagues and Parr and associates used a model in which stones were embedded in rubber tubing to simulate ureteral calculi and showed that as the longitudinal tension of the tubing was increased (mimicking increasing stone impaction), stone fragmentation decreased.[26,27]

As a result of these findings, many investigators advocated bypassing ureteral stones with a ureteral stent or pushing the stone back into the kidney prior to SWL. However, prospective, randomized clinical trials (RCTs) for SWL of proximal ureteral stones have failed to show a statistically significant difference in stone-free rates between patients treated with in situ SWL versus those treated with stent bypass or push-back.[28–31] Furthermore, the 1997 Ureteral Stone Clinical Guidelines Panel found no advantage in routine placement of a ureteral stent when treating ureteral calculi with SWL.[32] Median stone-free rates for patients with proximal ureteral calculi (above the iliac vessels) treated with push-back, stent bypass, or in situ SWL were 88%, 82%, and 82%, respectively. For distal ureteral calculi (below the iliac vessels), the corresponding stone-free rates were 79%, 86%, and 82%, respectively. These findings led the Panel to conclude as a Guideline that "Routine stenting to increase efficiency of fragmentation is not recommended as part of shock wave lithotripsy," and the 2007 Guideline reiterated this recommendation.[16,17]

The use of in situ SWL in the setting of an acutely obstructing ureteral calculus has been controversial. Cass and colleagues used in situ SWL to treat 13 patients with acutely obstructing ureteral calculi, associated hydronephrosis, and absence of contrast distal to the stone on intravenous urogram and reported a 92% success rate.[33] However, Srivastava and co-workers concluded that the degree of obstruction inversely correlates with the success rate of in situ SWL.[34] Among 51 patients with proximal ureteral stones treated with in situ SWL, those without impaction (minimal or no hydronephrosis) had a success rate of 93%, while those with impacted stones (moderate or severe hydronephrosis) had a success rate of only 35%. Likewise, Tligui and colleagues reported on 200 patients with obstructing ureteral stones (mean size 7 mm) and colic either refractory to medical therapy or recurring within 24 h, who underwent immediate SWL with the EDAP LT-02 lithotriptor.[35] At 3-month follow-up, 82% of patients (164/200) were stone free, including 38% of patients who required 2–3 SWL sessions. The authors concluded that immediate SWL for acute renal colic secondary to obstructing ureteral calculi yields acceptable stone-free rates with low associated morbidity.

In a recent RCT, Tombal and associates assessed the efficacy of emergency SWL on the short-term outcome of symptomatic ureteral stones.[36] Among 100 patients randomized to medical therapy alone or combined with SWL, the authors found that at 48 h after treatment, SWL was associated with a 13% incremental improvement in stone-free rate over medical therapy alone, with the greatest improvement occurring among patients with large proximal ureteral calculi (40% for

proximal stones >5 mm versus only 1.8% for distal stones <5 mm). Overall, the balance of the evidence suggests that SWL for acutely obstructing ureteral calculi is an acceptable therapeutic option.

40.3.2 Patient Factors

40.3.2.1 Body Habitus

Body habitus, particularly related to obesity, can impact the decision to perform SWL on patients with ureteral calculi. Weight limits on the lithotriptor table,[2] a skin-to-stone distance that exceeds the focal length of the lithotripter[37] and poor image quality (both fluoroscopy and ultrasound) due to excessive body fat, can all contribute to inability to treat, or poor outcomes with treatment, the obese patient. Other patient factors, such as severe scoliosis or contractures, may hinder the ability to properly position the patient or target the stone. In these cases, endoscopic stone management may be preferable.

40.3.2.2 Patient Positioning and Stone Localization

Patient positioning is critical to successful SWL of ureteral calculi. Adjacent hollow viscus structures merit consideration for stones in the proximal ureter, while the overlying pelvic bone presents a challenge for calculi in the middle and distal ureter. Goktas and co-workers randomized 48 patients with a single <1 cm proximal ureteral calculus to SWL in the supine or prone position.[38] They found no difference in stone-free rates in the two groups, although patients in the supine position better tolerated the procedure and required a fewer numbers of shocks for successful fragmentation. Hara and colleagues also compared 248 patients with proximal ureteral calculi treated in the supine position with 156 patients treated in the semilateral/rotated position.[39] The authors theorized that the transverse processes of the vertebrae could interfere with shockwave transmission in the supine position and that a semilateral approach might alleviate this problem. Although stone-free rates in the two groups were similar (94.8% versus 97.4%, respectively), the number of sessions required to render patients stone free who were treated in the semilateral position was less than that required for patients treated in the supine position (1.49 versus 1.74, $p = 0.023$). Similar positioning modifications have been proposed for distal ureteral calculi whereby patients are placed prone or the horse-riding position in order to allow the shock waves to enter the pelvis unimpeded by the pelvic bone.

Because of underlying bony structures, the administration of intravenous contrast, the instillation of contrast via a ureteral catheter, or placement of a ureteral stent may be necessary to facilitate identification of ureteral calculi (particularly in the middle ureter). Most third-generation lithotriptors are equipped with high-resolution fluoroscopy systems that permit reliable identification and in situ treatment of ureteral calculi, a significant improvement over the ultrasound-based second-generation lithotriptors.

40.3.3 Extrinsic Factors

40.3.3.1 Type of Lithotriptor

The original Dornier HM3 lithotriptor (Dornier Medical Systems, Marietta, GA) introduced in the 1980s used spark gap technology, a water bath coupler, fluoroscopic imaging, and general anesthesia. Subsequent generations of lithotriptors varied the shock wave generator (electromagnetic, piezoelectric), eliminated the water bath (water pool or cushion), added ultrasound imaging, provided a multifunctional table, and reduced anesthesia requirements. Furthermore, the shock wave aperture was broadened to reduce shock wave energy density at the skin, thereby decreasing treatment-associated pain and eliminating the need for general anesthesia. Nonetheless, increasing evidence suggests that stone-free rates are equivalent or have declined with newer generation lithotriptors. Few randomized trials have directly compared outcomes with different lithotriptors. Gerber and colleagues reported a prospective, randomized trial comparing patients with renal stones treated with SWL on the Dornier HM3 with those treated on the Siemens Lithostar Plus and additionally compared those patients to a matched consecutively treated series of 107 patients treated with the Modulith SLX.[40] On postoperative day 1, stone-free rates were superior in the HM3 group (91%) compared with the Lithostar Plus (65%) and SLX (48%) groups, and accordingly retreatment rates were progressively higher in the three groups (4%, 13%, and 38%, respectively). Similarly, Chan and associates prospectively randomized 198 patients with solitary renal ($n=132$) or ureteral calculi ($n=66$) to lithotripsy with the Dornier HM3 versus the MFL 5000 lithotriptor. At 12 weeks follow-up, there was no statistically or clinically significant difference in stone-free rates between the two lithotriptors for calculi in the kidney or ureter.[41]

In select patients with small distal ureteral calculi, good results have been reported with the use of office-based electromagnetic or piezoelectric SWL using ultrasound imaging and sedation. Jermini and colleagues reported that of 165 carefully selected patients with small distal ureteral calculi (of whom 97%

had stones <10 mm and none with stones >15 mm), 99% were stone free at 3 months and only 7% required retreatment.[42]

40.3.3.2 Treatment Parameters

Early lithotriptors were typically gated to the QRS complex of the electrocardiogram resulting in shock wave (SW) rates that rarely exceeded 60–80 SW per minute. Second- and third-generation lithotriptors were associated with a low risk of cardiac arrhythmias and thereby allowed nongated SWL and shorter treatment times. Both in vitro and animal studies, however, have suggested that slower SW rate during SWL is associated with superior calculus fragmentation.[43–45] The proposed mechanisms for these observations include decreased acoustic impedance mismatch and improved cavitation bubble production on the stone surface.

In the first clinical trial assessing outcomes according to SW rate, Pace and colleagues randomized 149 patients with >5 mm renal calculi to slow (60 SW/min) or fast (120 SW/min) SW rate and found that slow rate yielded better 3-month stone-free rates than fast rate (60% versus 44%, $p=0.064$), a difference that was further magnified for large ($\geq100^2$ mm) renal calculi (60% versus 28%, $p=0.015$).[46] To date, four published RCTs, comprising nearly 600 patients, have compared SWL outcomes with slow and fast SW rate. Semins and associates performed a meta-analysis of these 4 RCTs and found that patients treated at slow SW rate (60 SW/min) had a 10% higher likelihood of becoming stone free than patients treated at fast SW rate (120 SW/min) ($p=0.0002$).[47]

The only trial specifically addressing SW rate for the treatment of ureteral stones was reported by Pace and colleagues who randomized 157 patients with ≥5 mm proximal ureteral calculi to SWL at a rate of 60 SW/min or 120 SW/min.[48] The slower SW rate group had a higher stone-free rate (68% versus 51%, respectively, $p=0.03$), lower rate of auxiliary procedures (31% versus 47%, respectively, $p=0.03$), and required fewer cumulative shock waves (2,667 versus 2,938, respectively, $p<0.001$) than the fast SW group, although at a cost of longer operative duration (44 versus 24.5 min, respectively, $p<0.001$).

40.3.3.3 Adjuvant Medical Therapies

A variety of drugs have been tested for their effectiveness in promoting spontaneous stone passage. Among these, alpha (α) adrenergic antagonists and calcium channel blockers, with or without corticosteroids, have proven their benefit as medical expulsive agents that not only promote spontaneous stone passage but also reduce the time interval and associated pain of stone expulsion.[4] Based on the success of these agents in facilitating spontaneous stone passage, several investigators have explored their effectiveness in improving clearance rates after SWL of ureteral calculi.

Kupeli and co-workers reviewed 78 patients with distal ureteral stones, 30 of whom had stones <5 mm not requiring SWL and 48 who underwent SWL for calculi >5 mm (range 6–15 mm).[49] Half the patients in each group received analgesic alone, while the other half received tamsulosin 0.4 mg daily along with analgesic. At 15 days following treatment, patients who received tamsulosin after SWL had the highest stone-free rate (71%) of the four groups, particularly compared with the group undergoing SWL alone in whom the stone-free rate was only 33.3%. Gravas and colleagues performed a similar study whereby 61 patients with ≥6 mm distal ureteral calculi (mean 8.4 mm) treated with SWL were randomized to tamsulosin 0.4 mg or placebo for 1 month.[50] Unlike the previous study, these investigators failed to demonstrate a difference in stone-free rates or expulsion time between the two groups, although patients administered with tamsulosin did have a significantly reduced analgesic requirement. Finally, in an RCT involving 60 patients with a solitary renal or ureteral calculus undergoing SWL, Bhagat and colleagues treated patients with either 0.4 mg of tamsulosin or placebo until stone clearance or for a maximum of 30 days.[51] Compared to the placebo arm, the tamsulosin group showed a significantly higher clearance rate (97% versus 79%, $p = 0.04$). In addition, the average dose of analgesic used and rates of steinstrasse were also lower (albeit insignificantly) in the tamsulosin group.

Porpiglia and co-workers evaluated the effectiveness of nifedipine and corticosteroids versus no drug treatment in facilitating clearance of fragments after SWL on a Sonolith 4,000+ (EDAP, Technomed Medical Systems) in an RCT involving 80 patients with ureteral calculi.[52] The treatment arm demonstrated a higher stone-free rate (75% versus 50%, $p = 0.02$) and had lower pain medication requirements (37.5 mg versus 86.25 mg of diclofenac, respectively, $p = 0.02$) than the no-treatment control group.

Micali and colleagues also prospectively evaluated 113 patients with ureteral calculi undergoing SWL using a Dornier Lithotriptor S, in whom a subgroup comprised of those with upper or middle ureteral calculi was treated with nifedipine (30 mg/day for 14 days) and those with distal ureteral calculi was treated with tamsulosin (0.4 mg/day for 14 days).[53] The treatment groups were compared to a control group of 50 patients who received no adjuvant medical therapy. Stone-free rates were comparable between the two adjuvant therapy groups (86% for the nifedipine group and 82% for the tamsulosin group) and were significantly higher than the two control groups (upper and distal ureteral

calculi) for which stone-free rates were 52% and 57%, respectively.

Overall, these studies provide compelling evidence to recommend the use of medical expulsive agents to improve clearance of fragments after SWL treatment of ureteral calculi.

40.4 Clinical Efficacy

Despite extensive published series on SWL for patients with ureteral calculi, comparison between studies is problematic owing to nonuniform and/or poorly defined patient populations, different lithotriptors and treatment parameters, variability in reporting (i.e., stone-free versus "success" rates, single treatment versus retreatment rates, nonuniform definition of auxiliary procedure rates), and inconsistent use of adjuvant therapies. To date, the most comprehensive analysis of treatment outcomes for ureteral calculi was performed by the 2007 European Association of Urology (EAU)/Americal Urological Association (AUA) Ureteral Stones Clinical Guidelines Panel (Table 40.3).[16,17] These guidelines were derived from analysis of 348 published articles between 1996 and 2006 (the endpoint of the previous Guidelines report), of which 244 were ultimately found to have extractable data suitable for inclusion in the meta-analysis. The goal of this analysis was to compare treatment options for ureteral calculi, including medical expulsive therapy, SWL, URS, percutaneous nephrolithotomy (PCNL), and open and laparoscopic ureterolithotomy. Although randomized trials were distinctly uncommon in this analysis, the large numbers of patients treated in these retrospective and prospective series provide the best evaluable outcome data for these treatment modalities.

Outcome variables that were reviewed in these guidelines included stone-free rate, number of procedures required, spontaneous stone passage rate, and acute and long-term complications. Furthermore, outcomes were stratified by stone location – proximal (between the ureteropelvic junction and upper border of the pelvic bone), middle (overlying the pelvic bone), and distal (between the lower border of the pelvic bone and the ureteral orifice) ureter – and by stone size

Table 40.3 Stone-free rates for SWL of proximal, middle, and distal ureteral calculi according to the AUA/EAU Ureteral Stones Clinical Guidelines Panel[16,17]

Stone location	Stone size		
	overall	≤10 mm	>10 mm
Proximal	82%	90%	68%
Middle	73%	84%	76%
Distal	74%	86%	74%

(≤10 mm or >10 mm). We review the findings of the Guidelines Panel regarding SWL treatment of ureteral calculi.

40.4.1 Stone-Free Rates

Overall, median stone-free rates for proximal, middle, and distal ureteral calculi were 82%, 73%, and 74%, respectively. When stratified by stone size (≤10 mm and >10 mm), stone-free rates in the proximal, middle, and distal ureter were (90% versus 68%, 84% versus 76%, and 86% versus 74%, respectively). Such observations are consistent with an inverse relationship between stone-free rates and stone size. Additional procedures, including retreatments, secondary alternative procedures to remove stones and auxiliary, non-stone removal procedures, were relatively infrequently necessary: 0.62 procedures per patient for proximal ureteral stones, 0.52 for middle ureteral stones, and 0.37 for distal ureteral stones.

Interestingly, despite an evolution in lithotriptor technology, stone-free rates for ureteral stones have failed to improve substantially over time. Although in the 1997 Guidelines, ureteral stones were stratified into proximal and distal ureteral calculi only (stones above or below the iliac vessels, respectively) while the 2007 Guidelines stratified stones into proximal, middle, and distal ureteral calculi, there was no improvement in stone-free rates in the proximal ureter (83% in 1997 versus 82% in 2007) and stone-free rates for distal ureteral stones actually declined significantly. These findings are all the more significant since by the current definition of distal ureteral calculi, no middle ureteral stones, with their lower stone-free rates, would be included in the outcomes for distal ureteral stones.

40.5 Complications and Side Effects

In contrast to SWL for renal calculi, no parenchymal organs lie in the shock wave path for ureteral calculi. Consequently, many of the reported bleeding complications related to SWL of renal calculi are avoided when treating ureteral stones. The overall complication rate for SWL of ureteral calculi is approximately 7%, with most complications relating to infection or obstruction.[16,17,54] Ureteral injury is decidedly uncommon and thought to be related to stone manipulation or stent placement, occurring in 2%, 1%, and 1%, respectively, for proximal, middle, and distal ureteral stones. Accordingly, stricture rates are also low (<2%). Infectious complications (sepsis or urinary tract infection) occur with an incidence of 7%, 11%, and 7%, respectively for proximal, middle, and distal ureteral stones. Finally, rates of steinstrasse formation are 5%, 8%, and 4%, respectively.

40.6 Additional Considerations

40.6.1 Quality of Life

When evaluating the efficacy of therapies for stone management, the interval to stone-free status is an important variable for consideration. In a randomized trial comparing SWL and URS for the management of distal ureteral calculi, Peschel and colleagues reported that the time interval to become stone free after SWL was 10 days compared with 1.8 days for URS.[55] When questioned about satisfaction with their treatment modality and if they would undergo the same procedure again, patients responded according to the degree and timing of the success of treatment; 85% of SWL patients, including all but one of the patients rendered stone free, would repeat the procedure again. The remaining patient, who was successfully treated but required 6 weeks to clear the fragments, would not choose to repeat SWL. These findings underscore the importance of an early stone-free state since even patients who were free of symptoms said that the awareness and concern for residual stone fragments and fear of colic were an ever-present source of discomfort that restricted their ability to perform daily activities. In another RCT of patients with <15 mm distal ureteral calculi randomized to SWL or URS, 94% of SWL and 87% of URS patients were satisfied with their procedure, although 100% of patients in both groups were rendered stone free.[56]

Ultimately, treatment decisions must take into account not only procedure efficacy but also level of invasiveness and spectrum of complications.[54] The latter variables can be more difficult to define. Acceptable complication profiles and procedure tolerability may vary dramatically between patients and warrant discussion prior to any planned therapy.

40.6.2 Cost

Along with therapeutic efficacy and quality-of-life considerations, cost is another factor that can play into treatment algorithms. Lotan and colleagues used a decision analysis model to compare the cost of different treatment strategies for patients with ureteral calculi.[57] Using cost data derived from their own institution and outcome data derived from the literature, they determined that URS was less costly than SWL for stones in all locations in the ureter. A theoretical cost difference between URS and SWL of approximately $1,440, $1,670, and $1,750 was noted for proximal, middle, and distal ureteral calculi, respectively. Indeed, the cost of SWL would have to decrease by more than $1,489 overall to achieve cost equivalence with URS. Parker and associates also reviewed data from 220 patients with proximal ureteral calculi and compared success rates, cost effectiveness, and efficiency of URS versus SWL. These authors found that URS was associated with a significantly lower charge for the initial procedure ($7,575 versus $9,507, $p < 0.0001$) as well as cumulative charge for all procedures ($9,378 versus $15,583, $p < 0.0001$) compared with SWL.[58] However, charge data, rather than the cost data, should be viewed cautiously.

The cost differential between the two treatment modalities varies from one institution to the other depending on the cost of each treatment modality and the institutional success rates. Indeed, in countries other than the USA, SWL is a less costly treatment modality than URS. As such, Bierkins and colleagues from the Netherlands noted that for middle and distal ureteral calculi, SWL, despite a lower stone-free rate, was associated with lower overall costs than URS.[59]

40.6.3 Retreatment by SWL

In the event of SWL failure, options include SWL retreatment or an alternate treatment modality—usually URS. Pace and colleagues reported low success rates for repeat SWL of ureteral calculi following an initial failed treatment.[60] Among 1,588 patients with 1,593 calculi who underwent SWL with the Dornier MFL 5000 lithotriptor, the initial stone-free rate was 68%. After second and third treatments, the stone-free rates decreased to 46% and 31%, respectively. Accordingly, the overall success rate increased to 76% after two and 77% after three treatments. As such, the utility of repeat SWL after initial failure must be questioned.

40.7 Conclusions

With the increasing use of URS, the role of SWL for the management of ureteral calculi continues to evolve. Current evidence suggests that shock wave lithotripsy constitutes reasonable first-line therapy for non–cystine ureteral stones ≤10 mm in diameter that have a CT attenuation coefficient of <1,000 Hounsfield units. Furthermore, SWL is feasible in the setting of acute obstruction, and routine ureteral stenting is unnecessary in most cases. Adjuvant pharmacotherapy, including the use of alpha receptor antagonists or calcium channel blockers, appears to facilitate passage of stone fragments following SWL. Repeat SWL after initial treatment failure is largely unsuccessful and alternate endoscopic therapy (URS) should be considered.

References

1. Chaussy C, Brendel W, Schmiedt E. Extracorporeally induced destruction of kidney stones by shock waves. *Lancet.* 1980;2(8207): 1265-1268.
2. Ng CS, Fuchs GJ, Streem SB. Extracorporeal shock wave lithotripsy: patient, selection, and outcomes. In: Stoller ML, Gupta M, Bolton D, et al., eds. *Current Clinical Urology, Urinary Stone Disease: A Practical Guide to Medical and Surgical Management*, vol. 1. Totowa, NJ: Humana Press; 2007:555-569.
3. Pearle MS, Pierce HL, Miller GL, et al. Optimal method of urgent decompression of the collecting system for obstruction and infection due to ureteral calculi. *J Urol.* 1998;160(4):1260-1264.
4. Hollingsworth JM, Rogers MA, Kaufman SR, et al. Medical therapy to facilitate urinary stone passage: a meta-analysis. *Lancet.* 2006;368(9542):1171-1179.
5. Streem SB. Contemporary clinical practice of shock wave lithotripsy: a reevaluation of contraindications. *J Urol.* 1997;157(4): 1197-1203.
6. Asgari MA, Safarinejad MR, Hosseini SY, Dadkhah F. Extracorporeal shock wave lithotripsy of renal calculi during early pregnancy. *BJU Int.* 1999;84(6):615-617.
7. McCullough DL, Yeoman LD, Bo WJ, et al. Do extracorporeal shock waves affect fertility and fetal development? A study of shock wave effects on the rat ovary and fetus [abst]. *J Urol.* 1988;129:325A.
8. Vieweg J, Weber HM, Miller K, Hautmann R. Female fertility following extracorporeal shock wave lithotripsy of distal ureteral calculi. *J Urol.* 1992;148(3 Pt 2):1007-1010.
9. Abber JC, Langberg J, Mueller SC, Griffin JC, Thuroff JW. Cardiovascular pathology and extracorporeal shock wave lithotripsy. *J Urol.* 1988;140(2):408-409.
10. Vasavada SP, Streem SB, Kottke-Marchant K, Novick AC. Pathological effects of extracorporeally generated shock waves on calcified aortic aneurysm tissue. *J Urol.* 1994;152(1):45-48.
11. Carey SW, Streem SB. Extracorporeal shock wave lithotripsy for patients with calcified ipsilateral renal arterial or abdominal aortic aneurysms. *J Urol.* 1992;148(1):18-20.
12. Drach GW, Weber C, Donovan JM. Treatment of pacemaker patients with extracorporeal shock wave lithotripsy: experience from 2 continents. *J Urol.* 1990;143(5):895-896.
13. Streem SB, Yost A. Extracorporeal shock wave lithotripsy in patients with bleeding diatheses. *J Urol.* 1990;144(6):1347-1348.
14. Watterson JD, Girvan AR, Cook AJ, et al. Safety and efficacy of holmium: YAG laser lithotripsy in patients with bleeding diatheses. *J Urol.* 2002;168(2):442-445.
15. Turna B, Stein RJ, Smaldone MC, et al. Safety and efficacy of flexible ureterorenoscopy and holmium:YAG lithotripsy for intrarenal stones in anticoagulated cases. *J Urol.* 2008;179(4): 1415-1419.
16. Preminger GM, Tiselius HG, Assimos DG, et al. 2007 Guideline for the management of ureteral calculi. *Eur Urol.* 2007;52(6): 1610-1631.
17. Preminger GM, Tiselius HG, Assimos DG, et al. 2007 guideline for the management of ureteral calculi. *J Urol.* 2007;178(6): 2418-2434.
18. Stoller ML, Gupta M, Bolton D, Irby PB 3rd. Clinical correlates of the gross, radiographic, and histologic features of urinary matrix calculi. *J Endourol.* 1994;8(5):335-340.
19. Ng CS, Streem SB. Medical and surgical therapy of the cystine stone patient. *Curr Opin Urol.* 2001;11(4):353-358.
20. Bhatta KM, Prien EL Jr, Dretler SP. Cystine calculi–rough and smooth: a new clinical distinction. *J Urol.* 1989;142(4):937-940.
21. Kim SC, Burns EK, Lingeman JE, Paterson RF, McAteer JA, Williams JC Jr. Cystine calculi: correlation of CT-visible structure, CT number, and stone morphology with fragmentation by shock wave lithotripsy. *Urol Res.* 2007;35(6):319-324.
22. Williams JC Jr, Saw KC, Paterson RF, Hatt EK, McAteer JA, Lingeman JE. Variability of renal stone fragility in shock wave lithotripsy. *Urology.* 2003;61(6):1092-1096. discussion 1097.

23. Nakada SY, Hoff DG, Attai S, Heisey D, Blankenbaker D, Pozniak M. Determination of stone composition by noncontrast spiral computed tomography in the clinical setting. *Urology.* 2000;55(6): 816-819.

24. Sacco DE, Osman Cay O, Mueller PR, Dretler SP. Combining computerized tomography attenuation values with stone diameter predicts the success of extracorporeal shock wave lithotripsy ureteral stone clearance. American Urological Association 98th Annual Meeting; April 26–May 1, 2003; Chicago, Ill.

25. Pareek G, Armenakas NA, Fracchia JA. Hounsfield units on computerized tomography predict stone-free rates after extracorporeal shock wave lithotripsy. *J Urol.* 2003;169(5):1679-1681.

26. Mueller SC, Wilbert D, Thueroff JW, Alken P. Extracorporeal shock wave lithotripsy of ureteral stones: clinical experience and experimental findings. *J Urol.* 1986;135:831.

27. Parr NJ, Pye SD, Ritchie AW, Tolley DA. Mechanisms responsible for diminished fragmentation of ureteral calculi: an experimental and clinical study. *J Urol.* 1992;148(3 Pt 2):1079-1083.

28. Cass AS. Do upper ureteral stones need to be manipulated (push back) into the kidneys before extracorporeal shock wave lithotripsy? *J Urol.* 1992;147(2):349-351.

29. Chang SC, Kuo HC, Hsu T. Extracorporeal shock wave lithotripsy for obstructed proximal ureteral stones. A prospective randomized study comparing in situ, stent bypass and below stone catheter with irrigation strategies. *Eur Urol.* 1993;24(2):177-184.

30. Danuser H, Ackermann DK, Marth DC, Studer UE, Zingg EJ. Extracorporeal shock wave lithotripsy in situ or after push-up for upper ureteral calculi: a prospective randomized trial. *J Urol.* 1993;150(3):824-826.

31. Kumar A, Kumar RV, Mishra VK, Ahlawat R, Kapoor R, Bhandari M. Should upper ureteral calculi be manipulated before extracorporeal shock wave lithotripsy? A prospective controlled trial. *J Urol.* 1994;152(2 Pt 1):320-323.

32. Segura JW, Preminger GM, Assimos DG, et al. Ureteral Stones Clinical Guidelines Panel summary report on the management of ureteral calculi. The American Urological Association. *J Urol.* 1997;158(5):1915-1921.

33. Cass AS. In situ extracorporeal shock wave lithotripsy for obstructing ureteral stones with acute renal colic. *J Urol.* 1992;148(6): 1786-1787.

34. Srivastava A, Ahlawat R, Kumar A, Kapoor R, Bhandari M. Management of impacted upper ureteric calculi: results of lithotripsy and percutaneous litholapaxy. *Br J Urol.* 1992;70(3): 252-257.

35. Tligui M, El Khadime MR, Tchala K, et al. Emergency extracorporeal shock wave lithotripsy (ESWL) for obstructing ureteral stones. *Eur Urol.* 2003;43(5):552-555.

36. Tombal B, Mawlawi H, Feyaerts A, Wese FX, Opsomer R, Van Cangh PJ. Prospective randomized evaluation of emergency extracorporeal shock wave lithotripsy (ESWL) on the short-time outcome of symptomatic ureteral stones. *Eur Urol.* 2005;47(6): 855-859.

37. Hofmann R, Stoller ML. Endoscopic and open stone surgery in morbidly obese patients. *J Urol.* 1992;148(3 Pt 2):1108-1111.

38. Göktaş S, Peşkircioğlu L, Tahmaz L, Kibar Y, Erduran D, Harmankaya C. Is there significance of the choice of prone versus supine position in the treatment of proximal ureter stones with extracorporeal shock wave lithotripsy? *Eur Urol.* 2000;38(5):618-620.

39. Hara N, Koike H, Bilim V, Takahashi K, Nishiyama T. Efficacy of extracorporeal shockwave lithotripsy with patients rotated supine or rotated prone for treating ureteral stones: a case-control study. *J Endourol.* 2006;20(3):170-174.

40. Gerber R, Studer UE, Danuser H. Is newer always better? A comparative study of 3 lithotriptor generations. *J Urol.* 2005;173(6): 2013-2016.

41. Chan SL, Stothers L, Rowley A, Perler Z, Taylor W, Sullivan LD. A prospective trial comparing the efficacy and complications of the modified Dornier HM3 and MFL 5000 lithotriptors for solitary renal calculi. *J Urol.* 1995;153(6):1794-1797.

42. Jermini FR, Danuser H, Mattei A, Burkhard FC, Studer UE. Noninvasive anesthesia, analgesia and radiation-free extracorporeal shock wave lithotripsy for stones in the most distal ureter: experience with 165 patients. *J Urol.* 2002;168(2):446-449.

43. Greenstein A, Matzkin H. Does the rate of extracorporeal shock wave delivery affect stone fragmentation? *Urology.* 1999;54(3): 430-432.

44. Weir MJ, Tariq N, Honey RJ. Shockwave frequency affects fragmentation in a kidney stone model. *J Endourol.* 2000;14(7):547-550.

45. Paterson RF, Lifshitz DA, Lingeman JE, et al. Stone fragmentation during shock wave lithotripsy is improved by slowing the shock wave rate: studies with a new animal model. *J Urol.* 2002;168(5): 2211-2215.

46. Pace KT, Ghiculete D, Harju M, Honey RJ, University of Toronto Lithotripsy Associates. Shock wave lithotripsy at 60 or 120 shocks per minute: a randomized, double-blind trial. *J Urol.* 2005;174(2): 595-599.

47. Semins MJ, Trock BJ, Matlaga BR. The effect of shock wave rate on the outcome of shock wave lithotripsy: a meta-analysis. *J Urol.* 2008;179(1):194-197. discussion 197.

48. Pace KT, Ghiculete D, Harju M, Honey RJ. University of Toronto Lithotripsy Associates. Shock wave lithotripsy for upper ureteral stones: a randomized trial of 60 vs. 120 shocks/min. *J Urol.* 2007;4(supplement):431.

49. Küpeli B, Irkilata L, Gürocak S, et al. Does tamsulosin enhance lower ureteral stone clearance with or without shock wave lithotripsy? *Urology.* 2004;64(6):1111-1115.

50. Gravas S, Tzortzis V, Karatzas A, Oeconomou A, Melekos MD. The use of tamsulozin as adjunctive treatment after ESWL in patients with distal ureteral stone: do we really need it? Results from a randomised study. *Urol Res.* 2007;35(5):231-235.

51. Bhagat SK, Chacko NK, Kekre NS, Gopalakrishnan G, Antonisamy B, Devasia A. Is there a role for tamsulosin in shock wave lithotripsy for renal and ureteral calculi? *J Urol.* 2007;177(6):2185-2188.

52. Porpiglia F, Destefanis P, Fiori C, Scarpa RM, Fontana D. Role of adjunctive medical therapy with nifedipine and deflazacort after extracorporeal shock wave lithotripsy of ureteral stones. *Urology.* 2002;59(6):835-838.

53. Micali S, Grande M, Sighinolfi MC, De Stefani S, Bianchi G. Efficacy of expulsive therapy using nifedipine or tamsulosin, both associated with ketoprofene, after shock wave lithotripsy of ureteral stones. *Urol Res.* 2007;35(3):133-137.

54. Wolf JS Jr. Treatment selection and outcomes: ureteral calculi. *Urol Clin North Am.* 2007;34(3):421-430.

55. Peschel R, Janetschek G, Bartsch G. Extracorporeal shock wave lithotripsy versus ureteroscopy for distal ureteral calculi: a prospective randomized study. *J Urol.* 1999;162(6):1909-1912.

56. Pearle MS, Nadler R, Bercowsky E, et al. Prospective randomized trial comparing shock wave lithotripsy and ureteroscopy for management of distal ureteral calculi. *J Urol.* 2001;166(4):1255-1260.

57. Lotan Y, Gettman MT, Roehrborn CG, Cadeddu JA, Pearle MS. Management of ureteral calculi: a cost comparison and decision making analysis. *J Urol.* 2002;167(4):1621-1629.

58. Parker BD, Frederick RW, Reilly TP, Lowry PS, Bird ET. Efficiency and cost of treating proximal ureteral stones: shock wave lithotripsy versus ureteroscopy plus holmium:yttrium-aluminum-garnet laser. *Urology.* 2004;64(6):1102-1106.

59. Bierkens AF, Hendrikx AJ, De La Rosette JJ, et al. Treatment of mid- and lower ureteric calculi: extracorporeal shock-wave lithotripsy vs laser ureteroscopy. A comparison of costs, morbidity and effectiveness. *Br J Urol.* 1998;81(1):31-35.

60. Pace KT, Weir MJ, Tariq N, Honey RJ. Low success rate of repeat shock wave lithotripsy for ureteral stones after failed initial treatment. *J Urol.* 2000;164(6):1905-1907.

Percutaneous Nephrolithotomy

41

Mahesh Desai and Stephanie J. Symons

Abstract Percutaneous nephrolithotomy (PCNL) is now the established approach to a large stone burden in both adult and pediatric patients, allowing stone removal with less morbidity, cost, and a shorter hospital stay when compared with open procedures. As PCNL has developed, the technique has been adapted and successfully applied to the complex situations of obesity, bilateral stones, and ectopic kidneys. In all situations the planning and successful execution of the initial access into the kidney relies on a detailed understanding of renal anatomy and is critical to the outcome of PCNL. A successful puncture both decreases PCNL complications and increases stone clearance rates. Complete stone clearance should be the aim of each PCNL procedure. This chapter highlights tips and tricks that can be used to improve stone clearance rates and enhance outcomes in patients undergoing this challenging procedure.

41.1 Introduction

Percutaneous access to the kidney was described over 60 years ago, but it was not until 1976 that Fernström and Johansson first reported the use of a percutaneous tract specifically for stone removal.[1] Since then, the technique of percutaneous nephrolithotomy (PCNL) has continued to evolve worldwide, and it is now the established approach to a large stone burden in both adult and pediatric patients.[2,3] The percutaneous approach allows stone removal with less morbidity, lower cost, and a shorter hospital stay in comparison with open procedures. In addition, advances in instrumentation and technique have gradually decreased the complications of the percutaneous approach. For these reasons, PCNL has now replaced open surgery for the removal of large or complex renal calculi at most institutions.

41.2 Anatomical Considerations

The planning and successful execution of the initial access into the kidney is critical to the outcome of PCNL.[4] The ability to gain access to the desired renal calyx, with a minimum of complications, requires a thorough understanding of renal anatomy and the surrounding structures.

The kidneys lie in the retroperitoneum between the spinal levels T12 and L2/3 (Fig. 41.1). The right kidney is usually 2–3 cm lower than the left. Although a significant portion of each kidney is actually supracostal, the lower pole is almost always subcostal.[4] Each kidney lies obliquely, with its long axis parallel with the lateral border of the psoas, making the upper pole calyces more medial and posterior than the inferior pole. In the transverse plane, the kidneys are angled 30° posteriorly. In addition to this, each kidney moves in a craniocaudal direction with respiration; this movement is sometimes quite extensive and may be increased (but also controlled) under general anesthesia.

Renal calyceal anatomy has been accurately described by Sampaio after analyzing 140 three-dimensional resin endocasts of the pelvicalyceal system.[5] Calyceal anatomy is highly variable but understanding three important facets of

M. Desai (✉)
Department of Urology, Muljibhai Patel Urological Hospital, Nadiad, Gujarat, India
e-mail: mrdesai@mpuh.org

P.N. Rao et al. (eds.), *Urinary Tract Stone Disease*,
DOI 10.1007/978-1-84800-362-0_41, © Springer-Verlag London Limited 2011

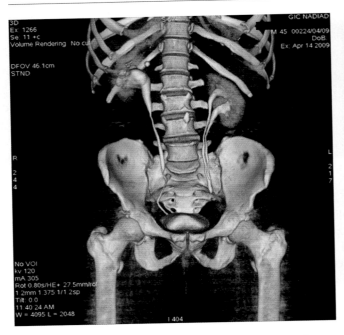

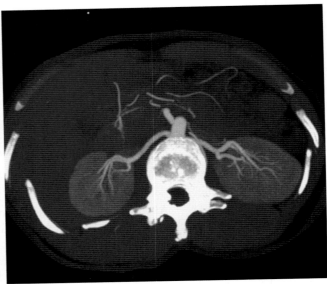

Fig. 41.3 Renal anatomy: CT angiogram of the renal vasculature; the anterior and posterior divisions of the renal artery are clearly seen bilaterally

Fig. 41.1 Renal anatomy: CT urogram reconstruction image, demonstrating renal positioning with a left duplex system

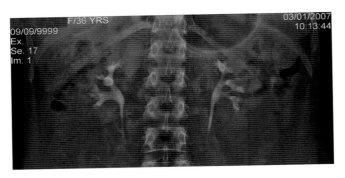

Fig. 41.2 Renal anatomy: 10 min post-contrast intravenous urogram film, demonstrating the middle calyceal groups draining into the lower calyceal groups bilaterally

their layout remain crucial to preoperative localization of any renal stone. First, there are three major calyceal groups: upper, middle, and lower, which then subdivide into minor calyces. Second, the upper and lower major calyces are generally compound, whilst the middle calyces are arranged in anterior and posterior sets. Finally, the major calyceal groups can drain into the renal pelvis in one of two ways. In the majority (62%), only the upper and lower major calyceal groups drain directly into the renal pelvis, with the middle calyceal group as an offshoot of either the upper or lower group (Fig. 41.2). In the remainder of kidneys (38%) the upper, middle, and lower major calyces each independently enter the renal pelvis.

Each main renal artery typically gives rise to an anterior and posterior division (Fig. 41.3). The anterior division further subdivides into four segmental branches, supplying the superior and inferior poles as well as the anterior upper and middle portions of the kidney. The posterior division supplies the remaining posterior area of the kidney. In more than 50% of kidneys, the posterior segmental artery is located in the middle or upper half of the posterior renal surface, and it may be damaged with an excessively medial needle puncture of an upper calyx.[6] Segmental arteries further subdivide into lobar, interlobar, arcuate, and finally interlobular arteries. Brödels line is an avascular plane running between the anterior and posterior blood supplies posterolaterally. A peripheral end-on puncture into a posterior calyx therefore minimizes the risk of bleeding during PCNL, simply because it minimizes the risk of vascular injury.

Structures surrounding the kidney must also be taken into consideration when planning PCNL access. On the right, the kidney is close to the adrenal, liver, ascending colon, and duodenum. On the left, the adrenal, spleen, descending colon, stomach, and pancreas must be considered. Both kidneys lie close beneath the diaphragm, and transgression of the pleural space is one of the greatest risks with a supracostal puncture. The pleura are attached to the medial half of the 12th rib and to the medial three-quarters of the 11th rib. Thus, a peripherally placed puncture that avoids going above the 11th rib will minimize the risks of pleural injury.

So, by taking these anatomical considerations into account, the urologist can minimize the risks of puncture for PCNL by choosing a path that will grant direct access to the stone with a straight instrument, whilst remaining posterolateral and if possible below the 12th rib.

41.3 Preoperative Assessment

41.3.1 Imaging

Radiological imaging is an essential part of PCNL tract planning. Intravenous urography (IVU) has historically been the mainstay of preoperative imaging for PCNL. However, the widespread and increasing presence of multiphase computed tomography (CT) scanners has now seen the demise of the IVU in many centers. A good IVU provides accurate information regarding the relationship of the kidney to the 12th rib and, with a thorough understanding of calyceal anatomy, will provide the urologist with a picture of stone position as well as pelvicalyceal dilatation and drainage. But a poorly performed IVU may provide only limited information. In comparison, the CT scan has the ability to scan during delayed phases of contrast excretion and to provide coronal and sagittal reconstruction images. But the main advantage of the CT scan is in showing the relationship of the kidney and stone to the surrounding structures, hence minimizing the risks of injury to an enlarged spleen or liver or to an unsuspected retrorenal colon. Three-dimensional reconstruction images are a further powerful tool in the future of percutaneous tract planning.[7]

Despite the advantages of the CT scan, for many urologists a preoperative CT is simply not a possibility for every patient. In some areas of the world endourologists will limit their requests for a CT to those patients in whom the anatomy is definitely abnormal, and continue to use IVU in the remainder of patients. A preoperative CT scan is certainly of benefit in patients with an ectopic, transplanted, or horseshoe kidney as well as those with orthopedic deformities.

In addition, radionucleotide scanning should be considered in patients with significant bilateral stone disease to show differential function. Differential renal function is also important in patients with a focally or globally thin renal parenchyma, where a partial or total nephrectomy may be preferable to PCNL.

41.3.2 Patient Assessment

All patients prior to PCNL should undergo routine laboratory investigation including renal function, hemoglobin, and a clotting profile. Medications potentially affecting the patient's coagulation status, including aspirin and nonsteroidal anti-inflammatory drugs (NSAIDs), should be discontinued 10–14 days prior to elective PCNL surgery. Blood cross-matching is not usually necessary preoperatively, but a group and save should be performed.

Urinary tract infection is a contraindication to PCNL. All urinary tract infections should be treated with culture-specific antibiotics prior to surgery. However, despite receiving a clear urine culture, it is well recognized that urinary stones serve as sanctuaries for urinary bacteria. Furthermore, even in cases of positive urine cultures, the pathogen grown may be different to the stone-colonizing pathogen found in the same patient.[8] There is evidence that preoperative treatment for 1 week with oral ciprofloxacin reduces the risk of urosepsis related to PCNL, regardless of urine culture results.[9] Despite a clear urine culture and prophylactic antibiotics, in some patients, needle puncture of the pelvicalyceal system may still reveal purulent urine, and the question arises as to whether it is safe to continue with the procedure in this circumstance. In the presence of thick or foul pus, placement of a nephrostomy tube is certainly the safe thing to do. But in the absence of known infection or thick pus, there is now evidence that with appropriate full antibiotic prophylaxis PCNL can be safely undertaken in the presence of purulent urine.[10,11]

41.3.3 Anesthetic Considerations

In the majority of cases, PCNL is performed in the prone position under general anesthesia. An anesthetic assessment will be necessary in any patient where fitness for this undertaking is uncertain. The prone position is a particular problem in the morbidly obese patient, where respiratory restriction may become critical. Patients with spinal or limb deformities may also cause a problem with prone positioning. Multiple authors have shown the safety and success of performing PCNL in the supine position for such patients.[12–15] For those patients where general anesthesia is felt to be unsafe, PCNL can also be successfully performed under local anesthesia and sedation.[16–18]

41.4 PCNL: Operative Technique

41.4.1 Ureteric Catheter Placement

Following prophylactic intravenous antibiotics and the administration of appropriate anesthesia as discussed, the first step in PCNL is to gain retrograde access to the pelvicalyceal system. The placement of a 5 Fr open-ended ureteric catheter provides the possibility of either saline contrast, or air injection to aid in both dilatation and visualization of the pelvicalyceal system, providing an optimal target for needle puncture. Patient positioning during guidewire and subsequent ureteric catheter insertion varies between surgeons. It is our practice to place the ureteric catheter over a guidewire with the patient in lithotomy position and then to fix it externally to a Foley catheter, prior to turning the patient prone. Other authors describe the use of flexible cystoscopy in the prone position for ureteric catheter placement, thus avoiding altering the patient's position and decreasing the risk of ureteric catheter dislodgement.[4]

Ureteric catheter placement is critically important, not just for gaining upper tract access, but for maintaining safe access. In some circumstances, stone burden or patient anatomy will prevent the antegrade passage of a guidewire for percutaneous tract stability. In such cases a guidewire can be safely passed retrograde and grasped from above for "through-and-through access" granting maximal tract stability. In addition, the ureteric catheter acts to discourage the passage of stone fragments into the ureter during PCNL. For this reason, when the stone burden is large or the ureter is dilated, some endourologists have described the routine use of either a 7 Fr occlusion balloon catheter or a stone entrapment device.[19,20]

Once the patient is placed prone, great care must be taken of the endotracheal tube and all pressure points must be padded. It is also vital that the patient is positioned on the operating table in such a way that there is clear access for the fluoroscopy C-arm to be placed below the table with access to the kidney, ureter, and bladder. Positioning the C-arm with free movement is critical to the subsequent surgery, and using a below-table tube greatly reduces the radiation exposure to the operating surgeon.

41.4.2 Antegrade Needle Access

When considering needle access for PCNL, three main questions need to be answered:

1. Who gains access: the urologist or the radiologist?
2. Under what imaging control is access gained: fluoroscopy or ultrasound?
3. Is the access to be gained in an antegrade or a retrograde fashion?

In answer to the third question, the vast majority of PCNLs are undertaken using antegrade access and this has become standard practice worldwide. The retrograde approach developed as a result of familiarity with transurethral procedures, but selection of the appropriate calyx is technically demanding and time consuming via this route.[21] Technological advances such as laparoscopic-assisted PCNL have resulted in a decrease in the indications for retrograde access, even in cases of ectopic and malrotated kidneys. Only antegrade access will be considered here.

41.4.3 Urologist or Radiologist?

In terms of who gains access, many modern endourologists believe strongly that the answer to this question should be the urologist. Certainly, in complex stone disease where there is a need for multiple-tract formation, the ability for the urologist to safely gain access to the kidney is a clear advantage in terms of manpower in the operating theater. It is readily apparent that urologists can be trained to safely perform percutaneous access, with studies suggesting competence after 60 procedures.[22,23] There is also some evidence that stone clearance rates may be improved and complication rates decreased when an experienced urologist is responsible for access.[24] In our practice, it is the urologist only who performs percutaneous renal puncture.

41.4.4 Fluoroscopy or Ultrasound?

The use of ultrasound or fluoroscopy for image control during needle puncture is a matter of equipment availability, training, and personal preference. Both modalities have been shown to work well for initial puncture purposes. However, the use of ultrasound scanning alone for full tract dilatation is generally not possible and this modality needs to be used in conjunction with fluoroscopy. Many ultrasound transducers are now available with lumens designed to accommodate the needle and it has been suggested that the increased accuracy of needle placement afforded by ultrasound-guided access may decrease the risks of complications associated with PCNL.[25] Ultrasound-guided access affords the urologist several advantages: real-time visualization of surrounding structures, easy identification of posterior and anterior calyces, and the absence of radiation (Fig. 41.4a and b). In a randomized trial of fluoroscopy versus ultrasound-guided access, Basiri demonstrated both modalities to be efficacious and noted that the use of ultrasound decreased the radiation exposure of the procedure overall.[26]

41.4.5 Percutaneous Puncture: Fluoroscopic Approach

Probably the easiest technique to learn using fluoroscopic guidance is the "bull's-eye technique." Initially, the appropriate calyx for puncture must be identified. If the calyx is stone bearing and the stone readily visualized on fluoroscopy this is straightforward. In other situations, such as a pelvic stone or upper pole access planned to target a pelvicalyceal/upper ureteric stone, identifying the appropriate calyx requires the retrograde injection of contrast. A posterior calyx will appear more medial with the C-arm at 0° and will not fill with as much contrast as an anterior calyx. Air can also be injected retrogradely as it will preferentially enter the posterior calyces to aid identification.

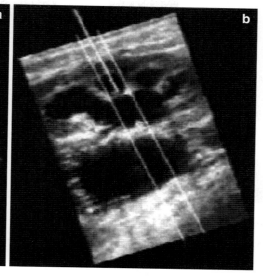

Fig. 41.4 Ultrasound-guided percutaneous renal access. (**a**) A direct path is seen from the punctured calyx to the renal pelvis for subsequent tract dilatation in an optimal puncture. (**b**) No direct path is visible from the punctured calyx to the renal pelvis in a suboptimal puncture

Once the target calyx is chosen, the C-arm is angled toward the surgeon at 30° from the vertical plane. With this orientation, the target calyx will be seen end-on and will appear circular. The position on the skin overlying the selected calyx is marked and a small puncture made in the skin with a blade. An 18G/15 cm long angiographic needle is then introduced through the skin at this position. The needle is advanced toward the calyx in the same trajectory as the orientation of the C-arm. Thus, the calyx, needle, and needle-hub are all in alignment creating a bull's-eye effect. The depth of needle advancement is then checked by reorienting the C-arm to 0°. In this orientation, the needle can be accurately advanced to reach the tip of the calyx only. It is important that needle placement, and subsequent tract dilatation, remains peripheral in order to minimize the risks of vascular injury to the kidney. Once the needle is seen to be accurately overlying the calyx in both the 0° and 30° planes, the stylet is removed from the center of the needle. Drainage of urine from the needle confirms its accurate placement within the calyx. A sample should always be taken for culture. In some instances, urine does not drain due to low pressure within the pelvicalyceal system. It is, therefore, worth injecting saline retrogradely via the ureteric catheter to test for a successful puncture. If there is still no drainage from the needle, it is possible that the needle has been advanced too far into the calyx and it should be withdrawn slowly using negative pressure with an attached syringe. If blood drains from the needle, it should simply be withdrawn and the puncture reattempted. The risk of significant hemorrhage caused by such a thin needle is negligible. In the presence of thick or foul pus, a nephrostomy should be inserted and the PCNL delayed to avoid sepsis.

Fluoroscopy-guided puncture may also be successfully undertaken without routine 30° orientation of the C-arm. With the C-arm at 0°, the target calyx is identified and the position marked on the overlying skin. This mark identifies the medial limit of the needle advancement. The needle is then withdrawn over the skin to a more lateral site for needle puncture (Fig. 41.5a and b). In exactly the same way as previously described, a nick is made in the skin and the needle advanced in a direct path to the tip of the desired calyx at a 30° angle from the horizontal axis. This method, the "triangulation" technique, relies on the surgeon's understanding of the renal orientation in order to accurately judge the horizontal angle of needle advancement. Just as in the bull's-eye technique, if the needle fails to hit the target calyx end-on, the C-arm is repositioned to 30° to confirm anterio-posterior positioning of the needle in relation to the target calyx.

The needle access is certainly the most critical step in the PCNL procedure as the safety of the tract and the effectiveness of subsequent stone removal relies upon it. Needle access is also the most technically challenging part of the procedure for the novice surgeon to master. In view of this, a variety of biological models have been suggested for puncture teaching and practice away from the operating theater.[27,28] A virtual reality simulator, the PERC Mentor, which enables surgeons to get to grips with needle punctures of varying degrees of difficulty, has also been developed.[29] A further technique for improving surgical accuracy has been suggested by Bruyère who reported the creation of a training model using the rapid prototyping technique based on abdominal CT images of a patient scheduled to undergo PCNL.[30] It was suggested that this technique be used not only to train urologists, but in preparing experienced surgeons facing a particularly difficult or complex

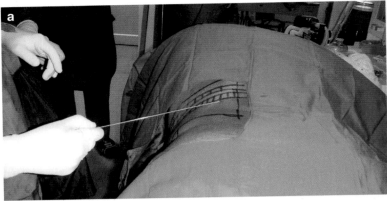

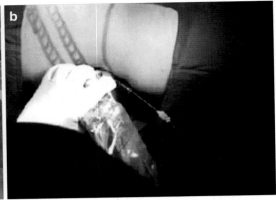

Fig. 41.5 Fluoroscopic needle access. (**a**) The target calyx is identified and the position marked on the overlying skin. This mark identifies the medial limit of the needle advancement. (**b**) The needle is then withdrawn over the skin to a more lateral site for needle puncture. Clear urine is seen draining from the needle following a successful puncture

procedure. Finally, in an attempt to remove an element of human error from the percutaneous access procedure altogether, robots have been trialed against humans to compare their accuracy with needle puncture. In this study, robots were shown to be more accurate, although slower, than their human counterparts.[31]

Out-of-theater experience with simulators is undoubtedly valuable in learning access techniques, but surgeons are also experimenting with ways of making the process of needle access easier to learn and more accurate within the operating theatre. Ko has demonstrated the use of a C-arm laser positioning device to facilitate percutaneous renal access for this purpose.[32]

41.4.6 Tract Dilatation: Placing the Guidewire

Tract dilatation can be achieved in several ways, using serial fascial dilators, metal coaxial dilators, or a balloon. However the dilatation is achieved, the main principle is that it should be performed over a guidewire that is stiff enough to support the dilatation. Ideally, the guidewire should be placed through the tract and down the ureter in order to enhance the stability of the tract during dilatation.

Thus, once accurate needle placement into the desired calyx has been achieved, a guidewire is passed gently through the needle, advanced into the renal pelvis and, if possible, down the ureter. Advancement of the guidewire into the ureter is often tricky and can be facilitated with the use of a Cobra catheter. It is our practice to then use a 0.035 in. J-tip guidewire to support dilatation of the nephrostomy tract. In the presence of a large stone burden, preventing advancement of the guidewire, it is worth using retrograde injection of saline to increase the space around the stone. A further

attempt at advancing the guidewire can be made during saline injection and this action may create enough space for satisfactory passage of the guidewire. In other situations, it will be impossible to advance the guidewire beyond the stone and a guidewire should, therefore, be advanced well into a neighboring calyx in order to grant some guidewire stability during tract dilatation. The stability of the guidewire must always be borne in mind by the operating surgeon, and in cases of an unstable tract the guidewire should be advanced to the ureter as soon as possible once stone fragmentation and clearance is underway.

41.4.7 Serial Dilators

Fascial dilators and Amplatz dilators are both designed to fit over a 0.038 in. guidewire. These serial dilators are both inserted in a screw type fashion in 2 Fr increments to the desired tract size, which is generally 28 or 30 Fr in adult patients. The advantage of these dilators over the metal coaxial dilators is that once the 8 Fr catheter is in place over the guidewire, the guidewire is unlikely to become kinked. In comparison, when using metal coaxial dilators, kinking of the guidewire during insertion can be a very significant problem and great care must be taken to avoid this. Metal dilators are inserted over a 58 cm long central hollow guide rod, and it is at the tip of the guide rod where kinking of the guidewire can occur. In order to improve control during insertion of these serial dilators the surgeon should rest an arm on the patient (Fig. 41.6) and avoid holding onto the central guide rod. The guidewire should be routinely tested for kinking by retracting and advancing it in small amounts during the dilatation process. Further control during the dilatation process can be gained by ensuring the smooth

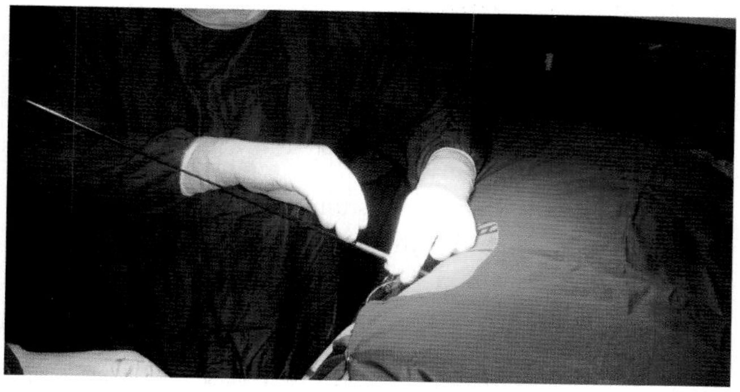

Fig. 41.6 Tract dilatation: improved control during insertion of rigid serial dilators is gained by the surgeon resting an arm on the patient

passage of one dilator over the next; avoiding unnecessary excess pressure exerted by the surgeon and therefore decreasing the risk of perforation caused by the dilators. As a routine, saline should be used to lubricate the dilators during tract dilatation to ensure smooth passage of each dilator over the last.

With all serial dilators, the dilatation should be performed from the skin to the tip of the desired calyx only, and not beyond. Serial dilators are an effective tool for nephrostomy tract dilatation, but all are associated with the risk of collecting system perforation if advanced too far into, or indeed beyond, the desired calyx during the dilatation process. When comparing metal dilators with sequential Amplatz dilators, the metal dilators have some advantages. During tract dilatation, metal dilators will provide a constant tamponade effect that is lost each time a serial Amplatz dilator is exchanged for the next, causing increased bleeding. Further, metal dilators may provide more effective tract dilatation in an undilated pelvi-calyceal system; Amplatz dilators have a conical tip that may not enter the calyx effectively causing under-dilatation. Of the serial dilator sets, the metal dilators are the most durable and cost effective in terms of their reusability.

41.4.8 Balloon Dilatation

Balloon dilatation was developed as a way of achieving tract dilatation in a single step, avoiding the need for serial dilators. A variety of high pressure balloons are available on the market. Balloon dilatation must be performed under fluoroscopic control to ensure accurate tract placement and also to demonstrate full tract dilatation. Each balloon has radiographic markers so that it can be successfully positioned over the guidewire prior to inflation. Just as in serial dilatation techniques, it is important to dilate a tract from the skin to the tip of the desired calyx in order to decrease

the risk of tearing a narrow infundibulum causing damage to the renal vasculature. Following full dilatation of the balloon, a working sheath is positioned over the balloon within the tract prior to deflation and removal of the balloon.

Where scarring is present, balloon dilatation may prove difficult. In some situations the tract may be successfully dilated except for one small area of "waisting." In this situation continued or increased pressure within the balloon may eventually dilate the area of scar tissue; otherwise incision of this area may be required, with care taken not to incise the balloon. Recently, newer balloons have been developed specifically to cope with the increased pressure required in the presence of renal scarring, although the literature evidence for the successful use of these devices is not yet available. In the presence of very dense scar tissue following prior renal surgery, balloon dilatation may not be possible. Under these circumstances, metal coaxial dilators are extremely useful. The inability to dilate dense scar tissue and the cost of the balloons are the two disadvantages to this excellent tract dilatation technique.

The technique of tract dilatation continues to develop in an attempt to make the procedure faster and to decrease the risks associated with it. A novel single step balloon dilatation system is currently under trial, which aims to eliminate the need for sheath placement over the balloon; this device has been shown to work satisfactorily in pigs.[33]

41.4.9 The "Mini-Perc"

As previously stated, tract dilatation with serial dilators or by balloon dilatation is generally to 28 or 30 Fr in adult patients. The "mini-perc" system was designed to reduce the morbidity associated with such large bore tract dilatation in children.[34] This system comprises a dual lumen catheter and a peel-away introducer providing tract sizes of 11–15 Fr. The reduced tract size works well in children in conjunction with pediatric instruments.[35,36] The mini-perc system has also been adapted for use in adult patients with smaller stones using tract sizes up to 18 Fr, with the same intention of reducing patient morbidity. However, the mini-perc technique requires longer operative time and the stone clearance results provided by such a reduction in tract size may not always be satisfactory. Both stone fragmentation technique and the size of stone fragments retrieved will be limited by the reduction in tract size. Giusti reported that, although hospital stay was reduced for patients undergoing mini-perc procedures, the stone-free rate was significantly reduced when compared with both standard and tubeless PCNL: 100% in the tubeless PNL group, 94% in the standard PNL group, and 77.5% in the mini-perc group.[37]

41.5 Stone Clearance: Tricks of the Trade

Throughout this chapter we have emphasized the importance of planning and establishing safe and appropriate percutaneous access for stone clearance. The aim of establishing access is always to be able to clear the maximum stone bulk from a single nephrostomy tract. The nephrostomy tract is always straight with the access sheath in situ; the only angulation available to the tract is afforded by the space within the pelvicalyceal system and the flexibility of the surrounding tissues. A dilated system will provide a large area of movement for the nephrostomy tract and therefore the nephroscope within the kidney. In this situation it is possible to reach stones in varying calyces and to clear stones from opposing renal poles with the use of a rigid nephroscope from a single nephrostomy tract. But in many cases the pelvicalyceal system is not dilated and the renal area within reach of the rigid nephroscope may be very limited. In such situations there are various tricks and techniques that the endourologist should be aware of, which may circumvent the need for multiple-tract formation.

The flexible nephroscope is an extremely valuable tool in the event of an "out-of-reach" stone, and one that many surgeons would advocate for use in every PCNL. A flexible nephroscope can be used in conjunction with the multitude of baskets and graspers that are available for mobilizing small stones and stone fragments within the urinary system overall. In addition, the flexible nephroscope can be used with laser lithotripsy, providing excellent stone fragmentation in situ. The disadvantage of the flexible scope lies in its cost and, in comparison with its rigid counterpart, its lack of durability. For these reasons, many urologists performing PCNL will not have a flexible scope available to them.

In the absence of a flexible scope, the use of a pediatric nephroscope will allow greater movement within the pelvicalyceal system than a standard 24 Fr adult nephroscope. A change in scope size may be enough to safely reach into an adjoining calyx that appeared previously out of sight. If a stone remains out of reach, a basket or a guidewire placed with the aid of an angulated catheter may be enough to dislodge a stone into the surgeon's direct line of vision.

If a small stone, or fragment, is lying within a calyx that is absolutely out of reach from the created nephrostomy tract, a "puncture wash" can be used. This requires a needle puncture into the stone-bearing calyx and the injection of saline to flush the stone out of the unreachable calyx hopefully into the renal pelvis from where it can be readily extracted. This technique of non-dilated puncture is also very useful in cases where a calyceal infundibulum is difficult to visualize. Methylene blue can be injected into the stone-bearing calyx in order to identify the infundibulum from within the renal pelvis. Similarly, a guidewire passed through the secondary needle puncture and into the renal pelvis will act as a guide

to the calyceal infundibulum. The guidewire may also be back-loaded onto a flexible scope if necessary to assist entry into the calyx for stone fragmentation or retrieval.

Despite all of these tricks for improving stone retrieval via a single nephrostomy tract, it is important to remember that in cases of a significant stone bulk in an out-of-reach calyx, a second nephrostomy tract remains the quickest and most effective method of stone clearance. In cases where the use of two or more tracts is anticipated, we would recommend initial puncture and guidewire placement to each calyx where access is planned, prior to dilatation of any tract (Fig. 41.7a–f). This approach helps significantly in multiple-tract PCNL by enabling the use of contrast under fluoroscopic guidance for each puncture. Contrast use becomes difficult following tract dilatation due to leakage from the Amplatz sheath and extravasation related to the tract. For any preplanned tract that is subsequently not required, the guidewire is simply removed at the end of the procedure.

The need to achieve complete stone clearance cannot be overemphasized. Endourologists continue to investigate new ways of ensuring that each PCNL is as complete as possible. Multiple tricks for enabling stone clearance from the antegrade approach have already been outlined. A combined approach using both antegrade and retrograde routes is also possible. Marguet described flexible ureteroscopy in combination with standard antegrade access for PCNL to enhance stone clearance and decrease the number of required nephrostomy tracts in complex stone disease with satisfactory results.[38] The quest for complete stone clearance has also led to PCNL being undertaken in an interventional radiology suite in order to investigate the use of high magnification rotational fluoroscopy in improved visualization of stone fragments.[39] Whatever equipment is available to the operating surgeon, the intention of each PCNL procedure should be to gain maximal stone clearance.

41.6 Nephrostomy

Following PCNL a nephrostomy drain is usually placed. The retrograde ureteric catheter that is placed intraoperatively may be left in place for 1 day after removal of the nephrostomy drain to ensure antegrade renal drainage. The nephrostomy drain is usually removed within 1–2 days postoperatively. Postoperative pain and analgesic requirements are greater in patients with large-bore nephrostomy tubes.[40,41] Analgesic requirements can be decreased with peritubal infiltration of bupivacaine at the time of nephrostomy insertion.[42,43] If prolonged drainage is indicated, such as in cases with significant collecting system perforation, residual stones, and impacted UPJ stones causing edema, an internal DJ stent is indicated and can be placed antegradely.

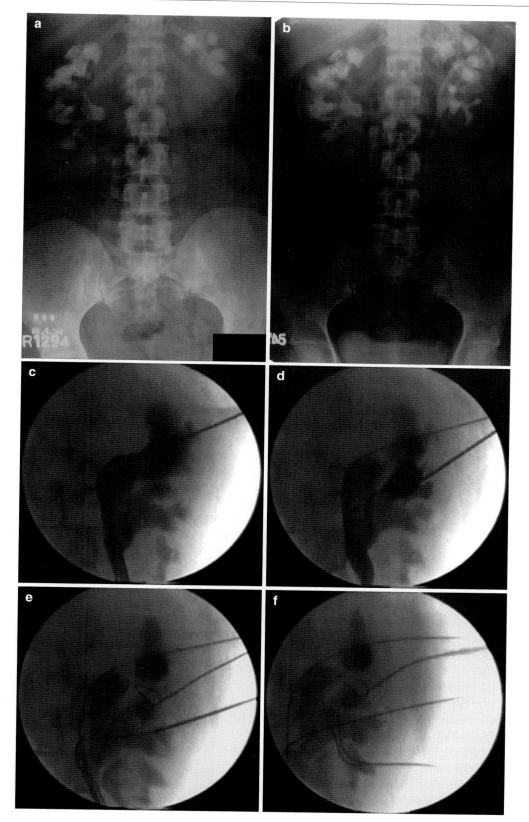

Fig. 41.7 Pre-dilatation guidewire placement for all potential tracts in a right Percutaneous nephrolithotomy (PCNL) for staghorn. (**a**) Plain KUB demonstrating bilateral staghorn calculus. (**b**) Intravenous urography (IVU) film.(**c**) Initial guidewire placement for right PCNL. (**d**) Second guidewire placement. (**e**) Third guidewire placement. (**f**) Fourth guidewire placement

In select situations, patients can be safely managed postoperatively without either nephrostomy drainage or an internal stent. So called "totally tubeless" PCNL should only be undertaken in straightforward cases without any intraoperative complications, bleeding, or collecting system perforations.[44] Complete stone clearance should also have been achieved in order to avoid ongoing percutaneous tract leakage secondary to ureteric obstruction.[45] In many situations, totally tubeless PCNL may not be advisable despite the absence of significant complications; for example, in patients with an impacted pelvic stone, where mucosal edema may be marked, limiting postoperative antegrade renal drainage. In such situations, an antegradely placed DJ stent may be left in situ, but no nephrostomy tube: a "tubeless" PCNL. When considering a tubeless PCNL, the exclusion criteria would generally be less rigid. However, exclusion criteria should still include the presence of infected hydronephrosis, matrix calculi, significant bleeding or residual stone burden, and the need for three of more percutaneous accesses.[46]

Instillation of hemostatic and tissue sealants into the tracts of "tubeless" patients does not appear to significantly decrease bleeding or extravasation.[47] However, one randomized controlled study has shown that fibrin sealants can reduce the postoperative pain and analgesic requirement.[48]

41.7 Complications

Common and significant complications associated with PCNL are systemic inflammatory response syndrome (SIRS), bleeding, pelvic perforation, and adjacent organ injury. Further complications include fluid overload, hypothermia, inward migration of working sheath, strictures of the collecting system, nephrocutaneous fistula, and mortality.

The incidence of SIRS after PCNL is common and has been reported as high as 23.4%, though progression to full sepsis is unusual (0.3–4.7%).[49] Risk factors for SIRS include the number of tracts, receipt of a blood transfusion, stone size, and presence of pyelocaliectasis. When full-blown sepsis does occur, successful management relies on a high index of suspicion, early intervention, and intensive treatment. The results of urine and stone cultures taken preoperatively, peroperatively, and during the febrile period hold great importance for decision making in terms of antibiotic changes during treatment.[8,50,51] There is evidence that PCNL-related sepsis can be reduced with the use of preoperative ciprofloxacin for 1 week.[9]

Bleeding can occur from the renal parenchyma (tract) or from an injury within the pelvicalyceal system (infundibular or pelvic tear). As discussed previously, in anatomical considerations, a tract that is too medial risks injury to major renal vessels. Venous bleeding can be controlled with placement of a wide bore nephrostomy tube; increased benefit is gained by clamping the nephrostomy tube for tamponade effect. If, despite these measures, bleeding continues and is bright red, an arterial bleed should be suspected. Arterial injuries may also manifest late (3–4 weeks post-procedure). The more common arterial injuries are arterio-venous fistula, pseudo aneurysm, and arterial laceration (Fig. 41.8). Profuse arterial bleeding requires urgent stabilization of the patient, followed by renal arteriography and super-selective angio-embolization of the bleeding arterial branch. Interventions to control bleeding are required in 0.6–1.4% of PCNL patients.[52] A very small number of patients may require open surgery with total or partial nephrectomy. Reported blood transfusion rates following PCNL range from 11.2% to 30.9%.[53,54] Diabetes, multiple-tract procedures, prolonged operative time, and the occurrence of intraoperative complications are all associated with significantly increased blood loss. Maneuvers that may reduce blood loss and transfusion rate include ultrasound-guided access, use of balloon dilatation systems, reduced operative time, and staged procedure in case of a large stone burden or intraoperative complications. Reducing the tract size in pediatric cases, non-hydronephrotic systems, and those with a narrow infundibulum, as well as secondary tracts in a multiple-tract procedure may also reduce blood loss during PCNL.[55] Staghorn stones, multiple tracts, the presence of diabetes, and large stones were associated with increased renal hemorrhage during PCNL on multivariate analysis.[56]

Collecting system perforations are not uncommon during PCNL and occur mainly during tract dilatation and occasionally during stone manipulation. These perforations are generally evident during nephroscopy and mostly resolve with nephrostomy drainage and ureteral DJ stenting (Fig. 41.9). A persistent perinephric urinoma may require ultrasound-guided percutaneous drainage.

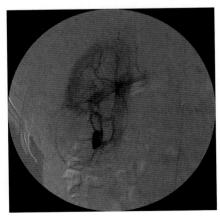

Fig. 41.8 PCNL complications: an angiogram demonstrating an arteriovenous fistula secondary to PCNL

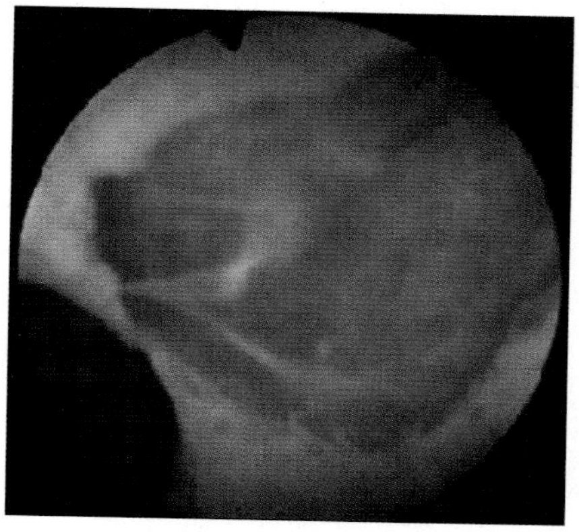

Fig. 41.9 PCNL complications: endoscopic view of the pelvicalyceal system during PCNL showing a pelvic wall perforation with a renal stone on the left

During PCNL, injury to structures adjacent to the kidney (pleural cavity, lung, colon, spleen, liver, and duodenum) can occur. Pleural and colonic injuries have been reported in 0–3.1% and 0.2–0.8% respectively of patients undergoing PCNL.[52] A significant pleural injury should be managed with tube thoracostomy drainage. A ureteral stent or prolonged nephrostomy drainage will satisfactorily treat a reno-pleural fistula. Colonic injury should be managed by placement of a ureteral DJ stent and by drawing the nephrostomy tube back into the colon at the point of perforation. In the absence of distal bowel obstruction, the colonic injury will generally heal. Bowel healing should be confirmed after approximately 1 week with a contrast study via the nephrostomy tube: in the absence of a colo-renal fistula, the colonic nephrostomy drain can be removed. Splenic injuries are rare during PCNL. Although splenic injuries may be managed conservatively, a splenectomy is occasionally required in cases of significant bleeding. Liver injury is also unusual and rarely requires surgical intervention.

PCNL-related fluid overload occurs as a result of irrigation fluid absorption through open venous channels or extravasation. Fluid absorption may cause clinically significant overload in patients with compromised cardiorespiratory or renal status and in pediatric patients. The use of a low-pressure system, reduction in nephroscopy time, and staging the PCNL procedure for large renal stone burdens, especially in the presence of complications such as perforation of the pelvicalyceal system, reduces fluid absorption and avoids volume overload. In addition, it is important to ensure that the operative tract sheath remains within the pelvicalyceal system during the PCNL procedure; if the tract sheath drifts peripherally, exposing the parenchymal or even extrarenal portion of the tract, fluid absorption and extravasation will increase exponentially. Fluid absorption may also be associated with both infective and noninfective pyrexia, necessitating adequate preoperative control of urinary infection.[57]

41.8 Special Situations

41.8.1 Bilateral Stone Disease

Simultaneous bilateral PCNL is a safe procedure that can be used effectively in adults as well as in children. In addition to being cost-effective, it involves only a single anesthetic with a shorter hospital stay and faster convalescence. However, patients with a large stone burden or complex pelvicalyceal anatomy should not be selected.[58] Following completion of one side, the decision to proceed with the contralateral PCNL should be based on time taken for the first side, blood loss, vital signs and blood parameters, any complications, and patient comorbidities. Despite the best of intentions, approximately 30% of anticipated simultaneous bilateral PCNL cases might be limited to single-sided PCNL, depending on intraoperative events.[59]

41.8.2 Ectopic Kidneys

PCNL, although an accepted treatment modality in anatomically normal kidneys, is still not universally performed for calculi in pelvic ectopic kidneys. Fear of inaccessibility and injury to abdominal viscera make it a technically challenging procedure.[60] Ultrasound-guided PCNL may be attempted if a clear ultrasound window is available from the skin to the target calyx, suggesting the absence of any intervening bowel loop. Technical factors that increase the safety of this procedure include ultrasound-guided puncture, use of a mature tract or an Amplatz sheath, routine postoperative double-J stenting, and nephrostogram prior to nephrostomy tube removal. With proper precautions and meticulous technique, PCNL is a safe and effective modality to treat calculi in pelvic ectopic kidney.[61] However, PCNL is perhaps more widely performed in pelvic ectopic kidneys with the assistance of laparoscopy.[62]

41.8.3 Horseshoe Kidneys

Urolithiasis is the most common complication of the horseshoe kidney, with a reported incidence of 21–60%, and PCNL is well recognized as being both safe and efficacious in these cases.[63] Despite this, just as in pelvic ectopic kidneys and other malrotated kidneys, there may be a fear of inaccessibility and injury to adjacent structures associated with PCNL in the horseshoe kidney. Therefore, it is worth noting one advantage of the horseshoe kidney anatomy over the normal kidney as regards PCNL. In patients with normal renal anatomy, access to the upper pole calyces during

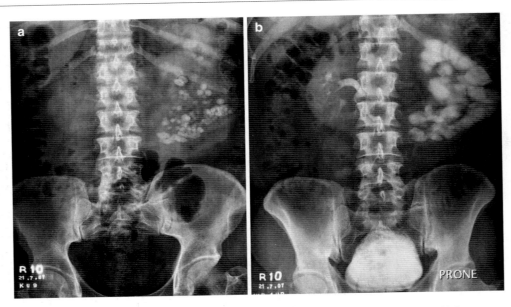

Fig. 41.10 Horseshoe kidneys. (**a**) Plain X ray KUB showing multiple left renal calculi in a horseshoe kidney. (**b**) Post contrast IVU film

PCNL often requires a supracostal approach, with the associated risk of pleural injury. In contrast, upper pole access in the horseshoe kidney is relatively safe due to the inferior displacement of the kidneys away from the pleura and a low reported incidence of associated pneumothorax.[64,65] Furthermore, upper pole access is a valuable aid to stone clearance, as the alignment of the nephroscope with the long axis of the kidney aids manipulation of the scope into the upper calyces, renal pelvis, lower calyces, pelviureteric junction (PUJ), and proximal ureter.

Two further factors make PCNL an attractive choice in the management of stones within horseshoe kidneys. These patients often have very significant stone burdens, making PCNL an effective technique for stone clearance with the minimal number of required procedures (Fig. 41.10a and b). In addition, ureteric insertion onto the renal pelvis tends to be both superiorly and laterally displaced, limiting the chances of stone fragment passage following extracorporeal shock wave lithotripsy.

of the PCNL procedure, especially in the morbidly obese patient where prone positioning will precipitate respiratory difficulties.

Supine positioning is one way to avoid the respiratory risks of a standard PCNL in the obese patient[12-15]; but brings with it the not-insignificant challenge of puncturing the kidney with limited access. An alternative to the supine position is the lateral decubitus position, which leaves the loin exposed, but still necessitates percutaneous renal puncture in an unusual position.[69,70] Both supine and lateral decubitus positioning can be used in conjunction with spinal anesthesia for PCNL. In a further attempt to minimize the risks of prone PCNL in the morbidly obese patient Wu et al. have recently reported the use of awake endotracheal intubation and prone patient self-positioning, with no increase in morbidity.[71] Despite the varied possibilities for minimizing the risks of general anesthetic PCNL, in the very high risk patient the technique of PCNL under local anesthesia with sedation should not be forgotten.

41.8.4 Obesity

Obesity is well recognized to increase the risks of anesthetic and surgical procedures. However, in the obese patient with a significant renal stone burden, surgery in the form of PCNL is often the most appropriate treatment as extracorporeal shock wave lithotripsy can prove ineffective. Although technically challenging, PCNL has been shown to be safe even in the morbidly obese patient with no difference in outcomes when compared to patients with lower body mass index.[66-68] However, patient positioning may be critical to the success

41.8.5 Pediatric PCNL

PCNL was first applied to the pediatric population in the 1980s using adult-size instruments. Although the technique is successful using adult-size instruments, even in young children, a reduction in the tract size is now recommended to decrease the risk of hemorrhagic complications.[55,72] The less invasive "mini-perc" procedure was developed as a method for performing PCNL, with the specific intent of decreasing the morbidity of the procedure in young children.[34]

Further technologic improvements, including miniaturization of endoscopes and advances in energy sources for stone fragmentation, has meant that PCNL can now be performed safely in children from just a few months old and with stones of all sizes. Stone-free rates in pediatric PCNL monotherapy are comparable to those of adult populations. Aron et al. reported complete stone clearance with PCNL monotherapy of 89% in preschool children with complete staghorn calculi.[72] Just as in adult patients, bilateral stone disease, compromised renal function, and renal anatomical abnormalities should not be viewed as contraindications to PCNL in the pediatric population.[73] However, comprehensive care of the pediatric patient undergoing PCNL requires close liaison between the urologist and nephrologist, as many of these patients will have metabolic abnormalities as a cause of their urolithiasis.

In view of the invasive nature of PCNL, there remains a concern of potential renal damage in relatively small kidneys. Several studies have tried to address this problem by determining the frequency of renal parenchymal damage following PCNL in children using technetium-99m dimercaptosuccinic acid (DMSA) scans. Samad et al. demonstrated focal damage in 5% of postoperative DMSA scans, but concluded that this may be an overestimate of renal injury since preoperative DMSA scans were not available in this study.[74] Others have shown no new renal scarring following PCNL in children, when preoperative and postoperative DMSA scans were compared.[75,76]

Needle puncture and antegrade access should be undertaken by the most appropriately trained person (urologist or radiologist) using either ultrasound or fluoroscopic guidance. Both techniques work well, but needle access remains technically challenging and out-of-theater experience with simulators is undoubtedly valuable in learning PCNL access. Ultrasound-guided access affords the advantages of real-time visualization of surrounding structures, easy identification of posterior and anterior calyces, and the absence of radiation. The aim of establishing access should always be to clear the maximum stone bulk from a single nephrostomy tract. To this aim, the use of flexible and pediatric scopes, puncture wash, and the use of second guidewires have been highlighted as techniques to improve stone clearance. In cases where the use of two or more tracts is anticipated, we would recommend initial puncture and guidewire placement to each calyx where access is planned, prior to dilatation of any tract. Complications associated with PCNL will be minimized through systematic preoperative patient preparation and access planning. A robust knowledge of the management of PCNL complications will further ensure that the technique remains as safe as possible in all situations, including the more technically challenging situations of ectopic kidneys, obesity, and pediatrics. Finally, although PCNL has now superseded open surgery in virtually all cases of large stone burden, it remains imperative to remember that occasionally a nephrectomy will be the better option for a patient with a very large stone burden in a poorly functioning kidney.

41.9 Conclusions

Since the initial use of a percutaneous tract for the specific purpose of stone removal in the mid-1970s, PCNL has become the surgical approach of choice in patients with a large renal stone burden. The technique has developed over time and now affords safe and effective stone clearance in patients of all ages, together with significant comorbidities and complexities of both renal and spinal anatomy. In all cases, the planning and successful execution of the initial access into the kidney is critical to the outcome of PCNL. The ability to gain access to the desired renal calyx, with a minimum of complications, requires a thorough understanding of renal calyceal and arterial anatomy as well as surrounding structures. The risks of PCNL puncture are minimized by choosing a path that will grant direct access to the stone with a straight instrument, whilst remaining posterolateral and, if possible, below the 12th rib. To this aim, CT scanning is now rapidly overtaking IVU as the preoperative planning radiological imaging of choice. Decisions regarding patient positioning and type of anesthesia will remain dependent upon patient body habitus and comorbidities.

References

1. Fernström I, Johansson B. Percutaneous pyelolithotomy. A new extraction technique. *Scand J Urol Nephrol.* 1976;10(3):257-259.
2. Al-Kohlany KM, Shokeir AA, Mosbah A, et al. Treatment of complete staghorn stones: a prospective randomized comparison of open surgery versus percutaneous nephrolithotomy. *J Urol.* 2005;173(2):469-473.
3. Shokeir AA, Sheir KZ, El-Nahas AR, et al. Treatment of renal stones in children: a comparison between percutaneous nephrolithotomy and shock wave lithotripsy. *J Urol.* 2006;176(2):706-710.
4. Ko R, Soucy F, Denstedt JD, et al. Percutaneous nephrolithotomy made easier: a practical guide, tips and tricks. *BJU Int.* 2007;101: 535-539.
5. Sampaio FJ, Mandarim-de-Lacerda CA. The kidney collecting system in man: systematization and morphometry based on 100 polyester resin casts. *Bull Assoc Anat.* 1985;69(207):297-304.
6. Sampaio FJ, Aragao AH. Anatomical relationship between the intrarenal arteries and the kidney collecting system. *J Urol.* 1990;143(4):679-681.
7. Thiruchelvam N, Mostafid H, Ubhayakar G. Planning percutaneous nephrolithotomy using multidetector computed tomography urography, multiplanar reconstruction and three-dimensional reformatting. *BJU Int.* 2005;95(9):1280-1284.
8. Margel D, Ehrlich Y, Brown N, et al. Clinical implication of routine stone culture in percutaneous nephrolithotomy – a prospective study. *Urology.* 2006;67(1):26-29.

9. Marriapan P, Smith G, Moussa SA, et al. One week of ciprofloxacin before percutaneous nephrolithotomy significantly reduces upper tract infection and urosepsis: a prospective controlled study. *BJU Int.* 2006;98:1075-1079.

10. Hosseini MM, Basiri A, Moghaddam SM. Percutaneous nephrolithotomy of patients with staghorn stone and incidental purulent fluid suggestive of infection. *J Endourol.* 2007;21(12):1429-1432.

11. Etemadian M, Haghighi R, Madineay A, et al. Delayed versus same-day percutaneous nephrolithotomy in patients with aspirated cloudy urine. *J Urol.* 2008;5(1):28-33.

12. Zhou X, Gao X, Wen J, et al. Clinical value of minimally invasive percutaneous nephrolithotomy in the supine position under the guidance of real-time ultrasound: report of 92 cases. *Urol Res.* 2008;36(2):111-114.

13. Steele D, Marshall V. Percutaneous nephrolithotomy in the supine position: a neglected approach? *J Endourol.* 2007;21(12):1433-1437.

14. Manohar T, Jain P, Desai M. Supine percutaneous nephrolithotomy: effective approach to high-risk and morbidly obese patients. *J Endourol.* 2007;21(1):44-49.

15. Shoma AM, Eraky I, El-Kenawy MR, et al. Percutaneous nephrolithotomy in the supine position: technical aspects and functional outcome compared with the prone technique. *Urology.* 2002;60(3):388-392.

16. Kanaroglou A, Razvi H. Percutaneous nephrolithotomy under conscious sedation in morbidly obese patients. *Can J Urol.* 2006;13(3):3153-3155.

17. Aravantinos E, Karatzas A, Gravas S, et al. Feasibility of percutaneous nephrolithotomy under assisted local anaesthesia: a prospective study on selected patients with upper urinary tract obstruction. *Eur Urol.* 2007;51(1):224-227.

18. Symons S, Biyani CS, Bhargava S, et al. Challenge of percutaneous nephrolithotomy in patients with spinal neuropathy. *Int J Urol.* 2006;13(7):874-879.

19. Springhart WP, Tan YH, Albala DM, et al. Use of Stone Cone minimizes stone migration during percutaneous nephrolithotomy. *Urology.* 2006;67(5):1066-1068.

20. Wosnitzer M, Xavier K, et al. Novel use of a ureteroscopic stone entrapment device to prevent antegrade stone migration during percutaneous nephrolithotomy. *J Endourol.* 2009;23(2):203-207.

21. McDougall EM, Liatsikos EN, Dinlenc CZ, et al. Percutaneous approaches to the upper urinary tract. In: Walsh PC, ed. *Campbell's Urology.* 8th ed. USA: Elsevier Science; 2002.

22. El-Assmy AM, Shokeir AA, Mohsen T, et al. Renal access by urologist or radiologist for percutaneous nephrolithotomy-is it still an issue? *J Urol.* 2007;178(3 Pt 1):916-920.

23. Allen D, O'Brien T, Tiptaft R, et al. Defining the learning curve for percutaneous nephrolithotomy. *J Endourol.* 2005;19(3):279-282.

24. Watterson JD, Soon S, Jana K. Access related complications during percutaneous nephrolithotomy: urology versus radiology at a single academic institution. *J Urol.* 2006;176(1):142-145.

25. Osman M, Wendt NG, Heger K, et al. Percutaneous nephrolithotomy with ultrasonography-guided renal access: experience from over 300 cases. *BJU Int.* 2005;96(6):875-878.

26. Basiri A, Ziaee AM, Kianian HR, et al. Ultrasonographic versus fluoroscopic access for percutaneous nephrolithotomy: a randomized clinical trial. *J Endourol.* 2008;22(2):281-284.

27. Häcker A, Wendt NG, Honeck P, et al. A biological model to teach percutaneous nephrolithotomy technique with ultrasound and fluoroscopy guided access. *J Endourol.* 2007;21(5):545-550.

28. Hammond L, Ketchum J, Schwartz BF. A new approach to urology training: a laboratory model for percutaneous nephrolithotomy. *J Urol.* 2004;172(5 Pt 1):1950-1952.

29. Stern J, Zeltser IS, Pearle MS. Percutaneous renal access simulators. *J Endourol.* 2007;21(3):270-273.

30. Bruyère F, Leroux C, Brunereau L, et al. Rapid prototyping model for percutaneous nephrolithotomy training. *J Endourol.* 2008;22(1):91-96.

31. Challacombe B, Patriciu A, Glass J, et al. A randomized controlled trial of human versus robotic and telerobotic access to the kidney as the first step in percutaneous nephrolithotomy. *Comput Aided Surg.* 2005;10(3):165-171.

32. Ko R, Razvi H. C-arm laser positioning device to facilitate percutaneous renal access. *Urology.* 2007;70(2):360-361.

33. Maynes LJ, Desai PJ, Zuppan CW, et al. Comparison of a novel one-step percutaneous nephrolithotomy sheath with a standard two-step device. *Urology.* 2008;71(2):223-227.

34. Jackman SV, Hedican SP, Peters CA, et al. Percutaneous nephrolithotomy in infants and preschool age children: experience with a new technique. *Urology.* 1998;52(4):697-701.

35. Schuster TK, Smaldone MC, Averch TD, et al. Percutaneous nephrolithotomy in children. *J Endourol.* 2009;23(10):1699-1705.

36. Manohar T, Ganpule AP, Shrivastav P, et al. Percutaneous nephrolithotomy for complex caliceal calculi and staghorn stones in children less than 5 years of age. *J Endourol.* 2006;20(8):547-551.

37. Giusti G, Piccinelli A, Taverna G, et al. Miniperc? No thank you! *Eur Urol.* 2007;51(3):810-814.

38. Marguet CG, Springhart WP, Tan YH, et al. Simultaneous combined use of flexible ureteroscopy and percutaneous nephrolithotomy to reduce the number of access tracts in the management of complex renal calculi. *BJU Int.* 2005;96(7):1097-1100.

39. Portis AJ, Laliberte MA, Drake S, et al. Intraoperative fragment detection during percutaneous nephrolithotomy: evaluation of high magnification rotational fluoroscopy combined with aggressive nephroscopy. *J Urol.* 2006;175(1):162-165.

40. Maheshwari PN, Andankar MG, Bansal M. Nephrostomy tube after percutaneous nephrolithotomy: large-bore or pigtail catheter? *J Endourol.* 2000;14(9):735-737.

41. Desai MR, Kukreja RA, Desai MM, et al. A prospective randomized comparison of type of nephrostomy drainage following percutaneous nephrostolithotomy: large bore versus small bore versus tubeless. *J Urol.* 2004;172(2):565-567.

42. Haleblian GE, Sur RL, Albala DM, et al. Subcutaneous bupivacaine infiltration and postoperative pain perception after percutaneous nephrolithotomy. *J Urol.* 2007;178(3 Pt 1):925-928.

43. Jonnavithula N, Pisapati MV, et al. Efficacy of peritubal local anesthetic infiltration in alleviating postoperative pain in percutaneous nephrolithotomy. *J Endourol.* 2009;23(5):857-860.

44. Aghamir SM, Hosseini SR, Gooran S. Totally tubeless percutaneous nephrolithotomy. *J Endourol.* 2004;18(7):647-648.

45. Crook TJ, Lockyer CR, Keoghane SR, et al. A randomized controlled trial of nephrostomy placement versus tubeless percutaneous nephrolithotomy. *J Urol.* 2008;180(2):612-614.

46. Shah H, Khandkar A, Sodha H, et al. Tubeless percutaneous nephrolithotomy: 3 years of experience with 454 patients. *BJU Int.* 2009;104(6):840-846.

47. Aghamir SM, Khazaeli MH, Meisami A. Use of Surgicel for sealing nephrostomy tract after totally tubeless percutaneous nephrolithotomy. *J Endourol.* 2006;20(5):293-295.

48. Shah HN, Hegde S, Shah JN, et al. A prospective, randomized trial evaluating the safety and efficacy of fibrin sealant in tubeless percutaneous nephrolithotomy. *J Urol.* 2006;176(6 Pt 1):2488-2492.

49. Chen L, Xu QQ, Li JX, et al. Systemic inflammatory response syndrome after percutaneous nephrolithotomy: an assessment of risk factors. *Int J Urol.* 2008;15(12):1025-1028.

50. Dogan HS, Guliyev F, Cetinkaya YS, et al. Importance of microbiological evaluation in management of infectious complications following percutaneous nephrolithotomy. *Int Urol Nephrol.* 2007;39(3):737-742.

51. Gonan M, Turan H, Ozturk B, et al. Factors affecting fever following percutaneous nephrolithotomy: a prospective clinical study. *J Endourol.* 2008;22(9):2135-2138.

52. Skolarikos A, de la Rosette J. Prevention and treatment of complications following percutaneous nephrolithotomy. *Curr Opin Urol.* 2008;18(2):229-234.

53. Michel MS, Trojan L, Rassweiler JJ. Complications in percutaneous nephrolithotomy. *Eur Urol.* 2007;51(4):899-906.

54. Singla M, Srivastava A, Kapoor R, et al. Aggressive approach to staghorn calculi-safety and efficacy of multiple tracts percutaneous nephrolithotomy. *Urology.* 2008;71(6):1039-1042.

55. Kukreja R, Desai M, Patel S, et al. Factors affecting blood loss during percutaneous nephrolithotomy: prospective study. *J Endourol.* 2004;18(8):715-722.

56. Turna B, Nazli O, Demiryoguran S, et al. Percutaneous nephrolithotomy: variables that influence hemorrhage. *Urology.* 2007;69(4):603-607.

57. Kukreja RA, Desai MR, Sabnis RB, et al. Fluid absorption during percutaneous nephrolithotomy: does it matter? *J Endourol.* 2002;16(4):221-224.

58. Desai M, Grover R, Manohar T, et al. Simultaneous bilateral percutaneous nephrolithotomy: a single-center experience. *J Endourol.* 2007;21(5):508-514.

59. Ugras MY, Gedik E, Gunes A, et al. Some criteria to attempt second side safely in planned bilateral simultaneous percutaneous nephrolithotomy. *Urology.* 2008;72(5):996-1000.

60. Rana AM, Bhojwani JP. Percutaneous nephrolithotomy in renal anomalies of fusion, ectopia, rotation, hypoplasia, and pelvicalyceal aberration: uniformity in heterogeneity. *J Endourol.* 2009;23(4):609-614.

61. Desai MR, Jasani A. Percutaneous nephrolithotripsy in ectopic kidneys. *J Endourol.* 2000;14(3):289-292.

62. El-Kappany HA, El-Nahas AR, Shoma AM, et al. Combination of laparoscopy and nephroscopy for treatment of stones in pelvic ectopic kidneys. *J Endourol.* 2007;21(10):1131-1136.

63. Yohannes P, Smith AD. The endourological management of complications associated with horseshoe kidney. *J Urol.* 2002;168:5-8.

64. Symons SJ, Ramachandran A, Kurien A, et al. Urolithiasis in the horseshoe kidney: a single-centre experience. *BJU Int.* 2008;102: 1676-1680.

65. Raj GV, Auge BK, Weizer AZ, et al. Percutaneous management of calculi within horseshoe kidneys. *J Urol.* 2003;170:48-51.

66. Bagrodia A, Gupta A, Raman JD, et al. Impact of body mass index on cost and clinical outcomes after percutaneous nephrostolithotomy. *Urology.* 2008;72(4):756-760.

67. Koo BC, Burtt G, Burgess NA. Percutaneous stone surgery in the obese: outcome stratified according to body mass index. *BJU Int.* 2004;93(9):1296-1299.

68. Nguyen TA, Belis JA. Endoscopic management of urolithiasis in the morbidly obese patient. *J Endourol.* 1998;12(1):33-35.

69. El-Husseiny T, Moraitis K, Maan Z, et al. Percutaneous endourologic procedures in high-risk patients in the lateral decubitus position under regional anesthesia. *J Endourol.* 2009;23(10): 1603-1606.

70. Gofrit ON, Shapiro A, Donchin Y, et al. Lateral decubitus position for percutaneous nephrolithotripsy in the morbidly obese or kyphotic patient. *J Endourol.* 2002;16(6):383-386.

71. Wu SD, Yilmaz M, Tamul PC, et al. Awake endotracheal intubation and prone patient self-positioning: anesthetic and positioning considerations during percutaneous nephrolithotomy in obese patients. *J Endourol.* 2009;23(10):1599-1602.

72. Aron M, Yadav R, Goel R, et al. Percutaneous nephrolithotomy for complete staghorn calculi in preschool children. *J Endourol.* 2005;19(8):968-972.

73. Samad L, Aquil S, Zaidi Z. Paediatric percutaneous nephrolithotomy: setting new frontiers. *BJU Int.* 2006;97(2):359-363.

74. Samad L, Qureshi S, Zaidi Z. Does percutaneous nephrolithotomy in children cause significant renal scarring? *J Pediatr Urol.* 2007;3(1):36-39.

75. Wadhwa P, Aron M, Bal CS, et al. Critical prospective appraisal of renal morphology and function in children undergoing shockwave lithotripsy and percutaneous nephrolithotomy. *J Endourol.* 2007;21(9):961-966.

76. Dawaba MS, Shokeir AA, Hafez AT, et al. Percutaneous nephrolithotomy in children: early and late anatomical and functional results. *J Urol.* 2004;172(3):1078-1081.

Ureteroscopy for Ureteric Stones

42

Amy E. Krambeck and James E. Lingeman

Abstract Ureteroscopy is a safe and effective treatment for both distal and proximal ureteral calculi. Significant advancements in scope design, intracorporeal lithotrites, stone retrieval devices, and assistive devices have greatly increased the safety of ureteroscopy. In this chapter we will review the history of ureteroscopy and indications for the procedure. We will also discuss the ideal use of flexible, semirigid, and rigid ureteroscopes. Appropriate applications of assistive devices, ureteral access sheaths, and stone retrieval devices will be reviewed. We will also assess applicability of different intracorporeal lithotrites. Finally, complications of ureteroscopy will be examined, as well as their appropriate treatment. Urologists with appropriate knowledge of and skill sets for ureteroscopy should consider this treatment modality a realistic first-line therapy for ureteral stone disease.

42.1 Introduction

As a result of technological advancements in not only ureteroscope design, but also intracorporeal lithotrites, ureteral access and stone retrieval devices, and postoperative stenting, ureteroscopy is fast becoming a preferred treatment for ureteral stone disease. In fact, with the introduction of current ureteroscopy techniques, open surgical manipulation for ureteral stones has become obsolete and the role of shock wave lithotripsy (SWL) for ureteral stone disease has decreased.

The first recorded surgical procedure performed specifically for ureteral stone disease was by Thomas Emmet in 1879. He reported surgical manipulation on three female patients with stones in the distal ureter. In one patient, a cystotomy was made and the stone extracted from the ureter using forceps via the ureteral orifice; in another patient, the stone was removed transvaginally using a cut down technique, thus the first recorded ureterolithotomy.[1] Shortly after Emmet's report, blind endoscopic removal of ureteral calculi was developed. The first successful endoscopic stone manipulation was reported by Gustav Kolisher in 1889. He located a distal ureteral stone with a metal-tipped catheter and injected sterile oil to displace the stone.[2] In 1912, Hugh Hampton Young introduced a pediatric cystoscope into a dilated ureter up to the level of the renal pelvis in a child with posterior urethral valves, performing the first documented ureteroscopy.[3] Due to technologic limitations, not until the development of fiberoptics did further advancements in the field of endourology take place. In 1957, Curtiss and Hirschowitz[4] created the first flexible endoscope, which was subsequently used clinically for ureteroscopy by Marshall in 1964.[1] Interestingly, it was not until 1977 that rigid ureteroscopy was clinically implemented by Goodman.[1]

The development of minimally invasive treatments for urinary calculi has been closely married to technologic advances in the fields of fiberoptics and radiographic imaging. Since the initial endoscope introduced by Hirschowitz, vast improvements have been made in ureteroscope design, mechanics, and optics. Early rigid ureteroscopes were large, 10–16 French (Fr), and utilized a rod-lens system making them inflexible. The smallest rod-lens ureteroscope was described by Huff with a diameter of 8.5 Fr.[5] Current rigid ureteroscopes are significantly smaller in size due to the replacement of the rod-lens system with fiberoptics. The flexibility of the fiberoptic bundles makes the previously rigid shaft bendable along its vertical axis without image distortion, hence the current term "semirigid." However, the image quality is not as clear as the rod-lens system. The first semirigid ureteroscope was introduced in 1989,[6] quickly followed by multiple other semirigid ureteroscope designs.[7]

A.E. Krambeck (✉)
Department of Urology, Mayo Clinic Rochester, Rochester, MN, USA
e-mail: Krambeck.amy@mayo.edu

P.N. Rao et al. (eds.), *Urinary Tract Stone Disease*,
DOI 10.1007/978-1-84800-362-0_42, © Springer-Verlag London Limited 2011

Original flexible ureteroscopes also had significant limitations and worked by passive deflection only. Furthermore, they lacked working and irrigation channels. Current flexible ureteroscopes are dual deflection and have one 3.5 Fr or greater working channel. In general, the tip of the scope ranges from 7.5 to 8.5 Fr and they range in length from 54 to 70 cm. The flexible ureteroscopes are tapered with maximal diameter proximally to allow slow dilation of the ureter as the device is passed retrograde.

In this chapter we will discuss the treatment goals for ureteral calculi. The role of modern rigid and flexible ureteroscopy for the treatment of ureteral calculi disease in both the lower and upper ureter, as well as the use of different lithotrites and assistive devices will also be explored. Finally, we will cover potential complications of ureteroscopy.

42.2 Ureteral Calculi

The treatment goal for ureteral calculi is to completely clear the patient of all stone disease while limiting morbidity. In general, most patients with ureteral calculi 4 mm or less in size do not require intervention.[8] Furthermore, stone location plays an important role as stones located in the distal ureter are more likely to pass spontaneously than those located more proximally.[8,9] The probability of spontaneous ureteral stone passage overall is directly related to the distance of the ureter to be traversed and inversely related to stone size. However, other factors must be considered, and in those patients with significant pain, bilateral ureteral stone disease, stone disease in a solitary kidney, unpassable stones larger than 5 mm, or smaller stones that do not pass after a trail of conservative management, immediate surgical intervention should be executed. Ureteral stones in patients with abnormal anatomy (ureteral ectopia, ureterocele, megaureter) may have impaired passage and thus, surgical intervention should be implemented early.[10–12] Calculi in the presence of urinary tract infections – that is, "infected stones" – should be considered an emergency condition and treated with ureteral stenting or percutaneous nephrostomy tube placement. Once the acute infection has been adequately treated, surgical stone manipulation should follow.

Although SWL is considered an accepted treatment modality for ureteral stones[8,9], studies have demonstrated that ureteroscopy is the most cost-effective treatment strategy for ureteral stones at all locations after observation fails.[13,14] Ureteroscopy can also be applied when SWL is contraindicated, such as patients on anticoagulation therapy.[15] Furthermore, ureteroscopy can be performed safely in patients with bilateral ureteral stone disease[9,16,17] or those with a solitary kidney.

Ureteroscopy was initially performed exclusively under general or regional anesthesia due to the large caliber of early ureteroscopes. With the introduction of fiberoptics and the progressive decrease in ureteroscope size, ureteroscopy can potentially now be performed under intravenous sedation or sedoanalgesia. Although most urologists still prefer to perform ureteroscopy under general anesthesia, several authors have reported success rates of ureteroscopy performed under sedoanalgesia equivalent to those of ureteroscopy under general anesthesia.[18–22] In our practice we prefer general anesthesia for ureteroscopy to limit patient discomfort. Most ureteral orifices will accommodate a 6–7 Fr device without dilation making rigid and flexible ureteroscopy possible, and using small-diameter Holmium:YAG fibers immediate treatment of ureteral calculi can be achieved. Since instrumentation (i.e., flexible versus rigid) can differ from upper to lower ureter, we will focus on these categories separately (Fig. 42.1).

42.3 Distal Ureteral Stones

Ureteroscopy for distal ureteral calculi is a highly successful, minimally invasive treatment associated with limited morbidity. It can be used to treat large or multiple stones of any composition and has a high immediate stone-free rate. Meta-analysis performed for the 2007 ureteral calculi American Urologic Association (AUA)/European Urologic Association guidelines noted ureteroscopy to be superior to SWL for the treatment of all sized distal ureteral stones.[23] Overall complication rates were similar in both the ureteroscopy and SWL-treated patients. A summary of ureteroscopy complications are presented in Table 42.1. The overall stone-free rate for distal ureteroscopy with one procedure was 94% (C.I. 86–96%). Ureteral injury occurred in 3% (C.I. 3–4%) and ureteral stricture development in 1% (C.I. 1–2%) of distal ureteroscopy patients. Based on these results, the AUA/EUA has recommended distal ureteroscopy as the first-line therapy for nonpassable distal ureteral calculi.

It is our preference to limit rigid or semirigid ureteroscopy to stones below the iliac vessels. In some cases, specifically female patients, it is possible to advance the ureteroscope to the renal pelvis; however, ureteroscope mobility is limited high in the ureter, making it difficult to efficiently retrieve all stone fragments. Meta-analysis has demonstrated a decrease in stone-free rates when rigid/semirigid ureteroscopes are used to treat proximal ureteral stones compared to flexible (77% versus 87%).[23] Furthermore, the risk of ureteral injury is not trivial in these cases. While the only statistically identifiable risk factors for ureteral injury during ureteroscopy are operative time and surgeon experience,[24] there has been a significant decrease in reports of ureteral injury secondary to ureteroscopy from 1989 to 2000 and this has been attributed to the use of more flexible instruments for ureteroscopy.[24–26] Based on these observations it is our opinion to limit rigid/semirigid ureteroscopy to distal ureteral stones.

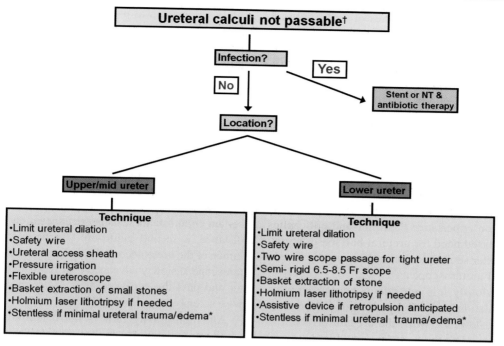

Fig. 42.1 Basic algorithm for ureteroscopic management of ureteral calculi. [†] This algorithm is for small calculi that have failed a trial of passage, larger calculi unlikely to pass spontaneously, bilateral calculi, calculi in a solitary kidney, or patients unable to tolerate conservative management. [*] Patients undergoing bilateral ureteroscopy, ureteroscopy in a solitary kidney, or renal insufficiency should have a temporary postoperative ureteral stent placed

Table 42.1 Summary of ureteroscopy complications reported in American Urologic Associated and European Urologic Association 2007 ureteral calculi guideline[23]

Complication	Distal ureter		Mid-ureter		Proximal ureter	
	Number of patients	% (CI)	Number of patients	% (CI)	Number of patients	% (CI)
Steinstrasse	[a]		[a]		109	0 (0–1)
Stricture	1,911	1 (1–2)	326	4 (2–7)	987	2 (1–5)
Ureteral injury	4,529	3 (3–4)	514	6 (3–8)	1,005	6 (3–9)
UTI	458	4 (2–7)	63	2 (0–7)	224	4 (1–8)
Sepsis	1,954	2 (1–4)	199	4 (1–11)	360	4 (2–6)

[a] Steinstrasse complication was not reported for distal and mid-ureteral calculi

In general, all attempts are made to avoid ureteral orifice dilation in our practice. The older rod-lens ureteroscopes provide excellent irrigant flow and visualization; however, they are large with diameters 8.5–16 Fr. Often the rod-lens ureteroscopes required balloon dilation of the ureteral orifice in patients that were not previously stented. With the introduction of the fiberoptic system, the diameter of the ureteroscope has been significantly downsized such that most patients undergoing ureteroscopy do not require balloon dilation of their ureteral orifice. Contemporary semirigid ureteroscope tip diameters range from 6.0 to 10 Fr with a length of 31 cm and working channel diameter of 2.1–6.6 Fr.[5] The majority of semirigid ureteroscopes have tapered oval or circular tips; however, American Cystoscope Manufacturers Incorporated (ACMI) has introduced the MR-6™, which is a triangular beveled tip thought to facilitate introduction into the ureteral orifice.[5]

Retrospective studies have compared the success rates and complications between rigid and semirigid ureteroscopes.

Francesca et al.[27] compared outcomes of 229 rigid to 44 semirigid ureteroscopy procedures. In the rigid ureteroscopy group, ureteral dilation was performed in 86.6% of cases with a success rate of 85.5%, ureteral perforation rates of 11.2%, and 1.6% rate of ureteral stenosis. In the semirigid group none of the patients required ureteral orifice dilation and the success rate was 89.8%, ureteral perforation rate 2%, and none developed ureteral stenosis. The authors concluded that ureteroscopy was safer using semirigid ureteroscopes without compromising success rates. Authors have also attributed the decrease in overall ureteroscopic complications from 20% to 12% over a 10-year interval to small ureteroscope sizes and increased surgeon experience.[25] Stoller and colleagues[28] reported a decreased need for ureteral balloon dilation of 16%, when smaller semirigid ureteroscopes were used as opposed to rigid ureteroscopes.

As stated previously, it is generally not necessary to perform ureteral dilation prior to insertion of the semirigid ureteroscope[29,30]; however, when the ureteral orifice is too narrow to accommodate the ureteroscope, dilation may be necessary. Ureteral dilation can be accomplished with serial dilators, balloon dilation, or with a smaller "mini" ureteroscope. There is controversy over the routine use of ureteral dilation when ureteroscopy is performed. Studies have demonstrated that ureteral dilation does not improve stone-free results of ureteroscopy nor does it protect against complications.[28,31] Furthermore, if ureteral dilation is avoided, ureteroscopy can potentially be performed without the necessity of postoperative ureteral stenting. Moneim and Khalaf[32] demonstrated that after ureteral dilation, unstented ureters were more likely to develop distal ureteral stricture disease compared to stented ureters. Therefore, if ureteral dilation is necessary, temporary postoperative stenting should be performed. If ureteral dilation is necessary to pass the ureteroscope, it is our preference to avoid balloon dilation and to instead use sequential ureteral coaxial dilators up to 10–12 Fr. This practice ensures that the ureter will not be dilated greater than what is necessary to complete the procedure. Although it is not our practice, it should be mentioned that some urologists prefer to dilate the ureteral orifice not to facilitate ureteroscope passage, but rather to allow for intact removal of larger distal ureteral calculi without fragmentation.

Recent tip miniaturization of semirigid ureteroscopes has allowed for the development of a 4.9 Fr distal tip ureteroscope with a 3 Fr working channel from Richard Wolf (Vernon Hills, Illinois, USA). Although data is limited, Gupta[33] reported on 25 patients treated with the "mini" ureteroscope. None of the patients required ureteral dilation. The procedure was performed under local anesthetic only in 8 patients, and 15 patients did not require a postoperative stent. Stone clearance at 1 week was 100% in Gupta's series. A ureteral safety guidewire was used in only three patients. Although the 4.9 Fr ureteroscope is not widely available to the general urologist, it is an excellent tool for use in the delicate ureter.

For distal ureteroscopy we advise placement of a ureteral guidewire before performing ureteroscopy. The ureteral guidewire opens the ureteral orifice to allow easier passage of the ureteroscope. Furthermore, should a complication occur during the procedure, the guidewire can act as a safety wire, allowing for quick placement of a ureteral stent. Most ureteral injuries, with the exception of complete avulsion, can be managed with ureteral stenting and the procedure can then be performed successfully and safely at a later date.[34] In certain circumstances where the ureter is narrow over a short distance, a second guidewire can be placed through the lumen of the ureteroscope. With direct visualization, the ureteroscope is slowly advanced over the wire to dilate the ureter and pass the narrowed area, at which point the second wire is removed.

Although gravity flow is not contraindicated, to avoid stone retropulsion and high intrarenal pressures we advise hand irrigation with normal saline through one of the working channels of the ureteroscope. If the stone can be removed intact, we prefer basket extraction; however, if the size of the stone does lend itself to easy extraction then Holmium:YAG laser lithotripsy is performed. All fragments larger than the safety wire (0.035 in.) are basket extracted, while the remainder is allowed to pass spontaneously. If significant ureteral edema or manipulation occurred during the procedure, then a temporary ureteral stent is inserted over the safety wire at the end of the case.

42.4 Upper/Proximal Ureteral Stones

The 2007 ureteral calculi AUA/EUA guidelines support either SWL in situ or flexible ureteroscopy for proximal and mid-ureteral stones. Meta-analysis demonstrated superior stone-free results using SWL for stones less than 10 mm in size, while ureteroscopy was superior for stones greater than 10 mm in size.[23] Outcome results of ureteroscopy for mid-ureteral calculi trended toward higher stone-free rates compared to SWL, but overall results were statistically similar. The overall stone-free rate for proximal ureteroscopy was 81%, with little difference noted based on stone size; 80% for stones less than 10 mm in size; and 79% for stones greater than 10 mm in size. For mid-ureteral stones, the overall stone-free rate was 86%, but it was size dependant; 78% stone-free with stones greater than 10 mm in size; and 91% with stones less than 10 mm in size. Unfortunately, the stone-free rates in this study included both flexible and rigid ureteroscopes to treat proximal- and mid-ureteral stones, and it is likely that if the study focused solely on flexible ureteroscopy, stone-free rates would have exceeded 90%. Overall complications for both mid- and proximal-ureteral stones treated with ureteroscopy were limited (Table 42.1). Based on these results, we prefer flexible ureteroscopy for most proximal- and mid-ureteral calculi.

Currently available flexible ureteroscopes are easily accommodated by even unstented ureteral orifices and allow immediate access to ureteral calculi. There has been significant downsizing of the tip and mid-shaft diameter of the flexible ureteroscope such that the average tip diameter is 6.9–7.5 Fr and mid-shaft diameter is 7.5–9.0 Fr,[30] making passage of the ureteroscope possible without dilation. The length of most available ureteroscopes range from 54 to 70 cm and have the ability to reach anywhere in the upper urinary tract.[5] The deflection capability of most current ureteroscopes allow for active deflection up to 270° in one (Olympus P5) or both directions (Storz FlexX2, Wolf Viper). Although this degree of deflection is generally not necessary for ureteroscopy of ureteral calculi, it has been found that the degradation in maximal deflection with the insertion of instruments through the working channel is less pronounced with the dual-deflection ureteroscopes[35] and this should be taken into account when choosing a ureteroscope.

In an attempt to improve image quality of flexible ureteroscopes, digital instruments have been developed. Digital ureteroscopes incorporate an optical chip – complementary metal oxide semiconductor (CMOS) or charge-coupled device (CCD) – at the tip of the scope. With this technology, internal optics are not required in the long shaft, which allows for stronger deflection cables to improve the durability of the instrument.[36] The camera is incorporated into the head of the scope, thus making digital ureteroscopes more lightweight and convenient. In 2006, Gyrus-ACMI (Southboro, Massachusetts, USA) introduced the DUR-D ureteroscope. This ureteroscope has a distal light-emitting diode (LED), as well as a CMOS. Several groups have published their experience with this device and all cite superior image quality compared to current flexible ureteroscopes.[37–40]

Robotic ureteroscopic applications have been explored in an attempt to decrease the complex skill sets necessary to perform flexible ureteroscopy effectively and expeditiously. A master-slave control system has been utilized to perform robotic ureteroscopy in the porcine model.[30,41] The procedure was successful and efficient in all cases. Robotic ureteroscopy has also expanded to human usage. Columbo and colleagues[42] recently presented their series of laser lithotripsy of renal calculi using the robotic ureteroscopy technology; however, the general applicability of this procedure remains to be seen.

For all flexible ureteroscopic cases performed in our practice, a ureteral guidewire is initially placed. We prefer a hybrid wire with a soft, lubricous tip and a kink-resistant body. The soft tip decreases the risk of ureteral perforation and allows for safe manipulation around the stone, while the strong body of the wire stabilizes and straightens the ureter. Examples of available wires of this type are the Sensor™ (Boston Scientific, Natick, MA) or the UroWIRE XF™ (Applied Medical, Rancho Santa Margarita, CA).[43] If there is difficulty in maneuvering the wire past the stone, a Glidewire® (Boston Scientific) or Roadrunner® (Cook Medical, Bloomington, IN) may be necessary. The Glidewire® or Roadrunner® is a soft, lubricous wire that can more easily maneuver around obstructions. Once the wire is positioned in the kidney, a 5 Fr ureteral catheter is advanced over the wire and used to perform a gentle retrograde pyelogram and/or to exchange the Glidewire® for a more sturdy wire.

Once the guidewire is in place, a ureteral access sheath is inserted over the wire. The access sheath facilitates the insertion and straight alignment of the ureteroscope in the upper urinary tract.[1,43,44] Kourambas and associates[45] reported a randomized controlled study comparing patients who underwent ureteroscopy with a 12–14 Fr ureteral access sheath and those who underwent ureteroscopy with no access sheath. They found a decrease in operating time and costs, as well as a simplification of ureteral reentry in those cases where the access sheath was utilized. The access sheath also allows efflux of irrigant out the distal end of the sheath, maintaining intrapelvic pressures below 20 cm of water despite irrigant fluid pressurized up to 200 cm of water.[46] Multiple different access sheaths are available, ranging from 10 to 16 Fr in diameter and 20–55 cm in length.[44] The diameter is generally presented as two numbers (e.g., 10/12) that represent the range of the outer diameter of the access sheath. Most contemporary flexible ureteroscopes are compatible with all access sheaths with a diameter of 10/12 Fr or larger. The Cook Flexor™ (Cook, Bloomington, IN) has been rated superior to the Applied Access Forte XE™ (Applied Medical) as well as the newer generation access sheaths with regard to buckling.[47,48]

A common criticism of the ureteral access sheath is inability to advance the sheath to the desired location; however, recent literature supports that the access sheath can successfully be deployed for all but 5–7% of cases.[44,45,49] If there is difficulty advancing the access sheath, ureteral dilation with sequential ureteral dilators or balloon dilation can be utilized, or a ureteral stent can be placed to allow the ureter to passively dilate and ureteroscopy is planned for a later date.[44,49] Authors have also suggested the administration of 1 mg of glucagon intravenously to stimulate ureteral smooth muscle relaxation and subsequent placement of the access sheath.[44] The administration of glucagon is controversial. When tested for the treatment of post-SWL ureteral colic in a randomized clinical controlled trial there was no apparent affect.[50] Of note, glucagon should not be given to patients with diabetes mellitus as significant hyperglycemia can develop. If ultimately the access sheath cannot be deployed, then ureteroscopy can be performed using two ureteral wires – one acting as a safety wire and the other used to facilitate ureteroscope insertion through the urethra and bladder – up the ureter to the desired location.

Pressurized normal saline irrigation up to 300 mmHg facilitates visualization when performing flexible ureteroscope. Although various systems are available, we preferred 1,000–3,000 ml standard pressure infusion bags. Pressurized irrigant has been found to be safe if a ureteral access sheath is in place[46]; however, if we are unable to place a ureteral access sheath, then we perform hand irrigation only. Once the stone is identified it should either be extracted or fragmented using an intracorporeal lithotrite and then removed. After the stone has been successfully treated, the ureter should be inspected as the ureteroscope and access sheath are withdrawn to assess for ureteral injury or edema. If significant ureteral edema or manipulation has occurred, a post-ureteroscopy stent should be placed over the safety wire to prevent colic and obstruction.

42.5 Stone Retrieval Devices

Multiple different stone retrieval devices have been developed. Retrieval devices should allow for visibility during stone manipulation, have enough radial force to open the ureter, and the ability to capture, retain, or disengage the stone.[43] In general, there are two broad categories of devices: graspers and baskets.

The alligator or rat tooth forceps is a grasper device not in common use for stone retrieval. The alligator forceps are used with an offset ureteroscope to allow for manipulation of the handle. Benefits of the alligator forceps is its reversible grasp and it is reusable, making it extremely cost-effective. Its large size of 3 Fr or greater and weak grasp has limited the effectiveness and wide applicability of the alligator forceps for stone manipulation. Another device, the disposable three-pronged grasper has been advocated by some as safe and effective. The three-pronged grasper is 2.4 Fr and flexible, thus producing minimal impact on ureteroscope deflection. The graspers also easily release the stone[51]; however, care should be taken to insure urothelium is not grasped with the stone.

Despite the benefits of the three-pronged graspers, the basket design has been found to be a more versatile and atraumatic stone retrieval device.[52–54] There are three main types of basket design: helical, flatwire, and tipless nitinol.

The helical basket contains cylindrical wires, each in the form of a helix. The larger the stone, the fewer number of wires are needed; and the smaller the stone, the more wires needed. Twisting of the basket is often needed to entrap the stone. The Dormia basket was once a popular general use helical basket, which is no longer manufactured. Currently, there are both stainless steel and nitinol helical baskets available.

Flatwire baskets contain flat, ribbon-like wires in a three- to six-wire configuration. The flatwire basket can be opened to radially open it and entrap both small and large diameter stones. Examples of the flatwire devices are the Segura Hemisphere® (Boston Scientific) and Bagley Helical® (Microvasive, Boston Scientific). These baskets have excellent radial opening force so are useful in tight quarters, but are not intended to be rotated due to significant shearing forces. Furthermore, the tip of the basket can inadvertently produce urothelial damage.

Tipless nitinol baskets are comprised of cylindrical wires that have memory, allowing the wires to conform to the shape of the ureter. The tipless feature minimizes trauma to the urothelium and papillae. Most endourologic companies make some form of the nitinol basket, and all of them are similar. In general, in vitro studies have shown the teardrop basket configuration and linear opening dynamics of the Cook NCircle™ 2.2 Fr (Cook Urological) basket best facilitates efficient stone capture.[54–56] The Cook NCircle™ also demonstrated the most rapid target basket width compared to 12 other baskets suggesting a more controlled view when opening.[57] The use of a 1.5 Fr ureteral basket is preferred in our practice when performing flexible ureteroscopy in order to increase irrigant flow and limit internal damage to the ureteroscope. There are multiple available baskets of this size. The 1.5 Fr Sacred Heart Halo™ (Sacred Heart Medical, Minnetonka, MN) has a unique design in that it allows rotation of an engaged stone via a rotary wheel in the basket handle.[58] The smallest basket available is a 1.3 Fr basket recently introduced from Boston Scientific.

More recently, the configuration of the nitinol basket has been manipulated in an attempt to increase efficiency and safety of stone basketing. The Cook NCompass™ (Cook Urological) is a 2.2 Fr basket that has a webbed configuration to capture stones as small as 1 mm in size.[43] The Bard Dimension™ (Bard Urological, Covington, KY) has a deflectable four-wire teardrop configuration, which has been reported to provide a greater ease of stone capture and release.[59] The Escape Tipless Nitinol™ basket (Boston Scientific) is a 1.9 Fr basket that allows the insertion of a 200 μm holmium laser fiber to fragment the stone in the basket should it become lodged in the ureter. Boston Scientific has also evaluated a basket with a unique design of two nitinol arms fused at the apex. With significant axial force the apex of the basket will break apart. This feature is to prevent ureteral avulsion should the stone and basket become lodged in the ureter.

42.6 Intracorporeal Lithotrites

Intracorporeal lithotripter devices have been effectively miniaturized to meet the improvements in ureteroscopic equipment. There are three categories of intracorporeal lithotrites available for the treatment of ureteral stones: electrohydraulic lithotripsy (EHL), ballistic lithotripsy, and laser lithotripsy. These can further be divided into flexible (laser lithotripsy and EHL) and rigid (ballistic).

The EHL probe acts as an underwater spark plug with two electrodes of different voltage separated by insulation. Spark discharge causes a hydraulic shock wave and formation of cavitation bubbles.[1] The EHL probe works effectively in normal saline solution,[60] and although the original probes were large, miniaturization of the probes to 1.6–5 Fr have allowed it to be used in flexible ureteroscopes without occluding the irrigation flow. A major disadvantage of the EHL is its propensity for ureteral mucosa injury and perforation. It is theorized that perforation is secondary to cavitation forces and does not require contact of the probe with the mucosa[61]; therefore, the risk of perforation is greatest with higher energies.[1] The risk of perforation using the EHL probe ranges from 40% to 8.5%.[1,62,63] Another shortcoming of EHL is stone retropulsion, which is more pronounced than with Holmium:YAG lithotripsy.[64] Although EHL is the least costly of all lithotrites,[65,66] it is capable of fragmenting 90% of stones[62] and is flexible. Unfortunately, the risk of perforation is not insignificant and therefore we do not use EHL for the treatment of ureteral stones in an effort to limit subsequent stricture formation.

Ballistic lithotripsy relies on energy generated by the movement of a projectile that is in direct contact with the stone. Probes for the rigid ballistic lithotrites range from 0.8 to 2.5 mm and there is a flexible nickel-titanium probe for the Swiss Lithoclast (Boston Scientific), which allows it to be used with a flexible ureteroscope.[67,68] Stone fragmentation with the ballistic lithotrites has been reported to range from 73% to 100% regardless of stone composition. The lower success rates have been reported when the device is inserted through a flexible or semirigid deflectable ureteroscope,[68–70] as bending can affect its internal mechanical function. One major advantage of the ballistic devices is an extremely low risk of ureteral perforation compared with EHL and laser lithotripsy.[71] In fact, the device can be placed directly on the urothelial without significant damage. The average risk of ureteral perforation during ureteroscopic ballistic lithotripsy is less than 1%.[1] Despite this benefit we limit the use of ballistic devices for ureteroscopy due to the high rate of stone retropulsion at 2–17%.[1] Most failures to fragment stones with these devices are related to inability to trap the stone and subsequent retropulsion.[72] Furthermore, proximal stones have a higher rate of migration compared to distal stones.[68,69]

Today, laser lithotripsy is the ureteroscopic intracorporeal lithotrite preferred by most endourologists. The Holmium:YAG laser is a 2140 nm laser that is highly absorbed by water. Since the majority of tissue is water the laser can cut and coagulate, as well as break stones of *any* composition. Fortunately, the depth of penetration is 0.5–1.0 mm and thus collateral damage is minimal.[73] Since the long pulse of the laser produces weak shock waves, stone fragments generated with the Holmium:YAG laser is primarily through photothermal mechanisms resulting in small fragments.[1,73,74] Teichman and colleagues[75] demonstrated that the Holmium:YAG laser produced smaller stone fragments than other intracorporeal lithotrites. The Holmium:YAG laser can be delivered through flexible 100–360 microfibers making it ideal for ureteroscopy. Furthermore, because of the weak shock wave produced by the Holmium:YAG laser retropulsion is the least likely of all the intracorporeal lithotrite devices.[76,77] Clinical results from high volume centers demonstrate excellent stone-free rates of 95–97% using the Holmium:YAG laser.[77,78] A major disadvantage of the holmium laser is the initial high cost of the device and the cost of the laser fibers. Another theoretical side effect of the Holmium:YAG laser is the production of cyanide when uric acid stones are treated, which has been reported in vitro. However, no significant cyanide toxicity has been reported in the literature to date.[1]

In an attempt to produce a cost-effective alternative to the Holmium:YAG laser, the frequency doubled, double-pulse ND:YAG (FREDDY) laser (World of Medicine, Berlin, Germany) has been developed. Two pulses are generated: one produces the bubble and the second heats it, resulting in a mechanical force.[78] The FREDDY has no tissue ablative properties. In vitro testing has shown improved stone fragmentation of the FREDDY laser compared to Holmium:YAG.[79] However, clinical studies have demonstrated inferior results compared to Holmium:YAG standards.[80,81] Another disadvantage to the FREDDY laser is that it cannot break cystine stones. Based on these limitations, the exact clinical role of the FREDDY laser remains to be seen; however, it may be a low cost second-line alternative to Holmium:YAG laser lithotripsy.

42.7 Assistive Devices

Proximal migration of stone fragments during ureteroscopy has been reported to occur in 40–50% of proximal ureteral stone cases and 5–10% of distal ureteral cases.[68,69,82] To prevent stone migration, different maneuvers have been utilized including reverse Trendelenberg position to optimize the effects of gravity. A variety of commercial devices have been introduced to prevent stone migration during intracorporeal lithotripsy in the ureter including backstops, stone cones, and gels.

Multiple commercially available backstop devices have been developed. The Cook NTrap™ is a currently available 2.8 Fr backstop device. It is composed of 24 interwoven nitinol wires that are deployed behind the stone like a cap. The device has been shown to prevent migration of particles as small as 1.5 mm in an ex-vivo model.[83] The Lithocatch Parachute™ (Boston Scientific, Boston, MA) is a 12 Fr balloon catheter that is placed over a wire behind the stone during lithotripsy.[84] The Percsys Accordion™ (Percutaneous Systems Inc., Mountain View CA) is also deployed behind the stone and expands like an accordion to again prevent fragment migration. The Stone Cone™ (Boston Scientific) has concentric coils that are positioned proximal to the stone to prevent fragment retropulsion.[82] Clinically, the Stone Cone™ has been shown to reduce the incidence of residual stone fragments of 3 mm or greater.[85] All these devices require that a wire be left in the ureter during the procedure.

In an attempt to limit the need for a safety wire, gel occlusive devices have been explored. Ali and colleagues[86] suggested instillation of lubricating jelly proximal to the stone, which was found to decrease rates of stone migration clinically.[87] However, stone-free rates and operative times were not impacted by this maneuver. Mirabile and colleagues[88] evaluated the feasibility of a thermosensitive polymer (UroJel, Fossa Medical, Boston, MA) in the porcine model. The gel is injected behind the stone where it solidifies. Once the stone is fractured, the gel can be dislodged.

Stone retropulsion is mainly an issue associated with rigid/semirigid ureteroscopy. Due to the minimal retropulsion produced during holmium laser lithotripsy, we do not routinely utilize the assistive devices during ureteroscopy. However, they are potentially of benefit if ballistic/pneumatic lithotripsy is utilized.[43]

42.8 Complications of Ureteroscopy

As modern ureteroscopes have become smaller and less traumatic, as safer intracorporeal lithotripters have become widely available, and as a better understanding of the technical principles of ureteroscopy has been developed, the number of complications associated with ureteroscopy has decreased. Overall complication rates range from 1% to 20%, with major complications reported from 0% to 6%.[1,24] Fortunately, most complications secondary to ureteroscopy respond favorably to simple ureteral stenting. As noted in Table 42.1, the 2007 AUA/EUA ureteral guidelines noted that ureteral complications occurred in less than 10% of cases regardless of location of the ureteral stone.[23]

Due to technologic advancements, the occurrence of ureteral perforation is decreasing; however, they do still occur and are a significant risk factor for future stricture formation. Ureteral perforation is most highly associated with the EHL device and the Holmium:YAG laser and pneumatic lithotrite.[1] Schuster and colleagues[24] also noted operative time as a significant risk factor for ureteral perforation in multivariate analysis. They further noted surgeon experience and stone location as risk factors for overall complications. The treatment of ureteral perforation consists of immediate termination of the procedure, placement of a ureteral stent for 2–4 weeks, and careful radiographic follow-up.

Ureteral strictures occur secondary to ureteral trauma, stone impaction, iatrogenic injury, or retained stone fragments in the ureteral wall. Roberts and colleagues[89] noted that duration of stone impaction and ureteral perforation were significant risk factors for ureteral stricture formation. A stricture rate of 24% was observed for stones impacted an average of 11 months, and four of the five patients who developed strictures experienced a ureteral perforation. If significant trauma occurs during ureteroscopy, placement of a ureteral stent for 4–6 weeks may prevent the development of a stricture.[1] If stricture occurs, they can potentially respond to incision and ureteral stent placement or balloon dilation with stent placement.[1,90]

Stones inadvertently displaced into the wall of the ureter (i.e., submucosal stones or stone granuloma) pose a high risk of stricture formation. Removal of these stones is difficult as ureteral perforation with urinoma can occur resulting in intense fibrosis. If submucosal stones are encountered, laser excision followed by ureteral stent placement is recommended. If laser excision fails, then open resection of the ureter should be considered. Stones that have been lost outside the collecting system are harmless and require no further intervention. If the stone is associated with infection, there is a potential for the development of a retroperitoneal abscess and, therefore, antibiotic therapy and close observation should be performed.

The risk of infection with ureteroscopy is not trivial and may occur via one of two methods: introduction of external pathogens by means of instrumentation or manipulation of potentially infected urinary calculi, or foreign bodies in the urinary tract. Because of the potential for infection or the presence of infected stones, antibiotic prophylaxis is indicated[91]. Fever in the early postoperative period is common and occurs in 1.2–6.9% of cases.[19,25,92,93] In most cases, the fever is thought to be secondary to chemically induced renal inflammation[94]; however, in one series where preoperative antibiotics were not routinely given, fever greater than 38°C occurred in 22% of patients, although infection was only documented in 3.7%. Overall, the incidence of sepsis associated with ureteroscopy is low, with culture positive infections occurring in 1–4% of cases[23,24] and sepsis in 0.3–2%.[23,24,94] A lack of uniformity in the definition of sepsis may be the cause of the variability in reporting.

Ureteral avulsion is the most dreaded and severe complication of ureteroscopy. It occurs when aggressive stone removal occurs in the presence of ureter entrapped in the basket or when excessively large stones are pulled through narrow areas of the ureter. Stoller and Wolf[94] reviewed 33 ureteroscopy series from 1984 to 1992 with more than 5,000 patients and noted a 0.3% incidence of ureteral avulsion. Grasso[93] reviewed three series from 1992 to 1998 with more than 1,000 patients and found no ureteral avulsions. If avulsion occurs, open repair is generally required. It is not unreasonable to attempt realignment of the ureter by placing a stent over the safety wire if one is present; however, ureteral stricture formation is often the result if continuity of the urothelium can be established. If no safety wire is in place or if the ureter is pulled out of the retroperitoneum (i.e., intussusception), immediate open repair is necessary.[1]

42.9 Conclusions

Although it is a more invasive technique than SWL, ureteroscopy with small, rigid, or flexible ureteroscopes is the most efficient technique for treatment and removal of ureteral stones. Advancements in scope design, size, assistive devices, lithotrites, and stone retrieval baskets have improved the overall safety profile of this procedure. Today ureteroscopy should be considered as a first-line treatment of ureteral calculi in patients desiring a single procedure with maximal efficacy.

References

1. Lingeman JE, Matlaga BR, Evan AP. Surgical management of upper urinary tract calculi. In: Kavoussi LR, Novick AC, Partin AW, Peters CA, Wein AJ, eds. *Campbell-Walsh Urology*. 9th ed. Philadelphia: Saunders-Elsevier; 2007.
2. Murphy LJT. *History of Urology*. Springfield: Charles C. Thomas; 1972.
3. Young HH, McKay RW. Congenital valvular obstruction of the posterior urethra. *Surg Gynecol Obstet*. 1929;48:509-535.
4. Hirschowitz BI, Peters CW, Curtiss LE. Preliminary reports on a long fiberscope for examination of the stomach and duodenum. *Univ Mich Med Bull*. 1957;23:178-180.
5. Basillote JB, Lee DI, Eichel L, et al. Ureteroscopes: flexible, rigid, and semirigid. *Urol Clin North Am*. 2004;31:21-32.
6. Dretler SP, Cho G. Semirigid ureteroscopy: a new genre. *J Urol*. 1989;141:1314-1316.
7. Ferraro RF, Abraham VE, Cohen TD, et al. A new generation of semirigid fiberoptic ureteroscopes. *J Endourol*. 1999;13:35-40.
8. Segura JW, Preminger G, Assimos D, et al. Ureteral stones clinical guidelines panel summary report on the management of ureteric calculi. *J Urol*. 1997;158:1915-1921.
9. Preminger G, Lindler T, Lamberton G, et al. A novel radial-dilating balloon-expandable ureteral access sheath: the initial human experience. American Urological Association; 2007; San Francisco, Abst 1448.
10. Diamond DA, Rickwood AMK, Lee PH, et al. Infection stones in children: a twenty-seven-year review. *Urology*. 1994;43:525-527.
11. Dretler SP. Management of the lower ureteral stone. *AUA Update Series*. 1995;14:62. lesson 8.
12. Kapoor DA, Leech JE, Yap WT, et al. Cost and efficacy of extracorporeal shock wave lithotripsy versus ureteroscopy in the treatment of lower ureteral calculi. *J Urol*. 1992;148:1095-1096.
13. Lotan Y, Gettman M, Roehrborn C, et al. Management of ureteral calculi: a cost comparison and decision making analysis. *J Urol*. 2002;167:1621-1629.
14. Watterson JD, Girvan AR, Cook AJ, et al. Safety and efficacy of holmium: YAG laser lithotripsy in patients with bleeding diatheses. *J Urol*. 2002;168:442-445.
15. Deliveliotis C, Picramenos D, Alexopoulou K, et al. One-session bilateral ureteroscopy: is it safe in selected patients? *Int Urol Nephrol*. 1996;28:481-484.
16. Hollenbeck BK, Schuster TG, Faerber GJ, et al. Safety and efficacy of same-session bilateral ureteroscopy. *J Endourol*. 2003;17:881-885.
17. Rittenberg MH, Bagley DH. Ureteroscopic diagnosis and treatment of urinary calculi during pregnancy. *Urology*. 1988;32:427-428.
18. Abdel-Razzak OM, Bagley DH. Clinical experience with flexible ureteropyeloscopy. *J Urol*. 1992;148:1788-1792.
19. Abdel-Razzak OM, Bagley DH. The 6.9 F semirigid ureteroscope in clinical use. *Urology*. 1993;41:45-48.
20. Grasso M, Bagley D. Small diameter, actively deflectable, flexible ureteropyeloscopy. *J Urol*. 1998;160:1648-1653.
21. Cybulski PA, Joo H, Honey JDA. Ureteroscopy: anesthetic considerations. *Urol Clin N Am*. 2004;31:43-47.
22. Preminger GM, Tiselius HG, Assimos DG, et al. 2007 Guideline for the management of ureteral calculi. *Eur Urol*. 2007;52:1610-1631.
23. Schuster TG, Hollenbeck BK, Faerber GJ, et al. Complications of ureteroscopy: analysis of predictive factors. *J Urol*. 2001;166:538-540.
24. Harmon WJ, Sershon PD, Blute ML, et al. Ureteroscopy: current practice and long-term complications. *J Urol*. 1997;157:28-31.
25. Brandes S, Coburn M, Armenakas N, et al. Diagnosis and management of ureteric injury: an evidence-based analysis. *BJU Int*. 2004;94:277-289.
26. Francesca F, Scattoni V, Nava L, et al. Failures and complications of transurethral ureteroscopy in 297 cases: conventional rigid instruments vs. small caliber semirigid ureteroscopes. *Eur Urol*. 1995;28: 112-115.
27. Stoller ML, Wolf JS Jr, Hofmann R, et al. Ureteroscopy without routine balloon dilation: an outcome assessment. *J Urol*. 1992;147:1238-1242.
28. Netto NR Jr, Lemos GC, D'Ancona CAL, et al. Is routine dilation of the ureter necessary for ureteroscopy? *Eur Urol*. 1990;17:269-272.
29. Canes D, Desai MM. New technology in the treatment of nephrolithiasis. *Curr Opin Urol*. 2008;18:235-240.
30. Rodrigues Netto N Jr, Caserta Lemos G, Levi D'Ancona CA, et al. Is routine dilatation of the ureter necessary for ureteroscopy? *Eur Urol*. 1990;17:269-272.
31. Moneim AA, Khalaf I. Critical evaluation of acute ureteral dilation: clinical and experimental study. *J Endourol*. 1988;2:345-353.
32. Gupta PK. Initial experience with a prototype ureteroscope. *J Endourol*. 2006;20:9-11.
33. Butler MR, Power RE, Thornhill JA, et al. An audit of 2273 ureteroscopies: a focus on intra-operative complications to justify proactive management of ureteric calculi. *Surg J R Coll Surg Edinb Irel*. 2004;2:42-46.
34. Shvartz O, Perry KT, Goff B, et al. Improved functional deflection with a dual-deflection flexible ureteroscope. *J Endourol*. 2004;18: 141-144.
35. Tan Y, Preminger G. Advances in video and imaging in ureteroscopy. *Urol Clin North Am*. 2004;31:33-42.

36. Leitao V, Haleblian G, Chandrashekar A, et al. The digital flexible ureteroscope: assessment of optics and technology. *J Endourol.* 2007;21(Suppl 1):A286.

37. Smith RD, Patel A. Impact of flexible ureterorenoscopy in current management of nephrolithiasis. *Curr Opin Urol.* 2007;17:114-119.

38. Traxer O, Thibault F, Beley S, et al. Evaluation of optical properties of the new digital flexible ureterorenoscope by comparison with 3 standard flexible ureterorenoscopes. *J Endourol.* 2007;21(Suppl 1): A242-A243.

39. Humphreys MR, Miller NL, Williams JC Jr, et al. A new world revealed: early experience with digital ureteroscopy. *J Urol.* 2008;179:970-975.

40. Desai MM, Monish A, Gill IS, et al. Flexible robotic retrograde renoscopy: description of novel robotic device and preliminary laboratory experience. *Urology.* 2008;72:42-46.

41. Colombo JR, Cocuzza M, Ganpule A, et al. Flexible ureteroscopic holmium YAG lithotripsy for upper tract stones: a multicentric analysis. *J Urol.* 2008;179:435. abstract.

42. Holden T, Pedro RN, Hendlin K, et al. Evidence-based instrumentation for flexible ureteroscopy: a review. *J Endourol.* 2008;22: 1423-1426.

43. Vanlangendonck R, Landman J. Ureteral access strategies: pro-access sheath. *Urol Clin N Am.* 2004;31:71-81.

44. Kourambas J, Byme RR, Preminger GM. Does a ureteral access sheath facilitate ureteroscopy? *J Urol.* 2001;165:789-793.

45. Rehman J, Monga M, Landman J, et al. Characterization of intrapelvic pressure during ureteropyeloscopy with ureteral access sheaths. *Urology.* 2003;61:713-718.

46. Monga M, Best S, Venkatesh R, et al. Prospective randomized comparison of 2 ureteral access sheaths during flexible retrograde ureteroscopy. *J Urol.* 2004;172:572-573.

47. Pedro RN, Hendlin K, Durfee W, et al. Physical characteristics of next-generation ureteral access sheaths: Buckling and kinking. American Urological Association; 2007; San Francisco, Abst 971.

48. Monga M, Gawlik A, Durfee W. Systematic evaluation of ureteral access sheaths. *Urology.* 2004;63:834-836.

49. Kahnoski RJ, Lingeman JE, Woods JR, et al. Efficacy of glucagon in the relief of ureteral colic following treatment by extracorporeal shock wave lithotripsy: a randomized double-blind trial. *J Urol.* 1987;137:1124-1125.

50. Bagley D, Ramsay K, Zeltser I. An update on ureteroscopic instrumentation for the treatment of urolithiasis. *Curr Opin Urol.* 2004;14:99-106.

51. Chenven E, Bagley D. In vitro retrieval and releasing capabilities of stone basket designs. *J Endourol.* 2002;16(Suppl 1):A11.

52. Honey RJ. Assessment of a new tipless nitinol stone basket and comparison with an existing flat-wire basket. *J Endourol.* 1998;12:529-531.

53. Monga M, Hendlin K, Lee C, et al. Systematic evaluation of stone basket dimensions. *Urology.* 2004;63:1043-1044.

54. Lukasewycz S, Hoffman N, Botnaru A, et al. Comparison of tipless and helical baskets in an invitro ureteral model. *Urology.* 2004;64: 435-438.

55. Lukasewycz S, Skenazy J, Hoffman N, et al. Comparison of nitinol tipless stone baskets in an in vitro caliceal model. *J Urol.* 2004; 172:562-564.

56. Hendlin K, Lee C, Anderson JK, et al. Radial dilation force of tipless and helical stone baskets. *J Endourol.* 2004;18:946-947.

57. Canales BK, Ramani A, Monga M. A new spin on the entrapped ureteral calculus. *J Endourol.* 2006;20:460-461.

58. Zeltser IS, Bagley DH. Basket design as a factor in retention and release of calculi in vitro. *J Endourol.* 2007;21:337-342.

59. Denstedt JD, Clayman RV. Electrohydraulic lithotripsy of renal and ureteral calculi. *J Urol.* 1990;143:13-17.

60. Vorreuther R, Corleis R, Klotz T, et al. Impact of shock wave pattern and cavitation bubble size on tissue damage during ureteroscopic electrohydraulic lithotripsy. *J Urol.* 1995;153(pt 1):849-853.

61. Raney AM. Electrohydraulic ureterolithotripsy. Preliminary report. *Urology.* 1978;12:284-285.

62. Hofbauer J, Hobarth K, Marberger M. Electrohydraulic versus pneumatic disintegration in the treatment of ureteral stones: A randomized prospective trial. *J Urol.* 1995;153(pt 1):623-625.

63. Teichman JM, Rao RD, Rogenes VJ, et al. Ureteroscopic management of ureteral calculi: Electrohydraulic versus holmium:YAG lithotripsy. *J Urol.* 1997;158:357-1361.

64. Elashry OM, DiMeglio RB, Nakada SY, et al. Intracoropreal electrohydraulic lithotripsy of ureteral and renal calculi using small caliber (1.9F) electrohydraulic lithotripsy probes. *J Urol.* 1996;156: 1581-1585.

65. Huang S, Patel H, Bellman GC. Cost effectiveness of electrohydraulic lithotripsy v Candela pulsed-dye laser in management of the distal ureteral stone. *J Endourol.* 1998;12:237-240.

66. Tawfiek ER, Grasso M, Bagley DH. Initial use of Browne pneumatic impactor. *J Endourol.* 1997;11:121-124.

67. Delvecchio FC, Kuo RL, Preminger GM. Clinical efficacy of combined lithoclast and lithovac stone removal during ureteroscopy. *J Urol.* 2000;164:40-42.

68. Knispel HH, Klan R, Heicappell R, et al. Pneumatic lithotripsy applied through deflection working channel of miniureteroscope: results in 143 patients. *J Endourol.* 1998;12:513-515.

69. Zhu S, Kourambas J, Munver R, et al. Quantification of the tip movement of lithotripsy flexible pneumatic probes. *J Urol.* 2000;164:1735-1739.

70. Piergiovanni M, Desgrandchamps F, cochand-Priollet B, et al. Ureteral and bladder lesions after ballistic, ultrasonic electrohydraulic, or laser lithotripsy. *J Endourol.* 1994;8:293-299.

71. Denstedt JD, Eberwein PM, Singh RR. The Swiss lithoclast: a new device for intracorporeal lithotripsy. *J Urol.* 1992;148(pt 2): 1088-1090.

72. Wollin TA, Denstedt JD. The holmium laser in urology. *J Clin Laser Med Surg.* 1998;16:13-20.

73. Dushinski JW, Lingeman JE. Urologic applications of the holmium laser. *Tech Urol.* 1997;3:60-64.

74. Teichman JM, Vassar GJ, Bishoff JT, et al. Holmium:YAG lithotripsy yields smaller fragments than Lithoclast, pulsed dye laser or electrohydraulic lithotripsy. *J Urol.* 1998;159:17-23.

75. Teichman JM, Vassar GJ, Glickman RD. Holmium:yttrium-aluminum-garnet lithotripsy efficiency varies with stone composition. *Urology.* 1998;52:392-397.

76. Sofer M, Watterson JD, Wollin TA, et al. Holmium:YAG laser lithotripsy for upper urinary tract calculi in 598 patients. *J Urol.* 2002;167:31-34.

77. Marks AJ, Teichman JM. Lasers in clinical urology: state of the art and new horizons. *World J Urol.* 2007;25:227-233.

78. Marguet CG, Sung JC, Springhart WP, et al. In vitro comparison of stone retropulsion and fragmentation of the frequency doubled, doubled pulse ND:YAG laser and the holmium:YAG laser. *J Urol.* 2005;173:1797-1800.

79. Yates J, Zabbo A, Pareek G. A comparison of the FREDDY and holmium lasers during ureteroscopic lithotripsy. *Lasers Surg Med.* 2007;39:637-640.

80. Dubosq F, Pasqui F, Girard F, et al. Endoscopic lithotripsy and the FREDDY laser: initial experience. *J Endourol.* 2006;20:296-299.

81. Dretler SP. The stone cone: a new generation of basketry. *J Urol.* 2001;165:1593-1596.

82. Holley PG, Sharma SK, Perry KT, et al. Assessment of novel ureteral occlusion device and comparison with stone cone in prevention of stone fragment migration during lithotripsy. *J Endourol.* 2005;19:200-203.

83. Tawfiek ER, Bagley DH. Management of upper urinary tract calculi with ureteroscopic techniques. *Urology.* 1999;53:25-31.

84. Desai MR, Patel SB, Desai MM, et al. The Dretler stone cone: a device to prevent ureteral stone migration – the initial clinical experience. *J Urol.* 2002;167:1985-1988.

85. Ali AA, Ali ZA, Halstead JC, et al. A novel method to prevent retrograde displacement of ureteric calculi during intracorporeal lithotripsy. *BJU Int.* 2004;94:441-442.

86. Mohseni MG, Arasteh S, Alizadeh F. Preventing retrograde stone displacement during pneumatic lithotripsy for ureteral calculi using lidocaine jelly. *Urology.* 2006;68:505-507.

87. Mirabile G, Phillips CK, Edelstein A, et al. Evaluation of a novel temperature-sensitive polymer for temporary ureteral occlusion. *J Endourol.* 2008;22:2357-2359.

88. Roberts WW, Cadeddu JA, Micali S, et al. Ureteral stricture formation after removal of impacted calculi. *J Urol.* 1998;159:723-726.

89. Singal RK, Denstedt JD. Contemporary management of ureteral stones. *Urol Clin North Am.* 1997;24:59-70.

90. Johnson DB, Pearle MS. Complications of ureteroscopy. *Urol Clin N Am.* 2004;31:157-171.

91. Blute ML, Segura JW, Patterson DE. Ureteroscopy. *J Urol.* 1988;139:510-512.

92. Grasso M. Complications of ureteropyloscopy. In: Taneja SS, Smith RB, Ehrlich RM, eds. *Complications of Urologic Surgery.* 3rd ed. Philadelphia: WB Saunders; 2001:268-276.

93. Stoller ML, Wolf JS. Endoscopic ureteral injuries. In: McAninch JW, ed. *Traumatic and Reconstructive Urology.* Philadelphia: WB Saunders; 1996:199-211.

94. Jeromin L, Sosnowski M. Ureteroscopy in the treatment of ureteral stones: over 10 years' experience. *Eur Urol.* 1998;34:344-349.

Indications for and Technique of Retrograde Intrarenal Surgery for Renal Stones

43

Gregory S. Rosenblatt and Gerhard J. Fuchs

Abstract Technologic advances over the past 3 decades have resulted in dramatic changes in the interventional management of kidney stones. Prudent application of minimally invasive surgical treatment modalities allows for the opportunity to achieve high stone-free rates with low morbidity and short recovery. Available modalities for the surgical management of kidney stones, including extracorporeal shock wave lithotripsy (ESWL), percutaneous renal surgery (PRS), and retrograde intrarenal ureterorenoscopic surgery (RIRS), obviate the need for open surgery in the vast majority of kidney stone patients. In this chapter, we review the differential indications when treating renal stones, and we review in detail the indications for and techniques of endoscopic RIRS. We discuss currently available stone fragmentation technology and examine in detail specific stone presentations, including stones of varying sizes located in any anatomic portion of the kidney (renal pelvis, superior versus inferior-pole calyces, calyceal diverticula). We also review the role of endoscopic retrograde surgical treatment for patients with anatomic abnormalities that include: fused/ectopic kidneys, allograft kidneys, prior upper urinary tract reconstruction, and body habitus abnormalities.

43.1 Introduction

Technologic advances over the past 3 decades have resulted in dramatic changes in the interventional management of kidney stones. Available modalities for the surgical management of kidney stones, including extracorporeal shock wave lithotripsy (ESWL), percutaneous renal surgery (PRS), and retrograde intrarenal ureterorenoscopic surgery (RIRS), obviate the need for open surgery in the vast majority of kidney stone patients. The minimally invasive surgical treatment modalities allow for the opportunity to achieve high stone-free rates with reduced morbidity and shortened recovery.

The introduction of ESWL in 1980 was a pivotal moment in the history of the surgical management of renal stones.[1,2] ESWL is now utilized by surgeons all over the world and is a first-line treatment for approximately 70%–80% of patients who have uncomplicated renal stone disease.[3,4] Approximately 25% of patients are treated with endoscopic surgery

(RIRS and PRS); only 1%–5% of patients with kidney stones will require treatment that involves an open surgical approach.[5–7] Thus, PRS or RIRS, sometimes in conjunction with ESWL, are minimally invasive surgical options for successful stone treatment in the majority of patients with more complex stones. Successful stone management hinges upon proper patient selection, acknowledging the limitations of the ESWL technology, and knowing the limits of one's own endourologic expertise. This chapter includes a review of the differential indications of renal stone treatment with special consideration of the role and surgical technique of RIRS.

43.2 Differential Indications for Renal Stone Treatments

The four main factors to consider when selecting the appropriate treatment for renal stones include stone burden, intrarenal and upper urinary tract anatomy (including patient body habitus), concomitant medical disease, and patient compliance. Provided there are no anatomic or physiologic hindrances to the spontaneous elimination of gravel, solitary stones or multiple stones of an added diameter

G.J. Fuchs (✉)
Department of Surgery, Cedars-Sinai Medical Center, Los Angeles, CA, USA
e-mail: fuchs@cshs.org

Table 43.1 Differential indications for endoscopic treatment of kidney stones

	ESWL	RIRS	RIRS-SWL	PCNL
Stone size (primary)	<2–2.5 cm	<1.5–2 cm	>1.5–2.5 cm Occ. staghorn	>2.5 cm Staghorn stone
Residual stones	5 mm and less No stent Anesthesia free Normal anatomy	All size <1.5 cm <50 fragments Abnormal anatomy OK	1.5–2.5 cm <50 fragments Normal anatomy	All size >2.5 cm Any number fragments Abnormal anatomy OK
Composition	Ca-ox. dihydrate Ca-ox. monohydrate Struvite	All compositions	All compositions	All compositions
Anatomy	Normal	Abnormal OK Urinary diversion OK	Normal Urinary diversion OK	Abnormal OK Urinary diversion OK
Physiology	Normal	Abnormal OK Size < 1.5 cm	Normal	Abnormal OK Size > 1.5 cm

ESWL extracorporeal shockwave lithotripsy, *RIRS* retrograde intrarenal surgery, *RIRS-SWL* concomitant use of RIRS and SWL in the same treatment session, *PCNL* percutaneous nephrolithotripsy and stone removal, fragment stone piece <4 mm size

of up to 2.5 cm are appropriate for initial treatment by ESWL alone, with an approximate 70% stone clearance rate (except inferior pole location greater than 1 cm).[8,9] Larger stone size and lower pole stone location are associated with lower stone-free rates when ESWL is used as monotherapy. In addition, with increasing stone burden, ESWL results in a larger amount of stone fragmentation product, and spontaneous passage may be complicated by ureteral obstruction, obstructive pyelonephritis, and a prolonged period of stone passage. Thus, larger stones, lower pole stones, and stones within kidneys that have abnormal or anomalous anatomy are better treated with endoscopic surgery. Of the two endoscopic approaches (percutaneous antegrade versus retrograde), RIRS is the best choice for moderately complex stone conditions, while more complex stone conditions may be better served by a percutaneous antegrade approach (Table 43.1).

43.3 The Evolution of Upper Tract Endoscopy and RIRS

In 1912, Hugh Hampton Young was the first person to use a rigid cystoscope to endoscopically visualize the upper urinary tract of a patient with urinary tract dilation, secondary to posterior urethral valve obstruction.[10] In 1962, McGovern performed the first flexible ureteroscopy, and it was not until the mid-1980s that a deflectable tip became available.[11] The first rigid rod-lens system ureteroscopes were developed in the late 1960s and became more widely used in the 1970s.[12] Fiber-optic technology eventually replaced the rod-lens system, and semirigid fiber-optic ureteroscopes became available in 1989.[13,14]

In the late 1980s, RIRS was predominantly used in the management of retained stones after failed ESWL treatment.

In general, two subsets of patients failed ESWL.[13,15] One subset was those who were found to have stone fragments retained in the lower calyces. Retrieval of the fragments with stone baskets or graspers was necessary to render these patients stone free. Other early RIRS patients were those who had failed ESWL treatment of stone contained within a calyceal diverticulum.

Technological refinements have resulted in smaller, yet sturdier instrument design, improvements in the working channel, greater degrees of active deflection, new energy sources, and improved stone retrieval devices. These improvements have allowed RIRS to evolve into what is now a routine diagnostic and/or therapeutic procedure for an increasing number of calculus-related and noncalculus-related conditions (i.e., stricture, tumor, bleeding) that occur within the upper urinary tract.

43.4 Current Indications for RIRS

As of 2009, the indications for primary RIRS at our institution are listed in Table 43.2. For these indications, RIRS has become a well-accepted treatment because as a minimally invasive outpatient procedure its success rates are superior to ESWL and the perioperative morbidity is low. Therefore, RIRS is the authors' primary choice for stone cases, where success with ESWL is doubtful and the stone burden and complexity too low to warrant the more invasive approach of PRS. This includes total stone burden of up to 2 cm at any location within the renal collecting system, especially when the stone composition is known to be calcium oxalate monohydrate (COMH), cystine, or uric acid (radiolucent). Stones in patients with nephrocalcinosis are also best addressed with RIRS, as are select patients with concomitant ureteropelvic junction (UPJ) or intrarenal stenosis. In patients with ureteral

Table 43.5 Essential procedural steps of retrograde intrarenal surgery (RIRS)

Steps	Goal	Execution	Equipment used
1	Evaluate bladder Assess upper tract anatomy for treatment planning Place safety guidewire	Cystoscopy Retrograde pyelogram under fluoroscopic control	Fluoroscopy X-ray table 19–21 F cystoscope 5 F straight angiocatheter 0.038 Bentson guidewire
2	Establish access to kidney	Optical dilation of ureter	9.5 F semirigid ureteroscope Second guidewire
3	Treat stone	Stone fragmentation and stone retrieval	Holmium/thulium laser Stone baskets/graspers Access sheath
4A	Treat stone (special situations) Larger stone	Combine RIRS with ESWL	Combination ESWL/fluoro X-ray table
4B	Treat stone (special situations) Lower calyx stone	Relocation technique (possible combination with ESWL)	Holmium/thulium laser Basket ("naked basket")
4C	Treat stone (special situations) Intrarenal stricture	 Identify access to stone Dilate/incise access to stone Fragment/remove stone	Holmium/thulium laser (possible ESWL combo) Hydrophilic guidewire Zero tip balloon dilator Zero tip nitinol basket
5	Safe exit from upper tract	Place indwelling ureteral drainage stent over safety wire	6/7 F ureteral double pigtail stent

43.5.4 Procedure Considerations

If the patient was treated for a UTI, confirm the sterility of the urine. Just prior to urinary tract instrumentation, a broad-spectrum antibiotic should be administered intravenously. As reflux of infected urine into the renal parenchyma and vasculature may result in serious septic complications, precautions should be taken to minimize this risk by keeping intrarenal pressures low. Once a safety wire is placed, forced diuresis with IV fluids and diuretic administration (furosemide, 10–20 mg) will produce increased flow and will thus decrease the chance of pyelorenal reflux. Additional measures at reducing infection risk are keeping a low intrarenal pressure environment through using irrigation prudently (gravity only, no pressurized irrigation), intermittent aspiration (three way system), and the use of an access sheath (especially for cases of longer duration) (Fig. 43.2a, b).

43.6 Upper Urinary Tract Access for RIRS

43.6.1 Technique

When possible, the patient should be positioned in low lithotomy. If lithotomy is not a feasible position (leg amputation, frozen hip, morbid obesity), RIRS can be performed when the patient is supine. If RIRS is to be part of a combined PRS procedure, the patient may be positioned prone. Initially, cystoscopy and a retrograde pyeloureterogram is performed for anatomic assessment. Next, a safety wire is placed into the kidney in a retrograde fashion under fluoroscopic control. This is to remain in place for the duration of the procedure, especially when repeat retrograde access to the kidney is necessary (i.e., basket removal of stone fragments). If a ureteral access sheath is utilized, the safety wire remains outside the access sheath. The role of the retrograde approach in the combination treatment of RIRS and PRS is to provide access to intrarenal areas that cannot be properly reached through the percutaneous access, such as certain upper- and mid-renal calyces. RIRS is utilized to fragment stone and reposition larger stone pieces from those calyces into the renal pelvis from where they can be readily retrieved via the PRS access (Table 43.5).

43.6.2 Upper Urinary Tract Dilation

Access to the kidney for diagnostic evaluation is usually feasible using a 7.5 F flexible instrument without prior/concurrent dilation. However, repeat access to the kidney and retrieval of stone particles will usually require some sort of upper tract preparation. Options include serial dilators, coaxial dilators, balloon dilators, "optical dilation," or the preparatory placement of an indwelling ureteral stent. An indwelling ureteral stent results in passive ureteral dilation that greatly facilitates

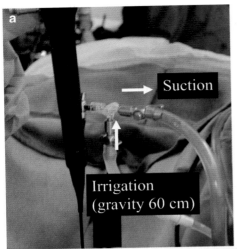

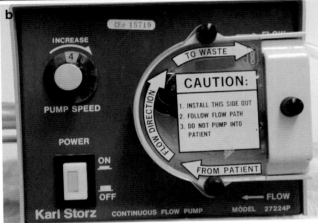

Fig. 43.2 (**a**) Three-way stop cock allowing for irrigation and intermittent suction to keep intrarenal pressure low and provide good visibility. (**b**) Suction pump allowing for graded suction (alternatively wall suction can be used)

43.7 Flexible Ureterorenoscopy: Technique

Commonly, a 7.5 F actively deflecting ureterorenoscope is used during RIRS. The instrument is introduced into the (empty) bladder and advanced under direct vision alongside a safety wire. Occasionally, we will utilize a second 0.038 in. "working" guidewire to facilitate access to the upper urinary tract (such as in male patients with enlarged prostates). Dilute contrast injection via the scope's working channel should be used to delineate ureteral and intrarenal anatomy. Risk of infectious and septic complications is minimized by forced diuresis (see previous section), frequent aspiration of fluid from the collecting system, and minimal (as needed) use of irrigant, in an effort to keep intrarenal pressure as low as possible.[5] We advise against the routine use of pressurized irrigant or forceful hand irrigation. Gravity irrigation at 60 cm H_2O and intermittent aspiration of fluid and/or vapor (holmium lithotripsy) is usually sufficient to allow for intraoperative visibility. We utilize a 3-way connector that allows for rapid switching between irrigation and suction (Fig. 43.2a). This method of intrarenal fluid volume exchange facilitates the maintenance of low intrarenal pressures. An additional method for improving visibility and decreasing intrarenal pressure is to use a ureteral access sheath.[7,11] If adequate visibility cannot be achieved, there is a higher risk for damage to the renal collecting system secondary to unmonitored activation of energy sources. In this situation, we recommend termination of the procedure with placement of an indwelling ureteral stent and subsequent return in 7–10 days (Table 43.5).

43.8 Retrograde Intrarenal Surgery (RIRS)

43.8.1 Stone Fragmentation: Electrohydraulic and Laser Technology

Electrohydraulic lithotripsy (EHL) was the first technique that was utilized for intracorporeal lithotripsy, and is still employed for RIRS when laser technology is not available.[17] A complete review of EHL technology is beyond the scope and aim of this chapter. In brief, EHL works by spark discharge from parallel electrodes that comprise the EHL probe. A hydraulic shockwave develops from vaporized water around the electrode, and this causes a cavitation bubble to form. Cavitation-bubble collapse results in a secondary shockwave and/or high-velocity microjets, both of which result in stone fragmentation when the stone is positioned appropriately close to the location of the generated shockwave. In most centers around the world, EHL has been replaced by newer holmium laser technology, as EHL carries a higher risk of upper urinary tract mucosal injury.

upper ureteral and intrarenal access, and this technique was routinely used in the early years of RIRS, when 10.4 F ureterorenoscopes were used. Since the downsizing of flexible scopes (currently, 6.9–7.9 F), RIRS is usually performed as a one-stage procedure, and the authors' first choice is "optical dilation," using a semirigid 9.5 F ureteroscope—a technique that is both efficient and cost-effective. The 9.5 F ureteroscope is introduced into the ureteral orifice over a second guidewire and advanced up the ureter as far as it can reach, thus dilating the ureteral orifice and distal two-thirds of the ureter. This approach allows access to the kidney in greater than 85% of cases in a one-stage procedure.[5] When access is not feasible in this fashion, an indwelling ureteral stent should be placed. Passive distention of the entire ureter will ensue over the following days, and intrarenal surgery can usually be performed as early as 7 days later. Other means of active dilation carry greater potential for ureteral damage and subsequent stricture formation, especially when multiple ureteral segments require dilation in order to gain access to the kidney.

Cavitation bubble diameter is controlled by the amount of energy used, but even low energy levels have been associated with ureteral perforation.[18] However, intrarenal EHL is still used in a number of countries where the expensive laser technology is not available as yet.

The holmium:YAG laser and, more recently, the thulium laser were developed, allowing for fragmentation as well as vaporization of stone material via a photothermal mechanism. Compared to EHL, the cavitation bubble produced by the holmium:YAG is elongated, resulting in a weaker shockwave. Thermal injury can occur up to 1 mm from the end of the holmium laser fiber, and thus, this is a safer method of achieving stone fragmentation. The holmium and thulium lasers can be used to fragment stones of any composition, whereas EHL may fail with more resistant stone compositions such as COMH and cystine.

Stones and stone fragments less than 4 mm size can usually be removed intact, whereas solid stones larger than 4 mm are fragmented first. Holmium laser energy is the authors' first choice for stone fragmentation. Stones of all composition can be fragmented and vaporized using holmium energy. Typically, the 200 µm fiber is used for ureteral and/or intrarenal stones. The basic energy setting is 0.6 J and 5 Hz (3 W) repetition rate and can be increased for larger or impacted stones. For large, bulky stones, we typically work at a higher energy settings up to 20 W (2 J and 10 Hz), and we decrease the energy down to 3 W (0.6 J and 5 Hz) as the stones are reduced in size/weight and for the final division of the smaller fragments. With the lower energy setting, the kinetic impact of the laser is reduced so that the smaller stones can be trapped against the mucosa for further disintegration and are not simply bouncing around without being fragmented.

43.8.2 Stone Composition

Holmium energy is the authors' first choice for treatment of intrarenal stones because of its ability to fragment and vaporize stones of all composition safely and efficiently. Stone compositions include (from least-to-greatest amount of required energy for fragmentation): uric acid, struvite, calcium oxalate dehydrate, calcium oxalate monohydrate, and cystine. Stones that are resistant to ESWL and/or EHL technology may contain a higher amount of calcium oxalate monohydrate or cystine, both of which are reliably treated using holmium energy. The same holds true for the newer thulium energy.

43.8.3 Renal Pelvis Stones

The endpoint of treatment is the reduction of all stone to fragments less than 4 mm. Fragments between 2–4 mm should be actively removed with the use of a stone basket. Fragments less than 2 mm may be left to pass spontaneously if they are in a nondependent portion of the kidney. We use a four-wire nitinol tipless basket for the majority of stone fragment retrieval (Cook Medical; Microvasive, Boston Scientific). The newer design of this basket allows for retrieval maneuvers even in small calyces. A ureteral access sheath allows for rapid repeated access to the kidney, and this is helpful when removing a large amount of fragments and gravel.[11]

For total stone burden less than 1.5 cm, RIRS monotherapy is generally our choice treatment, and is usually completed in a single outpatient session. Some of these stones may be amenable to ESWL monotherapy (stone composition known as CODH), but stone-free rates are higher when holmium laser and basket retrieval are employed. RIRS provides that advantage of a more predictable treatment outcome. As total stone burden increases, the chance of rendering a patient stone-free in a single session diminishes. When a patient's total stone burden is between 1.5 and 2.5 cm, concomitant use of ESWL can facilitate stone fragmentation. If the ureter is tight (too tight for optical dilation with the 9.5 F semirigid ureteroscope), consideration may be given to either percutaneous antegrade approach or preoperative stenting. Stone burden greater than 2.5 cm (i.e., staghorn stones) can be treated in select cases by combined RIRS/ESWL or by PRS. PRS should be employed for most complete, bulky staghorn stones, when progress is slow due to unfavorable renal anatomy or by a tight ureter that prevents expeditious retrieval of gravel or when the expectation is that a patient should be stone-free after one surgical session. If RIRS is used, the expectation is that more than one surgical session will be required to render a patient stone-free. The goal of the initial session is to divide the stone into fragments that are 4 mm or less and extract fragments using a basket retrieval device. A stent should be placed to allow for spontaneous passage of residual stone gravel. The patient is then scheduled for reevaluation 1–2 weeks later and—if deemed necessary—scheduled for a repeat surgery to clear the remaining fragments.

In select situations, we have employed simultaneous right and left RIRS for patients with bilateral stone burden. This will require two surgeons, two flexible ureterorenoscopes, and two laser sources. For patients with multiple medical comorbidities and in whom anesthesia time should be minimized, such an approach will allow for surgery to be performed in a shorter period of time.

Stone burden directly correlates to treatment time. Greater stone size may make the retrograde approach cumbersome and potentially traumatic. Prudence and experience should dictate how far to push the retrograde approach. At the conclusion of any RIRS procedure, a 7 F indwelling ureteral stent of appropriate length should be placed. The patient is typically discharged the same day of surgery. When we do not anticipate further surgery sessions in order to render a patient stone free, we schedule an outpatient visit approximately 5–10 days later, at which time renal ultrasound is performed to confirm the absence of large stone fragments or hydronephrosis, and the stent is removed using a flexible cystoscope under local anesthesia in the office setting. If significant hydronephrosis is noted, a KUB film is obtained to assess for any stone residual in the ureter that may need more time to pass or require a second look procedure.

43.8.4 Calyceal Stones

Stones within mid-kidney and superior pole calyces have a higher chance of unhindered passage of gravel after stone fragmentation, and ESWL monotherapy may be successful for treating stones in these positions. Although more invasive than ESWL, we offer patients the choice of RIRS in this setting, as this technique allows for a more predictable stone-free outcome. Stones within inferior pole calyces—especially when the stone burden is greater than 8 mm—typically will not clear well after ESWL therapy, and we, therefore, prefer a retrograde approach for stones up to 1.5 cm size. A 200 μm laser fiber will rarely inhibit deflection necessary for accessing the lower pole (Fig. 43.3a–f). In the interest of reducing stress to the scope by strenuous deflection and prolonged laser activation with the scope tip deflected, we employ the repositioning technique for lower pole stones. As soon as the stone is fragmented sufficiently to allow for entrapment in a basket, we grasp the stone, reposition it into the pelvis or upper pole location where it can be fragmented to completion with the scope being kept straight or nearly straight. If the lower pole stone cannot be reached with the laser fiber, simultaneous use of ESWL may be helpful to initiate breakage and then use the repositioning technique, as described previously (Fig. 43.4). Larger stones in the inferior-pole calyces are best treated by PRS (Table 43.6).

43.8.5 Stones Associated with Intrarenal Stenosis and Calyceal Diverticula

A special situation exists when patients have stone within a calyceal diverticulum. The stone-free rate after ESWL ranges from 4%–25%.[19–21] Percutaneous surgery, on the other hand, has a success rate greater than 90%. Lingeman reported on 26 patients initially treated with ESWL, and 10 of those (38%) went on to require PRS.[22] We have used RIRS in selected patients for more than 20 years.[5] Selected patients include those with diverticula located in either a superior pole or mid-kidney position. A retrograde pyelogram

at the time of surgery will usually delineate the upper tract anatomy. If there remains question as to the anatomy, endoscopic inspection of the renal collecting system can be performed.

Upper urinary tract access should be established in the manner we described earlier, with special care to avoid advancing the guidewire into the kidney prior to endoscopic evaluation of the collecting system (to avoid mucosal trauma that can inhibit proper identification of the narrowed infundibulum or neck of diverticulum). The point of interest may be as subtle as a small dimple in the mucosal surface. Once the opening is endoscopically identified, a guidewire is coiled (under fluoroscopic guidance) within the diverticulum. If the guidewire cannot be maneuvered through the opening, a hydrophilic glide wire should be tried. Once wire access is established, the scope is removed and a 5-F straight angiocatheter is passed over the wire and through the narrow segment. At this point, retrograde injection of diluted contrast may provide additional information on the anatomy of the collecting system proximal to the narrowed segment (Fig. 43.5a–d).

The technique for reconstructing the narrow segment will depend on the segment length and whether or not secure wire access to the cavity can be maintained. If the infundibulum is short (<0.5 cm), the obstruction may be negotiated by advancing the 7.5 F scope over a second guidewire and thereby dilate the access. Laser incision can be performed if the access is not sufficiently wide, provided the diverticulum can be accessed with the scope. Longer segments (>0.5 cm) are best managed first by formal dilation with a zero tip 3-F balloon. This should be advanced over the guidewire and inflated to 14 F under fluoroscopic control. If necessary, we will then utilize the holmium laser (energy of 10 W) to incise and sufficiently open the lumen. The incision is directed in the anatomic posterior direction so as to avoid the vascularity of the anterior aspect of the infundibulum.

Occasionally, the diverticulum will protrude into the collecting system, and the access point is not identifiable. Laser incision (holmium 10 W) is appropriate for marsupializing such a visually identifiable cavity into the collecting system. In cases where the cavity fills with contrast but the access point is not readily identified endoscopically, methylene blue can be injected retrograde (via the work channel of the flexible ureterorenoscope). Similar to the contrast, the methylene blue will find its way into the cavity. The collecting system is then washed clear of the blue dye, and under low-pressure conditions a trickle of blue will emanate from the cavity, thereby helping to identify the neck of the cavity. Access can then be gained using one of the aforementioned techniques.

Once access is gained, a stone may be retrieved by basket (stones less than 4 mm) or fragmented (stones greater than 4 mm). For larger or multiple stones, ESWL can be performed under the same anesthesia to accelerate and

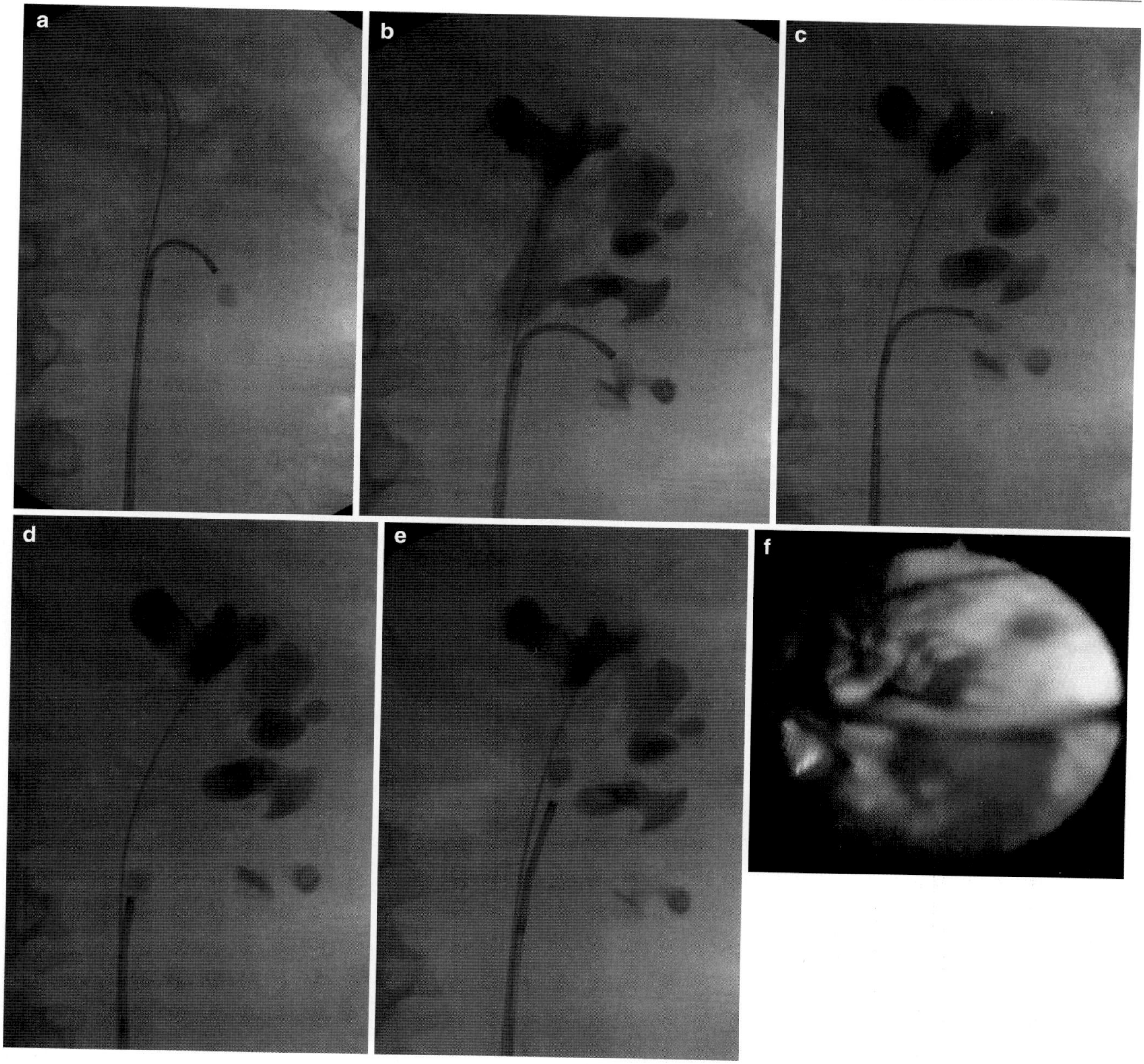

Fig. 43.3 (**a**) RIRS – repositioning technique for lower caliceal stone. (**b**) Contrast injection delineates renal collecting system. Stone is accessed in the lower pole and captured in zero tip Nitinol basket. (**c**) Stone retrieved from lower calyx for repositioning. (**d**) Ureteroscope with stone in basket straightened out to be advanced into upper pole calyx, (**e**) where it is released for laser fragmentation and basket retrieval of gravel. (**f**) Well-fragmented stone fragments are removed with the zero tip Nitinol basket

complete fragmentation (see earlier section). The endpoint of treatment is complete removal of all stone from the diverticulum/cavity and the "repair" of the narrow segment. Placement of an indwelling stent, preferably with the proximal tip inside the target calyx, is the final step of the procedure. A review of 96 patients with calyceal diverticula (treated over 10 years) found that the calyceal neck could be identified and dilated in 91 (95%).[23] Seven of the 96 patients had lower pole diverticula, and 4 of these patients could not be

treated with RIRS. If stones in inferior pole diverticula cannot be successfully treated with RIRS, percutaneous surgery is performed under the same anesthesia.

In summary, ESWL monotherapy carries a low success rate, and PRS—although highly successful—is quite invasive. Our primary approach to stones that form within calyceal diverticula consists, therefore, of retrograde access with endoscopic intrarenal correction of the outflow alteration, followed by holmium laser lithotripsy ± ESWL. This is best achieved

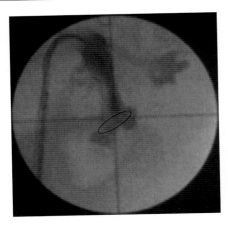

Fig. 43.4 Lower caliceal stone cannot be engaged in basket and cannot be readily accessed with ureterorenoscope for laser fragmentation (long caliceal neck, medial location). Therefore, E-SWL is employed (stone in center of cross hairs) for initial fragmentation. Then, stone fragments are repositioned for further laser fragmentation and active basket removal (see Fig. 43.3)

Table 43.6 Treatment algorithm for lower calyceal stones

	SWL	RIRS	PCNL
Stone size (primary)	<1.5 cm	<1.5 cm Need to be stone free	>1.5 cm Need to be stone free
Composition	Ca-ox. dihydrate Struvite	All compositions	All compositions
Anatomy	Normal	Abnormal Urinary diversion Size < 1.5 cm	Abnormal Urinary diversion Size > 1.5 cm
Physiology	Normal	Abnormal Size < 1.5 cm	Abnormal Size > 1.5 cm
Residual stones (secondary)	5 mm and less No stent Anesthesia free	All size <1.5 cm <10 fragments Abnormal anatomy	Abnormal anatomy All size >1.5 cm

when the diverticulum is in a superior pole or mid-kidney location. A percutaneous surgical approach is utilized when RIRS treatment cannot be accomplished. This typically includes diverticula that have a long narrow segment (>1.5 cm), those located in a dependent location relative to the infundibulum, or those that are located in the inferior pole of the kidney.[22,23] In these situations, given the higher failure rate of RIRS, one can consider primary percutaneous surgery. On occasion, a diverticulum with a large stone burden, especially when located on the anterior aspect of the kidney can be best managed with the laparoscopic approach.

43.9 Anatomical Abnormalities

43.9.1 Solitary Kidney

ESWL or RIRS may be employed; however, RIRS provides a more reliable outcome, as the goal is to render a patient free of all stone. If ESWL monotherapy is used, regular, frequent evaluation in the postprocedure setting is essential. The treatment of stones in a solitary kidney is tailored to reduce the risk of renal damage and ureteral obstruction. Renal ultrasound or abdominal radiography should be obtained at close intervals when a patient with a solitary kidney is being monitored for spontaneous stone passage (stones < 5 mm). The patient should be instructed to pay close attention to their urine output and volume and to report to the urologist if oliguria or anuria occurs, even if he/she is otherwise asymptomatic. Stone burden larger than 2 cm is best treated by PRS. If the risk of performing percutaneous surgery is too high (i.e., due to patient comorbidities), RIRS is the next-best alternative for larger stones. Overall, the risk attendant to multiple sessions with RIRS for larger stones in solitary kidneys is less than the risk of PRS.

43.9.2 Pelvic Kidney

When treating stones in a pelvic kidney, technical issues include: coupling the shock wave energy reliably on the stone with minimal absorption by bony structures and positioning the patient in such a way to allow for fluoroscopic stone localization and assessment of fragmentation. Prone patient position may be required to allow shock waves to treat the stone without attenuation by bony structures. These problems limit application and success of ESWL. RIRS, on the other hand, can be performed in the usual fashion.

43.9.3 Transplant Kidney

Kidney stones in a transplanted kidney are a special form of the solitary kidney scenario. Similar to the pelvic kidney situation, application of ESWL is technically more difficult due to the ectopic kidney location. Also, since the transplanted kidney is devoid of sensory innervation, pain from ureteral obstruction and hydronephrosis will not alert the patient to the potentially deleterious result of prolonged obstruction, and as such mandates closer monitoring of

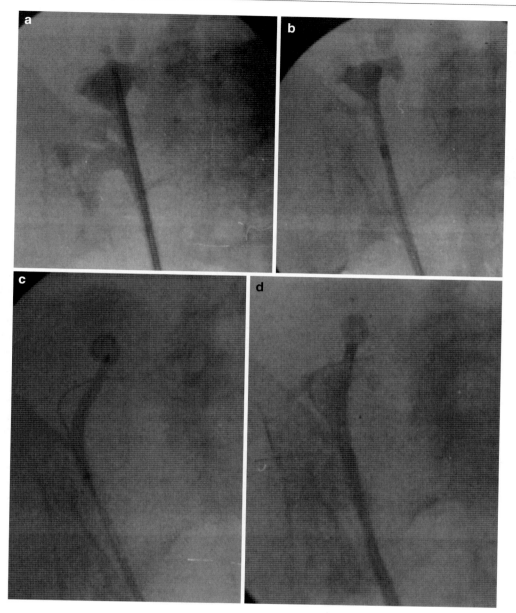

Fig. 43.5 (**a**) 7 mm stone in upper pole caliceal diverticulum in transplanted kidney; the semirigid ureteroscope cannot reach the stone bearing calyx. (**b**) With the flexible ureterorenoscope the stone bearing calyx can be identified and accessed. (**c**) A 14-F zero tip balloon dilator is in place for dilation of the narrow access to the stone bearing calyx. (**d**) After dilation of the caliceal neck the stone is fragmented with holmium laser and the fragments removed actively with a zero tip basket

these patients. Keeping in mind that retrograde access to the ureteral anastomosis can be technically challenging, our approach to treatment of stones in an allograft kidney is as follows. ESWL may be employed for stones 1 cm or smaller, when there is no associated anatomic abnormality and the stone can be properly localized. To avoid the scenario of having to place a ureteral stent into a transplanted ureter in order to relieve an obstructive complication, an indwelling ureteral stent is placed proactively at the time of surgery. RIRS is the treatment of choice for stones smaller than 1.5 cm. (Fig. 43.5). Even larger stones can be managed in this fashion, albeit with the need for multiple treatment sessions. Very large (staghorn) stones are best approached with percutaneous surgery while a large renal pelvic stone (>2.5 cm) may be treated with a laparoscopic pyelolithotomy.[24]

43.9.4 Fused/Ectopic Kidney

Crossed renal ectopia is an unusual congenital anomaly. The degree of anatomical abnormality varies, but any degree of malrotation can predispose to stone formation due to inefficient drainage of the collecting system. Knowledge of the upper urinary tract anatomy and functionality should be obtained by preoperative imaging with CT or magnetic resonance imaging (MRI) ± radionucleotide scan. Horseshoe kidneys represent the most common fused kidney scenario and stones are frequently encountered. Results with ESWL, RIRS, and PRS have been reported, with ESWL achieving the lowest stone-free rate (53% overall) and PRS achieving the highest overall stone-free rate. RIRS may be more technically challenging, as the ectopic kidney location may lead to altered anatomic relationships (i.e., relative UPJ obstruction, tortuous ureter, long infundibulum leading to the lower pole calyces). Basically, the RIRS technique for upper urinary tract access is the same as for the normotopically located kidney. It is important to remove all stone fragments, as drainage from the collecting system may be anatomically hindered (Fig. 43.6a–f). Usage of a ureteral access sheath has been reported to facilitate RIRS in the horseshoe kidney.

43.9.5 Obese Patients

RIRS may be the best method for the treatment of kidney stones in patients who are morbidly obese (BMI > 40). ESWL will not be effective if the stone cannot be radiographically located and/or positioned in the shockwave focal area. Access to the kidney for PRS can be tenuous, or even impossible if instruments are not long enough to reach the renal collecting system. Treatment of such patients is more demanding due to difficulties of patient positioning. If fluoroscopic guidance is not available due to patient weight exceeding the limitations of urologic X-ray tables, ultrasound may be employed to locate stones in the kidney and to verify the position of the proximal curl of the indwelling ureteral stent at the procedure conclusion.

43.9.6 Skeletal Abnormalities

Patients with severe skeletal abnormalities may not be physically able to be positioned in low-lithotomy position, the traditional position for RIRS. In most cases RIRS can still be successfully performed with the use of flexible scopes/ instruments and occasionally using ultrasound instead of X-ray for stone localization and stent position verification.

43.9.7 Upper Tract Reconstruction

Patients with upper urinary tract reconstruction or urinary diversion may develop stones secondary to reflux of infected urine. A conduit diversion or neobladder with reflexive ureter reimplantation can usually be navigated with a flexible cystoscope, and initially all mucous should be evacuated. Contrast/fluoroscopy and/or a guidewire can both be helpful when the bowel reservoir is tortuous. If the ureterointestinal anastomoses are of the refluxing-type, contrast/fluoroscopy may be helpful in identifying these areas (Fig. 43.7a–c). It is often helpful to have some knowledge of the implantation method that was used (previous operating report, imaging studies). We carefully search for sessile well-circumscribed areas in the reservoir/conduit wall, using a floppy-tipped guidewire to gently probe these areas. Intravenous methylene blue can also be useful to identify the ureteral insertion site/s. Once identified, the ureteral orifice should be cannulated with a safety wire preloaded in a 5-F angiocatheter. The wire should be advanced under fluoroscopic control and coiled in the kidney prior to advancing the angiocatheter up the ureter. Contrast may then be injected to define the upper tract anatomy, and a coaxial access set should then be used to place a second (working) wire. An access sheath will facilitate reaccess to the upper tract. RIRS treatment of kidney stones should follow the principles previously described in this chapter.

43.10 Complications of RIRS

43.10.1 Prevention

Complications of the RIRS procedure overall are rare with strict adherence to safe surgery guidelines. Medically, urinary tract infection with symptoms ranging from mild postoperative temperature elevation to full septic complications (very rare) can be encountered. Potential surgical complications of RIRS include: bleeding from instrumentation and use of energy sources, upper urinary tract injury and possible perforation, and postoperative ureteral stricture (Table 43.7a, b).

Awareness of preoperative urine culture results, the use of preoperative antimicrobial agents, and maintaining low pressures within the upper urinary tract during RIRS will

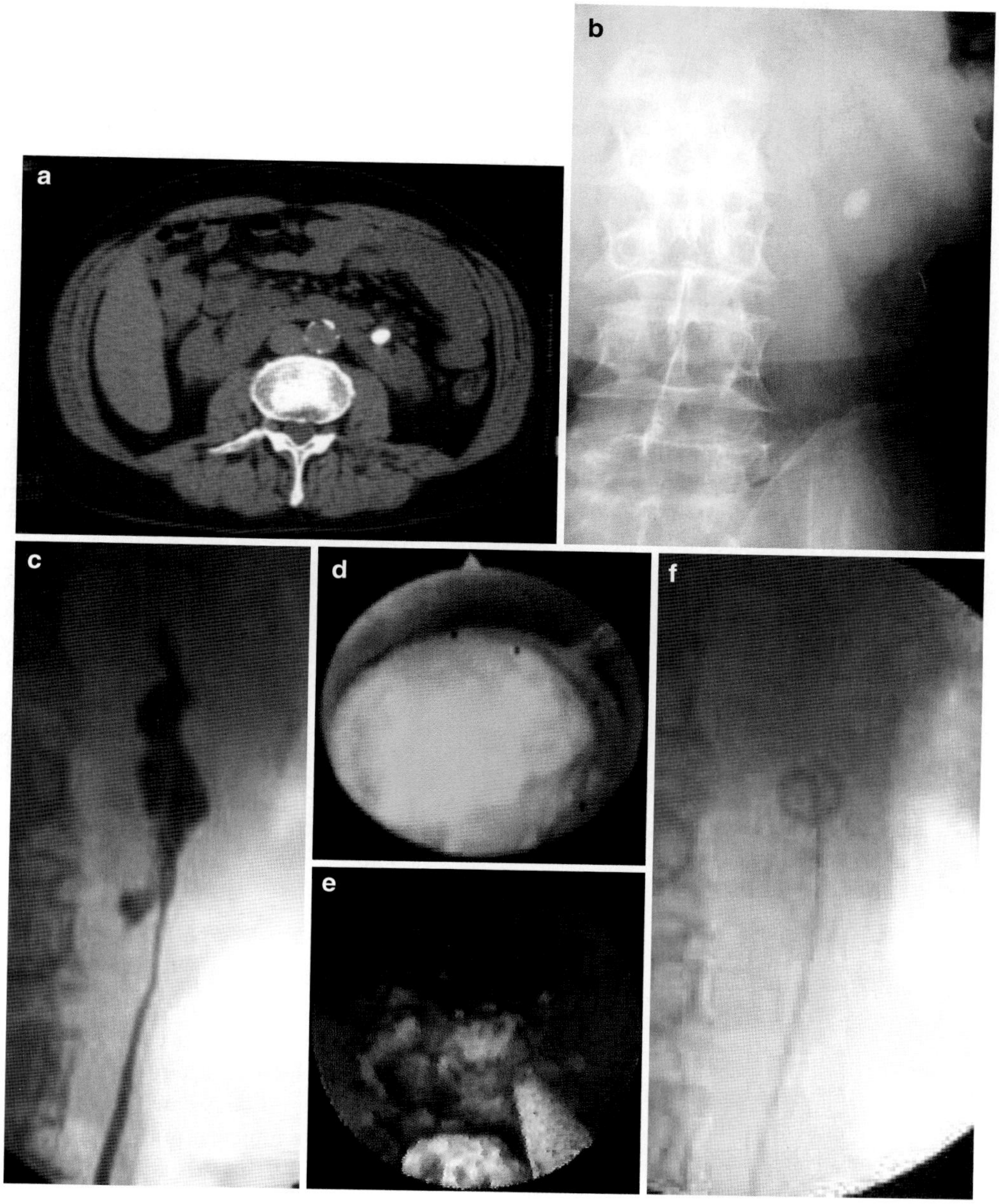

Fig. 43.6 (**a**) Renal pelvic stone in left moiety of horseshoe kidney. (**b**) KUB of 1.5 cm renal pelvic stone in left moiety of horseshoe kidney. (**c**) Retrograde pyelogram delineating anatomy of left upper tract of horseshoe kidney. (**d**) Endoscopic vision of intact stone. (**e**) Endoscopic vision of fragmented stone gravel before basket removal. (**f**) KUB after complete removal of the stone gravel

help to avoid infectious complications. As described earlier in this chapter, the routine use of a loop diuretic and keeping a low-pressure environment through avoidance of pressurized irrigation fluid flow and intermittent aspiration of intrarenal fluid by use of a suction pump will reduce the risk of postoperative infection. Furthermore, use of a ureteral access sheath—especially for prolonged cases and in patients with known or suspected infected stones—will also help to reduce intraoperative renal pelvis pressure.

Damage to the urinary tract can best be prevented by always visualizing the action of the ureteroscope, accessory instruments, and energy sources; avoiding blunt damage to the urothelium, either by the scope itself or by the sharp tips of accessories (guidewires, baskets, graspers) passed through the scope working channel. In addition, lithotripsy energy sources should never be fired unless the stone and energy fiber are directly visualized. Always maintaining a safety-wire access to the kidney will help in the management of most surgical RIRS complications, should one occur.

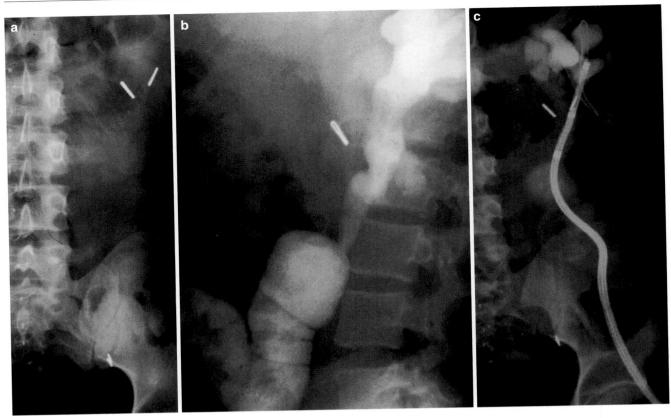

Fig. 43.7 (**a**) KUB of renal stone in solitary kidney with ileum conduit urinary diversion. (**b**) Retrograde pyelogram delineating anatomy of ileum conduit urinary diversion with ureteroenteric anastomosis refluxing into ureter. (**c**) Flexible cystoscope advanced all the way to kidney for stone treatment (fragmentation and active basket retrieval)

43.10.2 Management

Sepsis complications can be severe, especially after treatment of infectious stones. If patients exhibit signs or symptoms of sepsis (tachycardia, hypotension, temperature elevation), they should be closely monitored and treated with broad-spectrum antimicrobial agents. An appropriate intravenous access should be in-place, as blood pressure support may be required (Table 43.7b).

If bleeding from the use of energy sources and instrumentation occurs and vision is impaired, termination of the procedure with placement of an indwelling stent is the best course of action. Occasionally, a discrete bleeder can be identified and coagulated with the holmium or Nd:YAG Laser, but more commonly, bleeding is more of a generalized oozing nature involving multiple small areas and will self-terminate in short order; a second look procedure can usually be scheduled within 7–10 days. Breech of the integrity of the mucosa or perforation of the upper urinary tract rarely occurs. In such instances, the area of perforation should be examined, either endoscopically or fluoroscopically. In most situations, placement of an indwelling ureteral stent will allow the injury to heal, and the urologist can return at a later date to reassess the damaged area and complete the surgery. Severe injury, such as a circumferential ureteral tear or ureteral avulsion, is extremely rare and usually requires urgent operative intervention (Table 43.7a).

43.11 Conclusions

Retrograde intrarenal surgery for the management of renal stones and associated pathology (intrarenal strictures), using small caliber, actively deflecting instruments is a well-established minimally invasive treatment modality. Its role compared to ESLW and PRS is defined by a higher stone-free rate than ESWL and lesser invasiveness and risk than PRS.

A wide range of indications are now routinely performed at endourology subspecialty centers throughout the world and also an increasing number of community urologists are embarking on this safe, effective, and reproducible minimally invasive technique.

Table 43.7 (**a**) Intraoperative technical complications of ureteroscopic surgery and management. (**b**) Medical complications: prevention and management

Complications	Management
(a) Technical complications Ureteral injury • Mucosal tear with/without extravasation • False passage (guidewire) • Perforation (with extravasation), false passage • Ureteral bleeding (from scope or energy source) • Ureteral intussusception/avulsion • Damage to adjacent structures (vessels, bowel) **(b) Medical complications** • Acute urinary retention • Infection – Bacteremia, sepsis – Urethritis, prostatitis, cystitis • Periureteral fluid collection (extravasation) – Hematoma (sterile/infected) – Irrigation fluid • Positional – Nerve damage – DVT	Ureteral injury • Drainage ((1) stent, (2) stent + foley, (3) stent + foley + PCN) • Endoscopically correct guidewire placement and stent for 2 weeks • Drainage with stent (safety-wire!!), check with US/CT, PCN drainage of urinoma/hematoma • Observe, mostly will cease unless perforation or damage of large, adjacent vessel • Laparoscopic or open surgery required • Open surgery likely required – Avoid overdistention of bladder intraoperatively – Voiding trial for male patients with large prostates • Infection – Sterile urine preoperative, perioperative; IV antibiotics – Sterile technique, drainage (stent or PCN) – Antibiotics and symptomatic (anti-spasmodic) • Periureteral fluid collection (extravasation) – Observe (sterile); PCN drain (infected) – Observe (sterile); PCN drain (infected) • Positional – Proper positioning and cushioning – Evaluate, physical therapy – Proper positioning and cushioning, pulsatile stockings – Medical treatment

References

1. Chaussy C, Brendel W, Schmiedt E. Extracorporeally induced destruction of kidney stones by shock waves. *Lancet*. 1980;316(8207):1265-1268.
2. Chaussy C, Schmiedt E, Jocham D, et al. First clinical experience with extracorporeally induced destruction of kidney stones by shock waves. *J Urol*. 1981;127:417-420.
3. Chaussy C, Schmiedt E. Extracorporeal shock wave lithotripsy (ESWL) for kidney stones. An alternative to surgery? *Urol Radiol*. 1984;6:80-87.
4. Fuchs GJ, Chaussy CG. Extracorporeal shock wave lithotripsy of staghorn stones: reassessment of our treatment strategy. *World J Urol*. 1987;5:237-244.
5. Fuchs G, Fuchs A. Urinary stones which cannot be managed with extracorporeal shockwave lithotripsy. In: Andreucci VE, Fine LG, eds. *International Yearbook of Nephrology*. London: Springer; 1994.
6. Lingeman JE, Matlaga BR, Evan AP. Surgical Management of Upper Urinary Tract Calculi. In: Wein AJ et al., eds. *Campbell-Walsh Urology*. 9th ed. Philadelphia: Saunders Elsevier; 2007.
7. Rehman J, Monga M, Landman J, et al. Characterization of intrapelvic pressure during ureteropyeloscopy with ureteral access sheaths. *Urology*. 2003;61:713-718.
8. Fuchs G, Chaussy C. Patient selection for extracorporeal shock wave lithotripsy. In: McCullough D, ed. *Difficult Diagnoses in Urology*. Edinburgh: Churchill Livingstone; 1988.
9. Winfield HN, Clayman RV, Chaussy CG, et al. Monotherapy of staghorn calculi: comparative study between percutaneous nephrolithotomy and extracorporeal shock wave lithotripsy. *J Urol*. 1988;139:895-899.
10. Young HH, McKay RW. Congenital valvular obstruction of the prostatic urethra. *Surg Gynecol Obstet*. 1929;48:509-535.
11. Kourambas J, Byrne RR, Preminger GM. Does a ureteral access sheath facilitate ureteroscopy? *J Urol*. 2001;165:789-793.

12. Takayasu H, Aso Y. Recent development for pyeloureteroscopy: guide tube method for its introduction into the ureter. *J Urol*. 1974;112:176-178.
13. Bagley DH, Huffman JL, Lyon ES. Flexible ureteropyeloscopy: diagnosis and treatment in the upper urinary tract. *J Urol*. 1987;138:280-285.
14. Dretler SP, Cho G. Semirigid ureteroscopy: a new genre. *J Urol*. 1989;141:1314-1316.
15. Fuchs GJ, David RD. Flexible ureteroscopy, dilation of narrow caliceal neck, and ESWL: a new, minimally invasive approach to stones in caliceal diverticula. *J Endourol*. 1989;3:255-263.
16. Streem SB, Yost A, Domatch B. Combination 'sandwich' therapy for extensive renal calculi in 100 consecutive patients: immediate, long-term and stratified results from a 10-year experience. *J Urol*. 1997;158:342-345.
17. Angeloff A. Hydro electrolithotripsy. *J Urol*. 1972;108(6):867-871.
18. Begun FP. Modes of intracorporeal lithotripsy: ultrasound versus electrohydraulic lithotripsy versus laser lithotripsy. *Semin Urol*. 1994;12(1):39-50.
19. Lee MH, Lee YH, Chen MT, et al. Management of painful calyceal stones by extracorporeal shock wave lithotripsy. *Eur Urol*. 1990;18:211-214.
20. Psihramis KE, Dretler SP. Extracorporeal shock wave lithotripsy of caliceal diverticula calculi. *J Urol*. 1987;138:707-711.
21. Ritchie AW, Parr NJ, Moussa SA, et al. Lithotripsy for calculi in caliceal diverticula? *Br J Urol*. 1990;66:6-8.
22. Jones JA, Lingeman JE, Steidle CP. The roles of extracorporeal shock wave lithotripsy and percutaneous nephrostolithotomy in the management of pyelocaliceal diverticula. *J Urol*. 1991;146:72-77.
23. Fuchs GJ, Patel A, Tognoni P. Management of stones associated with anatomic abnormalities of the urinary tract. In: Coe FL et al., eds. *Kidney Stones: Medical and Surgical Management*. Philadelphia: Lippincott-Raven; 1996.
24. Desai RA, Assimos DG. Role of laparoscopic stone surgery. *Urology*. 2008;71(4):578-580.

Urolithiasis in Pregnancy

44

Chandra Shekhar Biyani, Mary Garthwaite, and Adrian D. Joyce

Abstract Management of urolithiasis during pregnancy is often challenging, requiring close cooperation between urologist, radiologist, and obstetrician. Physiological dilatation of the upper urinary tract occurs commonly in pregnancy due to altered uretero-dynamics. Ultrasonography is the preferred screening modality. X-rays present inherent risks of ionizing radiation and thus radiographic techniques including intravenous urography and computed tomography (CT) are best avoided. Magnetic resonance urography (MRU) offers a safe alternative to urography. If MRU fails to make the diagnosis, CT with a lower dose of ionizing radiation can be used in high-risk pregnancy. Fortunately, with conservative management, 70%–80% of symptomatic calculi pass spontaneously without any sequelae. We propose a logical, evidence-based, clinical management plan to enable the diagnosis, with the least possible risk to the patient and the fetus. During the first and second trimesters, sonographically guided PCN or internal ureteral stent placement is usually the first line of treatment. Specifically, ureteroscopic extraction is reserved for stones <1 cm. We believe that ureteroscopy should be avoided in the presence of sepsis and for stones >1 cm. However, we consider ureteroscopy as a useful option, since it combines a diagnostic procedure with definitive treatment. Patients with complicated stone disease should be delivered near full-term, and then, definitive measures should be planned for the postpartum period. Finally, for patients who are not near full-term, temporizing procedures appear to be valid alternatives. Management of stones in pregnancy must, therefore, be tailored to fit the individual patient.

44.1 Introduction

Loin pain in pregnancy poses a significant diagnostic and therapeutic challenge to all clinicians involved in the patient's care, including the general practitioner, obstetrician, urologist, radiologist, and anesthetist. Urolithiasis presenting during pregnancy is a major cause for concern considering the potential adverse effects of radiation exposure, surgical intervention, and anesthesia on both the mother and fetus. The incidence of urolithiasis during pregnancy varies between 0.026% and 0.531%;[1-3] causes complications in 1 in 200 to 1 in 2000 pregnancies[4] and may be a contributing factor in up to 40% of premature births.[3] Most studies have reported no difference in the incidence of symptomatic stones during pregnancy compared to nonpregnant women of childbearing age.[1,3,5] However, multiparous women seem to be affected more often than primipara by a ratio of approximately 3:1,[2,3,6-9] but the overall incidence in multiparous women is no greater when adjustment is made for age.[10,11] Folger[12] reported that pain resulting from urinary stones is the commonest cause of abdominal pain requiring hospitalization during pregnancy. Left and right side calculi occur with equal frequency and ureteric stones occur approximately twice as often as renal calculi. Interestingly, 80%–90% of patients present in the second or third trimester of pregnancy, while first trimester presentation is rare.[13,14]

Management of urolithiasis during pregnancy is often challenging and requires close cooperation between the urologist, radiologist, and obstetrician. Although 70%–80% of symptomatic calculi pass spontaneously with conservative management without any clinical sequelae they may rarely may initiate preterm labor.[3,11,13,15]

C.S. Biyani (✉)
Department of Urology, Pinderfields General Hospital, Wakefield, West Yorkshire, UK
e-mail: shekharbiyani@hotmail.com

P.N. Rao et al. (eds.), *Urinary Tract Stone Disease*,
DOI 10.1007/978-1-84800-362-0_44, © Springer-Verlag London Limited 2011

44.2 General Effects of Pregnancy on the Urinary Tract

Pregnancy is accompanied by numerous adaptive anatomical and physiological changes within the urinary tract (Table 44.1). Physiological hydronephrosis occurs in up to 90% of pregnancies, starting at 6–10 weeks of gestation, and generally resolves within 4–6 weeks of parturition.[16] The hydronephrosis of pregnancy is due to a combination of hormonal and mechanical effects. Progesterone affects the urinary smooth muscle during early pregnancy causing decreased peristalsis and dilatation of the ureter above the pelvic brim. The right is more affected than the left due to compression from the engorged right ovarian vein and uterine dextrorotation. Recent articles have suggested that mechanical compression may be the main cause for the dilatation, as several studies have demonstrated that dilatation is not seen when the ureter does not cross the pelvic brim, as in patients with pelvic kidneys or an ileal conduit.[17,18] A physiological state of absorptive hypercalciuria is observed during normal pregnancy, presumably caused by placental formation of 1,25-dihydroxycholecalciferol and suppressed production of parathyroid hormone.[19] However, in contrast, the filtered loads of antilithogenic substances like citrate, magnesium, and urinary glycosaminoglycans are also increased, reducing the risk of urinary lithogenesis.[20] Pathological calcium oxalate supersaturation has been reported during pregnancy, but crystalluria is no more common than in nonpregnant woman.[21] Thus, the relative percentage, type, and frequency of urinary stones occurring during pregnancy are similar to those in nonpregnant stone formers.[7,22]

44.3 Fetal Considerations in the Management of Urolithiasis in Pregnancy

44.3.1 Radiation Exposure

The most important factor complicating the radiological evaluation of stone disease in pregnancy is the risk of radiation exposure to the fetus. Diagnostic imaging during pregnancy carries the risk of ionizing radiation exposure to the fetus (Table 44.2).[23–26] The human body absorbs almost 90% of the exposed diagnostic radiation,[27] and the radiation dose absorbed (amount of energy deposited in the tissue by radiation) by a person is measured using the unit Rad or Gray (Gy). The Gy has replaced the Rad. The biological risk (risk that a person will sustain health effects from an exposure to radiation, dose equivalent and effective dose) of radiation exposure is measured using the unit Rem or Sievert (Sv) (1 rad = 1 rem = 0.01 Gy = 0.01Sv).

Table 44.1 Anatomical and physiological changes

	Anatomical	Physiological
Kidney	↑ in renal size ~1 cm	↑ renal plasma flow & GFR (30%–50%)
	↑ in renal volume ~30%	↑ creatinine and urea clearance
	Dilatation of the collecting system and pelvis	↑ protein and albumin excretion
	Dilatation of the renal vasculature	↑ uric acid, glucose, calcium, and citrate excretion
		Sodium retention
Ureter	Hydroureter (R > L)	↓ peristalsis
Bladder	Upward and anterior displacement	↑ bladder capacity
	Indentation of the bladder dome by the uterus	↑ bladder pressure
	Ureteric orifices are seen more cranially on cystoscopy	↑ vesicoureteric reflux (3.5%)

Table 44.2 Effects of gestational age and radiation dose on radiation-induced teratogenesis[23–26]

Gestational period	Estimated threshold dose	Effects	Spontaneous risk facing an embryo (0 rad exposure)
0–2 weeks	50–100 mGy	Death of embryo	350,000/10^6 pregnancies
2–8 weeks	200 mGy	Congenital malformation	30,000/10^6 pregnancies
	200–250 mGy	Growth retardation	30,000/10^6 pregnancies
8–15 weeks	60–310 mGy	Severe mental retardation (high risk [40%])	5000/10^6 pregnancies
		25–31 IQ point loss per 1000 mGy	
	200 mGy	Microcephaly	
16–25 weeks	250–280 mGy	Severe mental retardation (low risk)	
		13–21 IQ point loss per 1000 mGy	
After 26 weeks	>1000 mGy	Risk of stillbirth & neonatal death	20–2000/10^6 pregnancies

The principal effects of radiation on the mammalian fetus include teratogenesis, carcinogenesis, and mutagenesis.[23–26] The effects of radiation are categorized as either *nonstochastic* or *stochastic*. *Nonstochastic* effects are those that are cumulative with increasing dose and for which a threshold is believed to exist; for example, malformation, growth retardation, and cataract formation. *Stochastic* effects are those where the probability of the effect gets worse with increasing dose and where there appears to be no threshold; for example, the risk of malignancy and genetic effects.

The primary source of information on human data relies on studies from the 1945 atomic bomb survivors from Nagasaki and Hiroshima, who were irradiated with high doses in utero.[28,29] There is no doubt that regardless of gestational age, an acute exposure to radiation >0.5 Gy represents a major risk to the embryo.[1–3] The risk associated with radiation exposure is critically dependent on gestational age and the total amount of radiation delivered. The potential effects of radiation on a conceptus include prenatal death, intrauterine growth retardation, small head size, reduced IQ, organ malformation, and childhood cancer.

Radiation-induced fetal malformation (teratogenesis): The classical effects of radiation on the developing embryo are gross congenital malformation, intrauterine growth retardation (IUGR), and embryonic death. The frequency of severe mental retardation appears to be linearly related to the dose. During pregnancy, there is no apparent increased risk of severe mental retardation with radiation exposure before the 8th week or after 25th week of gestation.[26] Irradiation of the human fetus from diagnostic exposures of 50 mGy has not been observed to cause congenital malformations or IUGR.[30,31] In general, however, protected exposures have been shown to be less damaging than acute exposures, and the earlier the in utero exposure, the greater the effect.[32]

Radiation-induced malignancy (carcinogenesis): Various studies have demonstrated slightly increased risk of childhood cancer with radiation doses to the fetus of ≥10 mGy. However, this effect is not dependent on gestational age. The absolute risk for fatal cancer for ages 0–15 years following prenatal radiation exposure has been estimated to be 0.006% per 1 mGy. For the whole life span, this risk is about 0.015% per 1 mGy. ICRP Publication 90 suggests that an exposure of 30 mGy to a fetus doubles the risk of childhood cancer from 1 in 600 (general population) to 2 in 600.[33] The excess relative risk of developing childhood cancer has been reported to be ~0.28 at 1 mGy in the first trimester; and 0.03 at 1 mGy in the third trimester with an overall risk of 0.037 at 1 mGy during pregnancy.[34] It remains unclear as to whether the embryo is significantly more sensitive to the leukemogenic effects of radiation when compared with the child or adult. However, there is little disagreement with the concept that low doses of radiation present a carcinogenic risk to the embryo and adult, and that there may be different relative risks per mGy at different stages of development.[35]

Radiation-induced mutagenesis: Radiation exposure can result in germ-line mutations, potentially affecting future generations. In the general population, genetic diseases occur in ~11% of births and spontaneous mutations account for <3% of genetic disease.[32] The dosage required to double the baseline mutation rate is between 500 and 1000 mGy, far in excess of the radiation doses experienced in common radiographic studies.[30] Measurement of genetic effects is fraught with difficulties due to the high incidence of genetic birth defects inherent in the human population. The data from the children of the survivors of nuclear attacks on Hiroshima and Nagasaki indicates that radiation is weakly mutagenic and inherited mutations are rare, especially at low levels of exposure.[36,37]

The radiation dose delivered and its effect on the developing fetus depend upon the patient size, equipment, radiographic technique, duration of fluoroscopy, number of films, and the gestational age. For example, a kidneys-ureter-bladder (KUB) radiography delivers approximately 0.5 mGy to the fetus, a standard intravenous urography (IVU) exposes the fetus to 3 mGy and a limited IVU delivers about 2 mGy.[38] The National Radiological Protection Board (NRPB) reported mean and maximum fetal doses from the most recent surveys of diagnostic radiology practice (Table 44.3).[39,40] The lethal dose to fetal tissue is variable and increases from ~100 mGy after day 1 to 500 mGy at the end of the first trimester.[41] In the United Kingdom, it is recommended that an investigation resulting in an absorbed dose to the fetus of >0.5 mGy requires justification.[42] This dose gives a level of risk comparable with that due to variations in natural background radiation, found in the United Kingdom.[43] During the first month of pregnancy, spontaneous abortion is far more common than birth defects, and fortunately, first trimester presentation of urolithiasis is extremely rare. However, clinicians must carefully consider the risk-benefit ratio of an examination involving radiation during pregnancy during the first trimester.

44.3.2 Analgesics and Antibiotics

Small doses of morphine sulfate for episodic pain have demonstrated no adverse fetal effects, but chronic use of these agents can lead to fetal narcotic addiction, intrauterine growth retardation, and premature labor. Compounds containing codeine have been shown to have teratogenic effects when used in the first trimester, but may be used in the second and third trimester for short intervals with little fetal risk. Nonsteroidal anti-inflammatory drugs block prostaglandin synthesis and, therefore, may lead to premature closure of the ductus arteriosus in utero and, therefore, should be avoided in pregnancy. No evidence of teratogenicity has been reported for drugs such as ibuprofen and naproxen, and short courses would be appropriate if indicated; however, their chronic use may lead to

Table 44.3 Fetal doses following common diagnostic uroradiological procedure[39,40]

Examination	Fetal absorbed dose (mGy)		Effective dose (mSv)
	Mean	Maximum	
Abdomen X-ray	1.4	4.2	1.2
Intravenous urography	1.7	10	1.6
CT abdomen	8.0	49	10
CT pelvis	25	79	
99mTc Kidney scan (DTPA)	1.5	4.0	2.0
99mTc MAG 3		1.0	0.7
Physical quantity	*Non-SI unit*	*SI unit*	*Relationship*
Absorbed dose	rad	gray (Gy)	1 Gy = 100 rad 1 mGy = 0.1 rad 1 μ(micro)Gy = 0.1 mrad
Dose equivalent	rem	Sievert (Sv)	1 Sv = 100 rem 1 mSv = 0.1 rem 1 μ(micro)Sv = 0.1 mrem

"Background" radiation exposure: the average value for the United Kingdom is 2.7 mSv/year and the United States is 3 mSv/year

oligohydromnios and constriction of the fetal ductus arteriosus. Patients undergoing nonobstetric surgery may require antibiotic treatment and the antibiotics of choice are penicillins and cephalosporins, as neither group has been shown to have adverse effects on the fetus. Erythromycin is also well-tolerated without fetal morbidity. Aminoglycosides, tetracycline, chloramphenicol, the fluoroquinolones, and sulfa drugs are contraindicated in pregnancy due to adverse effects on the fetus.[44]

44.4 Clinical Presentation

The most common presenting symptoms and signs of urolithiasis are flank pain, gross or microscopic hematuria, and urinary tract infection.[45] The differential diagnosis of loin pain in pregnancy includes general abdominal conditions as well as the major obstetric complications of pregnancy (Table 44.4). Incorrect diagnoses, including appendicitis, diverticulitis, and placental abruption, have been reported in up to 28% of patients in whom a stone was subsequently confirmed. This is indicative of the diagnostic difficulties posed by patients presenting with urinary stone disease in pregnancy.[8] Hematuria is common in pregnant patients with stones, with microscopic hematuria reported in up to 75% of cases and gross hematuria in up to 15% of cases.[10] Patients may also present with urinary tract infection, irritative lower urinary tract symptoms, and rarely with preeclampsia.[10,11] Bladder stones are reportedly rare during pregnancy and their diagnosis during pregnancy can be difficult with stones often missed on ultrasound (US). Rare complications of bladder stones in pregnancy include vesicovaginal fistula.[46]

Table 44.4 The possible causes of loin pain in pregnancy

Obstetric causes	Nonobstetric causes	
	Nonurological	Urological
Accidental antepartum hemorrhage	Appendicitis	Urolithiasis
Torsion of the uterus	Cholecystitis	Acute pyelonephritis
Rupture of the uterus	Pancreatitis	Renal vein thrombosis
Uterine fibroids	Peptic ulcer disease	Urinary infection
Ovarian tumors	Intestinal obstruction	Renal rupture
Ectopic pregnancy		

44.5 Choice of Imaging Modalities

The most important factors to consider when presented with a pregnant patient with suspected urolithiasis are how to evaluate the problem with minimal risk to the fetus, then to determine the most appropriate management regimen, followed by if and when to intervene surgically. Kilpatrick and Monga[47] rightly stated, "Don't penalize her for being pregnant!". Anxiety regarding radiological procedures often generates undue fear and concern amongst obstetrician, urologist and radiologist, which may prompt the use of less sensitive alternatives for diagnosis with the potential for unnecessary delays in diagnosis, which may lead to untoward outcomes. Ultrasonography and magnetic resonance imaging (MRI) should be used when possible to avoid radiation exposure to the fetus, especially in the first trimester. If a modality with ionizing radiation is finally needed, the patient should be informed of the risks and benefits of the examinations.

44.5.1 Ultrasound (US)

Renal US is the diagnostic test of choice when assessing a pregnant patient with flank pain. It is inexpensive, readily available, and is believed to be safe to the unborn fetus because of its lack of ionizing radiation. However, US imaging has limitations in both pregnant and nonpregnant patients, including poor sound transmission through gas and bone, limiting the quality of the examination and its operator dependency. In the diagnostic evaluation of suspected renal colic in pregnancy, ultrasound is invaluable. However, it can be difficult to differentiate the physiological dilatation of pregnancy from ureteric obstruction and can miss up to 20% of patients with complete obstruction, so is, therefore, of limited value in cases of acute obstruction.[48] Stothers and Lee demonstrated a sensitivity rate of 34% and an 86% specificity rate for detection of abnormal findings in the presence of stones.[8] Evidence for the use of resistive index, presence or absence of ureteral jets, and measurement of pelvic diameter has been conflicting.[49] Nevertheless, ureteric dilatation below the pelvic brim is highly suggestive of pathological distal ureteric obstruction.[50] In addition, transvaginal US may help in elucidating the level of obstruction.[51]

44.5.2 MR Urography (MRU)

MR imaging during pregnancy has no known deleterious effects to the fetus and should be used when needed.[52] In a recent survey, most of the respondents (>90%) preferred to perform MRI in pregnant women with abdominal pain.[53] MRU can be used to evaluate the urinary tract without ionizing radiation and usually without administration of contrast medium. The test is performed in the supine position at field strength of 1.5 T (tesla). Safety or efficacy of a 3 T MRI machine during pregnancy has not been assessed. Acoustic injury to the fetus during pregnancy appears to be more hypothetical than a real concern.[54] Various MRI protocols for pregnant patients have been described, including rapid acquisition with relaxation enhancement (RARE), fast spin-echo (FSE), and half-Fourier acquisition single-shot turbo spin-echo (HASTE).[55–58] Roy et al. demonstrated excellent accuracy (sensitivity 100%) using RARE MRU.[57] MRU is able to differentiate a physiological from pathological ureteric dilatation during pregnancy, but it is an expensive technique and is of limited availability, thus, it should be reserved for special cases when US fails to provide a diagnosis. The RARE and HASTE techniques show ureteric caliber and level of obstruction but do not provide any information about the dynamics of the urinary system or the relationship of the ureter to any other retroperitoneal structures. Spencer et al. reported the use of gadolinium-enhanced, breath-hold

Table 44.5 Various definitions of a modified IVU

Authors	Protocol
Drago et al.[62]	Two exposure limited IVU, a second film at 30–60 min
Klein[63]	KUB + 20 min, ± delayed films
Waltzer[64]	KUB + 15 min, if obstruction then 60 min film
Boridy et al.[61]	KUB + 1 min + 15 min. Faint nephrogram on the 1-min film and no excretion on the 15-min film, delayed films at 120–180 min

Source: Adapted from Biyani and Joyce[49]

gradient echo MR excretory urography (MREU) to assess symptomatic hydronephrosis in pregnancy. They compared MREU with a gold standard isotope diuretic renography in 11 symptomatic pregnant women and noted a good correlation between assessment of excretion from symptomatic kidneys for isotope and MR studies.[59] However, potential fetal toxic effects with use of intravenous gadolinium contrast agents have been demonstrated in animal studies and the American College of Radiology's 2007 white paper emphasizes the need for a "well documented and thoughtful risk-benefit analysis" prior to the use of contrast agents.[60]

44.5.3 Intravenous Urogram (IVU)

As previously discussed, the use of radiation for diagnostic studies during pregnancy remains controversial. Various investigators have suggested that a modified or limited IVU[61–64] can be performed to decrease the radiation dose to the fetus. A modified IVU has been varyingly defined (Table 44.5).[49,61–64] A further limitation of IVU in pregnancy is the difficulty in differentiating delayed excretion of the contrast material associated with physiological dilation from that associated with obstruction due to calculus. Furthermore, an enlarged uterus and fetal skeleton may obscure small stones. Although, no adverse effects of contrast media on fetal development have been reported, exposure to contra media should be avoided. Depression of fetal thyroid function is a potential side effect due to exposure to free iodide.[65]

44.5.4 Computed Tomography (CT)

Traditionally, CT scanning has been avoided during pregnancy because of ionizing radiation. Interestingly, a study reported an unrealistically high perception of potential fetal harm by CT and routine X-rays in obstetricians.[66] In contrast, Lazarus et al.[67] reported that the number of pregnant women exposed to ionizing radiation has more than doubled in the last decade and the largest increase in imaging was with CT scan (25%). Furthermore, a recent survey of academic institutions in the United States suggested that 95% of respondents perform CT to assess pregnant woman presenting with abdominal pain when benefits are thought to outweigh the risks.[53] Various authors have reported the use of low-dose CT (LDCT).[68–70] White et al. performed CT scan in 20 patients during pregnancy.[70] In 19 patients, US scan demonstrated hydronephrosis with no calculi and a normal result in one patient. They observed >98% sensitivity and specificity with LDCT scan for detection of the renal calculi. The average radiation exposure was 7.0575 mGy. Another study[68] evaluated radiation dose resulting from MDCT of the chest, abdomen, and pelvis to the fetus at early gestation. The radiation doses to the fetus at 0 and 3 months for renal stone protocol was 8–12 mGy and 4–7 mGy; they concluded that doses are below the threshold dose thought to induce neurological detriment to the fetus. These doses are lower than those reported in Table 44.3. Angel et al.[71] used Monte Carlo simulations to investigate fetal radiation dose. They reported estimated normalized dose of 10.8 mGy/100 mAs (7.3–14.3 mGy). Fetal dose correlated well with patient size and fetal depth but not with gestational age. According to ICRP, significant neurological impairment is unlikely, unless a dose of 100 mGy or more has been delivered.[34] The radiation dose to the fetus from radiographic examination depends on the thickness of patient, the direction of the projection, X-ray technical factors, and the depth of the fetus from skin surface. McCollough et al. reported that the fetal radiation dose from CT is lower than that of limited IVU for a patient with an anteroposterior thickness of >25 cm.[72] As stated earlier, that radiation dose from CT scan of the pelvis could potentially double the risk of developing childhood cancer,[33] therefore, US and MRI should be used as alternative imaging modalities whenever possible.

44.5.5 Radionuclide Renography

The administration of a radioisotope to a pregnant woman will result in exposure of the fetus to radiation emitted from adjacent maternal organs and from any radioactivity transferred across the placenta.[42] Renography delivers about 10% of the radiation dose of an intravenous urogram. For ^{99m}Tc-labeled radiopharmaceuticals, the absorbed doses range from 0.2 to 1.8 mGy.[73] It is important to remember that the radioisotope is excreted in urine, and the bladder reservoir component will act as a significant source of exposure to the fetus. Therefore, to minimize the radiation risk to the fetus, the patient should be encouraged to maintain a high-fluid intake

and void as frequently as possible. Renography provides a physiological approach to diagnostic evaluation and its safety has been demonstrated.[74] However, physiological dilatation can be confused with pathological obstruction in 10%–20% of patients.[75]

44.6 Clinical Management Options

44.6.1 Conservative Treatment

There is a lack of evidence from randomized studies about the most appropriate treatment strategy for patients with stones during pregnancy. However, contemporary literature reflects that approximately 70%–80% of pregnant patients with symptomatic calculi will pass them spontaneously if treated conservatively with hydration, analgesia, and, if indicated, antibiotics.[1,7,9] Horowitz and Schmidt described it as "expectant therapy for the expectant mother."[13] However, this implies that intervention may be necessary in 20%–30% of patients. Indications for a more aggressive approach in pregnant patients include the following: (1) obstruction of a solitary kidney, (2) sepsis, (3) colic refractory to drug therapy, and (4) social and psychological reasons. Premature labor from renal colic is the most common obstetric complication of urolithiasis.[62] Standard tocolytic therapy with beta adrenergic agents halts premature labor and a single subcutaneous or intravenous dose of terbutaline sulfate 0.25 mg is often sufficient to arrest contractions. The risk of premature labor should cease completely with the passage or removal of the stone.

The initial management should be conservative, consisting primarily of rest, adequate hydration, analgesia, and antiemetics. The use of continuous segmental epidural block (T11 and L2) has been recommended and may even influence spontaneous passage of the calculi.[76]

44.6.2 Surgical Treatment

Various surgical interventions have been used to treat stones during pregnancy. Historically, pregnant patients with calculi underwent open surgery or blind basketry of the stone. Recent radiological advances, as well as technological improvements in new ureteral catheters, instrument design and energy sources, make the management of these patients potentially less invasive. The guiding philosophy in pregnant patients is to protect the mother and the fetus, therefore, the crux of therapy is minimal essential surgery. This should be based on the type of stone, timing of presentation, and availability of local expertise. Temporizing maneuvers in the third trimester may be appropriate because of the high risk of spontaneous abortion. In 1978, Meares suggested using a percutaneous nephrostomy (PCN) or internal ureteral stent(s) to manage complications of urolithiasis in pregnancy.[77]

44.6.2.1 Percutaneous Nephrostomy

The efficacy of PCN and retrograde ureteral stent(s) in decompressing the collecting system has been firmly established. Proponents of percutaneous drainage cite several advantages over retrograde ureteral stent placement: (1) PCN placement can be performed safely in acutely ill or septic patients with local anesthesia under US guidance; (2) it provides immediate drainage and allows culture of the urine for organism-specific antibiotic sensitivities; (3) PCN provides access for future percutaneous stone manipulation; (4) it avoids manipulation of the obstructed ureter with its potential for perforation and exacerbation of the infection; (5) if necessary, the nephrostomy tube can be irrigated to dissolve uric acid, cystine, or struvite stones; and (6) in addition, PCN is more cost effective than retrograde ureteral catheterization[78] and is successful in 91%–98% of patients.[79–81] Nevertheless, the disadvantages of nephrostomy tube insertion are well-recognized: (1) possibility of encrustation and tube obstruction requiring frequent tube replacement (6–8 weeks) to minimize encrustation, (2) infection, (3) possibility of bleeding from the track, (4) discomfort, (5) the procedure may be technically difficult in the third trimester, and (6) frustratingly, the ever-present risk of displacement of the nephrostomy tube.

44.6.2.2 Ureteral Stent

Insertion of internal ureteral stents can be performed with general/local anesthesia under transabdominal US guidance or with limited fluoroscopy. After the typical lower urinary tract issues, encrustation of the ureteric stent is the commonest complication, although no definite etiology of an increased tendency for the stent to encrust has been determined. However, pregnancy-related hyperuricosuria and absorptive hypercalciuria coupled with infection may be factors in stent encrustation, therefore, some investigators recommend hydration, dietary calcium restriction, and antibiotics.[80] Infection and migration are other complications of internal stent placement. Stent migration can be minimized by using double pigtail ureteral stents, which have a better memory or retentive design. As a consequence of such difficulties it has been suggested that ureteric stents should be reserved for the later stage (>22 weeks) of pregnancy.[82]

44.6.2.3 Ureteroscopy

Ureteroscopy has been widely used both in the diagnosis and treatment of urolithiasis, with advances in instrument design, flexibility, and downsizing having broadened both its diagnostic and therapeutic capabilities. Ureteroscopy has been safely employed during pregnancy and should always be performed by an experienced urologist.[83–86] Contraindications to the use of ureteroscopy during pregnancy are as follows: (1) stone size > 1 cm, (2) multiple calculi, (3) a solitary kidney, and (4) sepsis due to the increased risk of complications. Temporizing procedures should be considered in these situations. Most distal ureteric stones can be retrieved with a stone basket, but some may require fragmentation, which can be accomplished safely with pulse-dye laser, holmium:YAG laser or pneumatic lithotripsy.[83–86]

Percutaneous stone extraction should be deferred until the postnatal period because the necessity for prolonged anesthesia and radiation may pose a major hazard to the outcome of pregnancy. Extracorporeal shock wave lithotripsy (ESWL) is contraindicated in pregnancy because of the potential disruptive effects of the shock wave energy on the fetus.[87] Vieweg et al. reported a spontaneous miscarriage 24 h after ESWL treatment of a distal ureteric stone in the first trimester.[88]

Open surgery remains a viable alternative for the management of selected patients with urolithiasis in pregnancy. Shnider and Webster, who examined the risk of surgery, reported premature delivery in 6.5%, 8.6%, and 11.9% of patients, during the first, second, and third trimester, respectively.[89]

44.6.3 Algorithm for the Management of Stone Disease in Pregnant Women

Conservative management with bed rest, hydration, and analgesia results in spontaneous passage in two-third of patients (Level of Evidence 3, Strength of recommendations B). Surgical intervention is reserved for patients with urosepsis or renal failure or failure of expectant treatment. The availability of urological and radiological expertise will play an important role in the decision-making process, and, in addition, stone size and pregnancy status will also influence management. If conservative treatment fails in early pregnancy, temporary urinary diversion with percutaneous nephrostomy or an internal ureteric stent may be appropriate (Level of Evidence 3, Strength of recommendations B). The recent revolution in diagnostic technology and endoscopic instrumentation, resulting in high quality imaging and small caliber ureteroscopes, have made ureteric access a feasible and safe option (Level of Evidence 3, Strength of recommendations B). Ureteroscopic extraction is reserved for stones <1 cm, but should be avoided in the presence of sepsis or for stones >1 cm. Patients with complicated stone disease should be delivered near full-term and definitive measures planned for the postpartum period. Pregnancy remains an absolute contraindication for ESWL.

There is no universal consensus of agreement for a clinical algorithm for the management of a patient presenting with loin pain in pregnancy. The diagnostic and therapeutic dilemma presented by these patients is well recognized and the management of stones in pregnancy must, therefore, be tailored to fit the individual patient. Figure 44.1 presents a logical clinical management plan using the most appropriate investigations to reach a diagnosis with the least possible risk to the patient and the fetus.

44.6.4 Pregnancy Outcome and Complications

Information about the outcomes and complications of pregnancy in females with urolithiasis is limited. Swartz et al.[3] reported almost double the risk of preterm delivery compared with women without urolithiasis (OR 1.8, CI 1.5–2.1). In another study, Bánhidy et al.[1] reported no additional risk for adverse birth outcomes, especially congenital anomalies (OR 0.8, CI 0.6–1.0). Table 44.6 summarizes data on obstetric outcome.[1,3,8,90,91]

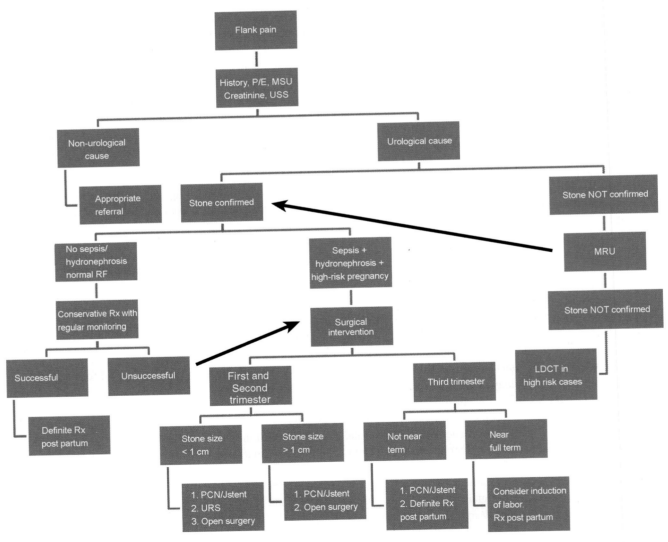

Fig. 44.1 Treatment algorithm. *P/E* physical examination, *MSU* mid stream urine, *MRU* magnetic resonance urography, *LDCT* low-dose computed tomography, *Rx* treatment, *RF* renal function, *PCN* percutaneous nephrostomy (Adapted from Biyani and Joyce[49])

Table 44.6 Kidney stones and pregnancy complications

References	Number of patients	Preeclampsia	Preterm labor	Preterm delivery	Premature rupture of membrane
Parulkar[91]	72		20%	2.9%	
Stothers and Lee[8]	80		–	2.5%	
Lewis et al.[90]	Cases 86	5.8%	12%	13%	7%
	Control 20,024	6.3%	9.9%		3%
Swartz et al.[3]	Cases 2,239		10.6%		2.9%
	Control 6,729		6.4%		3.2%
Bánhidy et al.[1]	Cases 69	14.5%	5.4%		
	Control 22,774	7.8%, $p = 0.04$	9.2%		

Table 44.7 Diagnostic imaging during pregnancy: recommendations

X-ray imaging

- *National Radiological Protection Board, Royal College of Radiologists, UK*: "Radiation doses resulting from most diagnostic procedures in an individual pregnancy present no substantial risk of causing fetal death or malformation or impairment of mental development"[41]
- *National Council on Radiation Protection*: "Fetal risk is considered to be negligible at 50 mGy or less when compared to the other risks of pregnancy, and the risk of malformations is significantly increased above control levels at dose above 150 mGy"[40]
- *American College of Obstetricians and Gynaecologists*: "Women should be counseled that x-ray exposure from a single diagnostic procedures does not result in harmful effects. Specifically, exposure to <50 mGy has not been associated with an increase in fetal anomalies or pregnancy loss"[95]
- *American College of Radiology*: After an exposure of 10 mGy to a newborn, the lifetime risk of developing childhood malignancy, particularly leukemia, might increase from a background rate of about 0.2–0.3% to about 0.3–0.7%, where the estimate varies depending on the methods used to assess the risk from statistical data[96]

Ultrasound imaging

- *American Institute of Ultrasound in Medicine*: "Mammalian bioeffects are not seen an unfocused beam having free-field spatial-peak temporal-average (SPTA) intensities below 100 mW/cm², or a focused beam having intensities below 1 W/cm², or thermal index values of less than 2"[98]
- *American College of Obstetricians and Gynecologists*: "There have been no reports of documented adverse fetal effects for diagnostic ultrasound procedures, including duplex Doppler imaging"[95]
- *United States Food and Drug Administration*: "Ultrasonic fetal scanning is generally considered safe and is properly used when medical information on a pregnancy is needed. But ultrasound energy delivered to the fetus cannot be regarded as completely innocuous. Laboratory studies have shown that diagnostic levels of ultrasound can produce physical effects in tissue, such as mechanical vibrations and rise in temperature. Although there is no evidence that these physical effects can harm the fetus, public health experts, clinicians, and industry agree that casual exposure to ultrasound, especially during pregnancy, should be avoided. Viewed in this light, exposing the fetus to ultrasound with no anticipation of medical benefit is not justified"[99]

Magnetic resonance imaging

- *ACR Guidance Document for Safe MR Practices: 2007*: Present data have not conclusively documented any deleterious effects of MR imaging exposure on the developing fetus. Therefore, no special consideration is recommended for the first, versus any other, trimester in pregnancy. MR contrast agents should *not* be routinely provided to pregnant patients[60]
- *Medicines and Healthcare Products Regulatory Agency*: The MHRA recommends that, where possible, the decision to scan should be made at the time by the referring clinician, an MR radiologist and the patient, based on the information above about risks weighed against the clinical benefit to the patient[54]

Radionuclide Scan

- *Administration of Radioactive Substances Advisory Committee*: "Special attention should be given to the optimization of the exposure, taking into account the exposure of the expectant mother and the unborn child"[97]

44.6.5 Clinical Management of Asymptomatic Stones in Patients Contemplating Pregnancy

It has been observed that renal stones tend to become symptomatic during pregnancy.[92] Therefore, the management of asymptomatic calculi in women of childbearing age must be considered in order to avoid the risks of subsequent management during a pregnancy (Level of Evidence 3, Strength of recommendations B). Mee and Thuroff[93] suggested that recurrent gross hematuria, documented stone growth, urinary tract infection, and recurrent renal colic associated with a mobile calyceal stone are all indications for prophylactic treatment in women of childbearing age who are contemplating future pregnancies. If possible, a careful metabolic workup should be performed prior to pregnancy. Management and genetic counseling of women with cystinuria should begin prior to conception. In patients with cystinuria, the mainstay of management is the assiduous maintenance of high-fluid intake.[94]

44.7 Conclusions

Although rare, symptomatic urolithiasis during pregnancy presents a challenging clinical problem that requires cooperation between the obstetrician, urologist, and radiologist. Flank pain and hematuria are the commonest presenting symptoms. The differential diagnosis of flank pain during pregnancy is expansive and, in this respect, a thorough medical history and physical examination is of vital importance. A fundamental part of the patient evaluation is urinalysis. In addition, US imaging is useful in resolving the diagnostic dilemma at the time of initial assessment. US combined with measurements of renal vascular resistance and ureteral jets appears to be the ideal imaging protocol. If the ultrasound fails to reveal a calculus in a symptomatic patient with hydronephrosis, isotope renography or MRU is useful in delineating the level and grade of obstruction. Many clinicians are concerned about suggesting imaging that involves radiation, however, the fact should be kept in mind that radiation-induced fetal abnormalities have not been reported below fetal absorbed dose level of 0.1 Gy. Ideally, radiographic techniques, including modified IVU and CT, are best avoided as they present inherent risks of ionizing radiation and contrast medium injection to the fetus. Judicious and selective use of LDCT appears to offer substantial diagnostic benefits (Table 44.7).[40,41,54,60,95–99] When the diagnosis is confirmed, a conservative approach is recommended in absence of hydronephrosis, sepsis, and abnormal renal function. Surgical intervention should be considered in patients with urosepsis or renal failure or failure of expectant treatment.

References

1. Bánhidy F, Acs N, Puhó EH, Czeizel AE. Maternal kidney stones during pregnancy and adverse birth outcomes, particularly congenital abnormalities in the offspring. *Arch Gynecol Obstet*. 2007;275:481–487.
2. Semmens JP. Major urologic complications in pregnancy. *Obstet Gynecol*. 1964;23:561.
3. Swartz MA, Lydon-Rochelle MT, Simon D, et al. Admission for nephrolithiasis in pregnancy and risk of adverse birth outcomes. *Obstet Gynecol*. 2007;109:1099–1104.
4. Gorton E, Whitfield HN. Renal calculi in pregnancy. *Br J Urol*. 1997;80(Suppl 1):4–9.
5. Coe FL, Parks JH, Lindhermer MD. Nephrolithiasis during pregnancy. *N Engl J Med*. 1978;298:324–326.
6. Byrd WE, Given FT. Urinary calculi associated with pregnancy. *Obstet Gynecol*. 1963;21:238–240.
7. Cass AS, Smith CS, Gleich P. Management of urinary calculi in pregnancy. *Urology*. 1986;28:370–372.
8. Stothers L, Lee LM. Renal colic in pregnancy. *J Urol*. 1992;148:1383–1387.
9. Strong DW, Murchison RJ, Lynch DF. The management of ureteral calculi during pregnancy. *Surg Gynecol Obstet*. 1978;146:604–608.
10. Jones WA, Correa RJ Jr, Ansell JS. Urolithiasis associated with pregnancy. *J Urol*. 1979;122:333–335.
11. Lattanzi DR, Cook WA. Urinary calculi in pregnancy. *Obstet Gynecol*. 1980;56:462–466.
12. Folger GK. Pain and pregnancy; treatment of painful states complicating pregnancy, with particular emphasis on urinary calculi. *Obstet Gynecol*. 1955;5:513–518.
13. Horowitz E, Schmidt JD. Renal calculi in pregnancy. *Clin Obstet Gynecol*. 1985;28:324–338.
14. Rittenberg MH, Bagley DH. Ureteroscopic diagnosis and treatment of urinary calculi during pregnancy. *Urology*. 1988;32:427–428.
15. Miller RD, Kakkis J. Prognosis, management and outcome of obstructive renal disease in pregnancy. *J Reprod Med*. 1982;27:199–201.
16. Peake SL, Rowburgh HB, Le Planglois S. Ultrasonic assessment of hydronephrosis in pregnancy. *Radiology*. 1983;146:167–170.
17. Harrow BR, Sloane JA, Salhanith L. Etiology of hydronephrosis of pregnancy. *Surg Gynecol Obstet*. 1964;119:1042.
18. Robert JA. Hydronephrosis of pregnancy. *Urology*. 1976;8:1–4.
19. Gertner JM, Coustan DR, Kliger AS, et al. Pregnancy as state of physiologic absorptive hypercalciuria. *Am J Med*. 1986;81:451–456.
20. Gambaro G, Cicerello E, Mastrosimone S, et al. Increased urinary excretion of glycosaminoglycans in pregnancy and in diabetes mellitus: a protective factor against nephrolithiasis. *(Letter) Nephron*. 1998;50:62–63.
21. Harris RE, Dunnihoo DR. The incidence and significance of urinary calculi in pregnancy. *Am J Obstet Gynecol*. 1967;99:237–241.
22. Coe FL, Parks JH, Asplin JR. The pathogenesis and treatment of kidney stones. *N Engl J Med*. 1992;327:1141–1152.
23. Brent RL, Gorson RO. Radiation exposure in pregnancy. In: Moseley RD, Baker DH, Gorson RO, eds. *Current Problems in Radiology*. Chicago: Year Book, Medical Publishers; 1972:1–48.
24. Brent RL. Utilization of developmental basic science principles in the evaluation of reproductive risks from pre- and postconception environmental radiation exposures. *Teratology*. 1999;59:182–204.
25. De Santis M, Di Gianantonio E, Straface G, et al. Ionizing radiations in pregnancy and teratogenesis: a review of literature. *Reprod Toxicol*. 2005;20:323–329.
26. Schull WJ. *Effects of Atomic Radiation: A Half-Century of Studies from Hiroshima and Nagasaki*. New York: Wiley-Liss; 1995.
27. Weissleder R, Wittenberg J, Harisinghani M. Medical physics. In: *Primer of Diagnostic Imaging*. 4th ed. St Louis: Mosby; 2007:1042–1052.
28. Brent RL. The effect of embryonic and foetal exposure to x-ray, microwaves, and ultrasound: counselling the pregnant and nonpregnant patient about these risks. *Semin Oncol*. 1989;16:347–368.
29. Yamazaki JN, Schull WJ. Perinatal loss and neurological abnormalities among children of the atomic bomb: Nagasaki and Hiroshima revisited, 1949 to 1989. *JAMA*. 1990;264:605–609.
30. Kinlen LJ, Acheson FD. Diagnostic irradiation, congenital malformations, and spontaneous abortion. *Br J Radiol*. 1968;41:648–654.
31. Tabuchi A. Foetal disorders due to ionising radiation. *Hiroshima J Med Sci*. 1964;13:125–173.

32. EUR 19603 European Advances in Radiological Protection. EC-NRPB agreement of association project coordinator reports for 1996–1999. Contract number F14P-CT95000. Electronically available at: http://www.nrpb.org.uk/Eur.htm).

33. ICRP Publication 90. *Biological Effects After Prenatal Irradiation (Embryo and Fetus)*. New York: Pergamon; 1991:143.

34. ICRP Publication 90. *Biological Effects After Prenatal Irradiation (Embryo and Fetus)*. New York: Pergamon; 2003:160–183.

35. Ek O, Faulkner K. Radiation risks from exposure to diagnostic x-rays during pregnancy. *Radiography*. 2000;6:131–144.

36. Brent RL. The effect of embryonic and foetal exposure to x-ray, microwaves, and ultrasound. *Clin Obstet Gynecol*. 1983;26:484–510.

37. Houston CS. Diagnostic irradiation of women during the reproductive period. *Can Med Assoc J*. 1977;117:648–651.

38. Swanson SK, Heilman RL, Eversman WG. Urinary tract stones in pregnancy. *Surg Clin North Am*. 1995;75:123–142.

39. ICRP Publication 90. *Biological Effects After Prenatal Irradiation (Embryo and Fetus)*. New York: Pergamon; 2003:122.

40. National Council on Radiation Protection and Measurement. *Medical Radiation Exposure of Pregnant and Potentially Pregnant Women*. NCRP Report no. 54, Bethesda, 1977.

41. National Radiological Protection Board (NRPB). Diagnostic medical exposure - advice on exposure to ionising radiation during pregnancy, Chilton, ISBN 0-85951-420-X. Available at: http://www.hpa.org.uk/web/HPAwebFile/HPAweb_C/1194947359535; 1998

42. Administration of Radioactive Substances Advisory Committee (1993) Notes for Guidance on the Administration of Radioactive Substances to Persons for Purposes of Diagnosis, Treatment or Research, Department of Health, London.

43. Hughes JS, óRiordan MC. *Radiation exposure of the UK population.- 1993 review, NRPB-R263*. London: HMSO; 1993.

44. Buhimschi CS, Weiner CP. Medications in pregnancy and lactation. In: Queenan JT, Spong CY, Lockwood CJ, eds. *Management of High-Risk Pregnancy - An Evidence Based Approach, Chap. 5*. 5th ed. Malden: Blackwell Science; 2007:38–58.

45. Cormier CM, Canzoneri BJ, Lewis DF, et al. Urolithiasis in pregnancy: current diagnosis, treatment, and pregnancy complications. *Obstet Gynecol Surv*. 2006;61:733–741.

46. Penning SR, Cohen B, Tewari D, et al. Pregnancy complicated by vesical calculus and vesicocutaneous fistula. *Am J Obstet Gynecol*. 1997;176:728–729.

47. Kilpatrick CC, Monga M. Approach to the acute abdomen in pregnancy. *Obstet Gynecol Clin North Am*. 2007;34:389–402.

48. Laing FC, Jeffrey RB Jr, Wing VW. Ultrasound versus excretory urography in evaluating acute flank pain. *Radiology*. 1985;154:613–616.

49. Biyani CS, Joyce AD. Urolithiasis in pregnancy. I: pathophysiology, fetal considerations and diagnosis. *BJU Int*. 2002;89:811–818.

50. MacNeily AE, Goldenberg SL, Allen GJ, et al. Sonographic visualisation of the ureter in pregnancy. *J Urol*. 1991;146:298–301.

51. Laing FC, Benson CB, DiSalvo DN, et al. Distal ureteral calculi: detection with vaginal US. *Radiology*. 1994;192:545–548.

52. Schwartz J, Crooks LE. NMR imaging procedures: no observable mutation or cytotoxicity in mammalian cells. *AJR*. 1982;139:583–586.

53. Jaffe TA, Miller CM, Merkle EM. Practice patterns in imaging of the pregnant patient with abdominal pain: a survey of academic centers. *Am J Roentgenol*. 2007;189:1128–1134.

54. MHRA: Safety Guidelines for Magnetic Resonance Imaging Equipment in Clinical Use DB2007(03). Available at: http://www.mhra.gov.uk/home/idcplg?IdcService=GET_FILE&dDocName=CON2033065; December 2007.

55. Hattery RR, King BF. Technique and application of MR urography. *Radiology*. 1995;194:25–27.

56. Pedrosa I, Zeikus EA, Levine D, Rofsky NM. MR imaging of acute right lower quadrant pain in pregnant and nonpregnant patients. *Radiographics*. 2007;27:721–743.

57. Roy C, Saussine C, Le Bras Y, et al. Assessment of painful ureterohydronephrosis during pregnancy by MR urography. *Eur Radiol*. 1996;6:334–338.

58. Tang Y, Yamasthita Y, Namimoto T, et al. The value of MR urography that uses HASTE sequences to reveal urinary tract disorders. *AJR*. 1996;167:1497–1502.

59. Spencer JA, Tomlinson AJ, Weston MJ, et al. Early reports: comparison of breath-hold MR excretory urography, doppler ultrasound and isotope renography in evaluation of symptomatic hydronephrosis in pregnancy. *Clin Radiol*. 2000;55:446–453.

60. Kanal E, Barkovich AJ, Bell C, et al. ACR Blue Ribbon Panel on MR Safety. ACR guidance document for safe MR practices: 2007. *AJR*. 2007;188:1447–1474.

61. Boridy IC, Maklad N, Sandler CM. Suspected urolithiasis in pregnant women: imaging algorithm and literature review. *Am J Roentgenol*. 1996;167:869–875.

62. Drago JR, Rohner TJ Jr, Chez RA. Management of urinary calculi in pregnancy. *Urology*. 1982;20:578–581.

63. Klein EA. Urologic problems of pregnancy. *Obstet Gynecol Surv*. 1984;39:605–615.

64. Waltzer WC. The urinary tract in pregnancy. *J Urol*. 1981;125:271–276.

65. Webb JA, Thomsen HS, Morcos SK. Members of Contrast Media Safety Committee of European Society of Urogenital Radiology (ESUR). The use of iodinated and gadolinium contrast media during pregnancy and lactation. *Eur Radiol*. 2005;15:1234–1240.

66. Ratnapalan S, Bona N, Chandra K, Koren G. Physicians' perceptions of teratogenic risk associated with radiography and CT during early pregnancy. *Am J Roentgenol*. 2004;182:1107–1109.

67. Lazarus E, Mayo-Smith W, Spencer P et al. *Utilisation of Radiological Examinations in Pregnant Women: A Ten Year Review – 1997–2006*. Chicago: RSNA Meeting; 2007:SSJ05–SSJ02.

68. Hurwitz LM, Reiman RE, Yoshizumi TT, et al. Radiation dose from contemporary cardiothoracic multidetector CT protocols with an anthropomorphic female phantom: implications for cancer induction. *Radiology*. 2007;245:742–750.

69. Katz DS, Venkataramanan N, Napel S, Sommer FG. Can low-dose unenhanced multidetector CT be used for routine evaluation of suspected renal colic? *Am J Roentgenol*. 2003;180:313–315.

70. White WM, Zite NB, Gash J, et al. Low-dose computed tomography for the evaluation of flank pain in the pregnant population. *J Endourol*. 2007;21:1255–1260.

71. Angel E, Wellnitz CV, Goodsitt MM, et al. Radiation dose to the fetus for pregnant patients undergoing multidetector CT imaging: Monte Carlo simulations estimating foetal dose for a range of gestational age and patient size. *Radiology*. 2008;249:220–227.

72. McCollough CH, Schueler BA, Atwell TD, et al. Radiation exposure and pregnancy: when should we be concerned? *Radiographics*. 2007;27:909–917.

73. Voigt R, Stoll W, Arndt J. The value of radio-isotope investigations of the urinary tract for the diagnosis of urinary tract calculi during pregnancy. *Geburtsh Frauenheilk*. 1980;40:863–867.

74. Tyden M-S, Goldstein HA, Zeissman HA, et al. Renal scans in pregnant transplant patients. *J Nucl Med*. 1988;29:1364–1367.

75. Brendler CB. Perioperative care. In: Walsh PC, Retik AB, Stamey TA, et al., eds. *Campbell's Urology, vol 3*. 6th ed. Philadelphia: W.B. Saunders; 1992:2351.

76. Maikranz P, Coe FL, Parks J, Lindheimer MD. Nephrolithiasis in pregnancy. *Am J of Kidney Dis*. 1987;9:354–358.

77. Meares EM Jr. Urologic surgery during pregnancy. *Clin Obstet Gynecol*. 1978;21:907–920.

78. Pearle MS, Lyle Pierce H, Miller GL, et al. Optimal method of urgent decompression of the collecting system for obstruction and infection due to ureteral calculi. *J Urol.* 1998;160:1260–1264.

79. Lee WJ, Patel U, Patel S, Pillari G. Emergency percutaneous nephrostomy: results and complications. *J Vasc Intervent Radiol.* 1994;5:135–139.

80. Rodriguez PN, Klein AS. Management of urolithiasis during pregnancy. *Surg Gynecol Obstet.* 1988;166:103–106.

81. Stables DP. Percutaneous nephrostomy: technique, indications, and results. *Urol Clin North Am.* 1982;9:15–29.

82. Denstedt JD, Razvi H. Management of urinary calculi during pregnancy. *J Urol.* 1992;148:1072–1075.

83. Akpinar H, Tüfek I, Alici B, Kural AR. Ureteroscopy and holmium laser lithotripsy in pregnancy: stents must be used postoperatively. *J Endourol.* 2006;20:107–110.

84. Carringer M, Swartz R, Johansson JE. Management of ureteric calculi during pregnancy by ureteroscopy and laser lithotripsy. *Br J Urol.* 1996;77:17–20.

85. Scarpa RM, De Lisa A, Usai E. Diagnosis and treatment of ureteral calculi during pregnancy with rigid ureteroscopes. *J Urol.* 1996;155:875–877.

86. Shokeir AA, Mutabagani H. Rigid ureteroscopy in pregnant women. *Br J Urol.* 1998;81:678–681.

87. Chaussy CG, Fuchs GJ. Current state and future developments of noninvasive treatment of human urinary stones with extracorporeal shock wave lithotripsy. *J Urol.* 1989;141:782–789.

88. Weber VJ, HM MK, Hautmann R. Female fertility following extracorporeal shock wave lithotripsy of distal ureteral calculi. *J Urol.* 1992;148:1007–1010.

89. Shnider SM, Webster GM. Maternal and fetal hazards of surgery during pregnancy. *Am J Obstet Gynecol.* 1965;92:891–900.

90. Lewis DF, Robichaux AG, Jaekle RK, et al. Urolithiasis in pregnancy. Diagnosis, management and pregnancy outcome. *J Reprod Med.* 2003;48:28–32.

91. Parulkar BG, Hopkins TB, Wollin MR, et al. Renal colic during pregnancy: a case for conservative treatment. *J Urol.* 1998;159:365–368.

92. Glowacki LS, Beecroft ML, Cook RJ, et al. The natural history of asymptomatic urolithiasis. *J Urol.* 1992;147:319–321.

93. Mee SL, Thuroff JW. Small calyceal stone: Is extracorporeal shock wave lithotripsy justified? *J Urol.* 1988;139:908–910.

94. Gregory MC, Mansell MA. Pregnancy and cystinuria. *Lancet.* 1983;2:1158–1160.

95. ACOG Committee Opinion #299. Guidelines for diagnostic imaging during pregnancy. *Obstet Gynecol.* 2004;104:647–651.

96. ACR Practice Guideline. *For Imaging Pregnant or Potentially Pregnant Adolescent and Women with Ionising Radiation (Resolution 26);* 2008:24–37.

97. ARSAC. Notes for guidance on the clinical administration of radiopharmaceuticals and use of sealed radioactive sources. Administration of Radioactive Substances Advisory Committee March 2006, Section 7: 7.5. Available at: http://www.arsac.org.uk/notes_for_guidence/documents/ARSACNFG2006Corrected06–11–07.pdf

98. American Institute of Ultrasound in Medicine. Available at: http://www.aium.org/publications/guidelinesStatementsX.aspx#statements. Accessed December 4, 2008.

99. US Food and Drug Administration, Center for Devices and Radiological Health, Diagnostic Devices Branch. Fetal keepsake videos. Available at: http://www.fda.gov/cdrh/consumer/fetal-videos.html. Accessed December 4, 2008.

Surgical Management of Urolithiasis in Transplanted Kidneys

Yehoshua Gdor and J. Stuart Wolf, Jr.

Abstract Urolithiasis is an uncommon complication in transplant kidneys. The use of computed tomography to evaluate living donors can detect calculi in kidneys and such kidneys should be avoided for transplantation, unless a small asymptomatic stone can be removed. Calculi may form de novo after transplant. The principles of treatment of calculi in transplant kidneys are similar to that of calculi in solitary kidneys. The major differences are the clinical manifestations and the anatomy. Since the treatment goal is stone-free status with one procedure with minimal morbidity and risk to the transplant kidney, advances in endoscopic equipment and techniques have shifted treatments from shockwave lithotripsy (SWL) to percutaneous nephrostolithotomy and ureteroscopy.

45.1 Introduction

Urolithiasis is an uncommon complication in transplant kidneys, with a reported incidence of 0.13%–3%. Calculi may already present in the donor kidney, or they may form de novo after transplantation.

45.2 Donated Kidney

When the diagnosis of renal calculi in a potential donor kidney is made before transplantation, the potential donor typically has been turned away. With the use of computed tomography for the evaluation of living donors, the diagnosis of asymptomatic renal calculi increasingly is being made. Concern for the safety for the donor and recipient suggest that donation of such a kidney should be avoided, but small renal calculi detected incidentally (as opposed to those that are detected with evaluation directed toward symptoms of urolithiasis) in other settings are rarely associated with clinical progression. As such, a variety of management plans have been proposed to facilitate transplantation of stone-bearing kidneys from living donors.

Devasia and associates reported one case of shockwave lithotripsy of a small renal calculus in a potential donor kidney; the kidney was removed and transplanted 6 weeks later with a residual fragment of 4 mm.[1] These same authors also reported a case of surgical nephrotomy to remove a known calculus from an ex vivo kidney under ultrasonographic guidance. Surgical pyelotomy and removal of the stone using a flexible cystoscope has also been reported.[2] In an effort to minimize risk to the donated kidney, our group prefers to remove renal calculi from the donor kidney ex vivo with a semirigid ureteroscope passed through the ureter after cold perfusion. We have reported such ex vivo ureteroscopy in 10 kidneys with small, solitary, unilateral, nonobstructing calculi. There were no complications owing to the stone removal. At mean follow-up of 36.4 and 33.2 months in donors and recipients, respectively, no new stones had formed.[3] Finally, other investigators have reported transplanting living donor kidneys with known small stones and following the recipient conservatively. Of 18 such cases reported in three series, none of the recipients has required treatment, although mean follow-up is less than 2 years in all reports.[1,4,5]

Regardless of the method elected for management of the renal calculus in an intended donor kidney, certain criteria should be met by the donor to protect against leaving a potential active stone former with only one kidney. Donors should be over 40 years of age, without a history of symptomatic calculi, with only one or two small stones in the affected kidney and no stones in the contralateral kidney. Additionally, a 24-h urine analysis for stone forming risks should be performed, and any potential donor with a significant metabolic risk factor for further stone formation should be excluded.

J.S. Wolf (✉)
Department of Urology, The University of Michigan,
Ann Arbor, MI, USA
e-mail: wolfs@umich.edu

P.N. Rao et al. (eds.), *Urinary Tract Stone Disease*,
DOI 10.1007/978-1-84800-362-0_45, © Springer-Verlag London Limited 2011

Unlike in living donors, preoperative renal imaging is not routinely performed for deceased donors.[2] Consequently, an unknown renal calculus may occasionally be transplanted along with the allograft. This may be the source of renal transplant calculi in up to 60% cases.[2,6] This finding notwithstanding, routine renal imaging prior to harvesting kidneys from deceased donors may not be merited given the infrequency of this occurrence.

45.3 De Novo Formation

There are several predisposing factors for stone formation among transplant patients Secondary hyperparathyroidism is commonly found in chronic renal failure patients, and may result in hypercalciuria. In some patients there may be a tendency to decreased fluid uptake, out of a habit developed after years of fluid restriction in patients on hemodialysis awaiting transplantation. Cyclosporine, an important immunosuppressant, can result in hyperuricosuria in about 50%–60% of patients.[7] Cyclosporine is also associated with a tubular effect that resembles distal renal tubular acidosis, such that it produces hypocitraturia.[8] Ureteral complications are the most common urologic complication of renal transplantation. If obstruction occurs gradually and is not detected, then urinary stasis might predispose to urinary calculi formation. Other potential causes of de novo formation of calculi in renal transplants include recurrent urinary tract infections and a foreign body nidus such as suture, staple, or forgotten stent.[9,10]

Despite the aforementioned potential risk factors for urolithiasis formation in transplant kidneys, the incidence remains low since other factors appear to outweigh the potential lithogenic aspects of renal transplantation. The encouragement of a generous fluid intake in transplant patients, the delivery of all glomerular filtration through one kidney rather than two, and some degree of impairment of urinary concentrating ability combine to reduce the risk of stone formation. Dumoulin et al. compared 24-h urine samples from 82 renal transplant patients on immunosuppressive treatment and good renal function with those from 82 healthy subjects.[11] Findings favoring renal stone formation included lower urinary citrate and greater urinary oxalate excretion in the transplant patients. As noted previously, the former owes to cyclosporine treatment. The latter is likely related to the excretion of significant body oxalate stores that developed over years of hemodialysis. Findings protecting against de novo stone formation were more numerous, however, including significantly greater urinary volumes, and lower levels of calcium and uric acid excretion. Overall, the calcium-oxalate saturation was not greater in renal transplant patients. These findings may explain, in part, the low de novo urolithiasis formation rate among patients with renal transplant.

45.4 Clinical Manifestations

Because the renal allograft is denervated, classic symptoms of renal colic are not expected, although some patients report mild discomfort in the iliac fossa containing the transplant kidney.[12] Diagnosis is suspected when signs of obstruction occur, such as decreased urine output, increased serum creatinine level, fever, and hematuria.[13] Presentation can be dramatic, with acute renal failure. These signs mimic those of acute rejection, which may delay the diagnosis of urolithiasis.[14]

Radiological diagnosis of urinary calculi in the transplant kidney can be difficult. The sensitivity of plain abdominal radiography may be reduced by the majority of the transplant kidney and ureter being positioned in the bony pelvic, but some renal (Fig. 45.1) or ureteral stones may be visible. Ultrasonography is limited in sensitivity for small stones, but has reasonable accuracy for stones >5 mm (Fig. 45.2). Just as in the nontransplant patient, noncontrast computed tomography is the best and safest means for the detection of urinary calculus, sensitive for

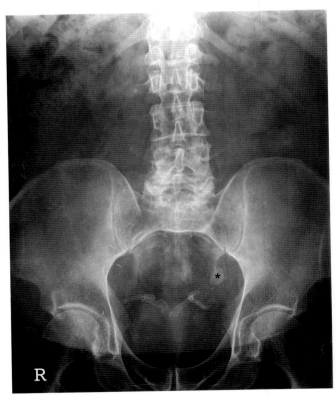

Fig. 45.1 A 2 cm pelvic stone in the lower pole of a transplant kidney in left iliac fossa (*black asterisk*)

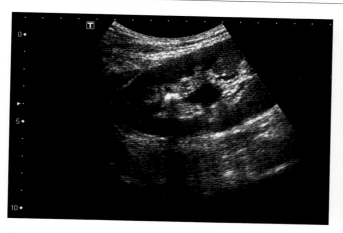

Fig. 45.2 An 11 mm stone in the lower pole of a transplant kidney visible on ultrasonography

small stones in any location in the transplant kidney and ureter (Fig. 45.3a, b).[14]

45.5 Treatment

In general, the treatment of transplant kidney stones is similar to that of single kidney stone. All treatment techniques are of use, and generally have success rates similar to their use in nontransplant patients, with some caveats related to the pelvic location of the kidney with a tortuous and abnormally inserted ureter.

45.5.1 Observation

Since transplant kidneys are solitary and vulnerable for obstruction, and since the anatomy of the ureter and ureterovesical anastomosis may not be predictable, observation in this setting is elected by only a few physicians. Klingler et al. justified the watchful-waiting approach, but only in patients with a known wide refluxed ureter, no signs of impaired function, and only for stones up to 4 mm in diameter. Close monitoring including urine output, weekly serum creatinine, and renal ultrasound is mandatory.[2] Results have been favorable in the series of known gifted urinary calculi noted previously,[1,4,5] but again, the follow-up is short. In another series of stones followed conservatively, one patient did require several treatments for stone growth.[4]

45.5.2 Shockwave Lithotripsy

Shockwave lithotripsy under close surveillance is a reasonable choice for small to medium size stones (5–15 mm), but

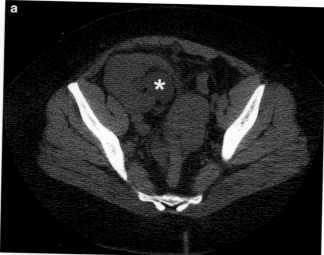

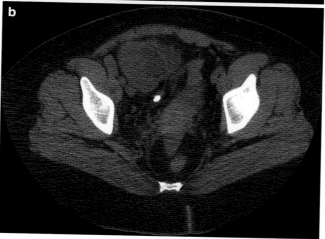

Fig. 45.3 Noncontrast computed tomography. (**a**) Hydronephrosis of a transplant kidney in the right iliac fossa (*white asterisk*). (**b**) Obstructing stone in the ureter of the same transplant kidney

there are technical challenges. Localization of the stone can be difficult due to the position of the kidney within the bony pelvis. The ureteral orifice can be difficult to access for placement of a stent or ureteral catheter, which some might consider. Additionally, potential complications of shockwave lithotripsy might be problematic in transplant kidney. Steinstrasse or other ureteral obstruction can be troublesome due to difficult retrograde cannulation of the ureter. The patient should be counseled that percutaneous access may be required if treatment fails or is complicated.[14] In patients with obstructing calculi smaller than 15 mm, if obstruction (or potential obstruction) can be quickly addressed with a ureteral stent or nephrostomy tube, then shockwave lithotripsy is reasonable to consider.

Challacombe and coworkers achieved a 100% stone-free rate on 13 patients with shockwave lithotripsy, eight of whom required multiple sessions. Of these patients, eight required ureteral stent insertion before a second procedure and four required a nephrostomy tube to relieve obstruction.[10] Klingler and associates treated seven patients with 5–15 mm stones by shockwave lithotripsy. Of the patients, three needed a nephrostomy tube, but all become stone free within 15 days.[2]

It appears that shockwave lithotripsy is an effective treatment for transplant kidney stones up to 15 mm in size, but intensive monitoring of these patients is mandatory since this procedure involves a considerable risk of ureteral obstruction.

45.5.3 Ureteroscopy

Retrograde ureteroscopy is an appealing technique for the first-line treatment of transplant ureteral stones, and for stones after failed shockwave lithotripsy in renal transplant kidneys. It is less invasive than percutaneous nephrostolithomy, and more controlled than shockwave lithotripsy. The major difficulties associated with performing ureteroscopy in transplanted kidneys are the neoureterocystostomy that is usually located in the anterior bladder dome, a location that is hard to find and negotiate, and the torturousity and redundancy of the transplant ureter, which causes difficulty in advancing the ureteroscope up to the transplant kidney.[15] The use of hydrophilic-coated guidewires through flexible cystoscopy and angled ureteral catheters are very helpful in gaining ureteral access. Antegrade (percutaneous) insertion of a guidewire can be used when retrograde access fails.[16] Once in the kidney, the unusual orientation of the kidney can make caliceal access challenging; flexible ureteroscopes with an active secondary deflection can be useful in gaining access to caliceal stones.

Del Pizzo and associates reported success in 13 of 14 (93%) transplanted patients with ureteroscopy, including 100% success in treating four patients with ureteral calculi. For diagnostic procedures these investigators used flexible ureteroscope and for stone treatment they used a semirigid ureteroscope. Ureteral perforation occurred in one patient.[13] Basiri and coworkers described their experience with ureteroscopic treatment of 28 renal transplant patients with ureteral complication. They had a 68% success rate in the identification of the neoureterocystostomy and guidewire insertion, and successfully treated four out of six ureteral calculi. The only minor complications were urine leakage and infection, which were treated conservatively.[15]

If the neoureterocystostomy can be accessed, then ureteroscopy appears to be a reasonable treatment for urinary calculi in transplant kidneys. The tortuous ureter precludes insertion of a ureteral access sheath, so the technique is primarily one of fragmentation to completion rather than fragment extraction.

45.5.4 Percutaneous Nephrostolithotomy

Because of the superficial position of the transplant kidney, nephrostomy drainage and percutaneous nephrostolithotomy are relatively straightforward. Percutaneous nephrostolithotomy is the treatment of choice for stone greater than 15 mm, mainly because it has the potential to remove all stone fragments in one procedure.[10] The authors consider it to be the preferred treatment for all stones in excess of 5–10 mm. There are several technical considerations when performing percutaneous nephrostolithotomy on transplant kidneys. Loops of bowel may be interposed over the transplant kidney and may be punctured with percutaneous access, so the use of ultrasonography (as a replacement for, or at least adjunct to, fluoroscopy) is crucial. Scar formation around the transplant kidney may cause difficulties in the initial needle puncture and with balloon dilation of the tract. Coaxial metal dilators may be required.[14] Finally, although "tubeless," percutaneous nephrostolithotomies appear to be supported by good clinical data in most patients, in the abnormal and high-risk transplant kidney postoperative percutaneous nephrostomy is recommended.

Klingler and associates performed percutaneous nephrostolithotomy in three transplant kidneys with large stones (mean 34 mm) using 27 F rigid nephroscopes and 14.5 F flexible cystoscopes. They reported a 100% stone-free rate with no complications.[2] Challacombe and coworkers reported their experience with three transplant patients with stones larger than 15 mm. Of the patients, two were rendered stone-free while one with a staghorn calculus required pyelolithotomy.[10] Zhaohui He and associates used "mini-perc" to address stones in seven transplanted kidneys, using 8.5/11.5 F semirigid ureteroscopes and 8/9.5 F flexible ureteroscopes through 16 F peel-away sheath.[17] The stones ranged in size from 0.6 to 40 mm. Stones were fragmented with a pneumatic lithotripter or the holmium:YAG laser. Larger fragments were extracted and smaller ones were flashed out. All patients were rendered stone-free at one procedure, and there were no intraoperative complications.

At our institution we have treated four patients with percutaneous nephrostolithotomy for renal stones, including a collection of eight 2–3 mm stones in one patient, two patients with solitary renal stones measuring 11 and 20 mm each, and one patient with a partial staghorn calculus. All patients were rendered stone-free with a single procedure (Fig. 45.4a, b). The only complication was ureteral obstruction in one patient, owing to a blood clot that occurred following removal of the nephrostomy tube on postoperative day 1, which required urgent ureteral stent placement.

The percutaneous approach is also an excellent technique for managing ureteral calculi, with antegrade ureteroscopy. Only minimal tract dilation is required to pass a standard

Fig. 45.4 Percutaneous nephrostolithotomy. (**a**) Percutaneous access being attained in lower pole calyx of transplant kidney bearing a 2 cm calculus (same patient as Fig. 45.1). (**b**) Completion of percutaneous nephrostolithotomy, and placement of 8 Fr nephrostomy tube

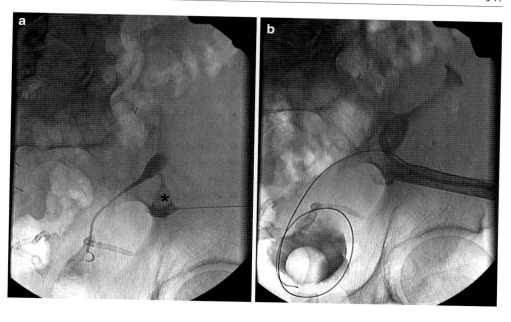

6.9 F flexible ureteroscope. Klingler et al. report on one patient that was successfully treated for distal ureteral stone using a flexible cystoscope through a percutaneous access site, after retrograde ureteroscopy failed.[2] At our institution, we have experience with antegrade ureteroscopic treatment of an 8 mm obstructing ureteral stone in a renal transplant patient, with stone-free result and no complications. Since nephrostomy tube placement is often the acute treatment for ureteral obstruction in transplant kidney, the percutaneous access (which is arguably the most morbid part of the procedure) is already in place and offers an excellent approach for flexible ureteroscopy and laser treatment of ureteral calculi.

Percutaneous nephrostolithotomy and antegrade ureteroscopy are excellent treatments for larger renal stones and obstructing ureteral stones. It offers the best strategy for complete stone removal, at the price of greater invasiveness. "Miniperc," dilating the tract to a smaller width, is an attractive option for smaller calculi in transplant kidneys or ureters.

45.6 Conclusions

The principles of treatment of calculi in transplant kidney are similar to that of calculi in solitary kidneys. The major differences are the clinical manifestations and the anatomy. Since the treatment goal is stone-free status with one procedure with minimal morbidity and risk to the transplant kidney, advances in endoscopic equipment and techniques have shifted treatments from SWL to percutaneous nephrostolithotomy and ureteroscopy, as has happened with stone treatment in the general population.

References

1. Devasia A, Chacko N, Gnanaraj L, Cherian R, Gopalakrishnan G. Stone-bearing live-donor kidneys for transplantation. *BJU Int.* February 2005;95(3):394-397.
2. Klingler HC, Kramer G, Lodde M, Marberger M. Urolithiasis in allograft kidneys. *Urology.* 2002;59(3):344-348.
3. Rashid MG, Konnak JW, Wolf JS Jr, et al. Ex vivo ureteroscopic treatment of calculi in donor kidneys at renal transplantation. *J Urol.* 2004;171(1):58-60.
4. Strang AM, Lockhart ME, Amling CL, Kolettis PN, Burns JR. Living renal donor allograft lithiasis: a review of stone related morbidity in donors and recipients. *J Urol.* 2008 Mar;179(3): 832-836.
5. Martin G, Sundaram CP, Sharfuddin A, Govani M. Asymptomatic urolithiasis in living donor transplant kidneys: initial results. *Urology.* 2007 Jul;70(1):2-5. discussion 5-6.
6. Yiğit B, Aydin C, Titiz I, Berber I, Sinanoğlu O, Altaca G. Stone disease in kidney transplantation. *Transpl Proc.* 2004;36(1): 187-189.
7. Harper JM, Samuell CT, Hallson PC, Wood SM, Mansell MA. Risk factors for calculus formation in patients with renal transplants. *Br J Urol.* 1994;74(2):147-150.
8. Stapenhorst L, Sassen R, Beck B, Laube N, Hesse A, Hoppe B. Hypocitraturia as a risk factor for nephrocalcinosis after kidney transplantation. *Pediatr Nephrol.* May 2005;20(5):652-656.
9. Benoit G, Blanchet P, Eschwege P, Jardin A, Charpentier B. Occurrence and treatment of kidney graft lithiasis in a series of 1500 patients. *Clin Transpl.* 1996;10(2):176-180.
10. Challacombe B, Dasgupta P, Tiptaft R, et al. Multimodal management of urolithiasis in renal transplantation. *BJU Int.* 2005;96(3): 385-389.

11. Dumoulin G, Hory B, Nguyen NU, et al. Lack of increased urinary calcium-oxalate supersaturation in long-term kidney transplant recipients. *Kidney Int*. 1997;51(3):804-810.

12. Crook TJ, Keoghane SR. Renal transplant lithiasis: rare but time-consuming. *BJU Int*. 2005;95(7):931-933.

13. Del Pizzo JJ, Jacobs SC, Sklar GN. Ureteroscopic evaluation in renal transplant recipients. *J Endourol*. 1998;12(2):135-138.

14. Rhee BK, Bretan PN Jr, Stoller ML. Urolithiasis in renal and combined pancreas/renal transplant recipients. *J Urol*. 1999;161(5):1458-1462.

15. Basiri A, Nikoobakht MR, Simforoosh N, Hosseini Moghaddam SM. Ureteroscopic management of urological complications after renal transplantation. *Scand J Urol Nephrol*. 2006;40(1):53-56.

16. Henderson A, Gujral S, Mitchelmore AE, Keeley FX Jr. Endo-urological techniques in the management of stent complications in the renal transplant patient. *Transpl Int*. 2002;15(12):664-666.

17. He Z, Li X, Chen L, Zeng G, Yuan J. Minimally invasive percutaneous nephrolithotomy for upper urinary tract calculi in transplanted kidneys. *BJU Int*. 2007;99(6):1467-1471.

Stents and Stenting

Reem Al-Bareeq and John D. Denstedt

Abstract Stents are typically placed to prevent or relieve ureteral obstruction caused by intrinsic or extrinsic etiologies. Stent design and biomaterials have improved in recent years from the first described double-J stent in 1978. The indications for placement of a ureteral stent include obstructing ureteral calculi, ureteral strictures, congenital anomalies such as ureteropelvic junction obstruction, retroperitoneal tumor or fibrosis, trauma and iatrogenic injury, and postoperative drainage.

Although stents have several advantages, they are not without potential associated complications. Recent advances in design and materials have been developed to produce an ideal urinary stent with minimal complications. The ureteral stent is a mainstay in the urologist's armamentarium, and understanding the properties, indications, and complications is very pertinent to providing optimal patient care. This chapter will address these issues along with recent advances for ureteral stents.

46.1 Introduction

The ureteral stent has been an essential tool in contemporary urologic practice for more than 3 decades. Stents are a common device in our daily urologic practice with numerous indications. They are typically placed to prevent or relieve ureteral obstruction caused by intrinsic or extrinsic etiologies. Stent design and biomaterials have improved in recent years from the first described double-J stent in 1978.[1] The word stent is defined as "a device used to support a bodily orifice" or "a slender thread, rod, or catheter inserted into a tubular structure, such as a blood vessel to provide support during or after anastomosis" in Webster's dictionary. It was Montie et al. who incorporated the word "stent" into the urologic literature when they defined the term: "an intraluminal device to maintain patency until healing has taken place."[2]

The indications for placement of a ureteral stent include obstructing ureteral calculi, ureteral strictures, congenital anomalies such as ureteropelvic junction obstruction, retroperitoneal tumor or fibrosis, trauma and iatrogenic injury, and postoperative drainage.

Although stents have several advantages, they are not without potential associated complications. Recent advances in design and materials have been developed to produce an ideal urinary stent with minimal complications. The ureteral stent is a mainstay in the urologist's armamentarium, and understanding the properties, indications, and complications is very pertinent to providing optimal patient care. This chapter will address these issues along with recent advances for ureteral stents.

46.2 History of Stents

Urinary tract stents and catheters were documented centuries ago in ancient Egypt using lead and papyrus catheters.[3] They were developed to facilitate upper tract drainage and maintain luminal patency. In the nineteenth century, Gustav Simon performed the first case of ureteral catheterization, which subsequently in the early 1900s, Joaquin Albarrano developed for specific use in the ureter.[4] The era of plastics allowed a vast array of materials to be considered for development of a "suitable" stent, which would be more rigid and easier to place. Tulloch reported using polyethylene tubes to allow healing of ureters and fistulas in patients.[5] However, these stents were not ideal as they were associated with

R. Al-Bareeq (✉)
Department of Urology, The University of Western Ontario, London, ON, Canada
e-mail: docreem@hotmail.com

P.N. Rao et al. (eds.), *Urinary Tract Stone Disease*,
DOI 10.1007/978-1-84800-362-0_46, © Springer-Verlag London Limited 2011

significant bladder irritation, infection, encrustation, and migration.[6]

Silicone stents were used in 1967 by Zimskind et al. for malignant ureteral obstruction and demonstrated less encrustation than other materials.[7] The problem of migration of these straight catheters was addressed by Gibbons et al. with their stents having distal flanges and sharply pointed barbs.[8] In 1978, the solution to migration was resolved by the development by Finney of the well-known double-J stent using proximal and distal J-shaped hooks.[1]

46.3 Stents: Design and Materials

Stent design and materials have continued to evolve due to the advances in technology and the creativity of surgeons and scientists. The ideal stent characteristically should be biocompatible, radiopaque, easy to insert, resistant to encrustation and infection, and cause little discomfort to the patient. Unfortunately, a stent that encompasses all these criteria has yet to be developed.

46.3.1 Stent Materials

A biomaterial is a natural or synthetic material that interfaces with human tissue during clinical treatment.[9] The modern ureteral stent is composed of synthetic polymeric biomaterials, which have biocompatible features. The basic attributes of a ureteral stent were outlined by Mardis et al. in their comparative study of materials for internal ureteral stents.[10] They concluded that ease of insertion, effective restoration and maintenance of flow, resistance to migration, significant biodurability, and biocompatibility are the most important properties of an ideal stent.

Indwelling ureteral stents are often associated with significant patient morbidity. However, the mechanism behind these problems is poorly understood and whether the physical properties of the stent play a role is still undetermined.[11]

The modern stents are commonly composed of synthetic polymeric compounds including polyurethane, silicone, Silitek® (ACMI, Southborough, Mass), C-Flex® (Consolidated Polymer Technologies, Clearwater, FL), Percuflex® (Microvasive Urology/Boston Scientific, Natick, MA), Tecoflex® (ACMI), and metals.[12]

C-Flex is a silicone-modified styrene/ethylene/butylene block thermoplastic copolymer. Silitek is a second-generation proprietary polyester copolymer that followed silicone and polyurethane. Percuflex is a proprietary olefinic block copolymer, which becomes soft and flexible at body

temperature, as well has great memory and strength. Various types of ureteral stents were developed to provide all the properties of strength, flexibility, low surface friction, radiopacity, biodurability, biocompatibility, and reasonable unit cost.[13] However, standardized testing of these materials has not been achieved, which creates difficulty when comparing the different types of stents. Hendlin et al. evaluated coil strength before and after urine exposure and the stiffness of commercially available double-J ureteral stents.[14] Twelve available 6F ureteral stents were tested for coil strength, and ten different stents were tested for tensile strength. A significant variability was found among the same type of stents from different lots with regard to stent stiffness.

Generally, it is perceived that polymers that are soft are better tolerated by patients. There are some data assessing the impact of stent composition on the degree of stent-related symptoms. Bregg and Riehle found no association between the degree of symptoms and stent composition, style, and length in 50 patients who had ureteral stents inserted for shock wave lithotripsy (SWL).[15] Pryor et al. compared four types of stents on 74 patients, which showed no difference in the incidence and severity of irritative symptoms among the different stent types.[16] The only prospective randomized study by Lennon comparing "firm" and "soft" ureteric stents demonstrated a higher incidence of renal pain, suprapubic pain, and dysuria with a firm stent.[17] However, Joshi et al. showed no difference in quality of life in their prospective randomized study between ureteral stents composed of firm or soft polymers in 130 patients.[18]

Metallic biomaterials for ureteral stents were introduced by Gort et al. for managing a ureteroileal stricture.[19] Metal stents were developed for long-term use in malignant extrinsic/intrinsic obstruction and strictures where encrustation and infection were a constant problem. Metallic stents are currently composed of superalloy titanium or nickel/titanium mixed alloys.[20] The alloy of nickel and titanium (nitonol) stent, the Memokath 051, has a special "shape memory" feature that allows it to soften at <10°C but regains its original shape when re-warmed to 55°C. This feature makes the stent easier to insert and remove, unlike the meshed counterparts. All the meshed stents allow urothelial ingrowth and would be incorporated into the wall of the ureter, leading to occlusion of the stent within weeks due to endothelial hyperplasia.[21]

A novel concept of using biodegradable materials for ureteral stents intended for short-term use has been introduced. The discomfort of stent-related symptoms and retrieval by endoscopy would be minimized by developing a material that would undergo a dissolution process followed by spontaneous expulsion. The most common materials used in biodegradable stents are high molecular weight polymers of polyactic and poly-L-glycolic acid. Lingeman et al. conducted a phase II clinical trial using a proprietary temporary ureteral drainage stent (TUDS, Microvasive/Boston Scientific) in 87 patients after uncomplicated ureteroscopy.[22] Stents maintained adequate positioning successfully for at least 48 h in 81% of patients. Eight patients had previous experience with a traditional stent in a prior procedure and were given questionnaires comparing the comfort levels of the standard and temporary stents. Traditional stents received a higher discomfort score than the temporary stents: 4.4 versus 7.4; scale 1 (extremely uncomfortable) to 10 (very comfortable). The issue needing further research is the variability in degradation times of these stents. In this study, three patients of 87 had retained fragments longer than 3 months, necessitating ancillary procedures such as SWL or ureteroscopy.

46.3.2 Stent Design

Finney developed the well-known double-J stent in 1978, and this design represents the original silicone closed-tipped stent.[1] Various stent manufacturers produce a basic double-J stent; however, designs and compositions differ with claims of better drainage, improved extraluminal flow, or less irritative symptoms, and reduced encrustation and infection. There are numerous novel stent designs that have been developed over the years, each of which is discussed as follows.

46.3.2.1 Grooved Stents

Grooved stents were developed to improve extraluminal flow in cases of post-lithotripsy or holmium laser fragmentation by incorporating grooves spiraling down the exterior length of the stent. Two examples of such stents are the Towers peripheral stent by Cook Urological and the Lithostent (ACMI).

46.3.2.2 Spiral Stents

The challenge of chronic ureteral obstruction due to tumor compression is achieving adequate internal drainage for the urinary tract. Spiral stents were developed using polyurethane with a built-in metal spiral wire to maintain patency. Tschada et al. developed the first spiral-reinforced ureteral stent and reported their initial clinical experience in 14 patients with chronic ureteral obstruction.[23] Stoller et al. assessed the flow through and around spiral stents with metal wire ridges on the exterior and smooth-walled double-J stents in an in vitro mechanical ureteral model and found that spiral-ridged JJ stents provided substantially greater flow along with markedly increased extraluminal flow.[24] The 7F spiral-ridged stents demonstrated greater drainage both around the stent and through the ureter compared with standard stents with the same diameter.

46.3.2.3 Meshed Stents

To overcome this issue of irritative symptoms that plague the patient with a stent and preserve adequate urinary drainage, the lightweight, self-expanding mesh stent was developed. Olweny et al. found that the flow rates through mesh stents were greater than standard stents at both 1 and 6 weeks in a porcine model.[25] However, the inflammation along the urinary tract was not significantly different between the two stents when blinded histopathologic analysis was performed on kidneys, ureters, and bladder.

46.3.2.4 Tail Stents

The design of the Tail® stent (Microvasive Urology/Boston Scientific) is similar to the standard pigtail stent with a 6F or 7F shaft that tapers to 3F closed tip tail at the distal end. The theory in developing this stent design was to reduce stent-related bladder irritability. Two randomized clinical studies have assessed the Tail stent in comparison to other drainage devices in regards to symptoms. Dunn et al. performed a randomized single-blinded trial comparing Tail stents to the standard 7F double-J stent in 60 patients.[26] Tail stents produced significantly fewer irritative voiding symptoms.

46.3.2.5 Dual-Durometer Stents

Dual-durometer stents are constructed of two different biomaterials. At the renal end, the stent is composed of a firm biomaterial that transitions to a soft biomaterial at the bladder end, which is believed to be better tolerated than harder stents.[11] The firm biomaterial at the renal end facilitates stent placement and reduces stent migration. Two stents developed with this design are the Sof-Curl (ACMI) and the Polaris (Microvasive Urology/Boston Scientific).

46.3.2.6 Magnetic-Tipped Stents

Retrieval of stents can be troublesome for most patients since it entails another endoscopic procedure if the stent is not tethered. Cost increases significantly when the additional procedure of removing the stent is necessary. Netto et al. determined the average cost per patient undergoing uncomplicated ureteroscopy without a stent was $1,830.89.[27] The cost increased to $2,445.31 in patients who underwent stent placement with a suture for self-removal. When cystoscopy was done for removal of the stent, the cost of ureteroscopy increased to $3,727.82 per patient.

To eliminate the morbidity associated with cystoscopic removal of stents, the magnetic stent, Magnetip (ACMI), was first developed in 1989 by Maculuso et al.[28] Recently, Taylor and McDougall revisited this concept by developing a more powerful rare-earth magnet attached to the retrieval catheter and a stainless steel bead on the stent.[29] The stent was successfully retrieved in 97% of patients with no complications.

46.3.2.7 Other Designs

Specialized stents used for upper tract drainage and ureteric healing after endoureterotomy/endopyelotomy have been developed, and incorporate a tapered diameter and no sideports to prevent ingrowth of the ureteral wall.

Lighted stents have been used for identification of the ureter in laparoscopic/open surgical procedures; i.e., general surgery and gynecology. The application of such stents prevents the iatrogenic ureteric injuries that potentially complicate these procedures.[30]

46.3.3 Stent Coatings

The principle of coating ureteral stents is to (1) prevent or minimize biofilm formation, (2) decrease stent-induced inflammatory reactions, (3) decrease stent-related symptoms to promote comfort in the patient, (4) easy insertion and retrieval, and (5) prevent encrustation deposition on the stent. Existing products do not encompass all of these features, although there has been substantial development in this area.[31–33]

A biofilm is a layer of extracellular matrix, protein, and glycocalyx that forms on the surface of all devices placed in the urinary tract. The biofilm facilitates adherence of bacteria to the stent. Up to 100% of patients with indwelling stents, depending on indwelling period, show ureteral stent colonization.[34] The common pathogens identified are *Escherichia coli* and *Enterococcus* species and to a minor extent, *Staphylococcus* species, *Pseudomonas*, and *Candida*.[34–36]

The most commonly used coating for ureteral stents is hydrogel, which is composed of a hydrophilic polymer that traps water within the polyanionic structure of its surface layers. The added surface water is very effective in reducing the coefficient of friction, which allows improved ease of insertion and increased biocompatibility by minimizing frictional irritation and cell adhesion at the biomaterial–tissue interface.[12]

Newer hydrophilic coatings have been developed such as polyvinylpyrrolidone coating applied to polyurethane.[37] The authors found a decrease in both hydroxyaptite encrustation and adherence of a hydrophobic *Enterococcus faecalis*

isolate in an in vitro model. Another similar coating shown to have less encrustation and colonization by bacterial biofilm is the phosphorylchorine group.[38] These novel coatings show promise in reducing the morbidity associated with infected and encrusted stents.

Heparin-coated stents/prostheses have been adopted from interventional cardiology to prevent biomaterial encrustation. Ureteral stents coated with heparin-like polysaccharides did not show any biofilm formation or encrustation after 6 weeks.[39]

Coating stents with oxalate-degrading enzymes derived from *Oxalobacter formigenes* have been evaluated by Watterson et al. in a rabbit implantation model.[40] The authors found less encrustation on enzyme-coated silicone disks compared to control disks after 30 days implantation in an infected rabbit bladder model.

A new strategy to improve the surface properties of ureteral stents incorporates plasma-deposited diamond-like amorphous carbon coatings (DLC) to decrease the formation of crystalline bacterial biofilm and stent-related side effects.[41] DLC is a thermodynamically meta-stable state of carbon with both diamond-like and graphite-like bonds and has exceptional biocompatibility. The advantages of this coating are the potential for reduced encrustation and less patient morbidity. DLC can be used to coat virtually any surface, and further investigation is warranted.

46.4 Indications

The indications for ureteral stent placement are constantly evolving with new trials evaluating specific circumstances. However, there are absolute indications for stent insertion which include relief of obstructed pyelonephritis, bilateral ureteral obstruction, obstruction of solitary functioning kidney, ureteric injuries (perforation/transection, avulsion or after repair) and post-treatment of urolithiasis (SWL or ureteroscopy) in patients with solitary kidney.

Relative indications include the relief of pain associated with ureteral obstruction and for relief of renal colic during pregnancy, significant ureteral edema evident at completion of ureteroscopy, or high expectancy of ureteral obstruction and pre-SWL to prevent ureteral obstruction from stone fragments.

There is increasing evidence supporting the idea that routine stent placement after uncomplicated ureteroscopy is unnecessary.[27,42–50] Routine stenting after ureteroscopy was commonplace since stones in the ureter can cause significant edema or mucosal inflammation at the location of a stone. Stents can prevent the expected edema-induced ureteral obstruction from the stone or instrumentation with balloon dilation. Balloon dilation of the ureter causes persistent edema and upper tract obstruction up to 96 h, as demonstrated in animal models. This section will delineate the use of stents in special circumstances and the controversies surrounding them.

46.4.1 Stent Use in SWL

The routine practice of placing ureteral stents before shock wave lithotripsy (SWL) for stones larger than 10 mm remains commonplace. The advantage of their placement would be to prevent obstruction from stone fragments that would potentially lead to pain and/or infection. The European Association of Urology (EAU) urolithiasis working party recommended the placement of a stent prior to SWL with stones >20 mm in diameter to obviate the possible obstruction by steinstrasse (street of stone).[51]

Stent placement accompanying SWL remains controversial with proponents advocating decreased complication rates in stented patients[52–54] while others found no difference.[55,56]

Al-Awadhi et al. advocated for beneficial effects of pre-SWL stenting in a study of 400 patients with a stone between 1.5 cm and 3.5 cm.[53] Patients were randomized to receive a stent or no stent and assessed for the rate of steinstrasse (13%) compared to the stented group (6%). In contrast, Preminger et al. and Bierkens et al. found no difference in the rate of steinstrasse following SWL in either stented or nonstented patients.[55,56]

Decreased stone-free rates for patients with stents undergoing SWL are debatable as well. Ryan et al. proposed in an experimental study that ureteral stents impair ureteral peristalsis, which impedes stone clearance.[56] This theory is further supported by Abdel-Khalek et al. study of 938 ureteral stones treated with in situ SWL.[57] The authors demonstrated a significant decrease in the stone-free rate in patients who had pre-SWL stenting. However, other studies comparing stented and nonstented patients for SWL showed no difference in stone-free rates.[59,60]

In situ SWL without stenting for obstructing ureteral stones has become an attractive treatment option. Several studies have demonstrated equivalent or better clearance rates in nonstented patients without stent-related morbidities.[61] Even moderately or severely obstructed urinary tracts with stones 2 cm or smaller can be managed without stenting and in situ-SWL, as demonstrated by El-Assmy et al. in a prospective randomized clinical trial. There was no statistical difference in re-treatment rate, flank pain, or temperature in 164 patients who were randomized to have a stent prior to shock wave lithotripsy and no stent for ureteral stone causing moderate or severe hydronephrosis.[62]

46.4.2 Stents for Drainage

One of the more urgent complications of calculus disease is obstructive pyelonephritis. It is a serious indication for ureteral stenting to avoid risk of renal loss and high mortality rate. The need for emergency decompression of the collecting system can be managed by ureteral stenting or percutaneous nephrostomy (PCN). However, the most efficient drainage method to relieve obstruction and drain infected urine is controversial.

Advocates of percutaneous drainage of the obstructed infected kidney propose several advantages over ureteral stent placement in that the larger external tube is suitable for monitoring urine output and avoids manipulation of the obstructed ureter that potentially can perforate, exacerbating the infection.[63,64] Another advantage is the procedure can be done under local anesthesia in an interventional radiology suite.

Proponents of ureteral stent placement cite greater patient comfort with an indwelling stent compared to the bothersome external tube of the nephrostomy. Mokhamalji et al. supported the opinion that PCN was superior to ureteral stents for drainage of hydronephrosis caused by stones.[65] A prospective randomized trial compared successful completion of procedure, X-ray exposure, analgesic requirement, and quality of life between patients with PCN and ureteral stents. The PCN group had a higher success rate for completion of procedure and shorter X-ray exposure. The stented group required more frequent analgesia and had more pronounced deterioration in quality of life. Only 80% of patients were stented successfully in the second group.

A randomized comparison to determine the optimal method of urgent decompression of the collecting system for obstruction and infection due to ureteral calculi by Pearle et al. noted that neither modality, PCN, or ureteral stent was superior in promoting more rapid recovery after drainage.[66] The authors demonstrated a higher cost value for ureteral stent placement (US $2,400 versus $1,110 for PCN), which is attributed to the general anesthesia and operating room costs. According to the findings, the authors suggested the choice of drainage procedure can be individualized according to the patient, institutional characteristics, and surgeon preference.

46.4.3 Stents Post-ureteroscopy

The standard of care has been to routinely place a ureteral stent following ureteroscopy to prevent the potential ureteral obstruction from stone fragments and edema or mucosal inflammation caused by the stone and instrumentation. Although stents have several possible advantages, they may be associated with significant morbidity. Several studies have questioned the routine practice of ureteral stent placement in uncomplicated ureteroscopy and assessed the related morbidities to the patient.

Two recent meta-analyses have addressed the issue whether the presence or absence of a stent is associated with postoperative complications after ureteroscopy.[67,68] Nabi et al. reviewed nine randomized controlled prospective trials with 831 participants to investigate the potential beneficial and adverse effects of routine ureteric stent placement after ureterscopy.[67] Outcome measures of interest were pain rated by patients on a validated scale, need for analgesia, lower urinary tract symptoms, unplanned medical visits or admission to hospital, complications related to the stent (e.g., migration, encrustation, fragmentation, ureteric erosion, and fistulas), return to normal physical activities, participants' satisfaction, health economics, and health-related quality of life. These trials were conducted in eight countries and published between 2001 and 2004. Seven studies had varying stone location, and most ureteroscopies were done on outpatient basis. There was heterogeneity in the trials in regards to ureteroscope sizes, intracorporeal lithotripsy devices, postoperative analgesia, and outcome assessment and reporting.

The authors' principal findings were that stenting after ureteroscopy is associated with increased lower urinary tract symptoms such as dysuria, frequency, or urgency. Unplanned medical visits and admissions to hospital were more common in the group without stents, though the difference was not significant. There was no significant difference between the groups with and without stents in the postoperative analgesic requirement, urinary tract infection, stone clearance rates, and ureteric stricture formation. They could not ascertain whether there was a difference in postoperative pain between the two groups since there were few studies reporting this.

These studies debate the necessity of stenting after ureteroscopy, the controversy continues until there is standardization in measurement outcomes and reporting methods. Also, the lack of a clear definition of uncomplicated ureteroscopy creates difficulty in distinguishing the appropriate setting for not placing a ureteral stent. Objective criteria to substantiate the edema after ureteroscopy are unavailable. Denstedt et al. have suggested that free flow of contrast into the bladder on retrograde pyelography will rule out any edema or perforation that would necessitate ureteral stent placement.[70]

Makarov et al. identified ten randomized trials with a total of 891 patients that examined the postoperative complications after ureteroscopy with and without stent placement.[69] The authors found a 4% lower occurrence of urologic complications in patients undergoing ureteral stent placement after ureteroscopy; however, this was not statistically significant due to the heterogeneity of the data.

A common problem for the two meta-analyses was the undefined term of "uncomplicated" ureteroscopy. There are no clear criteria to date that identify the suitable candidate for stentless ureteroscopy. Hollenbeck et al. retrospectively evaluated the clinical characteristics affecting postoperative morbidity in 219 unstented patients.[70] The authors found several factors including renal pelvic location, lithotripsy, bilateral procedures, history of urolithiasis, diabetes mellitus, recurrent/recent infection, operative time 45 min or greater plus lithotripsy or with ureteral dilation. This study creates a platform for future prospective trails to validate a suitable criteria for selection of patients for stentless ureteroscopy.

There still remains absolute indications for stent placement after ureteroscopy for stone extraction that include a history of renal failure, a solitary kidney, a transplant kidney, and a significant perforation or injury to the ureter during a procedure. Relative indications are significant ureteral edema at the completion of ureteroscopy, pregnancy, initial stone burden greater than 2 cm, a long-standing impacted stone, high-grade preoperative obstruction, balloon dilation of distal ureter, recent history of urinary tract infection or sepsis, and any patient with imminent postoperative travel plans.[70]

46.5 Complications

Although the ureteral stent has numerous advantages, it is not void of considerable morbidity to the patient. Major complications include infection, pyelonephritis, stent fracture, ureteral erosion, fistulas, hematuria, encrustation, flank pain, irritative voiding symptoms, suprapubic pain, and migration.[27,42–50] Up to 90% of patients will experience troublesome voiding symptoms related to the indwelling stent.[27,42–50] Several randomized studies demonstrated significantly more postoperative flank pain, bladder pain, lower urinary tract symptoms, and overall pain in the stented patients compared to nonstented patients following ureteroscopy.

The quality of life of stented patients is significantly affected by the indwelling ureteral stent. Joshi et al. developed and validated the Ureteral Stent Symptom Questionnaire consisting of 48 items and examines six criteria: pain, voiding symptoms, work performance, sexual health, overall general health, and additional problems. The authors demonstrated that 76% of patients had urinary symptoms, 70% had pain severe enough to require significant analgesics, 42% of patients had to reduce their activities by 50%, and patients felt less healthy in general.[72,73]

The stent-related symptoms have not been attributed to any certain factor such as stent characteristics or insertion techniques and positioning of the proximal and distal ends of the double-J stents.[74–76] However, Al-Kandari et al. demonstrated that the longer stents significantly caused more urgency and dysuria, so placing the correct length is essential[77]

To address the irritative bladder pain induced by ureteral stents, research has gone into instillation of intravesical drugs or intravesical submucosal injections. Beiko et al. assessed the safety and efficacy of intravesical instillation of oxybutynin, alkalinized lidocaine, or ketorolac compared to control solution of normal saline for ureteral stent symptoms.[77] These drugs were instilled immediately after insertion of stents in 42 patients who were randomized into four groups. Ketorolac appeared to be the most effective intravesical agent in reducing discomfort and could be further used as an agent that can be loaded on to ureteral stents. A recent randomized controlled study suggested that stent symptoms may be minimized by intravesical submucosal injection of ropivacaine before ureteroscopy in 22 patients requiring stents.[78] This novel idea was inspired by recent application of botulinum toxin to improve voiding dysfunction via cystoscopic intravesical injection.

The "forgotten" encrusted stent can be a challenge for the most skillful endourologist. Large stone formation around the stent can require a combination of approaches via percutaneous or ureteroscopic route. The dilemma is tackling this problem appropriately and not causing further damage such as breakage of the stent along with ureteral injury or ureteral avulsion. Some patients may need multiple procedures including SWL, ureteroscopy with or without laser lithotripsy, PCNL, and cystolitholapaxy.[79–81]

Usually encrustations associated with retained stents are only seen after 3 months of indwelling time.[82] Risk factors for an encrusted ureteral stent include long indwelling times, poor compliance, sepsis, pyelonephritis, chronic renal failure, recurrent or residual stones, lithogenic history, metabolic abnormalities, congenital renal anomalies, and malignant ureteral obstruction with associated chemotherapy and hyperuricosuria.[83]

The management costs of a "forgotten" stent are considerable and can be easily prevented by accurate tracking and recall of these devices. Recently, computerized stent monitoring software systems have been made to alert urologists when the stent is due for removal. McCahy and Ramsden reported a reduction in late stent removal from 3.6 to 1.1%.[84] Ather et al. had similar results with their computer database, which resulted in reduced rate of overdue stents from 12.5 to 1.2%.[85] Lynch et al. developed and implemented an electronic stent register (ESR) and a stent extraction reminder facility (SEFR) at St. Georges Hospital, UK.[86] The program utilized bar-code technology for stent registration and e-mail notification to the urologist when the maximum stent life (MSL) has been reached. In 251 stents recorded, 49% were removed after the intended removal date although it was before the date considered to be overdue (>4 weeks).

46.6 Recent Advances

The recent advances in ureteral stent biomaterial, design, and coating will be discussed in detail in this section.

46.6.1 Drug-Eluting Stents

The concept of incorporating stents with pharmacological agents that are released continuously was started in the field of cardiology using paclitaxel and sirolimus to reduce restenosis rates after angioplasty and stent insertion.[87,88] This principle was applied to ureteral stents using paclitaxel in the hope of reducing the hyperplastic reaction of the urothelium. Liatsikos et al. reported favorable results in paclitaxel-eluting stents in the ureter of a porcine model.[88] The stent demonstrated a mild inflammatory reaction without hindering ureteral patency compared to bare metal stents that caused more hyperplastic reaction.

Stents could be loaded with various active compounds such as antibiotics, analgesics, antispasmodics, or agents to reduce patients' symptoms.

Another recent development in combating stent encrustation and infection is the triclosan-loaded Triumph stent, an antimicrobial commonly found in antibacterial soaps, toothpastes, and plastic products. Cadieux et al. demonstrated significant decrease in *Proteus mirabilis* growth and survival in rabbit urinary tract infection model compared to those in controls.[90] A clinical trial using triclosan-eluting stents in patients requiring long-term stents has been completed, and further evaluation of this stent for short-term use is ongoing at the authors' institution. There is research being conducted into loading stents with analgesics such as Toradol and lidocaine to reduce the irritative symptoms related to stents.

46.6.2 Tissue-Engineered Stents

Although tissue-engineered stents is in its infancy, it has great potential to improve the biomaterials of ureteral stents. The main advantage of such a biomaterial is its excellent biocompatibility with ureteral tissue. Amiel et al. successfully created cartilaginous stents in vitro and in vivo using chondroyte-seeded polymer matrices.[91]

46.7 Conclusions

Further research and newer technology will allow refinements to the biomaterials for ureteral stents and improvements to its design. The ideal stent is still to be developed and efforts in this field are continuing toward this goal. Novel concepts have been developed although they are being further evaluated to implement them in the clinical setting.

References

1. Finney RP. Experience with new double J ureteral catheter stent. *J Urol.* 1978;120:678-681.
2. Montie JE, Stewart BH, Levin HS. Intravasal stents for vasovasostomy in canine subjects. *Fertil Steril.* 1973;24:877-883.
3. Bitschay J, Brodny ML. *A History of Urology in Egypt.* New York: Riverside Press; 1956:76.
4. Herman JR. *Urology: A View Through the Retrospectroscope.* Hagerstown, MD: Harper and Row; 1973.
5. Tulloch WS. Restoration of continuity of the ureter by means of a polyethylene tubing. *Br J Urol.* 1952;24:42-45.
6. Herdman JP. Polyethylene tubing in the experimental surgery of the ureter. *Br J Surg.* 1949;37:105-106.
7. Gibbons RP, Mason JT, Correa RJ Jr. Experience with indwelling silicone rubber ureteral catheters. *J Urol.* 1974;111:594-599.
8. Zimskind PD, Kelter TR, Wilkerson SL. Clinical use of long-term indwelling silicone rubber ureteral splints inserted cystoscopically. *J Urol.* 1967;97:840-844.
9. Chew B, Knudsen BE, Denstedt JD. The use of stents in contemporary urology. *Curr Opin Urol.* 2004; 14(2):111-115. (Review).
10. Mardis HK, Kroeger RM, Morton JJ, et al. Comparative evaluation of materials used for internal ureteral stents. *J Endourol.* 1993;7:105-115.
11. Thomas R. Indwelling ureteral stents: impact of material and shape on patient comfort. *J Endourol.* 1993;7:137-140.
12. Watterson JD, Cadieux P, Denstedt JD. Ureteral stents: which, when, and why? *AUA Update Series.* 2002;21(16):122.
13. Mardis HK, Kroeger RM, Hepperlen TW, et al. Polyethylene double-pigtail ureteral stents. *Urol Clin North Am.* 1982;9:95-101.
14. Lam JS, Gupta M. Update on ureteral stents. *Urology.* 2004;64:9-15.
15. Hendlin K, Dockendorf K, Horn C, et al. Ureteral stents: coil strength and durometer. *Urology.* 2006;68:42-45.
16. Bregg K, Riehle RA Jr. Morbidity associated with indwelling internal ureteral stents after shock wave lithotripsy. *J Urol.* 1989;141:510-512.
17. Pryor JL, Langley MJ, Jenkins AD. Comparison of symptom characteristics of indwelling ureteral catheters. *J Urol.* 1991;145:719-722.
18. Lennon GM, Thornhill JA, Sweeney PA, Grainger R, McDermott TE, Butler MR. 'Firm' versus 'soft' double pigtail ureteric stents: a randomised blind comparative trial. *Eur Urol.* 1995;28:1-5.
19. Joshi HB, Chitale SV, Nagarjan M, et al. A prospective randomized single blinded comparison of ureteral stents composed of firm and soft polymer. *J Urol.* 2005;174:2303-2306.
20. Gort HB, Mali WP, van Waes PF, et al. Metallic selfexpandable stenting of a ureteroileal stricture. *AJR Am J Roentgenol.* 1990;155:422-423.
21. Kulkarni RP, Bellamy EA. A new thermo-expandable shape-memory nickel–titanium alloy stent for the management of ureteric strictures. *BJU Int.* 1999;83:755-759.
22. Auge BK, Ferraro RF, Madenjian AR, et al. Evaluation of a dissolvable ureteral drainage stent in a swine model. *J Urol.* 2002;168(2):808-812.
23. Tschada RK, Henkel TO, Junemann KP, et al. Spiral-reinforced ureteral stent: an alternative for internal urinary diversion. *J Endourol.* 1994;8:119-123.
24. Stoller ML, Schwartz BF, Frigstad JR, et al. An in vitro assessment of the flow characteristics of spiral-ridged and smooth-walled JJ ureteric stents. *BJU Int.* 2000;85:628-631.
25. Olweny EO, Portis AJ, Sundaram CP, et al. Evaluation of a chronic indwelling prototype mesh ureteral stent in a porcine model. *Urology.* 2000;56:857-862.
26. Dunn MD, Portis AJ, Kahn SA, et al. Clinical effectiveness of new stent design: randomized single-blind comparison of tail and double-pigtail stents. *J Endourol.* 2000;14:195-202.
27. Netto NR Jr, Ikonomidis J, Zillo C. Routine ureteral stenting after ureteroscopy for ureteral lithiasis: is it really necessary? *J Urol.* 2001;166(4):1252-1254.
28. Macaluso JN Jr, Deutsch JS, Goodman JR, et al. The use of Magnetip double-J ureteral stent in urological practice. *J Urol.* 1989;142(3):701-703.
29. Taylor WN, McDougall IT. Minimally invasive ureteral stent retrieval. *J Urol.* 2002;168:2020-2023.
30. Chahin F, Dwivedi AJ, Paramesh A, et al. The implications of lighted ureteral stenting in laparoscopic colectomy. *JSLS.* 2002;6(1):49-52.
31. Beiko DT, Knudsen BE, Watterson JD, Cadieux PA, Reid G, Denstedt JD. Urinary tract biomaterials. *J Urol.* 2004;171:2438-2444.
32. Chew BH, Denstedt JD. Technology inside: novel ureteral stent materials and designs. *Nat Clin Pract Urol.* 2004;1:44-48.
33. Tolley D. Ureteric stents, far from ideal. *Lancet.* 2000;356:872-873.
34. Paick SH, Park HK, OH SJ, Kim HH. Characteristics of bacterial colonization and urinary tract infection after indwelling of double-J ureteral stent. *Urology.* 2003;62:214-217.
35. Shaw GL, Choong SK, Fry C. Encrustation of biomaterials in the urinary tract. *Urol Res.* 2005;33:17-22.
36. Keane PF, Bonner MC, Johnston SR, Zafar A, Gorman SP. Characterization of biofilm and encrustation on ureteric stents in vivo. *Br J Urol.* 1994;73:687-691.
37. Tunney MM, Gorman SP. Evaluation of a poly(vinyl pyrrolidone)-coated biomaterial for urological use. *Biomaterials.* 2002;23:4601-4608.
38. Stickler DJ, Evans A, Morris N, et al. Strategies for the control of catheter encrustation. *Int J Antimicrob Agents.* 2002;19:499-506.
39. Riedl CR, Witkowski M, Plas E, Pflueger H. Heparin coating reduces encrustation of ureteral stents: A preliminary report. *Int J Antimicrob Agents.* 2002;19:507-510.
40. Watterson JD, Cadieux PA, Beiko DT, et al. Oxalatedegrading enzymes from Oxalobacter formigenes: a novel device coating to reduce urinary tract biomaterial-related encrustation. *J Endourol.* 2003;17:269-274.
41. Laube N, Klienen L, Bradenahl J, et al. Diamond-like carbon coatings on ureteral stents- a new strategy for decreasing the formation of crystalline bacterial biofilm? *J Urol.* 2007;177:1923-1927.
42. Borboroglu PG, Amling CL, Schenkman NS, et al. Ureteral stenting after ureteroscopy for distal ureteral calculi: a multi-institutional prospective randomized controlled study assessing pain, outcomes and complications. *J Urol.* 2001;166:1651-1657.
43. Byrne RR, Auge BK, Kourambas J, Munver R, Delvecchio F, Preminger GM. Routine ureteral stenting is not necessary after ureteroscopy and ureteropyeloscopy: a randomized trial. *J Endourol.* 2002;16:9-13.
44. Chen YT, Chen J, Wong WY, Yang SS, Hsieh CH, Wang CC. Is ureteral stenting necessary after uncomplicated ureteroscopic lithotripsy? A prospective, randomized controlled trial. *J Urol.* 2002;167:1977-1980.
45. Cheung MC, Lee F, Leung YL, Wong BB, Tam PC. A prospective randomized controlled trial on ureteral stenting after ureteroscopic holmium laser lithotripsy. *J Urol.* 2003;169:1257-1260.
46. Damiano R, Autorino R, Esposito C, et al. Stent positioning after ureteroscopy for urinary calculi: the question is still open. *Eur Urol.* 2004;46:381-387.
47. Denstedt JD, Wollin TA, Sofer M, Nott L, Weir M, D'A Honey RJ. A prospective randomized controlled trial comparing nonstented versus stented ureteroscopic lithotripsy. *J Urol.* 2001;165:1419-1422.
48. Jeong H, Kwak C, Lee SE. Ureteric stenting after ureteroscopyfor ureteric stones: a prospective randomized study assessing symptoms and complications. *BJU Int.* 2004;93:1032-1035.
49. Netto NR Jr, Ikonomidis J and Zillo C. Routine ureteral stenting after ureteroscopy for ureteral lithiasis: is it really necessary? J Urol. 2001;166:1252.

50. Srivastava A, Gupta R, Kumar A, Kapoor R, Mandhani A. Routine stenting after ureteroscopy for distal ureteral calculi is unnecessary: results of a randomized controlled trial. *J Endourol.* 2003; 17:871-874.

51. EAU guidelines for urolithiasis, Preminger GM, Tiselius HG, Assimos DG, et al. 2007

52. Libby JM, Meacham RB, Griffith DP. The role of silicone ureteral stents in extracorporeal shock wave lithotripsy of large renal calculi. *J Urol.* 1988;139:15-17.

53. Sulaiman MN, Buchholz NP, Clark PB. The role of ureteral stent placement in the prevention of steinstrasse. *J Endourol.* 1999;13: 151-155.

54. Al-Awadhi KA, Abdul HH, Kehnide EO, AL Tawheed A. Steinstrasse: a comparison of incidence with and without J stenting and the effect of stenting on subsequent management. *BJU Int.* 1999;84:618-621.

55. Bierkens AF, Hendriz AJ, Lemmens WA, Debruyne FM. Extracorporeal shock wave lithotripsy for large renal calculi: the tole of ureteral stents. A randomized trial. *J Urol.* 1991;145(4): 699-702.

56. Preminger GM, Kettelhut MC, Elkins SL, et al. Ureteral stenting during extracorporeal shock wave lithotripsy: help or hinderance? *J Urol.* 1989;142:32-36.

57. Ryan PC, Lennon GM, Melean PA, Fitzpatrick JM. The effects of acute and chronic JJ stnet placement on uppper urinary tract motility and calculus transit. *Br J Urol.* 1994;74:434-439.

58. Abdel-Khalek M, Sheir KZ, Elsobky E, Showkey S, Kenawy M. Prognostic factors for extracorporeal shock-wave lithotripsy of ureteric stones: a multivariate analysis study. *Scand J Urol Nephrol.* 2003;37:413-418.

59. Mobley TB, Myers DA, Jenkins JM, Grine WB, Jordan WR. Effects of stents on lithotripsy of ureteral calculi: treatment results with 18, 825 calculi using the Lithostar lithotripter. *J Urol.* 1994;152:66-70.

60. Nakada SY, Pearle MS, Soble JJ, Gardner SM, McClennan BL, Claymen RV. Extracorporeal shock wave lithotripsy of middle ureteral stones: are ureteral stents necessary? *Urology.* 1995;46:649-652.

61. Cass AS. Ureteral stenting with extracorporeal shock-wave lithotripsy. *Urology.* 1992;39:446-448.

62. El-Assamy A, El-Nahas AR, Sheir KZ. Is pre-shock wave lithotripsy stenting necessary for ureteral stones with moderayte or severe hydronephrosis? *J Urol.* 2006;176:2059-2062.

63. Joshi HB, Obadeyi OO, Rao PN. A comparative analysis of nephrostomy, JJ stent and urgent in situ extracorporeal shock wave lithotripsy for obstructing ureteric stones. *BJU Int.* 1999;84:264-269.

64. St Lezin M, Hofmann R, Stoller ML. Pyonephrosis: diagnosis and treatment. *BJU Int.* 1992;70:360-366.

65. Zagoria R. In the management of a patient with non-malignant obstructive uropathy and known infection, isn't it safer and more prudent to attempt retrograde placement of a ureteral stent before percutaneous nephrostomy? *AJR Am J Roentgenol.* 1997;168:1616.

66. Mokhmalji H, Braun PM, Martinez Portillo FJ, Siegsmund M, Alken P, Kohrmann KU. Percutaneous nephrostomy versus ureteral stents for diversion of hydronephrosis casued by stones: a prospective, randomized clinical trial. *J Urol.* 2001;165:1088-1099.

67. Pearle MS, Pierce HI, Miller GL, et al. Optimal method of urgent decompression of the collecting system for obstruction and infection due to ureteral calculi. *J Urol.* 1998;160:1260-1264.

68. Nabi G, Cook J, N'Dow J, et al. Outcomes of stenting after uncomplicated ureteroscopy: systematic revew and meta-analysis. *BMJ.* 2007;334:572-578.

69. Makarov DV, Tock BJ, Allaf ME, Matlaga BR. The effect of ureteral stent placement on post-ureteroscopy complications: a meta-analysis. *Urology.* 2008;71(5):796-800.

70. Knudsen BE, Beiko DT, Denstedt JD. Stenting after ureteroscopy: pros and cons. *Urol Clin N Am.* 2004;31:173-180.

71. Hollenback BK, Schuster TG, Seifman BD, Faerber GJ, Wolf JS. Identifying patients who are suitable for stentless ureteroscopy following treatment of urolithiasis. *J Urol.* 2003;170:103-106.

72. Joshi HB, Stainthorpe A, MacDonagh RP, et al. Indwelling ureteral stents: evaluation of symptoms, quality of life and utility. *J Urol.* 2003;169:1065-1069.

73. Joshi HB, Newns N, Stainthorpe A, et al. Ureteral stent symptom questionnaire; development and validation of a multidimensional quality of life measure. *J Urol.* 2003;169:1060-1064.

74. candela JV, Bellman GC. Ureteral stents impact of diameter and composition on patient symptoms. *J Endourol.* 1997;11:45-47.

75. Rane P, Saleemi A, Cahill D, et al. Have stent-related symptoms anything to do with placement technique? *J Endourol.* 2001;15: 741-745.

76. Al-Kandari AM, Al-Shaiji TF, Shaaban H, et al. Effects of proximal and distal ends of double-J ureteral stent position on postprandial symptoms and quality of life: a randomized clinical trial. *J Endourol.* 2007;21:698-702.

77. Beiko Dt, Watterson JD, Knudsen BE, et al. Double-blind randomized controlled trial assessing the safety and efficacy of intravesical agents for ureteral stent symptoms after extracorporeal shockwave lithotripsy. *J Endourol.* 2004;18:723-730.

78. Sur RL, Haleblian GE, Cantor DA, Springhart WP, Albala DM, Preminger GM. Efficacy of intravesical ropivacaine injection on urinary symptoms following ureteral stenting: a randomized controlled study. *J Endourol.* 2008;22(3):473-478.

79. Borboroglu PG, Kane CJ. Current mangement of severly encrusted ureteral stents with a large associated stone burden. *J Urol.* 2000; 164:648-650.

80. Lam JS, Gupta M. Tips and tricks for the management of retained ureteral stents. *J Endourol.* 2002;16:733-741.

81. Bultitude MF, Tiptaft RC, Glass JM, Dasgupta P. Management of encrusted ureteral stnets impacted in upper tract. *Urology.* 2003; 62:622-626.

82. Damiano R, Oliva A, Esposito C, De Sio M, Autorino R, D'Armiento M. Early and late complications of double pig-tail ureteral stent. *Urol Int.* 2002;69:136-140.

83. Singh I, Gupta NP, Ak H, Aron M, Seth A, Dogra PN. Severely encrusted polyurethane ureteral stents; management and analysis of potential risk factors. *Urology.* 2001;58:526-531.

84. McCahy PJ, Ramsden PD. A computerized ureteric stent retrieval system. *Br J Urol.* 1996;77:147-148.

85. Ather MH, Talati J, Biyabani R. Physician responsibility for removal of implants: the case for a computerized program for tracking overdue double-J stents. *Tech Urol.* 2000;6:189-192.

86. Lynch MF, Ghani KR, Frost I, et al. Preventing the forgotten ureteric stent: results from Implementation of an electronic stent register. *BJU Int.* 2007;99:245-246.

87. Kastrati A, Mehilli J, von Beckerath N, et al. Sirolimus-eluting stent or paclitaxel eluting stent vs. balloon angioplasty for prevention of recurrences in patients with coronary in-stent restenosis: a randomized trial. *JAMA.* 2005;293:165-171.

88. Grube E, Buellesfeld L. Paclitaxel-eluting stents: current clinical experience. *Am J Cardiovasc Drugs.* 2004;4:355-360.

89. Liatsikos EN, Karnabatidis D, Kagadis GC, et al. Application of paclitaxel-eluting mesh stents within the pig ureter; an experimental study. *Eur Urol.* 2007;51:217-223.

90. Cadieux PA, Chew BH, Knudsen BE, et al. Triclosan loaded ureteral stents decrease Proteus mirabilis 296 infection in a rabbit urinary tract infection model. *J Urol.* 2006;175:2331-2335.

91. Amiel GE, Yoo JJ, Kim BS, et al. Tissue engineered stents created from chondrocytes. *J Urol.* 2001;165:2091-2095.

Flexible Ureterorenoscopy: Tips and Tricks

47

Olivier Traxer

Abstract Flexible ureterorenoscopy is rapidly becoming a major part of the urologist's therapeutic armamentarium. As with any sophisticated new technique, the operator must have a detailed knowledge of the features of the equipment, and perfect control of the instruments used. Over the past 2 decades flexible ureterorenoscopes (F-URS) continue to evolve and improve significantly including F-URS design, deflection capabilities, irrigation flow, imaging equipment, and durability. Due to these recent developments, endourologists have expanded the clinical indications for flexible ureterorenoscopy. The purpose of this chapter is intended to thoroughly familiarize the prospective user with tips and tricks for flexible ureterorenoscopy, step by step, through the setup for the procedure and the handling of the F-URS for the management of calculi, tumors of the upper urinary tract, caliceal diverticuli, and strictures.

47.1 Introduction

Flexible ureterorenoscopy is rapidly becoming a major part of the urologist's therapeutic armamentarium. As with any sophisticated new technique, the operator must have a detailed knowledge of the features of the equipment, and perfect control of the instruments used. Over the past 2 decades flexible ureterorenoscopes (F-URS) continue to evolve and improve significantly including F-URS design, deflection capabilities, irrigation flow, imaging equipment, and durability (Table 47.1). Due to these recent developments, endourologists have expanded the clinical indications for flexible ureterorenoscopy.[3,4,8,11,15,37,38,44,47]

The purpose of this chapter is intended to thoroughly familiarize the prospective user with tips and tricks for flexible ureterorenoscopy, step by step, through the setup for the procedure and the handling of the F-URS for the management of calculi, tumors of the upper urinary tract, caliceal diverticuli, and strictures.[21-23]

47.2 Theater Setup and Patient Positioning

As for all surgical procedures, setup is paramount and encompasses the patient, the equipment (laser, C-arm video tower), and the surgeon. The setup is the responsibility of the surgeon and should not be done by anybody else.

47.2.1 General Layout of the Operating Theater

The patient is usually put in the dorsal lithotomy position and patient's lower legs are bent outward (<90). Pressure points must be protected. The surgeon should stand between the legs of the patient, with his assistant behind him. The anesthetists are at the head of the patient. Intravenous sedation is possible in case of a diagnostic operation. Usually, it is recommended to work under general anesthetic. The urine must be sterile: Urinalysis to rule out a coexisting urinary tract infection (UTI) is an essential part of the preoperative workup. Prophylactic antibiotics should be administered.

Our usual setup (Fig. 47.1a):

- The instrument table (I) is placed under the patient's lower left leg at the same level as the buttocks. This allows the surgeon to align all the instruments and the ureteronoscope level with the patient, without having to involve his or her assistant.
- The endoscopy tower (V) and the fluoroscopy screens (R) are placed on the right of the patient (to the left of the surgeon).
- The screens V and R should be side by side.

O. Traxer (✉)
Department of Urology, Hôpital Tenon, Paris, France
e-mail: olivier.traxer@tnn.aphp.fr

P.N. Rao et al. (eds.), *Urinary Tract Stone Disease*,
DOI 10.1007/978-1-84800-362-0_47, © Springer-Verlag London Limited 2011

Table 47.1 Characteristics of new-generation flexible URS

	Length (cm)	Distal tip diameter (Fr)	Midshaft diameter (Fr)	Proximal Diameter (Fr)	Field of view (°)	Angle of visualization (°)	Working channel (F)	Deflection ventral/dorsal (°)
Olympus URFP5	67	5.9	8	8.9	85	0	3.6	275/180
Karl Storz FLEX-X2	67	6.5	7.5	8.4	88	0	3.6	270/270
WOLF Viper	68	6	7.5	8.8	85	0	3.6	270/270
Gyrus-ACMI DUR8 Elite	64	6.75	8.7–9.4	10.1	80	9	3.6	270/180
Gyrus-ACMI DUR-D	65	8.7	9.3	10.9	80	0	3.6	250/250
Olympus URF-V	67	9	9.5	10.9	85	0	3.6	275/180

- The C-arm control unit (A) is placed on the left of the patient (to the right of the surgeon).
- The X-ray tube is placed underneath the operating table.
- The C-arm, covered by a sterile drape, is placed just above the patient.
- The laser unit (L) is put behind and against the instrument table.

Figure 47.1b and c describes other types of setups.

If the standard setup is not possible due to the layout of the operating theater or due to a lack of space, it is possible to use the control screens V and R on either side of the patient. Or better still on a table above the patient. This allows the surgeon to keep right without moving the trunk.[7]

47.2.2 Position of the Surgeon

It is essential that the surgeon is as comfortable as possible. He can operate standing up or sitting down (Fig. 47.2). If he operates in the standing position, a right-handed surgeon is recommended:

- To keep his back propped up against the patient's right thigh.
- To stand up st458raight and fix the operating table at an appropriate height.
- To keep his elbows near his body.
- To stand less than 50 cm from the pubis.

The control pedals of the Fluroscopy (R) and the Laser (L) are placed under the Surgeon's right foot.[45]

47.2.3 Positioning the Patient in the Lateral Decubitus Position

Positioning the patient in the lateral decubitus position (Fig. 47.3) enables the movement of a stone or its fragments, by making it (them) move from the lower calyx toward the

infundibulum or better still, toward the renal pelvis. If it is the left kidney, the patient is positioned in the right lateral decubitus position. If it is the right kidney, the patient is positioned in the left lateral decubitus position.

47.2.4 Positioning the Patient in the Trendelenburg Position

Positioning the patient in the Trendelenburg position (Fig. 47.4) enables the movement of a lower-pole calculus or its fragments toward the infundibulum, or better still toward the renal pelvis.

47.2.5 Operating Table, Guide Wire, and Laser Unit

The instrument table is placed under the patient's lower left leg at the same level as the buttocks. This allows the surgeon to align all the instruments and the ureterorenoscope level with the patient, without having to involve his or her assistant.

A Safety Guide Wire is recommended for all flexible ureterorenoscopy procedures. It is inserted at the beginning of the operation during the cystoscopy and is secured to the patient's left inner thigh with a clip or sticky tape. It should be coiled (like a "snail") as shown in Fig. 47.5. Figure 47.6 shows the correct and incorrect positioning of the guide wire to the patient's left thigh.

By arranging the security guide wire in this way, the surgeon can prevent it from suddenly moving, particularly if he is using a hydrophilic guide wire.

The laser unit is put behind and against the instrument table (Fig. 47.5). The laser fiber is connected to the laser unit and immediately put down on the instrument table aligned with the laser, the table, and the patient (Fig. 47.5,

Fig. 47.1 (**a**) Our usual setup. (**b**, **c**) Other types of setups. R: X-ray screen. V: video tower. A: C-Arm. L: laser unit

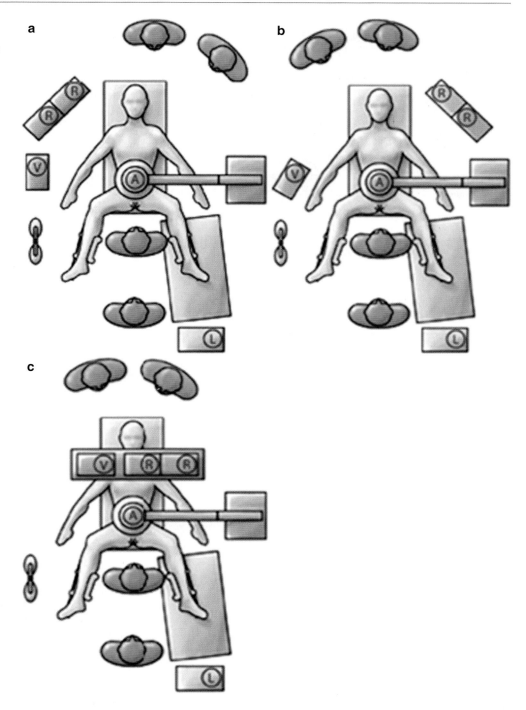

red arrow). It is recommended to fix the fiber to the table with saline-soaked compresses so that it does not fall off the instrument table(Fig. 47.7). The weight of the soaked compresses secures it without damaging it. The laser fiber should "run" freely on the instrument table, maintaining the largest curvatures as possible. Excessive torsion should not be placed on the laser fiber due to the risk of damaging it.

Respecting these two technical points:

- Place the laser unit close behind the instrument table (making contact with it).
- Secure the laser fiber (without pressure) on the instrument table with filled saline compresses.

This allows the surgeon to protect his laser fibers from all external damage. [45,54,55]

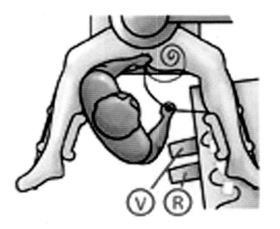

Fig. 47.2 Position of the surgeon. Control pedals of the fluoroscopy (R) and the laser (V) are placed under the surgeon's right foot

47.2.6 Setup of the Operating Area

The use of a sterile drape with irrigation bags allows measurement of the quantity of liquid irrigation during and after the operation. The irrigation bag is connected to a wall pump so that the irrigation liquid cannot accumulate there. To keep everything sealed in the operating area, it is advised to fix the irrigation bag to the end of the instrument table with sticky tape (Fig. 47.8, *red arrow*). To maintain the setup of the operating area, it is recommended never to dispose of items in the irrigation bag (camera, cystoscope, cold-light cable).

Fig. 47.3 Positioning the patient in the lateral decubitus position

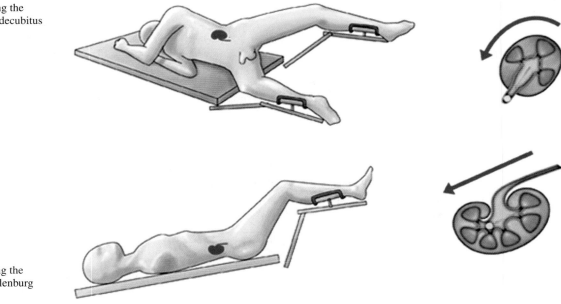

Fig. 47.4 Positioning the patient in the Trendelenburg position

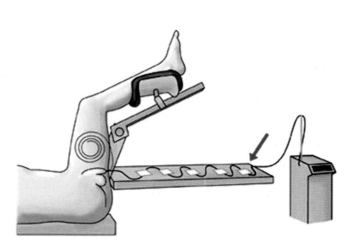

Fig. 47.5 Operating table, guide wire, and laser unit

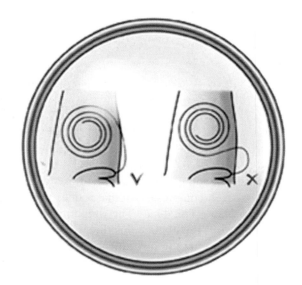

Fig. 47.6 Safety guide wire

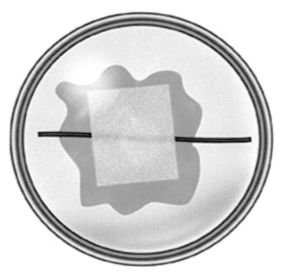

Fig. 47.7 Laser unit and laser fiber fixed with saline-soaked compresses

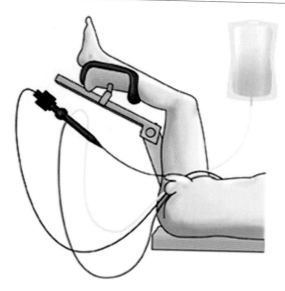

Fig. 47.9 Irrigation tube, light cord, and camera

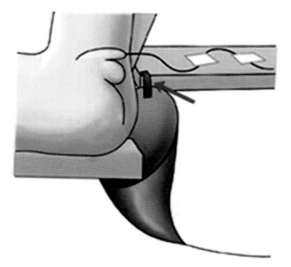

Fig. 47.8 Setup of the operating area

47.2.7 Irrigation Tube, Optic, and Camera

To enable the surgeon to move more freely, it is recommended to pass the cold-light cable, camera, and irrigation tubing together at the level of the fold of the patient's right groin (Fig. 47.9). It is also advisable to leave enough length for the three cords beyond the groin fold, to avoid all traction on the endoscope. The curve of the three wires should be large and untangled.

47.3 Irrigation Techniques

Irrigation still represents a major issue for flexible ureter-orenoscopy. Saline is the standard irrigant used for flexible ureterorenoscopy. In order to have the best visibility possible,

flexible laser ureterorenoscopy requires working with an optimal irrigation output and effective pressure. It is indispensable to know the following figures:[9,54–55]

- A fluid bag placed 60 cm above the patient creates an irrigation flow of 40 mL/min by the working channel free of a ureterorenoscope.
- This flow falls at 4 mL/min if an instrument of 3 Fr is introduced in the working channel, and at 10 mL/min if the instrument measures 2.4 Fr.
- These data show the importance of irrigation, which should not be compromised.

When the flexible ureterorenoscope is positioned in the renal caliceal cavities, the vision is often poor and blurred (blood, urine, contrast). Contrast can be injected through the working channel to opacify the collecting system for fluoroscopic imaging and determination of the position of the F-URS. However, mix irrigants cause distortion of the visual image due to different indices of refraction of irrigants with different densities (i.e., saline and contrast). To improve the initial vision and before starting the exploration of the renal cavities, it is strongly recommended to be patient and wait for the irrigation liquid to "wash" the renal caliceal cavities. It takes a few minutes before the vision improves considerably. If necessary, to speed up the process, a saline injection (syringe) can be used to insert the small amounts of liquid.

The use of a ureteral access sheath (UAS) avoids high intrarenal pressure (>150 cm H_2O) and allows an optimum irrigation of the cavities by draining the irrigation liquid with the stone fragments and the blood clots.

To obtain an optimum irrigation flow at the distal tip of the endoscope and not lose liquid at the point of entry level of the working channel (with the "teats"), it is recommended

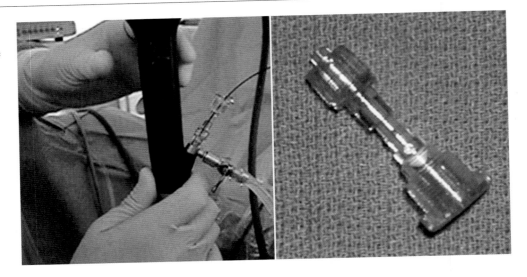

Fig. 47.10 Port seal fitted on the working channel of the flexible URS. The seal allows the operator to conserve irrigant by preventing leaks; to grip an instrument (such as a laser fiber)

to use a specific port seal enabling the use of a liquid irrigation instrument that does not leak. This is made of a silicone O-ring, which can adapt to all diameters of the instruments in the working channel. This ring provides a perfect seal (Fig. 47.10).

47.4 Different Possible Configurations for Irrigation in Flexible Ureterorenoscopy

47.4.1 Hydrostatic Pressure

The simplest way is to position the fluid bag between 60 and 100 cm above the patient (Fig. 47.11).

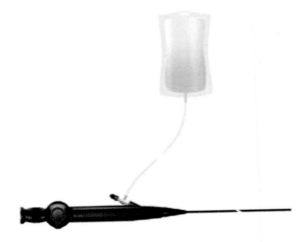

Fig. 47.11 Irrigation: hydrostatic pressure

47.4.2 Manual High Pressure

To increase temporarily the pressure in the renal caliceal cavities, it is possible to ask the theater nurse to apply manual pressure to the drip (Fig. 47.12).

47.4.3 Pressure Cuff

To increase the pressure in the renal caliceal cavities for a continuous period, it is possible to use a pressure cuff placed around the fluid bag (Fig. 47.13). However, in this case, it is difficult to know the exact pressure in the system despite the presence of a pressure gage. We do not recommend this method.

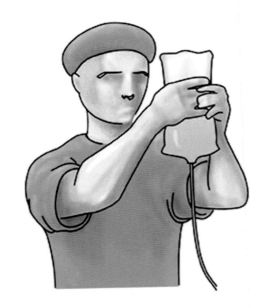

Fig. 47.12 Irrigation: manual high pressure

47.4.4 High Pressure with a Syringe

A very effective way to increase pressure temporarily is to use a connected syringe directly over the working channel of the flexible ureterorenoscope.[42]

- This syringe, controlled by the surgeon or his assistant, can be used in different ways.
- Isolated without a drip (in case of diagnostic flexible ureterorenoscopy) (Fig. 47.14a).
- Isolated without a drip but attached to a seal to allow the insertion of instruments (Fig. 47.14b).
- Linked to a drip. In this case, the syringe is fitted with an anti-reflux valve or a three-way tap, preventing the reflux in the drip (Fig. 47.14c).
- Linked to a drip, anti-reflux valve, and a seal to allow the insertion of instruments. This is the best method (Fig. 47.14d).

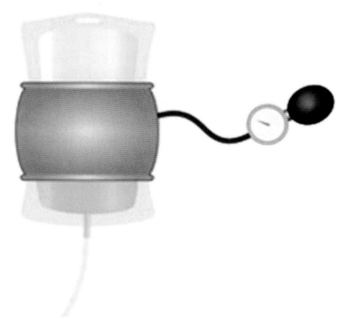

Fig. 47.13 Irrigation: pressure cuff

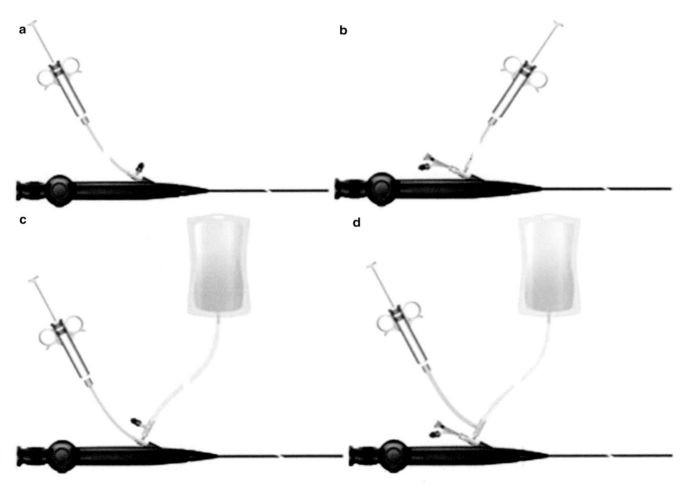

Fig. 47.14 Irrigation: high pressure with a syringe. (**a**) Syringe isolated without a drip. (**b**) Syringe isolated without a drip but attached to a seal to allow the insertion of instruments. (**c**) Syringe linked to a drip. In this case, the syringe is fitted with an anti-reflux valve or a three-way tap, preventing the reflux in the drip. (**d**) Syringe linked to a drip, with anti-reflux valve and a seal to allow the insertion of instruments. This is the best method

47.4.5 Automatic High-Pressure Machine

It is possible to use a more efficient and reliable system: an irrigation pump with a fluid control system (Fig. 47.15). These automatic pumps are programmed to increase the rate of flow in the drip without, importantly, increasing the intrarenal pressure. A control pedal allows temporary increase in pressure (+20 cm H_2O). Although they are expensive, these machines are the best way of achieving ideal perfusion.

47.5 Insertion of the Safety Guide Wire

Guide wires are essential for flexible ureterorenoscopy. Two 150-cm-long and 0.035- or 0.038-in. diameter guide wires (one safety, one working wire) should be used. The distal end (straight or curved) must be flexible and atraumatic. Standard floppy-tipped polytetrafluoroethylene (PTFE) wire could be used, but we strongly recommend using *stiff hydrophilic wires*. A safety wire should always be employed when the intended procedure involves placing and removing and then replacing the F-URS. The safety wire is fixed to the drape and remains in place for later use to replace the working wire or to place a stent at the end of the procedure.[29,39]

The positioning of the safety guide wire is one of the first stages to carry out. Its insertion is carried out during the cystoscopy after the retrograde ureteropyelography. A safety guide wire can be inserted in three different ways.

47.5.1 Use of a Cystoscope

The most simple and economic way is to insert the two guide wires, the safety wire and the working wire, at the beginning of the operation during the cystoscopy (Fig. 47.16). Consequently, the cystoscopy must be carried out twice in order to insert the two guide wires.

47.5.2 Use of a Dual-Lumen Catheter

The use of a dual-lumen catheter avoids one cystoscopy (Fig. 47.17). The dual-lumen catheter is a 10 Fr ureteral catheter with a flexible, atraumatic 6 Fr distal tip. Each lumen accepts a 0.038-in. diameter guide wire. The dual-lumen catheter allows the operator to insert a second guide wire, to inject contrast into the intrarenal collecting system with a

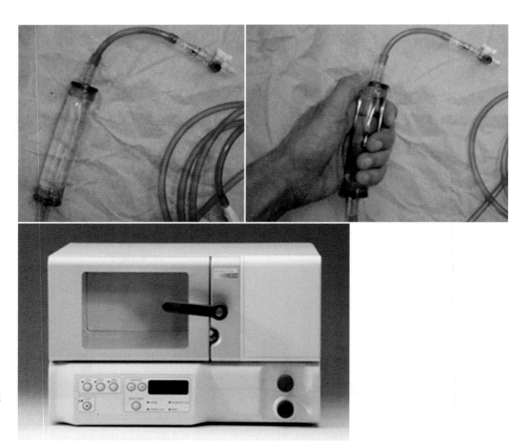

Fig. 47.15 Automatic high-pressure machine: Socomed Promepla. Irrigation tube with hand-assisted device and automated pressure pump

Fig. 47.16 Placement of safety guide wire with a cystoscope

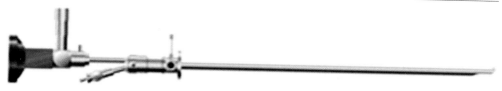

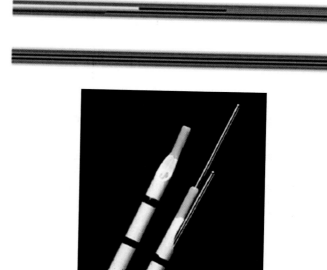

Fig. 47.17 Placement of a safety guide wire with a dual-lumen catheter (Cook Medical)

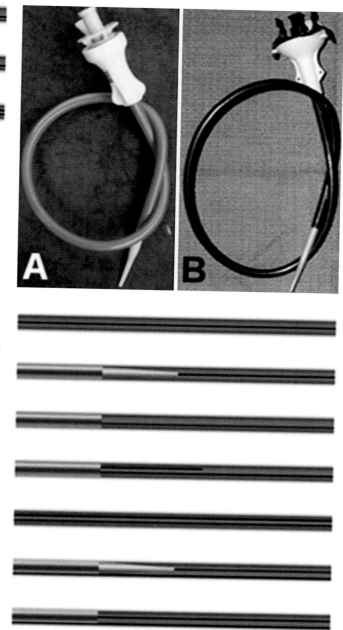

guide wire in situ, and to dilate the ureter in order to facilitate the passage of the flexible ureterorenoscope. After the positioning of the first guide wire during the cystoscopy, the dual-lumen catheter is positioned over the first guide wire as far as the ureter under fluoroscopic guidance or under visual control during cystoscopy. The second guide wire is introduced in the second channel of the dual-lumen catheter. The dual-lumen catheter is withdrawn, leaving in place the two guide wires: the working guide wire and the safety guide wire.

47.5.3 Use of a Ureteral Access Sheath

If the surgeon decides at the beginning of the operation that he/she will use a ureteral access sheath (UAS) (Fig. 47.18), it is possible for him/her to use it to insert the second guide wire (the safety guide wire).

- The first guide wire is inserted during the cystoscopy.
- The UAS is inserted over the first guide wire in the ureter under fluoroscopic control.
- Once in place the self-dilating introducer is withdrawn;

Fig. 47.18 Placement of a safety guide wire with a ureteral access sheath. (**a**) Navigator (Boston Scientific). (**b**) Flexor (Cook Medical)

the UAS and the first guide wire are left in place in the ureter.
- The second wire is introduced through the UAS under fluoroscopic control.

- Once in place, the UAS is withdrawn and the two guide wires are left in place. The security guide wire is fixed to the patient's inner left thigh. The self-dilating introducer is reinserted in the UAS and together they can be put back in place over the second guide wire: "the working guide wire."

47.6 Insertion of the Ureterorenoscope into the Ureteral Meatus

After inserting the two guide wires (the working guide wire and the safety guide wire), if the surgeon does not think it is necessary to use a ureteral access sheath, the insertion of the ureterorenoscope in the renal cavities is carried out according to the following sequence:

- The insertion of the ureterorenoscope in the renal cavities is done over the working guide wire and under fluoroscopic control. The ureterorenoscope is therefore without its cold-light cable, the camera, and irrigation.
- The surgeon must always keep the ureterorenoscope straight by using both hands to fix the distal tip of the ureterorenoscope, and the assistant must hold the handle of the ureterorenoscope.
- The surgeon carefully fits the ureterorenoscope over the guide wire so as not to damage the working channel and then slides the ureterorenoscope over the guide wire.
- In male patients, the penis is held upwards to straighten the ureter.
- The cold-light cable, the camera, and the irrigation are attached to the ureterorenoscope once the scope is inside the collecting system.
- The guide wire is withdrawn and the examination of the renal cavities can begin.

However, it can happen that the ureterorenoscope becomes fixed on the ureteral meatus and it is not possible to pass it (Fig. 47.19). We also see that under fluoroscopic control, the endoscope blocks and bends the ureteral meatus. It is said that the ureterorenoscope does "the big back." This situation occurs frequently when the ureteral meatus is stenosed or pin-point. The first cystoscopy allows evaluation of the appearance of the ureteral meatus. If it does not appear stenosed or pin-point, it is not necessary to dilate it without having first tried the "shoe-horn" technique. In the large majority of cases, this technique enables the ureteral meatus to be successfully negotiated.

To carry out the shoe-horn technique, it is necessary to fully understand what happens: The ureterorenoscope mounted over the working guide wire gets caught on the ureteral meatus. This is linked to the fact that the working channel of the ureterorenoscope is off center towards the lower part of the distal tip (opposite the bundles of optic fibers); it is therefore the top part of the distal tip containing the bundles of optic fibers that becomes caught on the ureteral meatus (Fig. 47.20a).

To resolve this problem, it is necessary to turn the distal tip of the ureterorenoscope 180° so that the top part, containing all the optic fibers, moves towards the bottom. In this position, the guide wire is going to lift the "roof" of the ureteral meatus, which can be flexed to follow the slope of the ureterorenoscope towards the renal caliceal cavities: This maneuver is called the shoe-horn technique (Fig. 47.20b).

To turn the distal tip, the surgeon should ask his assistant to turn the handle of the ureterorenoscope in his hands at least 180°. At the same time, the surgeon continues this rotational movement by also turning the body of the endoscope in his hands by pushing it over the working guide wire to negotiate the ureteral meatus. Sometimes the assistant has to turn the handle more than 360° in order to successfully negotiate the ureteral meatus. This is linked to the torque effect of the ureterorenoscope: A rotation of 180° of the handle enables you

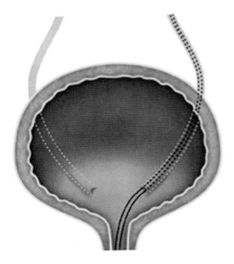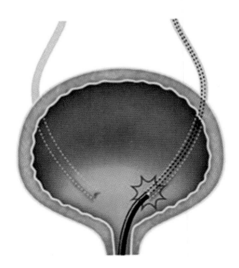

Fig. 47.19 Insertion of the ureterorenoscope into the ureteral meatus: "The Big Back"

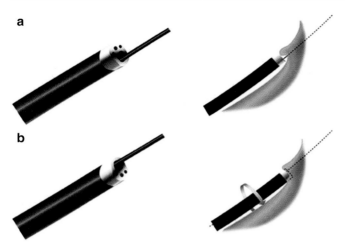

Fig. 47.20 (**a**) Insertion of the ureterorenoscope into the ureteral meatus. (**b**) Insertion of the ureterorenoscope into the ureteral meatus using the "shoe-horn technique"

to obtain a rotation of the distal tip at 180° if the torque effect is 100% (or 1 for 1). A good flexible ureterorenoscope presents a torque effect close to 100%. If the effect is less good, the handle is turned beyond 180° to obtain a 180° rotation of the distal tip. When the ureterorenoscope is caught on the ureteral meatus, the mechanical constraints that are placed on it are very important and profoundly change its natural torque effect. Therefore, the handle sometimes has to be turned beyond 360° to obtain a rotation of 180° of the distal tip.

If the shoe-horn technique fails, it is advisable to dilate the ureter or to insert a ureteral access sheath.

After the placement of the F-URS into the kidney, the intrarenal collecting system is explored, starting with the upper-pole calices, followed by the middle calices, and, finally, the lower-pole calices. The exploration is performed under endoscopic vision and fluoroscopic guidance.[40]

47.7 Insertion of the Ureteral Access Sheath

The insertion of a ureteral access sheath (UAS) is not a mandatory procedure in a flexible ureterorenoscopy. It is left to the surgeon's discretion to perform the procedure, in view of the patient's anatomy, the surgical strategy chosen, and any intraprocedural findings.

47.7.1 Roles and Advantages of the UAS

- It facilitates quick access to the ureter. The ureteral access sheath behaves like the equivalent of an Amplatz sheath for percutaneous kidney surgery, by enabling fast insertion

and removal of the ureterorenoscope from the renal cavities and the ureter.
- It dilates the ureter: the external diameter being at a minimum of 11 Fr.
- It facilitates the collection of fluid irrigation, improving the endoscopic vision.
- It avoids high pressure in the renal cavities.
- It facilitates the clearance of stone fragments.
- It protects the flexible ureterorenoscope.[57]

47.7.2 Insertion of the Ureteral Access Sheath

1. The UAS consists of a sheath and a self-dilating introducer and has a round section; it is reinforced to avoid it folding up and has an entrance that widens to facilitate the introduction of the ureterorenoscope (Fig. 47.21). The usual diameter of the sheath is 11/13 or 12/14 Fr.
2. The self-dilating introducer has a luer-lock tip to inject contrast agent in order to get retrograde imaging of the renal tract (ureteropyelography) without having to remove the UAS. This can prove very useful when the surgeon wants to see the configuration of the ureter (ureteral siphons and stitches) before progressing to the UAS.
3. Insertion of the UAS on the working guide wire under fluoroscopic control.
4. Withdrawal of the self-dilating introducer of the UAS by leaving the working guide wire in place (Fig. 47.22). When the self-dilating introducer is withdrawn, the surgeon must do the following steps:

   (a) Secure the sheath so that it cannot move back when the self-dilating introducer is withdrawn.
   (b) Fix the working guide wire in the access sheath.
   (c) Move the self-dilating introducer back to withdraw it.

To do these three movements with two hands, the surgeon must:

- Hold the working guide wire in his right hand.
- Block the access sheath at the level of the widened entrance with the little finger or the ring finger (fourth finger) of the left hand.
- Move the self-dilating introducer back over the working guide wire between the thumb and the index of his left hand.

After the placement of the F-URS into the kidney, through the UAS, the intrarenal collecting system is explored, starting with the upper-pole calices, followed by the middle calices and, finally, the lower-pole calices. The exploration is performed under endoscopic vision and fluoroscopic guidance.[41]

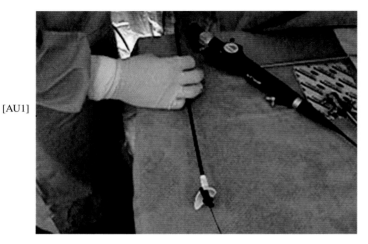

Fig. 47.21 Insertion of ureteral access sheath

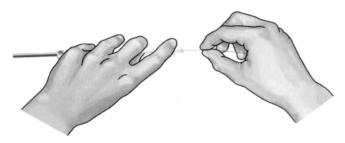

Fig. 47.22 Insertion of ureteral access sheath

47.8 Examination of the Renal Caliceal Cavities

An ureterorenoscope should always be held with two hands and both hands must work together so that the endoscope can move as a unit. There are three basic movements to mobilize a ureterorenoscope in the renal caliceal cavities:[10,12,25]

1. The dominant hand (right) moves in supination or in pronation to change the direction of the distal tip of the endoscope (Fig. 47.23a).
2. The movement of the thumb on the deflection control button enables a downward or upward deflexion of the distal tip of the ureterorenoscope (Fig. 47.23b, *red and green arrows*).
3. The non-dominant hand (left) pushes or withdraws the endoscope to move it forward or backward (Fig. 47.23c).

It is strongly advised against moving the ureterorenoscope by pushing it with the dominant hand, which holds the handle. Effectively, if the surgeon does this, he will see a forced curve of the proximal part of the body of the endoscope, which over time will be a source of damage. The movement forward or backward is therefore done with the non-dominant hand, which holds the body of the endoscope, accompanied by the dominant hand, which holds the handle (the two hands work as a unit).

47.8.1 Neutral Position of the Dominant Hand (Right Hand)

- The handle of the ureterorenoscope must be held with the dominant hand and the deflection control button must be moved by the thumb (neutral position) (Fig. 47.24).
- For a right-handed surgeon, the dominant hand is the right hand.
- The second hand (left hand, non-dominant) stabilizes the body of the endoscope in the ureteral meatus. For male patients, it also supports the penis.
- In this position (neutral position), it is not possible to accurately examine the renal caliceal cavities because the upward or downward deflection movements of the distal tip of the ureterorenoscope will be done in the patient's sagittal plane (anteroposterior). The orientation of the caliceal stems will not be in the sagittal plane but in oblique axis. So to insert a flexible ureterorenoscope in the different caliceal axes, it must be turned by using the dominant hand to move it by pronation-supination.

47.8.2 Examination of Right Renal Caliceal Cavities: Dominant Right Hand in Supination

- The entrances of the calyx groups – upper-pole, middle, and lower-pole calices – are seen on the left of the endoscopy screen.
- To insert the ureterorenoscope in one of three calyx groups, the surgeon must turn his hand in supination and at the same time perform a ventral deflection of the distal tip of the ureterorenoscope to position the chosen calyx entrance (upper-pole, middle, and lower-pole calices) at the center of the endoscopy screen. From then on, the left hand must push the ureterorenoscope so that it penetrates the calyx group (Fig. 47.24).

47.8.3 Examination of Left Renal Caliceal Cavities: Dominant Right Hand in Pronation

- The entrances of the calyx groups – upper-pole, middle, and lower-pole calices – are seen on the right of the endoscopy screen (Fig. 47.24).
- In order to insert the ureterorenoscope in one of three calyx groups, the surgeon must this time turn his hand in pronation and at the same time perform a ventral deflection of the distal tip of the ureterorenoscope to position the chosen

[AU1]

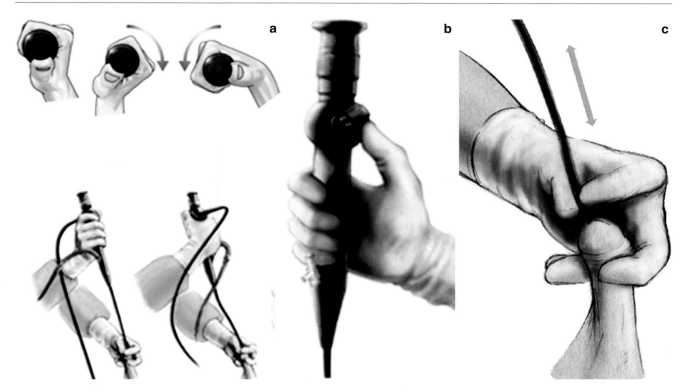

Fig. 47.23 Examination of the renal caliceal cavities. (**a**) The dominant hand (right) moves in supination or in pronation to change the direction of the distal tip of the endoscope. (**b**) The movement of the thumb on the deflection control button enables a downward or upward deflexion of the distal tip of the ureterorenoscope. (**c**) The non-dominant hand (left) pushes or withdraws the endoscope to move it forward or backward

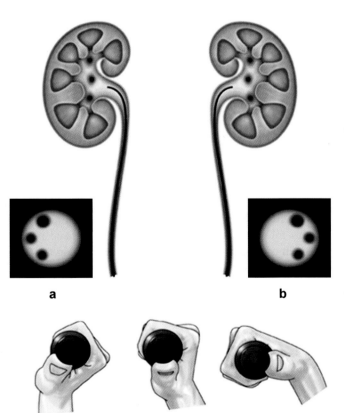

Fig. 47.24 Neutral position of the dominant hand (right hand). (**a**) Right kidney. (**b**) Left kidney

calyx entrance at the center of the endoscopy screen. Again, the left hand must push the body of the endoscope to penetrate the calyx group.[5,50–52,56]

47.9 Ureterorenoscope and Laser: Working Channel, Instrumentation, and Synergy Laser-Ureterorenoscope

All F-URS have a single 3.6 Fr working channel. Instruments can be passed through the working channel, and it is recommended to pass the instrument when the F-URS is straight, otherwise the working channel can be damaged. The working channel is particularly vulnerable to laser fibers, which are stiff with sharp tips. The recommendation is to straighten the tip of the F-URS before inserting a working instrument. When the instrument enters in the field of view, the F-URS could be deflected as necessary. Never force an instrument through the channel of the F-URS. The 3.6 Fr working channel accepts instruments up to 3–3.2 Fr (laser fibers, basket, and graspers). However, because the working channel is used also for irrigation, an instrument in the channel will reduce dramatically the flow rate. Use of smaller (1.5–1.9 Fr) caliber nitinol basket and 200 μ(micro) laser fibers has the least deleterious effects on the flow rate and deflecting capabilities of the F-URS.

The holmium-YAG laser is an indispensable tool for flexible ureterorenoscopy. We strongly advise against entering into a therapeutic flexible ureterorenoscopy procedure (stone or tumor) if the holmium-YAG laser is not available.[35]

47.9.1 The Holmium-YAG Laser

The holmium-YAG laser is a solid-state laser made from a rare element, holmium, and an yttrium-aluminum-garnet (YAG) crystal. It delivers pulsatile energy and operates at a wavelength of 2,100 nm (in the infrared part of the spectrum, which is invisible to the human eye). The laser allows intracorporeal lithotripsy to be performed, ureteral strictures to be managed, and urothelial tumors to be removed. This is a contact laser: For the system to work, the laser fiber must be placed right against the target (tissue or stone). A flexible ureterorenoscope requires two types of laser fibers: a small-diameter (150–200 μm) fiber and a large-diameter (365–600 μm) fiber. The large-diameter fibers will deliver more energy, but restrict the deflection of the scope. The reverse is true of the small-diameter fibers: they deliver less energy, but leave the scope free to deflect.

A red or green aiming beam shows where the fiber is in relation to the target. The holmium-YAG laser may cut through guide wires and nitinol instruments. This property may be put to good use when it comes to freeing a stone that has become blocked into a nitinol extraction basket. The holmium-YAG laser's penetrative power is very weak (<0.4 mm); so there is no risk of tissue perforation if the laser fiber comes into contact with the tissue. To perforate the ureteral mucous membrane, the surgeon must push the laser fiber through to the ureteral wall. One of the dangers of the holmium-YAG laser is the risk of damaging the ureterorenoscope due to the photo-thermal effects of the laser. Generally, this type of damage happens when the surgeon starts the fragmentation and simultaneously withdraws the laser fiber. To avoid this, a perfect synergy between the ureterorenoscope and the laser fiber is mandatory.[24]

47.9.2 Laser Fiber Not Fixed by Seal (Not Recommended)

- When the laser fiber is introduced in the working channel of the ureterorenoscope (Fig. 47.25), the laser unit must always be on "standby" mode (Inactive mode). So, if the surgeon accidentally starts the fragmentation at the wrong time or if the laser fiber moves in the working channel, nothing will happen.
- The laser fiber must protrude several millimeters at the distal tip of the ureterorenoscope (check the endoscopic images) and must be in contact with the target so that the laser unit is put in "ready" mode.

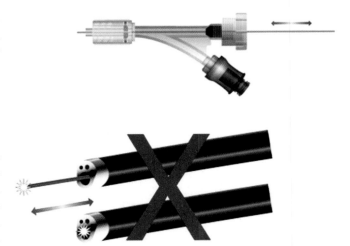

Fig. 47.25 Laser fiber not fixed by seal (not recommended)

- The fragmentation can start, but the surgeon must keep in mind that in this configuration, the slightest withdrawal of the laser fiber during the fragmentation will risk damaging the working channel. Because the laser fiber only protrudes a few millimeters beyond the distal end of the ureterorenoscope, it is very easy to move the fiber back without realizing, thus damaging the distal end of the ureterorenoscope. It is the most common cause of laser-perforation of ureterorenoscopes.
- It is strongly discouraged to work this way.

47.9.3 Laser Fiber Fixed by Seal (Strongly Recommended)

- To avoid the risk of distal perforation of the ureterorenoscope by an ill-timed withdrawal of the laser fiber at the moment of the fragmentation, it is recommended to fix it by holding the seal at its maximum (Fig. 47.26). Thus, the O-ring will block the laser fiber, preventing all movement forward and backward at the moment of the fragmentation.
- This trick also means that the surgeon's left hand is free, which no longer has to hold the laser fiber during the fragmentation. He can control his movement better by making use of his left hand to hold the body of the ureterorenoscope.

47.10 Management of Lower-Pole Calculi

When the lower-pole calculus is located, a nitinol basket (1.5–2.4 Fr) is inserted (with the endoscope kept undeflected) and the stone is captured. The stone is displaced to the upper caliceal system, or into the renal pelvis. The stone is released,

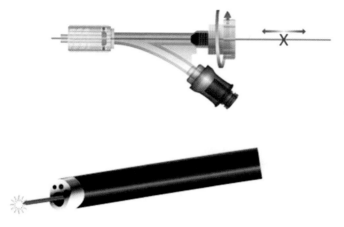

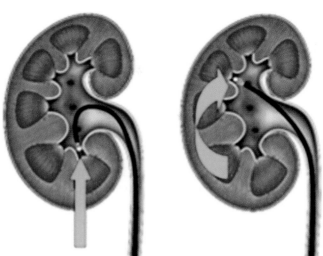

Fig. 47.26 Laser fiber fixed by seal (recommended)

and the nitinol grasper is withdrawn. A laser fiber (200–365 μm-diameter) is introduced into the working channel (Fig. 47.27).[53]

The fiber is advanced a few millimeters beyond the end of the working channel, and the red aiming beam is switched on. The laser fiber is fixed by using the port seal to avoid back movements of the laser fiber into the working channel. The F-URS with the fiber in place is placed against the stone, and fragmentation is started (initial setting: 5–6 Hz, 1–1.5 J corresponding to 5–9 W). When the fragmentation is obtained, the laser fiber is withdrawn, and the stone fragments are grasped and removed with the nitinol basket.

Displacing a lower pole stone into a more favorable location (upper pole, renal pelvis) before fragmentation has been shown to be more effective in stone-free rates.

If the stone cannot be displaced toward the upper pole or the renal pelvis (bulky stone, stricture of the caliceal stem), it may be fragmented in situ using a small-diameter (150–200 μm) laser fiber. For the introduction of the laser fiber, the F-URS must always be kept straight (undeflected). Deflection of the scope is not started until the fiber is at the tip of the endoscope. At the end of the procedure, a complete exploration of the intrarenal cavities is obtained to ensure that no fragments have been left behind.[6,27,31,36,43,46]

47.11 Fragmentation Techniques, Clotting Technique

When a stone has been identified but, due to its size, an extraction cannot be anticipated "in one piece," it must be broken up with the holmium-YAG laser by introducing in the working channel a laser fiber of variable size: 150–600 μm in diameter. The diameter of the laser fiber is chosen according to the location of the stone and the need or not to flex the distal tip of the ureterorenoscope to reach the stone. Whatever

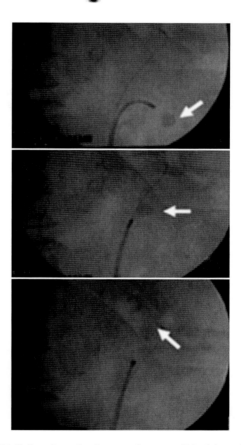

Fig. 47.27 Relocation of a lower pole stone. Principle and fluoroscopic control

its diameter, the laser fiber must be introduced into the working channel of the ureterorenoscope in a straight position (no deflection of the distal end) and the laser unit must be in "standby" mode (inactive mode).[48]

The laser fiber is advanced to the end of the working channel a few millimeters and, if needed, the distal tip of the ureterorenoscope is flexed to reach the stone and treat it. Switch on the red aiming beam to check that the fiber has made contact with the stone and set the laser unit to "ready" mode (active mode). Begin the laser fragmentation by touching the stone. (Parameters: 5–6 Hz, 1,000–1,500 mJ is 5–9 W).[16–20,26]

47.11.1 Fragmentation in a Stone Blocked Against a Renal Papillae

- The holmium-YAG laser has the important advantage of not moving back during the fragmentation. However, the small stones are likely to move during the fragmentation, which reduces the effectiveness of the laser fragmentation and lengthens the operating time.
- To minimize this inconvenience, it is recommended to wedge the stone between the laser fiber and a renal papule before starting the fragmentation (Fig. 47.28). This is described as "Trapped Fragmentation."
- If the stone's movements are close to the patient's breathing, it is possible to ask the anesthetists to put the patient in apnea for a few minutes or to make the patient breathe at "low frequency" (6–9/min) in order to reduce the movements of the diaphragm on the kidney and consequently on the stone.

47.11.2 "Postage Stamp" Fragmentation Technique

- The holmium-YAG laser fragmentation enables you to obtain tiny fragments comparable to grains of sand.
- To optimize this fragmentation, it is recommended to reach the stone by starting the fragmentation from the outside

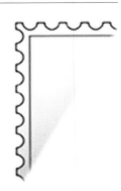
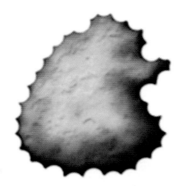

Fig. 47.29 "Postage stamp" fragmentation technique

toward the center and from the surface toward the bottom by making small holes all around the stone comparable to the outside edge of a postage stamp (Fig. 47.29).
- The sheer number of these little holes will enable a very fine fragmentation of the stone. This fragmentation technique has the advantage of not producing large fragments, necessitating that each one has a fragmentation or an extraction.

47.11.3 Clotting Technique

- During the laser fragmentation, a bit of blood often appears. The visibility at this point is compromised by the bleeding.
- By contrast, this bleeding can sometimes prove to be very useful, because at the end of the operation, it enables you to fix minimal stone fragments within the clot (Fig. 47.30).
- Therefore, it is easy for the surgeon to capture this clot and these stone fragments with the help of a nitinol basket and to extract them together.

47.12 Stone Removal Techniques

When a stone has been captured, it must be removed.[33] Classically, the ureterorenoscope is withdrawn by securing the stone trapped in the nitinol basket blocked at the distal tip of the ureterorenoscope. It is also possible to check whether the stone passes through the ureter without blocking it by endoscopically checking its "descent" toward the bladder. For that:

- The stone captured by the nitinol basket is placed a few millimeters in front of the end of the ureterorenoscope.
- The basket is blocked by the seal joint (like for the laser fiber) at the moment when the fragmentation is started.
- The ureterorenoscope is withdrawn by checking that the stone is moving without difficulty or without getting stuck.

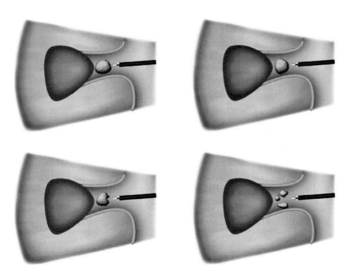

Fig. 47.28 Fragmentation in a stone blocked against a renal papillae

Fig. 47.30 Clotting technique

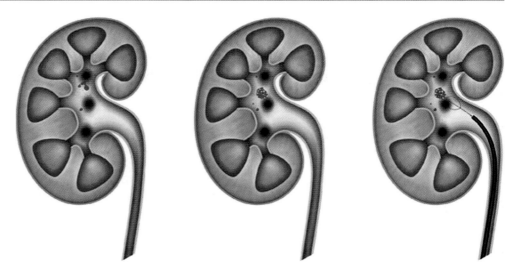

This is the ideal removal of a stone from the renal caliceal cavities. However, there are situations where the stone removal can be complicated. Here are the three most frequent:

- Figure 47.31a: The stone is too big to pass through the inside of a UAS.
- Figure 47.31b: The stone is blocked at the level of the ureter but re-released by the nitinol basket.
- Figure 47.31c: The stone is blocked at the level of the ureter and NOT re-released by the nitinol basket.

47.12.1 Removal by "Trapping" Stone on the Ureteral Access Sheath

If the surgeon has inserted a UAS at the beginning of the operation, the removal of fragments is done through this. Sometimes the stone fragment captured does not pass through the UAS and stays blocked at the end of the UAS. In this case, it is possible to remove everything in one step: ureterorenoscope, basket with the stone, and the UAS (Fig. 47.31a):

- The stone is kept trapped at the end of the UAS.
- The surgeon's right hand holds the ureterorenoscope and the nitinol basket with the stone.
- The left hand holds the UAS and the body of the endoscope. Both hands work in synergy, and it can be removed.

47.12.2 Release of a Stone Captured in a Nitinol Basket

When a stone remains blocked in the ureter during its descent, it is often possible to re-release it in order to be able to

withdraw the nitinol basket from the working channel of the ureterorenoscope (Fig. 47.31b). Once the basket is removed, a laser fiber must be introduced in the working channel of the ureterorenoscope to break up the stone and, secondarily, to extract its fragments. The maneuver to re-release the stone is the following:

- Open the basket fully.
- Push the basket toward renal caliceal cavities.
- At the same time, the basket must be put in the "open position."
- Usually, if these steps are followed, the stone is released from the basket, enabling the surgeon to continue with the procedure. If that is not the case, the process shown in Fig. 47.31a should be carried out.

47.12.3 Captured Stone Hemmed-In in the Ureter, Nitinol Basket in Place

When the stone remains blocked in the ureter, trapped in the nitinol basket, which cannot be withdrawn, the following sequence should be carried out (Fig. 47.31c):

- The handle of the nitinol basket must be taken off (proximal and distal screws).
- The handle is withdrawn, and the central structure in nitinol stays covered by its external sheath.
- Once the handle is withdrawn, the external sheath of the basket can also be removed by sliding over the central nitinol structure.
- The central structure in nitinol still contains the stone at the end, so it stays in place.
- The ureterorenoscope is withdrawn by sliding it outward over the central structure in nitinol.

Fig. 47.31 (**a**) Stone removal by "trapping" stone on the ureteral access sheath. (**b**) Release of a stone captured in a nitinol basket. (**c**) Captured stone hemmed-in in the ureter, nitinol basket in place

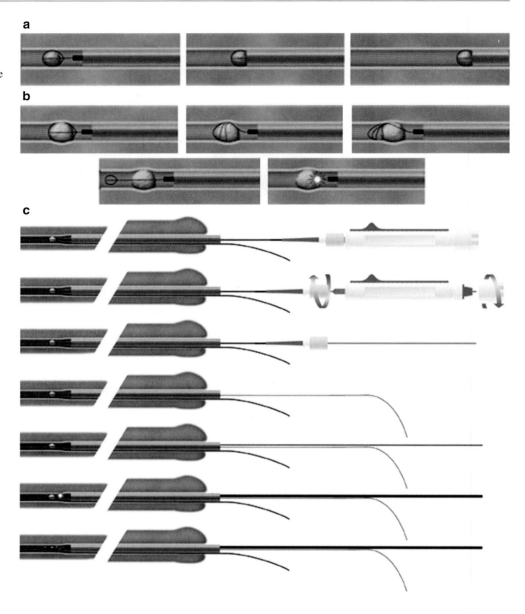

- The ureterorenoscope is repositioned over the guide wire, through the ureteral access sheath next to the central nitinol structure.
- Once the ureterorenoscope is in contact with the stone, a laser fiber is introduced in the working channel and the fragmentation of the stone can begin.
- During the fragmentation, it is possible to cut the central nitinol structure to free the stone, but this is not always necessary.
- If the central nitinol structure can be kept, the basket can be "shown again" in order to extract the residual fragments.

In order to avoid this sometimes complicated situation, it is highly recommended that for optimum results, it is best to fragment all renal stones rather than to attempt a risky extraction in one go, which will needlessly complicate the endoscopic movement.

The use of the *ESCAPE* system (Boston Scientific) enables you to introduce a nitinol basket of 1, 9 Ch and a laser fiber of 200 μm in the working channels of all flexible ureterorenoscopes. This system enables the fragmentation of a blocked stone in a nitinol basket without having to carry out the previous maneuver described.

47.13 Prevention of Stone Fragment Accumulation in Lower Calyx

If, at the end of the procedure, for any renal calculi regardless of location, many small stone fragments are left in the collecting system, there will be a major risk of fragment re-accumulation in the lower-pole calices. In order to avoid this risk, Fuchs and Patel described a technique to seal the lower pole with an autologous blood clot.[1,2] For this part of the procedure, the F-URS is placed in the lower pole. Saline is injected into the working channel of the F-URS, to flush the fragments toward the upper calices and the renal pelvis, and to clear any remaining contrast. Through the working channel of the scope, the operator injects 5–10 mL of autologous blood taken from a peripheral venous line. (This will completely obscure endoscopic vision, and the position of the F-URS in the lower pole will need to be checked with fluoroscopy.) When the injection is obtained, the F-URS is withdrawn, and the surgeon waits 5–10 min for the blood clots formation. Retrograde pyelogram is performed to check that the lower calyx is no longer visualized; i.e., that the clots are providing a seal (Fig. 47.32). At the end of the procedure, the surgeon may or may not decide to drain the ureter. If the ureter is to be drained, a ureteral catheter may be used for 24 h; alternatively, an internal stent may be left in the ureter for a few days.

47.14 Management of Caliceal Diverticula

A mixture of contrast and methylene blue or indigo carmine is injected through the working channel of the scope. A check is made with fluoroscopy to establish that the diverticulum is properly opacified. Opacification means that the neck of the diverticulum is patent. Saline is injected through the working channel of the scope, to flush the intrarenal collecting system. A detailed inspection of the collecting system is made, to see whether dye is leaking from the diverticular neck. Delayed emptying of the diverticulum would suggest a narrow neck (Fig. 47.33). Once the diverticulum has been identified, a laser fiber is passed through the working channel of the scope, to incise the neck of the diverticulum. Following incision of the diverticular neck, the F-URS is inserted into the diverticulum. Any stone or stones in the diverticulum may be fragmented in situ with the laser or extracted "in one piece" with the nitinol basket. Following treatment of the stone(s), the neck of the diverticulum is generously incised with the laser, to allow the diverticulum to be marsupialized into the collecting system. At the end of the procedure, a check is made to ensure that no fragments have been left behind. After this, the surgeon may or may not decide to drain the ureter. Ureteral drainage with an internal ureteral stent is strongly recommended. If possible, the renal pigtail of the stent should be placed inside the marsupialized cavity.[49]

47.15 Retrograde Endopyelotomy

Retrograde pyelogram is obtained to confirm the ureteropelvic junction (UPJ) obstruction. A safety guide wire is inserted through the dual-lumen catheter, and the safety guide wire is secured to the patient's left thigh. If required, a UAS is inserted. The F-URS is inserted over the working guide wire. The position of the F-URS is checked with the X-ray control: The F-URS could be in the renal pelvis, if the ureteropyelic junction (UPJ) is passable or the F-URS is distal to the UPJ if the junction is not passable. The working guide wire is withdrawn. The cold-light cable, the camera, and the irrigation system are attached. If possible, the intrarenal collecting system and the UPJ are explored. With the F-URS kept straight (distal tip undeflected), a 365-μm diameter laser fiber is introduced into the working channel of the scope. The fiber is advanced a few millimeters beyond the end of the working channel; the red aiming beam is switched on; and the laser is set at Ready. Power setting: 12–15 Hz, 1–1.5 J corresponding to 15–22 W. If the F-URS is in the intrarenal collecting system, the UPJ is incised as the scope is being withdrawn toward the ureter. If the ureterorenoscope is below the UPJ, the incision is made as the scope is being advanced toward the renal pelvis. Repeated passes with the laser fiber are made, until the periureteral fat appears. The F-URS is withdrawn. A high-pressure ureteral balloon catheter is inserted over the safety guide wire, and, under fluoroscopic guidance, the high-pressure balloon is inflated with contrast agent to dilate the incised area. The high-pressure ureteral balloon catheter is withdrawn. The dual-lumen catheter is inserted over the safety guide wire, and retrograde pyelogram is performed. If the endopyelotomy has been correctly performed, there will be an extravasation of contrast from the ureter. At the end of the procedure, an internal ureteral stent (8 Fr, or 12/8 Fr) should be inserted and left in place for 4–6 weeks; a urinary catheter should be left in place for 24 h.[14]

47.16 Antegrade Flexible Ureteroscopy

Flexible ureteroscopy may be performed using an antegrade approach; however, the procedure is rarely indicated. It may be considered where the retrograde route is ruled out. This would be the case in external and, above all, in internal urinary diversion. The technique is well established; however,

Fig. 47.32 Blood clots technique

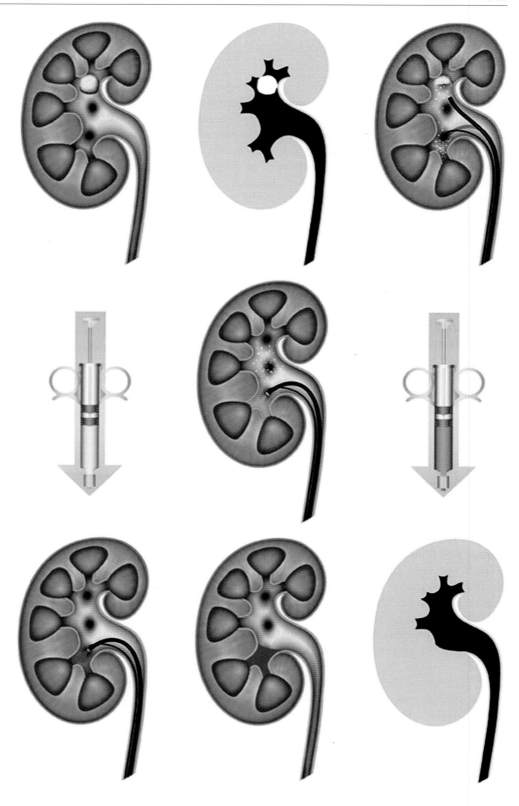

Fig. 47.33 Caliceal diverticulum. Methylene blue test

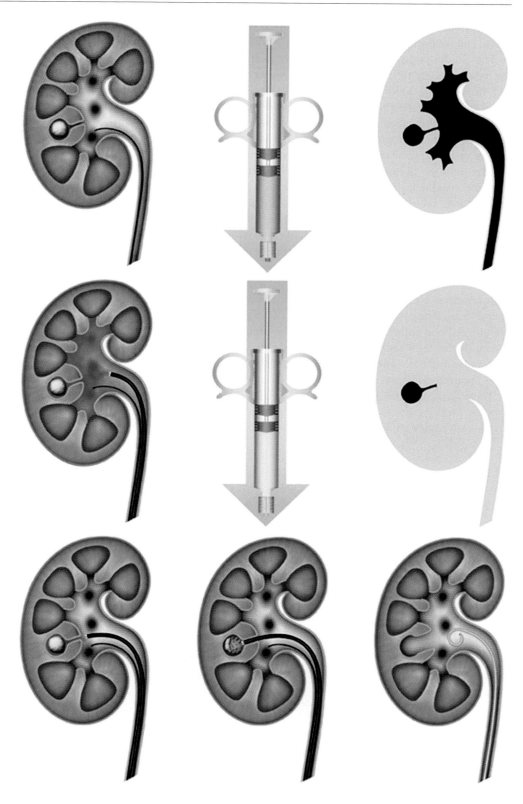

the antegrade approach places great mechanical stress on the scope, and weakens the equipment.

The patient is positioned prone. The intrarenal collecting system is identified and punctured, under ultrasound and fluoroscopic guidance. Preferentially, the middle or upper caliceal system should be punctured to ensure that the scope is aligned with the ureter. Contrast is injected through the puncture needle to opacify the intrarenal collecting system and the ureter; and the working guide wire is inserted into the ureter, under fluoroscopic guidance. The puncture needle is withdrawn. A dual-lumen catheter is inserted over the working guide wire, and the safety guide wire is inserted through the second channel of the dual-lumen catheter. The dual-lumen catheter is then withdrawn, and the safety guide wire is secured to the patient's body. The high-pressure ureteral balloon catheter is inserted over the working guide wire. Under fluoroscopic guidance, the high-pressure balloon catheter is inflated with contrast agent, to dilate the puncture needle tract. The high-pressure ureteral balloon catheter is withdrawn. The ureteral access sheath is inserted over the working guide wire, under fluoroscopic guidance. The dilating obturator is withdrawn from the ureteral access sheath.

Through the ureteral access sheath, the F-URS is inserted over the working guide wire, under fluoroscopic guidance. The working guide wire is withdrawn and the cold-light cable, the camera, and the irrigation system are attached. Antegrade exploration of the ureter is performed. Any calculi, tumors, or ureteral strictures are addressed in customary fashion.

At the end of the procedure, the ureterorenoscope is withdrawn. The ureteral access sheath is removed. Over the safety guide wire, a percutaneous nephrostomy tube is inserted, under fluoroscopic guidance. The safety guide wire is withdrawn, and the nephrostomy tube is secured to the skin.[30,34]

47.17 Management of Urothelial Tumors

A saline wash of the intrarenal collecting system may be obtained, and an aspiration sample is collected for cytopathology. If required, retrograde pyelogram may be performed to assist in the localization of the lesion. Retrograde pyelogram must not be performed prior to cytological sampling since the contrast agent will interfere with the cytolopathological examination. Once the tumor has been identified, the surgeon must decide which of the three ablation techniques available he would wish to use (Fig. 47.34):[13]

1. The first option consists in debulking the tumor by cold-cutting it with a tipless nitinol basket. This is followed by the collection of tumor stump tissue with biopsy forceps, and the vaporization of the tumor base with the holmium laser (settings: 10 Hz, 1–1.2 J, corresponding to 10–12 W).

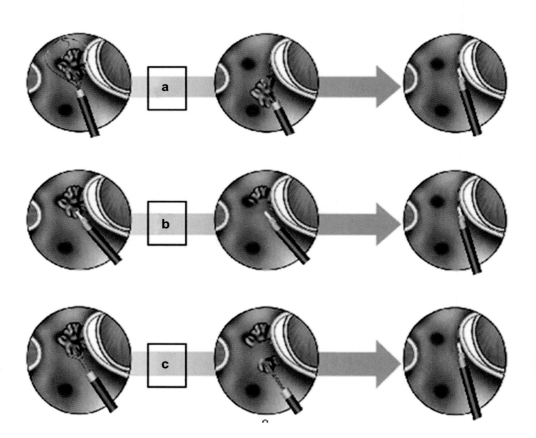

Fig. 47.34 Ablation techniques of urothelial tumors. (**a**) Nitinol basket cold cutting. (**b**) Laser ablation. (**c**) Biopsy forceps and laser ablation

2. The second option consists in taking biopsies and then vaporizing the entire tumor with the holmium-YAG laser, without any prior debulking.

3. The third option consists in completely resecting the tumor with the biopsy forceps, and then vaporizing the tumor base with the holmium laser.

With all of these techniques, a large-diameter laser fiber is used (generally 365 μm). However, for lesions in the lower pole, a small-diameter fiber (200 μm) has to be used in order to obtain maximum deflection of the scope. Once the renal urothelial lesion has been treated, the ureter is inspected carefully. To this end, the scope is gradually withdrawn, and all ureteral surfaces are inspected under endoscopic vision, right down to the ureteral orifice.

At the end of the procedure, the surgeon may or may not decide to drain the ureter. If the ureter is to be drained, a ureteral catheter may be used for 24 h; alternatively, an internal stent may be left in the ureter for a few days. Depending on the type of drainage chosen, adjuvant chemotherapy with instillation of a topical therapeutic agent may be started.[28,32]

47.18 Conclusions

Flexible URS combined with holmium-YAG laser is an effective, reproducible, and minimally traumatic diagnostic and therapeutic technique perfectly adapted to diseases of the upper urinary tract, and especially for the management of lower pole stone less than 15 mm. This technology must be part of the therapeutic armamentarium of any center involved in the management of urinary stones.

The equipment has improved dramatically over the past 2 decades in several areas in ureteroscope design, intracorporeal lithotripter, accessory devices, and especially video and imaging. Advances in electro-optics continue to improve the urologist's ability to perform minimally invasive procedures. While the development of flexible fiberoptic ureteroscopes (URS) has greatly facilitated upper tract procedures, distal sensor, digital technology may represent the next step in the evolution of endoscopy. Better image quality could translate into greater precision for diagnostic and treatment and shorter procedures. Tips and tricks are essential to improve the technique. Collectively, all these improvements allowed excellent results in the management of upper tract diseases, with high stone-free rate, particularly for the lower pole stone with lower morbidity.

References

1. Fuchs G, Patel A. Lower pole autologous blood clot occlusion: a technique to prevent stone fragments pooling in the lower calyx (LC). American Urological Association 98th Annual Meeting, April 26–May 1, 2003, Chicago.

2. Patel A. Lower calyceal occlusion by autologous blood clot to prevent stone fragment reaccumulation after retrograde intra-renal surgery for lower calyceal stones: first experience of a new technique. J Endourol. 2008;22:2501-2506.

3. Afane JS, Olweny EO, Bercowskye, et al. Flexible ureteroscopes: a single center evaluation of the durability and function of the new endoscopes smaller than 9Fr. J Urol. 2001;164:1164-1168.

4. Akpinar H, Tufek I, Alici B, et al. Ureteroscopy and holmium laser lithotripsy in pregnancy: stents must be used postoperatively. J Endourol. 2006;20:107-110.

5. Ankem MK, Lowry PS, Slovick RW, Munoz Del Rio A, Nakada SY. Clinical utility of dual active deflection flexible ureteroscope during upper tract ureteropyeloscopy. Urology. 2004;64:430-434.

6. Auge BK, Dahm P, Wu NZ, et al. Ureteroscopic management of lower pole renal calculi: technique of calculus displacement. J Endourol. 2001;15:835-838.

7. Bagley DH, Fabrizio M, El Gabry E. Ureteroscopic and radiographic imaging of the upper urinary tract. J Endourol. 1998;12: 313-324.

8. Beiko DT, Denstedt JD. Advances in ureterorenoscopy. Urol Clin N Am. 2007;34:397-408.

9. Blew BD, Dagnone AJ, Pace KT, et al. Comparison of Peditrol irrigation device and common methods of irrigation. J Endourol. 2005;19:562-565.

10. Bultitude MF, Dasgupta P, Tiptaft RC, Glass JM. Prolonging the life of the flexible ureterorenoscope. Int J Clin Pract. 2004;8:756-757.

11. Bultitude MF, Tiptaft RC, Dasgupta P, et al. Treatment of urolithiasis in the morbidly obese. Obes Surg. 2004;14:300-304.

12. Chiu KY, Cai Y, Marcovich R, Smith AD, Lee BR. Are new-generation flexible ureteroscopes better than their predecessors? BJU Int. 2004;93:115-119.

13. Chen GL, El-Gabry EA, Bagley DH. Surveillance of upper urinary tract transitional cell carcinoma: the role of ureteroscopy, retrograde pyelography, cytology and urinalysis. J Urol. 2000;164:1901-1904.

14. Conlin MJ, Bagley DH. Ureteroscopic endopyelotomy in a single setting. J Urol. 1998;159:727-731.

15. Dash A, Schuster TG, Hollenbeck BK, et al. Ureteroscopic treatment of renal calculi in morbidly obese patients: a stone matched comparison. Urology. 2002;60:393-397.

16. Del Vecchio F, Auge BK, Brizuela RM, Weizer AZ, Zhong P, Preminger GM. In vitro analysis of stone fragmentation ability of the Freddy Laser. J Endourol. 2003;17:177.

17. Denstedt JD. Preliminary experience with holmium YAG laser lithotripsy. J Endourol. 1995;9:255-258.

18. Diner EK, Rosenblum M, Patel SV, et al. Primary ureterorenoscopy and holmium laser lithotripsy for large renal stone and staghorn calculi. J Urol. 2005;173(Suppl 4):457.

19. Dubosq F, Pasqui F, Girard F, et al. Endoscopic lithotripsy and the FREDDY laser: initial experience. J Endourol. 2006;20:296-299.

20. Dubosq F, Pasqui F, Girard F, et al. Intérêt et place de la lithotritie endocorporelle Nd:YAG en urétéroscopie souple et semi-rigide: une alternative au laser holmium:YAG? Prog Urol. 2005;15:662-666.

21. Elashry OM, Elbahnasy AM, Rao GS, Nakada SY, Clayman RV. Flexible ureteroscopy: Washingtown University experience with the 9, 3F and 7, 5F flexible ureteroscopes. J Urol. 1997;157:2074-2080.

22. Fabrizio MD, Behari A, Bagley DH. Ureteroscopic management of intrarenal calculi. J Urol. 1998;159:1139-1143.

23. Gould DL. Retrograde flexible ureterorenoscopic holmium-Yag laser lithotripsy: the new gold standard. Tech Urol. 1998;1:22-24.

24. Grasso M, Chalik Y. Principles and applications of laser lithotripsy: experience with the holmium laser lithotrite. J Clin Laser Med Surg. 1998;16:3-7.

25. Grasso M, Bagley D. Small diameter, actively defectable flexible ureteropyeloscopy. J Urol. 1998;160:1648-1653.

26. Grasso M, Conlin M, Bagley DH. Retrograde ureteropyeloscopic treatment of large upper urinary tract (2 cm) and minor staghorn calculi. *J Urol*. 1998;160:346-351.

27. Grasso M, Ficazzola M. Retrograde ureteropyeloscopy for lower pole caliceal calculi. *J Urol*. 1999;162:1904-1908.

28. Grasso M, Fraiman M, Levine M. Ureteropyeloscopic diagnostis and treatment of upper urinary tract urothelial malignancies. *Urology*. 1999;54:240-246.

29. Johnson GB, Portela D, Grasso M. Advanced ureteroscopy: wireless and sheathless. *J Endourol*. 2006;20:552-555.

30. Kieran K, Nelson CP, Wolf S Jr, et al. Retrograde ureterosopy in patients with orthotopic ileal neobladder urinary diversion: an update. *J Urol*. 2006;175(Suppl 4):349.

31. Kourambas J, Delvecchio FC, Munver R, Preminger GM. Nitinol stone retrieval-assisted ureteroscopic management of lower pole renal calculi. *Urology*. 2000;20(56):935-939.

32. Lam JS, Gupta M. ureteroscopic management of upper tract transitional cell carcinoma. *Urol Clin N Am*. 2004;31:115-128.

33. Landman J, Monga M, El-Gabry EA, et al. Bare naked baskets: ureteroscope deflection and flow characteristics with intact and disassembled ureteroscopic nitinol stone baskets. *J Urol*. 2002;167:2377.

34. L'esperance Jo, Sung J, Marguet C, et al. The surgical management of stones in patients with urinary diversions. *Curr Opin Urol*. 2004;14:129-134.

35. Lobik L, Lopez Pujals A, Leveillee RJ. Variables affecting deflection of a new third-generation flexible ureteropyeloscope (DUR-8 Elite). *J Endourol*. 2003;17:733-736.

36. Michel M, Knoll T, Ptaschnyk T, Kohrmann KU, Alken P. Flexible ureterorenopyeloscopy for the treatment of lower pole calyx stones: influence of different lithotripsy probes and stone extraction tools on scope deflection and irrigation flow. *Eur Urol*. 2002;41:312.

37. Minevich E, Sheldon CA. The role of ureteroscopy in pediatric urology. *Curr Opin Urol*. 2006;16:295-298.

38. Minevitch E, Defoor W, Reddy P, et al. Ureteroscopy is safe and effective in prepubertal kids. *J Urol*. 2005;174:276-279.

39. Mostafavi MR. Clinical evaluation of differents wires in gaining access during ureteroscopy for ureteral stones disease. *J Endourol*. 2006;20(1):Abst A117.

40. Mugiya S, Ozono S, Nagata M, et al. Retrograde endoscopic management of ureteral stones more than 2 cm in size. *Urology*. 2006;67:1164-1168.

41. Parkin J, Keeley FX Jr, Timoney AG. Flexible ureteroscopes: a user's guide. *BJU Int*. 2002;90:640.

42. Pasqui F, Dubosq F, Tchala K, et al. Impact on active scope deflection and irrigation flow of all endoscopic working tools during flexible ureteroscopy. *Eur Urol*. 2004;45:58-64.

43. Preminger GM. Management of lower pole renal calculi: shock wave lithotripsy versus percutaneous nephrolithotomy versus flexible ureteroscopy. *Urol Res*. 2006;34:108-111.

44. Raza A, Smith G, Moussa S, et al. Ureteroscopy in the management of pediatric urinary tract calculi. *J Endourol*. 2005;19:151-158.

45. Saïdi A, Combes F, Delaporte V, Breton X, Traxer O, Lechevallier E. Urétéroscopie souple-Laser holmium:YAG. Matériel et technique. *Prog Urol*. 2006;16:19-24.

46. Schuster TG, Hollenbeck BK, Faerber GJ, et al. Ureteroscopic treatment of lower pole calculi: comparison of lithotripsy in situ and after displacement. *J Urol*. 2002;168:43-45.

47. Tan AH, Al-Omar M, Denstedt JD, et al. Ureteroscopy for pediatric urolithiasis: an evolving first line therapy. *Urology*. 2005;65:153-156.

48. Tawfiek ER, Bagley DH. Management of upper urinary calculi with ureteroscopic techniques. *Urology*. 1999;53:25.

49. Traxer O, Sebe P, Chambade D, et al. Comment repérer le collet d'un diverticule caliciel en urétérorénoscopie souple. *Prog Urol*. 2005;15:100-102.

50. Traxer O, Pasqui F, Dubosq F, Tchala K, Gattegno B, Thibault P. Urétérorénoscope souple à double déflexion active. Expérience initiale. *Prog Urol*. 2003;13:592-597.

51. Traxer O, Pasqui F, Dubosq F, et al. Etude comparative de deux urétérorénoscopes souples de dernière génération. *Prog Urol*. 2005;15:656-661.

52. Traxer O, Dubosq F, Jamali K, Gattegno B, Thibault P. New-generation flexible ureterorenoscopes are more durable than previous ones. *Urology*. 2006;68:276-279. discussion 280–281.

53. Traxer O, Thibault F, Niang L, et al. Inferior calyx stone and flexible ureterorenoscopy to mobilize the stone before fragmentation. *Prog Urol*. 2006;16:198-200.

54. Traxer O, Lechevallier E, Saussine E. Flexible ureteroscopy with holmium laser: technical aspects. *Prog Urol*. 2008;18:929-937.

55. Traxer O, Lechevallier E, Saussine E. Flexible ureteroscopy with holmium laser: the tools. *Prog Urol*. 2008;18:1164-1168.

56. Weizer AZ, Springhart WP, Ekeruo WO, et al. Ureteroscopic management of renal calculi in anomalous kidneys. *Urology*. 2006;67:1164-1168.

57. White MD, Moran ME. Fatigability on the latest generation ureteropyeloscopes: Richrad Wolf vs Karl Storz. *J Endourol*. 1998;12:182.

Aldrin Joseph R. Gamboa and Elspeth M. McDougall

Abstract The potential to learn in the operating room is becoming increasingly limited by factors such as resident work hour restrictions, the increased cost associated with trainee involvement in the operating room, the demands on clinicians to increase productivity, the increased complexity of patient diagnoses seen in tertiary care medical centers, and the overall goal to decrease patient morbidity and mortality. Surgical educators are seeking alternative methods of training and developing simulated teaching environments in an effort to address these educational challenges. Endourology poses unique challenges, with steep learning curves for the surgeon, as it creates a visual image of the operative site that has altered depth perception, decreased tactile feedback, increased dependence on video monitors, and increased demand on hand–eye coordination. The importance of creating standardized curricula for training programs is becoming increasingly important for minimally invasive technologies. Curriculum designed for technical skill education involves setting goals and objectives at the commencement, designing interventions targeted to these goals, and developing assessment tools that can certify competency in the desired skills. A variety of teaching strategies have been utilized in the development of curricula for endourology including material-based models, animate and cadaveric models, and virtual reality simulation. All of these have their advantages and disadvantages and in combination provide a robust and comprehensive skills training platform to complement the cognitive training that is required for mastering endourologic concepts and techniques. With computer-based surgical simulation, a trainee may be truly evaluated objectively in the absence of bias for race, sex, or age. The integration of simulation into the surgical training curriculum will allow the trainee to acquire the basic surgical skills foundation and obtain performance levels according to predetermined proficiency levels for each stage of the training program. This then allows the surgical educator to concentrate on teaching the judgment and professionalism of an expert surgeon, and to strengthen the knowledge and interpretation of what is observed in the clinical setting in order to create a competent surgeon at both the cognitive and skills performance levels.

48.1 Introduction

Surgical education has recently experienced considerable change as a result of the rapidly expanding technological developments in the field of surgery. The traditional method of acquiring surgical skills originated from the reforms of Dr. William Halsted, a century ago.[1,2] The Halstedian apprenticeship follows the principle of "see one, do one, teach one" and involves an extensive period of hands-on training with increasing responsibility for patient care.[3-5] The goal of this training has been to produce a well-rounded and technically competent surgeon, grounded in the basic principles of surgery.[6] The trainees' activities rely on supervised instruction by an expert clinician with gradual and progressive acquisition of skills as directed by the expert surgeon in observation of the trainee.[7-9] However, there are certain inherent risks with this type of training for the patient during the initial

A.J.R. Gamboa (✉)
Department of Urology, University of California, Irvine,
UCI Medical Center, Paranaque City, Philippines
e-mail: aldringamboa@yahoo.com

P.N. Rao et al. (eds.), *Urinary Tract Stone Disease*,
DOI 10.1007/978-1-84800-362-0_48, © Springer-Verlag London Limited 2011

stages of the trainees' learning curve, which may be more pronounced with the highly complex skills required for minimally invasive surgery.[10]

48.2 History of Surgical Training and Impact of Endourologic Teaching

The Halstedian model is limited by variability of experience during residency and difficulties with standardization of training programs.[11] The potential to learn in the operating room is becoming increasingly limited by factors such as resident work hour restrictions, the increased cost associated with trainee involvement in the operating room, the demands on clinicians to increase productivity, the increased complexity of patient diagnoses seen in tertiary care medical centers, and the overall goal to decrease patient morbidity and mortality.[11,12] In addition, medical errors are increasingly scrutinized by the profession and the public, thereby reducing the tolerance for errors while training surgeons in the operating room.[13–15] The public is demanding that trainees have documented proficiency in surgical skills before embarking on surgical procedures that may have morbidity associated with errors related to inexperience that could lead to complications and even death.[16]

For these reasons, the Halstedian method of teaching is becoming increasingly outdated. Surgical educators are seeking alternative methods of training in developing simulated teaching environments in an effort to address these educational challenges.[10,17,18] The concept of trial-and-error learning in the clinical environment has been revised for the benefit of both the learner and the patient.

Surgery has become a dynamic and technologically driven field of medicine. The widespread acceptance and growth of minimally invasive surgery has posed many challenges to the training of urology residents and to allowing postgraduate urologists to acquire difficult new surgical skills.[19,20] Endourology poses unique challenges to the surgeon as the visual field is now two dimensional rather than the three dimensional one seen at open surgery. The endoscope creates a visual image of the operative site that has altered depth perception, decreased tactile feedback, increased dependence on video monitors, and increased demand on hand–eye coordination. All of this contributes to a steep learning curve for many of the endourologic procedures.[21] For the inexperienced endourologic trainee, these technological features can translate into longer operative times and increased patient morbidity.[11,22–24]

In the last decade, the specialty of urology has witnessed an enormous growth of knowledge and innovation in the endourologic technologies.[25] The development of fiber optic instrumentation and miniaturization of endoscopes and ancillary equipment used for ureteral and renal endoscopic surgery have modified the way urinary stone disease is treated. The digital revolution continues to lead the way toward the development of new surgical treatment modalities, which will reduce patient morbidity and enhance surgical outcomes. Computerization has proven to be an essential part of many clinical routines, and serves as an interface in a multitude of medical procedures and patient management devices.[26–31] It is quite conceivable that all surgical procedures will become computer aided, or even completely robotic in the near future. However, the surgical procedures will continue to require expert professional guidance, supervision, and control. New technological approaches to surgical problems will require ongoing, advanced training for both the surgical resident and the practicing surgeon as these new techniques and devices are introduced and implemented.[32] Practicing surgeons and residents will need to learn together and support each others' educational activities in providing better care for their patients.[33,34]

As surgical technology and techniques advance, surgical educators recognize the importance of using new educational programs and teaching strategies for acquisition of technical skills outside the operating room to optimize the trainees' experience.[35–37] Some educational changes have resulted in an increase in the length of residency training programs or the necessity for subspecialty fellowship training programs such as in endourology.[38–40]

In the early 1980s, through the collaborative efforts of Dr. Arthur D. Smith, Ralph V. Clayman, Paul H. Lange, Kurt Amplatz, Keith W. Kaye, and Wilfrido R. Castenada-Zuniga, at the University of Minnesota, the initial development and investigation of minimally invasive surgical approaches for ureteral and renal stone disease was undertaken.[41] This group also created the first endourologic educational program to teach these new concepts and techniques in urologic surgery to community urologists. Concomitantly at this same time, the research efforts of Christian G. Chaussy, in Germany, led to the clinical application of extracorporeal shock-wave lithotripsy for the management of renal stone disease. The international work in these areas of minimally invasive urologic surgery led to the founding of the Endourological Society after three successful annual meetings held in London in 1983 under the directorship of John C. Wickham, in Germany in 1984 under the directorship of Dr. Peter Alken, and then New York City in 1985 under the directorship of Dr. Arthur D. Smith. The Endourologic Society was officially instituted on May 1, 1984 and incorporated on April 18, 1985. Since then, the society has played an instrumental role in encouraging research and education related to the subspecialty of endourology and the development of ureteroscopy, percutaneous renal access surgery, and extracorporeal shock-wave lithotripsy. In the early 1990s, the Endourological Society created a 1-year specific endourology fellowship training program with defined guidelines. This was designed to provide specialized training in endourology to cover all aspects of endourological surgery, including endourology of the lower and upper urinary tracts, extracorporeal shock-wave lithotripsy, and various laparoscopic procedures. Effective in 2009, this fellowship training became a required 2-year training program under the auspices of the Endourological Society. The goal of this endorsed fellowship training program has been to provide a foundation for training academic endourologists in research and education for the ongoing expansion of the subspecialty. The guidelines for this fellowship training have included minimum numbers of index cases such as percutaneous renal access procedures (30 cases/2 years), ureteroscopy procedures (60 cases/2 years), and laparoscopic procedures (60 cases/2 years), and encouragement to perform research in endourology and present academic findings at the international annual meeting.

Since the early days of endourologic training programs, held first at the University of Minnesota, the pig kidney and ureter were utilized as a comparable working model for the same human anatomy. This concept has formed the basis of innumerable endourological courses nationally and internationally over the past 2 decades.[41]

At the 2008 World Congress of Endourology, held in Shanghai, there were three live surgery cases related to endourology including two percutaneous nephrolithotomy (PCNL) procedures and one holmium laser management of bladder tumors. In addition, this meeting featured seven dedicated instructional courses related to percutaneous nephrolithotomy, ureteroscopy, and general endourologic procedures and principles.

The Endourological Society's mission has been to create a venue for scientific dialogue among endourologists worldwide through annual meetings, circulation of scientific literature, and surgical skill training courses and hands-on laboratory sessions. The Endourological Society has pioneered international relations through collaborative medical education of and by its members.[42] The development of the fellowship programs and postgraduate courses provides an opportunity for urologists worldwide to improve existing skills and acquire new endourologic techniques.[43] A large portion of these training formats are interactive and encompass all aspects of endourology. The fellowship training programs allow for continued mentoring and guidance of these young endourologists as they commence their own academic and private careers.

48.3 Creating the Curriculum for Teaching Endourology

Modern urologic practice has benefitted from the innovations and developments in the field of endourology. Although minimally invasive and associated with low morbidity, endourologic procedures comprise some of the most difficult

techniques to learn and master.[40,44] The safe and effective performance of endourologic procedures is dependent on the comprehensive skills training of the surgeon and the frequency with which these procedures are performed in the clinical practice. Many of the challenging surgical skills of endourology require repetitive practice with feedback in order to proficiently master these skills. The creation of endourological surgical skill centers may represent the wave of the future in dissemination of both knowledge and acquisition of these technical skills.[45] Both the American Urologic Association and the Endourological Society have recognized the importance of creating a standardized curriculum for application to resident and fellowship training programs, especially with regard to the minimally invasive technologies. As such, both of these societies are in the process of discussion and deliberative inquiry, in accordance with the Accreditation Council on Graduate Medical Education (ACGME), to create curricula that have a basic cognitive component, technical skills training guidelines, and an objective evaluation process. These curricula are aimed at facilitating surgeon training while complying with regulations for accreditation.[46] The random opportunities of our current apprenticeship system for surgical training need to be replaced by a curriculum or learning system that meets the needs of surgeons and their commitment to lifelong learning. Surgical simulation, whether modeled- or computer-based, provides the unique opportunity for repetitive skills training with the exploration of all possible outcomes in a risk-free environment that can maximize the educational experience and reduce the time of training for surgeons in complex surgical techniques.[47]

48.3.1 Learning with Practice

The operating room has always been considered a high-stress environment for education and may potentially compromise the learning of the trainee.[48–50] In a low-stress environment, such as a training laboratory, the trainee is provided with an opportunity for supervision and guidance by a dedicated expert endourologic surgeon especially in the initial basic training process.[51] This type of training potentially allows for a relaxed learning environment while focusing on repetitive performance of essential technical skills to understand the concepts and then master the appropriate basic clinical skills. The mentor plays an important role in this educational process, initially as an instructor and then later in developing judgment and strengthening the knowledge and interpretation of what is observed in order to create the truly competent surgeon.[10] Without the basic cognitive knowledge of the principles and practices of surgical skills, repetitive practice may only result in learning a poor technique well or acquisition of incorrect skills, which ultimately invalidates the main objective of proficiency through practice. In addition, the skills training laboratory is a unique venue for team building, especially for high reliability teams such as operating room and endourologic surgery teams as they work together in these complex surgical environments.[52] The concept of performance repetition can be traced to other high reliability team environments such as the military and commercial aviation.[53,54] Practice is also a well-accepted component in sports, music, and many other fine arts. The purpose of repetitive skills practice with feedback is to acquire technical proficiency, minimize performance error, and maximize performance quality. Military and commercial aviation training programs use complex flight simulators to reproduce routine and emergency contingencies on an ongoing basis to prepare pilots and their teams adequately for workplace competency.[55,56] The cornerstone of this type of training is exhaustive repetition in a practice setting that closely resembles the actual work environment, under expert supervision to foster proficiency in the performance of the optimal technique or procedure.[52,57,58]

Although specific levels of surgical proficiency may be difficult to define, the development of objective parameters will provide an opportunity to define a trainee's learning curve.[59–61] Well-delineated guidelines detailing the number of procedures that must be performed during training and the timing and extent of training are limited at this time. There are often individual variations in the level of skill acquisition at the different stages of surgical training despite the same training environment.[10] Some individuals may require more training time or additional expert supervision during training compared to other trainees. The duration of training would be individualized on the basis of the acquisition of individual proficiency, rather than training to a predetermined period of time. Training focused on the trainee's needs is an educational advantage that is not always possible in the operating room where the expert surgeon must first be focused on the patient.[50] As such, in a simulated setting, residents could complete training modules at their own pace, with the endpoint of reaching a specific, predetermined level of proficiency necessary to go into the operating room.[62,63]

48.3.2 New Developments in Urinary Stone Disease Education Strategies

With the constant growth and development of the field of minimally invasive urologic surgery, the profession will forever be in search of reliable and validated training systems.[3,64] A simulator is defined as "a device that enables the operator to reproduce or represent under test conditions, phenomena likely to occur in actual performance" and may apply to both physical and virtual models.[65] Therefore, the term *simulator* can be applied to any model used to represent surgery. One

way to categorize the various types of simulation is to focus on the concept of fidelity. *Low-fidelity* simulators are those that are not very lifelike, such as silicone or rubber representatives of tissues. The advantages of low-fidelity simulators include lower cost and portability. The main disadvantages are the lack of realism and the inability to teach entire operations. *High-fidelity* simulators are those that are more lifelike, often with the ability to move beyond simple skill or task training and simulate partial or whole operations. Traditional high-fidelity simulators have included animal models and cadavers and they allow for realistic tissue handling in a perfused tissue model. Unfortunately, animal models are costly, require veterinary assistance, raise social and ethical questions, and differ anatomically from the human. Cadaveric models, while anatomically ideal, are not always readily available and the tissues do not truly mimic the tissue compliance of live surgery. Commercially available high-fidelity simulators offer the advantage of reusability, realistic anatomy, and the ability to use real surgical instruments such as would be encountered in the operating room. These simulators are, however, significantly more expensive than low-fidelity models and require a considerable amount of maintenance.

No one model provides an all-encompassing platform on which to learn every endourologic skill. However, many provide valuable educational opportunities and together can be used to effectively train surgeons to acquire these challenging skills.[66–68] These models include mechanical latex models, animals, cadavers, and computer-based virtual reality surgical simulators. Herein, we describe some of these teaching methods and the advantages and disadvantages of each.

48.4 Material-Based Models

A variety of material-based models have been created for teaching ureteroscopy and percutaneous renal access. Some of the moderately high-fidelity bench trainers for teaching ureteroscopy and intrarenal surgery are currently available including the Uro-Scopic Trainer™ (Limbs and Things, Bristol UK, Fig. 48.1), the Scope Trainer™ (Mediskills Ltd., Edinburgh, UK), and the kidney-ureter-bladder (KUB) model LapED™ (www.laped.org, Irvine, CA, USA, Fig. 48.2). The Uro-Scopic Trainer consists of a mannequin of the male genitourinary tract including kidneys, ureter, and bladder through which standard endoscopic instruments may be utilized. The Scope Trainer offers similar features including a distensible bladder, ureteral orifices, and ureters that follow the natural course for an adult male. Standard procedures such as ureteral or renal intra-corporeal lithotripsy and ureteral tumor biopsy may be simulated with the Scope Trainer.

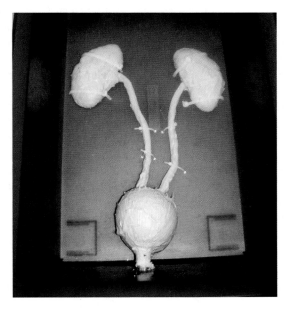

Fig. 48.1 Uro-Scopic Trainer™ by Limbs & Things, Ltd, Bristol, UK (Image kindly supplied by Limbs & Things, copyright 2009)

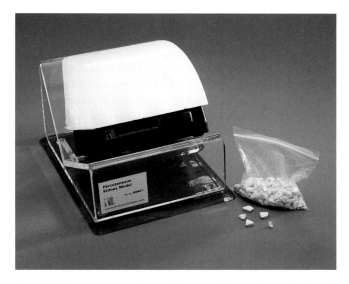

Fig. 48.3 Percutaneous Nephrolithotomy Trainer™ by Limbs & Things, Ltd, Bristol, UK (Image kindly supplied by Limbs & Things, copyright 2009)

Fig. 48.2 KUB Model™ developed at University of California, Irvine, CA (www.laped.org)

Recently at the University of California, Irvine, we developed a silicone kidney, ureter, and bladder (KUB) model using a cast from a human and pig kidney to create the intrarenal collecting system. This model has been used to teach ureteroscopy and intrarenal surgery procedures. Chou and colleagues examined the ability of two simulators, the high-fidelity bench model Uro-Scopic (Limbs and Things, Bristol, UK) and the virtual reality simulator UroMentor™ (Simbionix USA, Cleveland, OH), to teach basic ureteroscopic skills to inexperienced medical students.[10] Sixteen medical students received didactic training and video instruction by a single faculty member. Participants were

trained on either the bench model or the VR simulator until they were able to perform the ureteroscopic procedure independently. After a 2-month interval, the participants were graded on their ability to perform basic ureteroscopy on a pig model. These researchers found no significant difference between the two groups in their ability to perform the steps of the procedure and concluded that either of these training modalities may improve the initial clinical performance of urologic trainees.

Urologist-acquired percutaneous renal access has become more common, but it is still estimated that only 11% of urologists who perform percutaneous nephrolithotomy (PCNL) obtain their own renal access.[69] This may be due to lack of training, low level of comfort, or even perceived time constraints. As most urologists who perform PCNL do not obtain their own access, many residents may never learn this important skill. Surgical simulation is a possible answer to assist both practicing and training urologists to gain the necessary skills to obtain their own percutaneous renal access.[66]

Two nonbiological models offer training platforms for percutaneous renal access procedures. The Percutaneous Nephrolithotomy Trainer™ (Limbs and Things, Ltd, Bristol, UK) (Fig. 48.3) allows for simulated needle insertion, passage of guidewires, dilation of the nephrostomy tract, nephroscopy, and stone removal.[70] The model consists of a silicone slab that responds to insertion of wires, dilators, and sheaths. The slab contains multiple calices where stones may be placed for procedural variability. X-ray imaging is simulated, placing the translucent slab over a light box that is placed beneath the slab. The Perc Trainer™ (Mediskills, Ltd, Edinburgh, UK) is a bench model that simulates ultrasound- or fluoroscopic-controlled percutaneous renal access. This model also allows for percutaneous nephrostomy tract dilation, stone extraction, or fragmentation and nephrostomy tube placement.

The main advantage of the material-based models is that they allow the trainee to practice with actual endoscopic instruments used clinically in the model platform, mimicking the in vivo scenario. However, these models require the availability of other equipment such as the endoscopes, guidewires, catheters, stone baskets, grasping devices, and lithotripsy equipment for a complete training experience. The role of a dedicated, expert educator should also be factored into the initial stages of training to ensure the proper acquisition of the endourologic skills. The disadvantages of these model-based learning formats are the expense of the maintenance of the fragile endoscopes, replacement of the ancillary equipment, and the time the expert surgeon dedicates to providing feedback and guidance to the trainee. In addition, these models lack the realism of the reaction of normal tissue to the instrument manipulation, such as bleeding.[71,72]

48.5 Animals

Animal models have played a critical role in the field of medical research and surgical practice historically.[32,73] They have been used extensively to develop new surgical techniques and provide trainees with the necessary platform for expansion of skills. The advantage of using an anesthetized and ventilated animal model is that it allows realistic tissue conditions that more accurately simulate the human patient in terms of respect for handling tissues, issues of haptic feedback, anatomic relations, as well as bleeding and respiratory movements.[74]

Several animal models have been used to simulate the human anatomy. Although there are certain differences between animals and human anatomy, the porcine kidneys have been considered to most closely replicate that of the human for endourologic procedures.[75] Sampaio and colleagues have described in detail the differences between the porcine kidney and the human kidney.[75,76] The porcine kidney is slightly smaller and has a greater number of calices and intrarenal arteries compared to the human kidney. It also lacks the perinephric fat, which increases the pig kidney's mobility and poses further challenge to the training endourologist. The pig urinary tract has been used as an endourologic model because it is structurally and functionally similar to the human urinary tract.[77–80] This model has been used to train many procedures including shock-wave lithotripsy, percutaneous renal access procedures, and ureteroscopic procedures.

Biological bench models simulating percutaneous renal access surgery using pig kidneys have been described. Hammond and colleagues describe the use of porcine

kidneys containing pre-implanted artificial calculi inside intact chicken carcasses to simulate percutaneous nephrolithotomy using fluoroscopy.[40] Resident trainees subjected to this training format submitted anonymous questionnaires, and all the participants rated the exercise as worthwhile for improving comfort level with the procedures. Similarly, Strohmaier and colleagues utilized pig kidneys with intact ureters embedded in silicone to allow ultrasound-guided percutaneous renal access.[70] The researchers noted that simulation of all flexible and rigid endourologic techniques was possible with this model, which also provided a more realistic tissue handling than nonbiological models. Neither of these models has been rigorously validated, and comparisons to nonbiological models remained to be performed.

The main disadvantage of using live animals is the cost associated with this training model due to the handling and housing of the animals and the need for highly skilled personnel for intra-operative management. Possible bovine spongiform encephalopathy (BSE) contamination of health care workers has led some countries, such as Canada and Great Britain, to prohibit the use of animals for medical training programs.[54,81–84] However, it should be noted that the standardization of regulations for animal care, and supervision of animal facilities can minimize risks and maximize the opportunity of learning through this important teaching strategy.

An alternative to the living anesthetized animal has been utilization of a harvested animal organ, such as the pig kidney, to simulate the anatomic conditions of a defined procedure. The organ can in turn be modified by perfusing with a colored irrigant to provide the trainee a simulated experience with perfusion requiring attention to hemostasis.[85] The advantages of such a modification are its low cost, simplicity, availability, absence of anesthesia care, and minimization of ethical issues related to live animal use.

48.6 Cadaveric Anatomic Materials

Cadavers, whether fresh or embalmed, offer a very realistic surgical training environment and have been used for centuries to teach human anatomy. Cadavers have also been used as teaching models for endourologic procedures such as ureteroscopy and transurethral resection of the prostate.[86–91] While providing a realistic anatomic model, the cadaver eliminates the need for anesthesia care and there are no time constraints during the period of training.[92] The procedure can be performed similar to the clinical situation but is limited by the absence of bleeding and may be influenced by changes in the haptic feedback. The potential risk of transmission of communicable diseases is a concern when working with human cadavers and therefore requires the same protective procedures as clinical endourology.[93] Human cadaveric models may be limited in supply and may have associated legal and ethical issues in some societies. Different cultures and countries may have different views regarding the use of human cadavers for teaching and research purposes.[94] However, willed body donation is one of the most significant contributions to medical education and at all times donated tissues should be maintained with respect and utilized with only informed consent.[95]

48.7 Simulators for Teaching Endourology

Surgical simulation is increasingly playing a significant role in teaching surgical skills proficiency. This teaching strategy has been shown to aid in the acquisition of surgical skills, allow for objective assessment of trainees, and improve the ability to evaluate trainees' readiness for different levels of clinical responsibility.[96–98]

Several cystoscopic and ureteroscopic virtual reality simulators are currently available commercially. The best-studied urologic simulator is the UroMentor™ (Simbionix USA, Cleveland, Oh) (Fig. 48.4), a Windows-based virtual reality ureteroscopy simulator. Several investigators have independently tested groups of inexperienced medical students who were randomized to training or no training on the UroMentor and showed that the trained group outperformed the untrained group by both objective and subjective measures, thereby establishing face, content, and concurrent validity.[26,99] Construct validity was subsequently confirmed by Jacomides and colleagues who compared the performance of 16

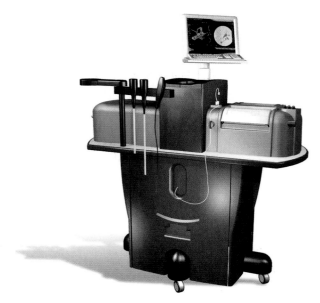

Fig. 48.4 UroMentor™ by Simbionix USA Corp., Cleveland, OH (Image courtesy of Simbionix)

medical students trained on the UroMentor with 16 VR-naïve urology residents and showed that the VR-trained students performed comparable to first year urology residents when tested on a UroMentor clinical scenario and that task completion times for the residents correlated inversely with their year of training.[23] Ogan and associates confirmed concurrent and predictive validity of the UroMentor by comparing the performance of VR-trained medical students with that of untrained residents during ureteroscopy in a cadaver model.[9] Student performance, but not resident performance, on the simulator correlated strongly with performance on the cadaver by some of the objective and subjective measures. Resident cadaver performance correlated strongly with level of training. The authors concluded that performance on the UroMentor can predict performance in the operating room for novices, but for more experienced endoscopists, clinical training and experience outweigh the contribution of VR training to overall operative proficiency.

Further study by Matsumo and colleagues compared the UroMentor to a previously validated high-fidelity bench trainer (Uro-Scopic Trainer) for the assessment of endourologic skills.[68] Urology residents of varying postgraduate years were assessed on their ability to perform endourologic tasks using a global rating scale. Senior residents scored significantly higher than junior residents and required less time to complete the VR simulator tasks. These researchers concluded that the performance on the VR simulator was comparable to performance on the high-fidelity bench model and that the UroMentor ureteroscopy simulator was a useful tool for the assessment of resident performance.

Recently, Reich and colleagues reported on a high-level VR simulator specifically designed for endourology procedures of the lower urinary tract.[100] The Uro-Trainer™ (Karl Storz, Gmb H Tuttlingen, Germany) features virtual reality images derived from digital video footage of hundreds of endourologic procedures. The authors note the potential benefit of this simulator for the teaching of lower urinary tract procedures as compared to the UroMentor, which focuses primarily on the upper urinary tract procedures. The Uro-Trainer provides the choice of four optical endoscopes (0°, 30°, 70°, and 120°) with realistic force feedback. Bleeding is responsive to fluid flow and blood loss can be recorded. Multiple procedures may be performed utilizing a variety of tools such as resection loops and laser fibers. During training, objective data such as percentage of bladder mucosa inspected, percentage of lesions treated, and blood loss are recorded. In this study, which included 24 medical students and 12 residents, exposure to the Uro-Trainer improved the performance of all groups, with more experienced participants showing greater aptitude, thus demonstrating construct validity. Further validation studies using the Uro-Trainer have been proposed.

Virtual reality simulation of percutaneous renal access has been demonstrated with the PercMentor™ (Simbionix USA,

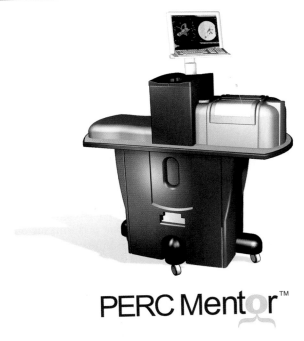

Fig. 48.5 PercMentor™ by Simbionix USA Corp., Cleveland, OH (Image courtesy of Simbionix)

faculty clinicians through the number of caseloads, intra-operative assessment, or recorded videos.[102] The limitations of these methods of assessment are susceptibility to subjectivity and possible bias since most faculty assessors are not specifically trained as evaluators. They may commit a "central tendency error" and not utilize the entire scale when evaluating resident performance. The assessment can also be influenced by the evaluators' overall impression of the trainee and may be further influenced by recall bias.[9]

Surgical simulation will play an important adjunct to traditional methods of education, especially in the formative and maintenance aspects of surgical proficiency.[86,95,103,104] As different clinical scenarios are being created, surgical simulation may eventually be used to evaluate clinical judgment of a trainee during testing of surgical skills performance. With computer-based surgical simulation, a trainee may be truly evaluated objectively in the absence of bias for race, sex, or age.[105,106] After establishing the content, construct, and predictive validity of the various simulators, these may be used in the future as part of the selection process of candidates for surgical training programs, assessment of trainees during their surgical training course, and as part of the certification and recertification process.[107–110]

Cleveland, OH) (Fig. 48.5). This percutaneous renal access simulator consists of a mannequin representing the human flank including simulated skin and palpable ribs. The access needle is designed so that its passage through the abdominal wall can be performed under simulated fluoroscopic guidance with real-time feedback including fluoroscopy times used, the ability to perform retrograde or antegrade pyelography, needle aspiration, and rotation of the C-arm. A computer interface provides multiple learning tasks designed to guide the student through components such as accessing various calices, passage of guidewires, and use of ureteral catheters to assist with guidewire passage. Face, content, and concurrent validity of the simulator have been established by Knudsen and colleagues who showed that inexperienced medical students and residents randomized to training on the PercMentor outperformed controls in a VR-case scenario by subjective and objective criteria.[9] The PercMentor-trained students and residents obtained percutaneous renal access in a porcine model faster and more accurately than their untrained counterparts, thereby demonstrating concurrent and predictive validity.[101]

48.9 Conclusions

Surgical simulation will not replace the need for well-designed, comprehensive educational curricula or reduce the importance of dedicated and committed educators, but will enhance and complement these efforts. The integration of simulation into the surgical training curriculum will allow the trainee to acquire the basic surgical skills foundation and attain performance levels according to predetermined proficiency levels for each stage of the training program. This will then allow the surgeon educator to concentrate on teaching residents the judgment and professionalism of being an expert surgeon, and strengthen the knowledge and interpretation of what is observed in the clinical setting in order to create a competent surgeon at both the cognitive and skills performance levels. Simulation must be used within an effective learning environment, underpinned by knowledge and professional attitudes.[47]

48.8 Assessment and Maintenance of Certification

Assessment of surgical competence has been based traditionally on evaluations of the trainee by senior surgeons or

References

1. Wallack M, Chao L. Resident work hours: the evolution of a revolution. *Arch Surg.* 2001;136(12):1426-1431.
2. Greenfield L. Limiting resident duty hours. *Am J Surg.* 2003;185(1): 10-12.
3. Matsumoto E, Hamstra S, Radomski S, et al. A novel approach to endourological training: training at the Surgical Skills Center. *J Urol.* 2001;166(4):1261-1266.

4. Anastakis D, Wanzel K, Brown M, et al. Evaluating the effectiveness of a 2-year curriculum in a surgical skills center. *Am J Surg*. 2003;185(4):378-385.

5. Dubrowski A, Backstein D. The contributions of kinesiology to surgical education. *J Bone Joint Surg Am*. 2004;86-A(12): 2778-2781.

6. Krizek T. Ethics and philosophy lecture: surgery…Is it an impairing profession? *J Am Coll Surg*. 2002;194(3):352-366.

7. Kopta J. The development of motor skills in orthopaedic education. *Clin Orthop*. 1971;75:80.

8. Khan M, Tiernan W. The increasing significance of how to learn motor skills. *Int J Surg*. 2004;2(2):124-125.

9. Knudsen B, Matsumoto E, Chew B, et al. Randomized, controlled, prospective study validating the acquisition of percutaneous renal collecting system access skills using a computer based hybrid virtual reality surgical simulator: phase I. *J Urol*. 2006;176(5): 2173-2178.

10. Chou D, Abdelshehid C, Clayman R, et al. Comparison of results of virtual-reality simulator and training model for basic ureteroscopy training. *J Endourol*. 2006;20(4):266-271.

11. Bridges M, Diamond D. The financial impact of teaching surgical residents in the operating room. *Am J Surg*. 1999;177(1):28-32.

12. Schneider J, Coyle J, Ryan E, et al. Implementation and evaluation of a new surgical residency model. *J Am Coll Surg*. 2007;205(3): 393-404.

13. Leape L. Error in medicine. *JAMA*. 1994;272(23):1851-1857.

14. Nuland S. Mistakes in the operating room: error and responsibility. *N Engl J Med*. 2004;351(13):1281-1283.

15. Way L. General surgery in evolution: technology and competence. *Am J Surg*. 1996;171(1):2-9.

16. Kohn L, Corrigan J, Donaldson M. *To err is human: building a safer health system*. Washington: National Academies Press; 2000.

17. Oliak D, Owens M, Schmidt H. Impact of fellowship training on the learning curve for laparoscopic gastric bypass. *Obes Surg*. 2004;14:197-200.

18. Corica F, Boker J, Chou D, et al. Short-term impact of a laparoscopic "mini-residency" experience on postgraduate urologists' practice patterns. *J Am Coll Surg*. 2006;203(5):692-8.

19. Vlaovic P, McDougall E. New age beyond didactics. *Sci World J*. 2006;6:2370-2380.

20. Morrison K, MacNeily A. Core competencies in surgery: evaluating the goals of urology residency training in Canada. *Can J Surg*. 2006;49(4):259-266.

21. Nicolaou M, Atallah L, James A, et al. The effect of depth perception on visual-motor compensation in minimal invasive surgery. *Lect Notes Comput Sci*. 2006;4091:156-163.

22. Rassweiler J, Fornara P, Weber M, et al. Laparoscopic nephrectomy: the experience of the laparoscopy working group of the German Urologic Association. *J Urol*. 1998;160(1):18-21.

23. Jacomides L, Ogan L, Cadeddu J, et al. Use of a virtual reality simulator for ureteroscopy training. *J Urol*. 2004;171(1): 320-323.

24. Daniels G, Garnett J, Carter M. Ureteroscopic results and complications: experience with 130 cases. *J Urol*. 1988;139(4):710-713.

25. de la Rosette J, Gravas S, Muschter R, et al. Present practice and development of minimally invasive techniques, imaging and training in european urology: results of a survey of the European Society of Uro-Technology (ESUT). *Eur Urol*. 2003;44(3): 346-351.

26. Watterson J, Beiko D, Kuan J, et al. A randomized prospective blinded study validating acqustion of ureteroscopy skills using a computer based virtual reality endourological simulator. *J Urol*. 2002;168(5):1928-1932.

27. Ballaro A, Briggs T, Garcia-Montes F, et al. A computer generated interactive transurethral prostatic resection simulator. *J Urol*. 1999;162(5):1633-1635.

28. Aydeniz B, Meyer A, Posten J, et al. The 'HysteroTrainer'—an in vitro simulator for hysteroscopy and fallopscopy. Experimental and clinical background and technical realisation including the development of organ modules for electrothermal treatment. *Contrib Gynecol Obstet*. 2000;20:171-181.

29. Berg D, Raugi G, Gladstone H, et al. Virtual reality simulators for dermatologic surgery: measuring their validity as a teaching tool. *Dermatol Surg*. 2001;27(4):370-374.

30. Bro-Nielsen M, Tasto J, Cunningham R, et al. PreOp endoscopic simulator: a PC-based immersive training system for bronchoscopy. *Stud Health Technol Inform*. 1999;62:76-82.

31. Edmond C, Heskamp D, Sluis D, et al. ENT endoscopic surgical training simulator. *Stud Health Technol Inform*. 1997;39:518-528.

32. Martin J, Regehr G, Reznick R, et al. Objective structured assessment of technical skills (OSATS) for surgical residents. *Br J Surg*. 1997;84(2):273-278.

33. Schmidt R. A schema theory of discrete motor skills learning. *Psycho Rev*. 1975;82:225-260.

34. Steinberg P, Merguerian P, Bihrie I, et al. The cost of learning robotic-assisted prostatectomy. *Urology* 2008; Epub ahead of print.

35. Steers W, Schaeffer A. Is it time to change the training of urology residents in the United States? *J Urol*. 2005;173(5):1451.

36. Martin R, Kehdy F, Allen J. Formal training in advanced surgical technologies enhances the surgical residency. *Am J Surg*. 2005;190(2): 244-248.

37. Chaudhry A, Sutton C, Wood J, et al. Learning rate for laparoscopic surgical skills on MIST VR, a virtual reality simulator: quality of human-computer interface. *Ann R Coll Surg Engl*. 1999;81(4):281-286.

38. Grillo H. To impart this art: the development of graduate surgical education in the United States. *Surgery*. 1999;125(1):1-14.

39. Gawande A. Creating the educated surgeon in the 21st century. *Am J Surg*. 2001;181(6):551-556.

40. Hammond DL, Ketchum J, Schwatz B. Accreditation council on graduate medical education technical skills competency compliance: urologic surgical skills. *J Am Coll Surg*. 2005;201(3):454-457.

41. Smith A. A personal perspective on the origins of endourology and the endourological society. *J Endourol*. 2002;16(10):705-708.

42. Kommu S, Dickinson A, Rane A. Optimizing outcomes in laparoscopic urologic training: toward a standardized global consensus. *J Endourol*. 2007;21(4):378-385.

43. Chung B, Matin S, Ost M, et al. Fellowship in endourology, the job search, and setting up a successful practice: an insider's view. *J Endourol*. 2008;22(3):551-557.

44. Brehmer M, Tolley D. Validation of a bench model for endoscopic surgery in the upper urinary tract. *Eur Urol*. 2002;42(2):175-179.

45. Dunnington G, Williams R. Addressing the new competencies for residents' surgical training. *Acad Med*. 2003;78(1):14-21.

46. Heard J, Allen R, Clardy J. Assessing the needs of residency program directors to meet the ACGME general competencies. *Acad Med*. 2002;77(7):750.

47. Wignall GR, Denstedt JD, Preminger GM, et al. Surgical simulation: a urological perspective. *J Urol*. 2008;179(5):1690-1699.

48. Edison M, Horgan S, Helton W. Using small-group workshops to improve surgical residents' technical skills. *Acad Med*. 2001;76(5): 557-558.

49. Goldman L, McDonough M, Rosemond G. Stresses affecting surgical performance and learning: I. Correlation of heart rate, electrocardiogram, and operation simultaneously recorded on videotapes. *J Surg Res*. 1972;12(2):83-86.

50. Mongin C, Dufour F, Lattanzio F, et al. Evaluation of stress in surgical trainees: prospective study of heart rate during laparoscopic cholecystectomy. *J Chir(Paris)*. 2008;145(2):138-142.

51. Hoznek A, Salamon L, de la Taille A, et al. Simulation training in video-assisted urologic surgery. *Curr Urol Rep*. 2006;7(2): 107-113.

52. Gawande AA. Creating the educated surgeon in the 21st century. *Am J Surg*. 2001;181:551-556.

53. Ericsson K. The road to excellence: the acquisition of expert performance in the arts and sciences, sports, and games. In: Ericsson KA, ed. *The Acquisition of Expert Performance: An Introduction to Some of the Issues*. Mahwah: Lawrence Erlbaum; 1996:1-50.

54. Hoznek A, Katz R, Gettman M, et al. Laparoscopic and robotic surgical training in urology. *Curr Urol Rep*. 2003;4(2):130-137.

55. Lancaster J, Casali J. Investigating pilot performance using mixed-modality simulated data link. *Hum Factors*. 2008;50(2):182-193.

56. Schmidt C, Ramsauer B, Witzel K. Risk management in hospitals: standard operating procedures in aviation as a model for structuring medical communication. *Z Orthop Unfall*. 2008;146(2):175-178.

57. Miller D, Montie J, Faerber G. Evaluating the Accreditation Council on Graduate Medical Education core clinical competencies techniques and feasibility in a urology training program. *J Urol*. 2003;170(4):1312-1317.

58. Edison M, Horgan S, Helton W. Using small-group workshops to improve surgical residents' technical skills. *Acad Med*. 2001;76(5):557-558.

59. Rouach Y, Timsit M, Delongchamps N. Laparoscopic partial nephrectomy: urology resident learning curve on a porcine model. *Prog Urol*. 2008;18(6):344-350.

60. Artibani W, Fracalanza S, Cavalleri S, et al. Learning curve and preliminary experience with da Vinci-assisted laparoscopic radical prostatectomy. *Urol Int*. 2008;80(3):237-244.

61. Haluck R, Krummel T. Computers and virtual reality for surgical education in the 21st century. *Arch Surg*. 2000;135(7):786-792.

62. Gates E. New surgical procedures: Can our patients benefit while we learn? *Am J Obstet Gynecol*. 1997;176:1293-1298.

63. Witzke D, Hoskins J, Mastrangelo M, et al. Immersive virtual reality used as a platform for perioperative training for surgical residents. *Stud Health Technol Inform*. 2001;81:577-583.

64. Brehmer M, Tolley D. Validation of a bench model for endoscopic surgery in the upper urinary tract. *Eur Urol*. 2002;42(2):175-189.

65. *Webster's Dictionary* (on-line); 2007.

66. Tanriverdi O, Boylu U, Kendirci M, et al. The learning curve in the training of percutaneous nephrolithotomy. *Eur Urol*. 2007;52(2):206-211.

67. Matsumoto E, Hamstra S, Radomski S, et al. The effect of bench model fidelity on endourological skills: a randomised controlled study. *J Urol*. 2002;167(2):1243-1247.

68. Matsumoto E, Pace K, Honey R. Virtual reality ureteroscopy simulator as a valid tool for assessing endourological skills. *Int J Urol*. 2006;13(7):896-901.

69. Bird VG, Fallon B, Winfield HN. Practice patterns in the treatment of large renal stones. *J Endourol*. 2003;17(6):355-363.

70. Strohmaier W, Giese A. Ex vivo training model for percutaneous renal surgery. *Urol Res*. 2005;33(3):191-193.

71. Oppenheimer P, Gupta A, Weghorst S, et al. The representation of blood flow in endourologic surgical simulations. *Stud Health Technol Inform*. 2001;81:365-371.

72. Strohmaier W, Giese A. Porcine urinary tract as a training model for ureterorenoscopy. *Urol Int*. 2001;66(1):30-32.

73. Zimmermann M. Ethical considerations in relation to pain in animal experimentation. *Acta Physiol Scand Suppl*. 1986;554:221-233.

74. Rowan A. Is justification of animal research necessary? *JAMA*. 1993;269(9):1113-1114.

75. Sampaio F, Pereira-Sampaio M, Favorito L. The pig kidney as an endourologic model: anatomic contribution. *J Endourol*. 1998;12(1):45-50.

76. Pereira-Sampaio M, Favorito L, Sampaio F. Pig kidney: anatomical relationships between the intrarenal arteries and the kidney collecting system: applied study for urological research and surgical training. *J Urol*. 2004;172(5):2077-2081.

77. Evan A, Willis L, Connors B, et al. Shock wave lithotripsy induced renal injury. *Am J Kidney Dis*. 1991;179(4):445-450.

78. Evan A, Connors B, Lingeman J, et al. Branching patterns of the renal artery of the pig. *Anat Rec*. 1996;246(2):217-223.

79. Watkin N, Morris S, Rivens I, et al. High-intensity focused ultrasound ablation of the kidney in a large animal model. *J Endourol*. 1997;11(3):191-196.

80. McDougall E. Validation of surgical simulators. *J Endourol*. 2007;21(3):244-247.

81. Cheong J. The use of animals in medical education: a question of necessity vs. desirability. *Theor Med*. 1989;10(1):53-57.

82. English D. Using animals for the training of physicians and surgeons. *Theor Med*. 1989;10(1):43-52.

83. Self D. The use of animals in medical education and research. *Theor Med*. 1989;10(1):9-19.

84. Scharmann W, Teutsch G. Ethical considerations on animal experiments. *ALTEX*. 1994;11(4):191-198.

85. Laguna M, Hatzinger M, Rassweiler J. Simulators and endourological training. *Curr Opin Urol*. 2002;12(3):209-215.

86. Pirkmajer B, Leusch G. A bladder-prostate model on which to practice using transurethral resection instruments. *Urologe A*. 1977;16(6):336-338.

87. Habib H, Berger J, Winter C. Teaching transurethral surgery using a cow's udder. *J Urol*. 1965;93:77-79.

88. Narwani K, Reid E. Teaching transurethral surgery using cadaver bladder. *J Urol*. 1969;101(1):101.

89. Fiddian R. A method of training in periurethral resection. *Br J Urol*. 1967;39(2):192-193.

90. Cervantes L, Keitzer W. Endoscopic training in urology. *J Urol*. 1960;84:585-586.

91. Trindale J, Lauenschlager M, de Araujo C. Endoscopic surgery: a new teaching method. *J Urol*. 1981;126(2):192.

92. Ogan K, Jacomides L, Shulman M, et al. Virtual ureteroscopy predicts ureteroscopic proficiency of medical students on a cadaver. *J Urol*. 2004;172(2):667-671.

93. Wines MP, Lamb A, Argyropoulos AN, et al. Blood splash injury: an underestimated risk in endourology. *J Endourol*. 2008;22(6):1183-1187.

94. Anderson R, O'Hare M, Balls M, et al. The availability of human tissue for biomedical research: the report and recommendations of the ECVAM workshop 32. *Altern Lab Anim*. 1998;26(6):763-777.

95. Gordinier M, Granai C, Jackson N, et al. The effects of a course in cadaver dissection on resident knowledge of pelvic anatomy: an experimental study. *Obstet Gynecol*. 1995;86(1):137-139.

96. Issenberg S, McGaghie W, Hart I, et al. Simulation technology for health care professional skills training and assessment. *JAMA*. 1999;282(9):861-866.

97. Anastakis D, Regehr G, Reznick R, et al. Assessment of technical skills transfer from the bench training model to the human model. *Am J Surg*. 1999;177(2):167-170.

98. Darzi A, Smith S, Taffinder N. Assessing operative skill. *BMJ*. 1999;318(7188):887-888.

99. Wilhelm DM, Ogan K, Roehrborn CG, et al. Assessment of basic ndoscopic performance using virtual reality simulator. *J Am Coll Surg*. 2002;195:675.

100. Reich O, Noll U, Gratzke C, et al. High-level virtual reality simulator for endourologic procedures of lower urinary tract. *Urology*. 2006;67:1144.

101. Margulis V, Matsumoto E, Knudsen B, et al. Percutaneous renal collecting system access: can virtual reality training shorten the learning curve? *J Urol suppl*. 2005;173:315. Abstract 1162.

102. Accreditation Council for Graduate Medical Education. *Urology Residency Case Log Report*. Chicago: ACGME; 2004.

103. de la Rosette J, Laguna M, Rassweiler J, et al. Training in percutaneous nephrolithotomy—a critical review. *Eur Urol* 2008; Epub ahead of print.

104. Tanriverdi O, Boylu U, Kendirci M, et al. The learning curve in the training of percutaneous nephrolithotomy. *Eur Urol.* 2007;52(1): 206-211.

105. Aucar J, Groch N, Troxel S, et al. A review of surgical simulation with attention to validation methodology. *Surg Laparosc Endosc Percutan Tech.* 2005;15(2):82-89.

106. Michel M, Knoll T, Kohrmann K, et al. The URO Mentor: development and evaluation of a new computer-based interactive training system for virtual life-like simulation of diagnostic and therapeutic endourological procedures. *BJU Int.* 2002;89(3):174-177.

107. Gallagher A, Ritter E, Satava R. Fundamental principles of validation, and reliability: rigorous science for the assessment of surgical education and training. *Surg Endosc.* 2003;17(10):1525-1529.

108. McDougall E, Corica F, Boket J, et al. Construct validity testing of a laparoscopic surgical simulator. *J Am Coll Surg.* 2006;202(5): 779-787.

109. Nedas T, Challacombe B, Dasgupta P. Virtual reality in urology. *BJU Int.* 2004;94(3):255-257.

110. Satava R. Historical review of surgical simulation- a personal perspective. *World J Surg.* 2008;32(2):141-148.

Abstract   In the age of shock wave lithotripsy and endoscopic stone therapy (percutaneous nephrolithotomy and retrograde [flexible] ureterorenoscopy), open stone surgery is only rarely performed and the indications are limited to a very low number of selected cases. In centers offering all stone treatment modalities, open stone removing procedures constitute around 1–5% of all procedures. However, despite that most situations can be handled by minimally invasive treatment, open stone surgery is still mandatory in special cases. It is therefore absolutely necessary that the skills of open stone removing procedures do not completely fall into oblivion. This chapter reviews current indications for open stone surgery and gives an overview on the applied techniques.

49.1 Introduction

During the last 30 years, the growing importance of minimally invasive treatment modalities has dramatically diminished the role of open stone surgery. Since the introduction of shock wave lithotripsy (SWL) and the endoscopic techniques of percutaneous nephrolithotomy (PNL) and retrograde (flexible) ureterorenoscopy (URS), very rare cases require open surgical stone removal. An analysis of US Medicare data revealed a decrease in open stone surgery from 12.5% in 1988 to 2% in 2000.[1] Other studies from Western centers report similar rates ranging from 1–5%.[2–5] In our institution, 26 open stone removing procedures were performed in the last 10 years, accounting for 0.4% of all stone-related procedures. In contrast to that, in developing countries with a high incidence of urolithiasis, the rate of open stone removal may still be higher. A recent survey from Pakistan reported an incidence of 26% for open stone surgery in the years 1987 to 1995, decreasing to 8% in the years 1996–1998.[6]

In 1979, the term "endourology" has been defined as "closed controlled manipulation within the genitourinary tract"[7] and summarizes most minimally invasive urological procedures. In times of increasing specialization, this development has led to dedicated "endourologists," who specialize in minimally invasive urinary tract stone treatment but may lack the skills to perform open stone removing procedures. This development creates potential problems. Although open stone surgery has become rare in most urological centers, it still is mandatory in special cases and even centers specializing in minimally invasive stone therapy report incidences of open stone surgery between 1% and 5%.[2–5] To be able to offer an adequate treatment to those selected patients, it is crucial that the techniques of open stone removal must not completely fall into oblivion. It is therefore desirable to train the new-generation urologists, who grew up with minimally invasive techniques, in the skill of open stone surgery. As patient numbers for open stone removal are low, this is often difficult to achieve in practice. In a recent survey, more than 90% of younger urologists (aged 30–40 years) considered themselves adequately trained in minimally invasive procedures, whereas only 55% considered themselves properly trained for open stone surgery. In contrast to that, almost all polled urologists older than 50 years were adequately trained in open stone removing procedures but lacked training in minimally invasive procedures during their residency.[8]

In this chapter, current indications and techniques of open stone surgery are reviewed and described.

49.2 Indications for Open Stone Surgery

Whereas open stone removal constituted a standard procedure until the 1980s, the introduction of shock wave lithotripsy and endourological techniques has limited the indications to exceptional cases today. Several contemporary studies report

P. Alken (✉)
Department of Urology, University Clinic Mannheim,
Heidelberg Medical School, Mannheim, Germany
e-mail: peter.alken@umm.de

P.N. Rao et al. (eds.), *Urinary Tract Stone Disease*,
DOI 10.1007/978-1-84800-362-0_49, © Springer-Verlag London Limited 2011

a rate of open stone surgery in interventional stone treatment to range from 1–5%.[2–5] Depending on the series, various reasons for open stone removal can be found.

In our institution, 26 open stone removal procedures were performed in the last 10 years, making up for 0.4% of all stone-related procedures. Indications were complete or partial staghorn stones (11 cases), concomitant open surgery for ureteropelvic junction obstruction, symptomatic renal cysts or tumors (6 cases), non-functioning stone-bearing lower poles requiring partial nephrectomy (3 cases), the desire to facilitate future stone passages in cystine stone formers receiving ileum-ureter replacement (2 cases), multiple stones in peripheral calyces (2 cases), a ventral diverticulum stone and failed minimally invasive procedures in 1 case, respectively.

In other series, main indications for open stone surgery included complex stone burden (55%), failed SWL or endourological procedures (29%), anatomical abnormalities like ureteropelvic junction obstruction, infundibular stenosis or renal caliceal diverticulum (24%), morbid obesity (10%) and comorbid medical diseases (7%).[5] Another series reported calculi in anterior caliceal diverticula (29%), large volume stones in non-functioning lower pole regions (29%), extremely large volume staghorn stones associated with infundibular stenosis (29%), and failed endoscopic interventions (14%) as indications for open stone removal.[4] Buchholz and colleagues reported among their open surgical cases nephrectomy for non-functioning stone-bearing kidney in 54%, Psoas-Hitch or Boari plasty in 23%, simultaneous pyeloplasty for ureteropelvic junction obstruction in 15%, and emergency nephrectomy for severe bleeding after PNL in 8%.[2]

The clinical guidelines by the European Association of Urology (EAU) and the American Urological Association (AUA) recommend either PNL or SWL or a combination for most renal stones, whereas indication for open stone removal is limited to very selected cases.[9,10]

Reviewing the EAU and AUA guidelines for open stone removal may be used in the following cases:

- *Complex stone burden* with a large stone mass in peripheral calices requiring multiple access tracts in a percutaneous approach or multiple staged procedures (see Fig. 49.1a, b)
- *Treatment failure* with SWL or endourological procedures
- *Patient choice* in complex stones preferring a single procedure over anticipated multiple minimally invasive procedures
- *Intrarenal anatomical abnormalities* requiring surgical correction or hampering endourological access like stones in caliceal diverticula (especially in an anterior calyx), ureteropelvic junction stricture, or infundibular stenosis
- *Concomittant open surgery*; for example, for renal tumors, symptomatic cysts, or ureteropelvic junction obstruction
- *Stones in ectopic or transplanted kidneys* where minimally invasive procedures may be difficult or impossible because of risk of damaging neighboring structures
- *Large stone burden in children* because of difficult endourological access to small sized anatomy, easy surgical access, and reducing the need to only one anesthetic procedure

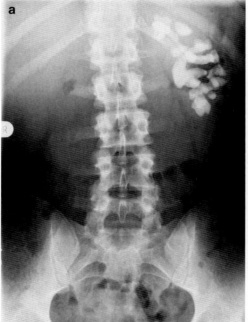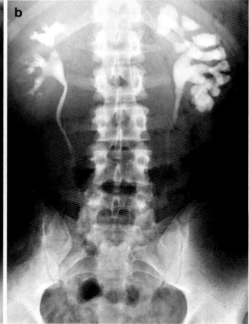

Fig. 49.1 (**a**) IVP of a patient with a large staghorn stone in the left kidney. (**b**) The relatively small central and large peripheral stone mass favors open stone removal as a percutaneous approach would require multiple access tracts and probably multiple staged procedures

Table 49.1 Current indications for open stone surgery

Major stone mass in multiple peripheral calices with narrow infundibula
Treatment failure of minimally invasive procedures
Patient choice preferring a single procedure to multiple minimally invasive procedures
Anatomical anomalies requiring surgical correction or hampering endourological access
Stones in ectopic or transplanted kidneys hampering endoscopic access
Morbid obesity (relative)
Concomitant open surgery
Large stone burden in children
Limited experience or limited access to minimally invasive techniques
Significant loss of renal function demanding partial or total nephrectomy

- Morbid obesity
- *Skeletal deformity*, like contractures or fixed deformities of hips or legs, hampering endourological access
- *Extent or complete loss of renal function* requiring partial or total nephrectomy
- *Limited experience or limited access* to minimally invasive techniques

Several of the aforementioned indications have to be regarded only as relative as percutaneous stone removal can be successfully performed in morbidly obese patients and those with ectopic, horseshoe, or transplanted kidneys.[11–13] Furthermore, children can be sufficiently treated by minimally invasive procedures in most cases,[14] and departments with limited experience with PNL should rather refer patients to more experienced centers than denying them the minimally invasive treatment option. Stones in anterior calyceal diverticula can be treated either minimally invasive by flexible URS or in a laparoscopic approach in most cases.[15–17]

Current indications for open stone surgery are listed in Table 49.1.

49.3 Preoperative Diagnostics

Besides assessing medical history and administering a thorough physical examination, the following diagnostic procedures should be performed prior to surgery to assess the exact stone mass and localization, renal anatomy, and function.

49.3.1 Sonography

By using an abdominal scanner, information about the renal anatomy, stone size, and localization as well as relation to neighboring organs can be obtained. Measuring the diameter of the renal parenchyma may give hints on the renal function as a chronic renal insufficiency leads to a reduction in the parenchymal diameter. An obstruction of the collecting system can be diagnosed as well as anatomical anomalies like ectopic kidneys, malrotation, horseshoe kidneys, cysts, or tumors.

49.3.2 Plain X-ray and Intravenous Urography

The combination of plain X-ray and intravenous (IV) urography gives information on the exact intrarenal stone localization, obstruction, and anatomical anomalies of the collecting system.

49.3.3 CT Scan

A computed tomography (CT) scan is not routinely required for preoperative diagnostic workup but can be useful in special situations. In the case of multiple peripheral stones and overprojection on plain X-ray, a CT scan is helpful for exact localization of the stone mass. Furthermore, in case of poor visualization of the stones on plain X-ray due to stone composition (uric acid or cystine stones), morbid obesity, or other hampering factors like overlying bowel, a CT scan is the method of choice for stone detection. Also, in case of unclear findings in sonography, a CT scan can be helpful in identifying anatomical anomalies of the kidney or adjacent organs.

49.3.4 Scintigraphy

The split renal function with region of interest has to be obtained by MAG3 scintigraphy prior to surgery if partial or total nephrectomy is considered.

49.3.5 Urine Culture

An existing urinary tract infection should be ruled out by urine culture. If bacteriuria is present, antibiotic treatment should be initiated and surgery be delayed until the urine is sterile. In case of infection stones, it may not always be possible to obtain sterile urine. In this case, surgery should be undertaken under antibiotic protection.

Based on these diagnostic findings, the patient has to be informed about the planned procedure in detail. The informed consent has to include all possible procedure-related risks and alternative treatment options.

49.4 Surgical Techniques for Open Stone Removal

49.4.1 Approach

In most cases, a flank incision offers the best surgical approach for stone removal from the kidney. The appropriate surgical approach may be varied depending on the location of the stone mass, potential hampering neighboring structures, or concomitant surgery.

For the flank incision, the patient should be positioned in a lateral position and overstretched. The skin is incised above the 12th to 10th rib. In case of previous surgery, the incision should be made always one rib above the last incision.

The renal fascia (Gerota's fascia) is incised over the lateral convex surface of the kidney. Afterward the perirenal fatty tissue (capsula adiposa) is dissected down to the renal capsule from upper to lower pole. After separating the ventral fatty tissue from the kidney surface, the ureter is located and a vessel loop is placed around it. Starting from the ureter, the renal pelvis is dissected. If necessary, the fatty tissue is further removed until the kidney is completely exposed. The hilum vessels are carefully dissected and also encircled by vessel loops. Intraoperative radiography and/or sonography using a 7 MHz scanner is used for exact localization of the calculi.

Next, the stones can be removed by one or a combination of the techniques described as follows.

49.4.2 Cold Ischemia

Several surgical interventions such as partial nephrectomy, anatrophic nephrolitotomy, or multiple radial nephrotomies may require temporary occlusion of the renal artery. As ischemic conditions can lead to enhanced vasoconstriction, reduction of medullary blood flow, endothelial and tubular cell injury, and consecutive loss of renal function[18]; arterial occlusion should be avoided or kept to a minimum whenever possible. Animal studies have shown that ischemic intervals of up to 30 min can be tolerated without persistent loss of renal function.[19] But a kidney with already reduced function may be more susceptible to ischemia. Several basic techniques help to improve the tolerance to the ischemic period. It has been shown that closing the renal artery alone leads to less functional impairment than closing both the artery and the vein.[20] Intermittent clamping of the renal artery allowing short periods of recirculation should be avoided as this also leads to increased renal damage.[21]

Several other adjunctive measures that can easily be employed increase the tolerance to the ischemic condition. Optimal pre-ischemic renal perfusion is achieved by generous pre- and intraoperative hydration and avoidance of hypotension. Renal plasma flow and osmotic diuresis are increased by applying mannitol solution 15 min prior to initiating ischemia.[22] Furthermore, the renin angiotensin system is suppressed by administration of an angiotensin-converting-enzyme (ACE) inhibitor; for example, enalapril. This prevents vasospasm and reduces the post-ischemic vascular resistance at reperfusion. ACE inhibitors have been shown to reduce post-ischemic tubular necrosis and lead to higher glomerular filtration rates.[23]

If the anticipated ischemic period exceeds 30 min, local hypothermia is most effective in limiting renal damage and provides protection for up to several hours.[19,24] The lower temperature leads to reduced energy-dependent metabolic activity with consecutive reduced oxygen consumption and adenosine triphosphate breakdown.[25] Based on animal studies, the optimal temperature for in vivo hypothermia was found to be 15°C.[19] As this is often difficult to achieve during an operation, a renal core temperature of 20°C is generally accepted.

Intraoperative hypothermia of the kidney can be achieved by various techniques described in experimental or clinical situations varying from surface cooling in ice, vascular perfusion, collecting system irrigation, cooling coils or plates. The most widely used technique for applying hypothermia is surface cooling in slush ice because of its simplicity. Immediately after clamping the renal artery, the mobilized kidney is surrounded by a plastic bag in which sterile ice slush is placed. It is important to completely imbed the kidney for 15 min into the ice to achieve an adequate temperature of 15–20°C at the core. During the operation on the kidney, care should be taken not to free large areas from the ice slush so that rewarming does not occur and the risk of ischemic injury is kept low.

This technique requires puncture of the renal vein and artery distal to the occluding clamp. It offers the advantage of a rapid and uniform development of hypothermia in the whole kidney, whereas topical cooling with ice leads to irregular hypothermia with lower temperatures at the surface and less effect at the core. The latter technique or transarterial cooling via an angiography balloon catheter that is preoperatively placed in the renal artery by the radiologist under fluoroscopic control offers an improved preservation of renal function compared to topical slush ice hypothermia in a comparative study.[26]

Disadvantages of this approach include a greater invasiveness and more technical equipment. A modern application of this technique has been described by Janetscheck for laparoscopic partial kidney resection.[27] As topical cooling with slush ice is technically easier to achieve and produces good functional results, this technique is generally preferred in open surgery.

49.4.3 Simple Pyelolithotomy

Indication: Renal Pelvic Stone

The renal pelvis is incised transversely in a U-shaped form with a Potts scissors sparing the ureteropelvic junction.

The loop around the ureter prevents small stones from migrating into the ureter. The stones are withdrawn from the renal pelvis with forceps. After removing all accessible calculi, a flexible nephroscope can be inserted to inspect the collecting system and remove remaining stones. Alternatively, the "coagulum pyelolithotomy" has been described, in which a coagulum mixture is injected into the closed renal pelvis. There it forms a cast containing the stones and can be extracted via a pyelotomy. Thorough irrigation of the collecting system is required. An 8 F catheter can be passed down the ureter to ensure that it is clear of stones. A nephrostomy tube may be placed and brought out through the lower pole, but is not necessary in an uncomplicated procedure. The pyelotomy is closed with running 4–0 absorbable sutures.[27]

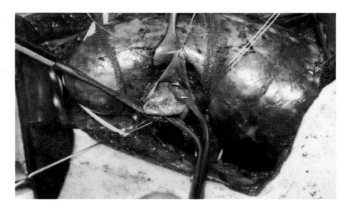

Fig. 49.3 Extended pyelolithotomy. Extraction of renal pelvic stone with stone forceps

49.4.4 Extended Pyelolithotomy (Gil-Vernet)

Indication: Staghorn Stones

For extended pyelolithotomy, complete mobilization of the kidney is necessary to control the renal artery and facilitate radiography. After removal of excess fatty tissue, the renal pelvis is completely dissected on the adventitia entering the renal hilum. The pelvis is separated bluntly from the hilum with moist cotton strips to expose the calyceal necks. The pelvis is then incised with Potts scissors in an open U-shape lengthened to reach the lowest and the highest calyx sparing the ureteropelvic junction (see Fig. 49.2). The stone is mobilized with stone hooks to free it from the pelvic urothelium and is pulled out with forceps under rotating movements (see Fig. 49.3). Where possible, the stone should be removed in a single piece. If necessary, the stone can be fragmented with cutting forceps, bone saw, or drill. Caliceal extensions of staghorn stones can be extracted with a rigid or flexible nephroscope. Radial nephrotomies (see below) may be used for complete stone removal if an extraction of caliceal stones with a nephroscope is not possible. After thorough irrigation of the collecting system, intraoperative radiography is used to document complete stone-free status. An 8 F catheter can be passed down the ureter to ensure that it is clear of stones. A nephrostomy tube may be placed and brought out through the lower pole, but is not necessary in an uncomplicated procedure. The pyelotomy is closed with running 4–0 absorbable sutures. For the complete removal of large staghorn stones with multiple caliceal extensions, it is often necessary to combine the extended pyelolithotomy with one or several radial nephrotomies.[27,28]

49.4.5 Pyelonephrolithotomy

Indication: Lower Caliceal Stone

After exposing the renal pelvis and vessels as described previously, an oblique incision extending into the infundibulum of the stone-bearing lower calyx is performed. The posterior segmental artery does not reach the lower pole, and the inferior segmental artery crosses the calyx neck at the ventral aspect from ventral to dorsal. Therefore, the renal parenchyma can be cut without damaging any relevant arterial blood vessels. The renal capsule over the infundibulum is incised and the parenchyma is bluntly separated with brain spatula or the knife handle. The pelvic incision is continued into the infundibulum and the affected calyx. After extracting the stone, bleeding vessels are ligated. After ensuring complete stone removal, the infundibulum and pelvis are closed with running 4–0 absorbable sutures.[27]

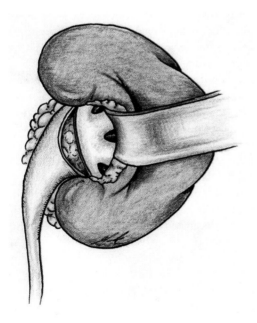

Fig. 49.2 Extended pyelolithotomy. The renal pelvis is dissected on the adventitia entering the renal hilum to expose the bases of the infundibula. The pelvis is incised in an open U-shape for stone removal

49.4.6 Anatrophic Nephrolithotomy

Indication: Staghorn Stones or Large Stone Mass Located in Multiple Peripheral Calices with Narrow Infundibula

As anatrophic nephrolithotomy requires clamping of the renal artery, hypothermia is always required to minimize renal injury (see Sect. 49.4.2). In this procedure, stone access is established by a renal longitudinal incision performed in an avascular area between the anterior and posterior arterial blood supply. As this demarcation line is very variable, it is necessary to identify the segment junction prior to the incision. Therefore, after complete exposure of the kidney and the renal vessels, the posterior segmental branch of the renal artery is clamped individually. Blanching of the posterior segment can be observed (see Fig. 49.4). Intravenous injection of methylene blue colors the remainder of the kidney and may so help to outline the incision area. The demarcation line between the ischemic and the blood-perfused area of the kidney surface is marked with a pen or the electrocauter.

After applying hypothermia and occluding the main renal artery, a longitudinal incision is performed in the previously identified area. The parenchyma is bluntly separated until the collecting system is reached. Depending on stone localization, the calices, the pelvis, or both are opened to extract the stones (see Fig. 49.5). If an extension of the initial incision is required, special attention has to be paid to the dorsal vessels crossing from dorsal to ventral at the cranial edge of the top calyx and from ventral to dorsal at the caudal edge of the lower calyx. Whenever possible, the stone should be extracted in a single piece. Intraoperative X-ray, sonography, or flexible

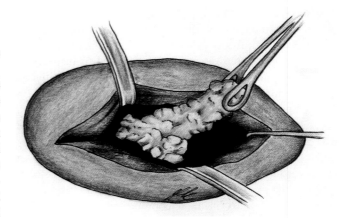

Fig. 49.5 Stone extraction via longitudinal anatrophic nephrolithotomy

nephroscopy is useful to check for complete stone removal. The collecting system is then closed with 5–0 absorbable sutures, and cut vessels are suture ligated. The parenchyma is approximated with 4–0 absorbable mattress sutures. Afterward, hypothermia is ended and the arterial clamp is released.[27,29,30]

49.4.7 Radial Nephrotomy

Indication: Caliceal Stones or Diverticulum Stones Not Extractable Via a Pyelotomy. Large Staghorn Stones with Multiple Caliceal Extensions that Require Several Radial Nephrotomies in Addition to an Extended Pyelolithotomy

An extended pyelolithotomy is initially performed, and as many stones as possible are removed by this least invasive access. Residual calculi detected by intraoperative pyeloscopy, radiography, or sonography can be removed by one or multiple small radial nephrotomies (see Fig. 49.6).

We prefer ultrasound-guided radial nephrotomies. The stone-bearing calyx and the intraparenchymal vessels are located exactly to assure the shortest transparenchymal access and prevent lesions to the arterial branches. The exact stone localization can be easily performed by intraoperative sonography using a small part 7 MHz scanner. The shortest transparenchymal access to the stone is determined to decide if an anterior or posterior incision is performed. By using the Doppler function in modern duplex sonography scanning probes in the estimated area of incision, an avascular area can be identified (see Fig. 49.7a, b).[31,32]

The renal capsule is radially incised over the stone at the predetermined site. The renal parenchyma is then bluntly separated with brain spatula until the stone-containing calyx is reached. After perforation of the calyx, the stone can be extracted with forceps (see Fig. 49.8a, b). Larger stones can be fragmented with a pneumatic drill or cutting forceps to

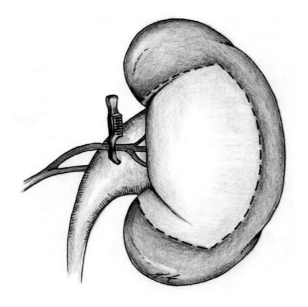

Fig. 49.4 Anatrophic nephrolithotomy. Vascular clamp on posterior segmental artery with resulting anatrophic demarcation

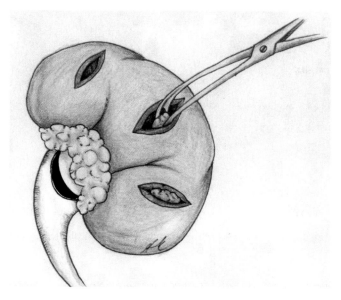

Fig. 49.6 Extended pyelolithotomy combined with radial nephrotomies. Multiple radial incisions of the renal parenchyma and removal of caliceal calculi with stone forceps

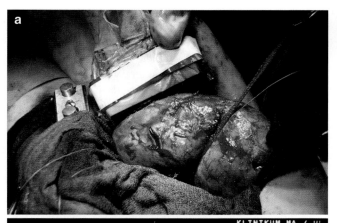

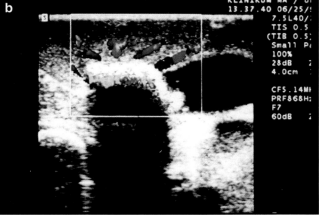

Fig. 49.7 (**a**) Sonography-guided radial nephrotomy. (**b**) By using modern duplex sonography scanners, all relevant structures including blood vessels can easily be identified. Even when multiple nephrotomies are performed, in most cases, no clamping of the renal artery is required

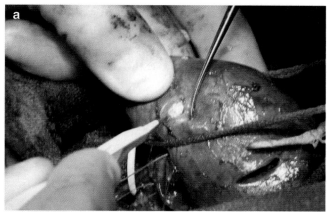

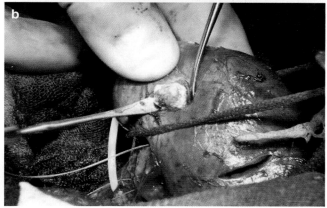

Fig. 49.8 Radial nephrotomy. Radial incision of renal parenchyma over the stone-bearing calyx (**a**) and stone extraction (**b**)

facilitate extraction. A dilation of the nephrotomy with a cold light–equipped nasal speculum may be useful for inspection of the collecting system. After removal of all stones and thorough irrigation of the calyx, the nephrotomy is closed with 4–0 absorbable sutures of the renal capsule.[27,33] Additional intraoperative radiography can help localize residual stones (see Fig. 49.9a, b).

If the technique of ultrasound-guided nephrotomy is properly mastered, temporary ischemia with or without hypothermia is not necessary even when multiple nephrotomies are performed (see Figs. 49.10 and 49.11). This helps in preserving the often already compromised renal function.

Alternatively, multiple radial nephrotomies can be performed under ischemia by clamping the renal artery and applying hypothermic conditions analogous to anatrophic nephrolithotomy.

49.4.8 Partial Nephrectomy

Indication: Partial or Complete Loss of Renal Function in the Stone-Bearing Area when Stone Removal Alone Is Not Expected to Improve the Function Significantly

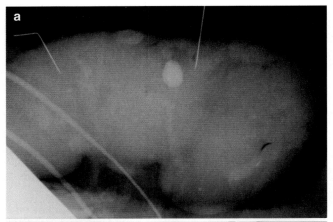

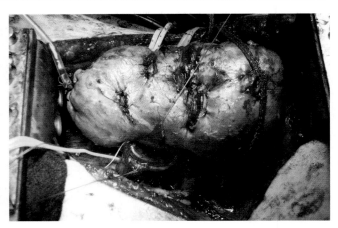

Fig. 49.11 Kidney after closure of multiple radial nephrotomies and insertion of nephrostomy tube

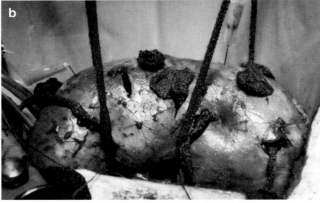

Fig. 49.9 (**a**) Intraoperative radiography. (**b**) A residual calculus is detected

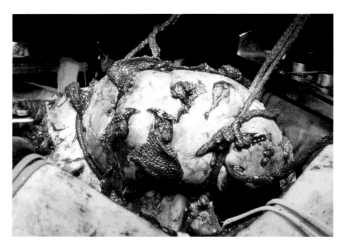

Fig. 49.10 Kidney after multiple sonography-guided radial nephrotomies without ischemia. Moist cotton strips are temporarily placed in the nephrotomies

The whole kidney is mobilized, and the renal vessels are exposed. In case of polar vessels supplying the segment to be resected, these are ligated and divided. If necessary, the renal artery is clamped to apply ischemia, and hypothermia is initiated, as described previously. The renal capsule is incised at the site of the proposed resection. The parenchyma is bluntly separated using brain spatula or the knife handle following the radial plane between the renal lobules. Arcuate vessels and caliceal infundibula are cut as distally as possible. After removing the specimen, vessels are suture ligated with 4–0 or 5–0 absorbable sutures and the collecting system is closed by running 5–0 absorbable sutures. Absorbable collagen or an argon-beam laser may be used for hemostasis if needed. The renal parenchyma including the capsule is closed using 3-0 absorbable mattress sutures. A ureteral stent is not necessary in the majority of cases. After releasing the clamp on the renal artery, a close inspection is necessary to detect bleeding.[27]

49.5 Conclusions

The widespread use of endourologic procedures and shock wave lithotripsy has limited the indications for open stone removing procedures dramatically. Today, open stone surgery is applied in patients mainly after failed minimally invasive treatment, in patients with anatomical renal or extrarenal abnormalities hampering or preventing minimally invasive treatment, in patients undergoing simultaneous open surgery for other reasons, or in patients with partial or complete loss of renal function.[2,5] In Western centers, open stone surgery constitutes 1–5% of stone removing procedures. Although this development toward less invasive stone treatment is generally favorable, it can lead to some problems as the reduced frequency of open stone surgery may influence the treatment outcome.

In this context, it is worth reviewing the results of the meta-analysis on interventional treatment of staghorn stones performed by the AUA Nephrolithiasis Guideline Panel in 2005. In this meta-analysis, a stone-free rate of 71% after open stone removing procedures was observed.[34] The significantly higher stone-free rate of 82% found in the meta-analysis

11 years earlier[35] may be regarded as an indication that the skill to perform open stone surgery is declining. However, as the data of the 2005 meta-analysis derive from only three patient groups including 51 patients, this reproach may not be completely justified. Today, a combination of PNL and SWL is considered treatment of choice for most staghorn calculi. However, whereas the stone-free rate of this approach was 81% in 1994, it also dropped to 66% in 2005.[34] Such a low treatment efficacy suggests that today complex cases are maltreated by minimally invasive technology and that in such cases, open stone surgery might offer a better alternative (compare Figs. 49.1a, b and 49.12a, b).

Generally, complex stone situations involving a large peripheral stone mass can be handled either by anatrophic nephrolithotomy or by extended pyelolithotomy combined with one or several radial nephrotomies. Both procedures require the complete mobilization of the kidney and the exposure of the renal vessels. Whereas anatrophic nephrolithotomy routinely requires ischemic conditions, extended pyelolithotomy and ultrasound-guided radial nephrotomies as described previously can be performed without clamping the renal artery in most situations. As transient ischemia bears the risk of further impairing the often already reduced renal function, this approach seems advantageous. Furthermore, as the renal vascular anatomy is very variable, it may become difficult to clearly identify a complete avascular area in which the longitudinal nephrotomy for anatrophic nephrolithotomy is performed. As damage to intraparenchymal arterial branches regularly leads to loss of nephron function, such an approach may further reduce the often already impaired renal function.

In contrast to this, extended pyelolithotomy and ultrasound-guided radial nephrotomies can be performed without applying ischemia in most situations. The exact position of the radial nephrotomy can be identified by using intraoperative ultrasonography to reliably localize the stone-bearing calyx and assess the shortest access to the stone. Furthermore, the Doppler function of modern duplex sonography probes visualizes intraparenchymal blood vessels and helps to identify an avascular area in which the incision can be performed with minimal harm to the kidney.

Although the points mentioned previously seem to favor the combination of extended pyelolithotomy over anatrophic nephrolithotomy, both procedures are equally performed leaving it to the individual urologist to decide which approach he prefers.

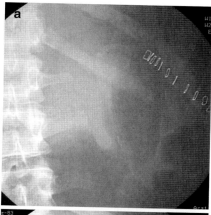
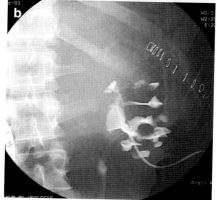

Fig. 49.12 (**a**) Postoperative radiography of the same patient as in Fig. 49.1 proving stone-free status after (**b**) a single open stone removing procedure (extended pyelolithotomy and multiple radial nephrotomies)

References

1. Kerbl K, Rehman J, Landman J, Lee D, Sundaram C, Clayman RV. Current management of urolithiasis: progress or regress? *J Endourol.* 2002;16:281-288.
2. Buchholz NN, Hitchings A, Albanis S. The (soon forgotten) art of open stone surgery: to train or not to train? *Ann R Coll Surg Engl.* 2006;88:214-217.
3. Kane CJ, Bolton DM, Stoller ML. Current indications for open stone surgery in an endourology center. *Urology.* 1995;45: 218-221.
4. Matlaga BR, Assimos DG. Changing indications of open stone surgery. *Urology.* 2002;59:490-493.
5. Paik ML, Wainstein MA, Spirnak JP, Hampel N, Resnick MI. Current indications for open stone surgery in the treatment of renal and ureteral calculi. *J Urol.* 1998;159:374-378.
6. Ather MH, Paryani J, Memon A, Sulaiman MN. A 10-year experience of managing ureteric calculi: changing trends towards endourological intervention–is there a role for open surgery? *BJU Int.* 2001;88:173-177.
7. Smith AD, Lange PH, Fraley EE. Applications of percutaneous nephrostomy. New challenges and opportunities in endo-urology. *J Urol.* 1979;121:382.
8. Bird VG, Fallon B, Winfield HN. Practice patterns in the treatment of large renal stones. *J Endourol.* 2003;17:355-363.
9. Preminger GM, Assimos DG, Lingeman JE, Nakada SY, Pearle MS, Wolf JS Jr. Chapter 1: AUA guideline on management of staghorn calculi: diagnosis and treatment recommendations. *J Urol.* 2005;173:1991-2000.
10. Tiselius HG, Ackermann D, Alken P, Buck C, Conort P, Gallucci M. Guidelines on urolithiasis. *Eur Urol.* 2001;40:362-371.
11. Francesca F, Felipetto R, Mosca F, Boggi U, Rizzo G, Puccini R. Percutaneous nephrolithotomy of transplanted kidney. *J Endourol.* 2002;16:225-227.

12. Koo BC, Burtt G, Burgess NA. Percutaneous stone surgery in the obese: outcome stratified according to body mass index. *BJU Int.* 2004;93:1296-1299.

13. Miller NL, Matlaga BR, Handa SE, Munch LC. Lingeman JE (2008) The presence of horseshoe kidney does not affect the outcome of percutaneous nephrolithotomy. *J Endourol.* 2008 Jun;22(6): 1219-1225.

14. Manohar T, Ganpule AP, Shrivastav P, Desai M. Percutaneous nephrolithotomy for complex caliceal calculi and staghorn stones in children less than 5 years of age. *J Endourol.* 2006;20:547-551.

15. Batter SJ, Dretler SP. Ureterorenoscopic approach to the symptomatic caliceal diverticulum. *J Urol.* 1997;158:709-713.

16. Canales B, Monga M. Surgical management of the calyceal diverticulum. *Curr Opin Urol.* 2003;13:255-260.

17. Miller SD, Ng CS, Streem SB, Gill IS. Laparoscopic management of caliceal diverticular calculi. *J Urol.* 2002;167:1248-1252.

18. Thadhani R, Pascual M, Bonventre JV. Acute renal failure. *N Engl J Med.* 1996;334:1448-1460.

19. Ward JP. Determination of the Optimum temperature for regional renal hypothermia during temporary renal ischaemia. *Br J Urol.* 1975;47:17-24.

20. Orvieto MA, Zorn KC, Mendiola F, et al. Recovery of renal function after complete renal hilar versus artery alone clamping during open and laparoscopic surgery. *J Urol.* 2007;177:2371-2374.

21. McLoughlin GA, Heal MR, Tyrell IM. An evaluation of techniques used for the production of temporary renal ischaemia. *Br J Urol.* 1978;50:371-375.

22. Collins GM, Green RD, Boyer D, Halasz NA. Protection of kidneys from warm ischemic injury. Dosage and timing of mannitol administration. *Transplantation.* 1980;29:83-84.

23. Krishan P, Sharma A, Singh M. Effect of angiotensin converting enzyme inhibitors on ischaemia-reperfusion-induced renal injury in rats. *Pharmacol Res.* 1998;37:23-29.

24. Wickham JE, Hanley HG, Joekes AM. Regional renal hypothermia. *Br J Urol.* 1967;39:727-743.

25. Harvey RB. Effect of temperature on function of isolated dog kidney. *Am J Physiol.* 1959;197:181-186.

26. Marberger M, Eisenberger F. Regional hypothermia of the kidney: surface or transarterial perfusion cooling? A functional study. *J Urol.* 1980;124:179-183.

27. Janetschek G, Abdelmaksoud A, Bagheri F, Al-Zahrani H, Leeb K, Gschwendtner M. Laparoscopic partial nephrectomy in cold ischemia: renal artery perfusion. *J Urol.* 2004;171:68-71.

28. Hinman F. *Atlas of Urologic Surgery.* 2nd ed. Philadelphia: W.B. Saunders; 1998.

29. Gil-Vernet J. New surgical concepts in removing renal calculi. *Urol Int.* 1965;20:255-288.

30. Assimos DG. Anatrophic nephrolithotomy. *Urology.* 2001;57:161-165.

31. Smith MJ, Boyce WH. Anatrophic nephrotomy and plastic calyrhaphy. *Trans Am Assoc Genitourin Surg.* 1967;59:18-24.

32. Alken P, Thuroff J, Riedmiller H, Hohenfellner R. Doppler sonography and B-mode ultrasound scanning in renal stone surgery. *Urology.* 1984;23:455-460.

33. Thuroff JW, Frohneberg D, Riedmiller R, et al. Localization of segmental arteries in renal surgery by Doppler sonography. *J Urol.* 1982;127:863-866.

34. Sleight MW, Gower RL, Wickham JE. Intrarenal access. *Urology.* 1980;15:475-477.

35. Preminger GM, Assimos DG, Lingeman JE, Nakada SY, Pearle MS, Wolf JS Jr. Chapter 1: AUA guideline on management of staghorn calculi: diagnosis and treatment recommendations. *J Urol.* 2005;173:1991-2000.

36. Segura JW, Preminger GM, Assimos DG, et al. Nephrolithiasis Clinical Guidelines Panel summary report on the management of staghorn calculi. The American Urological Association Nephrolithiasis Clinical Guidelines Panel. *J Urol.* 1994;151:1648-1651.

Autotransplantation and Ureteric Replacement: In Whom and How?

50

Jack M. Zuckerman and Dean G. Assimos

Abstract Patients with nephrolithiasis can develop ureteral stricture or sustain ureteral injury during attempts at stone removal. While some of these can be addressed with an endourologic approach, certain patients will need to undergo a major ureteral reconstructive procedure such as ileal ureter and other bowel substitution of the ureter, Boari flap, or autotransplantation. An extremely small number of patients may benefit from ileal ureter substitution to facilitate stone passage. The indications, techniques, and results of these various operations are reviewed in this chapter.

50.1 Introduction

Patients with nephrolithiasis may require ureteral replacement as a consequence of procedures utilized to remove stones, stricture due to stone impaction, congenital abnormalities of the ureter, and rarely to facilitate stone passage in the refractory stone former. The advent of minimally invasive stone removing techniques including ureteroscopy was associated with an increased incidence of ureteral injuries.[1] Endourological procedures, mainly ureteroscopy, are currently the most common cause of ureteral injury.[2] However, improvements in ureteroscopic technology and increasing surgical experience have resulted in low complication rates with ureteroscopic stone removal and stricture rates less than 1% at high volume centers.[3] Ureteral stricture associated with stone removal can be due to perforation of the ureter, thermal injury from intracorporeal lithotripsy, false passage of the ureter with endoscopes, guide wires, stents and endoscopic instruments, imbedded submucosal stone fragments, and devascularization during open or laparoscopic ureterolithotomy. Ureteral avulsion, an even rarer complication, is typically due to attempts at basket removal of large ureteral stones.[2,4,5] Other possible causes of this complication include intussusception of the ureter with manipulations of a ureteroscope or a ureteral access sheath.[6,7] Ureteral injury with endoscopic stone removal can occur during both antegrade and retrograde ureteroscopic stone removal. Inflammation of the ureter associated with stone impaction is thought to be a factor for development of stricture. Roberts and associates reported that strictures developed in 24% of patients after endoscopic stone removal of stones impacted greater than 2 months.[8] Patients with extreme levels of stone activity may benefit from ureteral replacement with bowel interposition to facilitate stone passage. This should only be undertaken if medical therapy for stone prevention fails or is not tolerated. Herein, the indications for ureteral replacement, patient selection and preparation, operative techniques, complications and their management, and reported results will be reviewed.

50.2 Indications and Contraindications

Ureteral replacement is a highly effective treatment for disorders leading to damage or disease of the ureter, and in some with normal ureteral function, a method of facilitating stone passage. A multitude of conditions besides stone-related problems have been treated surgically with ureteral replacement. Although the list of specific conditions leading to ureteral replacement is quite extensive, common themes emerge when looking at them together. The most common broad indication for replacement is ureteral stricture.

When evaluating a patient for ureteral replacement, it is important to determine that the targeted kidney has adequate function. If the disease process that has led to ureteral damage

D.G. Assimos (✉)
Department of Urology, Wake Forest University School of Medicine, Winston-Salem, NC, USA
e-mail: dassimos@wfubmc.edu

P.N. Rao et al. (eds.), *Urinary Tract Stone Disease*,
DOI 10.1007/978-1-84800-362-0_50, © Springer-Verlag London Limited 2011

is chronic rather than acute in nature, the renal function may have declined to such a degree that salvaging the kidney is not worthwhile. Nuclear renography is recommended, and reconstructive surgery is generally considered if the targeted renal unit contributes 10% or more of global renal function.

It is important to assess whether a minimally invasive or less extensive procedure could be effective. Endoureterotomy achieves reasonable success if the stricture is less than 1 cm, the involved renal unit has good function, and the targeted tissue has not been radiated.[9] Strictures in the middle and proximal ureter may be amenable to ureteroureterostomy if there is ample ureter above and below the stricture allowing performance of a tension-free anastomosis. Ureterocalicostomy is an option for patients with a proximal ureteral stricture at or just below the ureteropelvic junction, especially those with an intrarenal pelvis.[10] Renal mobilization may help in such cases. Similarly, distal ureteral strictures can be repaired with ureteral reimplantation.

Patients with middle and proximal ureteral strictures or those with avulsion injuries in these areas can be managed with a Boari flap procedure. This will depend on the distance of the ureteral gap, and capacity and condition of the bladder. The presence of a small, thickened, noncompliant bladder, or history of pelvic radiation may prohibit the performance of this procedure. This operation, though itself constituting major reconstruction, does not necessarily require entry into the peritoneum, and the use of bowel or vascular reconstruction is not needed, thereby limiting risks to the patient.

Large proximal lesions, especially those involving the renal pelvis, will often require a bowel interposition. Ileal ureter is usually preferred over interposition of the appendix or a Monti procedure as it better allows spontaneous passage of stones. This bowel segment is preferred to jejunum as the latter is associated with more electrolyte disturbances.[11] Ileal ureter replacement, however, is not appropriate for all patients. This procedure should be avoided in patients with certain degrees of renal insufficiency (serum creatinine greater than 2.0 mg/dL), or in those with anatomic or functional small bowel dysfunction such as inflammatory bowel disease, short gut syndrome, and radiation enteritis.

The decision to utilize a renal autotransplant is typically made when all other options have been exhausted. This procedure involves renal ischemia, both warm and cold, and therefore is best tolerated if the targeted renal unit has adequate function. Evaluation for autotransplant should include an assessment of the patient's vascular health. Since the renal artery and vein are commonly anastomosed to the iliac vessels, they should ideally be normal. Extensive plaque in the renal artery increases the complexity of the procedure. The iliac arteries should have no or limited atherosclerosis as the latter could compromise the arterial

anastomosis. In addition, the iliac veins need to be patent and free of clot.

50.3 Operative Technique

50.3.1 Ileal Ureter

Patient preparation is one of the foundations for success. The majority of patients should have a nephrostomy tube placed in the targeted renal unit. Urinary tract infection (UTI) is treated prior to embarking on this procedure. Patients are administered a mechanical bowel prep.

For replacement of ureteral defects with ileum, the patient is typically positioned supine. A 22-F Foley catheter is inserted into the bladder. This larger sized catheter is utilized to facilitate mucous passage during the postoperative period. A midline incision or one from the tip of the ipsilateral 11th or 12th rib extending to the midline is made and the peritoneal cavity is entered. Small bowel is retracted, and the ipsilateral colon is mobilized medially for access to the kidney and ureter. The ureter and renal pelvis are carefully exposed. During unilateral reconstruction, the bladder is mobilized and an ipsilateral psoas hitch is performed to limit the length of bowel used for reconstruction. This maneuver is not undertaken if bilateral separate ileal ureters are being created.

An appropriate piece of ileum is selected based on the patient's anatomy, mesenteric blood supply, and the length of ureteral replacement required. If possible, the segment should be at least 15 cm from the ileocecal junction. Once the bowel has been divided, the distal end should be marked to ensure proper orientation during ureteral anastomosis; the remaining ileum is anastomosed using a stapled or sutured technique. Succus is irrigated out of the isolated bowel segment. An opening in the colonic mesentery is made through which the isolated bowel segment is placed and positioned in the retroperitoneal space.

The urinary tract can be reconstituted in a number of ways, depending on the anatomy of the ureter and renal pelvis. Anastomosis of the ileum to the pelvis is preferred as this facilitates passage of any future stones. This is done using an end-to-side technique as this best preserves the blood supply of the renal pelvis. The ureter just below the ureteropelvic junction is ligated and a vertical pyelotomy is made; the length is based on the luminal size of the bowel. The bowel segment is oriented in an isoperistaltic direction. The bowel is then anastomosed to the renal pelvis using interrupted 3-0 or 4-0 absorbable suture (Fig. 50.1). If the patient has an intrarenal pelvis, an end-to-side anastomosis of the bowel to the anterior proximal ureter is made. Minimal dissection of the ureter is undertaken to preserve its vascular integrity. The ureter distal to the anastomosis is

50.3.4 Yang-Monti

Using the Yang-Monti technique, it is possible replace a larger defect in the ureter utilizing a relatively shorter segment of ileum. Depending on the length needed for reconstruction, a segment of ileum is transected and the free ends are reconnected. The isolated segment of ileum is then divided into equal segments of approximately 2–3 cm. Each segment is incised longitudinally near the mesenteric border and unfolded, with care to preserve the vasculature. The adjacent borders are approximated over a 16 French catheter and sewn; these segments are then combined to form the tubularized ureteral replacement. Alternatively, a "double" Monti procedure (Fig. 50.4) may be utilized in which a single segment of ileum is incised at the mesenteric border on opposing sides and unfolded. This technique also utilizes a catheter to aid in the creation of a tubular structure. The proximal end of the new ileal segment can be anastomosed end-to-end with the remaining healthy ureter. The distal end is implanted in the bladder with either a refluxing or antireflux technique.

50.3.5 Appendix

When utilizing the appendix for ureteral replacement, a midline abdominal incision is preferred. The diseased segment of ureter is located and controlled both proximal and distal to the lesion. The appendix is then located and evaluated for

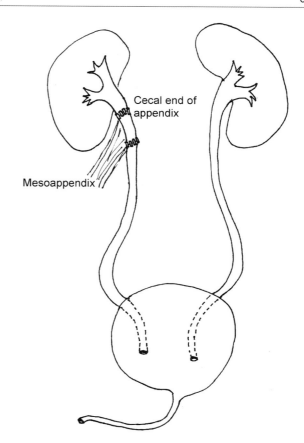

Fig. 50.5 Appendix. Schematic representation of a ureteral reconstruction utilizing the appendix. Note the intact mesoappendix and appropriate orientation

length, tissue viability, and vascular integrity. It is important to estimate the length of replacement required and ensure that the appendiceal interposition will be sufficient for a tension-free anastomosis. With care to preserve the appendicular arteries within the mesoappendix, the appendix is either stapled or tied and transected at the base of the cecum. The distal end of the appendix is opened obliquely, and the proximal end is spatulated. The isolated ureteral segment is then resected, and the free ends of healthy ureter are spatulated. The cecal end of the appendix, with its larger diameter, should be anastomosed to the more proximal ureter (Fig. 50.5). A ureteral stent is placed, and the distal anastomosis is completed. If the appendix is not of insufficient length for a tension-free anastomosis, additional ureter may be mobilized and, if necessary, a psoas hitch may be performed.

50.4 Results

50.4.1 Ileal Ureter

Ileal ureter is the most extensively reported form of ureteral replacement in the literature. We summated results of series

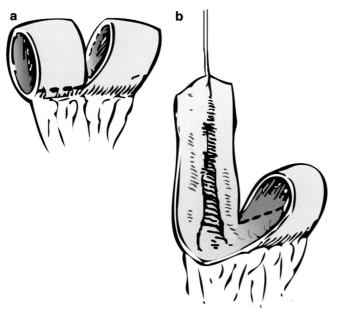

Fig. 50.4 (**a**) Division of the isolated ileal segment into two (**b**) The two segments are then opened at the anti-mesenteric side and then made into a tubular segment by suturing the edges longitudinally. The end of both the tubes are then anastamosed to make a long conduit

in which data on 5 or more patients subjected to this procedure were reported. We also attempted to avoid series where the majority of the patients had their ileum used as part of a urinary undiversion from a previous cutaneous stoma. However, we have included those studies where undiversion made up a minority of the cases performed. In addition, many of the cases were not performed in stone formers. When assessing "success" or "failure" rates for ileal ureters and other forms of replacement, we used each study's own self-determined criteria for determining success. For the majority of the series reviewed, success was based on stabilization or improvement in renal function.

Using these selection criteria, we found 16 case series published between 1959 and 2006 with a total of 491 patients.[12–27] A complete list, including patient number, age, gender, follow-up, indications, results, and complications, is found in Table 50.1. The number of patients in each study ranged from 5 to 89 with a mean of 31 patients per series. Of those studies reporting gender and age as part of their patient demographics, 56% of patients were male and 44% were female with an average age of 44.9 years. The follow-up periods ranged from 2 months to 23 years; the average follow-up duration for all series was 4.1 years. The average success rate for this group of studies was 86%. There were some series in which results were inferior. Tanagho reported a series in which all 5 patients had poor postoperative outcomes.[25] Bazeed and associates reported a success rate of only 57%; however, these procedures were done for schistosomiasis-associated ureteral stricture.[12] The remainder of the case series all reported success rates >80%. There were only two reported deaths in these series.

There were two large series in which ileal ureter reconstructions were undertaken in recurrent stone formers. Fritzsche and colleagues performed ileal ureter reconstruction in 24 patients with recurrent calculi.[18] They reported that many patients had recurrent calculi following the procedure; however, the number of stones decreased considerably over time. Additionally, no patients experienced symptomatic stone passage following ureteral replacement. Boxer and associates reported on 44 patients who underwent ileal ureteral replacement for stone disease.[15] In their series, 38 of the 44 patients had stable or improved renal function, improved radiographic appearance, and were asymptomatic.

50.4.2 Boari Flap

After ileal ureter, Boari flaps are the next most commonly reported form of ureteral replacement. We used the same selection criteria for these case series as we did with ileal ureters; a minimum of five cases were required for inclusion.

A total of 14 series (Table 50.2) with 358 patients met these criteria.[12,13,28–39] Publication dates ranged from 1966 to 2005. Only 6 studies reported gender in their analysis. Of these, 29% were male and 71% female. The average patient age was 42 years. Follow-up ranged from 1 month to 12 years with an average follow-up of 2 years. Success rates were higher for Boari flap compared to ileal ureters. Six series reported 100% success rates, and all had >70% success rates. The average success rate for all 14 series was 93%. Only two deaths were reported.

50.4.3 Renal Autotransplant

Between 1975 and 2005, 11 case series (Table 50.3) were published that reported data on renal autotransplant involving five or more patients.[40–50] Collectively, these series made up a total of 289 patients (40% male and 60% female) with an average age of 40.8 years. The mean follow-up after autotransplant was 3.2 years (10 months–16 years). The success rate for all series was 90%. Four patients required nephrectomy following autotransplant for complications related to the procedure: two for vascular compromise, one for renal vein thrombosis, one for infection. One patient died secondary to bowel infarction and septic shock.

50.4.4 Yang-Monti

There are very few published series with more than one patient looking at the Monti procedure for ureteral replacement. Two studies were found that reported on experience with at least two patients (Table 50.4). Ali-El-Dein and colleagues[51] published a series in 2003 with 10 patients, and in 2006, Castellan and associates[52] published their experience with another two patients. Of these 12 patients, 10 were male and 2 were female. The average age was 49.1 years. Follow-up ranged from 6 months to 4.5 years, with an average follow-up of 2.7 years. Both authors reported 100% success rates using the Yang-Monti technique for ureteral replacement in their patients, although one patient did require an exploratory laparotomy for small bowel obstruction.

50.4.5 Appendix

Using the appendix in ureteral replacement is infrequently reported in the literature. Only three studies were found,

Table 50.1 Ileal ureter

Ileal ureter

Study		Patients			Age (Years)		Follow-up		Indications	Results			Listed complications
Year of publication	First author	#	Male	Female	Mean	Range	Mean (Years)	Range	Descending order of frequency	Success	Failure	Death	
1959	Goodwin	16	NS	NS	NS	NS	NS	NS	Unspecified, urothelial malignancy, congenital	16	3	0	A nastomotic leak, fistula, incontinence, stenosis, uremia, acidosis
1975	Tanagho	5	3	2	26.8	14–64	NS	NS	Recurrent stones, ureteral stricture, pyelonephritis, congenital, ureterocele	0	5	0	Ileal dilation, persistent UTI, pyelonephritis, mucus plugging
1975	Fritzsche	47	NS	NS	NS	NS	NS	6 months–17 years	Recurrent stones, surgical complications, congenital, tuberculosis	44	3	0	Persistent bacteriuria
1978	Boxer	89	33	56	44.3	NS	NS	6 months–23 years	Recurrent stones, surgical complications, congenital, undiversion, tuberculosis, urothelial malignancy	72	17	1	NS
1981	Crooks	8	5	3	NS	NS	NS	NS	Bladder dysfunction, ureteral stricture, ureteral ischemia, undiversion, congenital	7	1	0	Small bowel obstruction, acidosis
1981	Skinner	23	NS	NS	NS	NS	NS	6 months–10 years	Undiversion, ureteral fistula, urothelial malignancy	20	3	0	Recurrent pyelonephritis, incontinence ureteral reflux, persistent UTI
1982	Bazeed	21	NS	NS	37.2	NS	2.3	6 months–6 years	Schistosomiasis	12	9	0	Ureteral reflux, persistent UTI
1990	Benson	10	5	5	51.0	22–77	4.8	3 months–6 years	Retroperitoneal fibrosis, surgical complications, recurrent stones, urothelial malignancy	10	0	0	Wound infection, incisional hernia
1995	Shokeir	50	45	5	42.0	NS	5.75	60–80 months	NS	43	7	0	Dessusception of nipple valve, bladder stones, urinary outflow obstruction, acidosis

(continued)

Table 50.1 (continued)

Ileal ureter

Study		Patients			Age (Years)		Follow-up		Indications	Results			Listed complications
Year of publication	First author	#	Male	Female	Mean	Range	Mean (Years)	Range	Descending order of frequency	Success	Failure	Death	
1997	Mattos	61	NS	NS	NS	NS	NS	NS	NS	54	6	1	29 total; Ileovesical stricture, renal deterioration, bacteriuria, pancreatitis, acidosis, diarrhea, hepatic encephalopathy
1997	Shokeir	9	6	3	35.0	18–58	5.2	2–7 years	Ureteral stricture, ureteral avulsion, ureteral fistula	9	0	0	Prolonged ileus, sepsis
1999	Waldner	19	NS	NS	52.0	38–72	4.75	4–6 years	Ureteral stricture, ureteral fistula, recurrent stones, retroperitoneal fibrosis, urothelial malignancy	19	0	0	NS
2002	Verduyckt	18	10	8	54.0	29–73	5.42	2 months–16 years	Retroperitoneal fibrosis, surgical complications, ureteral stricture, ureteral obstruction, urothelial malignancy	16	2	0	Post-op bleeding, prolonged ileus, urinary leakage, persistent hematuria, anastomotic obstruction requiring nephrectomy, anastomotic fibrosis
2003	Matlaga	16	10	6	49.4	25–72	1.55	7–59 months	Surgical complications, ureteral avulsion, congenital, ureteral stricture	18	0	0	Prolonged ileus
2004	Bonfig	43	23	20	45.6	5–73	3.4	1.5–109.5 months	Ureteral stricture, urothelial malignancy, bladder dysfunction, ureteral obstruction, undiversion, congenital, recurrent stones, ureteral fistula	42	1	0	Recurrent pyelonephritis, acidosis, ileal kinking, mucus plugging, ureteral dilation
2006	Chung	56	NS	NS	48.6	19–71	6.04	2 months–21 years	Surgical complications, recurrent stones, retroperitoneal fibrosis, ureteral obstruction, ureteral stricture, urothelial malignancy, unspecified	46	10	0	10 minor, 6 major; hernia, wound dehiscence, ileal obstruction, anastomotic stricture, chronic renal failure

NS not stated. Published series utilizing ileal ureteral replacement in ≥5 patients, according to date of publication.[12–27] Number of patients, male/female ratio, average age and range, follow-up intervals, indications, results, and complications are listed

Table 50.2 Boari flap

Study	First author	Patients			Age (Years)		Boari flap		Indications	Results			Listed complications
Year publication		#	Male	Female	Mean	Range	Follow-up mean (Years)	Range	Descending order of frequency	Success	Failure	Death	
1966	Williams	12	NS	NS	41.9	28–56	5	6 months–12 years	Ureteral stricture, ureteral fistula	9	3	0	Pyelonephritis
1970	Pearson	25	NS	NS	NS	NS	NS	NS	Surgical complication, ureteral stricture, retroperitonel fibrosis, megaureter, tuberculosis	25	0	0	Ureteral obstruction, hematoma
1975	Konigsberg	21	6	15	NS	9 months–62 years	2.25	1 months–11 years	Surgical complication, recurrent stones, urologic cancer, ureterocelectomy	15	6	0	Hydroneprosis, fistula, recurrent symptomatic urinary tract infection
1982	Bazeed	29	NS	NS	NS	NS	2.3	6 months–6 years	Schistosomiasis	27	2	0	Urinary tract infection
1982	Bowsher	54	13	41	46.0	2–71	NS	NS	Surgical complication, ureteral stricture, urologic cancer, other	52	1	1	Urinary tract infection, urinoma, pulmonary embolus
1986	Olsson	6	4	2	50.0	21–71	3.4	36–48 months	Recurrent stones, ureteral stricture, retroperitoneal fibrosis, ureteral fistula	6	0	0	No patient complications

(continued)

Table 50.2 (continued)

Study		Patients			Age (Years)		Boari flap		Indications	Results			Listed complications
First author	Year publication	#	Male	Female	Mean	Range	Follow-up mean (Years)	Range	Descending order of frequency	Success	Failure	Death	
Smith	1988	5	NS	NS	NS	NS	NS	NS	Procedure related ureteral stricture	5	0	0	NS
Benson	1990	6	2	4	53.0	38–71	5.1	2–6.5	NS	5	1	0	Persistent calicectasis, hydronephrosis
Mandal	1990	10	NS	NS	43.5	23–55	2	6–54 months	Ureteral fistula	10	0	0	No patient complications
Motiwala	1990	12	5	17	34.0	13–57	NS	NS	Surgical complication, ureteral stricture, retroperitoneal fibrosis, tuberculosis	12	0	0	Ureteral stent migration requiring open surgical removal
Onuora	1993	5	NS	NS	35.0	25–50	NS	NS	Ureteral fistula	4	1	0	Anastomotic stricture
Ravi	1993	150	NS	NS	35.0	4–80	NS	6 months–2 years	Schistosomiasis	148	1	1	Urosepsis, disseminated intravascular coagulation, urinoma, ureteral necrosis, persistent urinary tract infection
Pizzo	1998	15	NS	NS	NS	NS	NS	2–44 months	NS	15	0	0	Persistent hydronephrosis,
Castillo	2005	8	4	4	39.9	9–71	1.5	NS	Ureteral stricture	8	0	0	Gross hematuria, uroperitoneum requiring reoperation

NS not stated. Published series utilizing a Boari flap for ureteral reconstruction in ≥5 patients, according to date of publication.[12,13,28–39] Number of patients, male/female ratio, average age and range, follow-up intervals, indications, results, and complications are listed

Table 50.3 Renal autotransplant

| Autotransplant | | | | | | | | | | | | | |
| Study | | Patients | | | Age (Years) | | Follow-up | | Indications | Results | | Death | Listed complications |
Year of publication	First author	#	Male	Female	Mean	Range	Mean (Years)	Range	Descending order of frequency	Success	Failure		
1975	Lilly	14	9	5	40.6	6–63	NS	NS	Renovascular hypertension, urologic cancer, recurrent stones, congential, renal artery thrombosis	13	1	0	NS
1976	McLoughlin	5	1	4	47.0	35–66	NS	NS	Urologic cancer, renal artery aneurysm, abdominal aortic aneurysm	5	0	0	Pulmonary embolus, retroperitoneal hematoma, acute renal failure, respiratory distress
1982	Gil-Vernet	92	NS	NS	NS	10–65	NS	1–13	NS	87	5	0	False aneurysm, thrombosis, an astomotic infection, dvonephrosis
1987	Radomski	5	5	0	44.2	30–52	1.8	10–36 months	Urologic cancer, renovascular hypertension, surgical complication, schistosomiasis, congenital	5	0	0	Acute renal failure
1990	Merguerian	7	3	4	11.3	6–16	4.2	14 months–11 years	Renovascular hypertension	6	1	0	NS
1990	Novick	108	41	67	38.2	23–57	5.1	1–16 years	Renovascular hypertension, surgical complications, urologic cancer, recurrent stones, retroperitoneal fibrosis, urinary undiversion	25	2	0	Non-functioning autotransplant, hilar hemorrhage
1992	Van Der Velden	6	3	3	63.5	47–72	3.8	1–97 months	Urologic cancer	6	0	0	Gastrointestinal hemorrhage

(continued)

Table 50.3 (continued)

Study		Patients			Age (Years)		Follow-up		Indications	Results				
Year of publication	First author	#	Male	Female	Mean	Range	Mean (Years)	Range	Descending order of frequency	Success	Failure	Death	Listed complications	
1998	Perumalla	5	1	4	44.4	28–65	2.7	1–4.5 years	Ureteral ischemia/ necrosis, ureteral stricture, retroperitoneal fibrosis, surgical complication	5	0	0	Wound infection	
2003	Meng	7	2	5	46.0	32–59	1.4	10–25 months	Ureteral avulsion, UPJ disruption, ureteral stricture	6	1	0	Pneumonia, postoperative ileus	
2004	Wotkowicz	25	13	12	NS	NS	NS	NS	Renovascular hypertension, urologic cancer, ureteric complexities, congenital	20	5	0	Autotransplant nephrectomy; two kidneys never reimplanted because of extent of vascular and oncologic disease	
2005	Webster	15	4	11	32.1	4–59	NS	NS	Renovascular hypertension, surgical complication, ureteral avulsion	14	2	1	Acute tubular necrosis, suture abscess, bowel infarction (leading to sepsis and death), renal artery stenosis, renal vein thrombosis	

NS not stated. Published series utilizing renal autotransplantation in ≥5 patients, according to date of publication.[40-50] Number of patients, male/female ratio, average age and range, follow-up intervals, indications, results, and complications are listed

Table 50.4 Monti procedure

Monti														
Study			Patients			Age (Years)		Follow-up		Indications	Results			
Year of publication	First author		#	Male	Female	Mean	Range	Mean (Years)	Range	Descending order of frequency	Success	Failure	Death	Listed complications
2003	Ali-El-Dein		10	9	1	48.7	NS	0.8	6–13 months	Schistosomiasis, tuberculosis, urologic cancer	10	0	0	None
2006	Castellan		2	1	1	49.5	33–66	4.5	3.25–5.75 years	Recurrent stones, retroperitoneal fibrosis	2	0	0	Small bowel obstruction requiring exploratory laparotomy

NS not stated. Published series utilizing a Monti procedure during ureteral reconstruction, according to date of publication.[51,52] Number of patients, male/female ratio, average age and range, follow-up intervals, indications, results, and complications are listed

Table 50.5 Appendiceal replacement

Study		Patients			Age (Years)		Follow-up		Indications	Results				Listed complications
Year of publication	First author	#	Male	Female	Mean	Range	Mean (Years)	Range	Descending order of frequency	Success	Failure	Death		
1983	Goyanes	1	0	1	49.0	49	3.3	40 months	Retroperitoneal mass	1	0	0		None
2000	Richter	3	1	2	14.0	11–19	8.7	4–15 years	Urinary undiversion, ureteral obstruction	3	0	0		None
2003	Kaur	1	0	1	35.0	35	0.5	6 months	Ureteral stricture	1	0	0		Anastomotic stricture

Published series utilizing appendiceal ureteral reconstruction, according to date of publication.[53-55] Number of patients, male/female ratio, average age and range, follow-up intervals, indications, results, and complications are listed

reporting experience using the appendix in a total of 5 patients.[53–55] One patient was male, and four were female. The average age was 32.7 and the average follow-up was 4.2 years with a range of 6 months to 15 years. Of the five patients included, all five were determined to have successful outcomes at follow-up (Table 50.5).

50.5 Complications

Despite the often complex nature of ureteral reconstruction, there are surprisingly few postoperative complications. Although each procedure is accompanied by its own set of unique problems, ureteral replacement as a whole has certain complications in common. As with any surgical procedure, infection, bleeding, injury to adjacent structures, wound dehiscence, hernia, and thromboembolic events may occur with any of these procedures.

A ureteral or collecting system anastomosis is performed with any method of ureteral replacement. Therefore, an anastomotic leak or urinoma may occur in all forms of replacement. The causes include poor surgical technique or a lack of tissue viability on either or both sides of the anastomosis. Careful mobilization of the ureter and bladder and proper isolation of any bowel segment utilized limit their occurrence. Anastomotic stricture may develop for the same reasons. Postoperative stricture formation is less common with ileal ureter and may be due the larger lumen provided by this bowel segment.

Bowel-related complications may occur with any of these procedures including ileus, enterotomy and other forms of bowel injury, and bowel obstruction. Bowel anastomotic leak with ileal ureter and leak from the cecum may develop after appendiceal interposition. Patients subjected to these procedures frequently pass mucus in their urine but this is seldom problematic; new onset voiding dysfunction and urinary tract infection (UTI) occurr rarely. Metabolic acidosis may develop after bowel interposition; baseline renal insufficiency and the utilization of longer bowel segments are risk factors. This is treated with administration of oral alkalinizing agents.

Renal autotransplantation has risks not associated with other forms of replacement. Renal ischemia may lead to acute tubular necrosis and renal failure; typically transient events. Thrombosis of the arterial or venous anastomosis may occur, and, if not identified early and corrected, results in loss of the function of the involved renal unit. Stenosis of the arterial anastomosis can develop, which may lead to renovascular hypertension.

The bladder is reconfigured during Boari flap reconstruction. This may alter bladder capacity and lead to voiding dysfunction. This rarely occurs in patients with normal baseline bladder capacity and function.

50.6 Conclusions

The main goal of ureteral replacement is the establishment of good antegrade flow of urine and improvement or maintenance of renal function. A secondary aim may be to facilitate stone passage in those with active stone disease. Surgical approaches are tailored to the patient's needs and may be influenced by the adequacy and availability of autologous tissue. The best surgical option may not be apparent until the time of surgical exploration. Therefore, one must be prepared to alter their approach based on intraoperative findings. The chances of success are optimized with proper patient selection and preparation.

References

1. Assimos, D. G., Patterson, L. C., & Taylor, C. L. (1994). Changing incidence and etiology of iatrogenic ureteral injuries. *J Urol, 152*(6 Pt 2), 2240–2246.
2. Al-Awadi, K., Kehinde, E. O., Al-Hunayan, A., & Al-Khayat, A. (2005). Iatrogenic ureteric injuries: incidence, aetiological factors and the effect of early management on subsequent outcome. *Int Urol Nephrol, 37*(2), 235–241.
3. Harmon, W. J., Sershon, P. D., Blute, M. L., Patterson, D. E., & Segura, J. W. (1997). Ureteroscopy: current practice and long-term complications. *J Urol, 157*(1), 28–32.
4. Puppo, P., Ricciotti, G., Bozzo, W., & Introini, C. (1999). Primary endoscopic treatment of ureteric calculi. A review of 378 cases. *Eur Urol, 36*(1), 48–52.
5. Weinberg, J. J., Ansong, K., & Smith, A. D. (1987). Complications of ureteroscopy in relation to experience: report of survey and author experience. *J Urol, 137*(3), 384–385.
6. Bernhard, P. H., & Reddy, P. K. (1996). Retrograde ureteral intussusception: a rare complication. *J Endourol, 10*(4), 349–351.
7. Park, J., Siegel, C., Moll, M., & Konnak, J. (1994). Retrograde ureteral intussusception. *J Urol, 151*(4), 997–998.
8. Roberts, W. W., Cadeddu, J. A., Micali, S., Kavoussi, L. R., & Moore, R. G. (1998). Ureteral stricture formation after removal of impacted calculi. *J Urol, 159*(3), 723–726.
9. Razdan, S., Silberstein, I. K., & Bagley, D. H. (2005). Ureteroscopic endoureterotomy. *BJU Int, 95*(Suppl 2), 94–101.
10. Matlaga, B. R., Shah, O. D., Singh, D., Streem, S. B., & Assimos, D. G. (2005). Ureterocalicostomy: a contemporary experience. *Urology, 65*(1), 42–44.
11. Golimbu, M., & Morales, P. (1975). Jejunal conduits: technique and complications. *J Urol, 113*(6), 787–795.
12. Bazeed, M. A., Ashamalla, A., Abd-Alrazek, A. A., Ghoneim, M., & Badr, M. (1982). Management of bilharzial strictures of the lower ureter. *Urol Int, 37*(1), 19–25.
13. Benson, M. C., Ring, K. S., & Olsson, C. A. (1990). Ureteral reconstruction and bypass: experience with ileal interposition, the Boari flap-psoas hitch and renal autotransplantation. *J Urol, 143*(1), 20–23.
14. Bonfig, R., Gerharz, E. W., & Riedmiller, H. (2004). Ileal ureteric replacement in complex reconstruction of the urinary tract. *BJU Int, 93*(4), 575–580.
15. Boxer, R. J., Fritzsche, P., Skinner, D. G., et al. (1979). Replacement of the ureter by small intestine: clinical application and results of the ileal ureter in 89 patients. *J Urol, 121*(6), 728–731.

16. Chung, B. I., Hamawy, K. J., Zinman, L. N., & Libertino, J. A. (2006). The use of bowel for ureteral replacement for complex ureteral reconstruction: long-term results. *J Urol, 175*(1), 179–183. discussion 183-4.

17. Crooks, K. K. (1981). The use of antirefluxing intestinal segments in pediatric urinary reconstruction. *J Pediatr Surg, 16*(6), 801–805.

18. Fritzsche, P., Skinner, D. G., Craven, J. D., Cahill, P., & Goodwin, W. E. (1975). Long-term radiographic changes of the kidney following the ileal ureter operation. *J Urol, 114*(6), 843–847.

19. Goodwin, W. E., Winter, C. C., & Turner, R. D. (1959). Replacement of the ureter by small intestine: clinical application and results of the ileal ureter. *J Urol, 81*(3), 406–418.

20. Matlaga, B. R., Shah, O. D., Hart, L. J., & Assimos, D. G. (2003). Ileal ureter substitution: a contemporary series. *Urology, 62*(6), 998–1001.

21. Mattos, R. M., & Smith, J. J., 3rd. (1997). Ileal ureter. *Urol Clin North Am, 24*(4), 813–825.

22. Shokeir, A. A. (1997). Interposition of ileum in the ureter: a clinical study with long-term follow-up. *Br J Urol, 79*(3), 324–327.

23. Shokeir, A. A., & Ghoneim, M. A. (1995). Further experience with the modified ileal ureter. *J Urol, 154*(1), 45–48.

24. Skinner, D. G. (1982). Further experience with the ileocecal segment in urinary reconstruction. *J Urol, 128*(2), 252–256.

25. Tanagho, E. A. (1975). A case against incorporation of bowel segments into the closed urinary system. *J Urol, 113*(6), 796–802.

26. Verduyckt, F. J., Heesakkers, J. P., & Debruyne, F. M. (2002). Long-term results of ileum interposition for ureteral obstruction. *Eur Urol, 42*(2), 181–187.

27. Waldner, M., Hertle, L., & Roth, S. (1999). Ileal ureteral substitution in reconstructive urological surgery: is an antireflux procedure necessary? *J Urol, 162*(2), 323–326.

28. Bowsher, W. G., Shah, P. J., Costello, A. J., Tiptaft, R. C., Paris, A. M., & Blandy, J. P. (1982). A critical appraisal of the Boari flap. *Br J Urol, 54*(6), 682–685.

29. Castillo, O. A., Litvak, J. P., Kerkebe, M., Olivares, R., & Urena, R. D. (2005). Early experience with the laparoscopic Boari flap at a single institution. *J Urol, 173*(3), 862–865.

30. del Pizzo, J. J., Jacobs, S. C., Bartlett, S. T., & Sklar, G. N. (1998). The use of bladder for total transplant ureteral reconstruction. *J Urol, 159*(3), 750–752. Discussion 752–753.

31. Konigsberg, H., Blunt, K. J., & Muecke, E. C. (1975). Use of Boari flap in lower ureteral injuries. *Urology, 5*(6), 751–755.

32. Mandal, A. K., Sharma, S. K., Vaidyanathan, S., & Goswami, A. K. (1990). Ureterovaginal fistula: summary of 18 years' experience. *Br J Urol, 65*(5), 453–456.

33. Motiwala, H. G., Shah, S. A., & Patel, S. M. (1990). Ureteric substitution with Boari bladder flap. *Br J Urol, 66*(4), 369–371.

34. Olsson, C. A., & Norlen, L. J. (1986). Combined Boari bladder flap-psoas bladder hitch procedure in ureteral replacement. *Scand J Urol Nephrol, 20*(4), 279–284.

35. Onuora, V. C., al-Mohalhal, S., Youssef, A. M., & Patil, M. (1993). Iatrogenic urogenital fistulae. *Br J Urol, 71*(2), 176–178.

36. Pearson, B. S. (1970). Experiences with the Boari flap. *Br J Urol, 42*(6), 740.

37. Ravi, G., & Motalib, M. A. (1993). Surgical correction of bilharzial ureteric stricture by Boari flap technique. *Br J Urol, 71*(5), 535–538.

38. Smith, A. D. (1988). Management of iatrogenic ureteral strictures after urological procedures. *J Urol, 140*(6), 1372–1374.

39. Williams, J. L., & Porter, R. W. (1966). The Boari bladder flap in lower ureteric injuries. *Br J Urol, 38*(5), 528–533.

40. Gil-Vernet, J. M. (1982). Renal autotransplantation. *Eur Urol, 8*(2), 61–73.

41. Lilly, J. R., Pfister, R. R., Putnam, C. W., Kosloske, A. M., & Starzl, T. E. (1975). Bench surgery and renal autotransplantation in the pediatric patient. *J Pediatr Surg, 10*(5), 623–630.

42. McLoughlin, M. G., Williams, G. M., & Stonesifer, G. L. (1976). Ex vivo surgical dissection. Autotransplantation in renal disease. *JAMA, 235*(16), 1705–1707.

43. Meng, M. V., Freise, C. E., & Stoller, M. L. (2003). Expanded experience with laparoscopic nephrectomy and autotransplantation for severe ureteral injury. *J Urol, 169*(4), 1363–1367.

44. Merguerian, P. A., McLorie, G. A., Balfe, J. W., Khoury, A. E., & Churchill, B. M. (1990). Renal autotransplantation in children: a successful treatment for renovascular hypertension. *J Urol, 144*(6), 1443–1445.

45. Novick, A. C., Jackson, C. L., & Straffon, R. A. (1990). The role of renal autotransplantation in complex urological reconstruction. *J Urol, 143*(3), 452–457.

46. Perumalla, C., & Nicol, D. L. (1998). Renal autotransplantation for the management of complex ureteric defects. *Aust N Z J Surg, 68*(5), 376–379.

47. Radomski, J. S., Jarrell, B. E., Carabasi, R. A., & Yang, S. L. (1987). Renal autotransplantation and extracorporeal reconstruction for complicated benign and malignant diseases of the urinary tract. *J Cardiovasc Surg (Torino), 28*(4), 413–419.

48. van der Velden, J. J., van Bockel, J. H., Zwartendijk, J., van Krieken, J. H., & Terpstra, J. L. (1992). Long-term results of surgical treatment of renal carcinoma in solitary kidneys by extracorporeal resection and autotransplantation. *Br J Urol, 69*(5), 486–490.

49. Webster, J. C., Lemoine, J., Seigne, J., Lockhart, J., & Bowers, V. (2005). Renal autotransplantation for managing a short upper ureter or after ex vivo complex renovascular reconstruction. *BJU Int, 96*(6), 871–874.

50. Wotkowicz, C., & Libertino, J. A. (2004). Renal autotransplantation. *BJU Int, 93*(3), 253–257.

51. Ali-el-Dein, B., & Ghoneim, M. A. (2003). Bridging long ureteral defects using the Yang-Monti principle. *J Urol, 169*(3), 1074–1077.

52. Castellan, M., & Gosalbez, R. (2006). Ureteral replacement using the Yang-Monti principle: long-term follow-up. *Urology, 67*(3), 476–479.

53. Die Goyanes, A., Garcia Villanueva, A., Lavalle Echavarria, J. A., & Cabannas Navarro, L. (1983). Replacement of the left ureter by autograft of the vermiform appendix. *Br J Surg, 70*(7), 442–443.

54. Kaur, N., & Minocha, V. R. (2003). Ureteric stricture with a perirenal urinoma treated by ureteric replacement with appendix. *Int Urol Nephrol, 35*(1), 87–90.

55. Richter, F., Stock, J. A., & Hanna, M. K. (2000). The appendix as right ureteral substitute in children. *J Urol, 163*(6), 1908–1912.

Katharine V. Jamieson and Katharine A. Jamieson

Abstract The primary hyperoxalurias are a group of hereditary disorders characterized by overproduction and accumulation of the metabolic end product oxalate in the body. The heterogeneous nature of these disorders presents diagnostic and therapeutic challenges. While knowledge and understanding of these conditions are continually improving and may in the future yield further therapeutic modalities, at present the only strategy to correct the underlying metabolic defect is by replacement of the macroscopically normal recipient liver. Transplantation has developed to a point where it is accepted as a valuable treatment option for patients with primary hyperoxaluria type 1 (PH1), with good long-term results. However, controversies exist over the type and timing of transplantation. Furthermore, the long-term risks of immunosuppression cannot be ignored. This chapter will attempt to outline the different strategies and clinical considerations concerning this topic, illustrated with data collected by the European PH1 transplant registry.

51.1 Introduction

The primary hyperoxalurias are a heterogeneous disease group, characterized by increased synthesis and excretion of oxalate as a metabolic end product, with subsequent deposition of insoluble calcium oxalate. Two of the primary hyperoxalurias have thus far been well described – type 1 (PHI) and 2 (PH2) – both of which are inherited in an autosomal recessive fashion. Transplantation has thus far only been used as a treatment modality in the more common PH1, and therefore, this chapter will focus primarily on this topic.[1]

PHI results from low, absent, or mistargeted activity of the liver-specific peroxisomal enzyme alanine:glyoxylate aminotransferase (AGT, *AGXT* gene maps to 2p37.3).[2] The resulting decreased transamination of glyoxylate to glycine leads to a subsequent increase in its oxidation to oxalate in the cytoplasm – in humans, in the absence of an alternative metabolic pathway to allow breakdown of this oxalate, it is eliminated via the kidney, thus setting the scene for development of urinary stones, obstructive uropathy, nephrocalcinosis, and ultimately renal failure. Onset of symptoms occurs before the age of 5 in 50% of affected children, with end-stage renal failure occurring by 15 years of age in 50% of all PH1 patients, and by the third decade of life in 80%.[3] In the presence of renal failure with a glomerular filtration rate of less than 20–40 mL/min/1.73 m^2, overproduction of oxalate is compounded by decreasing renal excretion, with subsequent systemic oxalate accumulation and deposition (occurring in many tissues including bone, heart, retina, arteries, and nerves). Apart from the increased oxalate production, hepatic function remains entirely normal, even in late stages of the disease (Fig. 51.1).

The diagnosis can be established by measurement of plasma oxalate levels, and urinary oxalate and glycollate excretion in early cases with maintained renal function, but is more difficult in established renal failure.[4] It can be confirmed by measurement and localization of the enzymatic activity of AGT, which can be assessed using freshly frozen liver biopsy samples. Biopsy material was initially the corner stone of diagnosis but genetic techniques are advancing and can be used within families where the specific mutation has already been identified.[4]

K.V. Jamieson (✉)
Department of Transplantation Surgery, Addenbrooke's Hospital, Cambridge, Cambridgeshire, UK
e-mail: nvj1000@cam.ac.uk

Fig. 51.1 Diagramatic representation of oxalate metabolism in the human body

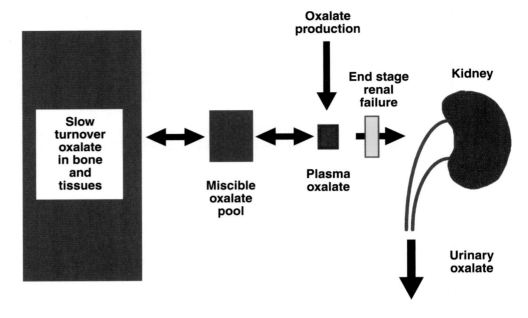

51.2 Clinical Management

If a diagnosis is established early in life before renal impairment has occurred, careful dietary management, high fluid intake (with the goal of maintaining a constant high urine output with dilute urine, and thus reduced risk of crystallization and stone formation)[5] and pharmacological manipulation (e.g., with administration of the AGT-coenzyme pyridoxine, or crystallization inhibitors)[6–8] may delay or avoid the development of stone disease. These measures together with optimal management of calculi are the essential features of early patient management, but can only be instituted after the diagnosis is established; as is evident from many previous publications and registry experience,[9] diagnosis is often delayed and renal failure is often the presenting problem precipitating diagnosis.[3,10,11] Even with highly motivated clinicians and patients, such management is difficult to sustain, particularly in children who tend to become noncompliant with the restrictions needed in adolescence.[12] In most cases where the diagnosis has been made before established renal impairment has occurred, there is a gradual decline in renal function over a period of years with the onset of chronic renal failure occurring in late childhood or early adult life. An infantile form is also recognized with an early rapid course, but disappointingly, the correlation between genotype and phenotype in terms of disease course is very variable and even within the same family, very different clinical patterns are seen with apparently the same genetic defect.[13,14] This heterogeneity, in combination with the rarity of the disease, makes decisions concerning timing and planning of intervention challenging.

Once the patient is in established renal failure, oxalate can no longer be excreted and systemic oxalosis rapidly develops

with deposition in muscles, bones, arteries, and nervous tissue, with progressive clinical deterioration and ultimately death. Production of oxalate by the liver ranges from 3.5–7.5 mmol/day, with an average tissue accretion rate of more than 50 μ(micro)mol/kg/day.[15] Daily prolonged hemodialysis or peritoneal dialysis may at best be able to remove oxalate sufficiently efficiently to slow the rate of accumulation, but is probably not able to balance the rate of production.[16,17]

51.3 Transplantation

For patients who progress to end-stage renal failure and in whom medical approaches can no longer compensate for the rate of oxalate production, three transplantation options have emerged:

1. Isolated renal transplantation to correct end-stage renal failure
2. Isolated liver transplantation as a preemptive strategy to correct the metabolic defect prior to significant renal damage
3. Combined hepato-renal transplantation

A registry of patients undergoing liver transplantation to correct the underlying metabolic defect in Europe has been maintained since the late 1980s and data from this registry will be used by way of illustration.

51.3.1 Isolated Renal Transplantation

Renal transplantation would seem a potential solution in replacing the diseased kidney with a functioning one to enable oxalate removal. The first reported renal transplant for PH1 was carried out in 1969. However, renal transplantation alone does not correct the underlying metabolic defect, and, in general, isolated renal transplant survival in PH1 patients has been disappointing.[18,19]

Prior to liver/kidney transplantation, 29 patients reported to the European registry had undergone 40 renal transplant procedures (4 were reported to be from living related donors). Eight patients received two grafts and one patient received four grafts. The survival of these grafts was generally poor and is illustrated in a report from the European Dialysis and Transplant Association (EDTA) registry with 5-year isolated kidney graft survival only being in the region of 10%,[18] which compares with a current anticipated isolated kidney graft survival of 70–80% for other indications. The same issue was examined in the European registry of patients receiving combined liver/kidney transplants who had often received previous failed isolated kidney grafts, showing that the majority of grafts were lost during the first 12 months and survival of isolated kidney grafts in these patients beyond 4 years was uncommon; although one patient who received a living related kidney did have satisfactory function for 12 years. Of these earlier cases, 40 kidney transplants showed definite evidence of recurrent oxalate deposits (both newly produced and that mobilized from tissue deposits), which was felt to have contributed to the loss of the graft in 30 cases.[20]

In selected cases, good outcomes may be achieved, but this requires living donors to ensure an optimal early graft function, appropriate timing, and careful postoperative medical management.[10,21,22] Isolated renal transplantation is currently only advocated in adult patients with late onset of a mild course of the disease or pyridoxine sensitivity. By contrast, cadaveric renal transplantation alone has little or no role to play in the management of patients with PH1, with generally poor outcomes. It is probably only appropriate to carry out cadaveric renal transplantation in conjunction with liver grafting to reverse the underlying metabolic defect.

51.3.2 Combined Liver/Kidney Transplantation

Early enzymatic evidence that the liver was the site of the metabolic defect[23] led to a patient receiving a combined liver/kidney grafting for PH1 in Cambridge in 1984.[24] Unfortunately, this first patient succumbed to postoperative sepsis, but oxalate dynamic studies confirmed the correction of the metabolic defect by the orthotopic hepatic allograft. Further proof of the liver as the site of the enzyme defect was provided by the transfer of PH1 to a patient who received a liver graft form a PH1 patient as part of a domino procedure.[25] Subsequent combined liver/kidney grafts were performed with long-term survival,[26] and the combined procedure has subsequently been widely applied, initially predominantly in European centers although now also applied increasingly commonly in North American centers. The transplant procedure itself is usually relatively straightforward. The liver graft is placed orthotopically, simply replacing the native liver; and as the liver is not otherwise abnormal, none of the usual technical liver transplantation problems (relating largely to portal hypertension in the more usual cirrhotic liver transplant recipient) arise. The kidney is usually placed in an extraperitoneal position in the iliac fossa with anastomosis of the renal vessels to the iliac vessels and of the ureter directly to the bladder in the conventional renal transplant fashion. The situation is somewhat more complex in children where it is usually necessary to use a reduced size graft (size-matched pediatric donors are rare), which can be obtained from either a cadaveric source or from a living related donor. The key issue, however, remains the complete excision of the oxalate-producing native liver.

Hepato-renal transplantation offers an attractive and potentially curative solution, in acting as a form of gene/enzyme therapy through replacing the enzyme-deficient organ (liver), as well as the irreversibly damaged end target organ (kidney). There is an additional potential immunological benefit in that the liver graft may protect the renal graft against rejection.[27] It is, however, important to remember that the enzymatically normal transplanted liver is simply a method of preventing further excess oxalate production and has no direct effect on oxalate deposits, which may have accumulated in patients who have gone on to develop renal failure. This oxalate load will only slowly be mobilized, and continuing care in maintaining a high urine output and dilute urine during the phase of mobilization is important if further problems with stone formation and oxalate deposition in the kidney are to be avoided.[28,29] This period of continuing supra-normal oxalate excretion has been poorly characterized in the patients reported in this registry, but may last for many months or even years, as suggested by some individual case reports in the European registry, particularly where there has been a long time period on dialysis.

Combined liver-kidney transplantation is currently recommended in patients with high levels of oxalate production that is resistant to pyridoxine therapy, with significant renal impairment, significant effects from systemic oxalosis deposition, or previous renal allograft failure due to oxalate deposition. It should also be noted that due to overlap of clinical findings in PH I and II, and uncertain benefits of liver transplantation in PH II (see later section), confirmation of the diagnosis by hepatic enzyme analysis or genetic testing is recommended prior to transplantation.

51.3.2.1 Timing of Transplantation

The timing of transplantation is influenced by several factors. The degree of systemic oxalosis has a direct effect on patient morbidity and mortality, and on graft survival. Early transplantation, before the accumulation of significant tissue oxalate deposits occurs, is thus advocated in cases not responsive to medical management. Oxalate elimination is dependent on renal function and thus decreases as renal function deteriorates. Oxalate dynamic studies suggest that the risk of increased plasma concentrations of oxalate, and by inference systemic deposition, occur with glomerular filtration rates (GFRs) of less than 40 mL/min/1.73 m², but can occur even at GFRs of 40–60.[30] After transplantation, plasma oxalate returns to normal within a few days as a result of decreased synthesis (Fig. 51.2). However, urinary oxalate secretion may remain elevated for weeks-months, a reflection of the length of time necessary for remobilization of tissue deposits of calcium oxalate – during this period, the renal graft remains vulnerable to renal calculi or nephrocalcinosis.[1] Attempts are thus made to perform transplantation when GFR is between 25 and 40mL/min/1.73 m², before the effects of oxalate retention become too pronounced.

Delaying hepatic transplantation with a prolonged duration of dialysis prior to transplantation worsens patient prognosis with decreased survival (Fig. 51.3), reflecting the more advanced level of oxalate deposition and decreased ability to withstand the operative procedure. Late transplant cases were more common in the earlier part of the experience and particular issues related largely to the complications of systemic oxalosis. Specific problems related to cardiomyopathy, bone deposits, and arterial deposits.

51.3.3 Liver Transplantation Alone

Preemptive isolated liver transplantation in the situation of preserved native renal function offers an attractive solution

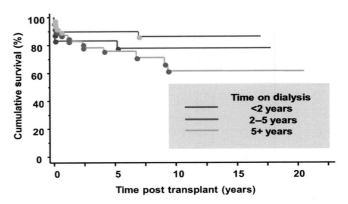

Fig. 51.3 A Kaplan–Meier survival plot to show the effect of time on dialysis prior to transplantation on post-transplant patient survival (Data from the European PH1 transplant registry, 1984–2007)

in treating the underlying problem prior to renal or systemic complications arising, and thus, avoids the need for renal replacement therapy. However, the potential morbidity and mortality of such an invasive intervention cannot be ignored, nor the effects of chronic immunosuppression including nephrotoxicity and malignancy.[31] Additionally, the timing of removal of a native liver in a disease with variable and unpredictable progression remains controversial.[32]

Results thus far do indicate that, as hypothesized, the correction of the metabolic defect is possible. The impact on renal function has been variable, seemingly dependent upon the degree of renal impairment at the time of transplantation. In some cases, renal function is improved; in others, the time needed before renal replacement therapy becomes necessary is significantly prolonged. Cases have been described in which preemptive liver transplantation was performed too late, with subsequent need for renal transplantation – such cases may be viewed as sequential combined transplantation, rather than truly preemptive. Currently, its use has been predominantly in carefully selected children with a severe, pyridoxine resistant form of the disease, in whom GFR is relatively preserved (generally agreed >40 mL/min/1.73 m², as below this the risk of systemic oxalosis increases). However, the lack of clinical, biochemical, or molecular markers to predict disease progression and the heterogeneous nature of the disease make recommendations difficult. The technical issues and complications are undoubtedly more favorable in isolated liver transplantation as compared to combined transplantation. However, the improving results for combined liver-kidney transplantation, and continually improving medical approaches including the emergence of alternative strategies to eliminate oxalate; e.g., treatment with *Oxalobacter* species[33] will continue to present arguments against preemptive liver transplantation. The lack of data directly comparing the different treatments makes objective evidence-based recommendations at this stage difficult.

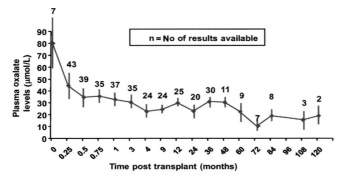

Fig. 51.2 A graph to show the changes in plasma oxalate levels following combined liver-kidney transplantation (Data from the European PH1 transplant registry, 1984–2007)

51.3.4 Other Forms of Transplantation

51.3.4.1 Sequential Transplantation

In some cases, sequential liver transplantation followed by kidney transplantation has been reported. Such procedures were carried out during earlier phases of the transplantation experience, or because clinical/physical considerations of the patient precluded simultaneous transplantation. The difficulties of such experiences have resulted from the fact that, in the absence of an adequately functioning kidney, oxalate elimination does not occur and systemic complications persist with subsequent detrimental effects upon the recipient. Even with concomitant dialysis, this is not an effective treatment strategy.

51.3.4.2 Auxiliary Liver Transplantation

Auxiliary liver transplantation has been proposed as a form of enzyme replacement therapy and is effective in a number of metabolic conditions in providing effective replacement of the deficient gene product. Unfortunately, as the underlying defect in PH1 is one of overproduction of a harmful product, this will persist in remaining native liver tissue (Fig. 51.4). The same theory presents an obstacle to the application of gene therapy techniques – these would require transfection of close to 100% of hepatocytes as any residual normal native hepatocytes would still be producing oxalate. This level of successful genetic manipulation is not currently achievable in human systems.

51.3.5 Transplantation in PH2

PH2 is caused by deficiency of glyoxylate reductase activity (GR, *GRHPR* gene location 9p11) – most of this enzyme is

found in hepatocytes, but it is also expressed in leukocytes and some other tissues.[9] Despite a different underlying genetic and enzymatic bases, both PH1 and 2 result in increased oxalate synthesis. However, due to the expression of the causative enzyme of PH2 in tissues other than the liver, it is not yet known whether liver transplantation would sufficiently correct the metabolic defect to justify the risks and morbidities associated with procedure. Additionally, the clinical course in PH2 tends to be more favorable, and for these reasons, isolated kidney transplantation (including cadaveric) is currently recommended if necessary in PH2.

51.3.6 Postoperative Supportive Therapy

Careful medical management is necessary both preceding and following transplantation. This includes intensive pre-transplantation dialysis to reduce plasma oxalate concentrations, maintenance of high-volume diuresis post-transplantation, and the introduction of neutral phosphates (to minimize supersaturation and crystallization) as soon as allograft function is established. Monitoring of plasma oxalate levels and urine oxalate concentrations should be initiated, with implementation of dialysis or additional hydration as needed to keep levels at 20–30 μ(micro)mol/L and <0.3 mmol/L respectively. Although the concentration of plasma oxalate does decrease following restoration of renal function, hyperoxaluria may persist for years after hepatic transplantation due to the length of time needed to mobilize and excrete accumulated tissue stores. A repeated error in patient care following transplantation has been to assume that the successful transplant procedure has immediately reversed all of the harmful effects of the underlying condition. This assumption is incorrect and the transplanted kidney remains at additional risk until normal urinary oxalate levels have been achieved. The nephrotoxic effects of immunosuppressive agents – particularly the calcineurin inhibitors cyclosporine and tacrolimus, which remain the mainstay of immunosuppressive protocols – remain problematic with an increasing emphasis on newer agents and calcineurin sparing strategies.

The problem is that the liver makes oxalate

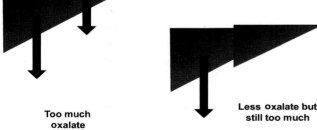

Too much oxalate

Less oxalate but still too much

Fig. 51.4 Diagrammatic representation of the difficulties with auxiliary liver transplantation as a treatment approach – the native liver continues to produce excess oxalate

51.4 Our Experience So Far: The European PH1 Transplant Registry

Thirty-five European centers currently carry out liver/kidney transplantation for the treatment of PH1. These centers established a PH1 study group and began to hold regular meetings to discuss their experiences. A voluntary registry was established to allow collation of the overall experience of the study group.

51.4.1 Patients

Between June 1984 and 2007, these centers reported 135 liver transplantations (in 126 patients), of varying types, the most common of which was combined kidney–liver transplants (Table 51.1).

The mean age at onset of first symptoms was 7.25 ± 9.9 years with a range from 0 to 47 years (Fig. 51.5). The age at which a diagnosis of PH1 was made ranged from 0 to 50 years, with a mean of 11.05 ± 12.4 years (Fig. 51.6). The mean interval from symptoms to diagnosis was 4.5 ± 7.7 years. Presentation was with one or more of the following features: nephrocalcinosis in 60% of cases, calculi in 71%, urinary tract infections in 40%, and uremia in 34%. The diagnosis was confirmed by liver biopsy-proven decreased AGT activity in 66% of cases, hyperoxaluria in 78%, hyperglycollicaciduria in 38%, and hyperoxalaemia in 48%. There was a positive family history in 41% of cases: 24 siblings having PH1, four cousins, and the history being reported as positive but not further specified in 24 cases. One parent has also received a combined transplant and four sets of parents were noted to be consanguineous.

Table 51.1 Types of transplants performed; data from the European PH1 transplant registry, 1984–2007

Type of transplant performed	Number of cases
Liver with simultaneous kidney	90
Reduced liver with simultaneous kidney	16
Liver alone	11
Liver with delayed kidney transplant	8
Reduced liver with delayed kidney transplant	2
Reduced liver alone	6
Auxiliary partial orthotopic living donor liver transplant	2
Total	135

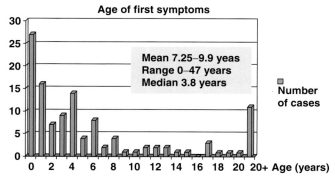

Fig. 51.5 Graphical representation of the age at which PH1 patients develop symptoms (Data from the European PH1 transplant registry, 1984–2007)

Patients were transplanted at a mean age of 17.36 ± 11.7 years following a period of dialysis of 3.5 ± 3.7 years (range 0–18 years) (Fig. 51.7).

The effects of the duration of dialysis on the patients' clinical condition at the time of transplant are shown in Table 51.2. Patients whose condition had worsened or was noted to be poor had been dialyzed for significantly longer, reflecting the poor removal of oxalate on dialysis and progression of systemic oxalosis in these cases (Table 51.3). The sites at which extra-renal oxalate was known to have accumulated are given in Table 51.4.

51.4.2 Results/Outcomes

A Kaplan–Meier cumulative survival plot shows patient and liver/kidney graft survival in Figs. 51.8, 51.9, and 51.10 with 1-, 5-, and 10-year patient survival values of 86%, 80%, and 69% respectively and fist liver graft survival rates of 80%, 72%, and 60 % at the same time intervals. There were ten retransplants, including two cases where third and fourth grafts were performed for chronic rejection related to non compliance with immunosuppressive medication, a recurring theme in patients transplanted in childhood who often become noncompliant with onerous treatment regimens during adolescence. There have been 25 deaths: 13 due to sepsis and multi-organ failure, 4 due to cardiac or thromboembolic events, 2 intra-operative deaths (at least one of which had cardiac failure as a contributing factor), 2 as a consequence of ongoing intra-abdominal bleeding, 1 with malignancy (astrocytoma), 1 with bleeding following a liver biopsy, 1 with a small bowel volvulus, and 1 with chronic rejection.

The patient's condition immediately prior to transplantation was ascribed by the physician in charge of their care to one of four categories (very good, good, fair, or poor). Five-year survival was 100% in those described as very good or good at the time of transplant, but only 73% in those described as fair and only 45% in those who were in poor condition with advanced systemic oxalosis.

The postoperative plasma oxalate levels are shown in Fig. 51.2. It should be noted that relatively few values are represented; plasma oxalate levels are often not measured postoperatively, reflecting the erroneous assumption that the transplant procedure immediately restores a normal situation. The evolution of the postoperative creatinine clearance in functioning kidney grafts is shown in Fig. 51.11. Function improves with time, suggesting that the initial function is impaired by the high early oxalate excretion rate. No figures are presented for 24-h urinary oxalate excretion as the data are very sparse.

The data from the registry on preemptive liver transplantation are limited, reflecting only five cases, of whom three have gone on to require subsequent renal replacement therapy.

Fig. 51.6 Graphical representation of the age at which diagnosis of PH1 is made (Data from the European PH1 transplant registry, 1984–2007)

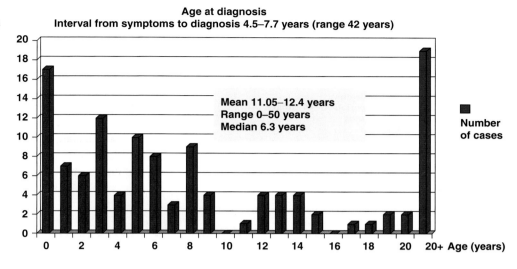

Age at diagnosis
Interval from symptoms to diagnosis 4.5–7.7 years (range 42 years)

Mean 11.05–12.4 years
Range 0–50 years
Median 6.3 years

Number of cases

Age at transplantation
Mean time from dialysis to transplantation 3.5–3.7 years
Range 0–18 years

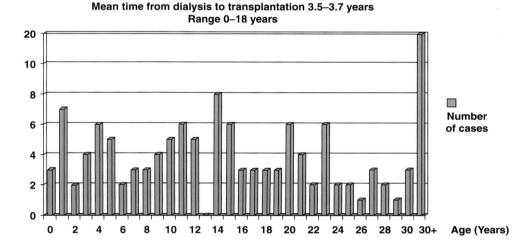

Number of cases

Fig. 51.7 Graphical representation of the age at transplantation (Data from the European PH1 transplant registry, 1984–2007)

Table 51.2 The clinical status at the time of transplantation and the time on dialysis; data from the European PH1 transplant registry, 1984–2007 – available for 104 cases

Status at transplantation	Number	Time on dialysis (years: mean ± SD)
Poor	27	3.6 ± 2.6
Fair	23	4.1 ± 4.4
Good	44	2.1 ± 2.8
Very good	10	1.4 ± 1.6

Table 51.4 Sites of extra-renal oxalate deposition; data from the European PH1 transplant registry, 1984–2007 – available for 126 cases

Organ/site	Percentage
Heart	14
Arteries	18
Skeleton	60
Nerves	11

51.5 Conclusions

Table 51.3 The effects of duration of dialysis on clinical course; data from the European PH1 transplant registry, 1984–2007 – available for 95 cases

Course on dialysis	Number	Time on dialysis (years: mean ± SD)
Improved	19	2.4 ± 2.6
Unchanged	36	2.7 ± 2.3
Worse	40	3.1 ± 2.6

From the initial 1984 case, combined liver/kidney transplantation has developed to the point where it has been accepted as a valuable treatment option for patients with PH1 with good long-term results.[13,22,24,26,29,34–36] Our growing understanding of the underlying genetic mechanisms[4,37–39] has improved our diagnostic abilities and can allow appropriate conservative measures to be instituted promptly to minimize renal damage, and may in the future present new therapies. It

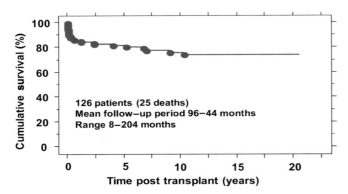

Fig. 51.8 A Kaplan–Meier cumulative survival plot to represent patient survival (Data from the European PH1 transplant registry, 1984–2007)

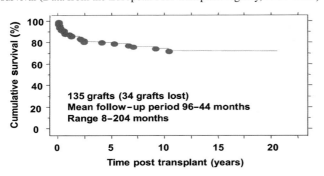

Fig. 51.9 A Kaplan–Meier cumulative survival plot to represent first liver graft survival (Data from the European PH1 transplant registry, 1984–2007. Note ten retransplants not included)

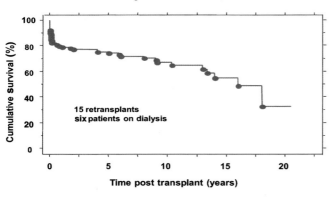

Fig. 51.10 A Kaplan–Meier cumulative survival plot to represent first kidney graft survival (Data from the European PH1 transplant registry, 1984–2007)

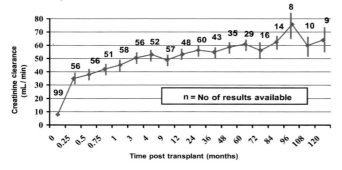

Fig. 51.11 A graph to show changes in creatinine clearance following combined liver–kidney transplantation (Data from the European PH1 transplant registry, 1984–2007)

has not as yet, however, allowed us to develop any clinical strategies to correct the underlying metabolic defect other than by the replacement of the macroscopically normal recipient liver with one from an unaffected donor. Controversies remain over the timing and type of transplantation. In order to maximize patient and graft survival, the pathophysiological characteristics of PH1 must be considered. Factors to consider include patient selection for the type of transplantation, timing of transplantation, and supporting clinical management, both at the time of transplantation and long term.

References

1. Cochat P, Gaulier JM, Koch Nogueira PC, et al. Combined liver-kidney transplantation in primary hyperoxaluria type 1. *Eur J Pediatr*. 1999;158(suppl 2):S75-S80.
2. Hoppe B, Latta K, von Schakenburg C, Kemper MJ. Primary hyperoxaluria - the German experience. *Am J Nephrol*. 2005;25(3): 276-281.
3. Cochat P, Deloraine A, Rotily M, Olive F, Liponski I, Deries N. Epidemiology of primary hyperoxaluria type 1. Societe de Nephrologie and the Societe de Nephrologie Pediatrique. *Nephrol Dial Transpl*. 1995;10 suppl(8):3-7.
4. Rumsby G. Biochemical and genetic diagnosis of the primary hyperoxalurias: a review. *Mol Urol*. 2000;4(4):349-354.
5. Scheinman JI. Primary hyperoxaluria: therapeutic strategies for the 90's. *Kidney Int*. 1991;40(3):389-399.
6. Leumann E, Matasovic A, Niederwieser A. Pyridoxine in primary hyperoxaluria type I. *Lancet*. 1986;2(8508):8699.
7. Milliner DS, Eickholt JT, Bergstralh EJ, Wilson DM, Smith LH. Results of long-term treatment with orthophosphate and pyridoxine in patients with primary hyperoxaluria. *N Engl J Med*. 1994;331(23): 1553-1558.
8. Leumann E, Hoppe B, Neuhaus T, Blau N. Efficacy of oral citrate administration in primary hyperoxaluria. *Nephrol Dial Transpl*. 1995;10(suppl 8):14-16.
9. Jamieson NV. A 20-year experience of combined liver/kidney transplantation for primary hyperoxaluria (PH1): the European PH1 transplant registry experience1984–2004. *Am J Nephrol*. 2005;25(3): 282-289.
10. Milliner DS, Wilson DM, Smith LH. Clinical expression and long-term outcomes of primary hyperoxaluria types 1 and 2. *J Nephrol*. 1998;11(suppl 1):56-59.
11. van Woerden CS, Groothoff JW, Wanders RJ, Davin JC, Wijburg FA. Primary hyperoxaluria type 1 in The Netherlands: prevalence and outcome. *Nephrol Dial Transpl*. 2003;18(2):273-279.
12. Gagnadoux MF, Niaudet P, Broyer M. Non-immunological risk factors in paediatric renal transplantation. *Pediatr Nephrol*. 1993;7(1):89-95.
13. Shapiro R, Weismann I, Mandel H, et al. Primary hyperoxaluria type 1: improved outcome with timely liver transplantation: a single-center report of 36 children. *Transplantation*. 2001;72(3):428-432.
14. Pirulli D, Marangella M, Amoroso A. Primary hyperoxaluria: genotype-phenotype correlation. *J Nephrol*. 2003;16(2):297-309.
15. Danpure CJ. *Scientific rationale for hepato-renal transplantation in primary hyperoxaluria type 1*. Amsterdam: Excerpta Medica; 1991.
16. Hoppe B, Graf D, Offner G, et al. Oxalate elimination via hemodialysis or peritoneal dialysis in children with chronic renal failure. *Pediatr Nephrol*. 1996;10(4):488-492.
17. Yamauchi T, Quillard M, Takahashi S, Nguyen-Khoa M. Oxalate removal by daily dialysis in a patient with primary hyperoxaluria type 1. *Nephrol Dial Transpl*. 2001;16(12):2407-2411.

18. Broyer M, Brunner FP, Brynger H, et al. Kidney transplantation in primary oxalosis: data from the EDTA registry. *Nephrol Dial Transpl.* 1990;5:332-336.

19. Hoppe B, Langman CB. A United States survey on diagnosis, treatment, and outcome of primary hyperoxaluria. *Pediatr Nephrol.* 2003;18(10):986-991.

20. Jamieson NV. The results of combined liver/kidney transplantation for primary hyperoxaluria (PH1) 1984–1997. The European PH1 transplant registry report. European PH1 Transplantation Study Group. *J Nephrol.* 1998;11(suppl 1):36-41.

21. Scheinman JI. Recent data on results of isolated kidney or combined kidney/liver transplantation in the U.S.A. for primary hyperoxaluria. *J Nephrol.* 1998;11(suppl 1):42-5.

22. Monico CG, Milliner DS. Combined liver-kidney and kidney-alone transplantation in primary hyperoxaluria. *Liver Transpl.* 2001;7(11):954-963.

23. Gibbs D, Watts R. The idientification of the enzymes that catalyse the oxidation of glyoxylate to oxalate in toe 100, 000 g supernatant fraction of human hyperoxaluric and control liver and heart tissue. *Clin Sci.* 1973;44:227-241.

24. Watts RW, Calne RY, Williams R, et al. Primary hyperoxaluria (type I): attempted treatment by combined hepatic and renal transplantation. *Q J Med.* 1985;57(222):697-703.

25. Donckier V, El Nakadi I, Closset J, et al. Domino hepatic transplantation using the liver from a patient with primary hyperoxaluria. *Transplantation.* 2001;71(9):1346-1348.

26. Watts RW, Calne RY, Rolles K, et al. Successful treatment of primary hyperoxaluria type I by combined hepatic and renal transplantation. *Lancet.* 1987;2(8557):474-475.

27. Rasmussen A, Davies HF, Jamieson NV, Evans DB, Calne RY. Combined transplantation of liver and kidney from the same donor protects the kidney from rejection and improved kidney graft survival. *Transplantation.* 1995;59(6):919-921.

28. Latta K, Jamieson NV, Scheinman JI, et al. Selection of transplantation procedures and perioperative management in primary hyperoxaluria type 1. *Nephrol Dial Transpl.* 1995;10(suppl 8):53-57.

29. Gagnadoux MF, Lacaille F, Niaudet P, et al. Long term results of liver-kidney transplantation in children with primary hyperoxaluria. *Pediatr Nephrol.* 2001;16(12):946-950.

30. Watts RW, Veall N, Purkiss P. Sequential studies of oxalate dynamics in primary hyperoxaluria. *Clin Sci (Lond).* 1983;65(6):627-633.

31. Ojo AO, Held PJ, Port FK, et al. Chronic renal failure after transplantation of a non-renal organ. *N Engl J Med.* 2003;349(10):931-940.

32. Cochat P, Schärer K. Should liver transplantation be performed before advanced renal insufficiency in primary hyperoxaluria type I? *Pediatr Nephrol.* 1993;7(2):212-218.

33. Hoppe B, Beck B, Gatter N, et al. Oxalobacter formigenes: a potential tool for the treatment of primary hyperoxaluria type I. *Kidney Int.* 2006;70(7):1198-1200.

34. Saborio P, Scheinman JI. Transplantation for primary hyperoxaluria in the United States. *Kidney Int.* 1999;56(3):1094-1100.

35. Ellis SR, Hulton SA, McKiernan PJ, de Ville de Goyet J, Kelly DA. Combined liver-kidney transplantation for primary hyperoxaluria type 1 in young children. *Nephrol Dial Transpl.* 2001;16(2):348-354.

36. Millan MT, Berquist WE, So SK, et al. One hundred percent patient and kidney allograft survival with simultaneous liver and kidney transplantation in infants with primary hyperoxaluria: a single-center experience. *Transplantation.* 2003;76(10):1458-1463.

37. Danpure CJ, Jennings PR, Fryer P, Purdue PE, Allsop J. Primary hyperoxaluria type 1: genotypic and phenotypic heterogeneity. *J Inherit Metab Dis.* 1994;17(4):487-499.

38. Cibrik DM, Kaplan B, Arndorfer JA, Meier-Kriesche HU. Renal allograft survival in patients with oxalosis. *Transplantation.* 2002;74(5):707-710.

39. Zhang X, Roe SM, Hou Y, et al. Crystal structure of alanine:glyoxylate aminotransferase and the relationship between genotype and enzymatic phenotype in primary hyperoxaluria type 1. *J Mol Biol.* 2003;331(3):643-652.

Chemolytic Treatment of Patients with Urinary Tract Stones

52

Hans-Göran Tiselius

Abstract The combined use of extracorporeal shock wave lithotripsy (SWL) and percutaneous irrigation with chemolytic agents has proven useful for providing an extremely low-invasive therapeutic approach. This form of treatment can be applied in patients with large infection stones, as well as in patients with stones composed of brushite, cystine, and uric acid. Although other treatment options might be less time consuming, the chemolytic method is a definite alternative in selected patients for whom other procedures are either excluded or associated with a greater risk. Chemolytic irrigation also can be of great importance to clear the renal collecting system from stone fragments after percutaneous stone removal. For stones composed of uric acid, an entirely oral treatment can be used to accomplish stone removal in a completely noninvasive way. The principles and possibilities of chemolytic treatment are outlined in this chapter.

52.1 Introduction

The remarkable technical achievements during the past decades have dramatically changed the principles for stone removal in the urinary tract, and, within a few years, a noninvasive or extremely low-invasive treatment has developed from an extensively invasive surgical approach. The ultimate goal to eliminate urinary tract stones by a purely pharmacological approach is, however, still remote and as yet possible essentially only for patients with stones composed of uric acid. For some stone salts, the solubility can be significantly influenced mainly by changes in the pH-level of the surrounding fluid/urine. This latter property has been used accordingly for designing chemolytic treatment regimens.[1,2] There are also other possibilities to increase the solubility of some stone constituents, for instance by administration of chelating agents,[3,4] but the clinical usefulness of such methods usually has been less successful because of undesirable side effects. Therefore, methods aiming to change environmental pH remain as the most powerful chemolytic tool. Several ways for administration of chemolytic agents have been advised, and percutaneous, transureteral, as well as oral routes will be discussed in this chapter.

In the continuous search for a stone removing method that is the least invasive and the least traumatic as possible, the various options for stone dissolution deserve serious consideration even though modern technology undoubtedly has made stone removal a much easier procedure than it used to be, both for the patient and for the treating surgeon. Chemolytic treatment probably was more important at a time when open surgery was the only way to remove stones actively from the kidneys and ureters. Nevertheless, and despite the successful development of noninvasive or low-invasive methods, the ultimate goal of stone removal ideally should be without any form of surgical or mechanical treatment and in this regard chemolytic treatment options still have a definite place. For the majority of stones requiring active removal, a completely nonsurgical approach, unfortunately, is not available, but chemolysis might be a very useful adjunct to efficiently eliminate residual stone fragments or stones, which might remain in the kidney after extracorporeal shock wave lithotripsy (SWL) and percutaneous nephrolithotripsy (PNL). Such an approach is particularly desirable in patients with infection stones as well as in patients with stones containing cystine, uric acid, and brushite, because of the very high recurrence risk seen with these stone constituents.[5]

A summary follows of the available tools for stone dissolution and how these methods can be used to improve and facilitate the treatment of our patients.

H.-G. Tiselius
Department of Urology, Karolinska University Hospital Huddinge, Stockholm, Sweden
e-mail: hans.tiselius@karolinska.se

P.N. Rao et al. (eds.), *Urinary Tract Stone Disease*,
DOI 10.1007/978-1-84800-362-0_52, © Springer-Verlag London Limited 2011

52.2 Chemolytic Treatment of Patients with Infection Stones

The crystalline components of the typical infection stone are magnesium ammonium phosphate (MAP; struvite), carbonate apatite (CarbAp), and usually also variable amounts of hydroxyapatite (HAP). Such triple phosphate stones can grow rapidly and often develop complete or partial staghorn morphology. The large stone burden and the great risk of recurrences seen in patients with such stones constitute a real treatment challenge for the urologist. A complete stone clearance is essential in order to eradicate the infection and thereby to counteract recurrent stone formation.[6] Small residual fragments harboring urease producing microorganisms very rapidly can grow into a new huge stone. Urease causes a splitting of urea that results in high urinary concentrations of ammonium and carbonate ions as well as an alkaline pH. Although some pharmacological methods are available for preventing recurrences, the fundamental principle is to eliminate all infection stone material from the urinary tract before a medical follow-up treatment program is instituted.[6]

The basic principle for dissolution of an infection stone is a reduction of the pH in the renal collecting system, because MAP, CarbAp, and HAP are highly soluble in acid solutions. The typical course of the change in urine supersaturation with changes in pH is shown in Fig. 52.1.

It is not possible to accomplish any clinically significant dissolution of infection stones by oral treatment and the only way to get such an effect is to establish contact between the crystalline material of the stone and an acid solution. Several different solutions have been described for the purpose of infection stone dissolution; the most well recognized and clinically used solutions are Suby G and hemiacidrin (Renacidin™).[4,7–19] There are also experimental reports of some other stone dissolving agents,[20] but their clinical application remains less well known.

Chemolytic treatment can be used for clearance of residual infection stone fragments in the kidneys or ureters following various kinds of stone removing procedures. By combining repeated SWL sessions and percutaneous irrigation with a chemolytic solution, it is possible to carry out a low-invasive removal of even large infection stones in an extremely low-invasive way.[16,19,21] Although such an approach sometimes might be time consuming it is definitely an alternative for certain risk patients and for patients in whom no other treatment alternative seems possible.

Before starting chemolysis of stones, assumed to be of infection origin, it is essential to confirm the diagnosis. An absolute reliable diagnosis can be obtained only by a stone analysis or by placing a stone fragment (if available) in a few milliliters of the chemolytic solution. Infection stones, amenable to the suggested treatment, thereby will be dissolved and replaced by a white salt within a period of 1–3 days. In the absence of stone material for in vitro test or for stone analysis, indirect evidence can be used to decide on the stone composition. An infection stone usually has a typical multi-layered appearance on the plain film of kidneys, ureters, and bladder (KUB). Positive urine cultures, with demonstration of urease-producing microorganisms, or a medical history of infections with such a microorganism are helpful indicators. The microscopic demonstration of typical MAP (struvite) crystals also can be used to confirm the diagnosis.

The combination of PNL and chemolysis can be used to eliminate residual infection stone fragments, whereas a combination of SWL and chemolysis can be used to remove infection staghorn stones. The author so far successfully has used the latter regimen for removal of more than 150 complete or partial infection staghorn stones according to the principles previously described.[16] In all patients, a 10% Renacidin™ solution was used to dissolve the stone material.

It is important that the solution of irrigation is introduced into the renal collecting system without a high pressure, and, for that purpose, two nephrostomy catheters should be used. One of these catheters is used for inflow and one for outflow of the irrigation solution Fig. 52.2. Several methods have been described for continuous control of the intrarenal pressure,[19,22] but the author has never encountered any problems without such devices provided that there is a free flow through the outlet nephrostomy tube and provided the patient is sufficiently educated to immediately report any kind of discomfort and instructed to stop the irrigation if problems are encountered.

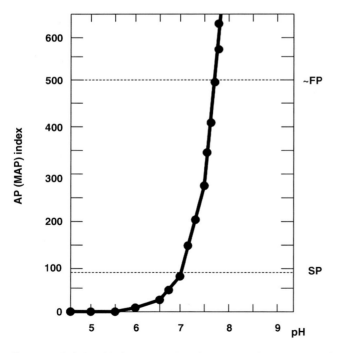

Fig. 52.1 Relationship between pH and the ion activity product of MAP expressed as AP(MAP) index. The approximate levels of solubility product (SP) and formation product (FP) are indicated.

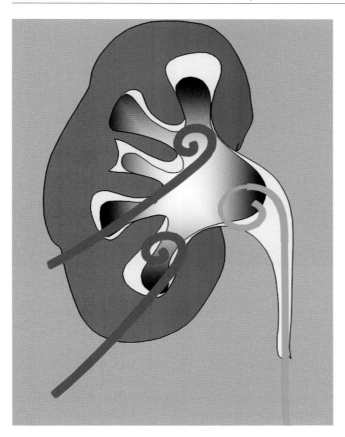

Fig. 52.2 For removal of a staghorn stone, two thin nephrostomy catheters and one internal stent should be inserted before the first shock wave lithotripsy (SWL) session. The chemolytic agent subsequently is administered through one of the nephrostomy catheters and allowed to drain freely through the other

For the combined SWL and chemolytic treatment, two thin nephrostomy catheters (usually 7 Fr) should be inserted into the kidney before stone disintegration. Ideally, the loops of these catheters should be in different parts of the kidney, but that goal is not always easy to reach. The idea is to use one of these catheters for inflow and the other one for outflow of the solution, and it is essential to eliminate the risk of high pressure and leakage of fluid. In addition, an internal ureteral stent should be used in order to avoid accumulation of large volumes of fragments in the ureter Fig. 52.2. Following SWL, which is undertaken to increase the contact surface area between the stone material and the surrounding medium (Renacidin or any other chemolytic solution), dissolution of the stone fragments can be started. It is important, however, to first test the system by irrigation with saline and always to collect any small fragment that passes during this procedure. This harvesting step is useful for enabling stone analysis as well as for an in vitro dissolution test. The irrigation with the chemolytic solution can be run at a speed that the patient tolerates without discomfort. This usually means a flow-rate up to about 120 mL/h. The patient should be instructed carefully to stop the irrigation at any sign of discomfort such as fever, shivering, or nausea. It is extremely essential to avoid a high intrarenal pressure, and steps must to be taken to avoid any leakage of the solution. Renacidin contains magnesium and absorption of magnesium is dangerous because a high magnesium concentration in blood can cause cardiac arrest. Such a complication has been reported, but the author has never encountered any problems of that kind. Daily measurements of serum electrolytes, creatinine, and magnesium should be made during the treatment period. It is, moreover, essential to cover the patients with antibiotics during the procedure. Although antibiotics can be administered orally when the procedure works smoothly, it is necessary to give appropriate antibiotics intravenously during the initial phase of the procedure and always when an SWL-session is carried out.

How frequently repeated SWL sessions can be carried out, to disintegrate solid stone residuals, depends on the type of lithotripter and the total SWL energy that has been used at the previous session. Intervals between successive SWL-sessions ideally should not be shorter than 7–10 days – an interval that also will allow sufficient time for fragment dissolution. Chemolytic irrigation between the sessions is continued until all small fragments have disappeared. The irrigation is stopped if the patient develops fever. The duration of the treatment depends on the size and density of the stones, but several weeks should be allowed for the treatment. For suitable patients it is the author's experience that the irrigation can be organized on an outpatient basis with chemolysis carried out during daytime. There are some reports that the irrigation has been carried out by the patient at home, but such an approach should be discouraged with regard to the potential risk of solution leakage and absorption. For the same reason it is the author's routine not to continue the irrigation during the night. The ideal outcome of the treatment is a completely stone-free kidney. It is, however, sometimes necessary to accept minor residual fragments that reside in the kidney despite aggressive irrigation. Fragments that remain insoluble are assumed to have a non-infection stone composition.

Figures 52.3 and 52.4 show two typical examples of the elimination of a complete and a partial staghorn stone. This treatment approach was chosen because of the medical condition of the patients.

This combined treatment also can be used successfully for removal of stents with encrustation of infection stone material. SWL disintegration of the encrustation followed by percutaneous irrigation with Renacidin is the method of choice in such cases, after which the stent can usually be extracted easily. It is of note, however, that when only one percutaneous nephrostomy catheter is used, it is extremely important to avoid over-pressure by using a very slow flow-rate or by intermittently injecting only small portions of Renacidin.

Of 118 patients, many of whom had both very complex stone situations and difficult medical conditions, SWL and

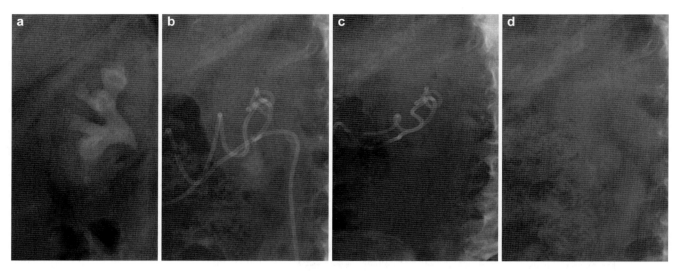

Fig. 52.3 This series of images shows the combined treatment of a complete staghorn stone in a 76-year-old medically weak woman. The stone was caused by urease producing microorganisms. Stone surface area was 2,175 mm². Disintegration was accomplished by a total of 10,800 shock waves given during four SWL sessions. The chemolytic irrigation required approximately 13 L of Renacidin. The situation in the kidney is shown before (**a**), during the initial part of the treatment (**b**), before removal of the nephrostomy catheters (**c**), and at late follow-up (**d**). The duration of the treatment was 21 days during the last 7 of which the patient was treated on an outpatient basis

chemolysis resulted in a stone-free rate of 60%.[16] In a consecutive and more representative series of patients with staghorn stones, a stone-free rate of 77% was achieved. The mean duration of the treatment for all our patients was long: 32 days. This makes the method less attractive as a standard procedure, but it is easy to use in high-risk patients. The rate of complications is very low. Other authors also have used this treatment approach successfully and Spirnak and coworkers recorded a stone-free rate of 90% (nine out of ten patients).[21]

In the follow-up of patients with infection stone disease, recurrence prevention with antibiotics and urine acidification is an essential part of the treatment. Some very problematic stone patients might benefit from treatment with urease inhibitors like acetohydroxamic acid, but the side effects of this form of treatment limit its use.[23]

52.3 Cystine Stone Dissolution

Cystine stone disease is encountered in less than 1–2% of all stone formers, but the rapid stone growth and frequent recurrences constitute a considerable clinical problem. A rational stone prevention should be based on an efficient clearance of stones and stone fragments from the renal collecting system. In view of a lifelong history of stone formation, it appears reasonable to be the least invasive as possible when choosing stone removing procedures.

Cystine stones form because of the poor solubility of cystine in urine. This type of stone is only seen in patients with the genetic disease cystinuria, because only patients with that disease have sufficiently high excretion levels of cystine to cause stone formation.

The basic principle for dissolution of cystine depends on its exponentially increased solubility in alkaline urine. It is, however, necessary to get a pH-level above 7.5–8 in order to accomplish dissolution, and oral treatment regimens with alkaline agents are thus not likely to be successful in terms of stone dissolution. The typical relationship between pH and the ion-activity product of cystine ($AP_{cystine}$) is shown in Fig. 52.5.

The formation product of cystine, $FP_{cystine}$, is approximately $1.3 \, 10^{-20}$ mol/L³ and the solubility product ($SP_{cystine}$) $1.0 \, 10^{-20}$ mol/L³.[24] Although a combination of pharmacological regimens theoretically can reduce $AP_{cystine}$ to levels below the $SP_{cystine}$, such a treatment is very demanding and usually of limited value because of side effects of the pharmacological agents. There are, however, reports of cystine stone dissolution with both penicillamine and tiopronin, but the author has never observed such an effect. A pharmacological approach of course has its given place in prevention of stone recurrences, but for stone elimination contact chemolysis with percutaneous irrrigation is preferable. Either the stones can be disintegrated and removed with PNL and any residuals subsequently dissolved with suitable agents, or the stone surface area can be increased with SWL treatment (as discussed previously for infection stones) and the stone material subjected to percutaneous chemolysis.

Percutaneous irrigation in order to dissolve cystine stones can be carried out with the alkaline solutions of tris(hydroxymethyl) aminomethane (THAM). Various concentrations of this solution

Fig. 52.4 A partial staghorn in the upper part of the kidney in a 69-year-old man with a CP-lesion. Percutaneous stone surgery was considered less appropriate for this patient. The stone surface area was measured to 3,022 mm². During a period of 6 weeks, and mostly in an outpatient setting, the stone was eliminated by four SWL sessions (10,900 shock waves) and 25 L of Renacidin. The gravel in the caudal cavity was not treated. The images show the situation before the first SWL session (**a**) 5 days, (**b**) 8 days (**c**), 19 days (**d**) later, as well as at the end of the treatment (**e**). At follow-up 2 months later (**f**), no residuals remained from the treated stone and there was also a reduction of the stone material in the lower part of the kidney

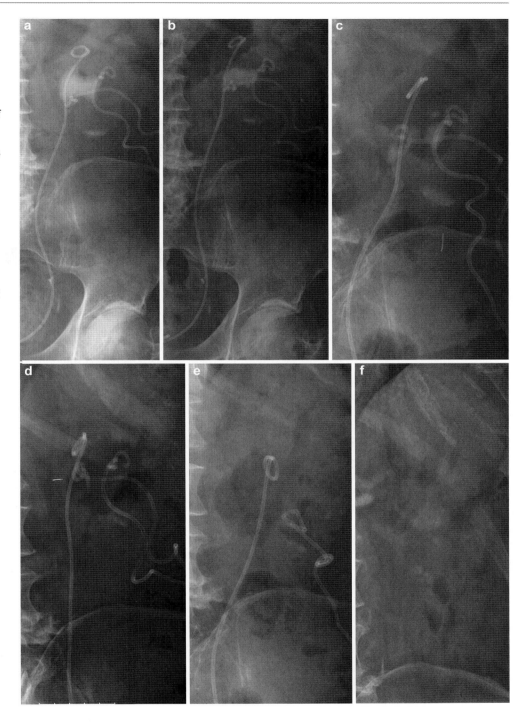

have been described and used.[2,14,25–30] The author uses either a 0.3 or a 0.6 mol/L THAM. To further augment the dissolving effect of THAM solutions, the combination with N-acetylcysteine has proven very successful.[14,25,31,32] N-acetylcysteine is an agent that forms highly soluble complexes with the cystine molecule. How THAM and N-acetylcysteine solutions can be prepared are shown in Tables 52.1 and 52.2. As for percutaneous irrigation of infection stones (Fig. 52.2), two nephrostomy catheters should

be inserted in the kidney. Also the use of an internal stent is recommended in order to avoid passage of cystine stone fragments to the ureter.

It is generally considered that cystine stones are SWL-resistant and although cystine stones might appear hard to disintegrate, most of them can be successfully treated with an appropriate SWL equipment. A combination of SWL and irrigation with the chemolytic solutions mentioned previously can

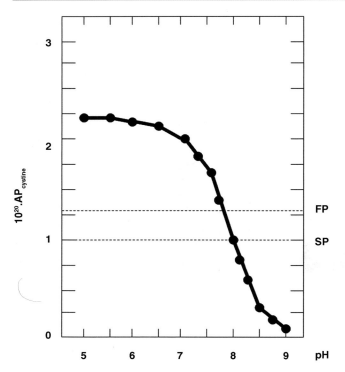

Fig. 52.5 Relationship between urine pH and the ion-activity of cystine ($AP_{cystine}$). The levels of the solubility product (SP) and the formation product (FP) are indicated

Table 52.1 Preparation of THAM solutions for dissolution of uric acid and cystine stone material

	THAM 0.3 mol/L	THAM 0.6 mol/L
Sterile water (mL)	800	800
Trometamol 3.3 mol/L (mL)	90	180
Sodium chloride (mmol)	30	30
Potassium chloride (mmol)	30	5

Table 52.2 Preparation of acetylcysteine solution for dissolution of cystine stone material

Acetylcysteine (200 mg/mL)	100 mL
Tribonate[a]	500 mL
Sterile water	400 mL

[a] The composition of tribonate is as follows: trometamol 36 g/L, sodium bicarbonate 13 g/L, acetic acid 2.8 g/L

be used for elimination of small to medium sized cystine stones (with a surface area up to 200–300 mm²).[28,29] For larger stones, a percutaneous stone removal or debulking is recommended because of the relatively slow dissolution of cystine. In a previously published algorithm it was concluded that cystine stones with a diameter up to 15 mm can be treated with SWL as monotherapy; those with a diameter 15–30 mm with SWL and chemolysis; whereas staghorn cystine stones will require removal with PNL, possibly combined with SWL and subsequently percutaneous dissolution with THAM/acetylcysteine.[33]

Attributable to the important role of complete fragment and crystal clearance for prevention of cystine stone recurrence, percutaneous irrigation with these dissolving agents always should be considered when a nephrostomy catheter is present or when residual stones or fragments are encountered.

Although stone dissolution has been described also by the transureteral route,[3,34,35] this approach is much less tolerable for the patient and the author has seldom been successful with such dissolution attempts.

An example of successful cystine stone dissolution is shown in Fig. 52.6. This patient, with multiple stones in the kidney, had a very poor compliance with all existing forms of pharmacological recurrence prevention.

In patients without known cystinuria, this stone diagnosis should be suspected when the density of the stone(s) on the KUB is lower than that of calcium stones with a similar size. The findings of hexagonal crystals at microscopic examination of a urinary sediment as well as demonstration of an increased excretion of cystine confirm the diagnosis. The workup of these patients should always include determination of the cystine excretion in urine.

An increased solubility of cystine can be anticipated following oral treatment with acetazolamide (Diamox®). When attempts are made to use oral chemolysis the effect on urine supersaturation should be assessed. The $AP_{cystine}$ can be calculated from the concentration of cystine ($C_{cystine}$) and pH by the following formula[24]:

$$AP_{cystine} = \frac{\left(10^{-pH}\right)^2 \cdot C_{cystine} \cdot 0.155}{\left[1 + \left(0.39 \cdot 10^9 \cdot 10^{-pH}\right) + \left(10^{-pH}\right)^2 \cdot 3.51 \cdot 10^{16}\right]}$$

Alkalinization of urine and administration of cystine complexing agents like tiopronin is the standard method for recurrence prevention. Aggressive alkalinization might result in calcium phosphate stone formation as replacement of cystine stones, but inasmuch as calcium phosphate stones are easier to manage from a stone removing point of view, this result is better than continuous cystine stone formation.[36]

52.4 Dissolution of Stones Composed of Uric Acid

Precipitation of uric acid occurs when the ion-activity product of uric acid (AP_{HU}) exceeds the formation product (FP_{HU}) of this salt at approximately $5\,10^{-9}$ mol/L². The most important determinants for an excessive saturation with uric acid are a high concentration of urate and a low pH.[24,37] The high urate concentration is either due to a small urine volume, a high urinary excretion of urate, or both. A reduced supersaturation accordingly can be achieved by increasing urine pH and by

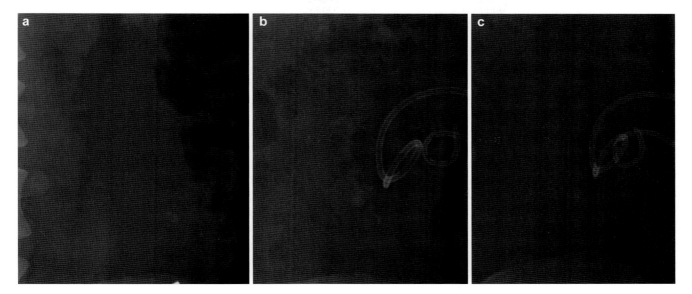

Fig. 52.6 An example of combined treatment with SWL and chemolysis of (**a**) multiple cystine stones in (**b**) a patient without compliance with any form of medical treatment. (**c**) Stone clearance was achieved with five SWL sessions (17,500 shock waves) and outpatient daytime chemolysis during 7 weeks with 24 L of acetylcystein and 23 L of THAM-solutions (in total 34 irrigation sessions)

decreasing the concentration of urate. Although prevention of uric acid stone formation can be accomplished by a reduction of AP_{HU} to a level below the formation product, it is necessary to get an AP_{HU} below the solubility product SP_{HU}, which is around $2 \cdot 10^{-9}$ mol/L^2.

Several studies have shown that *oral* chemolytic treatment of uric acid concrements is a very successful way of eliminating such stones from the urinary tract.[30,37–42] Such a therapeutic approach accordingly can be recommended as a first-line treatment for patients in whom uric acid stones are present.[1,2] In order to get a sufficiently low AP_{HU}, the first step is to alkalinize the urine. This is made by administration of an alkaline salt such as potassium citrate, sodium potassium citrate, or sodium bicarbonate.[42] How AP_{HU} changes with pH for an average urine composition is illustrated in Fig. 52.7.

Moreover, a reduction of the urate concentration should be made by combining a high fluid intake with the xanthine oxidase inhibitor allopurinol. An efficient reduction of AP_{HU} can be accomplished by the following regimen: allopurinol administered in a daily dose of 300 mg to decrease urinary urate also for patients in whom the urate excretion is not elevated. To increase pH it is the author's routine to give 6–10 mmol of potassium citrate three times daily. It is, however, possible also to use sodium potassium citrate in a similar dosage regimen or sodium bicarbonate. Theoretically, an increased sodium load can increase the risk of sodium urate precipitation, but there are no studies in support of such a risk. Others have suggested administration of 2–4 g of sodium bicarbonate three times daily.[43] The dose required needs to be decided from measurements of urinary pH and ideally also urate. Two cases of unsuccessful dissolution of

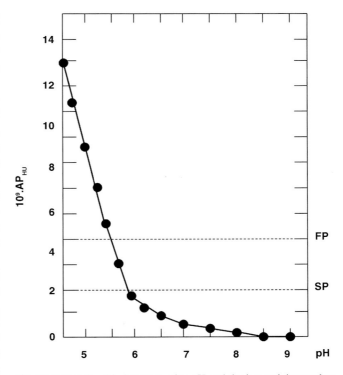

Fig. 52.7 Relationship between urine pH and the ion-activity product of uric acid (AP_{HU}). The levels of the solubility product (SP) and the formation product (FP) are indicated

uric acid despite treatment with alkali were explained by an insufficient increase in pH.[44]

In order to reduce the time for dissolution of *large* uric acid stones, a combination of SWL and oral chemolysis is advised. The stone disintegration with SWL thereby increases the contact surface area between the crystalline material and urine.

The problem before starting this kind of oral chemolytic regimen is to make certain that the patient really has a stone that is composed of uric acid. The most reliable clue is of course to analyze stone material that the patient hopefully has delivered. In addition, uric acid stones are usually not visible on KUB images, but clearly so on computed tomography (CT) examinations. For a patient who has delivered a uric acid stone or a stone fragment, its pronounced solubility in alkaline solutions can be clearly demonstrated by placing the material in a tube with THAM-solution. If dissolution is not observed within a few hours, the stone is not composed of pure uric acid and other options for stone removal should be considered. In order to further support the diagnosis, a high AP_{HU} is a useful indicator. AP_{HU} can be calculated from the urate concentration (C_{urate}) and urine pH by the following formula:

$$AP_{HU} = \frac{C_{urate} \cdot 10^{-pH} \cdot 0.53}{\left(1 + 1.63 \cdot 10^5 \cdot 10^{-pH}\right)}$$

Analysis of urine composition and calculation of AP_{HU} is also most useful for recording the effect of the pharmacological treatment to make certain that AP_{HU} is below SP_{HU}. Figure 52.8 shows a CT examination of a patient with a uric acid stone before and after 8 weeks of oral chemolytic treatment.

The time required for stone dissolution by oral treatment depends on the size and morphology of the stone, but several weeks or months usually are necessary to eradicate the stone. It is therefore essential that the patient is reasonably free of symptoms during the treatment period.

In symptomatic patients with stones in the kidneys or ureters, a more aggressive primary treatment is necessary, comprising SWL, ureteroscopic stone extraction/disintegration, or percutaneous surgery. In case residual stones or fragments, not causing obstruction, are left after such procedures, the clearance of the collecting system can easily be completed with oral chemolysis. For patients with a percutaneous nephrostomy catheter, contact dissolution with an alkaline solution administered percutaneously is a superb and usually much faster treatment alternative. Solutions of 0.3 or 0.6 mol/L THAM (tris[hydroxymethyl]aminomethane) (Table 52.1) can be used for the percutaneous irrigation and they have both proven to be effective and well tolerated by the patients. Other authors successfully have used 0.1 mol/L THAM together with 0.02% chlorhexidine.[30]

A low-invasive removal of large uric acid stones also can be accomplished by combining SWL with percutaneous chemolysis. It thereby is recommended that the patients are given two thin (7 Fr) nephrostomy catheters during the treatment period (as for dissolution of infection stones shown previously, Fig. 52.2). One of the catheters is used for inflow of the alkaline solution and the other one for outflow. In this way, a high intrarenal pressure can be avoided. For patients who experience local irritation by the chemolytic agent a local anesthetic can be administered through the percutaneous nephrostomy catheter before starting the irrigation.

Several reports have shown that oral as well as percutaneous chemolysis of uric acid stones is successful in most cases.[30,37-45] It needs to be emphasized, however, that stones composed of ammonium urate are formed during periods of a simultaneous infection and supersaturation with uric acid, and that there is no chemolytic agent available for that type of stone.

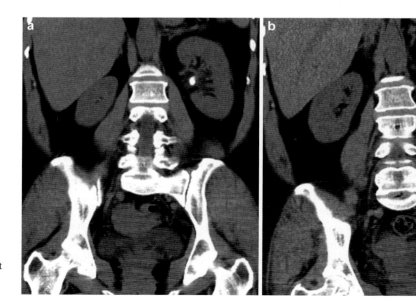

Fig. 52.8 CT examination of a patient with a renal pelvic uric acid stone (**a**) before and after 8 weeks (**b**) of daily oral treatment with 300 mg of allopurinol and 7 mmol × 3 of potassium citrate

52.5 Calcium Phosphate

There are several different crystal phases of calcium phosphate.[24] Usually calcium phosphate (hydroxyapatite, octacalcium phosphate, or carbonate apatite) occurs together with calcium oxalate and, in that combination, the stones are not particularly susceptible to chemolysis. Experimental studies showed that the presence of calcium oxalate in an amount exceeding 10% inhibited dissolution.[10]

Hydroxyapatite and octacalcium phosphate form in alkaline urine, and in pure form such stones can be dissolved by percutaneous irrigation with acid solutions of type hemiacidrin (Renacidin). This is a therapeutic option that deserves to be kept in mind, but percutaneous dissolution of the two mentioned types of stone is seldom used clinically and the author is not aware of any reports in the literature where this treatment alternative has been described.

A more useful application of chemolytic dissolution concerns brushite (calcium hydrogen phosphate). Also this calcium phosphate crystal phase is soluble in Renacidin. The compact morphology of brushite stones make the dissolution less rapid than is the case for infection stones, but Renacidin constitutes an excellent tool to clear the kidney from brushite stone residuals. The application of such a therapeutic step is justified by the very high risk of recurrences seen in patients with this kind of stone[5,13,46] for those patients it appears important to achieve a clearance of fragments as good as possible.

Figure 52.9 shows a patient with a huge brushite stone that was successfully eliminated by a combination of repeated SWL sessions and percutaneous chemolyisis with Renacidin. The technical details for this form of treatment are the same as for chemolytic treatment of infection stone (see previous).

Theoretically, acidification of urine by oral treatment should lead to dissolution of calcium phosphate stones, but a sustained low urine pH is not possible with continuous administration of an acidifying agent. Moreover, administration of acid drugs brings about a reduced excretion of citrate and consequently an increased risk of recurrent calcium stone formation. Citrate is an important inhibitor of that process and increased urinary citrate also reduces the ion-activity product of calcium phosphate crystal phases by complexation with urinary calcium.[47]

52.6 Calcium Oxalate

What has been discussed previously is applicable to only a fraction of stone-forming patients. Unfortunately, approximately 80% of all stones are composed either of pure calcium oxalate or mixtures of calcium oxalate and calcium phosphate. In the latter stone type, calcium oxalate usually dominates. For calcium oxalate containing stones, the principles for dissolution is not as straightforward as for the other stone constituents previously discussed.

Successful attempts to dissolve calcium oxalate stones were carried out and reported by Timmerman and Kallistratos many years ago.[3,35,48] They used solutions containing ethylenediaminetetraacetic acid (EDTA), which forms soluble complexes with calcium. The solution was usually administered through ureteral catheters or through percutaneous nephrostomy catheters and for obvious reasons this therapeutic approach was not easily tolerated by the patients. I have personally occasionally used ureteral catheters of administration of other chemolytic solutions to dissolve stones in the ureter. In most of those cases, that therapeutic approach was not particularly successful.

Experimental studies with various calcium chelating solutions have been reported.[4,49] The conclusion was that, albeit several of the solutions had favorable stone dissolving properties, the clinical usefulness was impossible because of toxic and irritative effects on the urothelium.[4,50–52]

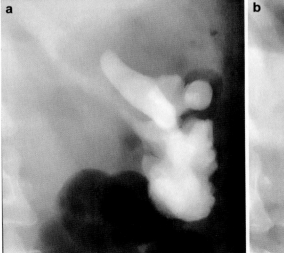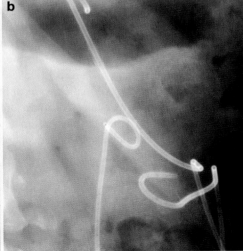

Fig. 52.9 A huge brushite stone (**a**) before and (**b**) after a series of SWL sessions and percutaneous irrigation with Renacidin

An anecdotic report suggested in a brief urologic letter that calcium oxalate stones could be dissolved successfully by percutaneous irrigation with coconut milk installed directly from the coconut. No similar report has subsequently been found in the literature and immersion of calcium oxalate stones in coconut milk did not result in any stone dissolution (unpublished data).

The solubility of calcium oxalate is essentially unaffected by variations in pH, within the physiological range, and in order to dissolve calcium oxalate it is necessary to reduce the pH to a level between 1 and 2. Such an acidification is not clinically feasible.

The author has no personal experience of dissolution of calcium oxalate stones. Neither are there any recent reports on such treatment modalities. It would indeed be great with a method that dissolved residual calcium oxalate fragments after SWL, but such a method probably requires a different mechanism of action. Enzymatic degradation of the stone matrix or any other method by means of which binding forces between different crystals can be broken is theoretically possible.[4] Further research in this area should indeed be useful, but efforts in that direction are not stimulated by the ease by means of which stones today can be removed from the urinary tract. Moreover, there is no consensus on the risk for new stone development from residual fragments.

52.7 Conclusions

Percutaneous chemolysis of urinary tract stones cannot be considered as a routine treatment modality. It is, however, an excellent and very low-invasive method for selected patients. Inasmuch as this treatment in combination with SWL can be carried out without regional or general anesthesia, it stands to reason that this gentle therapeutic approach constitutes a powerful tool for stone clearance, when other options for some reason are excluded. For stones composed of constituents fully soluble in the available solutions, a complete clearance of stone material can be expected. This property makes percutaneous chemolysis particularly suitable as an auxiliary step when residual fragments are present after other stone removing procedures for infection, brushite, cystine, and uric acid stones. This additional method definitely has a place in the treatment of those patients who will benefit from a meticulous clearance of fragments from the renal collecting system. For uric acid stones, oral stone dissolution is a superb noninvasive treatment option.

References

1. Tiselius HG, Ackermann D, Alken P, Buck C, Conort P, Gallucci M. Guidelines on urolithiasis. *Eur Urol.* 2001;141:753-758.

2. Tiselius HG, Alken P, Buck C, Gallucci M, Knoll T, Sarica K, Türk C. *Guidelines on Urolithiasis.* EAU publications, 2008.

3. Kallistratos G. Heutiger Stand der chemischen Niernesteinauflösung und - prophylaxe. *Ther Woche.* 1997;26:5920-5932.

4. Oosterlinck W, Veerbeeck R. Chemolysis of calcium containing urinary calculi. A review. *Acta Urol Belg.* 1994;62:31-37.

5. Leusmann DB, Niggermann H, Roth S, von Ahlen H. Recurrence rate and severity of urinary calculi. *Scand J Urol Nephrol.* 1995;29:279-283.

6. Lerner SP, Gleeson MJ, Griffith DP. Infection stones. *J Urol.* 1989;141:753-758.

7. Ries SW, Malment M. Renacidin: a urinary calculi solvent. *J Urol.* 1962;87:1979.

8. Blavia JG, Pais VM, Spellman RM. Chemolysis of residual stone fragments after extensive surgery for staghorn calculi. *Urology.* 1975;6:680-686.

9. Rodman JS, Reckler JM, Israel AR. Hemiacidrin irrigations to dissolve stone remnants after nephrolithomy. *Urology.* 1981;18:127-130.

10. Wall I, Tiselius HG, Larsson L. Hemiacidrin - a useful complement in the treatment of infectious renal stones. *Eur Urol.* 1988;15:26-30.

11. Wall I, Tiselius HG, Hellgren E. Minimally invasive treatment of hemiacaidrin soluble staghorn renal stones. *J Lithotr Stone Dis.* 1991;3:31-43.

12. Suby HI, Albright F. Dissolution of phosphatic calculi by the retrograde introduction of a citrate solution containing magnesium. *N Engl J Med.* 1943;81:228.

13. Heimbach D, Winter P, Hesse A. When is the indication of percutaneous chemolysis justified? *Urol Int.* 1995;54:157-161.

14. Pfister RC, Dretler SP. Percutaneous chemolysis of renal calculi. *Urol Radiol.* 1984;6:138-143.

15. Tiselius HG, Hellgren E, Wall I. Infected staghorn stones treated with ESWL and hemiacidrin. Proceedings of the 4th symposium on shock wave lithotripåsy: state of the art. Indianapolis, 1988. *Endourology.* 1988;2:137-139.

16. Tiselius HG, Hellgren E, Andersson A, Borrud-Ohlsson A, Eriksson I. Minimally invasive treatment of infection staghorn stones with shock wave lithotripsy and chemolysis. *Scand J Urol Nephrol.* 1999;33:286-290.

17. Dretler SP, Pfister RC, Newhouse JH. Renal-stone dissolution via percutaneous nephrostomy. *N Engl J Med.* 1979;300:341-343.

18. Weinrich W, Haas H, Alken P. Percutane chemolyse von Struvit-Steinen bei nierenbecken- und kelchhalsobstruction. *Aktuel Urol.* 1982;13:256-258.

19. Sheldon CA, Smith AD. Chemolysis of calculi. *Urol Clin N Am.* 1982;9:121-131.

20. Xiang-bo Z, Zhi-ping W, Jian-min D, Jian-zhong L, Bao-liang M. New chemolysis for urological calcium phosphate calculi - an in vitro study. *BMC Urol.* 2005;22:5-9.

21. Spirnak JP, DeBaz BP, Green HY, Resnick MI. Complex struvte calculi treated by primary extracorporeal shock wave lithotripsy and chemolysis with hemiacidrin irrigation. *J Urol.* 1988;140:1356-1359.

22. Angermeier K, Streem SB, Yost A. Simplified infusion method for 10% hemiacidrin irrigation of renal pelvis. *Urology.* 1993;41:243-246.

23. Lerner S, Malachy J, Gleeson J, Griffith DP. Infection stones. *J Urol.* 1989;141:753-758.

24. Tiselius HG. Solution chemistry of supersaturation. In: Coe FL, Favus MJ, Pak CYC, Parks JH, Preminger GM, eds. *Kidney Stones. Medical and Surgical Management.* Philadelphia: Lippincott-Raven; 1996:33-64.

25. Dretler SP, Pfister RC, Newhouse JH, Prien EL Jr. Percutaneous catheter dissolution of cystine calculi. *J Urol.* 1984;131:216-219.

26. Aabech J, Andersen JT. Treatment of cystine stones: comined approach using open pyelolithotomy, percutaneous pyelolithotipsy, extracorporeal shock wave lithotripsy and chemolysis. *Scand J Urol Nephrol.* 1993;27:415-417.

27. Tseng CH, Talwalker YB, Tank ES, Hatch T, Alexander SR. Dissolution of cystine calculi by pelvocaliceal irrigation with tromethamine-E. *J Urol.* 1982;128:1281-1284.

28. Schmeller NT, Kersting H, Schüller J, Chaussy C, Schmiedt E. Combination of chemolysis and shock wave lithotripsy in the treatment of cystien renal calculi. *J Urol.* 1984;131:434-438.

29. Ahlstrand C, Tiselius HG. Treatment of cystine urolithiasis by a combination of extracorporeal shock wave lithotripsy and chemolysis. *J Stone Dis.* 1993;5:32-38.

30. Lee YH, Chang LS, Chen MT, Huang JK. Local chemolysis of obstructive uric acid stone with 0.1 M THAM and 0.02% chlorhexidine. *Urol Int.* 1993;51:147-151.

31. Smith AD, Lange PH, Miller RP, Reinke DB. Dissolution of cystine calculi by irrigation with acetylcysteine through percutaneous nephrostomy. *Urology.* 1979;8:422-423.

32. Weinrich W, Ackermann D, Riedmiller H, Alken P. Die Auflösung von cystin-steinen mit N-acetylcystein nach perctaner nephrostomy. *Aktuel Urol.* 1981;12:224-226.

33. Kachel TA, Vijan SR, Dretler SP. Endourological experience with cystine calculi and a treatment algorithm. *Journal of Lithotripsy and Stone Disease.* 1991;145:25-28.

34. Dormia E, Dormia G, Malagola G, Minervini S. Experience with instrumental chemolysis for urolithiasis. *J Urol.* 2003;170:1105-1110.

35. Kallistratos G. Chemical dissolution of kidney stones. *Jpn J Urol.* 1973;64:555-576.

36. Koide T, Yoshioka T, Yamaguchi S, Utsunomiya M, Sonoda T. A strategy of cystine stone management. *J Urol.* 1992;147:112-114.

37. Rodman JS, Sosa E, Lopez MA. Diagnosis and treatment of uric acid calculi. In: Coe FL, Favus MJ, Pak CYC, Parks JH, Preminger GM, eds. *Kidney Stones. Medical and Surgical Management.* Philadelphia: Lippincott-Raven; 1996:973-989.

38. Moran ME, Abrahams HM, Burday DE, Greene TD. Utility of oral dissolution therapy in the management of referred patients with secondarily treated uric acidstones. *Urology.* 2002;59:206-210.

39. Norlén BJ, Hellström M, Nisa M, Robertson WG. Uric acid stone formation in a patient after kidney transplantation - metabolic and therapeutic considerations. *Scand J Urol Nephrol.* 1995;29:335-337.

40. Chutai MN, Khan FA, Kaleem M, Ahmend M. Management of uric acid stone. *J Pakistan Med Assoc.* 1992;42:153-155.

41. Rodman JS, Williams JJ, Petersen CM. Dissolution of uric acid calculi. *J Urol.* 1984;131:1039-1044.

42. Sharma SK, Inudhara R. Chemodissolution of urinary uric acid stones by alkali. *J Urol.* 1992;48:81-86.

43. Tung KH, Tan EC, Foo KT. Chemolysis of uric acid stones. *Ann Acad Med Singapore.* 1984;13:620-624.

44. Funahashi M, Yamada T, Murayama T. Two cases of uric acid unsuccessfully dissolved by oral chemolysis. *Hinyokika Kiyo.* 2006;52:47-48.

45. Lee YH, Chang LS, Chen MT, Huang JK, Chen KK, Lin AD. Experience with percutaneous nephrolithotomy, extracorporeal shock wave lithotripsy and chemolysis in the treatment of obstructive uric acid stones. *Eur Urol.* 1991;19:209-212.

46. Heimbach D, Jacobs D, Hesse A, Müller SC, Zhong P, Preminger GM. How to improve lithotripsy and chemolithoysis of brushitestones: an in vitro analysis. *Urol Res.* 1999;27:266-271.

47. Tiselius HG, Berg C, Fornander AM, Nilsson MA. Effect of citrate on the different phases of calcium oxalate crystallisation. *Scanning Microsc.* 1993;7:381-391.

48. Timmermann A, Kallistratos G. Modern aspects of chemical dissolution of human renal calculi by irrigation. *J Urol.* 1966;95:469-475.

49. Verplaetse H, Verbeeck R, Minnaert H, Oosterlinck W. Screeing of chelating agents for chemolysis. *Eur Urol.* 1986;12:190-194.

50. Oosterlinck W, Minnaert H, Varbaeys A, Verbeeck R, Verplaetse H, Cuvelier C. *Toxicity of EDTA-Chemolytic Solutions on the Urothelium.* Abstract 1414. European Association of Urology 7th Congress, Budapest, 1986.

51. Oosterlinck W, Verbeeck R, Cuvelier C, Bergauwe D. Rational for local toxicity of calcium chelators. *Urol Res.* 1992;19:19-21.

52. Oosterlinck W, Verbeeck R, Cuvelier C, Verplaetse H, Verbaeys A. Toxicity of litholytic ethylenediaminetetraacetic acid to the urothelium of the rat and dog. *Urol Res.* 1991;19:265-268.

Establishment and Management of a Stone Clinic

53

William G. Robertson

Abstract The incidence of upper urinary tract stone disease has risen steadily throughout the past 100 years and renal colic is now one of the commonest causes of admission to hospital. Spontaneous passage of the stones and the so-called "minimally invasive" procedures for their removal or fragmentation are the most frequent means of alleviating the patient's immediate problems. However, they do not cure the underlying abnormalities responsible for causing the stones to form in the first place and, as a result, patients often have further episodes of stone-formation if left without proper preventative treatment. Without subsequent biochemical screening and appropriate dietary and/or medical management, the patient will inevitably return for further stone removal at some point in the future.

53.1 Introduction

The incidence of upper urinary tract stone disease has risen steadily throughout the past 100 years and renal colic is now one of the commonest causes of admission to hospital. Spontaneous passage of the stones and the so-called "minimally invasive" procedures for their removal or fragmentation are the most frequent means of alleviating the patient's immediate problems. However, they do not cure the underlying abnormalities responsible for causing the stones to form in the first place and, as a result, patients often have further episodes of stone formation if left without proper preventative treatment. Without subsequent biochemical screening and appropriate dietary and/or medical management, the patient will inevitably return for further stone removal at some point in the future.[1,2]

Unfortunately, following the introduction of the various minimally invasive treatments to remove stones in the mid-1980s, many health authorities took the opportunity to save money by cutting out the detailed biochemical assessment of patients with stones on the assumption that if patients do have a recurrence of their stone problem after the removal of their first stone, then they can be easily re-treated at their local urology department to remove any subsequent stones. Not only is the failure to provide proper prophylactic treatment for the patient bad clinical management, in the long term it is economically more expensive. Financial analysis has shown that the projected costs of treating stone patients solely by removing their stones by minimally invasive procedures every time they form them is considerably more expensive than removing their initial stones and then screening them thoroughly to identify their risk factors in order to provide them with appropriate prophylactic management. The scheme that this chapter will describe, which includes a biennial biochemical screen, is more economical in terms of the management of recurrent stone formers than leaving the patients with no preventative treatment. In the UK, it has been calculated that every stone recurrence prevented in this way would save the local health authority concerned about £2,000.[1]

53.2 Stone Clinic

How then should we tackle the problem of investigating patients at a Stone Clinic to find out why they have formed their stones and what facilities should be available in such a clinic?

Ideally, a stone clinic should be designed to serve a number of functions.[2] Firstly, it must provide a service for diagnosing the presence or absence of stones in a given patient.

W.G. Robertson
Department of Physiology (Centre for Nephrology),
Royal Free and University College Medical School,
Rowland Hill Street, London NW3 2PF, UK
e-mail: w.robertson@ucl.ac.uk

P.N. Rao et al. (eds.), *Urinary Tract Stone Disease*,
DOI 10.1007/978-1-84800-362-0_53, © Springer-Verlag London Limited 2011

Calculi may occur at any point in the urinary tract, although more are located in the kidney and ureter than in the bladder. More than 60% of stones are small enough to be passed spontaneously in the urine. Within the kidney itself, concretions may be found in the calyces, in the renal pelvis, or extending from the calyces into the pelvis. They may be attached to the epithelial surfaces of the pelvi-calcyceal system, be encapsulated within the renal parenchyma, or lie free within the pelvis or lower pole of the kidney. Occasionally, they may occupy the entire pelvi-calcyceal space to form the so-called "staghorn" calculi.

Upper urinary tract stones may occur on either side and are often bilateral. There is a high rate of recurrence in patients who are not treated prophylactically. Moreover, the recurrence rate appears to be higher after the use of minimally invasive techniques for the disintegration and/or removal of stones than it was in the days of open kidney surgery (Fig. 53.1). This is particularly noticeable in patients treated with extracorporeal shock-wave lithotripsy (ESWL), which, by the nature of the technique, tends to leave behind fragments of stone that may act as foci for subsequent stone-formation. Percutaneous nephrostolithotomy (PCNL) is slightly less of a problem in this respect, as it is usually easier to ensure that most of the stone fragments are removed during the procedure. The newer technique of flexible ureteroscopy (FUR) may turn out to produce the best outcome of these three minimally invasive procedures since the stones and their fragments are usually more completely removed either by laser or by stone capture. However, since there is nothing inherent in the minimally invasive techniques that will treat the underlying cause(s) of stone formation in most cases, sole reliance on these procedures for the overall management of stone formers is inadequate and stones tend to recur unless dietary and/or medical treatment is instituted.

Concretions may also become lodged at any point in the ureter, but most commonly do so at the upper and lower ends.

There is a constriction at the pelvi-ureteric junction that often obstructs the passage of a small stone. Even if the stone negotiates this obstacle, it may pass down the ureter only to become lodged at the vesicoureteric junction. Ureteric calculi may produce partial or total obstruction to the flow of urine, usually giving rise to severe colic.

Finally, calculi may be found in the bladder, either lying free or lodged in a diverticulum in the vesical wall. Most probably, they originate in the upper urinary tract and continue to grow in their new location. Others may be initiated in the bladder. They occur almost exclusively in elderly males and usually consist of uric acid or are associated with infection following prostatic obstruction. The other main situation in which bladder stones are found is in patients who have had an enterocystoplasty.

The diagnosis of urolithiasis is rarely a major problem, since the stone behaves as a foreign body in the urinary tract and gives rise to symptoms that usually cannot be ignored for long, although about 3% of patients undergoing ultrasound or radiographic investigations for other abdominal problems have been found to have so-called "silent" or quiescent stones in their kidneys. A careful history of the pain may contain valuable diagnostic clues. A stone in the renal pelvis, for example, causes dull loin pain with occasional colic; in the ureter, it gives rise to agonizing pain radiating down into the groin; and in the bladder, to discomfort in the suprapubic and perineal regions. The patient may have hematuria, often microscopic, and episodes of frequency and dysuria caused by the passage of "sand" or "gravel." In addition, children and pregnant women often present with an atypical clinical picture. Diagnosis is usually confirmed by a combination of ultrasound, a plain abdominal X-ray and, particularly in the case of radiolucent stones (i.e., those consisting of uric acid, 2,8-dihydroxyadenine or xanthine), an intravenous pyelogram. Occasionally, a computed tomography (CT) or magnetic resonance imaging (MRI) scan can provide useful additional information.

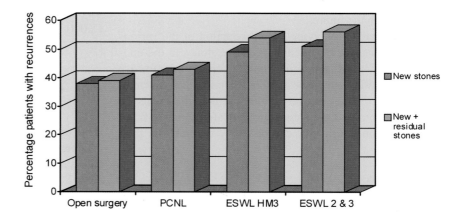

Fig. 53.1 Stone recurrence rates 3 years after various urological procedures for stone removal or disintegration

The full details of the diagnostic aspects of the investigations are set out in previous chapters of this book (see Chaps. 28–34).

Having established that the patient actually has a stone (or stones) in the urinary tract, it is essential that the clinic possesses the facilities to carry out the following detailed investigations to identify why the patient has formed his/her stone(s):

- Classification of the patient into one of the various types of the disorder, largely determined by the composition of the stone
- Identification of the demographic and epidemiological risk factors responsible for the stone-formation
- Identification of any lifestyle factors that might increase the risk of forming stones
- Determination of any metabolic and nutritional risk factors for stone formation
- Determination of the urinary risk factors for stone formation

The classification of stone patients according to stone type is shown in Table 53.1.

Once the patient is classified into whichever type of stone-forming group they belong, then the following process of management can be instituted:

- Institution and monitoring of the endourological and medical treatment of the disorder according to the risk factors for the disorder identified in the particular patient
- Follow-up of patients during their management period to ensure compliance with their treatment regime

All of these procedures have the following additional requirements for the successful running of the stone clinic:

- Training of the staff required for all of the procedures described previously.
- Establishment of a research environment with the aim of continually improving the overall management of patients with stone disease. (This is an ideal requirement but may not be possible in smaller hospitals.)

To achieve this, the ideal site for such a clinic should be within a general hospital with access to good facilities for uroradiology, endourology, lithotripsy, nephrology, and clinical biochemistry. Several other specialties within the general medical services may be occasionally required. Since many of the biochemical variables to be measured are diet dependent, the services of a good dietitian are essential and the clinic should be held in the morning so that blood and urine samples can be collected from the patient after a standardized overnight fast. The clinic should be conducted by trained physicians who appreciate the aims and limitations of stone management. The nursing staff should be well trained in the taking and handling of samples for analysis and the Chemical Pathology Laboratory should be equipped to perform the various analyses that are required for the assessment of the patient. It should be noted that some of the more specialized urine analyses (e.g., oxalate and citrate) might have to be performed by a commercial laboratory such as the Department of Chemical Pathology at University College London Hospitals.

Table 53.1 The classification of stone formers and their urinary risk factors for various types of stone formation

Stone type	Urinary risk factor	Chemical effect
Rare stones	↑Xanthine, ↑2,8-dihydroxyadenine	↑Supersaturation of relevant stone constituent
Iatrogenic stones	↑Silica, ↑sulfonamide, ↑indinavir, ↑triamterene, ↑sulfadiazine	↑Supersaturation of relevant drug
Cystine stones	↑Cystine	↑Cystine supersaturation
Uric acid stones	↓pH ↑Uric acid ↓Volume	↑Uric acid supersaturation
Infection stones	↑↑pH ↑Ammonium ions ↑Mucosubstances	↑Magnesium ammonium phosphate and +Calcium phosphate supersaturation ↑Agglomeration of crystals
Calcium stones	↓Volume ↑Oxalate ↑Calcium ↑pH ↓Citrate ↓Magnesium ↓Macromolecular inhibitors ↑Uric acid ↑Macromolecular promoters	↑Calcium oxalate and/or calcium phosphate supersaturation ↓Crystallization inhibitory activity ↑Crystallization promotive activity

53.3 Screening for the Risk of Stone Formation

Once the presence of a stone is confirmed and a decision is reached on the most appropriate urological procedure to relieve the patients of their stones, they should then be screened to identify the biochemical causes of their stones. It is usually best to carry out the screen at a time when the patients are eating and drinking "normally" in their free, home environment, but not when there is hematuria or immediately prior to the stone removal procedure. Once the procedure has been carried out, it is advisable to wait for 2–3 months before carrying out the screening process since during that period the patients are often consuming a diet that is different from "normal" and the risk of stone recurrence is relatively low – the so-called "Stone Clinic Effect."[3] If the patients do not form another stone within 3 months of the current episode, they usually return to their former "bad" dietary habits and the risk of stones increases again. The biochemical screening should *not* be carried out on in-patients since the hospital diet is likely to be very different from that consumed on their free, home diets.

Since urolithiasis is a multifactorial problem, there is no simple approach to the screening of patients. Gone are the days when a simple plasma calcium measurement and a dip-stick test for infection, hematuria, and pH were the key elements in the investigation of patients with stones. Not only is there a wide range of biochemical factors to be considered, there are also other factors that may lead to stones as a secondary problem, such as various metabolic disorders, lifestyle factors, a family history not only of stones but also of other medical disorders, epidemiological, demographic, genetic, and nutritional factors.

In the London Centre for Kidney Stone Research, a fully comprehensive system (Lithoscreen) has been developed over the past 10 years for the investigation of patients with stones.[4] A large database of patient information has been assembled using this system that, in turn, has thrown light on new risk factors, such as so-called "Metabolic Syndrome" or ethnic eating habits or practices, which are now known to influence the risk of stone formation in the ever-increasing obese populations of most Western societies (Fig. 53.2). The Lithoscreen system consists of the following.

53.3.1 Patientscreen

A complete demographic, lifestyle, and medical history of the patient should be recorded including:

- Date of birth, gender, weight, height, and body mass index (BMI)
- Blood pressure
- Ethnic origins including any details of cultural and religious habits or practices
- A detailed stone episode history including age at onset of stones
- A medical history not only of stones but also of other relevant disorders and a history of surgical procedures that might lead to stones as a secondary problem
- A lifestyle questionnaire including details of occupation, working or living in a hot environment, night-time sweating, strenuous exercise that leads to sweating, and air travel
- A history of urinary tract infections
- Details of any anatomical abnormalities in the urinary tract
- A history of past and current medication
- A family history of stones
- A family history of other medical problems that may influence the risk of stone formation such as hypertension,

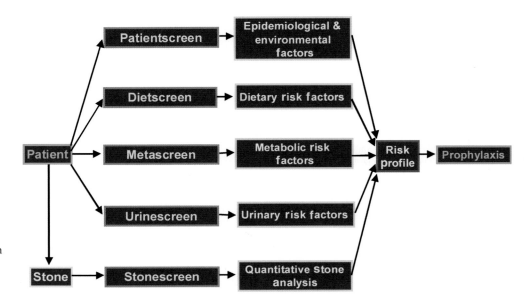

Fig. 53.2 Lithoscreen scheme for screening stone patients with a view to prescribing treatment to prevent recurrence of stone formation

type 2 diabetes, bowel disease, and any inborn errors of metabolism that are associated with stone formation

This aspect of the screening procedure can be carried out by a suitably trained clinical nurse practitioner.

From the previously listed information, it is often possible to make an initial diagnosis of why the patient has formed stones. Thus, patients with already identified medical conditions, such as primary hyperparathyroidism, distal renal tubular acidosis (dRTA), Dent's disease, hereditary or enteric hyperoxaluria, hyperuricemia, hypomagnesemia, metabolic syndrome, hypervitaminosis D, milk-alkali syndrome, various genetic disorders of purine metabolism, thalassemia

major, pancreatitis, or urinary tract infection, may be given a preliminary classification, although that may have to be modified after the metabolic screening, detailed later, is carried out. In addition, patients who have had operations such as small bowel resection, ileostomy, and enterocystoplasty, which may lead to changes in urinary biochemistry likely to cause urolithiasis, may be identified. A more complete list of all the main medical/surgical conditions that may lead to secondary stones is shown in Table 53.2.

The detailed Patientscreen also allows the identification of lifestyle factors that might increase the risk of forming stones from the regular passage of concentrated urine. Does

Table 53.2 The metabolic factors involved in secondary uric acid (UA) and calcium stone formation and their effects on urinary risk factors and stone type

Metabolic factor	Urinary risk factor(s)	Stone type
Gout	↑Uric acid	Uric acid
Glycogen storage disease	↑Uric acid	Uric acid
Lesch–Nyhan syndrome	↑Uric acid	Uric acid
Neoplastic disease	↑Uric acid	Uric acid
Secondary polycythemia	↑Uric acid	Uric acid
Anemia	↑Uric acid	Uric acid
Hemoglobinopathy	↑Uric acid	Uric acid
Psoriasis	↑Uric acid	Uric acid
Cystinuria	↑Uric acid, ↑cystine	Cystine/uric acid
Laxative abuse	↓Volume, ↑NH_4^+	NH_4 urate
Metabolic syndrome	↓pH (often + ↑oxalate, ↑uric acid, ↓ citrate)	Uric acid/CaOx
Ileostomy	↓Volume, ↓pH	Uric acid/CaOx
Primary hyperparathyroidism	↑↑Calcium, ↑pH	CaP/CaOx
Distal renal tubular acidosis	↑pH, ↑Calcium	CaP
Hereditary hyperoxaluria	↑↑Oxalate	CaOx
Enteric hyperoxaluria	↑Oxalate, ↓pH, ↓citrate, ↓magnesium	CaOx
Medullary sponge kidney	↑Calcium	CaOx/CaP
Cushing's disease	↑Calcium, ↑pH	CaOx/CaP
Sarcoidosis	↑Calcium	CaOx/CaP
Vitamin D intoxication	↑↑Calcium	CaOx/CaP
Milk-alkali syndrome	↑Calcium, ↑pH	CaP/CaOx
Immobilization	↑Calcium, ↑pH (from urinary tract infection)	CaP/MAP
Dent's disease	↑pH	CaP
Sjögren's syndrome	↑pH	CaP
Primary biliary cirrhosis	↑pH	CaP
Thalassemia major	↑↑Calcium (from excessive vitamin D)	CaOx/CaP
Betel-chewing	↑Calcium, ↑pH	CaP/CaOx
Hypomagnesemia	↑Oxalate	CaOx/CaP
Pancreatitis	↑Oxalate	CaOx/CaP
Corticosteroids	↑Calcium	CaOx/CaP
Acetazolamide	↑pH	CaP
$CaCO_3$ antacids	↑Calcium, ↑pH	CaP/CaOx
Small bowel resection	↑Oxalate, ↓pH, ↓citrate, ↓magnesium	CaOx
Jejunal-ileal by-pass	↑Oxalate	CaOx/CaP
Bariatric surgery	↑Oxalate	CaOx/CaP
Enterocystoplasty	↑Calcium, ↑pH, ↓citrate, ↓magnesium	CaP/CaOx

Table 53.3 Example of risk accumulation in an otherwise "normal-looking" urine from a CaOx/CaP stone former (AGW) compared with that in a normal subject with a similar, but with a lower risk, urine composition

Urine factor	Patient (AGW)	Normal (JHT)
Volume (L/day)	1.48	1.65
pH	6.20	6.00
Calcium (mmol/day)	6.05	5.50
Magnesium (mmol/day)	3.61	4.50
Oxalate (mmol/day)	0.41	0.35
Citrate (mmol/day)	2.01	2.50
Uric acid (mmol/day)	3.86	3.21
P_{SF} (CaOx)	0.86[a]	0.35
P_{SF} (CaOx/CaP)	0.91[b]	0.36
P_{SF} (CaP)	0.70[c]	0.42

[a]High risk of forming stones

[b]Very high risk of forming stones

[c]Moderately high risk of forming stones

the patient sweat a lot normally (particularly at night) or exercise strenuously and does not sufficiently replenish his/her water losses or live in a hot environment or travel to the Tropics on holiday or on business? The occupation of the patient – does he/she work in a hot or other dehydrating environment, such as chefs or kitchen workers in restaurants or airline pilots and air-crew? Does he/she have an intensive job where it is difficult to go to the toilet (and so they do not drink enough) such as taxi drivers or surgeons? Does he/she work as an over-pressed business executive who professes, "to be too busy to stop and have a drink or go to the toilet"? Does he/she work with metals or other chemicals that may damage the kidneys, such as cadmium, beryllium, and toluene and so lead to a secondary metabolic acidosis? Does he/she practice some ethnic habit that may lead to an increase in stone formation such as betel chewing? Does he/she regularly consume antacids, which contain high amounts of calcium and alkali? Is he/she a laxative abuser? Is he/she likely to form iatrogenic stones consisting of silica (from regular ingestion of magnesium trisilicate antacids), sulfonamide, triamterene, sulfadiazine, or indinavir? A detailed list of the lifestyle factors that may lead to stone formation is set out in Table 53.3.

53.3.2 Stonescreen

All patients (and the lithotripsy unit, endourological department, and urologists involved with the patients concerned) should be strongly encouraged to retain the stones or stone fragments for analysis after passage or removal. The stones should then be analyzed *quantitatively* by Fourier Transform Infra-Red (FTIR) spectroscopy (Stonescreen).[5] This is an important tool in the Lithoscreen scheme since it provides an additional clue as to the cause of the stone(s) in the patient

concerned. Unfortunately, the collection of stones is not well organized in many hospitals and, in any case, most do not have the facilities for quantitative analysis of the stones. However, a national commercial service for quantitative stone analysis is provided by the Department of Chemical Pathology at University College London Hospitals.

53.3.3 Metascreen

Metascreen provides a metabolic assessment of the patient in terms of identifying disorders that are likely to lead to the formation of secondary stones in the urinary tract.[4] This requires a blood and urine sample to be taken from the patient at their first appointment at the stone clinic *after an overnight fast* (see previous) and analyzed for the following:

- *Blood* – Urea, creatinine, sodium, potassium, bicarbonate, chloride, albumin, calcium, corrected calcium, magnesium, phosphate, alkaline phosphatase, uric acid, glucose, parathyroid hormone (PTH), and 25-hydroxyvitamin D_3. Plasma oxalate may also be required in patients with suspected hereditary hyperoxaluria but special precautions have to be taken in the sample collection and handling for this analysis.

- *Urine* – Osmolality, urea, sodium, potassium, calcium, phosphate, magnesium, uric acid, oxalate, and pH (measured by pH meter – not by dipstick). A sterile sample of urine should be sent for microbiological testing in cases of suspected urinary tract infection. In the light of the current interest in the role of "Metabolic Syndrome" and uric acid stone formation, it may also be useful to measure titratable acidity (TA), ammonium ion concentration (NH_4^+), and bicarbonate in order to assess the net acid excretion (NAE) of the patient.

From these analyses, it is possible to determine whether or not the patient is suffering from any underlying metabolic disorder that might lead to stones, such as primary hyperparathyroidism, distal renal tubular acidosis, Dent's disease, hereditary or enteric hyperoxaluria, hyperuricemia, hypomagnesemia, metabolic syndrome, hypervitaminosis D, and urinary tract infection. A full list of all the main metabolic disorders or conditions that might lead to secondary stone formation and the risk factors that lead to stones is presented in Table 53.2.

It is also possible to determine the renal handling of ions that are particularly involved in the formation of stones such as calcium, phosphate, uric acid, magnesium, citrate, and oxalate. Patients with renal leaks of calcium and/or phosphate can be identified and the cause of the renal leak related to their PTH and 25-OH vitamin D_3 status and to their renal throughputs of Na^+ and H^+ ions, high levels of which are known to cause calcium to leak out through the kidneys.

53.3.4 Urinescreen

This consists of two 24-h urine samples collected on consecutive days, the first into a plastic bottle already containing 50 mL of 2.2M hydrochloric acid as a preservative. (NB: Suitable warnings have to be given to the patient regarding the safe management of their acid-containing bottles.) This acidified urine collection is analyzed for volume, creatinine, calcium, magnesium, oxalate, citrate, and urea. (If the urinary oxalate excretion is high, then urinary glycollate should also be measured in the acidified sample.) On the following day, a second collection is made into a plain container and analyzed for volume, creatinine, pH (measured accurately by pH meter, *not* by dipstick), sodium, potassium, urate, protein, and a qualitative test for cystine (quantitative for cystine, lysine, ornithine and arginine if the qualitative test for cystine is positive).

From the combined analyses from these two urine samples, a number of algorithms can be employed to assess the overall biochemical risk (P_{SF}) of forming stones containing uric acid (UA), calcium oxalate (CaOx), or calcium phosphate (CaP), or various mixtures of these constituents.[6] This requires the use of seven of the aforementioned measurements in the 24-h urine samples (volume and pH and the urinary excretions of calcium, magnesium, oxalate, citrate, and uric acid). The P_{SF} values are calculated on a probability scale from 0 to 1. Values >0.5 are indicative of a significant risk of forming stones; values >0.9 are often found in urines from actively recurrent stone formers. In most patients, the high risk is rarely due to a single abnormal urinary constituent (except in the case of primary hyperoxaluria) but is more commonly due to a combination of between two and seven lesser "abnormalities" depending on the stone type. Indeed, it is possible to have a high P_{SF} value with every urinary risk factor within its "normal range" but with several of the risk factors lying toward the upper or lower limits of these ranges. This is an important feature of the model since it allows a risk assessment to be made of the patient who would have been previously described as "having no abnormalities in his/her urine" yet has an *abnormal combination* of the variables that lead to crystalluria and stones (Table 53.3). This risk factor model of stone formation can be used not only to assess the patient's probability of forming stones before treatment but can also be used to follow his/her progress during preventative treatment.

53.3.5 Dietscreen

During the week preceding the collection of the 24-h urine samples, the patient is requested to complete a diet diary (Dietscreen) of everything that he/she consumes each day on his/her free, home diet. The last 2 days of the diary should correspond to the days of the 24-h urine collections. The diary is analyzed for total fluid intake (including what is contained in the various foodstuffs), calories, total calcium and calcium derived from dairy products, magnesium, sodium, potassium, phosphate, oxalate, purine, total protein (and its various fractions, including animal protein, meat + fish + poultry protein, dairy protein, and fruit + vegetable + cereal protein), fiber, fat, refined sugars, and potential renal acid load (PRAL). Dietscreen allows an assessment to be made of the role of diet in the patient's risk of stones and can usually be correlated with the composition of the 24-h urine samples mentioned previously.

PRAL can be used to estimate the net acid excreted (NAE) by the patient, and the estimated 24-h urinary pH can be determined from previously published relationships between urinary pH and NAE.[7] The expected urinary pH estimated in this way can then be compared with the actual pH measured in the plain 24-h urine sample described previously. This can help in the diagnosis of acid–base disorders, such as dRTA, and renal buffering disorders, such as metabolic syndrome.[8] It can also identify those patients with urinary tract infections at the time of the investigations.

53.4 Epidemiological Factors in the Formation of Urinary Stones

There are three groups of epidemiological factors that have been found to be of importance in the formation of urinary stones – demographic, environmental, and pathophysiological. Each of these groups contains a number of categories, which are summarized in Tables 53.2 and 53.4. Each has

Table 53.4 The main demographic and lifestyle factors involved in uric acid (UA) and calcium stone formation and their effects on urinary risk factors

Epidemiological factor	Urinary risk factor(s)	Stone type
Age and gender	↑Calcium, ↑oxalate, ↑uric acid, ↑pH, ↓volume, ↓citrate, ↓magnesium, ↓inhibitors, ↑promoters	CaOx/CaP
Climate and season	↓Volume, ↑calcium, ↑oxalate, ↓pH	CaOx/UA
Stress	↑Calcium, ↑oxalate, ↑uric acid, ↓magnesium	CaOx/CaP
Low fluid intake	↓Volume, ↓pH	CaOx/UA or CaOx
Strenuous exercise	↓↓Volume, ↓pH	CaOx/UA or CaOx
Work/live in hot environment	↓Volume	CaOx/CaP
Frequent air travel	↓Volume	CaOx/CaP
Affluence and diet	↑Calcium, ↑oxalate, ↑uric acid, ↓citrate, ↓pH	CaOx/UA or CaOx or CaOx/CaP

been shown to increase the risk of stone formation through its effect on the balance between supersaturation, inhibitors, and promoters of crystallization in urine. For calcium stone formation, the most common form of the disorder, the main epidemiological factors are age, gender, season, climate, stress, occupation, affluence, diet (including fluid intake), and genetic/metabolic factors. The role of diet, in particular, has been studied in detail and this appears to explain much of the changing pattern of stone incidence over the past 100 years. As the composition of the diet becomes "richer" in a given population (owing to an increased consumption of protein, particularly animal protein, refined sugars, and salt), the incidence of stones increases. This often follows periods of economic expansion. During periods of recession, on the other hand, the incidence of stones has been noted to decrease in parallel with a return to a more healthy form of diet containing more fiber and fewer energy-rich foods.

53.5 Prevention of Stone Recurrence

The main aim in the prevention of stone recurrence is to decrease the likelihood of crystals forming in the urinary tract by reducing the supersaturation of urine with respect to the particular constituent(s) that occur in the patients' stones. Although most of the dietary and medical treatments are effective in reducing the risk of stone recurrence, the main problem in the long-term management of stone patients is compliance.[9–11] Generally, stone formers feel well for most of the time, except when they are experiencing an attack of renal colic. It is often difficult, therefore, to maintain their cooperation and motivation to adhere to their preventative treatment over a long period after their initial stone episode.

Indeed, if they do not have a recurrence of their problem within a few months of their episode, most stone formers will regress to their original abnormal pattern of urine biochemistry within 3–6 months and will eventually produce another stone.[12] Once they have had several episodes of renal colic, it is usually easier to motivate them on a more continuous basis. It is important, therefore, to review the patient regularly as an out-patient and to repeat the 24-h Urinescreen tests, preferably annually but at least biennially, to ensure that they are adhering to the prophylaxis prescribed and to check that their biochemical risk of stones remains low.

In order to try to improve patient compliance, a set of goals has been devised to minimize his/her risk of stone recurrence. These aims are based on the results obtained from the Lithoscreen procedure and take the form of "target diagrams," consisting of radar plots of (1) urinary risk factors for stone formation, (2) the biochemical risk of forming various types of stones, and (3) the dietary risk factors for stone formation.[13] The plots, which are in the form of colored concentric rings ranging from green at the center, through white, then pink, to red on the outside, are arranged such that the minimum risk of stones occurs when the data points of the radar plot are all located within the green "bull's eye." There is a slight risk of stones when the data are in the white ring, a moderate risk in the pink ring, and the highest risk occurs when the data lie situated in the outer red ring of the target. The target diagrams are used to show the patient where they are situated before treatment and how their observance of the prescribed treatment is progressing. The diagrams can be given to the patient in order to motivate them to adhere better to the particular form of prophylaxis and thereby increase the chances that they will experience fewer stone recurrences.

In the example shown in Fig. 53.3, a patient who had formed mixed CaOx/CaP stones was screened for risk

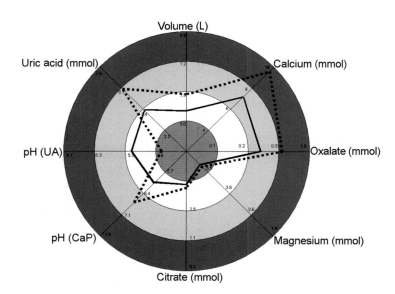

Fig. 53.3 A target diagram showing the urinary risk factor profile of a stone former before (*dashed line*) and after (*solid line*) treatment

factors and shown to have hypercalciuria (13.5 mmol/day), mild hyperoxaluria (0.52 mmol/day), mild hyperuricosuria (4.9 mmol/day), and a slightly raised urinary pH (6.7) as his main abnormalities. This combination put him at a high risk of forming any type of Ca-containing stone, but particularly those consisting of a mixture of CaOx and CaP. After dietary advice to reduce his urinary calcium, oxalate, and uric acid and to increase his fluid intake, the patient's urinary risk factors and overall biochemical probability of forming stones were markedly reduced (Fig. 53.4).

A similar target diagram has been constructed to show the patient's situation with respect to his dietary risk factors. This is shown in Fig. 53.5.

53.6 Conclusions

Target diagrams may be given to the patient in order to help them understand better whether or not they are reducing their risk of forming stones and, if not, which dietary factors they have to control in order to improve their risk. However, each follow-up consultation must be accompanied by a detailed explanation from the physician or clinical nurse practitioner of how to reduce the patient's risk of stones. Encouragement has to be given to adhere rigorously to the medical or dietary regimen prescribed at all times. In my experience, this can only be achieved by regular appointments at the stone clinic and at least biennial repeat 24-h urine collections and analysis.

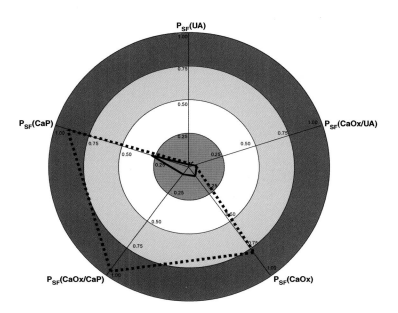

Fig. 53.4 A target diagram showing the relative probabilities of forming various types of stone in the same patient as shown in Fig. 53.3

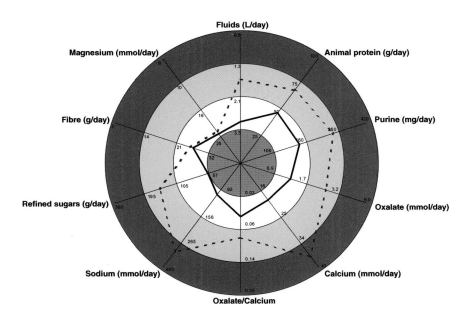

Fig. 53.5 A target diagram containing the dietary data in the patient shown in Fig. 53.3

References

1. Robertson WG. The medical management of urinary stone disease. *Eur Urol Update Ser*. 1998;7:139-144.

2. Peacock M, Robertson WG, Norman RW, Selby PL. Constitution and management of a stone clinic. In: Schwille PO, Smith LH, Robertson WG, Vahlensieck W, eds. *Urolithiasis and Related Clinical Research*. London: Plenum; 1984:259-266.

3. Hosking DH, Erickson SB, Van den Berg CJ, Wilson DH, Smith LH. The stone clinic effect in patients with idiopathic calcium urolithiasis. *J Urol*. 1983;130:1115-1118.

4. Robertson WG. A comprehensive screening procedure for the assessment of patients with recurrent stones. In: Borghi L, Meschi T, Briganti A, Schiani T, Novarini A, eds. *Kidney Stones*. Editoriale Bios: Cosenza; 1999:407-410.

5. Kasidas GP, Samuell CT, Weir TB. Renal stone analysis: why and how? *Ann Clin Biochem*. 2004;41:91-97.

6. Robertson WG. A risk factor model of stone-formation. *Front Biosci*. 2003;8:1330-1338.

7. Remer T, Manz F. Potential renal acid load of foods and its influence on urine pH. *J Am Diet Assoc*. 1995;95:791-797.

8. Robertson WG, Nair D, Laing C, Choong S, Jaeger P, Unwin RJ. The role of "Metabolic Syndrome" in the formation of uric acid-containing stones. *Urol Res*. 2008;36:177.

9. Borghi L, Meschi T, Amato F, Briganti A, Novarini A, Giannini A. Urinary volume, water and recurrences in idiopathic calcium nephrolithiasis: a 5-year randomized prospective study. *J Urol*. 1996;155:839-843.

10. Tiselius HG. Epidemiology and medical management of stone disease. *BJU Int*. 2003;91:758-767.

11. Pak CY. Medical stone management: 35 years of advances. *J Urol*. 2008;180:813-819.

12. Norman RW, Bath SS, Robertson WG, Peacock M. When should patients with symptomatic urinary stone disease be evaluated metabolically? *J Urol*. 1984;132:1137-1139.

13. Robertson WG. Is it possible to motivate patients with recurrent stones to adhere to their treatment regimen? In: Rodgers AL, Hibbert BE, Hess B, Khan SR, Preminger GM, eds. *Urolithiasis 2000*. Cape Town: University of Cape Town Press; 2000:624-627.

Medical Expulsive Therapy

54

Kim Davenport and Francis X. Keeley

Abstract Although large randomized controlled trials using medical therapy to promote stone passage in renal colic are lacking, the evidence to date would support the use of calcium channel antagonists or alpha-adrenoceptor antagonists during the initial period of conservative therapy for uncomplicated distal ureteral stones. Further studies are required to investigate their role in the treatment of proximal ureteral stones.

54.1 Introduction

The use of pharmacological agents in the treatment of renal colic stems from our understanding of ureteral smooth muscle physiology and urinary obstruction. Their use is becoming increasingly popular with the aim of increasing stone passage rates and reducing the time to stone passage.

Using ureteral smooth muscle relaxation to promote stone passage is not a new idea. Ross suggested potential benefits following his early work on ureteral physiology in 1972.[1] It is not completely understood how these agents act in vivo. It is assumed that ureteral peristalsis is essential to allow stone passage; however, in the presence of a ureteral stone, irritation and stretch stimulation of the ureter may result in increased, uncoordinated peristalsis,[2] which may actually hinder stone passage. In a canine in vivo model of acute obstruction, the mean peristaltic rate, baseline pressure, and peak pressures above the level of obstruction were all shown to increase significantly.[3] Conversely, below the level of obstruction, the mean peristaltic rate remained unchanged but the baseline and peak pressures generated were both significantly reduced. Control of this increased, uncoordinated ureteral activity may help to normalize peristalsis and promote spontaneous stone passage.[4]

There are many factors that influence the probability of spontaneous stone passage. Few may be modified, namely preventing ureteral smooth muscle spasm in the region of the stone and increasing proximal hydrostatic pressure by increasing fluid intake. This is supported by the slower progression of artificial ureteral concretions in the presence of proximal ureteral ligation or holes within the concretion.[5,6] Smooth muscle relaxant drugs and steroids may reduce ureteral muscle tone, edema, and inflammation, thereby increasing luminal diameter.

54.2 Effect of Pharmacological Agents on Ureteral Function

Many drugs in current use for alternative indications are capable of influencing normal ureteral physiology and reducing ureteral tone generation in vitro. The mechanism of action varies with each class of agents. The methods available include:

1. *Inhibition of prostaglandin synthesis by cyclooxygenase inhibition* (nonselective: NSAIDs or selective: cyclooxygenase II (COX II) inhibitors). These prevent stimulation of smooth muscle contraction by prostanoids (prostaglandins, thromboxanes, and prostacyclin).[7–10]
2. *Calcium channel antagonism*, which inhibits the calcium influx through voltage-sensitive calcium channels, essential for action potential generation.[11,12]
3. *Angiotensin-converting enzyme inhibition*, which inhibits smooth muscle contraction by inhibiting locally produced angiotensin II.[13]
4. *Potassium channel openers*, which hyperpolarize ureteral smooth muscle membranes and inhibit ureteral activity.[14]

K. Davenport (✉)
North Bristol NHS Trust, Bristol Urological Institute,
Bristol, Avon, UK
e-mail: drkimdav@aol.com

P.N. Rao et al. (eds.), *Urinary Tract Stone Disease*,
DOI 10.1007/978-1-84800-362-0_54, © Springer-Verlag London Limited 2011

5. *Nitrates*, which promote nitric oxide release, increasing cyclic guanosine monophosphate (cGMP) concentration resulting in smooth muscle relaxation.[15,16]

6. *Alpha-1-adrenergic receptor antagonism*, which blocks the sympathetic excitatory effect at alpha-adrenoceptors.[12]

7. *Beta-adrenergic agonism*, which promotes the sympathetic inhibitory effect at beta-adrenoceptors.[17–19]

8. *Phosphodiesterase inhibition*, which prevents the degradation of cGMP, promotes calcium uptake into intracellular storage sites and reduces the concentration available for smooth muscle contraction.[19–23]

9. *Calcitonin gene–related peptide agonism*, which opens adenosine triphosphate (ATP)–sensitive potassium channels, causing cell membrane hyperpolarization and blockage of the calcium channels necessary for action potential generation.[24]

Non-steroidal anti-inflammatory drugs (NSAIDs) provide excellent analgesia in renal colic. In the laboratory, these drugs appear to reduce ureteral activity and, in some cases, ablate all ureteral activity.[9,10] However, despite diclofenac and indomethacin being highly effective in reducing the number of new colic episodes and admissions to hospital, in clinical trials, they do not affect the time to stone passage or the stone passage rate[25–27] in renal colic (see Table 54.1).

The spasmolytic agents' phentolamine (α[alpha]-adrenergic antagonist) and orciprenaline (β[beta]-adrenergic agonist) have been shown to dilate the ureteral lumen at the level of an artificial concretion, permitting increased fluid flow.[28] However, these drugs have unacceptable significant circulatory side effects, as do the phosphodiesterase inhibitors (theophylline and papaverine),[20] and so would be unsuitable in the clinical setting. Nitrates stimulate the release of nitric oxide, which interacts with guanyl cyclase to increase cGMP, leading to vascular smooth muscle relaxation. They appear to have the same effect on ureteral smooth muscle, but unfortunately, they have a short duration of action and problematic side effects (flushing, headache, and postural hypotension) and so are not ideal for this indication. A clinical trial using nitrate patches has shown no beneficial effect in renal colic.[29] Although, Cox II inhibition reduces ureteral contractility as

effectively as indomethacin (NSAID) in porcine and human ureteral segments in vitro,[9,10] there is currently no data available regarding its use in the treatment of renal colic. However, they would be expected to have limited effects on stone passage rates similar to NSAIDs.

The most promising agents already in clinical use for alternative indications are calcium channel antagonists and alpha-1-adrenoceptor antagonists.

54.2.1 Calcium Channel Antagonists

Calcium is necessary for the development of action potentials and therefore contraction of the ureter. Calcium channel blockers interfere with the inward displacement of calcium ions through the slow channels of active cell membranes and so would be expected to have an inhibitory effect on ureteral function. Calcium channel blockers have been suggested to inhibit the stone-induced ureteral spasm seen as fast phasic contractions without influencing the tonic activity of the ureter based on animal and human studies.[30]

Verapamil, nicardipine,[31] diltiazem, and nifedipine[11,12] have all been shown to inhibit ureteral activity in animal models and in human ureter in vitro. Of these drugs, nifedipine appears to have the most effect on ureteral tone and is the safest for clinical use. In vitro, nifedipine at concentrations of 10^{-6}M suppressed spontaneous phasic and potassium induced tonic contractions.[11] In vivo, nifedipine allows ureteral peristalsis to continue and appears to have little effect on contraction frequency or tone.[4]

There have been many clinical studies investigating the use of nifedipine in renal colic.[32–35] Unfortunately, these studies combined the use of nifedipine with a steroid. Borghi et al.[32] randomized 76 patients with stones less than 15 mm to receive nifedipine 40 mg (group 1) versus placebo (group 2) in conjunction with 16-mg methylprednisolone (equivalent to 20 mg prednisolone) daily for a maximum of 45 days. The mean stone size was 6.7 ± 3 mm in group 1 and 6.8 ± 2.9 mm, hence there was no significant difference between the groups. Although stones at all levels were included, the

Table 54.1 The use of NSAIDs for the prophylaxis of acute renal colic

	Laerum[25]		Grenabo[26]		Kapoor[27]	
	Diclofenac 50 mg tds 7 days	Placebo tds 7 days	Indomethacin 25 mg PO bd + 100 mg PR nocte for 7 days	Placebo PO bd + PR nocte for 7 days	50 mg PR indomethacin tds	Placebo tds
Mean stone size	78% <6 mm	97% <6 mm	2.9 mm	2.8 mm	3.4 mm	3.1 mm
Readmission rate	10%	67%	11%	39%	0%	38%
Mean stone passage rate	68% at 3 weeks	74% at 3 weeks	59% at 1 week	61% at 1 week	N/A	N/A
Mean interval to passage	3 days	3.8 days	N/A	N/A	3.4 days	3.7 days

majority in both groups were distal ureteral. The study was randomized and double-blinded. Spontaneous stone passage occurred in 87% of patients in group 1 and 65% of group 2, which was statistically significant ($p = 0.021$). The time to passage reduced from 16.4 ± 11 days in group 2 to 11.2 ± 7.5 days in group 1 ($p = 0.036$).

Porpiglia et al.[33] recruited 96 patients with distal ureteral stones 1 cm or smaller in size. Group A ($n = 48$) was randomized to receive 30-mg deflazacort (equivalent to 25-mg prednisolone) for 10 days plus 30-mg nifedipine for a maximum of 4 weeks. Group B ($n = 48$) was used as the control group, but the patients were not given placebo preparations, and therefore, the study was neither placebo controlled nor blinded. The average stone sizes for each group were 5.8 ± 1.8 mm for group A and 5.5 ± 1.4 mm for group B (non significant). In group A, 79% of patients passed their stones at a mean time of 7 (range 2–10) days as compared with 35% at 20 (range 10–28) days in group B ($p < 0.05$ for both variables). This group also looked at the amount of diclofenac used during the trial period and showed that those receiving nifedipine used significantly less analgesia, mean diclofenac use per patient of 15 mg as compared with 105 mg ($p < 0.05$) (see Table 54.2).

Cooper et al.[34] used polypharmacy to improve stone passage. They randomized 70 patients with 2–6 mm stones at any level to receive standard treatment versus intensive management for 7 days. The standard arm received a NSAID (ketorolac), the analgesic acetaminophen, and the anti-emetic prochlorperazine. The intensive management arm received these in addition to nifedipine 30 mg, prednisolone 10 mg bd, and the antibiotic trimethoprim. These drugs increased stone passage from 56% in the control arm to 86% ($p = 0.001$). However, there was no difference in the mean time to stone passage (11.5 versus 12.6 days). Up to 40% of patients in the treatment arm and 60% in the control arm described symptoms that were considered drug side effects. This trial was totally unscientific. There were no attempts made to blind patients or provide a placebo group. Due to the large amounts of drugs prescribed, it remains unclear as to the relative benefits of each drug. There are also problems with patient compliance, increased side effects, and increased cost when prescribing this quantity of drugs concurrently. This study fails to provide any useful additional information.

Finally, Saita et al.[35] allocated 50 patients with stones less than 15 mm at any site to receive either 30-mg nifedipine and 25-mg prednisolone (group 1) or 25-mg prednisolone alone

(group 2) for 20 days. There was no indication as to how the patients were allocated treatment and again this study was neither placebo controlled nor blinded. The mean stone size was much larger than the other studies at 12 mm in group 1 and 12.8 mm in group 2. However, only 37 patients completed the study. The average time to stone expulsion in group 1 was 6 (range 2–10) days and in group 2, 10 (range 5–15) days. Stone passage occurred in 81% of group 1 patients and 68% of group 2. No statistical analyzes were performed, and therefore, it is not known whether these results were significant. In view of the small sample size, this study was unlikely to have yielded new information.

All four studies have indicated advantages to the use of nifedipine in renal colic. Since all have combined nifedipine with steroid, it is unclear as to the degree of benefit incurred with the use of nifedipine alone. Steroids not only have an anti-inflammatory effect on the ureter and so reduce edema at the level of the stone but they may also cause a degree of ureteral smooth muscle relaxation. All four studies have predominantly involved distal ureteral calculi, so it remains unclear as to whether the beneficial effects apply to stones at all levels or are limited to distal ureteral stones.

54.2.2 Alpha-1A-Adrenoceptor Antagonists

Within the sympathetic nervous system, alpha-1-adrenergic fibers are excitatory; therefore, by blocking the alpha-1-adrenergic receptors, smooth muscle relaxation and a reduction in contraction frequency should occur. Since the sympathetic nervous system only has a modulating role, pacemaker-driven peristalsis should continue. Reverse transcriptase–DNA studies have identified alpha-1A receptors along the length of the ureter; however, the distal ureter appears to have twice the number of receptors as compared with the mid or proximal ureter.[36]

There are many alpha-1-adrenoceptor antagonists available. They can be subdivided into selective and nonselective alpha-1-adrenoceptor antagonists. Tamsulosin is an alpha-1-adrenoceptor antagonist, which binds selectively and competitively to postsynaptic alpha-1-receptors, in particular to the subtype alpha-1A. This limits side effects.

In vitro, alpha-1-adrenoceptor antagonism results in a reduction in canine and human ureteral tone generation.[12,37]

Table 54.2 The effect of nifedipine ± steroid on stone passage rates, mean time to stone passage and analgesic use

	Borghi[32]			Porpiglia[33]		
	Group 1	Group 2	p value	Group 1	Group 2	p value
Spontaneous stone passage (%)	87.2 ($n = 34$)	64.9 ($n = 24$)	0.02	79 ($n = 38$)	35 ($n = 17$)	<0.05
Time to stone passage (days)	11.2	16.4	0.036	7	20	<0.05
Average total diclofenac use (mg)	N/A	N/A	N/A	15	105	<0.05

Animal and human in vivo studies have demonstrated that alpha-adrenoceptor antagonism allows ureteral contractions to continue but may reduce the contraction pressures.[4,19] Danuser showed that prazosin was able to prevent the increased activity seen following intravenous administration of the alpha-1-adrenoceptor agonist, phenylephrine.[19] This would further support the use of alpha-adrenoceptor antagonists in renal colic to prevent hyperperistalsis.

Tamsulosin has been used to promote stone passage in renal colic in many randomized controlled trials, but only in the treatment of distal ureteral calculi. Cervenakov et al.[38] published the first double-blind, randomized study using tamsulosin. Unfortunately, polypharmacy was used, making any interpretation of results extremely difficult. One hundred and two patients with juxtavesical ureteral stones up to 10 mm in size were randomized (method not stated) to receive standard treatment (group A) versus standard plus tamsulosin 400 mcg (group B) for 7 days. Standard treatment comprised diclofenac 50 mg tds and Yellon 40 mg tds (not widely available and action not known). No comment is made regarding the use of placebo in group A. There was no difference in stone size between the two groups. With the addition of tamsulosin, stone passage increased from 63% to 80%. The statistical significance is not stated for the difference in stone passage rates further devaluing the results from this study.

In a study by Dellabella et al.,[39] 60 patients with juxtavesical stones were randomized to receive the antispasmodic fluoroglucine-trimetossibenzene tds (group 1) or tamsulosin 400 mcg (group 2) for 4 weeks alongside the steroid deflazacort 30 mg (equivalent to 25 mg prednisolone) for 10 days and the antibiotic clotrimoxazole bd for 8 days. The mean stone size was 5.8 mm in group 1 and 6.7 mm in group 2 ($p = 0.047$). Group 2 were found to have a 100% expulsion rate compared with 70% in group 1 ($p = 0.001$). The mean time to expulsion was 65.7 h as compared with 111 h in group 1 ($p = 0.02$). Group 2 used less diclofenac analgesia and required fewer hospital admissions for intervention ($p < 0.0001$ for both). Again this study was not blinded. The use of polypharmacy and an active compound in group 1 as opposed to placebo makes interpretation of this data difficult as the effects of clotrimoxazole and fluoroglucine-trimetossibenzene on stone passage are also not known.

Dellabella et al. published results from a randomized study aiming to identify the role of steroids in conjunction with tamsulosin. Sixty patients with distal ureteral stones measuring 5–8 mm in diameter were randomized into two groups. Group 1 received tamsulosin 400 mcg alone for 28 days and group 2 received tamsulosin 400 mcg plus 30 mg deflazacort (equivalent to 25 mg prednisolone) for 10 days.[40] Unfortunately, there was no placebo-controlled group to compare true spontaneous stone passage rates. They found very high stone passage rates in both groups (90% versus 97%, $p = 0.6$). The use of steroid appeared to have the additional benefit of decreasing the time to stone passage (120 versus 72 h, $p = 0.036$). With stone passage occurring within 3–5 days, it is debatable as to whether these patients truly benefited from medical therapy; without a control group, the relevance of these results is unknown.

Autorino et al.[41] reported an improvement in distal ureteral stone passage rates of 28% (from 60% to 88%, $p = 0.01$) when tamsulosin was added to their current treatment regime of diclofenac 100 mg, aescin 80 mg (anti-inflammatory properties), omeprazole 20 mg, and levofloxacin 250 mg daily. However, the polypharmacy, absence of control, and small sample size of 32 in each group are again major issues with this study.

Yilmaz et al.[42] have reported results from a well-designed study with four groups comparing tamsulosin and two other alpha-1-adrenoceptor antagonists, terazosin and doxazosin, with a control group. None of the groups used steroids. A total of 114 patients with stones 10 mm or smaller located in the juxtavesical ureter or vesico-ureteral junction were included. The mean stone size was approximately 6 mm in all four groups. The patients were randomized (method not stated) as follows: 28 acted as controls (no placebo drug given), 29 received tamsulosin 400 mcg, 28 received terazosin 5 mg, and 29 received doxazosin 4 mg for 4 weeks. There were no statistically significant differences between the groups. The stone passage rates were 54%, 79%, 79%, and 76%, respectively. In groups 2, 3, and 4, this difference was significant compared with group 1 ($p = 0.03$, 0.03, 0.04 respectively). The average time to expulsion in days was 10.54 ± 2.12, 6.31 ± 0.88, 5.75 ± 0.88, and 5.93 ± 0.59, respectively. Again this difference was significant in groups 2, 3, and 4 compared with group 1 ($p = 0.04$, 0.03, 0.03 respectively). There was no statistically significant difference between the three drugs. The use of alpha-1-adrenoceptor antagonists significantly increases stone passage in the absence of steroid use. Since terazosin and doxazosin are nonselective alpha-1-adrenoceptor antagonists, these results would imply that selective alpha-1A-adrenoceptor antagonism is not essential for stone passage.

More recently, Hermanns et al.[43] have published conflicting results from their randomized, double-blind, placebo-controlled trial using tamsulosin 400 mcg versus placebo. One hundred patients were recruited, with 90 completing the trial. With a median stone size of 4.1 mm (tamsulosin arm) versus 3.9 mm (placebo arm), there was no statistically significant difference in stone passage rates (86.7% versus 88.9%, $p = 1.0$). However, the median time to stone passage was reduced by 3 days with tamsulosin (7 versus 10 days, $p = 0.36$) and requirements for analgesics were reduced ($p = 0.01$). This trial has provided the first evidence that tamsulosin may not be beneficial for all patients with ureteral stones. The predominant difference between this trial and the others previously discussed is the median stone size. Those showing benefit have a median stone size of 5–6 mm, whereas this trial has a smaller median stone size of 4 mm. The beneficial effects on time to stone passage and analgesic requirements do appear to hold true.

54.2.3 Direct Comparison between Nifedipine and Tamsulosin

These two drugs have been compared directly in vitro using human proximal and distal ureteral strips.[12] Nifedipine was found to have equal relaxant effects on proximal and distal ureter. Alpha-1-adrenoceptor antagonism had a slightly greater effect on distal ureter but, although a reduction in tone was seen in proximal ureter, this was to a lesser degree.

Two groups have directly compared nifedipine and tamsulosin in clinical trials. Porpiglia et al.[44] randomized 84 patients with juxtavesical or intramural stones less than 10 mm into three groups. The treatment groups received the steroid deflazacort 30 mg daily for 10 days plus misoprostol (a synthetic prostaglandin analogue) 200 mcg bd. In addition, group 1 received nifedipine 30 mg and group 2 received tamsulosin 400 mcg. Group 3 received none of these drugs and acted as the control. No blinding was performed in this trial. There was no difference in stone size between the groups ($p = 0.2$). After 4 weeks, both the nifedipine and tamsulosin groups produced similar stone expulsion rates (80% versus 85%, $p = 0.5$), which were significantly better than the 43% seen in the control group ($p < 0.01$ and $p < 0.001$ respectively). Tamsulosin was associated with a lower time to expulsion than the nifedipine and control groups, 7.9 days versus 9.3 days versus 12 days. The reduction in time to passage as compared with control was significant ($p = 0.02$) but not compared with nifedipine ($p = 0.2$). The difference between nifedipine and control was not significant ($p = 0.9$). This study would therefore indicate that tamsulosin has the additional benefit over nifedipine of reducing the time to stone passage.

The largest study to date performed by Dellabella et al.[45] compared tamsulosin (group 2) and nifedipine (group 3) with the control phloroglucinol (a synthetic agent with weak anti-cholinergic properties) (group 1) for 4 weeks. This randomized trial involved 210 patients with distal ureteral stones (below the common iliac vessels) greater than 4 mm. Each patient received the antibiotic clotrimoxazole for 8 days and the steroid deflazacort 30 mg for 10 days in addition to a trial drug. The mean stone sizes were 6.2, 7.2, and 6.2 mm. The expulsion rate was significantly higher in group 2 (97%) than in group 1 (64%, $p < 0.0001$) or group 3 (77%, $p < 0.0001$). The median time to stone passage was 120, 72, and 120 h in the phloroglucinol, tamsulosin, and nifedipine groups. In this study, tamsulosin resulted in significantly better outcomes as compared with nifedipine, despite the mean stone size being higher in this group and stones located proximal to the

intramural ureter being included. However, this study would have been improved by the use of placebo in group 1 as opposed to phloroglucinol and by omitting the concurrent use of clotrimoxazole and deflazacort. Again, the polypharmacy makes interpretation less clear.

54.2.4 Meta-Analysis of Clinical Trials Using Tamsulosin or Nifedipine

Hollingsworth et al.[46] published a meta-analysis including all randomized controlled trials in which calcium channel antagonists or alpha-adrenoceptor antagonists were used to treat ureteral stones. Only 9 of over 400 studies fit the inclusion criteria, which included published abstracts. Data from these nine trials ($n = 693$) were pooled.[33,34,42,44,47–51] Overall, patients given either drug had a 65% (absolute risk reduction = 0.31 95% CI 0.25–0.38) greater likelihood of stone passage than those not given such treatment (pooled risk 1.65; 95% CI 1.45–1.88). The pooled risk ratio for alpha-adrenoceptor antagonists was 1.54 (1.29–1.85) and for calcium channel antagonists with steroids was 1.90 (1.51–2.40). Figure 54.1 shows the study-specific risk ratios and the pooled estimate for the nine studies included, and for an additional five that did not have a true control.[32,38,39,45,52] When these five studies were analyzed with the previous nine, the overall risk ratio remained significant at 1.52 (1.39–1.65), $p < 0.0001$. The number needed to treat was calculated at 4.

Parsons et al.[53] performed a similar meta-analysis; however, they only analyzed those randomized controlled clinical trials using alpha-adrenoceptor antagonism. A total of 11 studies were analyzed ($n = 911$),[48,54] including two studies assessing the effect of alpha-adrenoceptor antagonism on stone passage rates post extracorporeal shock wave lithotripsy (SWL).[38,39,41,42,44,45,48–50,54,55] Patients receiving alpha-adrenoceptor antagonism were 44% more likely to spontaneously pass their stones (RR 1.44, 95% CI 1.31–1.59, $p < 0.001$). Exclusion of those receiving SWL resulted in only slight changes to the effect estimate ($n = 664$, RR 1.44, 95% CI 1.32–1.58).

54.2.5 The Role of Steroids

Steroids not only have an anti-inflammatory effect on the ureter but they may also cause a degree of ureteral smooth muscle relaxation. Studies on spontaneously contracting sheep ureter showed that the steroids methylprednisolone, dexamethasone, and hydrocortisone all dose-dependently inhibited ureteral motility, with dexamethasone being the most potent and hydrocortisone the least potent.[56] The action

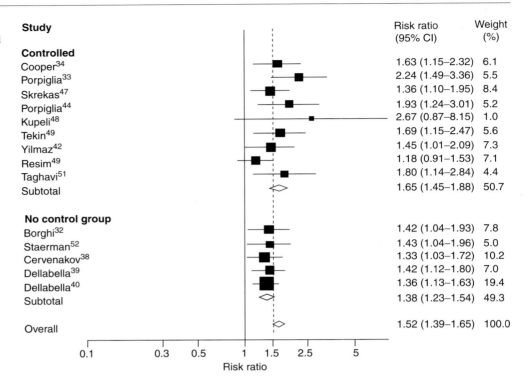

Fig. 54.1 Forest plot of risk ratios of stone passage, stratified by presence of control group (sizes of data markers are proportional to the weight of each study in the meta-analysis. Horizontal bars = 95% CI) (Adapted with permission from Hollingsworth et al.[46])

of steroids on the ureter is thought to be mediated via the synthesis of the anti-phospholipase protein, lipocortin, which inhibits phospholipase A2 enzymes necessary for prostanoid synthesis.

One study using placebo versus weekly methylprednisolone 40 mg intramuscularly (equivalent to 32 mg prednisolone) alongside tramadol and hydrochlorothiazide for 3 weeks reported improved stone passage from 44% to 88%.[57] Another study by Dellabella compared stone passage rates in 60 patients receiving tamsulosin 400 mcg alone (group 1), or in addition to 30 mg deflazacort (group 2) for a maximum of 28 days.[40] They found the two groups to have similar stone passage rates (90% versus 97%, $p = 0.6$); however, the time to stone passage was significantly reduced in group 2 (120 versus 72 h, $p = 0.036$). It would therefore seem feasible that steroids may have a beneficial effect on spontaneous stone passage by either reducing ureteral edema, reducing ureteral activity, or both.

Unfortunately, there are no studies to date comparing nifedipine, tamsulosin, and steroids separately with placebo alone ,and therefore, it is difficult to determine what proportion of benefit is solely due to these drugs. Despite the apparent beneficial effect of steroids, both nifedipine and tamsulosin do appear to improve stone passage rates and decrease analgesic requirements. In their meta-analysis, Hollingsworth et al.[46] compared studies using alpha-adrenoceptor antagonists versus control with those using alpha-adrenoceptor antagonists and corticosteroids versus control and found only a small additional benefit to using steroid.

54.3 Conclusions

Although large randomized controlled trials using medical therapy to promote stone passage in renal colic are lacking, the evidence to date would support the use of calcium channel antagonists or alpha-adrenoceptor antagonists during the initial period of conservative therapy for uncomplicated distal ureteral stones. Further studies are required to investigate their role in the treatment of proximal ureteric stones.

References

1. Ross JA, Edmond P, Kirkland IS. *Behaviour of the Human Ureter in Health and Disease*. Edinburgh: Churchill Livingstone; 1972.
2. Rose JG, Gillenwater JY. Pathophysiology of ureteral obstruction. *Am J Physiol*. 1973;225:830-837.
3. Crowley AR, Byrne JC, Darracott Vaughan E, et al. The effect of acute obstruction on ureteral function. *J Urol*. 1990;143:596-599.
4. Davenport K, Timoney AG, Keeley FX. Effect of smooth muscle relaxant drugs on proximal human ureteral activity *in vivo*: a pilot study. *Urol Res*. 2007;35:207-213.
5. Sivula A, Lehtonen T. Spontaneous passage of artificial concretions applied in the rabbit ureter. *Scand J Urol Nephrol*. 1967;1:259-263.
6. Kim HL, Labay PC, Boyarsky S, et al. An experimental model of ureteral colic. *J Urol*. 1970;104(3):390-394.
7. Cole RS, Fry CH, Shuttleworth KED. The action of the prostaglandins on isolated human ureteral smooth muscle. *Br J Urol*. 1988;61:19-26.
8. Mastrangelo D, Wizard M, Rohner S, et al. Diclofenac and NS398, a selective cyclo-oxygenase-2 inhibitor, decreases agonist induced contractions of the pig isolated ureter. *Urol Res*. 2000;28(6): 376-382.

9. Nakada SY, Jerde TJ, Bjorling DE, et al. Selective cyclooxygenase-2 inhibitors reduce ureteral contraction *in vitro*: a better alternative for renal colic? *J Urol*. 2000;163:607-612.

10. Jerde TJ, Calaman-Dixon JL, Bjorling DE, et al. Celecoxib inhibits ureteral contractility and prostanoid release. *Urol*. 2005;65:185-190.

11. Hertle L, Nawrath H. Calcium channel blockade in smooth muscle of the human upper urinary tract. 1. Effects on depolarisation-induced activation. *J Urol*. 1984;132:1265-1269.

12. Davenport K, Timoney AG, Keeley FX. A comparative *in vitro* study to determine the beneficial effect of calcium channel and alpha-$_1$-adrenoceptor antagonism on human ureteral activity. *BJU Int*. 2006;98:651-655.

13. Santis WF, Peters CA, Yalla SV, et al. Ureteral function is modulated by a local renin angiotensin system. *J Urol*. 2003;170(1):259-263.

14. Maggi CA, Giuliani S, Santicioli P. Effect of cromakalim and glibenclamide on spontaneous and evoked motility of the guinea-pig isolated renal pelvis and ureter. *Br J Pharmacol*. 1994;111:687-694.

15. Kekec Z, Yilmaz U, Sozuer E. The effectiveness of tenoxicam versus isosorbide dinitrate plus tenoxicam in the treatment of acute renal colic. *BJU Int*. 2000;85:783-785.

16. Mastrangelo D, Baertschi AJ, Roatti A, et al. Nitric oxide production within rat urothelial cells. *J Urol*. 2003;170(4):1409-1414.

17. Morita T, Wada I, Saeki H, et al. Ureteral urine transport: changes in bolus volume, peristaltic frequency, intraluminal pressure and volume of flow resulting from autonomic drugs. *J Urol*. 1987;137(1):132-135.

18. Yamamoto Y, Koike K. The effects of β-adrenoceptor agonists on KCL-induced rhythmic contraction in the ureter of guinea pig. *J Smooth Muscle Res*. 2000;36:13-19.

19. Danuser H, Weiss R, Abel D, et al. Systemic and topical drug administration in the pig ureter: effect of phosphodiesterase inhibitors, α$_1$, β and β$_2$ adrenergic receptor agonists and antagonists on the frequency and amplitude of ureteral contractions. *J Urol*. 2001;166(2):714-720.

20. Becker AJ, Stief CG, Meyer M, et al. The effect of the specific phosphodiesterase-IV-inhibitor rolipram on the ureteral peristalsis of the rabbit *in vitro* and *in vivo*. *J Urol*. 1998;160(3–1):920-925.

21. Stief CG, Taher A, Truss M, et al. Phosphodiesterase isoenzymes in human ureteral smooth muscle: Identification, characterization and functional effects of various phosphodiesterase inhibitors *in vitro*. *Urol Int*. 1995;55:183-189.

22. Sivrikaya A, Celik OF, Sivrikaya N, et al. The effect of diclofenac sodium and papaverine on isolated human ureteral smooth muscle. *Int Urol Nephrol*. 2003;35:479-483.

23. Tadayyon F, Shafiei L. Efficacy of theophylline in promoting ureteral stone passage. *Eur Urol*. 2005;4(3):A94.

24. Teele ME, Lang RJ. Stretch-evoked inhibition of spontaneous migrating contractions in a whole mount preparation of the guinea-pig upper urinary tract. *Br J Pharmacol*. 1998;123(6):1143-1153.

25. Laerum E, Omundsen OE, Gronseth JE, et al. Oral diclofenac in the prophylactic treatment of recurrent renal colic: a double blind comparison with placebo. *Eur Urol*. 1995;28:108-111.

26. Grenabo L, Holmlund D. Indomethacin as prophylaxis against recurrent ureteral colic. *Scand J Urol Nephrol*. 1984;18:325-327.

27. Kapoor D, Weitzel S, Mowad J, et al. Use of indomethacin suppositories in the prophylaxis of recurrent ureteral colic. *J Urol*. 1989;142:1428-1430.

28. Peters HJ, Eckstein W. Possible pharmacological means of treating renal colic. *Urol Res*. 1975;3:55-59.

29. Hussain HBKZ, Inman RD, et al. Use of glyceryl trinitrate patches in patients with ureteral stones: a randomized, double-blind, placebo-controlled study. *Urology*. 2001;58(4):521-525.

30. Andersson KE, Forman A. Effects of calcium channel blockers on urinary tract smooth muscle. *Acta Pharmacol Toxicol*. 1986;58(2):193-200.

31. Osca JM, Broseta E, Morera JF, et al. Effects of verapamil and nicardipine on the ureteral acetylcholine and depolarisation-induced contractions *in vitro*. *Br J Urol*. 1997;80(2):A1177.

32. Borghi L, Meschi T, Amato F, et al. Nifedipine and methylprednisolone in facilitating ureteral stone passage: a randomized, double-blind, placebo-controlled study. *J Urol*. 1994;152:1095-1098.

33. Porpiglia F, Destefanis P, Fiori C, et al. Effectiveness of nifedipine and deflazacort in the management of distal ureteral stones. *Urol*. 2000;56(4):579-582.

34. Cooper JT, Stack GM, Cooper TP. Intensive medical management of ureteral calculi. *Urology*. 2000;56(4):575-578.

35. Saita A, Bonaccorsi A, Marchese F, et al. Our experience with nifedipine and prednisolone as expulsive therapy for ureteral stones. *Urol Int*. 2004;72(1):43-45.

36. Sigala S, Dellabella M, Milanese G, et al. Evidence for the presence of alpha1 adrenoceptor subtypes in the human ureter. *Neurourol Urodyn*. 2005;24(2):142-148.

37. Weiss RM, Bassett AL, Hoffman BF. Adrenergic innervation of the ureter. *Invest Urol*. 1978;16(2):123-127.

38. Cervenakov I, Fillo J, Mardiack J, et al. Speedy elimination of ureterolithiasis in lower part of ureters with the α$_1$-blocker, Tamsulosin. *Int Urol Nephrol*. 2002;34(1):25-29.

39. Dellabella M, Milanese G, Muzzonigro G. Efficacy of tamsulosin in the medical management of juxtavesical ureteral stones. *J Urol*. 2003;170:2202-2205.

40. Dellabella M, Milanese G, Muzzonigro G. Medical-expulsive therapy for distal ureterolithiasis: randomised prospective study on role of corticosteroids used in combination with Tamsulosin – Simplified treatment regimen and health-related quality of life. *Urology*. 2005;66:712-715.

41. Autorino R, De Sio M, Damiano R, et al. The use of tamsulosin in the medical treatment of ureteral calculi: where do we stand? *Urol Res*. 2005;33:460-464.

42. Yilmaz E, Batislam E, Basar MM, et al. The comparison and efficacy of three different α$_1$-adrenergic blockers for distal ureteral stones. *J Urol*. 2005;173:2010-2012.

43. Hermanns T, Sauermann P, Rufibach K, Frauenfelder T, Sulser T, Stredel RT. Is there a role for tamsulosin in the treatment of distal ureteral stones of 7mm or less? Results of a randomised, double-blind, placebo-controlled trial. *Eur Urol*. 2009;56:407-412.

44. Porpiglia F, Ghignone G, Fiori C, et al. Nifedipine versus tamsulosin for the management of lower ureteral calculi. *J Urol*. 2004;172(2):568-571.

45. Dellabella M, Milanese G, Muzzonigro G. Randomized trial of the efficacy of tamsulosin, nifedipine and phloroglucinol in medical expulsive therapy for distal ureteral calculi. *J Urol*. 2005;174(1):167-172.

46. Hollingsworth JM, Rogers MAM, Kaufman SR, et al. Medical therapy to facilitate urinary stone passage: a meta-analysis. *Lancet*. 2006;368:1171-1179.

47. Skrekas T, Liapis D, Kalantzis A, et al. Increasing the success rate of medical therapy for expulsion of distal ureteral stones using adjunctive treatment with calcium channel blocker. *Eur Urol Suppl*. 2003;2:82.

48. Kupeli B, Irkilata L, Gurocak S, et al. Does tamsulosin enhance lower ureteral stone clearance with or without shock wave lithotripsy? *Urology*. 2004;64(6):1111-1115.

49. Tekin A, Alkan E, Beysel M, et al. Alpha-1 receptor blocking therapy for lower ureteral stones: a randomized prospective trial. *J Urol*. 2004;17(suppl 4):304.

50. Resim S, Ekerbicer H, Ciftci A. Effect of tamsulosin on the number and intensity of ureteral colic in patients with lower ureteral calculus. *Int J Urol*. 2005;12:615-620.

51. Taghavi R, Darabi MR, Tavakoli K, et al. Survey of the effect of tamsulosin and nifedipine on facilitating juxtavesical ureteral stone passage. *J Endourol*. 2005;19(suppl 1):A9.

52. Staerman F, Bryckaert PE, Colin J, et al. Nifedipine in the medical treatment of symptomatic distal ureteral calculi. *Eur Urol*. 2005;37:28.

53. Parsons JK, Hergan LA, Sakamoto K, et al. Efficacy of α-blockers for the treatment of ureteral stones. *J Urol*. 2007;177:983-987.

54. Resim S, Ekerbicer H, Ciftci A. Role of tamsulosin in treatment of patients with steinstrasse developing after extracorporeal shock wave lithotripsy. *Urology*. 2005;66(5):945-948.

55. De Sio M, Autorino R, Di Lorenzo G, et al. Medical expulsive treatment of distal ureteral stones using tamsulosin: a single center experience. *J Endourol*. 2006;20:12-16.

56. Angelo-Khattar M, Thulesius O, Cherian T. The effect of glucocorticosteroids on *in vitro* motility of the ureter of the sheep. *Br J Pharmacol*. 1989;96(3):527-530.

57. Salehi M, Fouladi MM, Shiery H et al. Does methylprednisolone acetate increase the success rate of medical therapy for passing distal ureteral stones? *Eur Urol*. 2005;4(3):25 (A92).

Metabolic Investigations: When and in Whom

55

David S. Goldfarb

Abstract There is little outcome-based evidence to guide the metabolic evaluation of stone formers. The existing guidelines are based on the experience and rational thought processes of investigators of stone disease. That stones are highly recurrent is always stressed in offering a rationale for diagnostic evaluation and preventive therapy. Recurrence affects about 30% of patients at 5 years, 50% at 10 years, and 80% at 20 years. Yet even these significant recurrence rates may fail to motivate patients to adhere to lifelong regimens of fluid intake, dietary modification, or medical therapy. Large stones, consequential stones requiring urologic intervention, stones complicated by comorbidities such as heart disease, diabetes, and concomitant urinary tract infections may warrant evaluation and prevention even if they are "first" kidney stones. History taking should focus on activities, diet, occupation, medications, and family history. Twenty-four hour urine collections offer rich data regarding the etiology of stones and provide insight into patients' metabolism, diet, and habits and allow both dietary and medical therapy to be prescribed based on the individual's own pathophysiology. Follow-up collections allow the practitioner to determine the effect of therapy and consider further dietary recommendations or changes in medication dosages. Characterizing the cause of hypercalciuria has not been demonstrated to favorably affect the rationale for treatment and has not been tested regarding its ability to produce improved outcomes. It is relatively expensive, time consuming, and inconvenient and is therefore not recommended.

55.1 Introduction

There is little outcome-based evidence to guide the metabolic evaluation of stone formers. The existing guidelines are based on the experience and rational thought processes of investigators of stone disease. These guidelines are in turn based on the current understanding of the pathophysiology of stone formation, a field that has advanced considerably in recent years. On the other hand, there is a paucity of randomized controlled trials that guide effective evaluation and treatment, and a dearth of new agents or strategies to effect stone prevention. Therefore, current practice cannot be said to be "evidence based." Alternate approaches that deviate from the guidelines offered by consensus panels or experts might reflect either common sense or newer pathophysiologic contributions to stone formation, but none of these innovative strategies to evaluate and treat patients have been compared to each other in trials designed to determine which is the superior diagnostic or therapeutic algorithm. It is therefore inevitable that a discussion of the application of diagnostic evaluative schemes will reflect the practice of the individual writer.

There are several variables that are often not considered in the proffered guidelines that must be considered when evaluating stone formers. That stones are highly recurrent is always stressed in offering a rationale for offering diagnostic evaluation and preventive therapy. Often cited figures are that recurrence will occur in 30% of patients at 5 years, 50% at 10 years, and 80% at 20 years.[1] Yet even these significant recurrence rates may fail to motivate patients to adhere to lifelong regimens of fluid intake, dietary modification, or medical therapy. The average stone, after all, is fortunately not as cataclysmic as a myocardial infarction, prevention of which requires patient compliance with every one of the treating physician's recommendations. Stones may be painful, time consuming, inconvenient, and expensive, but if

D.S. Goldfarb (✉)
Nephrology Section, New York Harbor VA Medical Center,
New York, NY, USA
e-mail: david.goldfarb@va.gov

P.N. Rao et al. (eds.), *Urinary Tract Stone Disease*,
DOI 10.1007/978-1-84800-362-0_55, © Springer-Verlag London Limited 2011

managed by a competent endourologist, they will be rarely life threatening today. Patients' motivations to adhere to prescribed regimens vary widely based on their age and experience with stone disease.

Algorithms for recommendations are often based on whether the patient has suffered a first stone or a recurrent one. Taking into account the relatively limited morbidity of most stones and the reasonable effectiveness of ensuing therapy, one influential, often cited paper concluded that since specific drug therapy with thiazides or allopurinol would not be warranted in most patients with a first kidney stone, "extensive metabolic evaluation is unnecessary."[2] While this opinion will often be appropriate, the classification of stones as either "first" versus "recurrent" as the basis for deciding whether to carry out metabolic evaluation is not necessarily apt in every instance. Stones in young people are often quickly forgotten since they fail to regard the future with seriousness. They seem less likely to make required modifications in weight, diet, and fluid intake. Older people recognize that staying out of the emergency department is a worthwhile goal and may find even spontaneous passage of smaller stones frightening and complicated by other morbidities. Anyone who requires urologic intervention, or has a solitary kidney, or recurrent and severe urinary tract infections may be impressed with the consequences of stones and seek metabolic evaluation and treatment more readily than the patient who spontaneously passes stones. It is therefore recommended that the patient's outlook regarding stone prevention and motivations for stone prevention be explored. Large stones, consequential stones requiring urologic intervention, stones complicated by comorbidities such as heart disease, diabetes, and concomitant urinary tract infections may warrant evaluation and prevention even if they are "first" kidney stones.

55.2 Evaluation of Stone Formers

55.2.1 History

The results of 24-h urine collections can only be understood in the context of a careful assessment of several aspects of the patient's history. The family history may frequently identify other stone formers, as up to 40% of stone formers seen in an emergency room have first-degree relatives with stones.[3] Though genetics may account for at least 50% of stone prevalence according to twin studies, the genetic basis for most calcium and uric acid stones is not understood.[4] Infrequently, a family history of specific etiologies such as autosomal dominant polycystic kidney disease or renal tubular acidosis may be revealed.

Occupational history is often a factor in stones, though its contribution has not been quantified. Workers in hot environments, athletes, drivers, and teachers may all have low urine volumes leading to stones. An increase in urine volume may be all that is needed to prevent stones in such cases, though this otherwise simple therapeutic effect may not be so easily achieved when these occupational variables are explored.

Other comorbidities are becoming increasingly more important to the assessment of stone formers with both diagnostic and therapeutic significance. Bowel disease may cause low urine volumes if diarrhea is present, as is the case with ileostomy, short bowel syndrome, or inflammatory bowel disease. Loss of base in stool leads to acid urine pH and low urine citrate excretion, predisposing the patient to both uric acid stones and calcium stones respectively. Inflammatory bowel disease and short bowel syndrome are also associated with enteric hyperoxaluria and reductions in glomerular filtration rate (GFR), constituting chronic kidney disease (CKD).[5] Such patients are difficult to treat and are at risk for progression of CKD.

More recently the links between stones, diabetes, hypertension, and metabolic syndrome are becoming more clear.[6–8] Diabetes is now recognized as a risk for both calcium and uric acid stones, though it notably increases the risk of the latter enormously. Patients with gout have more stones, probably more as the result of low urine pH associated with insulin resistance than due to abnormalities in uric acid excretion.[9] The links between weight gain, metabolic syndrome, and hypertension now mean that patients presenting with stones should be screened for these other comorbidities, diagnoses that may not have previously been identified.[10] Stones may be the first presentation of these disorders, particularly in younger people who are often not under the care of a physician. In addition, given the consequences of these disorders, they may offer more compelling motivations for patients to change diets, lose weight, and exercise. Blood pressure should be taken at every office visit, both because blood pressure control is important per se and because the use of thiazides to reduce calciuria may affect blood pressure so that establishment of baseline and response to therapy can be followed.

Medications may contribute to stone formation, and reviewing all the patient's prescriptions and over-the-counter supplements is important.[11] Vitamin C contributes to oxalate excretion and should be limited to no more than 500 mg/day.[12] Some protease inhibitors used to treat human immunodeficiency virus (HIV) – indinivir, nelfinavir, and saquinair – are poorly soluble and can cause stones and decreased GFR. Carbonic anhydrase inhibitors, such as acetazolamide, increase urine pH, reduce citrate excretion because of their associated metabolic acidosis, and can cause calcium phosphate stones. Triamterene is poorly soluble and can nucleate calcium stones; it is not the preferred means of reducing potassium losses induced by thiazides in stone formers. Recent antiepileptic medications associated with stones include the carbonic anhydrase inhibitor topiramate and the poorly soluble felbamate.[13] Calcium supplements (as opposed to increased dietary calcium intake) have variably been associated with increased risk for stones.[12,14]

A careful dietary history will include questions about the intake of protein, purines, sodium, fluids, oxalate, and calcium. The details of these factors are described elsewhere in this volume. Excessive intake of animal protein, such as the Atkins diet popular in recent years for weight loss, has often, but not always, been implicated in increasing the risk of stones through several mechanisms, including reductions in citrate excretion, and increases in oxalate, uric acid, and calcium excretion.[12,15] Despite this association, restriction of animal protein did not result in the expected benefit of reduced stones.[16] Increasing purine intake (e.g., sardines, organ meats) increases uric acid excretion, while increasing sodium intake leads to increased calcium excretion. The role of oxalate intake remains debated as oxalate restriction has not been studied with stone recurrence as an outcome. Increases in dietary calcium intake have generally been associated with fewer stones,[17,18] and higher calcium diets (with concomitant reductions in animal protein, oxalate, and salt intake) reduce stone recurrence.[19] Grapefruit juice has been associated with stones for unknown reasons.[20] While performing a dietary history is important, one must acknowledge that the evidence that such histories lead to therapeutic manipulations that successfully reduce stone recurrences is slim.

55.2.2 Laboratory Evaluation

All patients should have stones sent at least once, if not several times, for determination of composition by X-ray crystallography or infrared spectroscopy. For example, it is important to identify struvite stones, composed of magnesium-ammonium phosphate, often mixed with basic calcium phosphates, as there are critical implications for surgical and medical therapy. Cystinuria, in particular, may not be diagnosed if an inexpensive determination of stone composition is not made, leading to lost opportunities for effective therapy. Though even rarer, adenine phosphoribosyltransferase deficiency will be missed if its resultant 2,8-dihydroxy adenine stones are not analyzed.

Routine serum chemistries should be determined and urinalysis performed. Even normal serum calcium values greater than 10 mg/dL should lead to measurement of intact parathyroid hormone as stones may be a first presentation of primary hyperparathyroidism. Alternatively, hypercalcemia or hypercalciuria with stones may represent a first presentation of sarcoidosis. Examination for lymph node enlargement and a chest radiograph should be considered. The urinalysis is most useful for determination of pH, though the pH of the 24-h collection may be more helpful. A high urine pH greater than

7.5 or pyuria suggests urinary tract infection and struvite stones. Urine culture should follow, with *Proteus* species being typical, though many other bacterial species contain urease, the enzyme responsible for the high urine pH. If high urine pH is accompanied by low serum bicarbonate concentrations, renal tubular acidosis (RTA) may be present; these patients often make calcium phosphate stones.

Often accomplished during an emergency department visit, all patients should have at least a renal ultrasound to document the presence or absence of additional stones to gauge the severity of the stone-forming tendency. Polycystic kidney disease is suggested if more than four cysts are present.

55.3 Twenty-Four Hour Urine Collections

The consensus among urologists and nephrologists specializing in kidney stone prevention is that prevention regimens should be prescribed based on the results of 24-h urine collections. Much information about underlying risk factors and diet is to be gained from urine collections in stone formers. The last consensus statements issued from the National Institutes of Health, and the European Association of Urology guidelines, while not recent, concur.[21,22] Both guidelines suggest that 24-h collections be reserved for recurrent stone formers and children, but as discussed in the introduction, in many first-time stone formers and in varied circumstances, a complete evaluation may be warranted.

Despite the widespread consensus, one must concede that the superiority of basing therapy on the results of 24-h collections has not been compared to therapy based on stone composition or based on nothing other than the generic occurrence of renal colic. The strategy of choosing therapy based on urine collections is attractive as it appears to cater to the individual's specific results, but the causative nature of some of the results remains disputed, and the number of therapies proven to succeed based on the urine results remains low. Given the cost and inconvenience of performing the collections, one might ask, as patients often do, how important the results are. In the absence of the definitive randomized controlled trial on the subject, one would believe that patients enthusiastically appreciate knowing exactly what is in their urine and are usually willing to undergo the cost and inconvenience to understand their pathophysiology and view the results of their attempts to adhere to their medical regimens.

Basing therapy on random, spot urine collections instead of 24-h urine collections may be tempting in many instances, particularly in children. Significant variations throughout the day in urinary excretion of calcium, oxalate, citrate, pH, and volume are well known, especially given the variation that occurs in relation to meals and sleep. In those incapable of reliably collecting 24 h worth of urine in a container, spot collections may be the only data available. Expressing results normalized for urine creatinine content allows one to follow results in response to treatment and compare the results to published normal values.[23] An exception to the difficulty of using spot urine testing for diagnostic or therapeutic purposes is the case of uric acid stones. Since urine alkalinization is more important than reductions in uric acid excretion, spot samples that demonstrate an increase in urine pH to values greater than 6.0 are particularly predictive of successful stone prevention. Patients can test urine pH once a day at varying times to ascertain if alkalinization is adequate. Successfully increasing pH once a day or even every other day, and not around the clock, may be all that is necessary to prevent uric acid stone recurrences.[24] For treatment of existing uric acid stones, more persistent alkalinization is indicated.

Urine collections should be done on patients' self-selected or ad-lib usual diets. Particularly since urine results will be used to advise patients regarding suggested alterations in their dietary habits, it makes most sense to have urine collected on days that represent their usual dietary choices, and then longitudinally compare subsequent results to "pretreatment" urine collections in order to judge success with dietary manipulation. In the context of a research study, defined diets, food diaries, and provided meals dispensed by a study center may be appropriate. But in the course of clinical care, only the patient's chosen diet will allow patient and physician to monitor progress. Patients should not do collections while hospitalized, while having renal colic, or while recovering from urologic interventions. It is preferable to wait for removal of stents, treatment of infection, and resolution of hydronephrosis before proceeding with urine collections.

Various protocols for collecting the urine have been recommended. The superiority of specific approaches to the evaluation has not been conclusively demonstrated. The guidelines of the European Association of Urology suggest that two collections of 24 h be performed with one containing hydrochloric acid and one containing a preservative, sodium azide.[22] The addition of HCl ensures the dissolution of calcium oxalate and calcium phosphate; otherwise the poorly soluble crystals may precipitate and either be lost at the bottom of the collection container or not be measured while sequestered in insoluble crystals. This protocol, however, will not yield the patient's true urine pH value. Uric acid will be precipitated by the low pH from addition of HCl, necessitating the addition of a strong base like NaOH in order to solubilize precipitated and therefore unmeasurable uric acid. The alternative is to perform the collection without the addition of HCl or NaOH, determine the patient's true pH value, and treat aliquots with both HCl and NaOH in order to accurately measure both calcium salts and uric acid. Maintaining urine at room temperature also helps reduce crystallization and is preferable for most patients (and spouses) but requires the use of an antibacterial agent such as sodium

azide, thymol, or gentamicin.[25] The latter, as well as lithium or fluoride added to collection containers before the collection is performed, can also be used as determinants of urine volume, particularly if patients cannot accurately determine volume before removing aliquots of urine for study. They serve as checks on the patients' reported values. Patients should always shake up the collection container well before removing aliquots for measurement.

Most important is to measure the results of any dietary or pharmacologic manipulation. Demonstrating the efficacy of a treatment to a patient – whether the hypocalciuric effect of thiazides, the increase in citrate excretion with oral citrate supplementation, or the reduction in calcium excretion with restriction of dietary sodium – is always worthwhile. Without subsequent 24-h urine collections, patient and physician will be uncertain as to whether therapy is sufficient, requires intensification, or addition. Urine chemistry is a surrogate that hopefully will correlate with subsequent stone activity. Reductions of calculated supersaturation have not been proven to correlate with reductions in metabolic stone activity, but the author believes that they are very likely to be useful in that regard. On the other hand, the outcome of interest is not a change in urine chemistry but the prevention of stones. Ultimately, the patient's reduced experience of renal colic episodes or the failure of stone growth or recurrence on surveillance ultrasounds is more reassuring than a favorable urine profile.

For patients with hypercalciuria, evaluation focused on defining the patient's specific pathophysiologic abnormality was promoted in the past.[26] However, the protocol for defining "absorptive" versus "renal leak" hypercalciuria further increased the complexity of the evaluation and was not demonstrated to provide superior results. Calcium restriction, prescribed for those patients with "absorptive" hypercalciuria, appeared to be associated with more stone recurrence both in epidemiologic studies and in one randomized controlled trial.[19,27] Furthermore, although their hypercalciuria was termed "absorptive," patients with this syndrome also had decreased bone mineral density, possibly exacerbated and at least not addressed by restriction of dairy intake.[28] Finally, treatment of hypercalciuria with thiazides was successful regardless of the results of this classification scheme.[29] Even the originators of this classification eventually stopped promoting the cumbersome technique for clinical care outside of the Clinical Research Center.[30]

However, excessive "simplification" of the evaluation by not having 24-h collections done is often a missed opportunity to provide specific treatment recommendations. Despite significant improvements in the protocols for collecting urine by user-friendly laboratories, an evaluation is frequently avoided in the belief that prescribing generic therapy that does not specifically address the patients' urine chemistries is easier and satisfactory. To take an important example, increasing urine volume is nearly always appropriate for stone prevention as it is an inexpensive, safe, and effective therapy.[31] One might argue that telling patients to "drink more" does not require a 24-h urine collection. Urine volume, in fact, is one of the most important results of the collection as it identifies to what extent the patient is achieving or falling short of the goal of having 2.5 L of urine or more in order to dilute urinary stone-forming salts. The result makes concrete what has previously been a more abstract concept. Many patients who claim to be drinking "a lot" are rather poorly informed about what "a lot" is, and quite inaccurate as to what their daily urine volume is. Only with a prescription for 3 L (about 100 oz)/day and a measurement of urine volume can a successful result be visualized by the stone-forming patient.

The number of collections performed is no longer debated: the more collections, the more accurately one can assess what the patient's representative urine chemistry is. While some stone clinics have patients do three "pretreatment" collections to determine patients' baseline urine characteristics, more often two collections is a reasonable compromise.[32] Subsequent posttreatment collections done after several weeks to months following prescription of a prevention regimen, followed by a few yearly collections until stable, would be the usual practice. Patients may often be interested in performing collections both at home and at work, in order to identify differences resulting from varying access to toilet facilities, time, and availability of beverages, and dietary choices. One study demonstrated higher volumes at work than on weekends as the major difference in one small group of patients.[33]

Ideally, urine is analyzed by a laboratory that specializes in assessment of kidney stone risk factors.[34] Local laboratories are often unprepared to correctly process urine samples to account for crystallized salts that would be lost to measurement without manipulation of sample pH as described previously. Increasing urine pH to solubilize precipitated uric acid and lowering urine pH to 1 to solubilize precipitated calcium oxalate and phosphate are both required to reliably retrieve these otherwise unmeasurable crystals suspended in the urine or grounded at the bottom of the collection container. Calculation of supersaturation of the stone-forming salts calcium oxalate, calcium phosphate, and uric acid is extremely helpful for interpretation of urine chemistries. Based on computer programs that estimate supersaturation based on concentration of the critical components, pH, citrate, and other ionic constituents, all of the urine values are summarized in a single number that can help patients and clinicians understand the net impact of their treatment. Supersaturation can be a variable that patients understand from a practical, not a physicochemical, perspective. Diet changes produce sporadic results, and urine volume can be erratic as well. Supersaturation accounts for the complementary or offsetting effects to produce a value that expresses likelihood of precipitation of the relatively insoluble stone-forming salts. Different labs may calculate and express results in different manners. Supersaturation also makes clear that the most important variable determining likelihood of salt crystallization is concentration, not absolute solute excretion. Even low amounts of calcium excreted in 24 h may be associated with stone formation in a low urine volume and at a relatively high supersaturation. Supersaturation also strongly correlates with stone composition, though this relationship is imperfect.[35] Only a laboratory specializing in stone risk will provide the calculated values.

Table 55.1 offers an example of the results of collections in a man with hypercalciuria. The first two collections were done "pretreatment" and document hypercalciuria. Measurements of creatinine allow the clinician to be certain that the collection was performed correctly, without over- or under-collection. Men produce about 18–24 mg of creatinine per kilogram body weight, women 15–20 mg/kg. Creatinine values should be within 10–15% of each other. Expressing calcium excretion as milligram per gram of creatinine can salvage the data if miscollection has occurred. A commonly cited definition for hypercalciuria is 4 mg of calcium per kilogram body weight; this calculation can often demonstrate

Table 55.1 Results of 24-h urine collections in a 36-year-old man with calcium oxalate stones. Two collections were done "pretreatment" and one after initiation of thiazides

Date	24 h Vol	24 h Na	24 h Ca	24 h Ox	24 h Cit	24 h pH	24 h UA	SS CaOx	SS CaP	SS UA
3/22/08	2.4	229	222	42	446	5.6	727	5.5	0.3	1.2
11/29/07	1.9	212	336	44	501	5.9	643	10.1	1.5	0.8
11/28/07	1.2	188	344	28	447	5.9	512	11.6	2.9	1.0

Date	24 h NH4	24 h K	24 h Mg	24 h Phos	24 h Creat	Wt kg	Cr/kg	Ca/kg	Ca/Cr
3/22/08	44	31	126	1.0	1,633	77.3	21.1	2.9	136
11/29/07	37	49	99	1.3	1,721	75.0	22.9	4.5	195
11/28/07	25	39	96	1.1	1,607	75.0	21.4	4.6	214

Vol volume, L; *Na* sodium, mEq; *Ca* calcium, mg; *Ox* oxalate, mg; *Cit* citrate, mg; *UA* uric acid, mg; l *SS* supersaturation for *CaOx* calcium oxalate; *CaP* calcium phosphate; *UA* uric acid; NH_4 ammonium, mEq; *K* potassium, mEq; *Mg* magnesium, mg; *Phos* phosphorus, g; *creat* creatinine, mg; *Cr/kg* g creatinine/kg body weight; *Ca/kg* mg calcium/kg body weight; *Ca/Cr* mg calcium/g creatinine

Adapted from Litholink Corp, Chicago, IL

that a smaller absolute amount of calcium is in fact too high for a smaller person. However, the prior caveat offered about concentration of calcium being more important than the absolute amount still applies. In this case, thiazides were used to lower urine calcium and the patient successfully increased urine volume. The net effect of these two maneuvers can be seen in the markedly lowered supersaturation for calcium oxalate.

A similar concept is behind direct measurement of supersaturation of cystine in patients with cystinuria.[36] Changes in pH, cystine excretion, and urine volume can be integrated into a single value that should correlate with stone activity better than any individual variable alone. The test is available in the USA at present only from Litholink Corp (Chicago, IL, USA).

55.4 Conclusions

Twenty-four-hour urine collections offer rich data regarding the etiology of stones and provide insight into patients' metabolism, diet, and habits and allow both dietary and medical therapy to be prescribed based on the individual's own pathophysiology. Follow-up collections allow the practitioner to determine the effect of therapy and consider further dietary recommendations or changes in medication dosages. Characterizing the cause of hypercalciuria has not been demonstrated to favorably affect the rationale for treatment and has not been tested regarding its ability to produce improved outcomes. It is relatively expensive, time consuming, and inconvenient and is therefore not recommended.

Disclosure The author has served as a consultant for Takeda and Sanofi-Aventis, and participated in research with Amgen. This work was supported in part by the National Institutes of Diabetes and Digestive and Kidney Disease and the Office of Rare Disease Research, via grant 1U54DK083908–01.

References

1. Asplin J, Chandhoke PS. The stone-forming patient. In: Coe FL, Favus MJ, Pak CYC, Parks JH, Preminger GM, eds. *Kidney Stones: Medical and Surgical Management*. Philadelphia: Lippincott-Raven; 1996:337-352.
2. Uribarri J, Oh MS, Carroll HJ. The first kidney stone. *Ann Intern Med*. 1989;111:1006-1009.
3. Ljunghall S, Danielson BG, Fellstrom B, et al. Family history of renal stones in recurrent stone patients. *Br J Urol*. 1985;57:370-374.
4. Goldfarb DS, Fischer ME, Keich Y, et al. A twin study of genetic and dietary influences on nephrolithiasis: a report from the Vietnam Era Twin (VET) registry. *Kidney Int*. 2005;67:1053-1061.
5. Parks JH, Worcester EM, O'Connor RC, et al. Urine stone risk factors in nephrolithiasis patients with and without bowel disease. *Kidney Int*. 2003;63:255-265.
6. Obligado SH, Goldfarb DS. The association of nephrolithiasis with hypertension and obesity: a review. *Am J Hypertens*. 2008;21: 257-264.
7. Maalouf NM, Cameron MA, Moe OW, et al. Novel insights into the pathogenesis of uric acid nephrolithiasis. *Curr Opin Nephrol Hypertens*. 2004;13:181-189.
8. Taylor EN, Curhan GC. Body size and 24-hour urine composition. *Am J Kidney Dis*. 2006;48:905-915.
9. Kramer HJ, Choi HK, Atkinson K, et al. The association between gout and nephrolithiasis in men: the health professionals' follow-up study. *Kidney Int*. 2003;64:1022-1026.
10. Daudon M, Traxer O, Conort P, et al. Type 2 diabetes increases the risk for uric acid stones. *J Am Soc Nephrol*. 2006;17:2026-2033.
11. Daudon M, Jungers P. Drug-induced renal calculi: epidemiology, prevention and management. *Drugs*. 2004;64:245-275.
12. Taylor EN, Stampfer MJ, Curhan GC. Dietary factors and the risk of incident kidney stones in men: new insights after 14 years of follow-up. *J Am Soc Nephrol*. 2004;15:3225-3232.
13. Welch BJ, Graybeal D, Moe OW, et al. Biochemical and stone-risk profiles with topiramate treatment. *Am J Kidney Dis*. 2006;48: 555-563.
14. Jackson RD, LaCroix AZ, Gass M, et al. Calcium plus vitamin D supplementation and the risk of fractures. *N Engl J Med*. 2006;354: 669-683.
15. Rotily M, Leonetti F, Iovanna C, et al. Effects of low animal protein or high-fiber diets on urine composition in calcium nephrolithiasis. *Kidney Int*. 2000;57:1115-1123.
16. Dussol B, Iovanna C, Rotily M, et al. A randomized trial of low-animal-protein or high-fiber diets for secondary prevention of calcium nephrolithiasis. *Nephron Clin Pract*. 2008;110:c185-c194.
17. Taylor EN, Curhan GC. Oxalate intake and the risk for nephrolithiasis. *J Am Soc Nephrol*. 2007;18:2198-2204.
18. Curhan GC, Willett WC, Speizer FE, et al. Comparison of dietary calcium with supplemental calcium and other nutrients as factors affecting the risk for kidney stones in women. *Ann Intern Med*. 1997;126:497-504.
19. Borghi L, Schianchi T, Meschi T, et al. Comparison of two diets for the prevention of recurrent stones in idiopathic hypercalciuria. *N Engl J Med*. 2002;346:77-84.
20. Curhan GC, Willett WC, Speizer FE, et al. Beverage use and risk for kidney stones in women. *Ann Intern Med*. 1998;128:534-540.
21. National Institutes of Health Consensus Development Conference on Prevention and Treatment of Kidney Stones, Bethesda, Maryland, March 28–30, 1988; *J Urol*. 141:705–808.
22. Tiselius HG, Ackermann D, Alken P, et al. Guidelines on urolithiasis. *Eur Urol*. 2001;40:362-371.
23. DeFoor W, Minevich E, Jackson E, et al. Urinary metabolic evaluations in solitary and recurrent stone forming children. *J Urol*. 2008;179:2369-2372.
24. Rodman JS. Prophylaxis of uric acid stones with alternate day doses of alkaline potassium salts. *J Urol*. 1991;145:97-99.
25. Asplin J, Parks J, Lingeman J, et al. Supersaturation and stone composition in a network of dispersed treatment sites. *J Urol*. 1998;159:1821-1825.
26. Ruml LA, Pearle MS, Pak CY. Medical therapy, calcium oxalate urolithiasis. *Urol Clin N Am*. 1997;24:117-133.

27. Curhan GC, Willett WC, Rimm EB, et al. A prospective study of dietary calcium and other nutrients and the risk of symptomatic kidney stones. *N Engl J Med*. 1993;328:833-838.

28. Asplin JR, Donahue S, Kinder J, et al. Urine calcium excretion predicts bone loss in idiopathic hypercalciuria. *Kidney Int*. 2006;70: 1463-1467.

29. Pearle MS, Roehrborn CG, Pak CY. Meta-analysis of randomized trials for medical prevention of calcium oxalate nephrolithiasis. *J Endourol*. 1999;13:679-685.

30. Pak CY, Resnick MI. Medical therapy and new approaches to management of urolithiasis. *Urol Clin N Am*. 2000;27:243-253.

31. Borghi L, Meschi T, Amato F, et al. Urinary volume, water and recurrences in idiopathic calcium nephrolithiasis: a 5-year randomized prospective study. *J Urol*. 1996;155:839-843.

32. Parks JH, Goldfisher E, Asplin JR, et al. A single 24-hour urine collection is inadequate for the medical evaluation of nephrolithiasis. *J Urol*. 2002;167:1607-1612.

33. Norman RW. Weekend versus weekday urine collections in assessment of stone-formers. *J R Soc Med*. 1996;89:561-562.

34. Lingeman J, Mardis H, Kahnoski R, et al. Medical reduction of stone risk in a network of treatment centers compared to a research clinic. *J Urol*. 1998;160:1629-1634.

35. Parks JH, Coward M, Coe FL. Correspondence between stone composition and urine supersaturation in nephrolithiasis. *Kidney Int*. 1997;51:894-900.

36. Nakagawa Y, Asplin JR, Goldfarb DS, et al. Clinical use of cystine supersaturation measurements. *J Urol*. 2000;164: 1481-1485.

Medical Management of Idiopathic Calcium Stone Disease

56

Samuel P. Sterrett and Stephen Y. Nakada

Abstract Urolithiasis is a relatively common disorder with a high recurrence rate. Calcium-containing stones represent approximately 80% of all stones. Dietary and metabolic abnormalities can contribute to calcium stone formation and treatment options are tailored to address these abnormalities. Dietary factors that have been shown to reduce stone formation rates include fluids, sodium, animal protein, fruits and vegetables, calcium, and oxalate. If dietary measures are unsuccessful and metabolic defects persist, selective medical therapy along with dietary therapy may be instituted. Pharmacological agents used to address the metabolic defects of calcium stone disease include thiazides, potassium citrate, allopurinol, and orthophosphates. Dietary modifications with or without pharmacologic regimens are extremely effective and safe in the calcium stone former.

56.1 Introduction

The lifetime risk of stone formation in the USA exceeds 13% in men and 7% in women[1] with recurrence rates as high as 30–40% at 5 years if left untreated.[2] In addition, total annual medical expenditures for urolithiasis in the USA exceed $2 billion and indirect costs for lost wages is estimated at $139 million annually.[3,4] With comprehensive evaluation, dietary and metabolic abnormalities can be identified in more than 90% of stone formers, and the institution of preventative dietary and medical measures has resulted in substantial reduction in stone recurrence rates.[5]

Among the various stone compositions, calcium-containing stones represent approximately 80% of all stones. Calcium oxalate stones represent 60% of this number, and calcium phosphate hydroxyapatite and brushite represent 20%.[6] Calcium stones form as a result of many dietary and metabolic abnormalities. Identification of these factors is the key to successful treatment. In this chapter, we review the various dietary and pharmacological options for the medical management of calcium stone disease.

S.Y. Nakada (✉)
Department of Urology, University of Wisconsin School of Medicine and Public Health, Madison, WI, USA
e-mail: nakada@surgery.wisc.edu

56.2 Dietary Factors

Dietary measures have been well documented to reduce stone formation by reducing the excretion of stone constituents or increasing urinary inhibitors. In some stone patients, dietary modifications alone will be enough to prevent recurrence of disease. In others, dietary modifications will need to be supplemented with pharmacological therapy. A number of dietary factors have been shown to influence stone formation, including fluids, sodium, animal protein, fruits and vegetables, calcium, and oxalate.

56.2.1 Fluids

The general recommendation for all stone patients is to maintain a daily urine output of 2 l. In the calcium stone former, this fluid reduces urinary saturation of stone forming calcium salts and dilutes promoters of calcium oxalate crystallization. Several studies have demonstrated that a high fluid intake is inversely related to the risk of kidney stone formation.[7–9] In addition, Strauss and colleagues have demonstrated that failure to increase urine output is one of the three strong predictors of relapse for those patients observed in a dedicated stone clinic.[10]

P.N. Rao et al. (eds.), *Urinary Tract Stone Disease*,
DOI 10.1007/978-1-84800-362-0_56, © Springer-Verlag London Limited 2011

Not all beverages are comparable with regard to their beneficial effect. Carbonated beverages, alcohol, coffee, and tea have been shown in epidemiological studies to decrease the risks of nephrolithiasis.[11] Multiple studies have investigated the effect of citrus fruit juices on urinary stone risk factors. Lemonade and orange juice are two such juices that have proven to increase urinary citrate excretion.[12,13] Potassium-rich fruit juices such as orange juice provide organic anions that are metabolized to alkali, thereby increasing urinary pH and citrate. Lemonade, although replete with citric acid, does not provide these anions. In fact, Odvina demonstrated that despite comparable citrate content, orange juice has greater alkalizing and citraturic effects than lemonade.[14] Conversely, apple and grapefruit juice have been found to increase the risk of stone events.[15] Recent evidence also suggests that caffeine may increase the risk of stone recurrence in calcium stone formers by increasing the excretion of calcium. Caffeine increased urinary calcium/creatinine, magnesium/creatinine, citrate/creatinine, and sodium/creatinine but not oxalate/creatinine ratios in stone formers and controls. Furthermore, supersaturation calculations increased, despite the noted increases in the inhibitors citrate and magnesium.[16] Overall, most evidence suggests that the volume, not the type, of fluid ingested is more important for stone prevention.[17]

56.2.2 Sodium

Salt ingestion increases calcium stone risk by reducing renal tubule calcium reabsorption, thus increasing urinary calcium. Elevated urinary calcium results in an increased urinary saturation of monosodium urate and reduced urinary citrate. Consequently, inhibition of calcium oxalate and calcium phosphate stone formation is reduced, monosodium urate-induced calcium oxalate crystallization is enhanced, and urinary saturation of calcium oxalate and calcium phosphate is increased.

Sakhaee and colleagues confirmed the effects of salt loading in a clinical crossover study involving normal volunteers. Subjects given a high sodium diet were found to have not only increased calcium excretion but also increased urine pH and decreased citrate excretion.[18] Borghi and colleagues later showed that in combination with animal protein restriction and moderate calcium ingestion, a reduced sodium diet will decrease stone episodes by approximately 50%.[19] Given that the average American requires about 500 mg of sodium yet consumes 2,300–6,900 mg of sodium per day, we typically recommend a sodium intake range of less than 3,300 mg/day for those with moderate to severe hypercalciuria.[20]

56.2.3 Animal Protein

Animal protein provides an acid load because of the high content of sulfur containing amino acids. In turn, this reduces urine pH and citrate and enhances urinary calcium excretion via bone resorption and reduced renal calcium reabsorption. In addition, the purine load increases urinary uric acid as well as the risk of calcium oxalate stone formation. Meat, poultry, fish, seafood, cheese, and egg yolks are significant contributors to the acid load of the Western diet. Dairy, grains, and a few vegetables (corn, peas, lentils) also confer an acid load, albeit much lower, because of their higher concentration of phosphorus and sulfate.[21]

Clinical data supporting low animal protein diets for stone prevention is building. A positive correlation between animal protein consumption and new stone formation has been shown in men but not in women.[7,8] A lower rate of stone formation in hypercalciuric stone formers maintained on a normal calcium, low protein, and low sodium diet has also been demonstrated.[21] A recent study by Seiner and colleagues revealed that an increased intake of animal protein was identified as one of the most important dietary risk factors for stone formation in recurrent calcium oxalate stone patients.[22]

56.2.4 Fruits and Vegetables

Fruits and vegetables are potassium-rich foods and confer an alkali load. In addition, the citric acid contained in citrus fruits is metabolized to carbon dioxide and water, potentiating the alkali effect of these foods. A low intake of fruits and vegetables, coupled with a high intake of animal protein, confers an acid load that lowers urinary pH and citrate and may increase urinary calcium. Meschi and colleagues confirmed these findings by restricting fruits and vegetables in 12 normal adults over a 2-week period. They also found that addition of fruits and vegetables to the diet of hypocitraturic stone formers, not used to eating them, not only significantly increases citrate excretion without affecting oxalate excretion, but also decreases calcium oxalate and uric acid relative saturation.[23] We typically recommend at least five or more servings of fruits and vegetables per day.

56.2.5 Dietary Calcium

Historically, calcium restriction has been recommended to decrease urinary calcium and prevent stone formation. Current studies, however, show a protective effect of normal to high calcium intake in preventing stone formation.[11] The protective effect of high calcium intake in these studies was attributed to the decline in urinary oxalate that results from reduced intestinal oxalate absorption in the face of increased luminal calcium-oxalate complex formation. It is important to remember that urinary oxalate levels depend on a combination of dietary oxalate, calcium, and the state of intestinal calcium absorption. Decreasing both dietary calcium and oxalate can also produce low urinary calcium levels without the associated rise in urinary oxalate. Pak et al. demonstrated this eloquently in a large retrospective study of calcium stone formers. They found that a short-term program of dietary and calcium and oxalate restriction resulted in a significant decline in urinary calcium in hypercalciuric patients without a change in urinary oxalate.[24] Thus, hypercalciuric patients may be optimally treated with a program of modest calcium and oxalate restriction. Severe calcium restriction should be avoided to prevent a negative calcium balance.

There is ample evidence to suggest that calcium supplementation can be safe if attention is paid to preparation and timing. In a review of postmenopausal women, Domrongkitchaiporn et al. demonstrated that calcium supplementation does not have deleterious effects on urinary calcium, oxalate, or citrate levels. Furthermore, supplementation with a meal or combined calcium supplement and estrogen therapy was not associated with a significant increased risk of calcium oxalate stone formation in the majority of postmenopausal osteoporotic patients.[25] These authors later showed that supplementation with meals offered no increase in urine supersaturation of calcium oxalate, a protection that did not remain for patients taking a nighttime bolus ingestion.[26] Calcium citrate (350 mg three times daily) has proven to be an excellent choice for calcium supplementation as urinary citrate, in addition to urinary calcium, is increased. The protective effect of citrate provides reassurance to patients and physicians worried about the lithogenic potential of calcium supplements.[27] Vitamin D supplementation, required for optimal calcium absorption, has been shown to be safe without increasing urinary calcium excretion in healthy postmenopausal women.[28]

56.2.6 Dietary Oxalate

Dietary oxalate is believed to account for 10–50% of urinary oxalate, depending on dietary calcium and oxalate intake and the bioavailability of oxalate in foods.[29] Many plant foods contain oxalate, which is acquired through the soil during growth. A list of foods known to cause high urinary oxalate excretion is listed in Table 56.1. When dietary oxalate and calcium are consumed concurrently, urinary oxalate is

Table 56.1 Foods proposed to cause hyperoxaluria

Nuts (especially almonds, hazelnuts, cashews, and peanuts)
Tea (green and black)
Sesame seeds
Chocolate
Spinach
Swiss chard
Okra
Beets
Rhubarb
Soybeans (tofu and soy nuts)
Wheat bran
Buckwheat

decreased due to binding of oxalate in the gastrointestinal tract. Thus, a low calcium intake increases the oxalate absorbed. Magnesium is also capable of binding oxalate in the gastrointestinal tract. Increased oxalate absorption can lead to calcium oxalate stone formation. Patients with inflammatory bowel disease or fat malabsorption are at increased risk of calcium oxalate stone formation due to the precipitation of calcium and magnesium with fatty acids increasing oxalate absorption. In addition, calcium oxalate stone formers with mild hyperoxaluria have also been shown to have increased renal excretion and intestinal absorption of oxalate.[30] In general, a dietary restriction of oxalate rich foods is recommended for patients exhibiting urinary hyperoxaluria.

Vitamin C (ascorbic acid) ingestion is also considered a risk factor for calcium oxalate stone formation because of its conversion to oxalate. A large cohort study demonstrated a 41% increased risk of stone formation in men consuming 1 g or more of vitamin C daily compared to those consuming less than 90 mg daily.[31] Another study demonstrated a 20–33% increase in urinary oxalate with the consumption of 2 g of vitamin C daily.[32] We typically limit our stone patients to less than 500 mg of vitamin C supplementation daily.

56.3 Pharmacological Therapy

If dietary or conservative measures for calcium stone disease are unsuccessful and metabolic defects persist, selective medical therapy along with dietary measures may be instituted. The ideal drug should reverse any physiologic defect and be safe to the patient. A number of pharmacological agents have been used to target these metabolic abnormalities including thiazides, potassium citrate, allopurinol, and orthophosphates.

56.3.1 Thiazides

Thiazide diuretics are typically reserved for patients with severe renal hypercalciuria. This class of medications has been widely used to treat absorptive hypercalciuria because of its hypocalciuric action and high cost and inconvenience of alternative therapy. The hypocalciuric action of thiazides is attributed to enhanced calcium reabsorption in the distal tubule. In addition, thiazides promote sodium and calcium reabsorption in the proximal renal tubule, further reducing urinary calcium. Thus, a high sodium diet can attenuate the hypocalciuric effects of thiazide diuretics. Thiazides may also increase urinary excretion of zinc and magnesium.

Hydrochlorothiazide and chlorthalidone are the most commonly used thiazide diuretics. Recommended dosages are hydrochlorothiazide 25 mg once or twice daily or chlorthalidone 25–50 mg daily. Alternatively, indapamide (1.25–2.5 mg daily) is a non-thiazide diuretic that has a similar mechanism of action thiazides and has been shown in a randomized trial to be effective in preventing stone recurrence.[33] Side effects of thiazides are listed in Table 56.2. Side effects are common and occur in up to 30–35% of patients treated with thiazide. Many side effects are seen at the initiation of treatment but resolve with prolonged treatment. Thiazide-induced hypokalemia can lead to intracellular acidosis and hypocitraturia. The empiric use of potassium citrate can prevent both of these conditions.

Table 56.2 Possible side effects of thiazides

Hypokalemia
Fatigue
Drowsiness
Dizziness
Decreased libido
Impotence
Carbohydrate intolerance
Hyperuricemia
Musculoskeletal symptoms
Gastrointestinal complaints

Evidence also implies that thiazide-induced hypokalemia can result in sudden cardiac death in some hypertensive patients.[34] The addition of a potassium sparing diuretic may further reduce the mortality risk.

A number of randomized trials have demonstrated a benefit of thiazides in reducing the rate of stone recurrence in calcium stone formers (Table 56.3).[24,35–37] In a meta-analysis of randomized medical therapy trials, a 21% risk reduction in stone recurrence rates was demonstrated with the initiation of thiazides or indapamide.[38] We routinely prescribe Moduretic (hydrocholorothiazide and amiloride) to patients with persistent hypercalciuria unresponsive to dietary modifications.

56.3.2 Potassium Citrate

Potassium citrate increases urinary pH and citrate, thereby increasing urinary inhibitory activity, and reducing urinary calcium. Potassium citrate can be used for treatment of patients who have hypocitraturia, uric acid-induced calcium oxalate stone formation, hyperuricosuric calcium oxalate stone disease who are unable to tolerate allopurinol, and in conjunction with thiazides for patients with hypercalciuria to prevent thiazide-induced hypokalemia and hypocitraturia. In addition, potassium citrate can raise the urine pH in patients with enteric hyperoxaluria.

The typical dose of potassium citrate is 20 mEq twice per day, although higher doses may be required with severe hypocitraturia. Side effects of potassium citrate include gastrointestinal disturbances, weakness, mental status changes, or muscle pain. Close monitoring of urinary pH is needed in patients who form calcium phosphorus crystals, as these may precipitate at higher urine pH.

In a randomized trial, Barcello and colleagues have demonstrated a 75% reduction in stone recurrence rates among hypocitraturic stone formers.[39] Likewise, potassium citrate has been shown to be effective in reducing stone recurrence rates in hyperuricosuric calcium oxalate stone formers unable to tolerate allopurinol.[40]

Table 56.3 Randomized trials demonstrating a reduction in stone recurrence using thiazides

Author (date)	Study arms	Thiazide dose	Urinary calcium	Stone formation rates using thiazide
Pak (2003)[24]	Trichlormethiazide vs. indapamide	4 or 2 mg/day	Significantly decreased[a]	Significantly decreased[a]
Ohkawa (1992)[35]	Trichlormethiazide vs. no treatment	4 mg/day	N/A	Significantly decreased
Ettinger (1988)[36]	Chlorthalidone vs. magnesium hydroxide vs. placebo	25 or 50 mg/day	N/A	Significantly decreased
Laerum (1984)[37]	HCTZ vs. placebo	25 mg b.i.d.	N/A	Significantly decreased

[a] Urinary calcium and stone formation rates were significantly reduced in both groups compared to baseline

N/A not available, *HCTZ* hydrochlorothiazide

56.3.3 Allopurinol

Allopurinol is a xanthine oxidase inhibitor that prevents the conversion of hypoxanthine to xanthine, the precursor of uric acid. This blockade reduces the heterogenous nucleation of calcium oxalate by both uric acid and monosodium urate. In addition, uric acid and monosodium urate adsorb normally occurring macromolecular inhibitors of calcium oxalate crystallization. It is indicated in calcium stone formers who have moderate to severe hyperuricosuria and in whom dietary modification fails.[41] Allopurinol has been proven to reduce urinary uric acid levels and prevent recurrent stone formation. In the sole double-blinded, placebo-controlled study involving 29 calcium oxalate stone formers receiving allopurinol for 3 years, 51% had fewer recurrences than those treated with placebo.[42] A dosage of 100–300 mg/day is generally well tolerated, and the side effects are limited to irreversible liver enzyme elevation and skin rash. Monitoring uric acid levels as well as renal and hepatic function is recommended.

56.3.4 Orthophosphates

Orthophosphates have been shown to inhibit 1,25-dihydroxyvitamin D synthesis and are believed to reduce urinary calcium by directly impairing the renal tubular absorption of calcium and by binding calcium in the intestinal tract. Urinary phosphorus is markedly increased during treatment, a finding that reflects the absorbability of soluble phosphate. It is important to note that although orthophosphate reduces the urine saturation of calcium oxalate, it increases the urine saturation of brushite. Orthophosphates are typically prescribed for patients with absorptive hypercalciuria type 3. They are contraindicated in nephrolithiasis complicated by urinary tract infection because of the increased phosphorus load.

Orthophosphates are typically composed of a neutral or alkaline salt of sodium or potassium and a phosphorus component. They are associated with a high instance of gastrointestinal discomfort, which limits its efficacy. Newer slow release, neutral potassium phosphate formulas have been developed to limit this side effect. In addition, potassium avoids the use of sodium, which can offset the hypocalciuric action of the orthophosphate. Finally, this medication provides a lower pH than previously available orthophosphate preparations, making it less likely that crystallization of calcium phosphate may occur.

A randomized prospective double-blind trial was performed in 21 patients with documented stone formation and absorptive hypercalciuria type 1. Patients were randomized to either potassium phosphate or placebo. No significant side effects or increase in fasting serum potassium or phosphorus was seen in either group. Most importantly, potassium phosphate significantly reduced urinary calcium from 288 mg/day to 171 mg/day without altering oxalate excretion.[43]

56.4 Conclusions

Calcium stones are the most frequent type of kidney stone identified. The etiology of calcium stones is complex and multifactorial. Systematic identification of underlining metabolic abnormalities is essential in directing treatment protocols for these patients. Dietary modifications with or without pharmacologic regimens are extremely effective and safe for calcium stone formers.

References

1. Stamatelou KK, Francis ME, Jones CA, et al. Time trends in reported prevalence of kidney stones in the United States: 1976–1994. *Kidney Int.* 2003;63:1817-1823.
2. Johnson CM, Wilson DM, O'Fallon WM, et al. Renal stone epidemiology: a 25 year study in Rochester, MN. *Kidney Int.* 1979;16: 624-631.
3. Lotan Y, Pearle MS. Economics of stone management. *Urol Clin N Am.* 2007;34:1-13.
4. Clark JY, Thompson IM, Optenberg SA. Economic impact of urolithiasis in the United States. *J Urol.* 1995;154:2020-2024.
5. Park S, Pearle MS. Pathophysiology and management of calcium stones. *Urol Clin N Am.* 2007;31:323-334.
6. Pak CY. Etiology and treatment of urolithiasis. *Am J Kidney Dis.* 1991;18:624-637.
7. Curhan GC, Willett WC, Rimm EB, et al. A prospective study of dietary calcium and other nutrients and the risk of symptomatic kidney stones. *N Engl J Med.* 1993;328:833-838.
8. Curhan GC, Willett WC, Speizer FE, et al. Comparison of dietary calcium with supplemental calcium and other nutrients as factors affecting the risk for kidney stones in women. *Ann Intern Med.* 1997;126:497-504.
9. Borghi L, Meschi T, Amato F, et al. Urinary volume, water and recurrences in idiopathic calcium nephrolithiasis: a 5-year randomized prospective study. *J Urol.* 1996;143:240-247.
10. Strauss AL, Coe FL, Deutsch L, Parks JH. Factors that predict relapse of calcium nephrolithiasis during treatment: a prospective study. *Am J Med.* 1982;72:17-24.
11. Wein A. *Campbell's Urology.* Philadelphia: Elsevier; 2008:1411.
12. Seltzer MA, Low RK, McDonald M, et al. Dietary manipulation with lemonade to treat hypocitraturic calcium nephrolithiasis. *J Urol.* 1996;156:907-909.
13. Penniston KL, Steele TH, Nakada SY. Lemonade therapy increases urinary citrate and urine volumes in patients with recurrent calcium oxalate stone formation. *Urology.* 2007;70:856-860.
14. Odvina CV. Comparative value of orange juice versus lemonade in reducing stone-forming risk. *Clin J Am Soc Nephrol.* 2006;1: 1269-1274.
15. Curhan GC, Willett WC, Rimm EB, et al. Prospective study of beverage use and the risk of kidney stone. *Am J Epidemiol.* 1996;143:240-247.

16. Massey LK, Sutton RA. Acute caffeine effects on urine composition and calcium kidney stone risk in calcium stone formers. *J Urol.* 2004;172:555-558.

17. Stoller ML, Rubenstein JN. Rethinking urolithiasis. *J Urol.* 2005;173:1452.

18. Sakhaee K, Harvey JA, Padalino PK, et al. The potential role of salt abuse on the risk for kidney stone formation. *J Urol.* 1993; 150(pt 1):310-312.

19. Remer T, Manz F. Potential renal acid load of foods and its influence on urine pH. *J Am Diet Assoc.* 1995;95:791-797.

20. Penniston KL, Nakada SY. Preventive management of recurrent urolithiasis: medical and dietary approaches. *Sem Prev Alt Med.* 2007;3:67-73.

21. Borghi L, Schianchi T, Meschi T, et al. Comparison of two diets for the prevention of recurrent stones in idiopathic hypercalciuria. *N Engl J Med.* 2002;346:77-84.

22. Seiner R, Schade N, Nicolay C, et al. The efficacy of dietary intervention on urinary risk factors for stone formation in recurrent calcium oxalate stone patients. *J Urol.* 2005;173:1601-1605.

23. Meschi T, Maggiore U, Fiaccadori E, et al. The effect of fruits and vegetables on urinary stone risk factors. *Kidney Int.* 2004;66: 2402-2410.

24. Pak CY, Heller HJ, Pearle MS, et al. Prevention of stone formation and bone loss in absorptive hypercalciuria by combined dietary and pharmacological interventions. *J Urol.* 2003;169:465-469.

25. Domrongkitchaiporn S, Ongphiphadhanakul B, Stitchantrakul W, et al. Risk of calcium oxalate nephrolithiasis in postmenopausal women supplemented with calcium or combined calcium and estrogen. *Maturitas.* 2002;41:149-156.

26. Domrongkitchaiporn S, Sopassathit W, Stitchantrakul W, et al. Schedule of taking calcium supplement and the risk of nephrolithiasis. *Kidney Int.* 2004;65:1835-1841.

27. Sakhaee K, Poindexter JR, Griffith CS, Pak CY. Stone forming risk of calcium citrate supplementation in healthy postmenopausal women. *J Urol.* 2004;172:958-961.

28. Penniston KL, Nakada SY, Hansen KE. Vitamin D repletion does not alter urinary calcium excretion in postmenopausal women. AUA, Abstract 2008.

29. Holmes RP, Assimos DG. The impact of dietary oxalate on kidney stone formation. *Urol Res.* 2004;32:311-316.

30. Krishnamurthy MS, Hruska KA, Chandhoke PS. The urinary response to an oral oxalate load in recurrent calcium stone formers. *J Urol.* 2003;169:2030-2033.

31. Taylor EN, Stampfer MJ, Curhan GC. Dietary factors and the risk of incident kidney stones in men: new insights after 14 years of follow-up. *J Am Soc Nephrol.* 2004;15:3225-3232.

32. Massey LK, Liebman M, Kynast-Gales SA. Ascorbate increases human oxaluria and kidney stone risk. *J Nutr.* 2005;135:1673-1677.

33. Borghi L, Meschi T, Guerra A, et al. Randomized prospective study of a nonthiazide diuretic, indapamide, in preventing calcium stone recurrences. *J Cardiovasc Pharmacol.* 1993;22:S78-S86.

34. Grobbee DE, Hoes AW. Non potassium sparing diuretics and risk of sudden cardiac death. *J Hypertens.* 1995;13:1539-1545.

35. Ohkawa M, Tokunaga S, Nakashima T, et al. Thiazide treatment for calcium urolithiasis in patients with idiopathic hypercalciuria. *Br J Urol.* 1992;69:571-576.

36. Ettinger B, Citron JT, Livermore B, et al. Chlorthalidone reduces calcium oxalate calculous recurrence but magnesium hydroxide does not. *J Urol.* 1988;139:679-684.

37. Laerum E, Larsen S. Thiazide prophylaxis of urolithiasis. A double-blind study in general practice. *Acta Med Scand.* 1984;215: 383-389.

38. Pearle MS, Roehrborn CG, Pak CY. Meta-analysis of randomized trials for medical prevention of calcium oxalate nephrolithiasis. *J Endourol.* 1999;13:679-685.

39. Barcelo P, Wuhl O, Servitge E, et al. Randomized double-blind study of potassium citrate in idiopathic hypocitraturic calcium nephrolithiasis. *J Urol.* 1993;150:1761-1764.

40. Pak CY, Peterson R. Successful treatment of hyperuricosuric calcium oxalate nephrolithiasis with potassium citrate. *Arch Intern Med.* 1986;146(5):863-867.

41. Ettinger B. Hyperuricosuria and calcium oxalate lithiasis: a critical review and future outlook. In: Borghi L, Meschi T, Briganti A, Schianchi T, Novarini A, eds. *Kidney Stones.* Parma, Italy: Editoriale Bios; 1999:51-57.

42. Ettinger B, Tang A, Citron JT, et al. Randomized trial of allopurinol in the prevention of calcium oxalate calculi. *N Engl J Med.* 1986;315:1386-1389.

43. Breslau NA, Heller HJ, Reza-Albarran AA, et al. Physiological effects of slow release potassium phosphate for absorptive hypercalciuria: a randomized double-blind trial. *J Urol.* 1998;160:664-668.

Medical Management: Uric Acid and Cystine Stones

57

Khashayar Sakhaee

Abstract The main metabolic abnormality for uric acid stone formation is abnormally acidic urine (urinary pH < 5.5). The most important modalities of treatment in this condition include urinary alkalization to maintain a urinary pH between 6.0 and 6.5 and high fluid intake to ensure urine output above 2 L/day. Potassium alkali is the preferred treatment over sodium alkali treatment since it is effective in raising urinary pH, lowering urinary calcium excretion, and inhibiting sodium urate–induced calcium oxalate crystallizations. Cystinuria is an inherited disorder of dibasic amino acid transport, which clinically presents nephrolithiasis or bladder stones. Physicochemically, cystine has limited solubility in the urinary environment. Therefore, its precipitation solely depends on urinary cystine supersaturation. The early diagnosis of cystinuria is significant as early prevention and treatment measures may provide protection against renal function impairment. Prevention and treatment include the provision of high fluid intake and urine alkalinity in order to exceed a urinary cystine solubility threshold of 250 mg/L (1,000 μ[micro]mol/L). Specific treatment regimens are limited and only include chelation treatment with D-penicillamine or α(alpha)-mercaptopropionylglycine. These treatment regimens are usually effective, but a number of them confer side effects.

57.1 Introduction

It is well established that unduly acidic urine plays a major role in uric acid (UA) crystal deposition and stone formation. It has also become increasingly recognized that UA stones are accompanied by a cluster of features associated with the metabolic syndrome. Until now, the major effort in the treatment of this condition has been targeted at the correction of high urinary pH with alkalinizing agents. This treatment has been significantly effective in the reduction of UA stone incidence. With the recent advances in our understanding of the pathophysiologic basis of this disease, it is plausible to anticipate the development of novel drugs that not only correct urinary acidity but also reverse various features of the metabolic syndrome.

Cystinuria is an autosomal recessive disorder, which is caused by the defective transport of cystine and other dibasic amino acids in the kidney and intestine. This renal transport abnormality leads to the excessive excretion of poorly soluble cystine into the urine, which ultimately leads to cystine stone formation. These stones have been found to be present in both pediatric and adult populations, and may manifest as either kidney or bladder stones. However, the latter is more frequently encountered in childhood. The objective of treatment for this condition includes hydration and alkalinization in order to increase urinary cystine solubility. Pharmacological treatment may only be used if conventional treatment is insufficient.

57.2 Uric Acid

57.2.1 Clinical Presentation

UA stones may present as either pure UA or mixed UA and calcium oxalate.[1] With the exception of a few specific genetic mutations in UA metabolism which increase the risk of significant hyperuricemia (serum UA > 10 mg/dL), hyperuricosuria (urinary UA concentration > 1,000 mg/day), renal failure, and severe gout,[2] UA nephrolithiasis typically only affects adults. However, with increasing incidence of

K. Sakhaee
Department of Internal Medicine, University of Texas Southwestern Medical Center, Dallas, TX, USA
e-mail: khashayar.sakhaee@utsouthwestern.edu

obesity and diabetes, there has recently been a report of UA stones in pediatric populations.[3] Hyperglycemia, glucose intolerance, hypertension, dyslipidemia, hyperuricemia, and obesity are all factors associated with UA stones.[1]

57.2.2 Diagnosis

If available, the diagnosis of UA nephrolithiasis must first be confirmed by a stone analysis to document the presence of pure UA or mixed UA and calcium oxalate stones. The second step involves a complete metabolic evaluation to exclude the possibility of secondary influences.[4] Since stone analysis in the majority of instances may not be obtainable, physicians must then rely on full blood and 24-h urine profiles. The 24-h urinary profile should consist of the measurement of total volume, pH, creatinine, sodium, potassium, calcium, magnesium, oxalate, citrate, sulfate, and chloride. This full panel is required to segregate the endogenous metabolic abnormalities from environmental influences such as excessive protein intake. Urinary sulfate is a surrogate marker of acid ash consumption found in animal protein. In some instances, urinary urea is also used as a marker of protein ingestion. Computerized tomography (CT) examination is important since radiolucent uric acid stones can be readily shown with this technique.

57.2.3 Differential Diagnosis

In addition to UA stones, xanthine and 2,8-dihydroxyadenine (2,8-DHA) stones are radiolucent. Therefore, stone analysis is essential to differentiate these stones from UA stones. Xanthine stones are usually found in inherited UA pathway disorders, including Lesch–Nyhan Syndrome or in hereditary xanthinuria.[2] This stone may also occur infrequently in patients on allopurinol treatment. 2,8-DHA stones are seen in patients with adinine phosphoribosyl transferase deficiencies.[3,5] One important differential diagnosis, which is usually ignored by practicing physicians, is the differentiation between hyperuricosuric calcium oxalate nephrolithiasis and UA stones.[6,7] Urinary pH and urinary uric acid can be used to discern between these two conditions. Hyperuricosuria and urinary pH >5.5 are typically encountered in the former condition,[7] while acidic urine pH ≤ 5.5 is predominantly encountered in UA stone formers[1] (Table 57.1).

57.2.4 Treatment

57.2.4.1 Lifestyle Modifications

Similar to other kidney stone diseases, patients with UA stones must rigidly adhere to various lifestyle modifications. These measures include the administration of sufficient fluid intake in order to attain approximately 2 L of urine per day. One important factor in fluid repletion includes the consideration of extrarenal losses caused by hot environments and from strenuous physical exercise.[8] Dietary protein restrictions must be encouraged, and 24-h urinary sulfate measurements may be used to assess patient compliance. Generally, values less than 20–25 mmol/day are suggestive of low animal protein consumption. The recommended daily dietary protein allowance is 0.8 g/kg. To date, it remains unknown whether various other sources of dietary protein influence urinary pH and urinary UA.

57.2.4.2 Specific Pharmacological Treatment

Since urinary pH plays a key role in UA solubility, alkali treatment is essential in the treatment of this population.[9–11] It has been shown that potassium alkali treatment is preferred in the prevention of stone recurrence in these subjects.[9,10] Potassium alkali has also been shown to lower urinary calcium excretion, reducing the risk of calcium oxalate as well as UA stone formation. Sodium alkali must be used in those subjects with impaired renal function or gastrointestinal (GI) intolerance to potassium salt. The size of the patient usually dictates the

Table 57.1 Differential diagnosis of UA stones

Stone type	Radiographic findings	Urinary findings				Serum UA findings	Response to alkali therapy
		pH	UA	FE uric acid	Calcium		
UA stones	Radiolucent	Decreased	Normal	Decreased	Normal	Increased	Positive
Mixed UA/ calcium oxalate stones	Mixed radiolucent and radioopaque	Normal to decreased	Normal to increased	Normal to decreased	Normal to increased	Normal to increased	Positive
Hyperuricosuric calcium stones	Radioopaque	Normal	Increased	Normal	Normal	Normal	Positive
Xanthine stones	Radiolucent	Normal	Increased to normal	Normal	Normal	Decreased	Negative
2,8-DHA stones	Radiolucent	Normal	Normal	Normal	Normal	Normal	Negative

UA uric acid, *FE* fractional excretion

daily dosage of alkali treatment. Generally, 30–60 mEq of alkali is sufficient in raising urinary pH. It is crucial to monitor urinary pH at an interval of 6–12 months and maintain a urinary pH between 6.1 and 6.7 in order to avoid the complication of calcium phosphate stone formation.[12] In some instances, if alkalinization with sodium and/or potassium salts is not feasible, carbonic anhydrase inhibitor (Diamox®) may be used as an alternative agent. However, this drug can be complicated by the development of systemic metabolic acidosis, hypocitrituria, and highly alkaline urine. This may predispose the patient to calcium oxalate stone formation.[13–15] Hyperuricosuria in females (>600–700 mg/day) and in males (>700–800 mg/day) must be treated with allopurinol.

Hyperuricosuria is not commonly detected in patients with idiopathic UA nephrolithiasis. However, it is commonly encountered in patients with primary gout, in those with an inborn error in UA metabolism, and in patients in a state of high tissue turnover. Although the side effects of allopurinol treatment are minimal, it should not be used in patients with impaired kidney function or renal insufficiency. Typically, the dosage required is 300 mg/day. At this time, there is no alternate agent available to substitute for allopurinol. In preliminary studies, one possible agent, Febuxostat, has been shown to be effective in lowering serum urate concentrations and limit gouty attacks,[16] but it's effectiveness in hyperuricosuric calcium nephrolithiasis has not been demonstrated. Lastly, one may use rasburicase, a recombinant uricase, to convert UA to soluble allantoin and lower UA excretion. However, due to its serious side effects, the use of this agent is limited to patients with malignancies or in a high state of UA turnover (Table 57.2).

57.3 Cystine

57.3.1 Clinical Presentation

Cystine stones may affect both pediatric and adult populations, with over two-third of patients developing their first kidney stone within the first 2 decades of life.[17,18] Occurrence in infancy and in the elderly is infrequent. This stone may affect the kidney; however, the presence of bladder stones in children is suggestive of the presence of cystine stones. Although cystine stones affect both genders, male subjects display a more severe course with significant kidney stone burden.[18] More than half of cystinuric patients develop cystine stones during their lifetime. The course of this disease is aggressive with a high recurrence rate of approximately 60%, which usually leads to progressive renal function impairment.[19] Due to the high recurrence rate, these subjects are exposed to many invasive and noninvasive interventions.[20,21]

The most common clinical manifestations include gross hematuria, renal colic with or without stone passage, urinary tract infections, and back pain.[22,23] Hypertension also occurs frequently in cystinuric patients. Additionally, there has been a report on the rare association between hemophilia, retinitis pigmentosa, muscular dystrophy, mongolism, and hereditary pancreatitis.[24] The association between Wilson's disease and Faconi syndrome has also been reported with cystinuria.[25] In addition, mental disorders have been reported in cystinuric patients; however, the association to amino acid transport defects has not been experimentally supported.[26] Other physiologic abnormalities, including hypercalciuria, hyperuricosuria, and hypocitrituria, have been seen in cystinuric populations.[27] These abnormalities may likely be responsible for the occurrence of mixed calcium and cystine stones.[28] Hyperuricemia and UA stones have been seen in association with cystine stones.[29]

57.3.2 Diagnosis

The presumptive diagnosis of cystinuria should initially be based on its unique clinical presentation. This may include the occurrence of kidney stones during early childhood associated with a positive family history of kidney stone disease, and its recurrent course. This important step must be followed by a microscopic qualitative evaluation of fresh, first-voided urine for the presence of flat-hexagonal cystine crystals (benzene ring). In order to increase the

Table 57.2 A comparison of various treatments

Treatment type	Urine pH	Urinary citrate	Urinary uric acid	Undissociated uric acid	Urinary calcium	RSR calcium oxalate	Calcium stones
Potassium alkali	↑	↑	↔	↓	↓	↔	↓
Sodium alkali	↑	↑	↔	↓	↓	↑	↑
Diamox®	↑	↓	↔	↓	↑	↑	↑
Allopurinol	↔	↔	↓	↔	↔	↓	↓

↑ = Increased

↔ = No change

↓ = Decreased

RSR = Relative supersaturation

yield, one may incubate and refrigerate the urine overnight with glacial acetic acid at a pH of 4.0 to avoid urinary alkalinity, which is known to dissolve cystine crystals. In some instances, a qualitative cyanide-nitroprusside test may be performed on the urine.[30] The appearance of a purple-red color is suggestive of cystine excretion in excess of 75 mg/L. Although this test is sensitive, it is nonspecific, and the presence of homocystine and ketone in the urine may cause a false-positive result. At the present time, this test is not popular among practicing physicians.

Stone analyses to establish the presence of cystine is also an important step to diagnosis in this population. Cystine stones on kidneys-ureter-bladder (KUB) radiologic examination are typically radioopaque since the densities of sulfur and calcium are similar.[28] However, cystine stones are more rounded and homogenous in appearance. Occasionally, cystine stones are large and may attain a staghorn size. Other imaging techniques such as ultrasonography and CT examination have been used for the acute diagnosis of obstructive cystine stones.

The presumptive diagnosis should be followed by a quantitative cystine measurement to concretely establish this diagnosis. Ion exchange chromatography can reliably detect and quantify even small amounts of various amino acids, including cystine, in the urine.[31] Urinary cystine excretion exceeding 250 mg/g Cr usually indicates the diagnosis of homozygous cystinuria (Fig. 57.1).

57.3.3 Physicochemistry of Cystine

It is well known that cystine solubility is pH dependant[32] and increases with urinary alkalinity. At a urinary pH of 7.0, the cystine solubility is 250 mg/L (1 mmol/L). This solubility increases to 500 mg/L (2 mmol/L) at a pH of 7.5. Traditionally, the solubility curve described by Dent et al. is widely used in the estimation of urinary cystine saturation (Fig. 57.2). However, it has been shown that urinary cystine solubility is not as predictable. This is largely due to the complex urinary composition that is comprised of various electrolytes that are known to change the ionic strength of whole urine specimens.[33] Urinary supersaturation with respect to cystine is the measured determinant of cystine crystallization. To date, there is no reported specific promoter or inhibitor playing a role in this process. The solubility limit of 250 mg/g Cr (1 mmol/L) is usually exceeded in homozygous cystinuric subjects who excrete between 600 and 1,400 mg/day (2.5–5.8 mmol/day). Although mixed stones have also been reported in association with cystine stones,[28] cystine does not play any role in the heterogenous nucleation of calcium oxalate, brushite, or hydroxyapatite crystals.[33]

Diagnosis of cystine stones

Clinical presentation:

- Kidney stones during early childhood
- Positive family history
- Recurrent course

Qualitative evaluation:

- Flat-hexagonal cystine crystals in urine
- Purple-red cyanide- nitroprocide test
- Stone analysis

Quantitative analysis:

- Ion exchange chromatography
- Cystine excretion exceeding 250 mg/g Cr

Fig. 57.1 Diagnosis of cystine stones

57.3.4 Treatment

57.3.4.1 Lifestyle Modifications

The treatment of cystine stones must be aimed at reducing urinary cystine concentration and lowering urinary cystine excretion. This goal may first be attained by increasing fluid intake, a conservative measure that targets lowering cystine concentrations. Decreased cystine excretion may also be attained through dietary protein restrictions, which lower substrates for cystine synthesis (Table 57.3).

A high fluid intake plays a key role in the urinary undersaturation of cystine. This may be attained by drinking 3 L of fluid in children and 4–5 L of fluid in adults. Fluid intake should be homogenously distributed throughout the day, and the patient must be instructed to drink at bedtime in order to maintain consistent urinary dilution.[34,35] Almost all fluids are useful for this purpose. However, one should avoid drinking milk, which may increase urinary cystine excretion due to its high methionine content. Fruit juices are generally useful because they not only provide urinary dilution but also increase urinary pH due to their alkali content. Usually, two glasses of orange juice increase urinary pH by 0.5 units.[36]

A low protein diet has been recommended to lower urinary cystine excretion. This may be attained by restricting meat and meat products, which contain methionine, a principal substrate responsible for cystine production.[37] One obstacle is that such dietary restrictions may be met with poor patient compliance in adult patients.[36] Moreover, restricted protein intake is not recommended in pediatric populations.[25] In addition, sodium intake may also affect urinary cystine excretion.[38] It has been shown that a decline in dietary sodium intake of 150 mEq/day may reduce urinary cystine by 156 mg/day (650 mmol/day).[38] Salt restrictions are also useful in lowering the urinary cystine excretion in pediatric populations.[39]

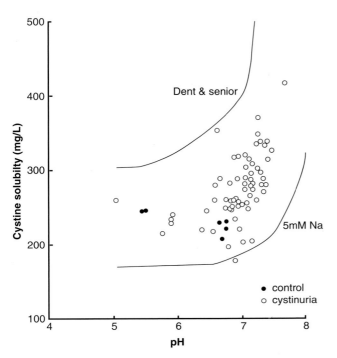

Assessment of urinary cystine solubility

Fig. 57.2 Assessment of urinary cystine solubility (Reprinted from Pak and Fuller[33]. With permission of Elsevier)

57.3.5 Specific Pharmacological Treatment

57.3.5.1 Oral Alkali Treatment

Following the original work by Dent et al.,[32] which reported that cystine solubility is pH dependant, oral alkali treatment has been widely used in the treatment of cystinuric subjects. However, due to cystine's high pKa of 8.5, a large dose of alkali is necessary to achieve optimal solubility. The attainment of a urinary pH exceeding 7.5 is very difficult in clinical practice, mainly due to poor patient compliance to such high doses of alkali. More significantly, there is a risk of urinary monohydrogen phosphate saturation coupled with an increased risk of calcium phosphate stone formation.[40] Due to these limitations, the main objective is maintaining a urinary pH between 6.5 and 7.0. Both sodium and potassium alkali have been shown to be equally effective in raising urinary pH. However, increasing sodium intake poses the risk of increasing urinary cystine excretion.[38] Therefore, the preferred alkali treatment is potassium citrate. The starting dose for adults is 15–20 mEq twice a day, and the dosage must be incrementally adjusted to attain optimal urinary pH (Table 57.3).

Table 57.3 Treatment of cystine stones

Treatment type	Mechanism of action	Indication	Side effects
Fluid	Reduces urinary cystine concentrations	All cystinuric (urinary cystine >250 mg/day)	None
Diet (low salt and low protein)	Limits substrate for cystine production and reduces cystine excretion	Limited owing to poor dietary compliance	Reduces cystine solubility owing to solvent action
Oral alkali	Increases cystine solubility	All cystinuric (urinary cystine >250 mg/day)	Urinary pH >7.5 increases the risk of calcium phosphate stones
First-generation chelating agents (D-penicillamine)	Thiol-disulfide exchange with cystine	Severe cystinuria (>500 mg/day) and moderate cystinuria (250–500 mg/day) when fluid and alkali are ineffective	Dermatologic, hematologic, and renal side effects
Second-generation chelating agents (Thiola)	Thiol-disulfide exchange with cystine	Severe cystinuria (>500 mg/day) and moderate cystinuria (250–500 mg/day) when fluid and alkali are ineffective	Less frequent dermatologic, hematologic, and renal side effects
Captopril	Thiol-disulfide exchange with cystine	Controversial	Unproven effectiveness
Glutamine	Reduces cystine excretion by competitive inhibition	Controversial, may be useful with high sodium intake	High sodium intake increases urinary cystine
Ascorbic acid	Reduction of cystine to cysteine	Adolescents and adults with homozygous cystinuria	Increased risk of calcium oxalate stones

57.3.5.2 Chelating Agents

Chelating agents such as D-penicillamine (di-methyl cysteine) and α(alpha)-mercaptopropionylglycine must be used in subjects who are nonresponsive to conservative management or urinary alkalization and in those with severe cystinuria (>500 mg/day). Both of these agents are thiol derivatives, which cleave a single cystine molecule into two cysteine molecules to make a highly soluble disulfide compound consisting of the respective drug and cysteine molecules. Such a reaction lowers the excretion of sparingly soluble cystine.[41,42]

Originating approximately 4 decades ago, D-penicillamine was the first chelating agent found to lower urinary cystine excretion in complicated cystinuric subjects.[42] In 1977, it was further shown that new stone recurrence, stone passage, and stone growth were significantly lowered when D-penicillamine was added to a conservative treatment.[23] The results of these studies were later confirmed during the long-term follow-up of 62 cystinuric patients. During this follow-up, it was shown that chelating treatment with D-penicillamine significantly decreased stone episodes from 1.2 episodes per patient per year before treatment to 0.22 episodes per patient per year following the treatment[43] (Table 57.3).

Despite its clinical efficacy, D-penicillamine treatment is known to be accompanied by various dermatological (pemiphigus), hematologic (agranulocytosis, thrombocytopenia), renal (nephritic syndrome), and rheumatological (polymyocitis) complications.[44] The dosage of this medication must be adjusted to reduce the urinary cystine concentration below its solubility limit (<250 mg/L). Generally, the dosage of approximately 1,000 mg/day reduces the urinary cystine excretion by 360 mg/day.[45] It has also been shown that each incremental dosage of 250 mg/day of D-penicillamine decreases urinary cystine by 75–100 mg/day.[36] The recommended dosage for children is 20–40 mg/kg/day.[35] This drug should preferably be administered in divided dosages before meals to allow for its optimal intestinal absorption. It has been suggested that cystine excretion is higher at night; therefore, it is preferable to administer one dose at bedtime.[35] In instances in which complications to the drug ensue, one may select an incremental dosage of this treatment over 3-day intervals starting with a low dose of 10–20 mg/day with a gradual increase over a 1-month period until the optimal dosage is attained. Since a vitamin B6 deficiency may occur with D-penicillamine, vitamin B6 supplementation at the dosage of 50 mg/day is beneficial.

Alpha(α)-mercaptopropionylglycine (Thiola®) is a useful substitute for D-penicillamine in the treatment of cystinuric patients. In various clinical studies, it has been shown that both drugs are equally effective in reducing kidney stone incidence. However, at the present time, α(alpha)-mercaptop ropionylglycine is the preferred drug among practicing physicians since it presents lower incidences of side effects.[43,45] The mechanism of action of this drug is similar to that of D-penicillamine. Upon the oral administration of this drug, it has been shown that one-fourth of the administered dose appeared unchanged in the urine. Mediated by a thiol-disulfide exchange mechanism, this participates due to the interaction with cystine, which leads to lowered urinary cystine excretion.[45] A previous long-term study has shown that Thiola is effective in causing stone remission and reducing the individual stone formation rates in patients with and without prior D-penicillamine treatment. In patients with stone relapse on D-penicillamine, Thiola was shown to significantly decreased new stone formation by 71%, and 61.5% of the patients remained in remission. Side effects – including skin reactions, oral ulcers, and GI intolerance – were shown to be frequent with Thiola treatment. However, only 43% of cystinuric patients displayed multiple adverse reactions to this drug compared to a distinctly higher number of patients (67%) on D-penicillamine[45] (Table 57.3).

Subsequently, two independent studies also supported these findings. One study in a total of 27 adult patients with cystine stones reported a significant decrease in stone episodes and urological procedures when thiol drugs (D-penicillamine and Thiola) were added to conservative management, including hydration and alkali treatment.[46] Moreover, a study conducted on 16 patients with cystinuria, who were followed for 7–141 months, showed the stone event per patient-year decreased significantly from 1.58 to 0.52 when D-penicillamine or Thiola was added to those patients who were nonresponsive to conservative management. This finding suggests a 65% decrease in yearly stone event rate during thiol treatment compared to conservative management.[47] The recommended dosage for thiol treatment ranges between 400 and 1,200 mg/day.

As a third-generation cheating agent, bucillamine (Rimatil®) was assumed to be more effective in reducing urinary cystine excretion than D-penicillamine and α(alpha)-mercaptopropionylglycine due to its possession of dithiol components.[22] However, this effectiveness was not verified in phase-II clinical trials despite its initial success. In addition, captopril (Capoten®) is an angiotensin-converting enzyme inhibitor, which is commonly used in the treatment of hypertension. This agent also possesses a thiol component, which has been suggested to form a thiol-cysteine mixed disulfide and reduces urinary cystine excretion.[48] In an initial report, a dose of 75–100 mg/day of captopril was shown to significantly reduce urinary cystine excretion.[49] However, the result of this study was not further verified by other investigators.[46,50] The lack of efficacy of captopril treatment was an expected finding considering that 2 mol captopril is required to bind 1 mol of cystine. Therefore, a sufficient amount of captopril could not be safely administered to adequately lower urinary cystine excretion.

57.3.6 Other Pharmacological Treatments

Ascorbic acid has been suggested to be useful in the treatment of cystinuria and was first tested in a pediatric population.[51] When used at high dosages, this agent is known to convert cystine to cysteine. The recommended doses are 3 g/day for children and 5 g/day for adults.[52] The European Association of Urology recommends this treatment for patients with elevated urinary cystine excretion. However, it has been argued that the efficacy of this treatment is due to the provision of alkali from the effervescent ascorbic acid tablet containing bicarbonate.[53,54] Additionally, excessive ascorbic acid ingestion may increase the risk of calcium oxalate stone formation since this acid is one of the major precursors of oxalate formation.[55]

When given to cystinuric patients, oral and intravenous glutamine were shown to lower urinary cystine excretion. This action was suggested to be a result of increased renal tubular cystine reabsorption or reduced renal tubular cystine secretion.[56] However, the result of this study also remained unverified by other investigators[57] and the efficacy of this drug remains unclear since its effectiveness is sustained by high sodium consumption[38] (Table 57.3).

57.4 Conclusions

Lifestyle modifications are important but not sufficient for the effective management of both recurrent UA and cystine stone formation. The primary abnormality responsible for UA stone formation is unduly acidic urine as a result of defective urinary ammonium excretion. Treatment with potassium alkali has been used successfully to correct this abnormality and lower stone incidence. The high recurrence and associated morbidity rates of cystine stones substantiate the use of pharmacological agents to lower urinary cystine excretion. Thiol compounds such as D-penicillamine and α(alpha)-mercaptopropionylglycine confe similar biological activity and are known to significantly lower stone incidence. However, due to serious side effects, patient compliance remains low with both of these agents. Future direction in the management of these conditions should be targeted at the development of novel therapeutic agents that correct the underlying pathophysiologic and molecular genetic basis of these disorders.

Acknowledgment The author would like to acknowledge the editorial support of Ms. Hadley Armstrong.

The author was supported by the National Institutes of Health Grant R01-DK081423–01A1.

References

1. Sakhaee K, Adams-Huet B, Moe OW, Pak CY. Pathophysiologic basis for normouricosuric uric acid nephrolithiasis. *Kidney Int.* 2002;62(3):971-979.
2. Moe OW, Abate N, Sakhaee K. Pathophysiology of uric acid nephrolithiasis. *Endocrinol Metab Clin N Am.* 2002;31(4):895-914.
3. Cameron JS, Moro F, Simmonds HA. Gout, uric acid and purine metabolism in paediatric nephrology. *Pediatr Nephrol.* 1993;7(1):105-118.
4. Cameron MA, Pak CY. Approach to the patient with the first episode of nephrolithiasis. *Clin Rev Bone Miner Metab.* 2004;2: 265-278.
5. Riese RJ, Sakhaee K. Uric acid nephrolithiasis: pathogenesis and treatment. *J Urol.* 1992;148(3):765-771.
6. Sorensen CM, Chandhoke PS. Hyperuricosuric calcium nephrolithiasis. *Endocrinol Metab Clin N Am.* 2002;31(4):915-925.
7. Pak CY, Poindexter JR, Peterson RD, Koska J, Sakhaee K. Biochemical distinction between hyperuricosuric calcium urolithiasis and gouty diathesis. *Urology.* 2002;60(5):789-794.
8. Sakhaee K, Nigam S, Snell P, Hsu MC, Pak CY. Assessment of the pathogenetic role of physical exercise in renal stone formation. *J Clin Endocrinol Metab.* 1987;65(5):974-979.
9. Sakhaee K, Nicar M, Hill K, Pak CY. Contrasting effects of potassium citrate and sodium citrate therapies on urinary chemistries and crystallization of stone-forming salts. *Kidney Int.* 1983; 24(3):348-352.
10. Pak CY, Sakhaee K, Fuller C. Successful management of uric acid nephrolithiasis with potassium citrate. *Kidney Int.* 1986;30(3): 422-428.
11. Freed SZ. The alternating use of an alkalizing salt and acetazolamide in the management of cystine and uric acid stones. *J Urol.* 1975;113(1):96-99.
12. Coe FL, Evan A, Worcester E. Kidney stone disease. *J Clin Invest.* 2005;115(10):2598-2608.
13. Gordon EE, Sheps SG. Effect of acetazolamide on citrate excretion and formation of renal calculi. *N Engl J Med.* 1957;256(26): 1215-1219.
14. Lamb EJ, Stevens PE, Nashef L. Topiramate increases biochemical risk of nephrolithiasis. *Ann Clin Biochem.* 2004;41(Pt 2):166-169.
15. Kuo RL, Moran ME, Kim DH, Abrahams HM, White MD, Lingeman JE. Topiramate-induced nephrolithiasis. *J Endourol.* 2002;16(4):229-231.
16. Becker MA, Schumacher HR Jr, Wortmann RL, et al. Febuxostat compared with allopurinol in patients with hyperuricemia and gout. *N Engl J Med.* 2005;353(23):2450-2461.
17. Leusmann DB, Blaschke R, Schmandt W. Results of 5, 035 stone analyses: a contribution to epidemiology of urinary stone disease. *Scand J Urol Nephrol.* 1990;24(3):205-210.
18. Dello SL, Pras E, Pontesilli C, et al. Comparison between SLC3A1 and SLC7A9 cystinuria patients and carriers: a need for a new classification. *J Am Soc Nephrol.* 2002;13(10):2547-2553.
19. Gambaro G, Favaro S, D'Angelo A. Risk for renal failure in nephrolithiasis. *Am J Kidney Dis.* 2001;37(2):233-243.
20. Pras E. Cystinuria at the turn of the millennium: clinical aspects and new molecular developments. *Mol Urol.* 2000;4(4): 409-414.
21. Pierides AM. Clinical aspects of cystinuria. *Contrib Nephrol.* 1997;122:167-172.
22. Sakhaee K. Pathogenesis and medical management of cystinuria. *Semin Nephrol.* 1996;16(5):435-447.

23. Dahlberg PJ, Van den Berg CJ, Kurtz SB, Wilson DM, Smith LH. Clinical features and management of cystinuria. *Mayo Clin Proc.* 1977;52(9):533-542.

24. Their SO, Segal S. Cystinuria. In: Stanbury JB, Wyngaarden JB, Fredrickson DS, eds. *Metabolic Basis of Inherited Disease.* New York: McGraw Hill; 1972:1504-1519.

25. Sakhaee K, Sutton RAL. Pathogenesis and medical management of cystinuria. In: Coe FL, Favus MJ, Pak CY, Parks JH, Preminger G, eds. *Kidney Stones: Medical and Surgical Management.* Philadelphia: Lippincott-Raven; 1996:1007-1017.

26. Scriver CR, Whelan DT, Clow CL, Dallaire L. Cystinuria: increased prevalence in patients with mental disease. *N Engl J Med.* 1970;283(15):783-786.

27. Sakhaee K, Poindexter JR, Pak CY. The spectrum of metabolic abnormalities in patients with cystine nephrolithiasis. *J Urol.* 1989;141(4):819-821.

28. Their SO, Halperin EC. Cystinuria. In: Coe FL, ed. *Nephrolithiasis.* New York: Churchill Livingstone; 1980:208-230.

29. Vergis JG, Walker BR. Cystinuria, hyperuricemia and uric acid nephrolithiasis. Case report. *Nephron.* 1970;7(6):577-579.

30. Brand E, Harris MM, Biloon S. The excretion of a cystine complex which decomposes in the urine with the liberation of free cystine. *J Biol Chem.* 1930;86:315-331.

31. Spackman DH, Stein WH, Moore S. Automatic recording apparatus for use in chrmoatography of amino acids. *Annal Chem.* 1958;30(7):1190-1206.

32. Dent CE, Senior B. Studies on the treatment of cystinuria. *Br J Urol.* 1955;27(4):317-332.

33. Pak CY, Fuller CJ. Assessment of cystine solubility in urine and of heterogeneous nucleation. *J Urol.* 1983;129(5):1066-1070.

34. Monnens LA, Noordam K, Trijbels F. Necessary practical treatment of cystinuria at night. *Pediatr Nephrol.* 2000;14(12):1148-1149.

35. Fjellstedt E, Denneberg T, Jeppsson JO, Christensson A, Tiselius HG. Cystine analyses of separate day and night urine as a basis for the management of patients with homozygous cystinuria. *Urol Res.* 2001;29(5):303-310.

36. Pak CY. Cystine Lithiasis. In: Resnick LM, Pak CY, eds. *Urolithiasis: A Medical and Surgical Reference.* Philadelphia: W.B. Saunders; 1990:133-143.

37. Kolb FO, Earll JM, Harper HA. "Disappearance" of cystinuria in a patient treated with prolonged low methionine diet. *Metabolism.* 1967;16(4):378-381.

38. Jaeger P, Portmann L, Saunders A, Rosenberg LE, Thier SO. Anticystinuric effects of glutamine and of dietary sodium restriction. *N Engl J Med.* 1986;315(18):1120-1123.

39. Rodriguez LM, Santos F, Malaga S, Martinez V. Effect of a low sodium diet on urinary elimination of cystine in cystinuric children. *Nephron.* 1995;71(4):416-418.

40. Vega D, Maalouf NM, Sakhaee K. Increased propensity for calcium phosphate kidney stones with topiramate use. *Expert Opin Drug Safety.* 2007;6(5):547-557.

41. Lindell A, Denneberg T, Jeppsson JO. Urinary excretion of free cystine and the tiopronin-cysteine-mixed disulfide during long term tiopronin treatment of cystinuria. *Nephron.* 1995;71(3):328-342.

42. Crawhall JC, Scowen EF, Watts RW. Effect of penicillamine on cystinuria. *Br Med J.* 1963;1(5330):588-590.

43. Linari F, Marangella M, Fruttero B, Bruno M. The natural history of cystinuria. In: Smith LH, Robertson WG, Finlayson B, eds. *Urolithiasis: Clinical and Basic Research.* New York: Plenum; 1980:145-154.

44. Halperin EC, Thier SO, Rosenberg LE. The use of D-penicillamine in cystinuria: efficacy and untoward reactions. *Yale J Biol Med.* 1981;54(6):439-446.

45. Pak CY, Fuller C, Sakhaee K, Zerwekh JE, Adams BV. Management of cystine nephrolithiasis with alpha-mercaptopropionylglycine. *J Urol.* 1986;136(5):1003-1008.

46. Barbey F, Joly D, Rieu P, Mejean A, Daudon M, Jungers P. Medical treatment of cystinuria: critical reappraisal of long-term results. *J Urol.* 2000;163(5):1419-1423.

47. Chow GK, Streem SB. Medical treatment of cystinuria: results of contemporary clinical practice. *J Urol.* 1996;156(5):1576-1578.

48. Sloand JA, Izzo JL Jr. Captopril reduces urinary cystine excretion in cystinuria. *Arch Intern Med.* 1987;147(8):1409-1412.

49. Perazella MA, Buller GK. Successful treatment of cystinuria with captopril. *Am J Kidney Dis.* 1993;21(5):504-507.

50. Dahlberg PJ, Jones JD. Cystinuria: failure of captopril to reduce cystine excretion. *Arch Intern Med.* 1989;149(3):713-717.

51. Lux B, May P. Long-term observation of young cystinuric patients under ascorbic acid therapy. *Urol Int.* 1983;38(2):91-94.

52. Knoll T, Zollner A, Wendt-Nordahl G, Michel MS, Alken P. Cystinuria in childhood and adolescence: recommendations for diagnosis, treatment, and follow-up. *Pediatr Nephrol.* 2005;20(1):19-24.

53. Birwe H, Schneeberger W, Hesse A. Investigations of the efficacy of ascorbic acid therapy in cystinuria. *Urol Res.* 1991;19(3):199-201.

54. Ragone R. Medical treatment of cystinuria with vitamin C. *Am J Kidney Dis.* 2000;35(5):1020.

55. Traxer O, Huet B, Poindexter J, Pak CY, Pearle MS. Effect of ascorbic acid consumption on urinary stone risk factors. *J Urol.* 2003;170(2 Pt 1):397-401.

56. Miyagi K, Nakada F, Ohshiro S. Effect of glutamine on cystine excretion in a patient with cystinuria. *N Engl J Med.* 1979;301(4):196-198.

57. Van Den Berg CJ, Jones JD, Wilson DM, Smith L. Glutamine therapy of cystinuria. *Invest Urol.* 1980;18(2):155-157.

Medical Management of Struvite Stones

58

Tarık Esen and Tayfun Oktar

Abstract Struvite stones, which have also been referred to as "infection stones," are commonly encountered and constitute a significant group. The presence of urinary tract infection with a urease-producing organism is necessary for these stones to form. If left untreated, struvite calculi pose a significant risk to kidney and also to the patient's life. For this reason, the mainstay of treatment is complete removal of stones. Medical management is also an essential part of the treatment, especially due to the increased risk of recurrence. The aim of this chapter is to review the medical management options for struvite stones.

58.1 Introduction

Struvite stone is the earliest type of stone afflicting humans. Because of their strong association with urinary tract infections caused by urease positive bacteria, struvite calculi are also referred to as infection stones. These stones constitute a significant group in urolithiasis because of their tendency to cause serious morbidities, to lead to staghorn calculi as well as to pose treatment difficulties.

The oldest struvite renal calculus has been found in a late Bronze Age burial mound in Hungary.[1] In 387 BCE, Hippocrates documented the association between urinary tract infection and urinary stone disease. Approximately 2,000 years later, Marcet recognized the combination of phosphate calculi with alkaline, ammoniacal urine, and putrefaction.[2,3] In the early 1800s, Ulex, a Swedish geologist discovered magnesium ammonium phosphate in guano and named it "struvite" after his mentor, HCG von Struve, a Russian diplomat and naturalist.[3] In 1901, the theory of bacterial splitting of urea as a promoter of stone formation was first proposed by Brown, in a study of six patients' stone analysis, who all suffered from urinary tract infections with *Proteus vulgaris*.[4] This was a significant contribution to the understanding of the origin of infection stones. In 1925, Hager and Magath suggested that a bacterial enzyme hydrolyzed urea, and Sumner isolated urease from *Canavalia ensiformis*.[5]

58.2 Pathogenesis

Struvite stones are composed of magnesium ammonium phosphate ($MgNH_4PO_4.6H_2O$) and varying amounts of carbonate apatite ($Ca_{10}[PO_4]_6CO_3$).[6] Normal urine is undersaturated with ammonium phosphate. An alkaline urinary environment with pH greater than 7.2 and the presence of ammonia are required for struvite stone formation.[6,7] In the presence of urinary tract infection with urease-producing bacteria, ammonia production is elevated and urinary pH is increased, which lead to struvite stone formation. Urea is first hydrolyzed to ammonia and carbon dioxide in the presence of bacterial urease through the following reaction[6,7]:

$$\left(NH_2\right)_2 CO + H_2O \rightarrow 2NH_3 + CO_2$$

These products alkalinize the urine (pH > 7.2) and this favors the formation of ammonium;

$$NH_3 + H_2O \rightarrow NH_4^+ + OH^-$$

In the presence of urease, ammonia continues to be produced despite alkaline urine, further increasing urinary pH.[7] The alkaline environment leads to the formation of carbonic acid, which then dissociates into HCO_3 and H. Further dissociation of HCO_3 yields carbonate and two hydrogen ions:

$$CO_2 + H_2O \rightarrow H_2CO_3$$
$$H_2CO_3 \rightarrow H^+ + HCO_3^-$$
$$HCO_3^- \rightarrow H^+ + CO_3^{2-}$$

T. Esen (✉)
Department of Urology, Istanbul Faculty of Medicine, Istanbul University, Istanbul, Turkey
e-mail: tarikesen@doruk.net.tr

P.N. Rao et al. (eds.), *Urinary Tract Stone Disease*,
DOI 10.1007/978-1-84800-362-0_58, © Springer-Verlag London Limited 2011

Under alkaline conditions, the dissociation of hydrogen phosphate provides phosphate, and this completes the generation of constituent ions for infection stone formation:

$$H_2PO_4^- \rightarrow H^+ + HPO_4^{2-}$$

$$HPO_4^{2-} \rightarrow H^+ + PO_4^{3-}$$

These chemical processes, with the presence of magnesium, lead to the formation of struvite precipitation.[7]

Urinary supersaturation of the ions comprising struvite stones leads to particle formation. Subsequently, particles grow into crystals. Crystallization may occur both intra and peribacterially.[6] Crystals growing peribacterially may form a phosphate cover on the bacteria, and bacteria enclosed within the stone may lead to recurrent infections.[8] Consequently, crystals aggregate to larger crystals and then full-sized stones form if retained in the urinary tract.

The ammonium produced by the bacteria induces damage to the protective urothelial glycosaminoglycan (GAG) layer.[3] The ammonium has an affinity for the charged sulfate groups of the glycosaminoglycan layer. Thus, hydrophilic activity of the GAGs is altered and adhesion of struvite crystals to the urothelium enhances.[9] Crystal adhesion with supersaturation may lead to rapid development of large stones. Formation of an exopolysaccharide biofilm is also a pathologic factor for stone growth.[10]

58.3 Bacteriology

The members of the *Enterobacteriaceae* comprise the majority of urease-producing pathogens (Table 58.1).[3,11] The most common causative organism is *Proteus mirabilis*.[12] These bacteria use urease to meet their nitrogen requirement. *Klebsiella*, *Pseudomonas*, and *Staphyloccus* species are the other important urease-producing organisms.[2] The most common uropathogen, *E. coli*, only rarely produces urease.[6] Ureaplasma urealyticum has an obligate growth requirement for urea and may be a causative factor for struvite stones.[3] The urease is plasmid encoded and may be transmitted from one organism to another. The Urea-Rapid test, a urea-indol medium from Bio-Merieux, can be used to detect bacterial urease.[6]

58.4 Epidemiology – Clinical Manifestations

Struvite calculi account for 10–15% of all urinary calculi.[13,14] They occur more commonly in women than in men, in a ratio of 2:1.[15]

Table 58.1 Organisms that may produce urease (Adapted from Gleeson et al.[11] and Wong HY et al.[3])

Organisms		Usually (>90% of isolates)	Occasionally (5–30% of isolates)
Bacteria			
Gram-negative		*Proteus mirabilis*	*Klebsiella pneumoniae*
		Proteus morgagnii	*Klebsiella oxytoca*
		Proteus rettgeri	*Serratia marcescens*
		Providencia stuartii	*Haemophilus parainfluenza*
		Haemophilus influenzae	*Bordetella bronchiseptica*
		Bordetella pertussis	*Aeromonas hydrophilia*
		Bacteroides corrodens	*Pseudomonas aeruginosa*
		Yersinia enterocolitica	*Pasteurella spp*
		Brucella spp	
		Flavobacterium spp	
Gram-positive		*Corynebacterium hofmanii*	*Staphylococcus epidermidis*
		Corynebacterium ovis	*Bacillus spp*
		Corynebacterium renale	*Corynebacterium murium*
		Corynebacterium ulcerans	*Corynebacterium equi*
		Micrococcus varions	*Peptococcus asaccharolyticus*
		Staphylococcus aureus	*Clostridium tetani*
			Mycobacterium rhodochrous group
Mycoplasma		T-strain mycoplasma	
		Ureaplasma urealyticum	
Yeast		*Candida humicola*	
		Cryptococcus	
		Sporobolmyces	
		Rhodotorula	
		Trichosporon cutaneum	

Patients with recurrent or persistent urinary tract infection (UTI) are predisposed to struvite calculi. The risk factors include urinary tract obstruction, chronic indwelling catheter, urinary diversion, and neurogenic bladder dysfunction.[6] These stones afflict 8% of spinal cord–injured patients and 4.7–30% of patients with ileal conduit.[3,16–18] Children with congenital urinary tract malformations and premature infants are also at risk for infection stones. In addition, as the number of UTIs correlates with age, elderly men and women are prone to struvite stones.[19]

The clinical presentation is usually more insidious. The typical renal colic may not be observed, and patients may present with recurrent urinary tract infection, hematuria, vague abdominal pain, fever, and even with urosepsis. Acute pyonephrosis with perirenal abscess formation and xanthogranulomatous pyelonephritis may occasionally occur.[3] An alkaline urine (pH 7.1) is detected on urine analysis, and magnesium ammonium phosphate crystals are frequently observed.

Mostly, these stones are detected on abdominal plain films as they are radiopaque. However, poorly mineralized stones may be faintly radiopaque or even radiolucent. Computed tomography (CT) investigation of the staghorn stone may be useful before surgical treatment, and renal scintigraphy may be warranted in chronically obstructed kidneys. The average absolute CT values for struvite stones range from 651 to 944 hounsfield units between different series.[20,21]

58.5 Medical Management

The goal of medical management in patients with struvite stones is generally to maximize the effects of other therapies and to prevent stone recurrence. Dissolution therapy may be an alternative for selected patients who are poor candidates for other surgical treatment options. Medical management options include dissolution therapy, urease inhibitors, urinary acidification, antibiotics, and dietary modifications.

58.5.1 Dissolution Therapy (Chemolysis)

The dissolution of calculi with lavage chemolysis is a part of medical management of struvite stones. The use of chemolysis or dissolution therapy has dated back to the 1930s. Hellstrom and Albright reported their initial experience with combination of antiseptics and acidifying agents.[22,23] In 1943, the first application of direct chemolysis to struvite calculi was described by Suby and Albright.[24] This initial solution was too irritating to the epithelium. For this reason, the solution was modified to Suby's G solution by addition of magnesium in order to reduce mucosal irritability. In 1959, Mulvaney reported their experience with a new solvent: 10% hemiacidrin (renacidin).[25] This solution is similar in composition to Suby's G but contains additional magnesium salts and D-gluconic acid. Acids provide hydrogen ions and citrate to form soluble complexes with phosphate and calcium from the stone. The clinical effectiveness of these solutions is dependent on their acidic pH because the solubility of struvite is markedly increased at pH below 5.5.

Early studies reported severe complications including sepsis, electrolyte abnormalities, and even death. In response to these reports, the US Food and Drug Administration (FDA) withdrew approval for the use of hemiacidrin above the bladder. However, the detailed investigation of these complications by Nemoy and Stamey concluded that the deaths were likely caused by urosepsis rather than the irrigation solution.[26] So, the treatment is contraindicated in the presence of urinary tract infection.

There are several precautions recommended when chemolysis is planned. These are maintenance of sterile urine, unobstructed inflow and outflow, maintenance of intrapelvic pressure below 25 cm H_2O, absence of extravasation, and monitoring of serum magnesium levels.[8,27] Hypermagnesium should be avoided due to potentially fatal complication.[28] This treatment should not be used during the immediate postoperative period and should only be applied when the renal tract has completely healed following surgery due to the risk of absorption of magnesium.[29] Broad-spectrum antibiotics should be started before the treatment, continued during, and after completion of chemolysis for a period of 10 days.[8] Frequent (every 24–48 h) surveillance cultures should be obtained throughout therapy.

The procedure can be performed through a nephrostomy tube that is left in place during surgery or after insertion of a nephrostomy catheter if no operation is performed. The ideal system includes a dual nephrostomy tube (inflow and outflow) together with a ureteral catheter securing unobstructed passage of fragments.[13]

Several investigators reported the results of direct dissolution of struvite calculi, whereas others used dissolution as an adjuvant to residual fragments after a debulking procedure. Prophylactic irrigation has also been used in the absence of residual calculi. Although there was significant variability of methodology, technique of stone irrigation, and adjunctive procedures, overall, the success of adjuvant therapy (77%) was found to be slightly more successful than primary chemolysis (68%).[13,30–33] In a recent study of 118 patients with staghorn stones, Tiselius et al. reported a stone-free rate of 60% with combined shock wave lithotripsy (SWL) and percutaneous chemolysis with hemiacidrin.[34] Although a low complication rate was reported, the patients required a long hospital stay, with a mean of 32 days. Therefore, the authors advocated this treatment for high-risk patients and for those patients in whom other procedures are impossible. The major advantage of this procedure is that it can be carried out without anesthesia; therefore, it may be an option for high-risk patients. Today, the introduction of modern endourological techniques and extracorporeal shock wave lithotripsy (ESWL) limited the applications of chemolysis to treat selected cases with residual stone fragments and to decrease stone recurrence.

58.5.2 Urease Inhibitors

Since struvite stones form in the presence of urease, inhibition of this enzyme retards the growth of existing stones and probably helps to prevent the formation of new stones. Acetohydroxamic acid (AHA) is an approved urease inhibitor designed to inhibit struvite stone formation. It was first identified in 1964 and causes an irreversible inhibition of the enzyme urease.[27] It is easily absorbed from the gastrointestinal tract and reaches peak plasma levels after 1 h. The half-life is 3.5–10 h in normal subjects.[19] It has high renal clearance and has the ability to penetrate the bacterial cell wall. AHA also works synergistically with several antibiotics, facilitating the sterilization of urine. The initial trial consists of 250 mg twice daily and if this is tolerated, the dosage is then increased to 250 mg three times daily.[3] In three double-blind, placebo-controlled trials, a significant reduction in stone growth was detected with AHA treatment compared to placebo.[35–37] In a double-blind, placebo-controlled clinical trial of acetohydroxamic acid in 210 male spinal cord–injured patients with chronic urea-splitting urinary infection, Griffith and colleagues reported that the acetohydroxamic acid patients with stones had decreases in urinary ammonia while the placebo patients had increases in ammonia.[35] Also, patients with stones treated with acetohydroxamic acid were found to exhibit significantly longer intervals from randomization to first stone growth than patients treated with placebo ($p < 0.005$, medians 15 versus 9 months) and AHA reduced significantly the proportion of patients with stone growth at 12 months (33% versus 60%, p equals 0.017). However, this decrease was diminished at 24 months (42% versus 60%, p equals 0.260) in the same study. In a randomized double-blind study, Williams and colleagues compared 18 patients who received acetohydroxamic acid with 19 patients who received placebo.[36] No patient who received acetohydroxamic acid had a doubling of stone size whereas seven patients showed a 100% increase in the two-dimensional surface area of their stones. Similarly, in a prospective study of 94 patients with chronic urinary infection, Griffith and colleagues reported a stone growth in 17% of the AHA group and in 46% of the placebo group ($p < 0.005$).[37] However, a major disadvantage of AHA treatment is that 20–30% of patients were unable to tolerate AHA because of side effects.[37] The side effects include gastrointestinal upset, neurological symptoms such as headache, tremulousness, loss of taste, anxiety, hallucinations, deep vein thrombosis, and hemolytic anemia.[3,13] These effects were shown to reverse on termination of AHA therapy. The administration of AHA is contraindicated in patients with severe renal insufficiency (serum creatinine > 2.5 mg/dL, creatinine clearance < 20 mL/min) because the risk of toxicity increases and the effectiveness of the AHA decreases.[13]

In general, urease-inhibiting drugs should be considered palliative rather than therapeutic and due to the side effects, its clinical use remains limited.

58.5.3 Acidification

Struvite stone cannot form in a urinary pH of less than 7.19 or in the absence of ammonia because alkaline urine is required for supersaturation of struvite and carbonate. Therefore, urinary acidification increases the solubility of struvite and carbonate. Additionally, antibiotic efficacy is improved in an acidic environment, increasing the antimicrobial success. Several oral agents to acidify urine have been studied. Ascorbic acid and ammonium chloride have not succeeded for long-term urinary acidification.[19,23] Oral L-methionine has been studied for acidification. It is metabolized in the liver via L-cysteine to sulfate and hydrogens. A reduction in the urinary pH to values of 6.0–6.2 was observed over an 8-h period after a single dose of 1,500-mg L-methionine.[38] Jarrar and colleagues observed 19 active struvite stone formers on L-methionine therapy over a period of 10 years.[39] In these patients, urine was acidified with L-methionine (Acimethin) using a dose of three to six tablets 500 mg/day. During therapy, the mean pH values decreased significantly from 7.5 to 5.5. Recurrent stones were detected in only 10% of cases (two patients). Jacobs and colleagues demonstrated in vitro that the dissolution rate of struvite stones in artificial urine rose with a decreasing pH-value.[40] They reported that the diminution of the pH-value from 6.5 to 5.75 led to an increase of the dissolution rate of more than 35% and stated that the intake of 1,500–3,000 mg L-methionine may lead to a sufficient acidification for a good dissolution of struvite stones.

58.5.4 Antimicrobials

The goal of antimicrobial treatment is to eradicate infection, thus eliminating the formation and potential growth of struvite calculi by destruction of urease-producing bacteria. It is warranted in virtually all patients with struvite calculi. Culture-specific antimicrobials are the drugs of choice and may decrease the frequency and magnitude of urinary tract infections. Griffith and Osborne have shown that a reduction of bacterial colony from 10^7 to 10^5 decreases the urease production by 99%.[2] Although antibiotics may suppress bacteriuria, in the presence of remnant fragments, their effectiveness in eliminating infection is compromised. For this reason, long-term antibiotics are not recommended as monotherapy for patients with infection stones. Rather, they should be used to prevent stone recurrences or growth after operative procedures as an adjunct to therapy. The duration of therapy may vary according to different treatment protocols. In general, an antimicrobial course for up to 3 months may be an option and if urine sterility is maintained, antibiotics are discontinued.[3] Urine cultures should be routinely collected at each follow-up visit for 1 year.

58.5.5 Diet

Dietary manipulation has been proposed to limit the amount of substrate for struvite stone formation. The goal of this approach was to reduce urinary phosphate, magnesium, and ammonia. In 1945, Shorr recommended a low-phosphorus, low-calcium diet supplemented with aluminum hydroxide gel.[41] Aluminum hydroxide binds with phosphate in the gut to form insoluble aluminum phosphate; therefore, urinary phosphate levels decrease. This regimen resulted in partial or complete dissolution in 23% of patients in their series.[42] However, prolonged use of aluminum hydroxide preparations carries a significant risk of calcium abnormalities (hypercalciuria) and possible aluminum toxicity.[43] For this reason, its use has been limited. In general, the avoidance of foods and vitamin supplements high in phosphorus and magnesium may be recommended.[8]

58.6 Conclusions

Struvite stones are best managed by complete clearance of all infected stone materials. Medical treatment is adjunctive in nature, and is mainly used for prevention of recurrence. Culture-specific antibiotics, urease inhibitors, chemolytic dissolution, and urinary acidification are medical treatment options. Potential significant side effects are of clinical concern.

References

1. Scheneider HJ. Epidemiology of urolithiasis. In: Scheneider HJ, ed. *Urolithiasis: Etiology Diagnosis*. Berlin: Springer; 1985: 137–184.
2. Griffith DP, Osborne CA. Infection (urease) stones. *Miner Electrolyte Metab*. 1987;13:278–285.
3. Wong HY, Riedl CR, Griffith DP. Medical management and prevention of struvite stones. In: Coe FL, Favus MJ, Pak CYC, Parks JH, Preminger GM, eds. *Kidney Stones: Medical and Surgical Mangement*. Philadelphia: Lippincott-Raven; 1996:941–950.
4. Brown TR. On the relation between the variety of microorganisms and the composition of Stone in calculous pyelonephritis. *JAMA*. 1901;36:1395–1397.
5. Hagar BH, Magath TB. The etiology of encrusted cystitis with alkaline urine. *JAMA*. 1925;85:1352–1355.
6. Bichler KH, Eipper E, Naber K, Braun V, Zimmermann R, Lahme S. Urinary infection stones. *Int J Antimicrob Agents*. 2002 Jun;19(6):488–498.
7. Pearle MS, Lotan Y. Urinary lithiasis: etiology, epidemiology, and pathogenesis. In: Wein AJ, Kavuossi LR, Novick AC, Partin AW, Peters CA, eds. *Campbell-Walsh Urology*. Philadelphia: Saunders-Elsevier; 2007:1386–1387.
8. Healy KA, Ogan K. Pathophysiology and management of infectious staghorn calculi. *Urol Clin N Am*. 2007 Aug;34(3):363–374.
9. Grenabo L, Hedelin H, Pettersson S. Adherence of urease-induced crystals to rat bladder epithelium. *Urol Res*. 1988;16(1):49–52.
10. Choong S, Whitfield H. Biofilms and their role in infections in urology. *BJU Int*. 2000 Nov;86(8):935–941.
11. Gleeson MJ, Kobashi K, Griffith DP. Noncalcium nephrolithiasis. In: Coe FL, Favus MJ, eds. *Disorders of Bone and Mineral Metabolism*. New York: Raven Press; 1992:801–827.
12. Silverman DA, Stamey TA. Management of infection stones: the Stanford experience. *Medicine (Baltimore)*. 1983;62:44–51.
13. Freid RM, Smith AD. Chemolysis of urinary calculi. In: Smith AD, Badlani GH, Bagley DH, Clayman RV, Docimo SG, Jordan GH, Kavoussi LR, Lee BR, Lingeman JE, Preminger GM, Segura JW, eds. *Smith's Textbook of Endourology*. Ontario: BC Decker; 2007:148–158.
14. Levy FL, Adams-Huet B, Pak CY. Ambulatory evaluation of nephrolithiasis: an update of a 1980 protocol. *Am J Med*. January 1995;98(1):50–59.
15. Resnick MI. Evaluation and management of infection stones. *Urol Clin N Am*. 1981 Jun;8(2):265–276.
16. Comarr Ae, Kawaichi Gk, Bors E. Renal calculosis of patients with traumatic cord lesions. *J Urol*. 1962 May;87:647–656.
17. Kracht H, Büscher HK. Formation of staghorn calculi and their surgical implications in paraplegics and tetraplegics. *Paraplegia*. 1974 Aug;12(2):98–110.
18. Koff SA, Lapides J. Altered bladder function in staghorn calculus disease. *J Urol*. 1977 May;117(5):577–580.
19. Wang LP, Wong HY, Griffith DP. Treatment options in struvite stones. *Urol Clin N Am*. 1997 Feb;24(1):149–162.
20. Zarse CA, McAteer JA, Tann M, et al. Helical computed tomography accurately reports urinary stone composition using attenuation values: in vitro verification using high-resolution micro-computed tomography calibrated to fourier transform infrared microspectroscopy. *Urology*. 2004 May;63(5):828–833.
21. Mostafavi MR, Ernst RD, Saltzman B. Accurate determination of chemical composition of urinary calculi by spiral computerized tomography. *J Urol*. March 1998;159(3):673–675.
22. Hellstrom J. The significance of staphylococci in the development and treatment of renal and ureteric Stones. *Br J Urol*. 1938;10:348–378.
23. Albraight F, Sulkowitch HW, Chute R. Non-surgical aspects of the kidney stone problem. *JAMA*. 1939;113:2049–2053.
24. Suby HI, Albraight F. Dissolution of phosphatic urinary calculi by the retrograde introduction of a citrate solution containing magnesium. *N Engl J Med*. 1943;228:81–91.
25. Mulvaney WP. A new solvent for certain urinary calculi: a preliminary report. *J Urol*. 1959 Oct;82:546–548.
26. Nemoy NJ. Stamey TA use of hemiacidrin in management of infection stones. *J Urol*. 1976 Dec;116(6):693–695.
27. Bernardo NO, Smith AD. Chemolysis of urinary calculi. *Urol Clin N Am*. 2000 May;27(2):355–365.
28. Tiselius HG, Alken P, Buck C, Gallucci M, Knoll T, Sarica K, Türk CHR. *EAU Guidelines on Urolithiasis*, 2008.

29. Cato AR, Tulloch AG. Hypermagnesemia in a uremic patient during renal pelvis irrigation with renacidin. *J Urol.* 1974 Mar;111(3): 313–314.

30. Dretler SP, Pfister RC. Percutaneous dissolution of renal calculi. *Annu Rev Med.* 1983;34:359–366.

31. Blaivas JG, Pais VM, Spellman RM. Chemolysis of residual stone fragments after extensive surgery for staghorn calculi. *Urology.* 1975 Dec;6(6):680–686.

32. Palmer JM, Bishai MB, Mallon DS. Outpatient irrigation of the renal collecting system with 10 per cent hemiacidrin: cumulative experience of 365 days in 13 patients. *J Urol.* 1987 Aug;138(2): 262–265.

33. Spirnak JP, DeBaz BP, Green HY, Resnick MI. Complex struvite calculi treated by primary extracorporeal shock wave lithotripsy and chemolysis with hemiacidrin irrigation. *J Urol.* 1988 Dec;140(6):1356–1359.

34. Tiselius HG, Hellgren E, Andersson A, Borrud-Ohlsson A, Eriksson I. Minimally invasive treatment of infection staghorn stones with shock wave lithotripsy and chemolysis. *Scand J Urol Nephrol.* October 1999;33(5):286–290.

35. Griffith DP, Khonsari F, Skurnick JH, James KE. A randomized trial of acetohydroxamic acid for the treatment and prevention of infection-induced urinary stones in spinal cord injury patients. *J Urol.* 1988 Aug;140(2):318–324.

36. Williams JJ, Rodman JS, Peterson CM. A randomized double-blind study of acetohydroxamic acid in struvite nephrolithiasis. *N Engl J Med.* 1984 Sep 20;311(12):760–764.

37. Griffith DP, Gleeson MJ, Lee H, Longuet R, Deman E, Earle N. Randomized, double-blind trial of Lithostat (acetohydroxamic acid) in the palliative treatment of infection-induced urinary calculi. *Eur Urol.* 1991;20(3):243–247.

38. Hesse A, Heimbach D. Causes of phosphate stone formation and the importance of metaphylaxis by urinary acidification: a review. *World J Urol.* October 1999;17(5):308–315.

39. Jarrar K, Boedeker RH, Weidner W. Struvite stones: long term follow up under metaphylaxis. *Ann Urol (Paris).* 1996;30(3): 112–117.

40. Jacobs D, Heimbach D, Hesse A. Chemolysis of struvite stones by acidification of artificial urine–an in vitro study. *Scand J Urol Nephrol.* 2001 Oct;35(5):345–349.

41. Shorr E. The possible usefulness of estrogen and aluminum hydroxide gels in the management of renal stone. *J Urol.* 1945;53:507.

42. Shorr E, Carter Ac. Aluminum gels in the management of renal phosphatic calculi. *J Am Med Assoc.* 1950 Dec 30;144(18): 1549–1556.

43. Lotz M, Zisman E, Bartter FC. Evidence for a phosphorus–depletion syndrome in man. *N Engl J Med.* February 22, 1968;278(8): 409-415.

Dietary Assessment and Advice

59

Roswitha Siener and Albrecht Hesse

Abstract Among the prerenal risk factors of stone disease, diet plays an important role. Various interventional studies have provided evidence that appropriate dietary modifications can reduce the risk of stone formation and recurrence rate. Individualized dietary recommendations should be offered to patients according to their stone type, specific metabolic, and dietary risk profile. The reduction of overweight, risk-adapted dietary modifications based on a comprehensive dietary assessment as well as appropriate changes in lifestyle are the basis of a successful metaphylaxis in urinary stone disease.

59.1 Introduction

Stone recurrence rates may be as high as 30–50% after 5 years without intervention.[1] Unfavorable nutritional patterns are considered to be important risk factors for stone formation. Various interventional studies have provided evidence that appropriate dietary modifications can reduce the risk of stone formation and recurrence rates.[2–5] To prevent stone recurrence, dietary recommendations should be tailored based on stone type, dietary assessment, and metabolic risk profile. As the stone composition has significant therapeutic importance in the evaluation of the stone-forming patient, all urinary stones should be analyzed for composition.[6]

59.2 Dietary Assessment

The assessment of dietary habits is part of the basic evaluation program and, next to stone history, the most important basis for the prevention of stone recurrences. Specific dietary assessment provides fundamental information for the evaluation of nutritional risk factors for urinary stone formation. Effective dietary recommendations depend on accurate assessments of habitual intakes of food and nutrients in stone formers.

A dietary assessment is a comprehensive evaluation of the food intake of the stone-forming patient. It is one of four parts of a nutritional assessment in a clinical setting. The four parameters of assessment include: (1) an assessment of anthropometric data, e.g., height, weight, body mass index, waist circumference; (2) dietary assessment, which includes retrospective and prospective methods; (3) a physical examination with a medical history; and (4) metabolic examination.

Two main categories of methods are employed in diet assessment.[7] The first is retrospective and the most usual of these are 24-h recall, diet history, food frequency questionnaire, and diet inventory. The advantages of retrospective methods of dietary assessment are that they are quick, cheap, and make limited demands on subjects. The major problem of these methods is largely inaccurate memory, and this can only be overcome by using a prospective methodology.

The two main prospective methods that are commonly employed are weighed food inventory and estimated food inventory. Seven-day weighed dietary records are currently accepted as the most accurate technique for assessing habitual dietary intake. However, errors in estimating food intake may occur, arising from inexact application of the seven-day weighed intake technique. The technique should therefore be applied by trained personnel. With estimated inventory, foods are unweighed but portion sizes are estimated with reference to food photos, models, or by replicating descriptions of portions and weighing. Again, patients need training on recording, and records must be checked by a dietitian for legibility, completeness, and missing entries. If nutrient intake is of interest, then foods have to be coded for computer analysis and analyzed using an appropriate computer program,

R. Siener (✉)
Department of Urology, University of Bonn, Bonn, Germany
e-mail: roswitha.siener@ukb.uni-bonn.de

P.N. Rao et al. (eds.), *Urinary Tract Stone Disease*,
DOI 10.1007/978-1-84800-362-0_59, © Springer-Verlag London Limited 2011

e.g., PRODI. An interventional trial in calcium oxalate stone formers has demonstrated that the described procedure is useful in the assessment of dietary habits of stone patients in both clinical practice and scientific evaluation.[5]

An additional effect of weighing and recording food intake is that many patients find that the exercise itself is a stimulus to change eating habits. The use of food records reveals unhealthy eating habits to the stone former and increases the motivation and compliance of patients to adhere to dietary modifications.

Providing nutrition education and counseling to stone patients of different ages and from different backgrounds requires a good understanding of diet quality and eating behaviors, and profound knowledge of dietary risk factors for urinary stone disease and management of diet-related diseases associated with urolithiasis. Individualized dietary recommendations should be offered to patients according to their metabolic and dietary risk profile. Dietitians are trained to do this and should therefore be involved in the nutrition education and counseling of the patient.

The primary goal of metaphylaxis of urinary stone disease is the correction of individual biochemical risk profile. A reduction in the risk of stone formation and recurrence rate can already be achieved by appropriate dietary treatment.

Table 59.1 General dietary metaphylaxis of stone disease

Body weight	• Reduction of overweight • Avoid fasting or high-protein weight-loss diets; e.g., Atkins diet • Sufficient physical activity
Fluid intake	• Urine volume: at least 2.0 L/24 h • Specific weight of urine <1.010 • Neutral beverages • Circadian drinking
Balanced diet	• Consume a variety of nutrient-dense foods from all food groups • Meet recommended nutrient intakes within energy needs by adopting a balanced eating pattern • Consume a variety of vegetables, salads, fruits, and whole-grain products each day • Limit intake of meat, fish, and poultry • Select lean meat, meat products, milk or dairy products • 0.8 g protein/kg body weight/day • Consume about 1,000–1,200 mg calcium daily • Limit sodium chloride intake to no more than 6 g/day • Limit intake of fats and oils high in saturated fatty acids, and choose fats coming from sources of polyunsaturated and monounsaturated fatty acids, such as vegetable oils • Choose and prepare foods and beverages without added sugars

59.3 General Dietary Metaphylaxis

General dietary metaphylaxis is suitable as basic treatment for all stone patients irrespective of stone composition. The general dietary metaphylactic measures specified in Table 59.1 aim at normalization of the dietary habits and lifestyle factors that are known to be important risk factors for urinary stone formation. General metaphylactic measures are the reduction of overweight, the consumption of a balanced diet according to the recommendations for stone patients, and a sufficient circadian fluid intake accomplished with neutral beverages. Any excess should be avoided including an excessive intake of energy. Moreover, sufficient physical activity is recommended as a general metaphylactic measure for stone formers.

A balanced diet should be composed of a selection of varied, healthy, and natural foodstuffs.[8] A variety of vegetables, salads, fruits, and whole-grain cereals should be part of the daily diet. Fresh or frozen products without additional sauce should be preferred instead of canned foods. The intake of meat, fish, and poultry should be limited. Low-fat meat and dairy products (i.e., milk, yoghurt, and cheese) should be chosen. The intake of products with a high content of sugar or salt should be avoided. Fat from vegetable sources (i.e., plant oils) should be preferred. In addition to general metaphylactic measures, specific dietary recommendations should

be followed if stone composition is known or particular abnormalities have been discovered.

59.4 General Recommendations for Fluid Intake

A sufficient circadian fluid intake accomplished by suitable beverages is one of the most effective dietary measures irrespective of stone composition or the cause of stone formation. An adequate urine dilution is an important goal to avoid urinary supersaturation with lithogenic substances and to reduce the risk for stone formation. Findings from observational and interventional studies support evidence that high fluid intake to assure a consistent urine volume of at least 2 L/24 h is the initial therapy for the prevention of stone recurrences.[2,9–12] Depending on the environmental temperature and the degree of physical activity, it is usually necessary to drink ≥2 L/day to achieve this urine flow.

The stone patient must learn to drink. Therefore, dietary treatment should start with a comparison between the daily fluid intake and 24-h urine volume and density.[8] The fluid intake should be evenly distributed over the day. It is particularly important to drink before going to bed at night to avoid urine concentration during the sleeping period. Patients with severe stone disease should be encouraged to have nocturia at least once per night. Patients exposed to chronic dehydration – caused by hot and/or dry environments, extensive physical activity, or diarrhea – are recommended to replace extrarenal fluid losses.

The type of beverage should be selected cautiously. When the stone composition is unknown, the preferred beverages should be urine neutral. Neutral beverages – fluids that dilute urine without affecting its composition – include tap water, mineral water with a low mineral content, fruit and herbal teas (Table 59.2). Less suitable beverages are coffee[13] and black or green tea.[14] All types of alcoholic beverages including beer, as well as soft drinks, including cola, are unsuitable for stone-forming patients.[15,16] Alkalizing beverages – fluids that additionally increase urinary pH and citrate excretion – are bicarbonate-rich mineral water and citrus juices (i.e., orange and lemon juices).[17–19] Neutral and alkalizing beverages are suitable for metaphylactic treatment of the majority of urinary stones, i.e., calcium oxalate, uric acid, and cystine. Urinary acidification, for example in calcium phosphate and infection stone disease, can be achieved with acidifying beverages. Suitable beverages are cranberry juice and mineral water rich in sulfate and low in bicarbonate and

calcium.[20,21] It should be emphasized that fruit juices have a considerable content of energy and should be diluted before ingestion.

59.5 Calcium Oxalate Stone Disease

Specific metaphylactic measures for calcium oxalate stone formers should be directed toward any abnormalities that have been recorded in urine composition in order to reduce the risk of recurrent stone formation. Risk factors for calcium oxalate stone formation include hyperoxaluria, hypercalciuria, hyperuricosuria, a reduced urinary excretion of inhibitors magnesium and citrate, and a low urine volume (Table 59.3).

59.5.1 Hyperoxaluria

Hyperoxaluria is a primary risk factor for calcium oxalate stone formation. An elevated oxalate excretion can result from an increased dietary intake, an increased intestinal absorption of oxalate from the diet, or an increased endogenous production of oxalate from ingested or metabolically generated precursors. It has been suggested that up to 50% of the urinary oxalate is derived from the diet.[22] Some foodstuffs,

Table 59.2 General recommendations for fluid intake

General measures
- Urine volume: at least 2.0 L/24 h
- Specific weight of urine <1.010
- Fluid intake should be evenly distributed over the day
- Drink before going to bed and drink again before each voiding
- Avoid dehydration by sauna, sunbathing, excessive exercise, use of laxatives
- Adjust fluid intake to ambient temperature and physical activity

Neutral beverages
- Mineral water with a low content of bicarbonate, calcium, and sulfate
- Tap water (cave: pay attention to sterility of drinking water)
- Herbal tea, fruit tea, kidney tea, bladder tea

Unsuitable beverages
- Caffeinated coffee, black tea, green tea (max. 0.5 L/day),
- Soft drinks, including sugar-sweetened cola
- Alcoholic beverages, including beer

Alkalizing beverages
- Mineral water with a high bicarbonate content and a low-calcium content (at least 1,500 mg HCO_3^-/L, max. 150 mg calcium/L)
- Citrus juices (diluted with water)

Acidifying beverages
- Mineral water with a low bicarbonate and calcium content and a high sulfate content (max. 350 mg HCO_3^-/L, max. 150 mg Ca/L, at least 400 mg SO_4^{2-}/L)
- Cranberry juice (diluted with water)

Table 59.3 Dietary recommendations for calcium oxalate stone patients

Risk factor	Dietary recommendations
Low urine volume	- Fluid intake at least 2.5 L/day - Alkalizing and neutral beverages
Hypercalciuria	- 1,000–1,200 mg calcium/day - 0.8 g protein/kg body weight/day; 50% of protein intake from vegetable origin - Max. 6 g sodium chloride/day
Hyperoxaluria	- Avoidance of oxalate-rich foodstuffs - Adaptation of dietary calcium intake - Magnesium administration
Hyperuricosuria	- Restriction of purine intake - Avoidance of fructose-sweetened foods and soft drinks - Avoidance of alcoholic beverages, especially beer
Hypocitraturia	- 0.8 g protein/kg body weight/day; 50% of protein intake from vegetable origin - Fruits and vegetables (cave: oxalate-rich foods)
Hypomagnesuria	- Fruits, vegetables, and cereals (cave: oxalate-rich foods)

particularly vegetables and cereals, contain high amounts of oxalic acid, for example spinach, rhubarb, sorrel, and wheat bran.[14,23,24] The consumption of small amounts of these food-stuffs can significantly increase urinary oxalate excretion already in healthy individuals without disturbances in oxalate metabolism.[15,25] Moreover, an increased absorption of oxalate has been demonstrated in 46% of patients with calcium oxalate stone disease.[26]

59.5.2 Hypercalciuria

Hypercalciuria is a common identifiable abnormality in patients with calcium oxalate stone disease. Findings from studies revealed an elevated urinary calcium excretion as an independent risk factor for relapse in patients undergoing preventive treatment.[2,27,28] Patients should strive to meet the recommended daily intake for calcium, which ranges from 1,000 to 1,200 mg/day. A balanced diet without dairy products contains about 500 mg/day of calcium. The remaining calcium supply of 500–700 mg/day should be fulfilled with milk or dairy products, which are the most important calcium-containing foodstuffs. A restriction of dietary calcium can cause a negative calcium balance, leading to osteopenia in the long term. Moreover, a reduction in dietary calcium increases intestinal absorption and urinary excretion of oxalate.[29]

Other nutritional factors known to increase urinary calcium excretion by different mechanisms are an increased dietary protein and sodium intake.[30–32] The increase in urinary calcium excretion and the decrease in urinary pH and citrate excretion with increasing protein intake are mainly attributed to the acidifying effect of phosphoproteins and sulfur-containing amino acids (methionine, cystine) that are in a higher proportion in animal than in vegetable protein. Moreover, a high ingestion of sodium may promote urinary calcium excretion.[30] A randomized prospective trial showed that a low-calcium diet, accomplished by abolishing milk and dairy products, is less efficacious in the prevention of stone recurrences in calcium oxalate stone patients with hypercalciuria than a diet with a normal calcium but low salt and animal protein content.[3] Increasing buffering capacity by increasing fruit and vegetable intake with a balanced diet counteracts the acidity generated by the dietary protein, reduces calciuria, and consequently improves calcium balance.[33]

59.5.3 Hyperuricosuria

Hyperuricosuria may promote calcium oxalate stone formation probably through its inhibitory action on glycosaminoglycans, inhibitors of calcium oxalate stone crystallization. A high dietary purine intake is associated with an enhanced endogenous production and urinary excretion of uric acid. Patients should therefore restrict the intake of foodstuffs rich in purine (see Sect. 59.6).

59.5.4 Hypocitraturia and Hypomagnesuria

Hypocitraturia and hypomagnesuria are two important risk factors for calcium oxalate stone formation. Urinary citrate inhibits calcium stone formation by forming a soluble complex with calcium and by effects on nucleation, agglomeration, and crystal growth. Magnesium is suggested to reduce oxalate absorption and urinary excretion nearly as effectively as calcium by binding oxalate in the intestine.[34] A rise in the intake of fruits and vegetables is associated with an increase in urinary pH, magnesium, and citrate excretion.[33,35,36] The favorable changes in urinary risk profile associated with the supplementation of vegetables and fruits are likely due to their high content in potassium, magnesium, bicarbonate, and citrate and their low sulfate content.

In addition to the general recommendations for fluid intake, neutral and alkalizing beverages should be recommended (Table 59.2).

59.6 Uric Acid Stone Disease

Hyperuricosuria, acidic urinary pH levels (<pH 6.0), and a low urine volume promote uric acid stone formation. Hyperuricemia may be present, but is not mandatory related with stone formation.[37] Uric acid is the end product of purine metabolism and is derived from dietary sources, de novo synthesis, and tissue catabolism.

59.6.1 Hyperuricosuria

The most common etiological factor for hyperuricosuria is the overconsumption of dietary purines. Because urinary uric acid excretion strongly depends on the daily dietary purine intake, uric acid stone patients should be placed on a low-purine diet (max. 500 mg uric acid/day) (Table 59.4). Dietary purines are present in foodstuffs either of animal or vegetable origin. Purine-rich foods are mainly meat and meat products, innards, fish, and seafood. Foodstuffs from vegetable sources usually have lower purine contents than foods from animal sources. Among vegetable foods, legumes, including soy products, beans and peas, contain considerable

Table 59.4 Dietary recommendations for uric acid stone patients

Risk factor	Dietary recommendations
Low urine volume	• Fluid intake at least 2.5 L/day • Alkalizing and neutral beverages
Hyperuricosuria	• Ovo-lacto-vegetarian diet • Reduction of purine intake • Restriction of meat, meat products, poultry, and fish to max. 4 meals/week • Avoidance of innards, seafood, skin from fish, poultry, and roast pork • Avoidance of fructose-sweetened foods and soft drinks • Avoidance of alcoholic beverages, especially beer
Low urinary pH	• 0.8 g protein/kg body weight/day; 50% of protein intake from vegetable origin • Fruits and vegetables

quantities of purines. Furthermore, yeast and yeast products are purine rich.

Moreover, it has been suggested that fructose increases the risk of stone formation by effects on uric acid metabolism.[38,39] Uric acid stone patients should be advised to limit fructose intake, especially with fructose-sweetened foods and soft drinks.

59.6.2 Low Urinary pH

An acidic urinary pH promotes uric acid stone formation. Urinary pH is abnormally low in a significant number of patients with uric acid nephrolithiasis.[40] The lower the urinary pH and the higher the uric acid concentration, the greater is the risk for uric acid precipitation. Alkalization of urine increases the solubility of uric acid. The dissolution of uric acid stones requires urinary pH levels between 6.5 and 7.2. Ingestion of dietary protein, mainly from animal origin, has an acidifying effect, whereas fruits and vegetables have an alkalizing effect.[41] Uric acid stone patients should therefore prefer a balanced ovo-lacto-vegetarian diet.

59.6.3 Low Urine Volume

A low urine volume should be corrected preferably with alkalizing beverages (Table 59.2). Ethanol is suggested to increase uric acid production, a factor that is expected to increase the risk of uric acid stone formation.[42,43] Moreover, beer is the only alcoholic beverage acknowledged to have a large purine content, which is predominantly guanosine.[44] In healthy subjects, the consumption of beer resulted in a

reduction of urinary pH and an increase in urinary uric acid excretion.[15] Alcoholic beverages, especially beer, are therefore unsuitable for uric acid stone patients.

59.7 Calcium Phosphate Stone Disease

The most important calcium phosphates involved in urinary stone disease are carbonate apatite and brushite. Although both minerals contain calcium and phosphate, carbonate apatite and brushite are two completely different kinds of stones. Brushite crystallizes in weakly acidic urine (pH optimum 6.5–6.8) at high concentrations of calcium and phosphate. Carbonate apatite stones develop at pH levels greater than 6.8 with high calcium and low citrate concentrations.

Diet plays a limited role in the prevention of stone recurrences in patients with calcium phosphate stone disease (Table 59.5). Patients are advised to eat a varied, balanced mixed diet and to assure a sufficient urine dilution. Whereas foods from animal sources have an acidifying effect, foods from vegetable origin display an alkalizing effect. Due to strong alkalizing effects, the intake of citrus fruits and juices should thus be restricted.

59.7.1 Hypercalciuria

Patients with hypercalciuria should strive to meet the recommended daily intake for calcium, which ranges from 1,000 to 1,200 mg/day (see Sect. 59.5). Moreover, an increased intake of dietary protein and sodium is known to increase urinary calcium excretion. A moderate intake of protein and sodium is therefore recommended.

Table 59.5 Dietary recommendations for calcium phosphate stone patients

Risk factor	Dietary recommendations
Low urine volume	• Fluid intake at least 2.5 L/day • Acidifying and neutral beverages
High urinary pH	• No pure vegetarian diet • Avoidance of alkalizing foods and beverages, such as citrus fruits and juices
Hypercalciuria	• 1,000–1,200 mg calcium/day • 0.8 g protein/kg body weight/day; 50% of protein intake from vegetable origin • Max. 6 g sodium chloride/day
Hyperphosphaturia	• Restriction of meat intake • Avoidance of foodstuffs with a high phosphate content

59.7.2 Hyperphosphaturia

For patients with hyperphosphaturia, it is important to reduce the consumption of foodstuffs with high phosphate content such as hard, soft, and processed cheeses, legumes, nuts, cocoa, and liver. Cheese and nuts have also a relatively high content of protein and calcium. Restriction of the intake of these foods will thus contribute to a decreased excretion of both phosphate and calcium.

59.7.3 High Urinary pH

Urinary acidification should be achieved with acidifying beverages. Suitable beverages are mineral water with a high sulfate content and a low content of bicarbonate and calcium. A high sulfate content of water has been found to be capable of providing sustained urinary acidification. Moreover, cranberry juice has an acidifying and bacteriostatic effect.[20,21,45] Due to the high-energy content, it is recommended to drink cranberry juice diluted with water. Moreover, the oxalate content of cranberry juice has to be taken into account.

59.8 Cystine Stone Disease

Cystine stones are caused by an autosomal recessive hereditary transport defect for the amino acids cystine, arginine, ornithine, and lysine. Because the habitual diet may promote cystine stone formation, dietary modification is an integral part of treatment. A reduction of urinary cystine excretion, urine alkalization, and extensive urine dilution are the cornerstones of metaphylactic treatment of cystine stone disease.

59.8.1 Cystinuria

Cystine is derived from the essential amino acid methionine. A high methionine or protein content, respectively, of the diet may contribute to increased urinary cystine excretion. Methionine is contained in considerable quantities in meat, fish, sausages, eggs, dairy products, and soybeans.[8] Unfortunately, a dietary restriction of methionine-containing products is not practical and can seriously reduce the quality of life. Therefore, cystine stone patients are advised to maintain a balanced diet with moderate protein content, which should not exceed 0.8 g protein/kg body weight/day

Table 59.6 Dietary recommendations for cystine stone patients

Risk factor	Dietary recommendations
Low urine volume	• Fluid intake at least 3.5 L/day • Alkalizing and neutral beverages
Cystinuria	• 0.8 g protein/kg body weight/day; 50% of protein intake from vegetable origin • Restriction of methionine-rich foodstuffs • Max. 6 g sodium chloride/day
Low urinary pH	• 0.8 g protein/kg body weight/day; 50% of protein intake from vegetable origin • Fruits and vegetables

(Table 59.6). A mainly vegetarian diet has a relatively low content of methionine and brings about an alkalization. Vegetables, salads, fruits, and cereals should form the major content of the diet. In children, such a diet may not sufficiently meet the demand of iron and iodine. Children should therefore be given one to two meat and one fish meals weekly.[8]

Moreover, dietary sodium has been suggested to increase cystine excretion.[46] Therefore, the sodium chloride intake with the diet should be limited. This can be accomplished by preferring fresh foodstuffs and by restricting the use of salt during cooking. Notably, much of the salt intake comes from "hidden sources," such as fast food, canned foods, pickled and smoked products.

59.8.2 Low Urine Volume

A high urine volume is one of the most important measures in cystine stone disease. Whereas for the majority of stones, fluid intake should be adjusted to achieve a consistent urine volume of at least 2 L/24 h, excessive urine dilution is necessary for a successful metaphylaxis in patients with cystine stone disease. To remain below the critical limit of 1.33 mmol cystine/L with a cystine excretion of >4.2 mmol/24 h, urine volume must be at least 3.5 L/24 h.[8] Depending on the extent of physical activity and the ambient temperature, a fluid intake of 3.5 to 4.0 L/day is required. Particularly throughout the night, appropriate hydration to maintain urine volume of 1.5 L is recommended. Hydration should mainly be satisfied with alkalizing beverages as the solubility of cystine clearly increases with rising urinary pH.

59.9 Conclusions

Diet plays an important role in urinary stone formation. Specific dietary assessment provides fundamental information for the evaluation of nutritional risk factors for urinary stone formation. General dietary metaphylaxis is suitable as basic treatment for all stone patients irrespective of stone composition. Unspecific metaphylactic measures are the reduction of overweight, the consumption of a balanced diet according to the recommendations for stone patients and a sufficient circadian fluid intake accomplished with neutral beverages. Specific metaphylactic measures for stone formers should be based on the stone type and the biochemical risk profile of the patient. Dietary modification can reduce or even prevent stone recurrences.

References

1. Coe FL, Keck J, Norton ER. The natural history of calcium urolithiasis. *J Am Med Assoc*. 1977;238:1519-1523.
2. Borghi L, Meschi T, Amato F, Briganti A, Novarini A, Giannini A. Urinary volume, water and recurrences in idiopathic calcium nephrolithiasis: a 5-year randomized prospective study. *J Urol*. 1996;155:839-843.
3. Borghi L, Schianchi T, Meschi T, et al. Comparison of two diets for the prevention of recurrent stones in idiopathic hypercalciuria. *N Engl J Med*. 2002;346:77-84.
4. Nomura K, Ito H, Masai M, Akakura K, Shimazaki J. Reduction of urinary stone recurrence by dietary counseling after SWL. *J Endourol*. 1995;9:305-312.
5. Siener R, Schade N, Nicolay C, von Unruh GE, Hesse A. The efficacy of dietary intervention on urinary risk factors for stone formation in recurrent calcium oxalate stone patients. *J Urol*. 2005;173: 1601-1605.
6. Hesse A, Kruse R, Geilenkeuser WJ, Schmidt M. Quality control in urinary stone analysis: results of 44 ring trials (1980–2001). *Clin Chem Lab Med*. 2005;43:298-303.
7. Anderson AS. An overview of diet survey methodology. *Br Food J*. 1995;97:22-26.
8. Hesse A, Tiselius HG, Siener R, Hoppe B. *Urinary Stones. Diagnosis, Treatment, and Prevention of Recurrence*. Basel: Karger; 2009.
9. Curhan GC, Willett WC, Rimm EB, Stampfer MJ. A prospective study of dietary calcium and other nutrients and the risk of symptomatic kidney stones. *N Engl J Med*. 1993;328:833-838.
10. Curhan GC, Willett WC, Speizer FE, Spiegelman D, Stampfer MJ. Comparison of dietary calcium with supplemental calcium and other nutrients as factors affecting the risk for kidney stones in women. *Ann Intern Med*. 1997;126:497-504.
11. Curhan GC, Willett WC, Knight EL, Stampfer MJ. Dietary factors and the risk of incident kidney stones in younger women. *Arch Intern Med*. 2004;164:885-891.
12. Taylor EN, Stampfer MJ, Curhan GC. Dietary factors and the risk of incident kidney stones in men: new insights after 14 years of follow-up. *J Am Soc Nephrol*. 2004;15:3225-3232.
13. Massey LK, Sutton RAL. Acute caffeine effects on urine composition and calcium kidney stone risk in calcium stone formers. *J Urol*. 2004;172:555-558.
14. Hönow R, Hesse A. Comparison of extraction methods for the determination of soluble and total oxalate in foods by HPLC-enzyme-reactor. *Food Chem*. 2002;78:511-521.
15. Hesse A, Siener R, Heynck H, Jahnen A. The influence of dietary factors on the risk of urinary stone formation. *Scanning Microsc*. 1993;7:1119-1128.
16. Rodgers A. Effect of cola consumption on urinary biochemical and physicochemical risk factors associated with calcium oxalate urolithiasis. *Urol Res*. 1999;27:77-81.
17. Hönow R, Laube N, Schneider A, Keßler T, Hesse A. Influence of grapefruit-, orange- and apple-juice consumption on urinary variables and risk of crystallization. *Br J Nutr*. 2003;90:295-300.
18. Keßler T, Hesse A. Cross-over study of the influence of bicarbonate-rich mineral water on urinary composition in comparison with sodium potassium citrate in healthy male subjects. *Br J Nutr*. 2000;84:865-871.
19. Seltzer MA, Low RK, McDonald M, Shami GS, Stoller ML. Dietary manipulation with lemonade to treat hypocitraturic calcium nephrolithiasis. *J Urol*. 1996;156:907-909.
20. Gettman MT, Ogan K, Brinkley LJ, Adams-Huet B, Pak CYC, Pearle MS. Effect of cranberry juice consumption on urinary stone risk factors. *J Urol*. 2005;174:590-594.
21. Keßler T, Jansen B, Hesse A. Effect of blackcurrant-, cranberry- and plum juice consumption on risk factors associated with kidney stone formation. *Eur J Clin Nutr*. 2002;56:1020-1023.
22. Holmes RP, Goodman HO, Assimos DG. Contribution of dietary oxalate to urinary oxalate excretion. *Kidney Int*. 2001;59: 270-276.
23. Siener R, Hönow R, Seidler A, Voss S, Hesse A. Oxalate contents of species of the Polygonaceae, Amaranthaceae and Chenopodiaceae families. *Food Chem*. 2006;98:220-224.
24. Siener R, Hönow R, Voss S, Seidler A, Hesse A. Oxalate content of cereals and cereal products. *J Agr Food Chem*. 2006;54: 3008-3011.
25. Jahnen A, Heynck H, Gertz B, Claßen A, Hesse A. Dietary fibre: the effectiveness of a high bran intake in reducing renal calcium excretion. *Urol Res*. 1992;20:3-6.
26. Voss S, Hesse A, Zimmermann DJ, Sauerbruch T, von Unruh GE. Intestinal oxalate absorption is higher in idiopathic calcium oxalate stone formers than in healthy controls: measurements with the $[^{13}C_2]$oxalate absorption test. *J Urol*. 2006;175:1711-1715.
27. Siener R, Glatz S, Nicolay C, Hesse A. Prospective study on the efficacy of a selective treatment and risk factors for relapse in recurrent calcium oxalate stone patients. *Eur Urol*. 2003;44: 467-474.
28. Strauss AL, Coe FL, Deutsch L, Parks JH. Factors that predict relapse of calcium nephrolithiasis during treatment. *Am J Med*. 1982;72:17-24.
29. Von Unruh GE, Voss S, Sauerbruch T, Hesse A. Dependence of oxalate absorption on the daily calcium intake. *J Am Soc Nephrol*. 2004;15:1567-1573.
30. Muldowney FP, Freaney R, Moloney MF. Importance of dietary sodium in the hypercalciuria syndrome. *Kidney Int*. 1982;22: 292-296.
31. Reddy ST, Wang CY, Sakhaee K, Brinkley L, Pak CYC. Effect of low-carbohydrate high-protein diets on acid-base balance, stone-forming propensity, and calcium metabolism. *Am J Kidney Dis*. 2002;40:265-274.
32. Robertson WG, Heyburn PJ, Peacock M, Hanes FA, Swaminathan R. The effect of high animal protein intake on the risk of calcium stone-formation in the urinary tract. *Clin Sci*. 1979;57:285-288.
33. Siener R, Hesse A. The effect of different diets on urine composition and the risk of calcium oxalate crystallisation in healthy subjects. *Eur Urol*. 2002;42:289-296.
34. Liebman M, Costa G. Effects of calcium and magnesium on urinary oxalate excretion after oxalate loads. *J Urol*. 2000;163:1565-1569.
35. Meschi T, Maggiore U, Fiaccadori E, et al. The effect of fruits and vegetables on urinary stone risk factors. *Kidney Int*. 2004;66: 2402-2410.
36. Siener R, Hesse A. Influence of a mixed and a vegetarian diet on urinary magnesium excretion and concentration. *Br J Nutr*. 1995;73: 783-790.

37. Straub M, Strohmaier WL, Berg W, et al. Diagnosis and metaphylaxis of stone disease – Consensus concept of the National Working Committee on Stone Disease for the Upcoming German Urolithiasis Guideline. *World J Urol*. 2005;23:309-323.

38. Choi HK, Curhan G. Soft drinks, fructose consumption, and the risk of gout in men: prospective cohort study. *Br Med J*. 2008; 336:309-312.

39. Emmerson BT. Effect of oral fructose on urate production. *Ann Rheum Dis*. 1974;33:276-280.

40. Cameron MA, Sakhaee K. Uric acid nephrolithiasis. *Urol Clin N Am*. 2007;34:335-346.

41. Siener R, Hesse A. The effect of a vegetarian and different omnivorous diets on urinary risk factors for uric acid stone formation. *Eur J Nutr*. 2003;42:332-337.

42. Choi HK, Atkinson K, Karlson EW, Willett W, Curhan G. Alcohol intake and risk of incident gout in men: a prospective study. *Lancet*. 2004;363:1277-1281.

43. Zechner O, Scheiber V. Alcohol as an epidemiological risk in urolithiasis. In: Smith LH, Robertson WG, Finlayson B, eds. *Urolithiasis Clinical and Basic Research*. New York: Plenum Press; 1981.

44. Gibson T, Rodgers AV, Simmonds HA, Toseland P. Beer drinking and its effect on uric acid. *Br J Rheumatol*. 1984;23:203-209.

45. Kontiokari T, Nuutinen M, Uhari M. Dietary factors affecting susceptibility to urinary tract infection. *Pediatr Nephrol*. 2004;19: 378-383.

46. Norman RW, Manette WA. Dietary restriction of sodium as a means of reducing urinary cystine. *J Urol*. 1990;143:1193-1195.

Stone Management in the Presence of Morbid Obesity

60

Aaron Potretzke and Manoj Monga

Abstract Obesity is an overwhelming epidemic with implications for all aspects of medicine. Urology is no exception, and specifically obesity has had a pronounced effect on stone disease. Obese patients are at a greatly increased risk for all stones, but particularly uric acid stones. The understanding of the physiology of urolithiasis in obese patients will improve both the prevention and medical treatment of stones. Currently, surgery is the definite treatment, but obstacles exist that complicate surgery in obese persons. A review of the literature, experience of urologists, and current recommendations for accommodations for obese patients are described here within.

60.1 Introduction

Obesity is an overwhelming epidemic with implications for all aspects of medicine. Urology is no exception, and specifically obesity has had a pronounced effect on stone disease. Obese patients are at a greatly increased risk for all stones, but particularly uric acid stones. The understanding of the physiology of urolithiasis in obese patients will improve both the prevention and medical treatment of stones. Currently, surgery is the definite treatment, but obstacles exist that complicate surgery in obese persons. A review of the literature, experience of urologists, and current recommendations for accommodations for obese patients are described here within.

60.2 Epidemiology of Obesity

60.2.1 Obesity in the United States

The obesity epidemic continues to expand across the USA and the world. Its impact on personal and public health is irrefutable. Obesity is strongly associated with, or a risk factor for, diabetes

M. Monga (✉)
Department of Urologic Surgery, University of Minnesota, Minneapolis, MN, USA
e-mail: mongam@ccf.org

mellitus, hypertension, dyslipidemia, stroke, and ischemic heart disease. It is also associated with increased risks for certain cancers, including endometrial, ovarian, cervical, breast, and gallbladder in women, and prostate and colorectal in men.[1]

The definitions of overweight and obese are based on a unit of measure termed Body Mass Index (BMI). BMI is calculated by dividing weight in kilograms by the square of height in meters. In the adult population, overweight, obesity, and extreme obesity are defined by BMIs greater than or equal to 25.0, 30.0, and 40.0.[2]

Unfortunately, the increases in obesity prevalence over the last 25 years have been marked. According to the studies conducted in the National Health and Nutrition Examination Survey (NHANES), the prevalence of obesity in those aged 20–74 has doubled from 1976–1980 to 1999–2000 (15.0% and 30.9%, respectively). The most recent publication from NHANES reports that in 2003–2004, of adults over 20 years of age, 66.3% were either overweight or obese, 32.2% were obese, and 4.8% were considered extremely obese.

When these data are stratified by race/ethnicity, overall 30% of Caucasians, 45% of African-Americans, and 36.8% of Hispanics were obese.[3] These epidemiologic numbers are projected to increase steadily, as current estimates for the year 2010 are that 35% of white men, 36% of white women, 33% of black men, and 55% of black women will be obese.[4] Further indication of the magnitude and significance of the obesity epidemic is the projected "years of life lost" (YLL); for 20-year-olds with a BMI >45, the YLL are 20 years for white males, 13 years for black males, 8 years for black females, and 5 years for white females.[5]

P.N. Rao et al. (eds.), *Urinary Tract Stone Disease*,
DOI 10.1007/978-1-84800-362-0_60, © Springer-Verlag London Limited 2011

60.2.2 Obesity Worldwide

The people of both developed and developing nations across the world are also increasingly plagued by obesity. Recent estimates suggest that between 1 and 1.5 billion adults are overweight and that at least 300 million are obese.[6,7] Prevalence ranges from less than 5% in China and some parts of Africa to greater than 75% in the urban areas of Samoa.[7] Other publications report estimated prevalence rates in developed countries range between 9% (women in Sweden) to 25% (women in Japan).[8]

60.2.3 Obesity in Children and Adolescents

The prevalence of childhood obesity is similarly a growing problem. For children and adolescents (ages 2–19 years), the definition of overweight is a BMI that is greater than the 95th percentile for age, adjusted for sex. As in the adult population, increases in the prevalence of obese children and adolescents have been progressive, as the percentage of overweight children roughly doubled from 1971–1974 to 1988–1994. The data from the 2003–2004 NHANES survey show that obesity was present in 13.9%, 18.8%, and 17.4% for children and adolescents aged 2–5, 6–11, and 12–19.[9] Significant differences in overweight prevalence are demonstrated between racial/ethnic groups in persons aged 6–19 years. African-American and Hispanic girls were significantly more overweight than Caucasian girls. In contrast, Hispanic boys exhibit a significantly higher prevalence of overweight than Caucasian and African-American boys.[10]

Like their adult counterparts, children are affected by obesity worldwide. Estimates in 2007 propose that 22 million children (age 5 or less) are overweight. It is notable that 75% of these children live in impoverished nations.[11] Developed nations such as Japan, Northern Ireland, and England have childhood obesity prevalence rates of 10.7%, 8.5%, and 29.5%, respectively.[8]

60.3 Epidemiology of Stones in the Obese Population

60.3.1 Calcium Oxalate and Uric Acid Stones

It is well reported that the incidence and prevalence of renal stone disease has been increasing in developed nations, including the USA.[12] In fact, even across the time period of 1997–2002, hospital discharges for renal calculi increased by 18.9%, although ureteral calculi were not significantly changed. It has been suggested that the increase in overall stone disease may be related to an increase in the number of obese persons and their associated increased risk of stones.[13]

Obesity is associated with an increase in both calcium oxalate and uric stones, although oxalate stones are related to a lesser degree.[14] Obese persons are at a particularly increased risk of forming uric acid stones.[15,16] As evidence, Ekeruo demonstrated in a small study that 63% of stones in obese people were composed of uric acid.[17] Others have found that men and women with a normal BMI have uric acid stones 7.1% and 6.1% of the time, while those who were obese by BMI had uric acid stones in much greater proportions (28.7% and 17.1%). It is noteworthy that it was also found that the proportion of uric acid stones in obese patients increased significantly with age.[18] Negri et al. conducted a study of the characteristics of people suffering from stone disease. They found that those stone formers who, on stone analysis, were affected by "pure" uric acid stones were significantly heavier and had greater BMIs than those participants with "pure" calcium oxalate stones. In fact, 43.3% of uric acid stone patients were obese compared to only 16.1% of those who form calcium oxalate stones.[19]

The effect that uroliths have on the kidney is not insignificant. In a study using the NHANES III data, Gillen et al. showed that a relationship between kidney stones and decreased renal function was present, and greatly dependent on BMI.[20] More precisely, of patients with kidney stones and BMIs ≥ 27, the decrease in glomerular filtration rate (GFR) was 3.4 mL/min/1.73 m² greater than that seen in similarly overweight patients without stone disease. Patients in this group had roughly twice the chance of having a GFR of between 30 and 59, a level indicative of kidney failure. Kidney stone disease is only one of a number of serious renal diseases that are influenced by obesity. Although it will not be specifically addressed here, it is important to note that obesity-related glomerulopathy is increasingly common and associated with significant morbidities.

60.4 Risk Factors for Stones in the Obese Population

The metabolic syndrome, of which obesity is a criterion, is associated with urinary tract stone disease. This topic is discussed in Chap. 9.

60.4.1 General Risk Factors

Obesity itself predisposes to stone occurrence. Additionally, obesity is a predictor of recurrent stones in first-time stone formers.[15,17,21] Typically, obese persons with stone-forming tendencies excrete higher levels of sodium, calcium, uric acid, and citrate. Statistically significant and positive correlations have been found between BMI and urinary uric acid, sodium, ammonium, and phosphate, along with serum uric acid and creatinine. The risk of stone formation has been found to be significantly correlated with BMI[22]; the relative risk of developing a stone is 1.33 in men with BMI ≥ 30 compared to BMIs of 21–22.9. Furthermore, the median number of stone occurrences is significantly higher in men with BMI ≥ 25.[14]

Curhan et al. reported an effect of gender on the association of obesity and nephrolithiasis.[23] They reported that the odds ratio for stone formation for BMIs ≥ 32 compared to BMIs 21–22.9 was 1.76 for women, but only 1.38 for men. The risk of stone disease in obesity is inversely associated with urinary pH.[24] As such, an acidic urine environment is a marked risk factor for both uric acid and calcium oxalate stones.

Paralleling the advancement of understanding in other clinical fields, recent observations suggest a genetic influence on stone disease in overweight and obese people. Although the exact mechanism has not been clarified, research suggests that a disorder in calcium metabolism amongst families may account for some of the aggregation of pathologies such as obesity, hypertension, and stone disease.[25]

60.4.2 Urinary Metabolic Factors

The most recent and direct study of metabolic factors influencing stone disease in the obese population was conducted by Duffey et al.[26] Unique to this study is that the investigators evaluated a random sample of patients not presenting with an incident stone event. In this study, 45 morbidly obese patients (BMI = 49.5) about to undergo bariatric surgery were examined for both environmental and metabolic qualities. Diets were recorded and considered for differences in sodium, calcium, and protein. In sum, 97.8% of these obese patients had at least one stone risk factor, while 80% had three or more risk factors. The most common urine abnormality noted was a low urine volume, affecting 71% of subjects. More than 50% of the study group also had elevated relative supersaturation of uric acid. When males and females were compared, it was found that men had significantly greater excretion of oxalate, sodium, phosphate, and sulfate. It is also worth mentioning that 23% of the males were hyperoxaluric. Additionally, increasing BMI was associated with lower magnesium excretion and brushite relative supersaturation.

Ekeruo et al. compared metabolic disturbances in obese versus non-obese stone formers, and reported that obesity increased the risk of high urine sulfate (70% versus 24%), hypercalciuria (59% versus 48%), gouty diathesis (54% versus 18%), hyperuricosuria (43% versus 20%), and hyperoxaluria (31% versus 10%).[17] These results have been echoed by other authors who found a significant difference in metabolic factors such as oxalate, uric acid, sodium, and phosphate.[27]

60.4.3 Dietary Risk Factors

Some of the most common risk factors for stone disease, both in the obese and non-obese, are low urine volume (secondary to low fluid intake or increased fluid losses) and high animal protein intake, termed by some investigators as "purine gluttony."[12,17] Those persons eating ≥77 g/day of animal protein have a 33% elevation in relative risk when compared to those who eat little animal protein (≤50 g/day).[28]

Increases in dietary fat are correlated with increased urinary oxalate.[29] There is some level of debate as to whether increased sugared colas and other specific types of beverages increase the risk of stone disease. Rodgers found that sugared-cola consumers had increased urinary oxalate and thereby an increased risk of stones.[30] It may be inferred that obese persons may be more inclined to such types of beverages. However, Curhan et al. reported that soda had no effect on stone incidence. They reported that caffeinated and decaffeinated coffee, tea, beer, and wine all decreased the risk of stones. Others suggest that diets with less alcohol lead to a decrease in the risk of calcium oxalate stones.[31] Interestingly, apple and grape juice increased stone risk.[32] It is believed that tea, especially green tea, may be protective against calcium oxalate stones as a result of its anti-oxidative properties.[33]

60.4.4 Mechanism

The physiology of increased urinary acid concentration in obesity and the metabolic syndrome has been described by Sakhaee and Maalouf.[34] They explain that a net increase in renal acid excretion combined with maladapted urinary ammonium excretion leads to an impairment in buffering capacity, ultimately resulting in lower urinary pH. They also note that future research will focus on the relationships that insulin signaling and insulin resistance have with these defects. Thus far, it has been reported that increasing insulin resistance has correlated to decreasing urinary pH.[35,36] Urinary pH, in fact, correlates to other measures of insulin resistance, such as a depressed glucose metabolism. Current biochemical knowledge proposes that the action of insulin on the sodium-hydrogen exchanger 3 receptor influences ammonia synthesis and excretion. Insulin is also thought to have effects on ammonium synthesis and excretion by the proximal tubule.[24] Abate et al. demonstrated that low insulin sensitivity was significantly associated with acidic 24-h urinary pH values.[37] They went on to describe that those patients with recurrent uric acid stones aggregated at the highest levels of insulin resistance. Finally, they demonstrated that those who were most insulin resistant not only had the lowest pH values but also had lower levels of urinary ammonium. This implies that the protons excreted in urine as titratable acids are insufficiently buffered by ammonia.

Increased animal protein consumption can be another cause of lower urinary pH as it stimulates endogenous acid production in the body. As the increased acid burden requires buffering for homeostasis, bone is reabsorbed and with it calcium. In concordance, glomerular filtration rate is accelerated while calcium reabsorption in the nephron is decreased. Ultimately, these conditions predispose to uric acid stones preferentially, but also to calcium oxalate stones.[12]

Further evidence of uric acid stone predispositions comes from Negri et al. The authors assert that clear differences can be seen in the serum and urine analyses of calcium oxalate versus uric acid stone formers. Calcium oxalate stone formers have elevated serum uric acid and low uric acid clearance (typical of a gout patient), uric acid fractional excretion, and UA/creatinine ratio. The average urinary pH in patients with uric acid stones was 5.17 compared to 5.93 in calcium oxalate patients.[19] As indicated previously, low urinary pH is undeniably the most common and important predisposing factor to uric acid stones and also contributes to mixed uric acid/calcium oxalate stones.[36]

Hypertension, a common comorbidity in obese patients, has been shown to play an independent role in low urinary pH.[38] In a review of the relationship between hypertension and nephrolithiasis, Obligado and Goldfarb discuss the likely impact that obesity (and the metabolic syndrome) has had on the increase in stone incidence observed in Western society.[38] They propose an interesting notion that a common pathophysiology may be responsible for obesity, components of the metabolic syndrome, hypertension, and stone disease. They also suggest that since a clear etiologic relationship is not evident for hypertension and nephrolithiasis, it may instead be a common factor of obesity that relates the two pathologies. Epidemiologic data seem to support this assumption. An in-depth discussion on proposed mechanisms is provided by the authors, but can be summarized in stating that volume expansion (often present in hypertension) causes decreased sodium and calcium reabsorption, as the two are closely coupled. Also, there is some evidence in animal models that suggests a genetic influence on calcium leak in the nephron that may predispose to these conditions.[38]

60.5 Conservative Therapy for Stone Disease

A comprehensive approach to conservative, medical management of stone disease is provided in the previous chapters in the section on "Medical Management." Some of the basics are summarized here, with an emphasis on indications and efficacy in obesity.

60.5.1 Medication

The objective of medical and dietary treatment of urolithiasis is to correct the metabolic defect noted on stone and/or urine analysis that is predisposing the patient to stone formation. Generally, treatment of patients of normal weight is the same as for those who are overweight. There is a general lack of knowledge of treatment efficacy in obese patients. In patients with hypercalciuria, thiazide diuretics can be started; in hyperuricosuria, allopurinol can be used to decrease production of uric acid.[39] For both entities, however, conservative therapy is a reasonable first-line alternative.

The typical conservative treatment for uric acid stones is multi-focused. Increasing the urinary pH with bicarbonate salts or citrates is considered effective, as is increasing fluid intake and decreasing protein consumption. In the specific case of a patient with known hyperuricemia, medical therapy is indicated to lower the uric acid concentration.[16]

Ekeruo et al. showed that in a group of obese stone formers, the incidence of recurrent stones decreased from 1.8 to 0.2 stones per patient per year on appropriate medical therapy and conservative dieting.[17] In this particular study, medical therapy consisted of potassium citrate, allopurinol, hydrochlorothiazide, and/or chlorthalidone depending on the condition identified on metabolic assessment. All patients were also offered guidelines for a diet that would lower animal protein consumption. Congruent to the decrease in stone recurrence, many of the baseline abnormal urinary metabolic parameters showed appropriate response, including an increase in pH, urinary volume, and citrate, and a decrease in urine calcium, urate, and sulfate.

In greater detail, Ekeruo and colleagues report excellent response of their patients to potassium citrate therapy. Citrate corrects the simple hypocitraturia present in the acidic urine of obese patients. Moreover, citrate inhibits the formation of stones in scenarios common to obese patients such as hypocitraturic calcium nephrolithiasis, uric acid stone disease, and gouty diathesis. Overall, it decreases the relative saturation of calcium oxalate by decreasing urinary calcium and increasing urinary pH. Alkalinization of urine with bicarbonate or organic anions decreases the calcium excretion in urine by mollifying the effect of sodium on calcium excretion. Additionally, the serum bicarbonate will prevent calcium reabsorption from bone, also lowering the calcium burden on the kidney.[38]

Ekeruo et al. claim "the importance of dietary modifications decreasing purine intake cannot be overemphasized." Obese kidney stone patients who are unable to control stone risk factors with diet are candidates for allupurinol therapy, especially in cases where hyperuricemia also is present. The conclusion of the aforementioned discussion is that in obese patients, metabolic evaluation and appropriately tailored therapy may be an effective approach to stones.[17]

Less conservative and complementary therapy has been explored in recent years. Drugs for expedited expulsion of stones, such as α(alpha)-blockers and calcium-channel blockers, have been used with encouraging success. Analgesia for acute renal colic has been addressed with nonsteroidal anti-inflammatory drugs (NSAIDs), opioids, and antimuscarinics.[40] These therapies are mentioned here only to note that the response to anti-inflammatory and spasmolytic drugs for the relief of renal colic is similar between obese and non-obese patients.[41] However, obese patients may not present with classic flank pain, due to ill-defined body landmarks, but rather may present with vague complaints.[42]

60.5.2 Diet

Diet is frequently purported to be the most important environmental factor predisposing to urolithiasis. Logically, dietary recommendations are made to persons suffering from stone disease in an effort to decrease the risk of recurrence. In non-obese patients with known urine abnormalities or metabolic disturbances, certain dietary recommendations have become standard. For patients with low urine volume, an increase in fluid intake to between 2.5 and 3 L/day (or quantity sufficient to support 2 L of urine) should be suggested. In hypercalciuria, patients restrict sucrose and sodium (<2.4 g/day), decrease consumption of non-dairy animal protein, and also make sure to take 1,000 mg of calcium a day. Hyperoxaluric patients should limit oxalate in their diets, avoid high doses of vitamin C supplementation, and assure adequate calcium intake.[39] Supplementation with vitamin B6 may also help to lower oxalate by increasing oxalate metabolism and decreasing synthesis. Those with hypocitraturia should begin citrate supplementation by either organic means – fruits and vegetables – or through supplementation (i.e., potassium citrate). Patients with hyperuricosuria (most obese stone formers are hyperuricosuric) should restrict purine intake by adhering to a low-animal-protein diet. Those with elevated urinary sodium excretion should be mindful to restrict salty foods. Finally, diligent follow-up by both physician and patient should be a priority to ensure that the desired changes in metabolic activity have occurred.[39,43]

Research has been conducted on the effects of diet on risk of stone disease, although a thorough understanding of how diet may affect obese patients with stones has yet to be fully elucidated. In a representative population, Siener et al. found that risk factors for stone disease, largely metabolic abnormalities, decreased significantly after patients adapted their intake to a more "nutritionally balanced diet," that is one with less protein and alcohol and more fluid.[31] Hesse and Siener investigated the use of a vegetarian diet for treatment of oxalate-based stone disease. It has been thought that a vegetarian diet, by decreasing animal protein and thereby amino acids that generate purines, would decrease oxalate concentrations in urine. These authors studied two comparable, isoenergetic nutrient rich diets, one consisting of an ovo-lacto-vegetarian menu and the other a typical mixed diet. The ovo-lacto-vegetarian diet showed a significant *increase* in oxalate excretion. Despite this, the risk of calcium oxalate stones was effectively unchanged, likely as a result of an associated increase in urinary pH.[29] Obligado and Goldfarb suggest that adhering to a diet of more fruits and vegetables, low-fat dairy and non-dairy products, and low sodium may protect against obesity and subsequently hypertension and nephrolithiasis. A low sodium diet is intuitively beneficial as naturesis causes obligate calciuria. As well, diets rich in potassium, magnesium, and citrate have been shown to decrease calciuria.

As with all treatments, dieting as part of a weight-loss program should be done with some discretion. In particular, patients and doctors should take care when embracing current trends that support low-carbohydrate, high-protein approaches such as the Atkins and South Beach diets. A study of ten subjects undergoing a 6-week diet, of which 2 weeks consisted of a very-low carbohydrate/high-protein diet and then 4 weeks of a moderately low carbohydrate/high-protein diet, were actually found to have increased risks for stones. The increased risk resulted from lower urinary pH and citrate levels, and increased net acid excretion, undissociated uric acid excretion, and calcium excretion.[44] When recommending these types of diets to overweight and obese patients, it is important to remember these risks as well as the risk of bone loss without proper calcium supplementation.

While dietary modifications and weight loss are widely recommended for multiple medical conditions associated with obesity,[45] supportive evidence is lacking to substantiate the hypothesis that weight loss would positively impact stone incidence. In fact, and to the contrary, Taylor et al. found that there was no reduction in stone risk after weight loss, although the authors note that few patients in their study population actually lost weight and so the results are not significant or convincing.[22]

60.5.3 Imaging in Obesity

Imaging modalities are generally affected by patient body habitus and weight. Nephrolithiasis is most routinely and sensitively imaged by non-contrast computed tomography (NCCT).[46] The same can be said for those who are obese, although specific considerations will be mentioned later. Kidney-ureter-bladder (KUB) X-ray radiography may also be used as a screening tool for stones, as it is quick to use and relatively inexpensive; but with a strong clinical suspicion, NCCT should be used as a definitive study. It bears mentioning here that KUB X-rays and ultrasound are thought to be less sensitive in diagnosing urolithiasis in obesity, although evidence exists to the contrary.[41]

The weight limit established for computed tomography (CT) scanner tables is, for most medical centers with 16- or 64-slice scanners, 450 lb. Newer CT scanners have improved and may allow up to 680 lb. Another limitation is the diameter of the gantry, which is typically 70 or 90 cm for older and newer scanners, respectively. The tables themselves are able to withstand more than this weight; however, the current restrictions are based on the ability of the table motor to reliably move the table through the gantry at constant pace.

Radiation exposure is another concern in the imaging of obese patients with CT. In order to adequately penetrate subcutaneous tissues and depict intra-abdominal organs, the amount of radiation dosed is increased intentionally to remove artifact and develop clear radiographs. When combined with longer exposure times, which also accompany increased body size, obese patients are exposed to incrementally more radiation per study than their leaner counterparts.[47]

60.5.4 Bariatric Surgery and Stone Disease

Hyperoxaluria and nephrolithiasis are known complications of early bariatric surgeries, such as the jejunoileal bypass. Recently, an interesting correlation between modern bariatric surgery and urinary metabolic changes has come to light. Durrani et al. found that of 972 patients undergoing gastric bypass, 8.8% had stones preoperatively, 3.2% developed stones postoperatively, and 31.4% of those with stones before surgery had recurrent stones thereafter.[48] Similarly, Nelson et al. observed in a retrospective study that many of their bariatric patients receiving Roux-en-Y gastric bypass were developing oxalate nephrolithiasis postoperatively.[49] They noted that some patients had developed enteric hyperoxaluria after, on average, 29 months and 46 kg of weight loss. The authors concluded that hyperoxaluria, nephrolithiasis, and even oxalate nephropathy should be considered potential complications of Roux-en-Y bypass surgery.

A subsequent retrospective study of stone formers by Asplin and Coe showed that in 132 patients who had undergone modern bariatric surgery, average 24-h urine oxalate levels were 83 mg/day.[50] This compared with 39 mg/day for the average kidney stone patient and 34 mg/day in the

normal, control patient. The urinary oxalate excretion was, however, lower than had been seen in jejunoileal bypass, which had a historical average of 102 mg/day. Furthermore, the supersaturation of calcium oxalate in urine was higher in bariatric patients than in the average person afflicted with stones. What is particularly concerning, and is a common theme in this so-called new epidemic[51] of bariatric surgery and hyperoxaluria, is the risk of developing oxalate levels high enough to cause renal failure.

Sinha et al. echoed these findings in a cross-sectional study of 60 patients who developed urolithiasis 2.9 years following Roux-en-Y surgery.[52] They found that hyperoxaluria was common 6 months after the operation, however, the increase in relative supersaturation was noted only after 12 months. Recently, a prospective longitudinal cohort study has demonstrated that these urinary findings occur earlier in the time course following bariatric surgery. Duffey et al. conducted a prospective study of 24 patients undergoing Roux-en-Y bypass and found that at only 3 months postoperatively these patients had significantly increased urinary oxalate excretion (41 versus 31 mg/day preoperatively, $p = 0.030$) and increased relative supersaturation of calcium oxalate in urine (3.47 versus 1.73, $p = 0.030$).[53]

In order to study further the effects of bariatric intervention on non-stone formers, a group of patients with no known history of stones were assessed 6 months after Roux-en-Y surgery. When compared to normal adult controls, mean urinary oxalate levels were nearly double (62 and 33 mg) in the bariatric patients.[54] Finally, though presented with much less convincing data, new urolithiasis was also reported as a complication of pediatric bariatric (gastric banding) surgery.[55]

Although still undefined, the likely mechanism for hyperoxaluria and renal stone disease following bypass surgery is a malabsorption of fats and bile salts, which leads to saponification of calcium and a reciprocal increase in the absorption of intestinal oxalate. It has also been proposed that gut flora such as *Oxalobacter formingenes*, and other oxalate-metabolizing bacteria, may be decreased following bypass surgery and thereby increasing the levels of oxalate available for absorption in the gut.[51,53]

The current recommendations for prophylactic treatment of hyperoxaluria and calcium oxalate stones following bariatric surgery are to decrease oxalate and fat consumption, increase calcium and citrate supplementation, alkalinize urine, and maintain adequate urine production through fluid intake. Longitudinal studies of urinary abnormalities suggest that the most effective strategy to prevent hyperoxaluria and stone formation would be to increase fluid intake to at least 2 L/day in order to promote excretion of dilute urine and prevent supersaturation of calcium oxalate.[53] In addition, decreasing consumption of spinach, tea, nuts, and cocoa may help.

Unfortunately, each of these strategies has its limitations. Though limiting dietary oxalate is theoretically an excellent first step, only 10–20% of renally excreted oxalate is from dietary sources; therefore, it is difficult to make a large impact on oxalate levels through diet.[53] Indeed, in an early study, a decrease in urinary oxalate following jejunoileal bypass of only 1.1–0.7 mmol/24 h was observed in an at-home low-oxalate diet.[56]

Some studies question the relative importance of dietary oxalate on stone risk. Siener et al. studied 186 calcium oxalate stone formers, half with hyperoxaluria and half without, and found that the dietary intake of oxalate was not different in the two groups. Instead, they found that ascorbate and fluid consumption were correlated positively, and calcium intake was inversely related.[57] Therefore, providing the patient with calcium supplementation (1,000–1,200 mg/day) may be intuitive to bind oxalate in the gut, though increased levels of fatty acids may saponify much of this calcium, limiting its bioavailability to complex with oxalate. Despite this, Hylander et al. found that a 2,000 mg/day supplementation of calcium, given to a small group of jejuenoileal bypass patients, lowered renal oxalate significantly.[58] As an additional note, treatment with a lactic acid bacteria probiotic has been tried, although with minimal, short-lived success.[59] The future will certainly hold further research on the treatment of this condition as it becomes increasingly commonplace.

60.6 Surgical Therapy for Stone Disease

60.6.1 General Considerations

The morbidly obese patient is at an increased risk for many complicated medical problems – such as diabetes, obesity hypoventilation, sleep apnea, hypertension, and heart disease – that contribute to an increased risk of perioperative morbidity and mortality (see Table 60.1).[61–64] Obese patients are more likely to experience the following perioperative complications: longer operating times, wound dehiscence,[65] incisional hernias, recurrent hernias,[66] readmission to intensive care units, longer hospital times, prolonged ventilation,[67] atelectasis, pneumonia,[68] thromboembolism,[69] and nosocomial infections,[70] among other comorbidities.

Table 60.1 Rates of postoperative complications in obese patients

Postoperative complication	Rate for obese patients (%)	Rate for non-obese patients (%)
Wound infection	11.2	5.8
Wound dehiscence	1.7	0
Pulmonary embolism	6	0.1
Thrombophlebitis	4.3	0.7
Mortality (trauma only)	42	5

Adapted from Flancbaum and Choban[60]

Though endourologic procedures for stones may carry a lower risk for certain wound complications, hospital stays are longer and complication rates higher for obese patients following stone surgery.[71] Some of the complications encountered by the urologist operating for stone on an obese person may include inability to reach stones percutaneously, intraoperative rhabdomyolysis, temporary renal failure, and wound infection.[42] Additionally, the potential operative complications for a nonobese person are exaggerated in the obese patient. They include bleeding (minor or major), infection, deep vein thrombosis (DVT), difficulty with anesthesia, and inadvertent organ injury. Consequently, special care needs to be taken for DVT prophylaxis and anesthetic preparation. Unique issues arise in the surgical arena: patients may exceed the weight limits of the standard surgical table or have skin-to-stone distances that exceed the length of standard endoscopic equipment.

To counter the multitude of possible perioperative morbidities for the obese patient, a multi-disciplinary approach to preoperative assessment, intraoperative monitoring, and peri- and postoperative care should be taken. Preoperative evaluation for clotting risks, heart dysfunction (left ventricular dysfunction or arrhythmias), sleep apnea or hypoventilation, and metabolic conditions should be conducted. The anesthesia team is vitally involved in pre- and intraoperative care and so should be well prepared for the specific needs and monitoring of the obese patient. Because of the variations in orotracheal anatomy in the obese patient, intubation and ventilation may be problematic, and may require fiberoptic assistance.[60] Nursing personnel are invaluable in postoperative care as early ambulation or rotation in bed is crucial to prevent DVT, PE, or decubitus ulceration. The position of the obese surgical patient in bed may be important for oxygenation early in the postoperative period. Vaughn et al. suggest that the patient be positioned in the semirecumbent posture for the first 48 h after surgery.[72] The modern health care system also has increasing responsibility to have the capacity to provide larger beds, transportation modalities, and operating tables and radiologic equipment capable of supporting greater weights.[73]

Non-invasive procedures should be the first choice for the obese patient as their unique surgical risk factors increase the potential value of a minimally invasive procedure. With modifications of current noninvasive and minimally invasive procedures for urolithiasis, the approach to the morbidly obese patient can be successfully planned.

60.6.2 Extracorporeal Shock Wave Lithotripsy (SWL)

Extracorporeal shock wave lithotripsy (SWL) has been shown to be an effective treatment of large renal stones, but is limited as a technique in the obese patient to those patients in whom the skin-to-stone distance (SSD) is equal to or less than the focal depth of the SWL machine.[42] Table weight restrictions limit the size of the patient who can be treated on each individual lithotripter (see Table 60.2). Difficulty with imaging and targeting of stones before intervention has also presented a problem. Increased subcutaneous and visceral thickness leads to the distance between lithotriptor and stone exceeding the focal length of the lithotripter.[74]

In fact, skin-to-stone distance (SSD), or the distance from the surface of the skin to the center of the stone – as measured at $0°$, $45°$, and $90°$ – has become an important predictor of SWL success. Pareek et al. first used non-contrast computed tomography to assess SSD and discovered that SSD was a significant predictor of post-SWL stone-free rates. Any SSD greater than 10 cm is considered a poor indicator for success.[75] El Nahas and colleagues found that SSD had a significant predictive value for treatment failure ($p = 0.033$), although this relationship did not hold up to multivariate analysis.[76] Clinical experience with SWL and morbidly obese patients has shown it to be a safe and effective technique without increased rates of complications.[77] Unfortunately, the rate of failure significantly increases with BMI in the obese range; El-Nahas et al. reported success rates of 80% for obese (BMI > 30) patients compared to 93% for non-obese, in a prospective study using CT imaging to determine a successful treatment.[76]

Ackermann et al. found in a study of 246 patients that BMI had a significant impact on stone-free rates at 3 months. Analysis showed that those patients with a BMI of 20–28 had the greatest chance of successful outcomes.[78] Similarly, Pareek et al. reported that the average BMI for patients rendered stone-free following SWL was 27, while the average BMI for those with residual fragments was 31.[79] Even newer-generation lithotripters have been susceptible to the increased treatment failure rates associated with BMI. Indeed, some authors would suggest that newer-generation lithotripters have lower success rates in overweight/obese patients (47%) compared to first-generation machines (87%). The overall success rates of the two lithotripters were 58% and 79% for the newer and traditional models.[80]

This has led some investigators to recommend percutaneous nephrolithotomy (PCNL) as an initial approach to patients with a BMI > 50, in patients with an otherwise unfavorable body habitus, or in those patients who have failed two courses

of ESWL with a remaining stone burden of >2 cm.[77,81] As with nonobese patients, ESWL should not be performed in patients who have an uncontrolled coagulopathy, ureteral obstruction, untreated urinary tract infection, or are pregnant.

60.6.3 Ureteroscopy

Ureteroscopic stone surgery is often the treatment of choice for the morbidly obese. To paraphrase the late Joseph Segura, "The ureter is never fat." Fortunately, ureteroscopic approaches and equipment need no modification in obese persons. The additional considerations for ureteroscopic stone removal in obesity are the presence of an anesthesiologist with experience in administering anesthesia to obese patients and a table with sufficient weight capacity. Intraoperative fluoroscopic imaging may not be possible due to the size of the patient, though recent advances in operating room tables and C-arm technology have for the most part addressed this issue.

Success rates for ureteroscopic lithotripsy and stone extraction vary from 50% to 92%.[74] Though obesity is commonly referenced as an indication for ureteroscopy, only one case-matched study has been reported to support favorable outcomes. Dash et al. found in a group of 16 morbidly obese patients that 83% had successful ureteroscopy; this success was equivalent to that seen in their non-obese patient population, and trended toward superiority for specifically larger stones >1 cm in size.[82]

Indications for ureteroscopy in obese patients are identical to those for the nonobese and include qualities of renal anatomy, specific qualities of the patient making other techniques unfeasible (i.e., inability to tolerate the prone position for PCNL), and characteristics of the stone(s) (i.e., ureteral location or cystine composition). Indeed, the limitations of SWL in the morbidly obese and the limitations pertaining to PCNL (see the next section) lead to an expanded role for ureteroscopy in this patient population.

The complications of ureteroscopic stone surgery are usually minor and include pain and urinary tract infection. Rarely, a major complication is reported, such as retroperitoneal hemorrhage (in a patient with uncorrected coagulopathy) or ureteral stricture, perforation or avulsion.[74] There is no indication that procedure-specific complications are higher in the morbidly obese.

Table 60.2 Lithotripter specifications

Manufacturer	Model	Focal length (mm)	Table weight limit
Siemens	Lithostar Modular	155	300
Karl Storz	Modulith	165	300
Medstone	STS	153	350
HealthTronics	Lithotron	150	350
Dornier	DoLi S	150	300

60.6.4 *Percutaneous Nephrolithotomy (PCNL)*

PCNL is generally an option pursued in those patients who have failed other minimally invasive approaches or have a stone type (cystine, calcium oxalate monohydrate) or size (>2 cm, staghorn) that dictates the use of PCNL. Patients, obese and nonobese, who are pregnant or have an untreated coagulopathy are not candidates for PCNL. PCNL has been described in morbidly obese patients with complication rates similar to the non-obese patient.[83-85] The complications that potentially arise in PCNL include failed access, thoracic complications (pneumo/hydro/hemothorax), residual stone, postoperative pyrexia, prolonged nephrostomy drainage, hemorrhage (minor or major), ureteric obstruction, urinary retention, deep vein thrombosis, septic shock, and perforation of the renal collecting system.[84]

In 1988, Carson et al. showed that PCNL could be used effectively in morbidly obese patients who surpassed the weight or size limit for the ESWL machine.[86] The same has been reported by other authors in recent studies.[85,87,88] There does not appear to be as strong a correlation between BMI and PCNL failures as compared to ESWL failures.[83] El-Assmy et al. stratified 1,121 patients undergoing PCNL by BMI and found no association with success rates and complication rates. Pearle et al. reported on 96 PCNLs in patients with a BMI > 30, and reported an 88% success rate, with 14% complication and 9% blood transfusion rates. However, Faerber and Goh reported that though success rates were similar between obese and non-obese patients (82% versus 89%), hospital stays were longer (4.4 versus 3.5 days) and complication rates were higher (37% versus 16%).

PCNL may fail for reasons similar to ESWL. The skin-to-stone distance may be greater than the standard nephroscope, making dissolution of the stone impossible without risk to the surrounding tissue.[81] Therefore, this approach requires accurate measurement of the skin-to-stone distance using either ultrasound or computed tomography to allow the surgeon to make an informed decision about accessing the stone.[81] In many obese patients, the standard method of percutaneous access may be sufficient, but the skin-to-stone distance in other patients may be too great for standard equipment.

Various methods of improving access to renal calculi in an obese patient have been described. Curtis et al. described a "cut down" method in which a 12-cm skin incision is made through the subcutaneous tissue to the muscle sheath, thereby decreasing the distance from surface to stone.[89] After placement of an Amplatz sheath, the stone can then be accessed with a standard nephroscope. Grasso et al. has recommended the use of simultaneous retrograde flexible ureteroscope to facilitate placement of the percutaneous guide wires under direct visualization.[90] Another technique uses a two-stage approach in which a 10–12 F nephrostomy tube is initially placed and the tract is allowed to mature for 1 week. A flexible cystoscope is then used for secondary PCNL.[81]

Although these techniques have been successful, the development of new equipment to address the issues of skin-to-stone distance now allows for a simpler approach. After obtaining renal access, an Amplatz sheath with a standard diameter (30 F) but increased length (24 cm) is used to maintain access. Sutures may be placed on the external tip of the sheath for retrieval of the sheath as it is advanced into the subcutaneous fat. All manufacturers have replaced their standard nephroscope working length (17–20 cm) with 25-cm working lengths to adapt to the increase in body habitus of our patients. The increased distance facilitates access to stones in most locations for the vast majority of morbidly obese patients and allows passage of standard ultrasonic lithotripters for efficient fragmentation and extraction. Stone basket extraction of larger fragments is usually performed utilizing a Cook Perc-circle tipless nitinol basket on a rigid handle (Cook Urological, Spencer, IN). Flexible cystonephroscopes are particularly useful in the obese patient due to the additional working length. We prefer to use the holmium laser in conjunction with a tipless nitinol stone basket when using the flexible cystonephroscope. At the conclusion of the procedure, a Cope loop nephrostomy tube is left – Malecot type drainage tubes are prone to inadvertent dislodgement in obese patients.

60.6.5 *Recent Developments in Endourology in Obesity*

There are several reasons why obese patients may not tolerate surgery such as PCNL or ureteroscopy, as have been mentioned previously. However, due to continued innovation in thought and technology, many of these concerns have been addressed. Previously, some obese patients had trouble in tolerating the prone position necessary for PCNL. Manohar et al. have recently described successful cases of PCNL performed in the supine position in morbidly obese patients.[91] Also, obese patients with large renal stones formerly had difficulty in undergoing multiple procedures or having complete resolution of stone burden. Mariani has described 16 cases, of which 13 patients were obese, in which staged electrohydraulic and holmium:YAG laser ureteroscopic nephrolithotripsy was performed. Flexible ureteroscopes were employed in these operations and were thought to function well for such cases. Outcomes were 100% successful and complications minimal (three patients with fever and one with pneumonia postoperatively).[92] For those obese patients at high risk for perioperative morbidity, simultaneous bilateral retrograde intrarenal surgery can be performed by two urologists so as to decrease operating time and potential anesthesia side effects.[93] Finally, Kanaroglou and Razvi report two cases of PCNL under intravenous (IV) and local anesthesia in order to remove risk of cardiorespiratory compromise in two morbidly obese males.[94]

60.7 Conclusions

Obesity is likely to continue to affect an increasing number of patients throughout the world. Urologists will need to make advancements in diagnosis and in both conservative and surgical management of obese patients with stones. There are many promising prospects on these fronts, however, and research moves these possibilities steadily forward.

References

1. Soloman CG, Manson JE. Obesity and mortality: a review of the epidemiologic data. *Am J Clin Nutr.* 1997;66(suppl):1044S-1050S.
2. Flegal KM, Carroll MS, Ogden CL, Johnson CL. Prevalence and trends in obesity among US adults, 1999–2000. *JAMA.* 2002; 288(14):1723-1727.
3. Ogden CL, Carroll MD, Curtin LR, McDowell MA, Tabak CJ, Flegal KM. Prevalence of overweight and obesity in the United States, 1999–2004. *JAMA.* 2006;295(13):1549-1555.
4. Wang CY, Colditz GA, Kuntz KM. Forecasting the obesity epidemic in the aging U.S. population. *Obesity.* 2007;15:2855-2865.
5. Fontaine KR, Redden DT, Wang C, Westfall AO, Allison DB. Years of life lost due to obesity. *JAMA.* 2003;289(2):187-193.
6. Rigby N, Baillie K. Challenging the future: the Global Prevention Alliance. *Lancet.* 2006;368(9548):1629-1631.
7. World Health Organization. Obesity and overweight; 2003. Available at: http://www.who.int/dietphysicalactivity/publications/facts/obesity/en/. Accessed May 5, 2008.
8. Crombie IK, Irvine L, Elliott L, Wallace H. (2008) Targets to tackle the obesity epidemic: a review of twelve developed countries. *Public Health Nutr.* 2008; 1–8 [Epub ahead of print].
9. Centers for Disease Control. Obesity and overweight: childhood overweight: overweight prevalence; 2007. Available at: http://www.cdc.gov/nccdphp/dnpa/obesity/childhood/index.htm. Accessed May 5, 2008.
10. Hedley AA, Ogden CL, Johnson CL, Carroll MD, Curtin LR, Flegal KM. Prevalence of overweight and obesity among US children, adolescents, and adults, 1999–2002. *JAMA.* 2004;291(23): 2847-2850.
11. World Health Organization. Childhood overweight and obesity; 2008. Available at: http//www.who.int/dietphysicalactivity/childhood/en/. Accessed May 5, 2008.
12. Siener R. Impact of dietary habits on stone disease. *Urol Res.* 2006;34:131-133.
13. Scales CD Jr, Curtis LH, Norris RD, et al. Changing gender prevalence of stone disease. *J Urol.* 2007;177(3):979-982.
14. Siener R, Glatz S, Nicolay C, Hesse A. The role of overweight and obesity in calcium oxalate stone formation. *Obes Res.* 2004;12(1): 106-113.

15. Lee SC, Kim YJ, Kim TH, Yun SJ, Lee NK, Kim WJ. Impact of obesity in patients with urolithiasis and its prognostic usefulness in stone recurrence. *J Urol.* 2008;179(2):570-574.
16. Liebman SE, Taylor JG, Bushinsky DA. Uric acid nephrolithiasis. *Curr Rheumatol Rep.* 2007;9(3):251-257.
17. Ekeruo WO, Tan YH, Young MD, et al. Metabolic risk factors and the impact of medical therapy on the management of nephrolithiasis in obese patients. *J Urol.* 2004;172:159-163.
18. Daudon M, Lacour B, Jungers P. Influence of body size on urinary stone composition in men and women. *Urol Res.* 2006;34(3):193-199.
19. Negri AL, Spivacow R, Del Valle E, et al. Clinical and biochemical profile of patients with "pure" uric acid nephrolithiasis compared with "pure" calcium oxalate stone formers. *Urol Res.* 2007;35:247-251.
20. Gillen DL, Worcester EM, Coe FL. Decreased renal function among adults with a history of nephrolithiasis: a study of NHANES III. *Kindey Int.* 2005;67(2):685-690.
21. Sakhaee K. Nephrolithiasis as a systemic disorder. *Curr Opin Nephrol Hypertens.* 2008;17:304-309.
22. Taylor EN, Stampfer MJ, Curhan GC. Obesity, weight gain, and the risk of kidney stones. *JAMA.* 2005;293(4):455-462.
23. Curhan GC, Willett WC, Rimm EB, Speizer FE, Stampfer MJ. Body size and risk of kidney stones. *J Am Soc Nephrol.* 1998;9(9): 1645-1652.
24. Maalouf NM, Sakhaee K, Parks JH, Coe FL, Adams-Huet B, Pak CY. Association of urinary pH with body weight in nephrolithiasis. *Kidney Int.* 2004;65(4):1422-1425.
25. Mente A, Honey JD, McLaughlin JM, Bull SB, Logan AG. High urinary calcium excretion and genetic susceptibility to hypertension and kidney stone disease. *J Am Soc Nephrol.* 2006;17(9):2567-2575.
26. Duffey BG, Pedro RN, Kriedberg C, et al. Lithogenic risk factors in the morbidly obese population. *J Urol.* 2008;179:1401-1406.
27. Taylor EN, Curhan GC. Body size and 24-hour urine composition. *Am J Kidney Dis.* 2006;48(6):905-915.
28. Curhan GC, Willett WC, Rimm EB, Stampfer MJ. A prospective study of dietary calcium and other nutrients and the risk of symptomatic kidney stones. *N Engl J Med.* 1993;328(12):833-838.
29. Hesse A, Siener R. Current aspects of epidemiology and nutrition in urinary stone disease. *World J Urol.* 1997;15:165-171.
30. Rodgers A. Effect of cola consumption on urinary biochemical and physicochemical risk factors associated with calcium oxalate urolithiasis. *Urol Res.* 1999;27:77.
31. Siener R, Schade N, Nicolay C, von Unruh GE, Hesse A. Efficacy of dietary intervention on urinary risk factor for stone formation in recurrent calcium oxalate stone patients. *J Urol.* 2005;173:1601-1605.
32. Curhan GC, Willett WC, Rimm EB, Spiegelman D, Stampfer MJ. Prospective study of beverage use and the risk of stone disease. *Am J Epidemiol.* 1996;143(3):240-247.
33. Itoh Y, Yasui T, Okada A, Tozawa K, Hayashi Y, Kohri K. Preventative effects of green tea on renal stone formation and the role of oxidative stress in nephrolithiasis. *J Urol.* 2005;173(1):271-275.
34. Sakhaee K, Maalouf NM. Metabolic syndrome and uric acid nephrolithiasis. *Semin Nephrol.* 2008;28(2):174-180.
35. Maalouf NM, Cameron MA, Moe OW, Adams-Huet B, Sakhaee K. Low urine pH: a novel feature of the metabolic syndrome. *Clin J Am Soc Nephrol.* 2007;2(5):883-888.
36. Sakhaee K, Adams-Huet B, Moe OW, Pak CYC. Pathophysiologic basis for normouricosuric uric acid nephrolithiasis. *Kidney Int.* 2002;62:971-979.
37. Abate N, Chandalia M, Cabo-Chan AV Jr, Moe OW, Sakhaee K. The metabolic syndrome and uric acid nephrolithiasis: novel features of renal manifestation of insulin resistance. *Kidney Int.* 2004;65:386-392.
38. Obligado SH, Goldfarb DS. The Association of nephrolithiasis with hypertension and obesity: a review. *Am J Hypertens.* 2008; 21(3):257-264.

39. Finkielstein VA, Goldfarb DS. Strategies for preventing calcium oxalate stones. *CMAJ*. 2006;174(10):1407-1409.

40. Micali S, Grande M, Sighinolfi MC, De Carne C, De Stefani S, Bianchi G. Medical therapy of urolithiasis. *J Endourol*. 2006; 20(11):841-847.

41. Tentolouris N, Charamoglis S, Anastasiou I, Serafetinides E, Mitropoulos D. The impact of body mass on management of patients with renal colic. *Int Urol Nephrol*. 2003;35(1):79-82.

42. Hofmann R, Stoller ML. Endoscopic and open stone surgery in morbidly obese patients. *J Urol*. 1992;148:1108-1111.

43. Taylor EN, Curhan GC. Diet and fluid prescription in stone disease. *Kidney Int*. 2006;70:835-839.

44. Reddy ST, Wang CY, Sakhaee K, Brinkley L, Pak CYC. Effect of low-carbohydrate high-protein diets on acid base balance, stone-forming propensity, and calcium metabolism. *Am J Kidney Dis*. 2002;40(2):265-274.

45. Meschi T, Schianchi T, Ridolo E, et al. Body weight, diet and water intake in preventing stone disease. *Urol Int*. 2004;72(suppl 1):29-33.

46. Potretzke AM, Monga M. Imaging modalities for urolithias: impact on management. *Curr Opin Urol*. 2008;18(2):199-204.

47. Uppot RN. Impact of obesity on radiology. *Radiol Clin North Am*. 2007;45(2):231-246.

48. Durrani O, Morrisroe S, Jackman S, Averch T. Analysis of stone disease in morbidly obese patients undergoing gastric bypass surgery. *J Endourol*. 2006;20(10):749-752.

49. Nelson WK, Houghton SG, Milliner DS, Lieske JC, Sarr MG. Enteric hyperoxaluria, nephrolithiasis, and oxalate nephropathy: potentially serious and unappreciated complications of Roux-en-Y gastic bypass. *Surg Obes Relat Dis*. 2005;1(5):481-485.

50. Asplin JR, Coe FL. Hyperoxaluria in kidney stone formers treated with modern bariatric surgery. *J Urol*. 2007;177:565-569.

51. Miller N. Modern bariatric surgery and nephrolithiasis – are we on the verge of a new epidemic? *J Urol*. 2008;179:403-404.

52. Sinha MK, Collazo-Clavell ML, Rule A, et al. Hyperoxaluric nephrolithiasis is a complication of Roux-en-Y gatric bypass surgery. *Kidney Int*. 2007;72:100-107.

53. Duffey BG, Pedro RN, Makhlouf A, et al. Roux-en-Y gastric bypass is associated with early increased risk factors for the development of calcium oxalate nephrolithiasis. *J Am Coll Surg*. 2008; 206(6):1145-1153.

54. Patel BN, Passman CM, Fernandez A, Asplin JR, Coe FL, Lingeman JE et al. Prevalence of hyperoxaluira after modern bariatric surgery. Presented at: 25th World Congress of Endourology & SWL, October 30–November 3, 2007; Cancun, Mexico.

55. Nadler EP, Youn HA, Ginsburg HB, Ren CJ, Fielding GA. Short-term results in 53 obese pediatric patients treated with laparoscopic adjustable gastric banding. *J Pediatr Surg*. 2007;42(1):137-141.

56. Nordenvall B, Backman L, Burnman P, Larsson L, Tiselius HG. Low-oxalate, low-fat dietary regimen in hyperoxaluria following jejunoileal bypass. *Acta Chir Scand*. 1983;149(1):89-91.

57. Siener R, Ebert D, Nicolay C, Hesse A. Dietary risk factors for hyperoxaluria in calcium oxalate stone formers. *Kidney Int*. 2003;63:1037-1043.

58. Hylander E, Jarnum S, Nielsen K. Calcium treatment of enteric hyperoxaluria after jejunoileal bypass for morbid obesity. *Scand J Gastroenterol*. 1980;15(3):349-352.

59. Lieske JC, Goldfarb DS, De Simone C, Regnier C. Use of a probiotic to decrease hyperoxaluria. *Kidney Int*. 2005;68(3):1244-1249.

60. Flancbaum L, Choban P. Surgical implications of obesity. *Ann Rev Med*. 1998;49:215-234.

61. Drenick EJ, Bale GS, Seltzer F, Johnson DG. Excessive mortality and causes of death in morbidly obese men. *JAMA*. 1980;243(5): 443-445.

62. Hubert HB, Feinleib M, McNamara PM, Castelli WP. Obesity as an independent risk factor for cardiovascular disease: a 26-year follow-up of participants in the Framingham Heart Study. *Circulation*. 1983;67(5):968-977.

63. Pemberton LB, Manax WG. Relationship of obesity to postoperative complications after cholecystectomy. *Am J Surg*. 1971;121(1): 87-90.

64. Strauss RJ, Wise L. Operative risk of obesity. *Surg Gynecol Obstet*. 1978;146(2):286-291.

65. Erkanli S, Kayaselcuk F, Bagis T, Kuscu E. Impact of morbid obesity in surgical management of endometrial cancer: surgical morbidity, clinical and pathological aspects. *Eur J Gynaecol Oncol*. 2006;27(4):401-404.

66. Sugerman HJ, Kellum JM Jr, Reines HD, DeMaria EJ, Newsome HH, Lowry JW. Greater risk of incisional hernia with morbidly obese than steroid-dependent patients and low recurrence with pre-fascial polypropylene mesh. *Am J Surg*. 1996;171(1):80-84.

67. Yap CH, Mohajeri M, Yii M. Obesity and early complication after cardiac surgery. *Med J Aust*. 2007;186(7):350-354.

68. Flier S, Knape JT. How to inform a morbidly obese patient on the specific risk to develop postoperative pulmonary complications using evidence-based methodology. *Eur J Anaesthesiol*. 2006; 23(2):154-159.

69. Benotti PN, Wood GC, Rodriguez H, Carnevale N, Liriano E. Perioperative outcomes and risk factors in gastric surgery for morbid obesity: a 9-year experience. *Surgery*. 2006;139(3):340-346.

70. Choban PS, Heckler R, Burge JC, Flancbaum L. Increased incidence of nosocomial infections in obese surgical patients. *Am Surg*. 1995;61(11):1001-1005.

71. Faerber GJ, Goh M. Percutaneous nephrolithotripsy in the morbidly obese patient. *Tech Urol*. 1997;3(2):89-95.

72. Vaughan RW, Bauer S, Wise L. Effect of position (semirecumbent versus supine) on postoperative oxygenation in markedly obese subjects. *Anesth Analg*. 1976;55(1):37-41.

73. DeMaria EJ, Carmody BJ. Perioperative management of special populations: obesity. *Surg Clin N Am*. 2005;85:1283-1289.

74. Busby JE, Low RK. Ureteroscopic treatment of renal calculi. *Urol Clin N Am*. 2004;31:89-98.

75. Pareek G, Hedican SP, Lee FT Jr, Nakada SY. Shock wave lithotripsy success determined by skin-to-stone distance on computed tomography. *Urology*. 2005;66(5):941-944.

76. El-Nahas AR, El-Assmy AM, Mansour O, Shier KZ. A prospective multivariate analysis of factors predicting stone disintegration by extracorporeal shock wave lithotripsy: the value of high-resolution noncontrast computed tomography. *Eur Urol*. 2007; 51(6):1688-1694.

77. Ruiz-Deya G, Buckley FP, Thomas R. Extracorporeal shock wave lithotripsy and the morbidly obese patient. *J Endourol*. 1998;Suppl 1:P11-P13.

78. Ackermann DK, Fuhrimann R, Pfluger D, Studer UE, Zingg EJ. Prognosis after extracorporeal shock wave lithotripsy of radiopaque renal calculi: a multivariate analysis. *Eur Urol*. 1994;52(2): 105-109.

79. Pareek G, Armenakas NA, Panagopoulos G, Bruno JJ, Fracchia JA. Extracorporeal shock wave lithotripsy success based on body mass index and Hounsfield units. *Urology*. 2005;65(1): 33-36.

80. Portis AJ, Yan Y, Pattaras JG, Andreoni C, Moore R, Clayman RV. Matched pair analysis of shock wave lithotripsy effectiveness for comparison of lithotripters. *J Urol*. 2003;169(1):58-62.

81. Giblin JG, Lossef S, Pahira JJ. A modification of standard percutaneous nephrolithotripsy technique for the morbidly obese patient. *Urology*. 1995;46(4):491-493.

82. Dash A, Schuster TG, Hollenbeck BK, Faerber GJ, Wolf JS Jr. Ureteroscopic treatment of renal calculi in morbidly obese patients: a stone-match comparison. *J Urol*. 2002;60(3): 393-397.

83. Buckley FP, Ruiz-Deya G, Thomas R. Percutaneous management of urolithiasis: a reliable option in the morbidly obese patient. *J Urol.* 1998;159(Suppl):1234.

84. Koo BC, Burtt G, Burgess NA. Percutaneous stone surgery in the obese: outcome stratified according to body mass index. *BJU Int.* 2004;93(9):1296-1299.

85. Pearle MS, Nakada SY, Womack JS, Kryger JV. Outcomes of contemporary percutaneous nephrolithotomy in morbidly obese patients. *J Urol.* 1998;160(3 pt 1):669-673.

86. Carson CC 3rd, Danneberger JE, Weinerth JL. Percutaneous lithotripsy in morbid obesity. *J Urol.* 1988;139(2):243-245.

87. El-Assmy AM, Shokeir AA, El-Hahas AR, et al. Outcome of percutaneous nephrolithotomy: effect of body mass index. *Eur Urol.* 2007;52(1):204-205.

88. Sergeyev I, Koi PT, Jacobs SL, Godelman A, Hoenig DM. Outcome of percutaneous surgery stratified according to body mass index and kidney stone size. *Surg Laparosc Endosc Percutan Tech.* 2007;17(3):179-183.

89. Curtis R, Thorpe AC, Marsh R. Modification of the technique of percutaneous nephrolithostomy in the morbidly obese patient. *Brit J Urol.* 1997;79:138-140.

90. Grasso M, Lang G, Taylor FC. Flexible ureteroscopically assisted percutaneous renal access. *Tech Urol.* 1995;1(1):39-43.

91. Manohar T, Jain P, Desai M. Supine percutaneous nephrolithotomyL effective approach to high-risk and morbidly obese patients. *J Endourol.* 2007;21(1):44-49.

92. Mariani AJ. Combine electrohydraulic and homium:YAG laser ureteroscopic nephrolithotripsy of large (greater than 4 cm) renal calculi. *J Urol.* 2007;177(1):168-173.

93. Chung SY, Chon CH, Ng CS, Fuchs GJ. Simultaneous bilateral retrograde intrarenal surgery for stone disease in patients with significant comorbidities. *J Endourol.* 2006;20(10):761-765.

94. Kanaroglou A, Razvi H. Percutaneous nephrolithotomy under conscious sedation in morbidly obese patients. *Can J Urol.* 2006;13(3):3151-3155.

Index

P.N. Rao et al. (eds.), *Urinary Tract Stone Disease*,
DOI 10.1007/978-1-84800-362-0, © Springer-Verlag London Limited 2011